Stedman's
GI & GU WORDS
Includes Nephrology
FOURTH EDITION

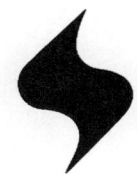

Stedman's
GI & GU WORDS
Includes Nephrology

FOURTH EDITION

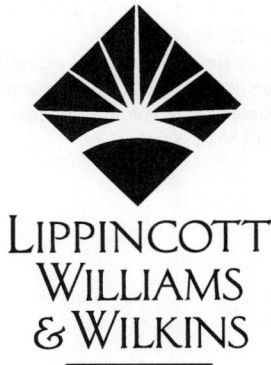

LIPPINCOTT
WILLIAMS
& WILKINS

Publisher: Julie K. Stegman
Senior Product Manager: Eric Branger
Associate Managing Editor: Steve Lichtenstein
Production Coordinator: Jason Delaney
Typesetter: Peirce Graphic Services, LLC.
Printer & Binder: Malloy Litho, Inc.

Copyright © 2005 Lippincott Williams & Wilkins
351 West Camden Street
Baltimore, Maryland 21201-2436

All rights reserved. This book is protected by copyright. No part of this book may be reproduced in any form or by any means, including photocopying, or utilized by any information storage and retrieval system without written permission from the copyright owner.

Printed in the United States of America

2005

Library of Congress Cataloging-in-Publication Data
Stedman's GI & GU words : includes nephrology.—4th ed.
    p. ; cm. — (Stedman's word books)
  Includes bibliographical references.
  ISBN 0-7817-5524-7
  1. Gastroenterology—Terminology. 2. Urology—Terminology.
I. Title: Stedman's GI and GU words. II. Title: GI & GU words.
III. Stedman, Thomas Lathrop, 1853–1938. IV. Series.
[DNLM: 1. Gastrointestinal Diseases—Terminology—English.
2. Gastroenterology—Terminology—English. 3. Nephrology—Terminology—
English. 4. Urogenital Diseases—Terminology—English. 5. Urology—
Terminology—English. WI 15 S812 2005]
RC802.S68 2005
616.3'3'0014—dc22

                                                                2004019889
                                                                04 05 06
                                                  1 2 3 4 5 6 7 8 9 10

Contents

ACKNOWLEDGMENTS vii

EDITOR'S PREFACE ix

PUBLISHER'S PREFACE x

EXPLANATORY NOTES xi

A-Z WORD LIST 1

APPENDICES A1
    1. Anatomical Illustrations A1
    2. Normal Lab Values A45
    3. Herbs Used to Treat GI/GU Conditions A47
    4. Sample Reports A51
    5. Common Terms by Procedure A59
    6. Drugs by Indication A62

Acknowledgments

An important part of our editorial process is the involvement of medical transcriptionists—as advisors, reviewers, and/or editors.

We extend special thanks to Kathy Hess, CMT, and Harriet R. Stewart, CMT, FAAMT, for editing the manuscript, helping resolve many difficult questions, and contributing material for the appendix sections. We are grateful to our MT Editorial Advisory Board members, including Marty Cantu, CMT; Ava George; and Robin Koza, who were instrumental in the development of this reference. They recommended sources and shared their valuable judgment, insight, and perspective.

We also extend thanks to Jeanne Bock, CSR, MT, for working on the appendix. Additional thanks to Helen Littrell for performing the final prepublication review. Other important contributors to this edition include Shemah Fletcher; Tina Whitecotton, MT; and, Mary Chiara Zaratkiewicz.

And, as always, Barb Ferretti and Lisa Fahnestock played an integral role in the process by reviewing the content files for format and providing a final quality check.

As with all our *Stedman's* word references, this resource incorporates the suggestions and expertise of our many contacts in the medical transcriptionist community. Thanks to all of our advisory board participants, reviewers, and editors; AAMT meeting attendees; and others who have written us with requests and comments—keep talking, and we'll keep listening.

Editor's Preface

In this Olympic year, the news has been full of stories of athletes training for and performing in the Athens games. These athletes trained daily and continually challenged themselves in an effort to be chosen for this year's team. Likewise, as medical transcriptionists, we must continue to train (though not physically, but that wouldn't be a bad idea, either!) and challenge ourselves constantly in order to stay at the top of our game. To this end, we are fortunate to have excellent resources such as those provided by *Stedman's,* specifically *Stedman's GI & GU Words, Includes Nephrology, Fourth Edition.* I count myself doubly fortunate to be a part of the editing process by which these resources are updated and improved. Being able to hone my skills and learn new words while I work seems to me to be a win-win situation under the best possible circumstances!

As I stated in a prior Editor's Preface (in which I served as second editor), as a perfectionist, I find myself editing everything I read, and I find that it is very difficult sometimes to get through novels and other publications that contain misspelled words and other editing blunders. Having used *Stedman's* products since I began working in this business, I can trust that that is not the case with their publications because of their meticulous attention to detail. While attempting to improve on some of the finest word books in the business is a painstaking process, it is a very rewarding one, and I hope you are as pleased as I am with the end result. Not only are the A-Z entries the best they have ever been thanks to the addition of new terms from current journals, books, and web sites, there are also sample reports and other appendices that should make our jobs as medical transcriptionists easier.

I have enjoyed working with Harriet Stewart and appreciate her attention to detail on this edition. Thank you, Harriet! It has also been my pleasure to work with Steve Lichtenstein at Lippincott Williams and Wilkins, and I appreciate his patience with all my questions. Thank you, Steve! It is truly a privilege to be associated with a company that continually publishes some of the best resources in our industry.

Kathy Hess, CMT

Publisher's Preface

Stedman's GI & GU Words, Includes Nephrology, Fourth Edition, offers an authoritative assurance of quality and exactness to the wordsmiths of the healthcare professions—medical transcriptionists, medical editors and copyeditors, health information management personnel, court reporters, and the many other users and producers of medical documentation.

The specialties of gastroenterology, urology, and nephrology have evolved significantly over the past several years. Gastroenterology-related terminology includes: GI endoscopy, hepatology, and clinical nutrition. Urology-related terminology includes: genitourinary surgery, laparoscopic urology, endourology, urolithology and lithotripsy, renography, ultrasonography, male infertility, urogynecology, and fluorodynamics.

In *Stedman's GI & GU Words, Fourth Edition*, users will find thousands of words that relate to the specialties of gastroenterology, urology, and nephrology. Users will also find terms for protocols, diagnostic and therapeutic procedures, new techniques, lab tests, clinical research terms, as well as equipment names, and abbreviations with their expansions. The appendix sections provide anatomical illustrations with useful captions and labels, sample reports, and common terms by procedure.

This compilation of more than 90,000 entries, fully cross-indexed for quick access, was built from a base vocabulary of approximately 66,000 medical words, phrases, abbreviations, and acronyms. The extensive A-Z list was developed from the database of *Stedman's Medical Dictionary, 27th Edition,* and supplemented by terminology found in current medical literature (please see list of References on page xv).

We at Lippincott Williams & Wilkins strive to provide you with the most up-to-date and accurate word references available. Your use of this word book will prompt new editions, which we will publish as often as updates and revisions justify. We welcome your suggestions for improvements, changes, corrections, and additions—whatever will make this *Stedman's* product more useful to you. Please complete the postage-paid card in this book for future suggestions and recommendations, or visit us online at www.stedmans.com.

Explanatory Notes

Medical transcription is an art as well as a science. Both approaches are needed to correctly interpret the dictation of a physician, whose language is a product of education, training, and experience. This variety in medical language means that there are several acceptable ways to express certain terms, including jargon. *Stedman's GI & GU Words, Includes Nephrology, Fourth Edition*, provides variant spellings and phrasings for many terms. These elements, in addition to complete cross-indexing, make *Stedman's GI & GU Words, Includes Nephrology, Fourth Edition*, a valuable resource for determining the validity of terms as they are encountered.

Alphabetical Organization

Alphabetization of main entries is letter by letter as spelled, ignoring punctuation, spaces, prefixed numbers, or other characters. For example:

cesium
cesium-137 wire
CE-SM gastric lesion staging by endoscopy
Cestoda **tapeworm**

In subentry alphabetization, the abbreviated singular form or the spelled-out plural form of the noun main entry word is ignored.

Format and Style

All main entries are in **boldface** to expedite locating a sought-after term, to enhance distinction between main entries and subentries, and to relieve the textual density of the pages.

Irregular plurals and variant spellings are shown on the same line as the singular or preferred form of the word. For example:

diagnosis, pl. **diagnoses**
CA-125, CA125

Hyphenation

As a rule of style, multiple eponyms (e.g., Mears-Rubash approach) are hyphenated. Also, hyphens have been added between a manufacturer and one or more eponyms (e.g., Vital-Metzenbaum dissecting scissors). Please note that in many cases, hyphenation is a question of style, not of accuracy, and thus is a matter of choice.

Possessives

Possessive forms have been dropped in this reference for the sake of consistency and conformance with the guidelines of the American Association for Medical Transcription (AAMT) and other groups. Please note, however, that in many cases, retaining the possessive, like hyphenating, is a question of style, not of accuracy, and thus is a matter of choice. To form the possessive of a word, simply add the apostrophe or apostrophe "s" to the end of the word.

Cross-indexing

The word list is in an index-like main entry-subentry format that contains two combined alphabetical listings:

(1) A *noun* main entry-subentry organization, which is typical of the A-Z section of medical dictionaries like *Stedman's*:

fibroblast
    human synovial f.
    interstitial f.
    perivascular f.

muscle
    circular m.
    pelvic m.
    smooth m.

(2) An *adjective* main entry-subentry organization, which lists words and phrases as you hear them. The main entries are the adjectives or modifiers in a multiword term. The subentries are the nouns around which the terms are constructed and to which the adjectives or modifiers pertain:

anterior
    a. abdominal wall
    a. axillary line
    a. nephrectomy

intestinal
    i. decompression
    i. endoscopy
    i. hemorrhage

This format provides the user with more than one way to locate and identify a multiword term. For example:

Ellik
    E. kidney stone basket

basket
    Ellik kidney stone b.

cautery
    blind c.
    Bovie c.

Bovie
    B. cautery
    B. holder

It also allows the user to see together all terms that contain a particular descriptor, as well as all types, kinds, or variations of a noun entity. For example:

lavage
    l. bowel preparation
    colonic l.
    l. cytology
    gastric l.

treatment
    t. morbidity
    Murphy t.
    t. protocol
    suppression t.

Wherever possible, abbreviations are separately defined and cross-referenced. For example:

IBD
    inflammatory bowel disease

inflammatory
    i. bowel disease (IBD)

disease
    inflammatory bowel d. (IBD)

References

In addition to the manufacturers' literature we gather at various medical meetings, scientific reports from hospitals, and the lists of our MT Editorial Advisory Board members (from their daily transcription work), we used the following sources for new terms in *Stedman's GI & GU Words, Fourth Edition*.

Books

Agur, AMR, Lee, MJ. Grant's Atlas of Anatomy, 10th edition. Baltimore: Lippincott Williams & Wilkins, 1999.

Blaser MJ. Inflections of the Gastrointestinal Tract. 2nd Edition. Philadelphia: Lippincott Williams & Wilkins, 2002.

Blumenthal M, Goldberg A, Brinckmann J. Herbal Medicine: Expanded Commission E Monographs. Newton, MA: Integrative Medicine Communications, 2000.

Drake E. Sloanes's Medical Word Book, 4th Edition. Philadelphia: Saunders, 2001.

Eastwood G, Avunduk C. Manual of Gastroenterology, 2nd Edition. Baltimore: Lippincott Williams & Wilkins, 1994.

Eisenberg RL. Gastrointestinal Radiology: A Pattern Approach. 4th Edition. Philadelphia: Lippincott Williams & Wilkins, 2003.

Gartner H. Color Atlas of Histology. 3rd Edition. Philadelphia: Lippincott Williams & Wilkins 2001.

GI Words and Phrases. Modesto, CA: Health Professions Institute, 1989.

Gilinsky NH, Forbes A. Self-Assessment Color Review of Gastroenterology. Baltimore: Lippincott Williams & Wilkins, 1999.

Gomella LG. The 5-Minute Urology Consult. Baltimore: Lippincott Williams & Wilkins, 2000.

Graham SD, Jr. Glenn JF. Glenn's Urologic Surgery. 5th Edition. Philadelphia: Lippincott Williams & Wilkins, 1998.

Hardy, NO. Westport, CT. From Stedman's Medical Dictionary, 27th edition. Baltimore: Lippincott Williams & Wilkins, 2000.

Hollinger FB. Viral Hepatitis. Philadelphia: Lippincott Williams & Wilkins, 2002.

Kelsen DP. Gastrointestinal Oncology: Principles and Practices. Charlottesville, VA: Lippincott, Williams & Wilkins, 2002.

Lance LL. 2001 Quick Look Drug Book. Baltimore: Lippincott Williams & Wilkins, 2000.

Massry SG, Glassock RJ. Massry and Glassock's Textbook of Nephrology, 4th Edition. Baltimore: Lippincott Williams & Wilkins, 2000.

Moore KL and Agur A. Essential Clinical Anatomy. 2nd Edition. Philadelphia: Lippincott Williams & Wilkins, 2002.

Moore KL and Dalley AF II. Clinical Oriented Anatomy. 4th Edition. Baltimore: Lippincott Williams & Wilkins, 1999.

References

Nettina, SM. The Lippincott Manual of Nursing Practice. 7th Edition. Philadelphia: Lippincott Williams & Wilkins, 2001

Peters DC. Treatment Options in Gastroenterology. Baltimore: Lippincott Williams & Williams, 2000.

Prakash C. A Therapeutic Guide to Common Problems in Gastroenterology. Philadelphia: Lippincott Williams & Wilkins, 2003.

Premkumar K. The Massage Connection Anatomy and Physiology. Baltimore: Lippincott Williams & Wilkins, 2004.

Pyle V. Current Medical Terminology, 9th Edition. Modesto: Health Professions Institute, 2003.

Sauerland, E. Grant's Dissector, 12th Edition. Baltimore: Lippincott Williams & Wilkins, 1999.

Schenk M, Jackson, MS. From Stedman's Medical Dictionary, 27th edition. Baltimore: Lippincott Williams & Wilkins, 2000.

Schiff ER. Schiff's Diseases of the Liver. 9th Edition. Philadelphia: Lippincott Williams & Wilkins, 2002.

Schrier RW. Diseases of the Kidney and Urinary Tract. 7th Edition. Philadelphia: Lippincott Williams & Wilkins, 2001.

Schrier RW. Essential Atlas of Nephrology. Philadelphia: Lippincott Williams & Wilkins, 2001.

Schrier RW. Manual of Nephrology, 5th Edition. Baltimore: Lippincott Williams & Wilkins, 1999.

Seldin DW, Giebisch G. The Kidney: Physiology and Pathophysiology, 3rd Edition. Baltimore: Lippincott Williams & Wilkins, 2000.

Senkarik M, San Antonio, TX. From Stedman's Medical Dictionary, 27th edition. Baltimore: Lippincott Williams & Wilkins, 2000.

Siorky MD. Handbook of Urology. Philadelphia: Lippincott Williams & Wilkins, 2004.

Stedman's Medical Dictionary, 27th Edition. Baltimore: Lippincott Williams & Wilkins, 2001.

Tessier C. The AAMT Book of Style. Modesto: AAMT, 1995.

Walsh PC, Retik AB, Vaughan ED, Wein AJ. Campbell's Urology, 7th Edition. Philadelphia: Saunders, 1998.

Yamada T. Atlas of Gastroenterology. 3rd Edition. Philadelphia: Lippincott Williams & Wilkins, 2003.

Images

LifeART Nursing 2, CD-ROM. Baltimore, Lippincott Williams & Wilkins.

LifeART Pediatrics 1, CD-ROM. Baltimore, Lippincott Williams & Wilkins.

References

LifeART Super Anatomy Collection 3, CD-ROM. Baltimore, Lippincott Williams & Wilkins.

LifeART Super Anatomy Collection 4, CD-ROM. Baltimore, Lippincott Williams & Wilkins.

UpToDate Clinical Reference Library on CD, Version 8:3. Wellesley, MA: UpToDate, 2000.

Yamada T, Alpers DH, Laine L, Owyang C, Powell DW. Textbook of Gastroenterology, 3rd Edition on CD-ROM. Philadelphia: Lippincott Williams & Wilkins, 1999.

Journals

American Journal of Gastroenterology. Baltimore: Lippincott Williams & Wilkins, 1998, 2000–2004.

AUA News. Baltimore: Lippincott Williams & Wilkins, 1996–2000.

Contemporary Dialysis and Nephrology. Philadelphia: Lippincott Williams & Wilkins, 1996.

Contemporary Gastroenterology. Philadelphia: Lippincott Williams & Wilkins, 1999–2000.

Contemporary Urology. Philadelphia: Lippincott Williams & Wilkins, 1996, 1999–2000.

Current Opinion in Gastroenterology. Philadelphia: Lippincott Williams & Wilkins, 1999–2004.

Current Opinion in Nephrology and Hypertension. Philadelphia: Lippincott Williams & Wilkins, 1999–2001.

Current Opinion in Urology. Philadelphia: Lippincott Williams & Williams, 1999–2004.

Dialysis & Transplantation. Van Nuys, CA: Creative Age Publications, Inc., 1996.

Diseases of the Colon & Rectum. Philadelphia: Lippincott Williams & Wilkins, 1999–2001.

Gastroenterology Nursing. Philadelphia: Lippincott Williams & Wilkins, 1996.

Gastrointestinal Endoscopy. St. Louis: Mosby-Yearbook, Inc., 1996–2004.

Inflammatory Bowel Disease. Philadelphia: Lippincott Williams & Wilkins, 1999–2001.

Journal of Clinical Gastroenterology. Philadelphia: Lippincott Williams & Wilkins, 1999–2001.

Journal of the American Society of Nephrology. Philadelphia: Lippincott Williams & Wilkins, 1996–2004.

Journal of Urology. Baltimore: Lippincott Williams & Wilkins, 1997–2001.

Latest Word. Philadelphia: Saunders, 1999–2001.

Ostomy/Wound Management. Wayne, PA: HMP Communications, 1999–2000.

Techniques in Urology. Philadelphia: Lippincott Williams & Wilkins, 1999–2000.

Urology Times. Cleveland: Advanstar Communications, 1996.

References

Websites

http://gastroenterology.medscape.com/Home/Topics/gastroenterology/gastroenterology.html

http://urology.medscape.com/Home/Topics/urology/urology.html

http://www.acg.gi.org/

http://www.asge.org/index.jsp

http://www.asn-online.com/

http://www.betterworld.com/BWZ/9608/act.htm#Gas

http://www.centerwatch.com

http://www.duj.com

http://www.fascrs.org

http://www.fda.gov

http://www.gastro.org

http://www.herbalremedies.com/cinnamon1.html

http://www.hort.purdue.edu/newcrop/med-aro/factsheets/DILL.html

http://www.hpisum.com

http://www.kcweb.com/herb/goldenseal.htm

http://www.kidney.org

http://www.mtdaily.com

http://www.mtdesk.com/newterms.shtml

http://www.niddk.nih.gov

http://www.observations.org/Healing2/Articles/GastIntestHerbs.html

http://www.pdrhealth.com/drug_info/nmdrugprofiles/herbaldrugs/100620.shtml

http://www.physci.org/1/herb/urgen.html#Ap

http://www.spwb.saunders.net

http://www.virtualdrugstore.com/druglist.html

A

A
    A antigen
    A Bayesian nomogram
    A bile
    A ring
    A ring of esophagus
A_4
    leukotriene A_4
A28 immunological study
A-4 protein
A2008 ABGII hemodialysis machine
AA amyloid
AAA
    abdominal aortic aneurysm
    aromatic amino acid
AAC
    antibiotic-associated colitis
AAD
    antibiotic-associated diarrhea
AAG
    antral atrophic gastritis
Aagenaes syndrome
A-a gradient
AAH
    atypical adenomatous hyperplasia
AAL
    anterior axillary line
AAPBDS
    anomalous arrangement of pancreaticobiliary ductal system
AAPC
    antibiotic-associated pseudomembranous colitis
AAPMC
    antibiotic-associated pseudomembranous colitis
Aaron sign
Aarskog-Scott syndrome
Aarskog syndrome
AAS
    acute abdominal series
AASK
    African-American Study of Kidney Disease and Hypertension
AASLD
    American Association for the Study of Liver Diseases
AAT
    androgen ablation therapy
AATD
    alpha-1-antitrypsin disease
AAV
    adenoassociated virus

AAWM
    American Academy of Wound Management
abacterial pyuria
Abadie enterostomy clamp
abarelix
abarelix-depot-F
abate
Abbe
    A. intestinal anastomosis
    A. small bowel operation
Abbe-McIndoe vaginal construction
Abbott
    A. AxSYM antibody to hepatitis C virus lab test
    A. esophagogastroscopy
    A. esophagogastrostomy
    A. HCV EIA 2nd generation kit
    A. HCV 2.0 test kit
    A. IMx PSA assay
    A. LifeCare pump
    A. Lifeshield needleless system
    A. TDx monoclonal fluorescence polarization immunoassay
    A. tube
Abbott-Miller tube
Abbott-Rawson double-lumen gastrointestinal tube
ABC
    avidin-biotin complex
    alkaline phosphatase Vectastain ABC
    ABC reagent
ABD
    adynamic bone disease
abdomen
    acute surgical a.
    boardlike rigidity of a.
    boat-shaped a.
    carinate a.
    diffusely tender a.
    distended a.
    doughy a.
    dull to percussion a.
    exquisitely tender a.
    flabby a.
    flat plate of a.
    hyperresonant a.
    navicular a.
    nondistended a.
    a. obstipum
    pendulous a.
    plain film of a.
    protuberant a.
    resonant a.

abdomen *(continued)*
    rigid a.
    rotund a.
    scaphoid a.
    silent a.
    soft a.
    splinting of a.
    surgical a.
    tight a.
    tympanitic a.

abdominal
    a. abscess
    a. angina
    a. aorta
    a. aortic aneurysm (AAA)
    a. aortography
    a. apoplexy
    a. apron
    a. ballottement
    a. bruit
    a. canal
    a. cavity
    a. circumference (AC)
    a. colectomy
    a. compartment syndrome (ACS)
    a. compression (AC)
    a. compression belt
    a. contents
    a. crisis
    a. cryptorchidism
    a. cutaneous nerve entrapment syndrome
    a. decompression
    a. desmoid tumor
    a. distention
    a. dropsy
    a. ectopic pregnancy
    a. fasciocutaneous flap
    a. fat
    a. fat pad
    a. fistula
    a. fluid wave
    a. fullness
    a. ganglion block
    a. girth
    a. guarding
    a. incision dehiscence
    a. inguinal ring
    a. kidney
    a. laparotomy pad
    a. lavage
    a. leak-point pressure (ALPP)
    a. membrane
    a. migraine
    a. muscle deficiency syndrome
    a. nephrectomy
    a. nephrotomy
    a. pain
    a. paracentesis
    a. part of esophagus
    a. partitioning
    a. patch electrode
    a. peritoneum
    a. pool
    a. pressure technique
    a. procedure
    a. pulse
    a. radiography
    a. rectopexy
    a. region
    a. retropexy
    a. rigidity
    a. sacrocolpopexy
    a. section
    a. situs inversus
    a. stoma
    a. surgery
    a. tap
    a. testis
    a. tomodensitometric examination
    a. tympany (AT)
    a. typhoid
    a. ultrasonography
    a. ultrasound
    a. ureter
    a. vascular accident
    a. viscus
    a. wall
    a. wall hernia
    a. wall lift technique
    a. wall mass
    a. wall venous pattern
    a. zone

abdominalgia
    periodic a.

abdominalis
    angina a.
    facies a.
    pulsus a.
    purpura a.

abdominis
    angina a.
    diastasis rectus a.
    hydrops a.
    rectus a.

abdominocentesis

abdominocystic

abdominogenital

abdominopelvic
    a. cavity
    a. orocecal transit time

abdomino-Peña pull through procedure

abdominoperineal
    a. excision
    a. resection (APR)

abdominoplasty
    Ehrlich a.

Monfort a.
Randolph a.
abdominosacral resection
abdominoscopy
abdominoscrotal hydrocele
abdominothoracic
abdominovaginal
abdominovesical pouch
abenteric
Aberdeen knot
aberrans
    vas a.
    vasculum a.
aberrant
    a. crypt focus (ACF)
    a. mRNA splicing
    a. obturator vein
    a. pancreas
    a. suprarenal cortex
    a. umbilical stomach
    a. ureter
aberrantes
    ductuli a.
aberration
    genetic a.
    a. by scintigraphy
aberratio testis
abetalipoproteinemia
ABG
    arterial blood gas
ABH blood group
ability
    a. to form solid stool
    a. of glucocorticoid receptor
    impaired urinary concentrating a.
    renal autoregulatory a.
Ablaser laser delivery catheter
ablate-and-chip method
Ablatherm HIFU system
ablation
    androgen a.
    carbon dioxide laser plaque a.
    cold forceps a.
    cold snare a.
    cryogenic a.
    cryosurgical a.
    endoscopic thermal a.
    homogenous a.
    laser a.
    a. model
    needle a.
    neoadjuvant total androgen a.
    percutaneous radiofrequency a.
    photochemical a.
    photothermal laser a.
    prostate gland needle a.
    sphincter of Oddi a.
    thermal a.
    transurethral needle a. (TUNA)
    tumor a.
    ultrasound a.
    valve a.
    visual laser a.
ablative
    a. adrenalectomy
    a. laser therapy
abluminal
ABM
    adjusted body mass
abnormal esophageal test
abnormality
    amino acid a.
    atherosclerotic a.
    CHARGE a.'s
    chromosomal a.
    clotting a.
    coloboma, heart disease, atresia choanae, retarded growth, genital hypoplasia, and ear a.'s (CHARGE)
    congenital urologic a.
    crystallization a.
    diminished branching a.
    electrolyte a.
    hematologic a.
    hepatic a.
    a. of hepatic artery
    immunologic a.
    laboratory a.
    metabolic a.
    mucosal a.
    ocular a.
    omphalocele, exstrophy of bladder, imperforate anus, and spinal a.'s (OEIS)
    platelet a.
    pruning a.
    rectosphincteric a.
    spinal cord injury without radiographic a. (SCIWOA)
    urogenital a.
    vascular a.
ABO
    ABO barrier

NOTES

ABO *(continued)*
    ABO blood group
    ABO incompatible
Abocide disinfectant
ABO-incompatible living donor kidney transplantation
aboral migration
AB/PAS
    Alcian blue and periodic acid-Schiff
Abrams-Griffith nomogram
abrasion
    mucosal a.
Abrikosov tumor
abrupt pulse
abscess
    pericolic a.
Abscession biliary drainage catheter
absence
    a. of comorbid disorders
    a. of diluted duct
    enuretic a.
    protein in vitamin K a. (PIVKA)
absent
    a. ankle jerk
    a. bowel sounds
    a. gag reflex
    a. peristalsis
    pneumobilia a.
Absidia
    A. capillata
    A. coerulea
    A. corymbifera
    A. ramosum
absolute
    a. alcohol
    a. alcohol sclerosant
    a. dehydration
    a. diet
    a. erythrocytosis
    a. sterility
absorbable
    a. clip
    a. gelatin sponge
    a. staple
    a. suture
absorbent padding
absorptiometer
    QDR 1000 densitometer a.
absorptiometry
    dual-energy x-ray a. (DEXA, DXA)
    dual-photon a.
absorption
    alcohol a.
    antibiotic a.
    DEXA a.
    dual-energy x-ray a.
    enteral a.
    fluorescent treponemal antibody a. (FTA-ABS)
    gastrointestinal a.
    impaired gastric a.
    internal a.
    intestinal a.
    oxalate intestinal a.
    paracetamol a.
    reservoir mucosal a.
    transcellular a.
    xenobiotic a.
absorptive
    a. cell
    a. hypercalciuria
    a. hyperoxaluria
abstinence
ABT-627
abuse
    alcohol a.
    ethanol a.
    intravenous drug a.
    ipecac a.
    laxative a.
    phencyclidine a.
    salicylate a.
    sexual a.
    substance a.
ABV
    doxorubicin, bleomycin sulfate, vinblastine
ABVD
    doxorubicin, bleomycin sulfate, vinblastine, dacarbazine
ABW
    actual body weight
AC
    abdominal circumference
    abdominal compression
    activated charcoal
    acute cholecystitis
    adenylate cyclase
    alcoholic cirrhosis
    Pepcid AC
ACA
    adenocarcinoma
    anticardiolipin antibody
    anticentromere autoantibody
acalculous
    a. cholecystitis
    a. cholesterolosis
    a. gallbladder disease
Acanthocephala
acanthocytosis
acanthosis
    glycogenic a.
    a. nigricans
acarbose
acathectic
acathexia

Acationox
ACBE
    air-contrast barium enema
accelerated
    a. hypertension
    a. senescence
    a. transplant rejection
acceleration
    cavernous artery blood flow a.
accelerator
    serum thrombotic a.
    a. urinae
Accellon Combi cervical biosampler
access
    arteriovenous a.
    endoscopic a.
    hemodialysis vascular a.
    a. papillotomy
    peritoneal a.
    a. psychomotor skill
    reliable percutaneous renal a.
    vascular a.
    venovenous a.
accessorium
    pancreas a.
accessorius
    ductus pancreaticus a.
    lien a.
accessory
    a. adrenal gland
    a. adrenals
    Assura irrigation a.
    a. diaphragm
    a. duct of Luschka
    a. duct of Santorini
    a. obturator artery
    a. pancreas
    a. pancreatic duct
    a. parotid gland
    a. phallic urethra
    a. portal system of Sappey
    a. saphenous vein
    a. sex gland
    a. spleen
    a. superior colic artery
    a. thyroid gland
    a. trocar
    a. vessel
accident
    abdominal vascular a.
accordion-like bunching
accordion sign

Accu-Chek III
Accu-Dx test
AccuMeter
    ChemTrak A.
accumulation
    gamma-aminobutyric acid a.
    glomerular a.
    glycoprotein a.
    lysosomal a.
    tubular iron a.
AccuPrep
accuracy
    optimal diagnostic a.
accurate
    A. catheter
    A. Surgical and Scientific Instruments (ASSI)
Accuratome precurved papillotome
AccuSharp endoscope
Accuson-128 color flow Doppler machine
Accutorr oscillometric device
ACD
    adult celiac disease
ACE
    angiotensin-converting enzyme
    antegrade colonic enema
    antegrade continence enema
    BICAP silver ACE
    ACE gene polymorphism
    ACE inhibitor
    ACE procedure
ACEI
    angiotensin-converting enzyme inhibitor
acetaldehyde (Ach)
acetaminophen
    a. hepatotoxicity
    a. overdose
    a. toxicity
acetate
    anaritide a.
    buserelin a.
    calcium a.
    chlormadinone a.
    cortisone a.
    Cortone A.
    cyproterone a. (CPA)
    desmopressin a.
    free a.
    goserelin a.
    hydrocortisone a.
    Hydrocortone A.

NOTES

acetate *(continued)*
    leuprolide a.
    mafenide a.
    medroxyprogesterone a.
    megestrol a.
    methylprednisolone a.
    octreotide a.
    phorbol myristate a. (PMA)
    roxatidine a.
    uranyl a.

acetazolamide
acetic acid
acetohydroxamic
    a. acid
    a. acid irrigation

acetomorphine
acetonemic
acetonitrile eluate
acetonuria
acetowhite lesion
acetylation
acetylcholine
acetylcholinesterase
acetyl coenzyme hypoglycin A
acetylcysteine
acetylsalicylic
    a. acid (ASA)
    5-a. acid

acetylsulfadiazine
acetylsulfaguanidine
acetylsulfathiazole
acetyltransferase
    choline a. (ChAT)

***N*-acetyltransferase 2**
acetyltriglycine renal scan
ACF
    aberrant crypt focus

ACG
    American College of Gastroenterology

Ach
    acetaldehyde

achalasia
    a. balloon dilation
    a. cardia
    classic a.
    cricopharyngeal a.
    a. dilator
    esophageal a.
    idiopathic a.
    pelvirectal a.
    secondary a.
    sphincteral a.
    vigorous a.

achalasia-like esophagus
ache
Achiever
    A. balloon dilation catheter
    A. balloon dilator

achlorhydria
    a. apepsia
    gastric a.
    histamine-resistant a.
    medically induced a.
    watery diarrhea, hypokalemia, and a. (WDHA)

achlorhydric
acholangic
    a. biliary cirrhosis
    a. biliary fibrosis

acholia
acholic stool
acholuria
acholuric jaundice
achoresis
achromaturia
Achromycin V
achylia
    a. gastrica
    a. gastrica haemorrhagica
    a. pancreatica

achylous
achymia
achymosis
acid
    acetic a.
    acetohydroxamic a.
    acetylsalicylic a. (ASA)
    5-acetylsalicylic a.
    amino a.
    aminocaproic a.
    aminolevulinic a. (ALA)
    5-aminolevulinic a. (5-ALA)
    4-aminosalicylic a. (4-ASA)
    5-aminosalicylic a. (5-ASA)
    amoxicillin and clavulanic a.
    arachidonic a.
    aromatic amino a. (AAA)
    ascorbic a.
    benzoic a.
    benzoyl-tyrosyl-paraaminobenzoic a. (BT-PABA)
    7-beta-epimer of chenodeoxycholic a.
    bile a. (BA)
    branched-chain amino a. (BCAA)
    caustic a.
    a. cell
    chenodeoxycholic a. (CDA, CDCA)
    choleic a.
    cholic a. (CA)
    cinnamic a.
    citric a.
    clavulanic a.
    a. clearance test (ACT)
    cocarcinogenic fecal bile a.
    complementary deoxyribonucleic a. (cDNA)

conjugated bile a.
conjugated linoleic a. (CLA)
cyclooxygenase messenger ribonucleoprotein a.
cysteine sulfinic a.
delta-aminolevulinic a. (d-ALA)
deoxycholic a.
deoxyribonucleic a. (DNA)
Diagnex Blue test for gastric a.
diatrizoic a.
diethylenetriamine pentaacetic a. (DTPA)
dihydroxyeicosatrienoic a.
diisopropyliminodiacetic a. (DISDA, DISIDA)
dimercaptosuccinic a. (DMSA)
a. dyspepsia
eicosapentaenoic a. (EPA)
epoxyeicosatrienoic a. (EET)
epsilon-aminocaproic a.
essential amino a.
essential fatty a. (EFA)
esterified fecal a.
ethacrynic a.
ethylenediaminetetraacetic a. (EDTA)
ethyleneglycoltetraacetic a. (EGTA)
fatty a.
fecal bile a. (FBA)
folic a.
folinic a.
free fatty a.
free fecal bile a.
gamma-aminobutyric a.
gastric a.
genomic deoxyribonucleic a.
a. gland
glutamic a.
a. guanidine thiocyanate-phenol-chloroform method
guanidinosuccinic a. (GSA)
a. hematin method
a. hemolysis test
hepatoiminodiacetic a. (HIDA)
hippuric a.
homovanillic a. (HVA)
hyaluronic a.
hydrochloric a. (HCl)
hydroxyeicosatetraenoic a. (HETE)
20-hydroxyeicosatetraenoic a.
hydroxyindoleacetic a. (HIAA)
5-hydroxyindoleacetic a. (5-HIAA)

a. hypersecretion
hypervariable deoxyribonucleic a.
ibotenic a.
iminodiacetic a. (IDA)
a. indigestion
a. infusion
a. ingestion
a. injury
intravesical hyaluronic a.
iocetamic a.
iopanoic a.
iothalamic a.
^{131}I paraaminohippuric a.
isovaleric a.
keto a.
a. labile
lactic a.
Lewis a.
linoleic a.
lithocholic a. (LCA)
long-chain fatty a. (LCFA)
luminal a.
mandelic a.
medium-chain fatty a. (MCFA)
mefenamic a.
2-mercaptoethanesulfonic a. (mesna)
messenger ribonucleic a. (mRNA)
methylaminoisobutyric a. (MeAIB)
2-methylcitric a.
methylmalonic a.
a. microclimate
mucosal fatty a.
nalidixic a. (NA)
N-benzoyl-L-tyrosyl-P-aminobenzoic a.
nitroblue tetrazolium-paraaminobenzoic acid (NBT-PABA)
nonsulfated bile a.
Novamine amino a.
nucleic a.
okadaic a.
oleic a.
oral bile a. (OBA)
oxalic a.
PAH a.
p-aminohippuric a.
pantothenic a.
paraaminobenzoic a. (PABA)
paraaminohippuric a.
paraisopropyliminodiacetic a. (PIPIDA)

NOTES

acid (*continued*)
- a. peptic ulcer
- a. perfusion test
- phenazopyridine hydrochloric a.
- a. phosphate osteoclast
- polyglycolic a.
- polyprenoic a.
- pteroylglutamic a.
- a. pump
- a. reflux
- a. reflux test
- a. regurgitation
- renal excretion of a.
- renal messenger ribonucleic a.
- renal messenger ribonucleoprotein a.
- reptilase a.
- retinoic a.
- ribonucleic a. (RNA)
- saponifiable fecal bile a.
- saturated fatty a. (SFA)
- secondary bile a.
- a. secretion
- a. secretory disorder
- seminal plasma citric a.
- serum hyaluronic a.
- serum uric a.
- short-chain fatty a. (SCFA)
- sialic a.
- sulfuric a.
- a. suppression
- a. suppression therapy (AST)
- a. suppressive agent
- tannic a.
- taurocholic a.
- technetium-99m diethylenetriamine pentaacetic a.
- technetium-99m diisopropyl iminodiacetic a.
- technetium-99m iminodiacetic a.
- total bile a. (TBA)
- tranexamic a.
- Travasol amino a.
- tricarboxylic a. (TCA)
- trichloroacetic a. (TCA)
- trihydrocoprostanic a. (TCA)
- unsaturated fatty a.
- uric a.
- ursodeoxycholic a. (UDCA)
- valproic a.
- vanillacetic a. (VLA)
- vanillylmandelic a. (VMA)
- zoledronic a.

acid-ash diet

acid-base
- a.-b. balance
- a.-b. disorder
- a.-b. disturbance
- a.-b. equilibrium
- a.-b. imbalance
- a.-b. map

acidemia
- a. defect
- isovaleric a.
- a. of stool test

acid-fast bacillus (AFB)

acidic
- a. environment
- a. epididymal glycoprotein
- a. fibroblast growth factor
- a. sialomucin
- a. sulfomucin

acidification
- a. defect
- duodenal a.
- a. of stool test
- urine a.

acid-inhibitory factor

acidity
- circadian gastric a.
- gastric a.
- intracellular a.
- intragastric a.
- titratable a.
- urinary a.

acid-neutralizing capacity (ANC)

acidopathy
- specific organic a.

acidophilic
- a. body
- a. degeneration
- a. PAS-positive granule

acidophilus
- a. capsule
- *Lactobacillus a.*
- a. milk

acidosis
- acute a.
- a. after urinary intestinal diversion
- anion gap a.
- bicarbonate wastage renal tubular a.
- carbon dioxide a.
- chronic metabolic a.
- congenital lactic a.
- distal renal tubular a. (dRTA)
- generalized distal renal tubular a.
- high anion gap metabolic a.
- hyperchloremic metabolic a.
- hypokalemic renal tubular a.
- lactic a.
- long-term effects of metabolic a.
- metabolic a.
- nonanion-gap metabolic a.
- proximal renal tubular a.
- Rector-Gordon-Healey-Mendoza-Spitzer type IV renal tubular a.
- renal hyperchloremia a.

renal tubular a. (RTA)
renal tubular metabolic a.
renal tubular type I–IV a. (RTA-I–IV)
respiratory a.
uremic a.
winter a.
acidotic
acid-pepsin reflux esophagitis
acid-peptic
    a.-p. condition
    a.-p. disease
    a.-p. esophagitis
    a.-p. juice
acid-provoked spasm
acid-related disorder (ARD)
acid-Schiff
    Alcian blue and periodic a.-S. (AB/PAS)
    periodic a.-S. (PAS)
    a.-S. stain
acid-suppressed stomach
Acidulin
aciduria
    L-glyceric a.
    3-hydroxy-3-methylglutaric a.
acification
    intracellular a.
acinar
    a. adenocarcinoma
    a. cell
    a. cell carcinoma
    a. defect
    a. gradient
    a. hepatocellular carcinoma
    a. tissue
acinarization of pancreas
Acinetobacter
    A. calcoaceticus
    A. lwoffi
acini (*pl. of* acinus)
acinic cell
aciniform
acinitis
acinose
acinotubular
acinous
    a. adenoma
    a. cell
acinus, pl. **acini**
    liver a.
    pancreatic a.

    a. renalis malpighii
    a. renis malpighii
Aciphex
acipimox
acivicin
ACKD
    acquired cystic kidney disease
ackee fruit poisoning
ACL
    anal canal length
ACLA
    anticardiolipin antibody
aclacinomycin A
Acme One Time enteral feeding bag
ACMI
    A. cystourethroscope
    A. endoscope
    A. fiberoptic colonoscope
    A. fiberoptic esophagoscope
    A. fiberoptic proctosigmoidoscope
    A. gastroscope
    A. Martin endoscopy forceps
    A. monopolar electrode
    A. T-915, TX-915 fiberoptic sigmoidoscope
    A. ulcer measuring device
acnes
    Propionibacterium a.
acne vulgaris
aconitine
acontractile detrusor
acontractility
    bladder a.
    detrusor a.
aconuresis
acoprosis
acoprous
acorn-tipped
    a.-t. bougie
    a.-t. catheter
acorn treatment
acoustically transparent cradle
acoustic blink
ACP-ASIM
    American College of Physicians-American Society of Internal Medicine
acquired
    a. chordee
    a. cystic kidney disease (ACKD)
    a. diverticulosis
    a. functional megacolon
    a. gastric ectopia

NOTES

acquired *(continued)*
    a. hernia
    a. hyperlipoproteinemia
    a. hyperoxaluria
    a. immunity
    a. immunodeficiency
    a. immunodeficiency syndrome (AIDS)
    a. lactose deficiency
    a. neutrophil chemotaxis defect
    a. pancreatitis
    a. renal artery aneurysm
    a. renal cystic disease (ARCD)
    a. ureteropelvic junction obstruction

acquisita
    epidermolysis bullosa a.
    hypertrichosis lanuginosa a.

acquisition
    endoscopic data a.

acraturesis

Acrobacter
    A. butzleri
    A. nitrofigilis
    A. skirrowii

acrobystia
acrobystiolith
acrobystitis
acrocephalopolydactylous dysplasia
acrochordon
acrocyanosis
acrodermatitis enteropathica
acrolein
acromegalic gigantism
acromphalus
acrophase
acroposthitis
acrosin
acrosomal granule

acrosome
    a. reaction
    a. reaction assay

acrosome-reacted spermatozoon
acrylate

ACS
    abdominal compartment syndrome

ACT
    acid clearance test

ACTH
    adrenocorticotropic hormone

Acticoat
    A. composite dressing
    A. foam dressing

Acticon neosphincter
Actidose-Aqua
Actigall

actin
    a. filament
    smooth muscle isoform a.

acting
    long a. (LA, L.A.)

Actinomyces naeslundii
actinomycin C, D

actinomycosis
    biliary a.
    gastric a.
    intraabdominal a.

actinomycotic
    a. appendicitis
    a. esophageal disease

actinomycotica
    perityphlitis a.

action
    cytolytic a.
    immunomodulatory a.
    snake venom-converting enzyme-inhibiting a.
    viruslike a. (VLA)

Action-II
Actis venous flow controller (VFC)

activated
    a. alkaline glutaraldehyde
    a. capsule endoscope
    a. charcoal (AC)
    a. partial thromboplastin time (aPTT)
    a. protein C resistance (APCR)
    a. thromboplastin time

activation
    antibody-independent complement a.
    B-lymphocyte a.
    complement a.
    nuclear transcriptional a.
    platelet a.
    a. of programmed cell death pathway
    selective bladder a.
    T-cell a.
    T-lymphocyte a.
    very late a. (VLA)

activator
    continuous erythropoiesis receptor a. (CERA)
    plasminogen a. (PA)
    tissue plasminogen a. (TPA, tPA)
    tissue-type plasminogen a.
    urokinase plasminogen a.
    vascular plasminogen a. (v-PA)

active
    a. bowel sounds
    bowel sounds normal and a. (BSNA)
    a. chronic gastritis
    a. chronic hepatitis
    a. congestion
    a. duodenal ulcer
    A. Living incontinence pad
    A. Living incontinence shield

a. renin
a. schistosomiasis
a. source of bleeding
a. systemic bacterial infection
a. transport
actively bleeding varix
activin A
activity
    adenosine deaminase a.
    antiandrogenic a.
    antiproliferative a.
    a. assay
    ATPase a.
    beta galactosidase a.
    brush-border disaccharidase specific a.
    brush-border enzyme a.
    brush-border hydrolase a.
    cavitation bubble a.
    clinical a.
    complement hemolytic a.
    disaccharidase enzyme a.
    efferent renal sympathetic nerve a. (ERSNA)
    endogenous peroxidase a.
    fibrinolytic a.
    gastric myoelectrical a.
    gastric urease a.
    hepatic uroporphyrinogen decarboxylase a.
    hourly scratching a. (HSA)
    hyaluronidase a.
    intrinsic enzymatic a.
    Knodell criteria for histology a.
    mitotic a.
    motor a.
    muscarinic a.
    myoelectric a.
    NA+/H+ antiporter a.
    Na/K-ATPase a.
    necroinflammatory a.
    nonstrenuous a.
    opsonic a.
    oxidoreductase a.
    phasic contractile a.
    phospholipase A2 catalytic a.
    plasma renin a. (PRA)
    postheparin lipolytic a. (PHLA)
    protein serine/threonine kinase a.
    PyNPase a.
    renal sympathetic a.
    renal vein renin a. (RVRA)
    renal xanthine oxidase-xanthine dehydrogenase a.
    respiratory burst a.
    a. score
    serum cholinesterase a.
    single potential analysis cavernous electrical a.
    specific a.
    spermidine uptake a.
    spike-burst electrical a.
    sympathetic nervous system a.
    thermic effect of physical a. (TEPA)
    tumorigenesis a.
    tyrosine kinase a.
    xanthine oxidoreductase a.
Actril disinfectant
actual
    a. body weight (ABW)
    a. gastric myoelectric uncoupling
    a. intraprostatic temperature
    a. weight (AW)
Acucise
    A. access sheath
    A. balloon
    A. balloon catheter
    A. balloon cutting device
    A. endopyelotomy
    A. endopyelotomy catheter
    A. retrograde procedure
    A. RP outpatient procedure
acuity
acuminatum, pl. **acuminata**
    condyloma a.
    Dinophysis acuminata
    esophageal condyloma a.
    giant anorectal condyloma a.
AcuNav steerable phased vector-array ultrasound catheter probe
acupuncture
AcuSnare polypectomy device
acute
    a. abdominal series (AAS)
    a. abdominal vascular disease
    a. acalculous cholecystitis
    a. acidosis
    a. alcoholic hepatitis
    a. appendicitis
    a. cellular rejection
    a. cholecystitis (AC)
    a. colonic pseudoobstruction
    a. corrosive esophagitis

NOTES

acute *(continued)*
- a. diverticulitis
- a. drug-induced cholestasis
- a. edematous pancreatitis (AEP)
- a. epididymitis
- a. erosive gastritis (AEG)
- a. esophageal food impaction (AEFI)
- a. extrarenal obstruction
- a. fatty liver
- a. fatty liver of pregnancy (AFLP)
- a. febrile neutrophilic dermatosis
- a. flank pain
- a. flank pain syndrome
- a. focal bacterial nephritis (AFBN)
- a. gallstone pancreatitis (AGP)
- a. gastric anisakiasis
- a. gastric ischemia
- a. gastric mucosal lesion
- a. gastroenteritis (AGE)
- a. glomerulonephritis (AGN)
- a. graft-versus-host disease
- a. hemorrhagic cystitis (AHC)
- a. hemorrhagic gastritis
- a. hemorrhagic pancreatitis
- a. hepatic coma
- a. hepatic failure
- a. hepatic rupture
- a. hepatic toxicity
- a. hepatitis (AH)
- a. hepatocellular degeneration
- a. humoral rejection (AHR)
- a. humoral renal allograft rejection
- a. hydramnios
- a. hypokalemic nephropathy
- a. idiopathic inflammatory bowel disease
- a. idiopathic scrotal edema
- a. infectious colitis
- a. infectious diarrhea
- a. infectious nonbacterial gastroenteritis
- a. infundibulopelvic angle
- a. intermittent porphyria (AIP)
- a. interstitial nephritis (AIN)
- a. intrinsic renal failure
- a. juvenile cirrhosis
- a. lead poisoning
- a. leukopenia
- a. liver failure (ALF)
- a. lymphoblastic leukemia
- a. lymphocytic leukemia
- a. megacolon
- a. mercury poisoning
- a. mesangial proliferative glomerulonephritis
- a. methanol intoxication
- a. mononucleosis-like hepatitis
- a. MVT
- a. myelomonocytic leukemia
- a. necrotizing esophagitis
- a. nephritic syndrome
- a. nephrosis
- a. nonobstructive pyelonephritis
- a. nonocclusive bowel infarction
- a. nonvariceal upper gastrointestinal hemorrhage
- a. obstructive suppurative cholangitis (AOSC)
- a. occlusive mesenteric ischemia
- a. on chronic liver disease (AOCLD)
- a. pancreatitis prevention
- a. parenchymatous hepatitis
- a. phase of neurogenic bladder
- a. phase protein
- a. physiology, age and chronic health evaluation (APACHE)
- a. polycystic disease
- a. poststreptococcal glomerulonephritis (APSGN)
- a. proctitis
- a. recurrent pancreatitis (ARP)
- a. rejection of liver transplant
- a. relapsing pancreatitis
- a. renal failure (ARF)
- a. renal insufficiency (ARI)
- a. renal transplant vasculopathy
- a. schistosomiasis
- a. sclerosing hyaline necrosis (ASHN)
- a. scrotum
- a. self-limited colitis (ASLC)
- a. self-limited hepatitis
- a. serum sickness nephritis
- a. suppurative cholangitis (ASC)
- a. suppurative nephritis
- a. surgical abdomen
- a. tubular necrosis (ATN)
- a. tubular necrosis backleak
- a. urate nephropathy
- a. ureteric colic
- a. urethral syndrome
- a. urethritis
- a. uric acid nephropathy
- a. urinary retention (AUR)
- a. variceal bleeding
- a. vascular rejection
- a. viral hepatitis (AVH)
- a. yellow atrophy
- a. yellow atrophy of the liver

acute-phase response element (APRE)
AcuTrainer handheld electronic device
Acutrim
acyclic retinoid
acyclovir sodium
acyltransferase
    lecithin-cholesterol a. (LCAT)

acystia
acystinervia, acystineuria
A-D
    antidiarrheal
        Imodium A-D
A/D
    arthritic dose
        Ascriptin A/D
ADA
    American Diabetes Association
        ADA diet
Adair-Allis forceps
Adalat CC
Adamantiades-Behçet syndrome
Adapin
adaptation
    failed a.
    intestinal a.
adapter, adaptor
    camera a.
    C-mount a.
    Cook plastic Luer Lok a.
    friction-fit a.
    Olympus a.
    Polaroid SX-70 with ACMI a.
    Ralks a.
    swivel a.
    Tuohy-Borst a.
    Y a.
adaptic
    a. colitis
    A. dressing
    A. packing
adaptive
    a. gastroprotection
    a. immunity
    a. relaxation
    a. thermogenesis (AT)
adaptor (*var. of* adapter)
ADC
    antral diverticulum of colon
ADCC
    antibody-dependent cell-mediated cytotoxicity
    antibody-dependent cellular cytotoxicity
Adcon-P adhesion barrier solution
ADD
    angled delivery device
Add-A-Cath
    Lawrence A.-A-C.
add-back treatment

Addis
    A. count
    A. method
Addison
    A. clinical planes
    A. crisis
    A. disease
    A. point
    A. syndrome
addisonian syndrome
addisonii
    melasma a.
additional unproven role
addressin
ADD'Stat laser
adduct
    malondialdehyde-acetaldehyde a.'s (MAA)
adduction
    arytenoid a.
adductor
    a. brevis muscle
    a. longus muscle
ADE
    apparent digestive energy
adefoir dipivoxil
adefovir dipivoxil
adelomorphous cell
adenasthenia gastrica
adenemphraxis
Aden fever
adenine
    a. phosphoribosyltransferase (APRT)
    a. phosphoribosyltransferase deficiency
adenitis
    mesenteric a.
    phlegmonous a.
    syphilitic inguinal a.
adenoacanthoma
adenoassociated virus (AAV)
adenocarcinoma (ACA)
    acinar a.
    annular a.
    appendiceal a.
    bladder mesonephric a.
    clear cell a.
    colloid-producing a.
    colonic a.
    colorectal a.
    duodenal a.
    esophageal a.

NOTES

adenocarcinoma *(continued)*
    exophytic a.
    flat rectal a.
    gastric a.
    giant cell a.
    hepatoid a.
    a. of infantile testis
    infiltrating a.
    invasive a.
    metachronous small bowel a.
    metastatic a.
    mucinous a.
    mucin-producing a.
    mucosal a.
    papillary a.
    Paris renal a.
    peritoneal a.
    prostatic a.
    renal a.
    rete testis a.
    scirrhous a.
    seminal vesicle a.
    a. in situ
    testicular a.
    ulcerating a.
    urachal a.
adenofibromyoma
    testicular a.
adenoid cystic carcinoma
adenoleiomyofibroma
adenolysis
adenoma, pl. **adenomas, adenomata**
    acinous a.
    adrenal cortex a.
    adrenocortical a.
    aggressive a.
    aldosterone a.
    bile duct a. (BDA)
    bladder nephrogenic a.
    Brunner gland a.
    carcinoma ex pleomorphic a.
    chromophobe a.
    colonic a.
    colonoscopic view of a.
    colorectal villous a.
    cortical a.
    depressed a.
    a. destruens
    duodenal a.
    embryonal a.
    flat a.
    gastric a.
    hepatic a.
    hepatocellular a. (HCA)
    incidental a.
    islet cell a.
    kidney a.
    Leydig cell a.
    liver cell a. (LCA)
    mesonephric a.
    metachronous a.
    moderately differentiated a.
    monopolypoid a.
    mucinous a.
    nephrogenic a.
    nonhyperfunctioning
        adrenocortical a.
    nonpolypoid a.
    papillary a.
    periampullary a. (PAA)
    Pick testicular a.
    Pick tubular a.
    pituitary a.
    poorly differentiated a.
    prostatic a.
    rectal villous a.
    renocortical a.
    a. sebaceum
    serrated a.
    sessile a.
    sheetlike a.
    synchronous a.
    testicular tubular a.
    tubulovillous a.
    undifferentiated a.
    villoglandular a.
    villous colorectal a.
    well-differentiated a.
adenoma-associated antigen
adenoma-carcinoma sequence
adenoma-hyperplastic polyp ratio
adenoma-nonadenoma ratio
adenomas (*pl. of* adenoma)
adenomata (*pl. of* adenoma)
adenomatoid tumor
adenomatosis
    multiple endocrine a. type I, II
        (MEA-I, II)
adenomatous
    a. colorectal polyp
    a. epithelium
    a. gastric polyp
    a. hyperplasia (AH)
    a. polyp (AP)
    a. polyp-cancer sequence
    a. polyp of colon (APC)
    a. polyposis
    a. polyposis coli (APC)
    a. polyposis coli gene
    a. polyp of stomach
adenomucinosis
    disseminated peritoneal a.
adenomyoepithelioma of stomach
adenomyoma of gallbladder
adenomyomatosis
    gallbladder a.
adenomyosarcoma
    embryonal a.

adenomyosis
adenopapillomatosis
    gastric a.
adenopathy
    axillary a.
    inguinal a.
    lymph node a.
    palpable a.
    paraductal a.
    posterior mediastinal a.
adenosarcoma
    embryonal a.
adenosine
    a. deaminase
    a. deaminase activity
    a. diphosphatase (ADPase)
    a. diphosphate (ADP)
    a. monophosphate (AMP)
    a. nucleotide
    a. signal
    a. triphosphatase (ATPase)
    a. triphosphate (ATP)
adenosis
    sclerosing a.
adenosquamous cell carcinoma
adenovirus
    a. colitis
    enteric a.
    human a. 12
    a. infection
    subgroup F a.
adenovirus-12 viral protein
adenylate
    a. cyclase (AC)
    a. cyclase complex
adenyl cyclase stimulation
adequacy
    dialysis a.
    urea a.
ADF
    aortoduodenal fistula
ADH
    alcohol dehydrogenase
    antidiuretic hormone
adherence
    a. assay
    bacterial a.
adherent
    a. clot
    a. invasive *Escherichia coli*
adhesin
    bacterial a.

adhesion
    antigen-independent a.
    attic a.
    bacterial a.
    banjo-string a.
    cell-cell a.
    coronal a.
    dense a.
    a. dyspepsia
    fibrous a.
    filmy a.
    a. formation
    freeing up of a.
    hard a.
    hepatic a.
    intraabdominal a.
    intraperitoneal a.
    lysis of a.
    mannose-specific a.
    a. molecule
    omental a.
    pelvic a.
    perihepatic a.
    peritoneal a.
    postcholecystitis a.
    postoperative a.
    preputial a.
    taking down of a.
    T-cell a.
    thick a.
    thin a.
    tight perirectal a.
    tuft a.
    violin-string a.
adhesive
    a. band
    a. base
    Comfeel skin a.
    a. dressing
    fibrin tissue a.
    a. ileus
    Indermil a.
    Mastisol liquid surgical a.
    a. peritonitis
    a. protein receptor
    a. tape
    Uro-Bond skin a.
ADHF
    American Digestive Health Foundation
Adipex-P
adiphenine
adipocele

NOTES

adipohepatic
adipolytic
adipopectic
adipopexis
adipose
    a. arteries of kidney
    a. capsule of kidney
    a. tissue
adiposogenital dystrophy
adiposum
    hepar a.
adiposuria
adiposus
    ascites a.
adjacent hepatic artery
adjunctive nephrectomy
adjustable silicone gastric banding (ASGB)
adjusted body mass (ABM)
adjustment
    risk a.
adjuvant
    a. alpha blockade
    anesthesia a.
    a. drug therapy
    Freund a.
    a. hepatic arterial infusion chemotherapy
    a. nephrectomy
    a. treatment
ADL 8-2698
    alvimopan
Adlone
adminiculum, pl. **adminicula**
    a. lineae albae
administration
    intravesical electromotive drug a. (EMDA)
    percutaneous bacille Calmette-Guérin a.
adnexa
    hepatocellular a.
adnexal
    a. fullness
    a. mass
    a. tenderness
    a. torsion
    a. tumor
adolescent
    a. genitalia
    a. genitourinary examination
    a. incontinence
    a. penis
    a. spina bifida
    a. stress hematuria
    a. urologic evaluation
adoptive immunotherapy
ADP
    adenosine diphosphate
ADPase
    adenosine diphosphatase
ADPKD
    autosomal-dominant polycystic kidney disease
    oligosymptomatic ADPKD
ADPKD1
    ADPKD1 gene
    ADPKD1 genotype
ADPKD2 genotype
ADR
    Adriamycin
adrenal
    accessory a.'s
    a. artery
    a. catecholamine
    a. cortex
    a. cortex adenoma
    a. cortex androgen
    a. cortex carcinoma
    a. cortex estrogen-secreting tumor
    a. cortex fine-needle biopsy
    a. cortex ganglioneuroma
    a. cortex hyperfunction
    a. cortex testosterone-secreting tumor
    a. cortex zone
    a. corticoadenoma
    a. crisis
    a. cryptococcosis
    a. disease
    a. gland
    a. gland atrophy
    a. gland composition
    a. gland cyst
    a. gland incidentaloma
    a. gland innervation
    a. gland laparoscopic excision
    a. gland mass
    a. gland melanoma
    a. gland metastatic tumor
    a. gland microscopic section
    a. gland myelolipoma
    a. hemorrhage
    a. hirsutism
    a. insufficiency
    Marchand a.'s
    a. medulla
    a. rest
    a. rest tumor
    a. scintigraphy
    a. steroid
    a. tuberculosis
    a. vein
    a. vein aldosterone sampling
    a. venography
    a. virilism
    a. zona glomerulosa hyperplasia

adrenalectomy
    ablative a.
    endoscopic a.
    flank approach a.
    ipsilateral a.
    laparoscopic a.
    needlescopic a.
    open a.
    partial a.
    retroperitoneoscopic a.
    thoracoscopic transdiaphragmatic a.
    transperitoneal laparoscopic a. (TLA)
adrenalin
    a. chloride
    a. injection
    a. injection therapy
adrenalinuria
adrenal-sparing surgery
adrenergic
    a. neuron
    a. receptor
    a. signal
adrenergic-cholinergic agonist
adrenoceptive
adrenocortical
    a. adenoma
    a. macrocyst
adrenocorticohyperplasia
adrenocorticotropic
    a. hormone (ACTH)
    a. hormone infusion test
adrenogenital syndrome
adrenomedullin 52-amino acid peptide
adrenoreceptor
    alpha-1 a.
adrenostatic
adrenotoxin
adrenotropic
adrenotropin
adrenotropism
Adriamycin (ADR)
    cisplatin, cyclophosphamide, A. (CISCA)
    A. glomerulopathy
    A. nephropathy
    A. PFS
Adriamycin-induced nephrosis
Adrucil
Adson
    A. clamp
    A. dissecting hook
    A. needle holder
    A. suction tube
    A. tissue forceps
Adson-Brown tissue forceps
adsorption
adult
    a. celiac disease (ACD)
    a. familial hyaline membrane disease
    a. hypolactasia
    a. intersexual
    a. lactase deficiency
    a. phimosis
    a. polycystic kidney disease (APKD)
    a. polycystic liver disease (APLD)
    a. respiratory distress syndrome (ARDS)
    a. sigmoidoscope
adult-onset
    a.-o. nocturnal enuresis
    a.-o. obesity
advance
    A. formula
    postoperative a.
    preoperative a.
    a. to regular diet
    technical a.
advanced
    A. Care cholesterol test
    a. glycation end (AGE)
    A. surgical suture applier
    a. therapeutic endoscopy
Advanced-RF Natal Care
advancement
    Duckett meatal a.
    Glenn-Anderson a.
    meatal a.
    a. of rectal flap
    sleeve a.
    a. sleeve flap
Advanta bed
advantage
    GE RT 3200 A. II
Advantx digital system
adventitia
    fibrofatty a.
    tunica a.
adventitial fibroplasia
adventitious
    a. albuminuria
    a. cyst

NOTES

adverse prognostic factor
Advicor
adynamic
    a. bone
    a. bone disease (ABD)
    a. ileus
    a. intestinal obstruction
adysplasia
    kidney a.
Adzorbstar
AEC
    American Endosonography Club
    AEC Study
AEFI
    acute esophageal food impaction
AEG
    acute erosive gastritis
AELT
    ascites euglobulin lysis time
AEP
    acute edematous pancreatitis
AER
    albumin excretion rate
    alcohol elimination rate
    automatic endoscopic reprocessor
AERD
    atheroembolic renal disease
aerobic
    a. culture
    a. glycolysis
aerobilia
Aerochamber pediatric spacer device
Aerococcus
aerocystography
aerocystoscope
aerocystoscopy
aerodigestive
aerogastria
    blocked a.
aerogenes
    Enterobacter a.
aeroginosum
    sputum a.
Aeromonas
    A. bestiarum
    A. caviae
    A. diarrhea
    A. hydrophila
    A. liquefaciens
    A. media
    A. punctata
    A. salmonicida
    A. sobria
    A. trota
Aeromonas-**associated enterocolitis**
aeroperitonia
aerophagia, aerophagy
aerosialophagy
aerosis

aerosol
    hydrocortisone acetate rectal a.
    inhalation a.
    ^{99m}Tc DTPA a.
aerourethroscope
aerourethroscopy
aeruginosa
    Pseudomonas a.
AES
    anal endosonography
    anterior esophageal sensor
AESOP
    automated endoscopic system for optimal positioning
aethoxysclerol
AFB
    acid-fast bacillus
AFBN
    acute focal bacterial nephritis
afferent
    a. arteriolar vasoconstriction
    a. glomerular arteriole
    a. ileal limb
    a. innervation
    a. jejunal limb
    a. limb nipple stenosis
    a. loop
    a. loop syndrome
    mechanosensitive a.
    a. nerve fiber
    a. neuron
    a. projection
    a. renal nerve
    splanchnic primary a.
    a. terminal
    a. tubular isoperistaltic segment
    a. vessel of glomerulus
afferentia
    vasa a.
affinity-avidity hypothesis
aflatoxin
AFLP
    acute fatty liver of pregnancy
AFP
    alpha fetoprotein
African
    A. hemochromatosis
    A. iron overload
African-American
    A.-A. Study of Kidney Disease
    A.-A. Study of Kidney Disease and Hypertension (AASK)
africanum
    Pygeum a.
AFTP
    ascitic fluid total protein
A/G
    albumin-globulin ratio
    antigen

antiglobulin
   Trial AG
AGA
   American Gastroenterological
     Association
   antigliadin antibody
     IgG AGA
agalactiae
   Streptococcus a.
agalactosuria
agammaglobulinemia
   Bruton-type a.
   X-linked infantile a.
aganglionic
   a. bowel
   a. megacolon
   a. segment of colon
aganglionosis
   congenital intestinal a. (CIA)
agar
   brain-heart infusion a.
   a. bridge
   a. dilution
   EMB a.
   eosin-methylene blue a.
   a. gel
   MacConkey a.
   phenylethyl alcohol a.
   Sabouraud glucose a.
   sorbitol-MacConkey a.
   thiosulfate-citrate-bile salts-sucrose a. (TCBS)
   vancomycin/nalidixic acid a.
   Wilkins-Chalgren a.
agarose
   a. gel
   a. gel electrophoresis
agastria
agastric
AGE
   acute gastroenteritis
   advanced glycation end
agency
   Regional Organ Procurement A. (ROPA)
agenesis
   bladder a.
   corpus callosum a.
   kidney a.
   pancreatic a.
   renal a.
   sacral a.

   scrotal a.
   seminal vesicle a.
agenitalism
agenosomia
agent
   acid suppressive a.
   Albunex imaging/contrast a.
   antiadhesive a.
   anticholinergic a.
   antidiarrheal a.
   antidiuretic hormonelike a.
   antifungal a.
   antihypertensive a.
   antimicrobial a.
   antimotility a.
   antimuscarinic a.
   antisecretory a.
   antispasmodic a.
   5-ASA a.
   azole antifungal a.
   benzamide prokinetic a.
   beta-sympathomimetic tocolytic a.
   bulk a.
   bulking a.
   carbon dioxide trapping a.
   central adrenergic a.
   chemotherapeutic a.
   contrast a.
   cyanocobalamin radioactive a.
   cytotoxic a.
   distal tubular acting a.
   Durasphere injectable bulking a.
   embolic a.
   gallstone-solubilizing a.
   gastrokinetic a.
   Hawaii a.
   hemostatic a.
   imidoacetic acid radioactive a.
   immunosuppressive a.
   interleukin-2 receptor-blocking a.
   iodinated contrast a.
   iopamidol contrast imaging a.
   Levovist contrast a.
   Macroplastique soft tissue synthetic bulking a.
   motility a.
   mucolytic a.
   nonsteroidal antiinflammatory a. (NSAIA)
   Norwalk a.
   parasympathomimetic a.
   peripheral adrenergic a.

NOTES

agent *(continued)*
    periurethral bulking a.
    pharmacological a.
    progestational a.
    progesteronal a.
    prokinetic a.
    renoprotective a.
    rose bengal sodium ^{131}I radioactive a.
    Rubratope-57 radioactive a.
    sclerosing a.
    selenomethionine radioactive a.
    Sethotope radioactive a.
    test-yolk buffer cryopreservation a.
    thrombolytic a.
    vanilloid a.
    virucidal a.
    Yoshi-864 antineoplastic alkylating a.

age-related nocturia
ageusia
ageusic
agglutination test
agglutinin
    febrile a.'s
    peanut a. (PNA)

aggregate
    lymphoid a.

aggregated lymphatic follicles of Peyer
aggregati
    folliculi lymphatici a.

aggregation
    bile salt a.
    erythrocyte a.
    familial a.

aggressive
    a. adenoma
    a. fibromatosis
    a. therapeutic trial

agilis
    Lactobacillus a.

aging
    Baltimore Longitudinal Study of A. (BLSA)
    chemoprevention of a.

aglomerular
AGN
    acute glomerulonephritis

agona
    Salmonella a.

agonadal
agonadism
agonic intussusception
agonist
    adrenergic-cholinergic a.
    alpha-1 a.
    alpha-adrenergic a.
    alpha-2-adrenergic a.
    Bay K 8644 channel a.
    beta-2, 3 a.
    beta-adrenergic a.
    cholinergic a.
    dopamine a.
    dopaminergic a.
    5-HT4 a.
    kappa receptor opioid a.
    muscarinic cholinergic a.
    nicotinic a.
    nonpeptidyl a.
    opioid receptor a. (ORA)

Agoral
AGP
    acute gallstone pancreatitis

agranulocytic ulcer
AGUS
    atypical glandular cells of unknown significance

AH
    acute hepatitis
    adenomatous hyperplasia
    alcoholic hepatitis

ahaustral
AHC
    acute hemorrhagic cystitis

7a-HCO
AHLT
    auxiliary heterotopic liver transplantation

AHO
    Albright hereditary osteodystrophy

AHR
    acute humoral rejection

A-Hydrocort
Aichi virus
AID
    artificial insemination donor

AIDS
    acquired immunodeficiency syndrome

AIDS-related complex (ARC)
AIH
    artificial insemination husband
    autoimmune hepatitis

AIN
    acute interstitial nephritis
    anal intraepithelial neoplasia

AIO
    all-in-one
        AIO parenteral solution

AIP
    acute intermittent porphyria
    aldosterone-induced protein

AIPRI
    Angiotensin-Converting Enzyme Inhibition in Progressive Renal Insufficiency
        AIPRI trial

air
    biliary a.
    blood gas on room a.

a. cushion
a. cyst
a. cystogram
a. embolism
free a.
a. insufflation
intramural colonic a.
intraperitoneal a.
a. pressure enema reduction
a. pyelography
a. swallowing
a. thermometer
a. tightness test
air-contrast barium enema (ACBE)
air-filled
    a.-f. balloon
    a.-f. loop
airflow obstruction
air-fluid level
airfuge
    Beckman a.
Airlift balloon retractor
airway
    double-lumen gastric laryngeal mask a.
    a. epithelium
    esophageal gastric tube a. (EGTA)
    esophageal obturator a. (EOA)
    gastric laryngeal mask a. (GLMA)
    a. obstruction
    patent a.
airway-arterial fistula
AJCC
    American Joint Committee on Cancer
    AJCC TNM tumor classification
AJCC/UICC
    American Joint Committee on Cancer/International Union Against Cancer
    AJCC/UICC staging system
Ajmalin
    A. liver disease
    A. liver injury
AJPBD
    anomalous junction of pancreaticobiliary ducts
Akerlund
    A. deformity
    diverticulum of A.
akinesia
    rectal a.

ALA
    aminolevulinic acid
5-ALA
    5-aminolevulinic acid
Alagille syndrome
Alagille-Watson syndrome
AL amyloid
alanine aminotransferase (ALT)
alanine-glyoxylate aminotransferase
alarm
    bed-wetting a.
    a. clock voiding
    enuresis a.
    glutaraldehyde a.
    a. symptom
    a. therapy
alascence
    Diphyllobothrium a.
Alaxin
Alazide
alba, pl. **albae**
    adminiculum lineae albae
    linea a.
Albarran
    A. deflecting level
    A. disease
    A. gland
    A. laser cystoscope
    A. mechanism
    A. reflecting bridge
    A. test
    A. tubule
albendazole
albensis
    Vibrio cholerae biotype *a.*
Albert-Lembert
    A.-L. method
    A.-L. suture
Albert suture
albicans
    Candida a.
albiduria, albinuria
Albright
    A. hereditary osteodystrophy (AHO)
    A. solution
    A. syndrome
Albuferon
albuginea
    a. penis
    a. testis
    tunica a.
albugineotomy

NOTES

albugineous
albuginitis
albumin
 ^{125}I a.
 Bence Jones a.
 bovine serum a. (BSA)
 diethylenetriamine-pentaacetic acid-galactosyl-human serum a.
 a. excretion rate (AER)
 fatty acid-free bovine serum a.
 glycated a.
 a. gradient
 human serum a.
 intravenous a.
 macroaggregated a. (MAA)
 a. messenger RNA
 a. metabolism
 nonglycated a.
 plasma a.
 a. plasma concentration
 serum a.
 sonicated a.
 a. synthesis
 technetium-99m galactosyl-human serum a.
 technetium-99m macroaggregated a.
albuminaturia
albumin-coated resin hemoperfusion
albumin-globulin ratio (A/G)
albuminocholia
albuminoid liver
albuminorrhea
albuminous nephritis
albuminuria
 adventitious a.
 Bamberger hematogenic a.
 globular a.
 nephrogenous a.
 postrenal a.
 residual a.
albuminuric retinitis
albumosuria
 Bence Jones a.
Albunex
 A. imaging/contrast agent
 A. injection
albus
 Staphylococcus a.
Albustix test
alcalifaciens
 Providencia a.
Alcian
 A. blue
 A. blue dye
 A. blue and periodic acid-Schiff (AB/PAS)
 A. blue stain

Alcock
 A. canal
 A. syndrome
Alcock-Timberlake obturator
alcohol
 absolute a.
 a. absorption
 a. abuse
 a. consumption
 a. cooling bath
 a. dehydrogenase (ADH)
 a. dehydrogenase inhibition
 a. diuresis
 a. elimination rate (AER)
 ethyl a.
 graded a.
 a. injection of tumor
 a. intoxication
 isoamyl a.
 polyvinyl a.
 a. potentiation
 a. sclerosis
 a. thermometer
alcohol-fixed gastric biopsy
alcoholic
 a. cirrhosis (AC)
 a. diarrhea
 a. fatty liver
 a. fibrosis
 a. hemorrhagic gastritis
 a. hepatitis (AH)
 a. hyalin
 a. liver disease (ALD)
 a. pancreatitis
 a. prognostic factor
 a. varix
alcohol-induced
 a.-i. extracellular volume contraction
 a.-i. gastric injury
 a.-i. gastrointestinal symptom
 a.-i. hypoglycemia
 a.-i. pancreatitis
alcoholism
 American Medical Society on A. (AMSA)
alcoholuria
Alconefrin
ALD
 alcoholic liver disease
Aldactazide
Aldactone
Aldara
aldehyde dehydrogenase (ALDH)
Alden loop gastric bypass
aldesleukin
ALDH
 aldehyde dehydrogenase
Aldoclor

aldolase
    fructose a.
Aldomet
Aldoril
aldose reductase (AR)
aldosterone
    a. adenoma
    a. deficiency
    a. synthase
    a. synthase polymorphism
aldosterone-induced protein (AIP)
aldosterone-sensitive distal nephron
aldosterone-to-renin ratio
aldosteronism
aldosteronoma
aldosteronopenia
aldosteronuria
Aldrich-Mees line
Aldridge operation
alendronate
Aleo meter
alert
    Sears Wee A.
Alexander-Adams operation
Alexander elevator
alexandrite
    a. laser
    a. laser lithotripsy
    a. and rhodamine
alexithymia
aleydigism
ALF
    acute liver failure
    American Liver Foundation
alfa
    darbepoetin a.
    epoetin a.
    recombinant interferon a. (rIFN-alfa)
alfa-2a, 2b
    interferon a.-2a, 2b
    PEG-interferon a.-2a, 2b
    recombinant interferon a.-2a, 2b
    teceleukin and interferon a.-2a, 2b
alfacon-1
    interferon a.-1
Alfa-gliatest
    ELISA Kit A.-g.
alfa-interferon therapy
alfa-n1
    interferon a.-n1

alfa-n3
    interferon a.-n3
alfaxalone
alfentanil
Alferon N
alfuzosin HCl
Algenic Alka
algesimeter
    Boas a.
Al-Ghorab
    A.-G. modification
    A.-G. modification shunt
    A.-G. procedure
Algicon
algidicarnis
    Clostridium a.
algid malaria
alginate spray
alginolyticus
    Vibrio a.
alginuresis
Alglucerase
algoid cell
algorithm
    current a.
    a. of diagnosis
    imaging a.
    management a.
    specific a.
Alibra
alicaforsen
alimentary
    a. apparatus
    a. bolus
    a. canal
    a. diabetes
    a. edema
    a. glycosuria
    a. hyperinsulinism
    a. obesity
    a. system
    a. therapy
    a. tract
    a. tract duplication
alimentation
    central venous a.
    enteral a.
    forced a.
    parenteral a.
    peripheral intravenous a.
    rectal a.
    total parenteral a.

NOTES

Alimentum
aliquot
AlitraQ
Alka
    Algenic A.
alkali
    caustic a.
    a. ingestion
alkaline
    a. citrate therapy
    a. injury
    a. milk drip
    a. phosphatase (ALP, AP)
    a. phosphatase-antialkaline phosphatase (APAAP)
    a. phosphatase isoenzyme
    a. phosphatase test
    a. phosphatase Vectastain ABC
    a. protease inhibitor (API)
    a. reflux esophagitis
    a. reflux gastritis
alkaline-ash diet
alkalinity
alkalinization
    oral a.
    a. test
    urinary a.
alkalitherapy
alkaloid
    ergot a.
    indolalkylamine a.
    Veratrum a.
alkalosis
    hypochloremic hypokalemic metabolic a.
    hypokalemic metabolic a.
    metabolic a.
    respiratory a.
    watery diarrhea with hypokalemic a. (WDHA)
Alka-Mints
alkane
    breath a.
alkaptonuria
Alka-Seltzer
Alken approach
Alkets
allantoic
    a. cyst
    a. tract
allantois
allele
    carrier of a.
    HLA-DP a.
    I1307K a.
allelic
    DC locus a.
allelotyping
    p53 a.

Allemann syndrome
Allen
    A. anastomosis clamp
    A. intestinal clamp
    A. intestinal forceps
    A. stirrups
    A. strap
    A. test
Allen-Brown shunt
Allen-Kocher clamp
Allen-Masters syndrome
allergen
    food a.
allergic
    a. colitis
    a. cystitis
    a. dermatitis
    a. enteropathy
    a. interstitial nephritis
    a. proctitis
    a. reaction
    a. vasculitis
allergy
    cow's milk a. (CMA)
    cow's milk protein a.
    food a.
    gastrointestinal a.
    latex a.
    medication a.
all four quadrants
ALLHAT
    Antihypertensive and Lipid-Lowering Treatment to Prevent Heart Attack Trial
Alliance integrated inflation system
alligator jaws Olympus FG 6L grasping forceps
alligator-type grasping forceps
Allingham
    A. colotomy
    A. fissure
    A. operation
    A. rectum excision
    A. ulcer
all-in-one (AIO)
Allis
    A. catheter
    A. clamp
    A. forceps
    A. inhaler
    A. tooth grasper
Alliston GE reflux repair
allium vegetable
alloantibody
    donor-specific a.
alloantigen-dependent
    postoperative a.-d.
alloantigen response
alloantigen-specific
allocating cadaveric kidney

allocation
    Eurotransplant kidney a.
allochezia
allodynia
allogeneic
    a. mixed leukocyte culture
    a. MLC
allogenic
    a. kidney transplant
    a. liver perfusion
allograft
    clinically stable human renal a.
    hepatic a.
    human leukocyte antigen renal a.
    injured a.
    kidney a.
    long-term survival of renal a.
    nephrectomy a.
    outcome of cadaveric renal a.
    a. parenchyma
    a. rejection
    renal a.
    Repliform dermal a.
    a. survival
    a. survival rate
allograft-mediated hypertension
alloplast
    bioactive antimicrobial coated solid a.
alloplastic
    a. biomaterial
    a. prostatic bladder
    a. spermatocele
allopurinol
allotransplantation
allowance
    recommended daily a. (RDA)
alloy
    shape memory a. (SMA)
all-purpose capsule (APC)
All-Silicone Side-Eye EPT feeding tube
allylamine
Almacone II
aloe
    cascara sagrada and a.
Aloka MP-PN ultrasound probe
alopecia
alosetron
    a. HCl
    a. HCl tablet
    a. hydrochloride
Aloxi

ALP
    alkaline phosphatase
alpha
    5-a.-androstane-3-alpha 17-beta-diol
    5-a.-androstane-3-beta 17-beta-diol
    a. blockade
    a. chain disease
    estrogen receptor a. (ER alpha)
    a. fetoprotein (AFP)
    a. fetoprotein level
    a. gene
    a. glycerylphosphorylcholine
    a. heavy-chain disease
    A. I inflatable penile prosthesis
    interferon a.
    a. interferon
    a. interferon treatment
    A. I penile implant
    a. ketoglutaramate
    lymphoblastoid interferon a.
    a. motor neuron
    a. *Streptococcus viridans*
    a. sympathetic blockade
    transforming growth factor a. (TGF-alpha)
alpha-1
    a.-1 adrenoreceptor
    a.-1 agonist
    a.-1 blocker
    a.-1 globulin
alpha-1-acid glycoprotein
alpha-1-adrenoceptor antagonist
alpha-adducin
alpha-adrenergic
    a.-a. agonist
    a.-a. antagonist
    a.-a. receptor
alpha-1-adrenergic receptor
alpha-2-adrenergic
    a.-2-a. agonist
    a.-2-a. receptor
alpha-amylase
    pancreatic a.-a.
alpha-21 antiplasmin
alpha-1-antitrypsin
    a.-1-a. deficiency
    a.-1-a. deficiency disease
    a.-1-a. disease (AATD)
    a.-1-a. disease-related emphysema
    a.-1-a. globulin
    a.-1-a. level
alpha-2b

NOTES

alpha-2-beta-1 integrin cell-surface
  collagen
alpha-3-beta-1 integrin
alpha-blocker
  a.-b. therapy
  a.-b. treatment
alpha-3, -4, -5 chain
alpha-delta-mannosidase
alpha-dextrinase
9-alpha-fluorohydrocortisone
alpha-galactosidase A
alpha-gliadin fraction
alpha-glucosidase inhibitor
alpha-1-glycero-monooctanoin
alpha-hemolytic streptococcus
alpha-hydroxylase
  17-a,-h. deficiency
alpha-ketoacid dehydrogenase
alpha-loop maneuver
alpha-methylparatyrosine
Alphamul
alphaprodine
alpha-receptor
  a.-r. antagonist
  a.-r. blockade therapy
5-alpha-reductase
  5-alpha-reductase inhibition
  5-alpha-reductase inhibitor
alpha-sigmoid loop
alpha-TGI
Alport syndrome
ALPP
  abdominal leak-point pressure
alprazolam
alprostadil/prazosin HCl
alprostadil urethral suppository
Alprox-TD
ALR cystoresectoscope
Alseroxylon-Alkavervir
Alstrom disease
Alstrom-Edwards syndrome
ALT
  alanine aminotransferase
  ALT test
Altace
Altemeier
  A. perineal rectosigmoidectomy
  A. procedure
  A. repair
alteplase
alteration
  genetic a.
  molecular genetic a.
  nuclear matrix a.
altered sperm motility
ALternaGEL
alternate-day treatment
alternate mRNA splicing
alternating calculus

alternative
  a. cell attachment domain
  a. endourological procedure
Altertome
  Microvasive A.
Althausen test
Altmann pulse
Altracin
ALTRA-FLUX hemodialyzer
ALT-RCC
  autolymphocyte-based treatment for renal
  cell carcinoma
altretamine
Alu-Cap
Aludrox
alum
  a. curd
  intravesical a.
aluminum
  a. carbonate
  a. hydroxide
  a. hydroxide, magnesium hydroxide,
  and simethicone
  a. hydroxide and magnesium
  trisilicate
  a. phosphate
  a. toxicity
Alupent
Alutabs
alvei
  Hafnia a.
alveolar
  a. hydatid cyst
  a. hydatid disease
  a. rhabdomyosarcoma
AlveoSampler
  QuinTron A.
alverine citrate
alvi
  incontinentia a.
alvimopan (ADL 8-2698)
alvine calculus
alvus
Alzer Model 2001 osmotic minipump
AMA
  antimitochondrial antibody
  AMA inflatable cylinder
Amadori product
AMAG
  autoimmune metaplastic atrophic gastritis
amalonaticus
  Citrobacter a.
Amanita
  Amanita phalloides mushroom
  poisoning
  A. mushroom
  A. mushroom hepatotoxicity
amantadine
Amaryl

amasesis
amastigote
amatoxin
amaurosis
    Leber a.
ambenonium chloride
Ambicor penile prosthesis
ambigua
    Shigella a.
ambiguous external genitalia
ambiguus
    nucleus a.
Ambilhar
AmB-induced reduction GFR
ambiothermic
AmBisome
amblygeustia
ambulation
ambulatory
    a. blood pressure
    a. hemorrhoidectomy
    a. intraesophageal bilirubin monitoring
    a. intraesophageal pH monitoring
    a. manometry
    a. probe
    a. urodynamic monitoring
    a. urodynamics
amebiasis
    a. of bladder
    hepatic a.
    indigenous a.
    intestinal a.
amebic
    a. appendicitis
    a. colitis
    a. dysentery
    a. granuloma
    a. hepatitis
    a. lectin antigen
    a. liver abscess
    a. ulcer
amebicidal
amebism
ameboma mimicking carcinoma
ameliorated vasodilating response
ameliorate pain
America
    Crohn and Colitis Foundation of A. (CCFA)

American
    A. Academy of Wound Management (AAWM)
    A. ACMI (S3565, TX-915) flexible fiberoptic sigmoidoscope
    A. Anorexia/Bulimia Association
    A. Association for the Study of Liver Diseases (AASLD)
    A. College of Gastroenterology (ACG)
    A. College of Physicians-American Society of Internal Medicine (ACP-ASIM)
    A. Diabetes Association (ADA)
    A. Digestive Health Foundation (ADHF)
    A. Dilation System dilator
    A. Endoscopy automatic reprocessor
    A. Endoscopy dilator
    A. Endoscopy mechanical lithotriptor
    A. Endosonography Club (AEC)
    A. Endosonography Club Study
    A. Gastroenterological Association (AGA)
    A. Joint Committee on Cancer (AJCC)
    A. Joint Committee on Cancer/International Union Against Cancer (AJCC/UICC)
    A. Liver Foundation (ALF)
    A. Medical Society on Alcoholism (AMSA)
    A. Medical Systems (AMS)
    A. Society for Gastrointestinal Endoscopy (ASGE)
    A. trypanosomiasis
    A. type culture collection
    A. Urological Association (AUA)
    A. Urological Association symptom index
americanus
    Necator a.
Amerlex-M second antibody
Ames
    A. Hemastix reagent strip semiquantitative agglutination SERA-TEK A.
    A. test
A-Methapred
AMF
    autocrine motility factor

NOTES

Amicar
Amicon D-20 filter
amicrobic cystitis
amicrofilaremic filariasis
amidation
    carboxyl-terminal a.
amidolytic assay
amifloxacin
amifostine
amikacin
Amikin
amiloride hydrochloride
amiloride-sensitive, electroneutral Na+/H+ antiporter
Amin-Aid powdered feeding
amine
    aromatic a.
    biogenic a.
    a. precursor uptake and decarboxylation (APUD)
    a. precursor uptake and decarboxylation cell
amino
    a. acid
    a. acid abnormality
    a. acid-based dialysate solution
    a. acid excretion in neonate
    a. acid-glucose mixture
    28-a. acid peptide
    A. Mel Hepa
    a. terminus
aminoacetate
    dihydroxyaluminum a.
aminoacidopathy
    dibasic a.
aminoaciduria
    hyperdibasic a.
    imidazole a.
    a. in neonate
    overflow a.
    renal a.
    transport a.
aminobenzoate
    butyl a.
    a. potassium
4-aminobiphenyl
aminobiphosphonate gastrotoxic drug
aminocaproic acid
Aminofusin L Forte amino acid solution
aminoglutethimide
aminoglycoside
aminoguanidine
aminoisobutyricaciduria
    beta a.
5-aminolevulinic
    5-a. acid (5-ALA)
    5-a. acid-induced fluorescence endoscopy
aminolevulinic acid (ALA)
aminonucleoside
    glomerular epithelial cell toxin puromycin a.
    puromycin a.
aminopenicillin
aminopeptidase
    leucine a. (LAP)
aminophylline
aminopromazine
aminopropionitrile
    beta a.
aminopyrine
    a. breath test
    a. clearance
aminorex
aminosalicylate
5-aminosalicylic
    5-a. acid (5-ASA)
    5-a. acid enema
4-aminosalicylic acid (4-ASA)
amino-terminal undecapeptide
aminothiol concentration
aminotransferase
    alanine a. (ALT)
    alanine-glyoxylate a.
    aspartate a. (AST)
amiodarone
Amipaque
Amitone
amitriptyline hydrochloride
AML
    angiomyolipoma
amlodipine besylate
ammonia
    arterial a.
    blood a.
    a. level
    plasma a.
    a. production
    serum a.
    a. toxicity
ammonia-13 (^{13}N)
ammoniagenesis
ammoniagenic coma
ammonium
    a. acid urate calculus
    a. acid urate urolithiasis
    a. hydroxide
amnesia
    antegrade a.
    procedural a.
    retrograde a.
amnion
amodiaquine
amoeba
Amogel PG

amorphous filling defect
amoxicillin
    a. and clavulanic acid
    luminal a.
    a. trihydrate
amoxicillin-clavulanate
amoxicillin-omeprazole treatment
amoxicillin-tinidazole-ranitidine therapy
Amoxil
AMP
    adenosine monophosphate
        AMP level
        urinary cyclic AMP
amperage
amphetamine
amphibolic fistula
amphibolous fistula
amphipathic bile salt
amphiregulin
Amphocin
Amphojel
Amphotec
amphotericin
    a. B
    a. B-induced reduction glomerular filtration rate
    a. B nephropathy
    a. B resistance
    a. B therapy
ampicillin
Ampicin
Amplatz
    A. catheter
    A. fascial dilator
    A. sheath
    A. Super Stiff guidewire
    A. TractMaster system
Amplicor HCV 2.0 RNA test
amplification refractory mutation system-polymerase chain reaction (ARMS-PCR)
amplitude
    esophageal body contraction a.
    high-energy a.
    mean distal contraction a. (MDCA)
amplitude-acrophase vector
amplitude-coded color Doppler sonography
ampulla, pl. ampullae
    a. ductus deferentis
    duodenal a.
    Henle a.
    a. hepatopancreatica
    invagination of the a.
    Lieberkühn a.
    rectal a.
    a. recti
    a. of rectum
    a. of vas deferens
    a. of Vater
ampullary
    a. ablative therapy
    a. carcinoma
    a. granulation tissue
    a. hamartoma
    a. lesion
    a. stenosis
    a. stone
    a. tumor
ampullectomy
    endoscopic snare a.
ampulloma
ampullopancreatic carcinoma
amputation
    penile a.
AMS
    American Medical Systems
        AMS controlled-expansion penile prosthesis
        AMS 700CX penile prosthesis cylinder
        AMS Hydroflex penile prosthesis
        AMS inflatable 700 penile prosthesis
        AMS malleable 600 penile prosthesis
        AMS ProstaJect ethanol injection system
        AMS 700-series double-cuff Silastic artificial urinary sphincter
        AMS 800-series double-cuff Silastic artificial urinary sphincter
        AMS Sphincter 800 Urinary Prosthesis
        AMS three-piece inflatable penile prosthesis
        AMS Ultrex penile prosthesis
AMSA
    American Medical Society on Alcoholism
    amsacrine
amsacrine (AMSA)
Amsterdam
    A. biliary stent

NOTES

Amsterdam (continued)
    A. criteria
    A. criteria for hereditary nonpolyposis colorectal cancer
Amsterdam-type prosthesis
Amussat
    A. incision
    A. operation
    A. valve
    A. valvula
amygdala
amylacea
    corpora a.
amylase
    ascitic a.
    a. concentration
    pancreatic a.
    P-type a.
    salivary a.
    serum a.
    S-type a.
    a. unit
    urinary a.
amylase/creatinine clearance ratio
amylase-resistant starch (ARS)
amylin
amyl nitrite
amylo-1,6-glucosidase deficiency
amyloglucosidase
amyloid
    AA a.
    AL a.
    a. kidney
    a. nephropathy
    a. nephrosis
    serum a. P (SAP)
amyloidlike glomerulopathy
amyloidoma
amyloidosis
    a. of bladder
    cutaneous lichen a.
    hepatic a.
    kidney a.
    localized a.
    rectal a.
    renal a.
    secondary a.
    systemic a.
    type IV a.
amyloidotic glomerulus
amylopectinosis
amylorrhea
amylosuria
AN
    anorexia nervosa
AN69 membrane dialyzer
ANA
    antinuclear antibody

anabolic
    a. steroid
    a. steroid spermatogenesis impairment
    a. steroid treatment
Anacardium occidentale L
anacidic stomach
anacidity
ANAD
    anorexia nervosa and associated disorders
anadenia ventriculi
anaerobe
    obligate a.
anaerobic
    a. culture
    a. glycolysis
anal
    a. abscess
    a. anastomosis
    a. atresia
    a. bulging
    a. canal
    a. canal hypertonia
    a. canal length (ACL)
    a. column
    a. condyloma
    a. crypt
    a. dilation
    a. dilator
    a. discharge
    a. disk
    a. effluent
    a. electrical stimulation
    a. EMG PerryMeter sensor
    a. encirclement
    a. endoscopy
    a. endosonography (AES)
    a. epidermoid carcinoma
    a. fascia
    a. fibrosis
    a. fissure
    a. fistula
    a. foreign body
    a. ileostomy with preservation of sphincter
    a. incontinence
    a. intersphincteric groove
    a. intraepithelial neoplasia (AIN)
    a. intramuscular gland
    a. mapping
    a. margin
    a. neoplasm
    a. pecten
    a. pit
    a. pitting
    a. plate
    a. pouch
    a. procidentia
    a. prolapse

a. protrusion
a. reflex
a. sepsis
a. sinus
a. sphincter (AS)
a. sphincter contraction
a. sphincter dysfunction
a. sphincter function
a. sphincter reconstruction
a. sphincter repair
a. sphincter squeeze pressure
a. sphincter tone
a. squamous dysplasia
a. squamous intraepithelial lesion
a. stenosis
a. stricture
a. surgery
a. transitional zone (ATZ)
a. transitional zone dysplasia
a. triangle
a. ulceration
a. valve
a. vector manometry
a. verge
a. wart
a. wink
a. wound
analeptic enema
anales
   columnae a.
   sinus a.
   valvulae a.
analgesia
   patient a.
   patient-controlled a.
analgesic
   a. effect
   narcotic a.
   a. nephropathy
   a. requirement
analgesic-antipyretic
analgosedation
analis
   pecten a.
analog, analogue
   arginine a.
   prostaglandin a.
   somatostatin a.
Analpram-HC anorectal cream
analysis, pl. **analyses**
   anthropometric a.
   bioelectrical impedance a. (BIA)

Bland-Altman a.
body composition a.
CFTR gene a.
cineradiographic a.
contexture a.
cosinor a.
cost effectiveness a.
crude cost a.
cytogenetic a.
cytometric a.
Diacyte DNA ploidy a.
DNA ploidy a.
electrophoresis immunoblot a.
encrustation a.
energy dispersive x-ray a.
enzymatic spectrophotometric a.
fecal a.
flow cytometric a.
flow cytometry a.
fluid a.
fluorescent image a.
Fourier transform a.
gastric a.
gene-linkage a. (GLA)
heteroduplex a.
histochemical-ultrastructural a.
image a.
Kaplan-Meier a.
logistic regression a.
monoclonality by genetic a.
multivariable logistic regression a.
multivariate a.
Northern blot a.
ploidy a.
prefreeze semen a.
pressure flow a.
p53 tumor-suppressor gene a.
pulse-width a.
real-time spectral a.
reflectance a.
regression a.
renal morphometric a.
retrospective a.
semen a.
sequencing a.
serum cytokine a.
single-parameter DNA a.
single strand conformation
   polymorphism a.
Southern blot a.
spectral a.
spectrophotometric a.

NOTES

analysis *(continued)*
    stepwise regression a.
    survival a.
    trace-gas a.
    two-dimensional flow cytometric a.
    univariate a.
    urine cytokine a.
    Vindelov method flow cytometry a.
    a. of virulence factor
    Western blot a.
    x-ray a.

analyzer
    automatic chemical a.
    Beckman ion-selective a.
    Cell Soft 2000 semen a.
    C-Trak a.
    GastrograpH Mark III pH a.
    Hamilton-Thorn motility a.
    Hitachi 717 a.
    IMMULITE 2000 anti-HBc IgM a.
    IMMULITE 2000 anti-HBs a.
    IMMULITE HBsAg immunoassay a.
    MicroLyzer Gas a.
    Olympus SP-series image a.
    Orion model EA 940 ion a.
    Packard Auto-Gamma 5650 a.
    reflectance TS-200 spectrum a.
    RJL Model 10 bioelectrical impedance a.
    sequential multiple a. (SMA)
    Siemens Somatom DRH CT a.
    SYNCHRON CX-5, CX-7 automated a.
    Ultrasound Bone A.
    wave a.

Anandron
anaphylactica
    enteritis a.
anaphylactic reaction
anaphylactoid
    a. food sensitivity
    a. purpura
    a. purpura nephritis
anaphylaxis
anaplasia
anaplastic
    a. malignant teratoma
    a. seminoma
    a. Wilms tumor
Anaprox
anaritide acetate
anasarca
anascitic
Anaspaz
anastalsis
anastomose
anastomosis, pl. **anastomoses**
    Abbe intestinal a.
    anal a.
    antecolic a.
    antiperistaltic a.
    aseptic a.
    bilioenteric a.
    Billroth I, II a.
    bladder neck-to-urethra a.
    Brackin ureterointestinal a.
    Braun a.
    Carrel aortic patch a.
    cervical esophagogastric a.
    circular stapled a.
    a. clamp
    Coffey ureterointestinal a.
    coloanal a. (CAA)
    colocolonic a.
    colorectal a.
    Cordonnier technique ureterocolonic a.
    Couvelaire ileourethral a.
    crunch stick a.
    curved end-to-end a. (CEEA)
    delayed a.
    diseased organileal pouch-anal a.
    dismembered a.
    dog-ear of a.
    double-stapled ileal pouch-anal a.
    Duhamel laparoscopic pullthrough a.
    end-to-end a. (EEA)
    end-to-side a.
    enteroenteric a.
    esophagocolic a.
    esophagojejunal a.
    extracorporeal a.
    extravesical a.
    fishmouth a.
    Furniss ureterointestinal a.
    Gambee a.
    Goodwin technique ureterocolonic a.
    Halsted a.
    handsewn a.
    hepaticojejunal a.
    Hofmeister a.
    Hofmeister-Pólya a.
    homocladic a.
    Horsley a.
    H-shaped ileal pouch-anal a.
    ileal pouch-anal a. (IPAA)
    ileal pouch-distal rectal a.
    ileoanal a.
    ileocolic a.
    ileorectal a. (IRA)
    ileosigmoid a.
    ileotransverse colon a.
    ileovesical a.
    intestinal a.
    intracorporeal a.

intravesical a.
isoperistaltic a.
J-shaped ileal pouch-anal a.
Kocher a.
Leadbetter and Clarke ureteral a.
LeDuc ureteral a.
Lich-Gregoire a.
low anterior resection in combination with coloanal a. (LAR/CAA)
low coloanal a.
magnetic compression a.
mechanical a.
mesocaval a.
mucosa-to-mucosa a.
Navy single-layer everting a.
neobladder-urethra a.
Nesbit technique ureterocolonic a.
nondismembered a.
Pagano technique ureterocolonic a.
Pagano ureteral a.
pancreaticogastric a.
Parks ileoanal a.
peristaltic a.
Politano-Leadbetter a.
Pólya a.
portacaval a.
pouch-anal a.
primary a.
pyeloileocutaneous a.
rectosigmoid a.
reniportal a.
retrocolic a.
right-angle end-to-side a.
Roux-en-Y a.
Roux-type gastroduodenal a.
Schoemaker a.
side-to-side a.
single-layer continuous intestinal a.
small bowel a.
spatulated overlap a.
splenorenal venous a.
S-shaped ileal pouch-anal a.
stapled end-to-end ileoanal a.
stapled intestinal a.
stapled pouch-anal a.
State end-to-end a.
Strickler technique ureterocolonic a.
Strickler ureteral a.
sutureless bowel a.
tension-free a.
transanal a.
transureteroureteral a.
two-layer interrupted intestinal a.
ultralow a.
ureteral a.
ureterocolonic a.
ureteroileal a.
ureterointestinal a.
ureterosigmoid a.
ureterotubal a.
ureteroureteral a.
urethrovesical a.
vascular a.
vesicourethral a.
Von Haberer-Finney a.
Wallace a.
wide elliptical a.
wide-lumen stapled a.
W-shaped ileal pouch-anal a.
Z-plasty a.

anastomotic
   a. complication
   a. leak
   a. leakage
   a. material
   a. recurrence
   a. repair
   a. stoma
   a. stricture
   a. suture
   a. ulcer
   a. ulceration
   a. urethroplasty

anastomotic-stomal ulcer

anatomic
   a. fundoplication failure
   a. stress incontinence

anatomical
   a. anomaly
   a. approach
   a. characteristic
   a. findings
   a. radical retropubic prostatectomy

anatomically correct fundoplication

anatomy
   anomalous a.
   aortoiliac a.
   Billroth II a.
   congenitally altered a.
   distal ureteral a.
   normal a.
   pelvic a.
   peritoneal a.

NOTES

Anatrast barium sulfate paste
anatrophic
    a. nephrolithotomy
    a. nephroscopy
    a. nephrotomy
ANC
    acid-neutralizing capacity
ANCA
    antineutrophil cytoplasmic antibody
ANCA-associated systemic vasculitis
Ancalixir
ANCA-SVV
    antineutrophilic cytoplasmic autoantibody-small vessel vasculitis
Ancef
anchor
    Cope viscerotomy a.
    esophageal Z stent with a.'s
    Mainstay urologic soft tissue a.
    Mitek bone a.
    transvaginal bone a.
anchoring
    a. balloon
    a. suture
Ancobon
Ancure abdominal aortic aneurysm system
Ancylostoma, Ankylostoma
    A. duodenale
ancylostomiasis
Andersen
    A. disease
    A. syndrome
    A. triad
Anderson
    A. classification
    A. gastric tube
Anderson-Hynes dismembered pyeloplasty
Andractim
Andresen diet
Andrews
    A. operation
    A. suction tip
androblastoma
Androderm testosterone transdermal patch
AndroGel
androgen
    a. ablation
    a. ablation therapy (AAT)
    a. ablative monotherapy
    adrenal cortex a.
    a. blockade
    a. deficiency
    a. deprivation
    a. deprivation therapy
    exogenous a.
    a. gonadotropin feedback control
    a. insensitivity syndrome
    plasma a.
    a. precursor
    a. priming
    a. receptor
    a. receptor element
    a. suppression
    a. withdrawal endocrine therapy
androgen-binding protein
androgen-independent prostate cancer
androgenital syndrome
androgenization
androgenize
androgeny
    infertility a.
    sexual dysfunction a.
andrology
andropause
androstenedione
    basal a.
androstenedione-to-testosterone ratio
androsterone
anechoic
anejaculation
Anemagen OB Gelcaps
anemia
    autoimmune hemolytic a.
    B_{12} a.
    Banti splenic a.
    a. of chronic renal failure
    copper-deficiency a.
    deficiency a.
    Faber a.
    febrile pleomorphic a.
    folate a.
    hemodialysis-associated a.
    hemolytic a.
    homozygous sickle cell a.
    hypochromic microcytic a.
    hypovolemic a.
    iron-deficiency a.
    macroangiopathic hemolytic a.
    megaloblastic a.
    pernicious a.
    posthepatitis aplastic a.
    refractory sideroblastic a.
    sickle cell a.
anemic urine
anephric
anepiploic
Anergan
anergy
    clonal a.
aneroid manometry
Anestacon 2% lidocaine hydrochloride jelly
anesthesia
    a. adjuvant
    general endotracheal a. (GETA)

local a.
methoxyflurane a.
pharyngeal a.
Ponka technique herniorrhaphy a.
Ponka technique for local a.
preperitoneal a.
spinal a.
topical oropharyngeal a. (TOPA)
anesthetic
Cetacaine topical a.
EMLA a.
a. hepatitis
a. hepatotoxicity
lidocaine topical a.
topical a.
Xylocaine topical a.
aneuploid cell
aneuploidy
DNA a.
mucosal a.
AneuRx stent graft system
aneurysm
abdominal aortic a. (AAA)
acquired renal artery a.
aortic a.
arterial a.
arteriosclerotic a.
berry a.
bilobate false a.
cirsoid a.
congenital renal artery a.
cricoid a.
Dieulafoy cirsoid a.
dissecting abdominal a.
dissecting renal artery a.
embolization of a.
extravisceral a.
false a.
fusiform renal artery a.
gastric a.
GDA a.
hepatic artery a.
hypogastric artery a.
iliac artery a.
intramural a.
intrarenal renal artery a.
mycotic a.
perforating a.
renal artery a.
ruptured abdominal aortic a. (RAAA)
saccular a.

splenic artery a. (SAA)
thoracoabdominal aortic a. (TAAA)
aneurysmal dilation
aneurysmatic
aneurysmectomy
ANF
atrial natriuretic factor
Angelchik
A. antireflux prosthesis
A. ring prosthesis
Angeles
Los A. (LA)
Anger scintillation camera
angiectasia
angiitis
hypersensitivity a.
angina
abdominal a.
a. abdominalis
a. abdominis
a. dyspeptica
intestinal a.
Schultz a.
anginal attack
anginiform
anginose, anginous
angioarchitecture of arterial supply of diverticulum
angioblast
angiocatheter
Angiocath PRN catheter
angiocholecystitis
angiocholitis proliferans
Angiocol
angiodysplasia
bleeding colonic a.
diffuse a.
gastric a.
gastroduodenal a.
pedunculated a.
submucosal endothelial a.
submucosal fibromuscular a.
angiodysplastic lesion
angioedema
hereditary a. (HAE)
angiofibroma
nasopharyngeal a.
a. of penis
angiogenesis
tumor a.
angiogenic factor
Angiografin

NOTES

angiogram
  celiac a.
  cystic duct a.
  mesenteric a.
  splenic a.
angiographic
  a. assessment
  a. end-hole catheter
  a. intervention
  a. portacaval shunt
  a. variceal embolization
angiographically
angiography
  biliary a.
  a. catheter
  celiac a.
  computed tomographic a. (CTA)
  computerized tomographic hepatic a. (CTHA)
  3-D gadolinium-enhanced MR a.
  diagnostic a.
  digital venous subtraction a. (DSA)
  Doppler ultrasonography a.
  dynamic fluorescein a.
  fluorescence a.
  intraarterial digital subtraction a.
  intraoperative a.
  intravenous renal a.
  magnetic resonance a. (MRA)
  mucosal a.
  quantitative a.
  renal a.
  selective mesenteric a.
  subtraction a.
  superior mesenteric a.
  therapeutic a.
  visceral a.
  Wilms tumor a.
angioinfarction
AngioJet Xpeedior catheter
angiokeratoma
  a. corporis diffusum
  a. corporis diffusum universale
  diffuse a.
  a. of Fordyce
  scrotal a.
  a. of scrotum
angioma, pl. **angiomata**
  bleeding a.
  cherry angiomas
  gastric a.
  littoral cell a.
  petechial a.
  spider a.
  telangiectatic a.
  testicular a.
  umbilicated a.
  upper gastrointestinal a.
angiomatoid tumor

angiomatosis
  hepatic a.
angiomatous lymphoid hamartoma
Angiomed
  A. blue stent
  A. Puroflex stent
angiomyolipoma (AML)
  gastric a.
  kidney a.
  renal a.
  tuberous sclerosis a.
angioneurectomy
angioneurotic
  a. anuria
  a. edema
  a. hematuria
angioplasia
angioplasty
  a. balloon
  a. balloon catheter
  balloon percutaneous transluminal a.
  percutaneous transluminal a. (PTA)
  percutaneous transluminal balloon a.
  percutaneous transluminal renal a. (PTRA)
  renal percutaneous transluminal a.
angiosarcoma
  bladder a.
  hepatic a.
  radiation-induced a.
angiosclerosis
  radiation-induced a.
angiosclerotica
  dyspragia a.
angiostatin
AngioStent
angiostrongyliasis
angiotensin
  a. I-converting enzyme insertion/deletion polymorphism
  a. I, II, III
  a. II infusion test
  a. II receptor
  proximal tubular secretion of a.
  a. receptor blocker (ARB)
angiotensin-converting
  a.-c. enzyme (ACE)
  a.-c. enzyme gene
  a.-c. enzyme gene polymorphism
  A.-c. Enzyme Inhibition in Progressive Renal Insufficiency (AIPRI)
  A.-c. Enzyme Inhibition in Progressive Renal Insufficiency trial
  a.-c. enzyme inhibitor (ACEI)
angiotensin-dependent hypertension
angiotensinogen
Angiovist

AngioZyme
angle
    acute infundibulopelvic a.
    anorectal a.
    Camper a.
    cardiohepatic a.
    duodenojejunal a.
    epigastric a.
    a. formed
    hepatorenal a.
    a. of His
    a. of incidence
    infundibulopelvic a.
    LIP a.
    lower infundibulopelvic a.
    mesangial a.
    splenorenal a.
angled
    a. delivery device (ADD)
    a. dissecting forceps
angle-tip Glidewire
angular
    a. notch of stomach
    a. velocity
angularis
    a. body
    incisura a.
angulation
angulus
    a. on lesser curve
    a. of stomach
anhaustral colonic gas pattern
anhemolytic streptococcus
anhepatic stage of liver transplantation
anhydrase
    carbonic a. (CA)
    carbonic a. II
anhydrosis
anhydrous
    sodium phosphate dibasic a.
ani (*pl. of* anus)
anicteric
    a. sclerae
    a. skin
    a. viral hepatitis
anidulafungin
anileridine
anion
    a. exchange
    a. exchange resin
    a. gap
    a. gap acidosis

anionic
    a. ferritin
    a. IgG 4 fraction
aniridia
anisakiasis
    acute gastric a.
    gastric a.
Anisakis marina
anismus
anisocoria
anisocytosis
anisokaryosis
anisonucleosis
anisotropine methylbromide
anisoylated plasminogen-streptokinase activator complex
anistreplase
anitidine
ankle jerk
ankyloproctia
ankylosing spondylitis
Ankylostoma (*var. of Ancylostoma*)
ankylostomiasis
ankylurethria
anlage
    a. of pancreas
    splenic a.
anlagen
    prepancreatic a.
Ann
    A. Arbor cancer staging
    A. Arbor classification
ANNA
    antineuronal nuclear antibody
annexin
annular
    a. adenocarcinoma
    a. esophageal stricture
    a. pancreas
annulus, anulus, pl. **annuli**
    a. urethralis
ano
    fissure in a.
    fistula in a.
anococcygeal raphe
anococcygeus
anocutaneous
    a. line
    a. reflex
    a. stimulation
anoderm
Anogesic

NOTES

anomalotrophy
anomalous
    a. anatomy
    a. arrangement of pancreaticobiliary ductal system (AAPBDS)
    a. calix
    a. genitalia
    a. junction of pancreaticobiliary ducts (AJPBD)
    a. pancreaticobiliary communication
    a. pancreaticobiliary duct (APBD)
    a. pancreaticobiliary ductal union (APBDU)
    a. pancreaticobiliary union (APBU)
    a. pancreatobiliary duct junction (APBDJ)
anomaly
    anatomical a.
    Cruveilhier-Baumgarten a.
    Dieulafoy a.
    DiGeorge a.
    duplication a.
    fixation a.
    pan-bud a.
    penile a.
    ureter duplication a.
    urinary tract a.
    urogenital sinus a.
    vitelline duct a.
    a. of Zahn
anoplasty
    cutback a.
    dermal island-flap a.
    House advancement a.
    Martin a.
    posterior sagittal and three-flap a.
    a. treatment
    Y-V a.
anorchia
    bilateral a.
anorchism
anorectal
    a. abscess
    a. angle
    a. atresia
    a. band
    a. carcinoma
    a. disease
    a. dressing (ARD)
    a. dysgenesis
    a. endosonography
    a. examination
    a. fistula
    a. flexure
    a. foreign body
    a. function test
    a. herpes
    a. imaging
    a. junction
    a. line
    a. malformation
    a. manometry
    a. measurement
    a. mobilization
    a. myectomy
    a. nomenclature
    a. physiology
    a. physiology testing
    a. ring
    a. sensorimotor dysfunction
    a. sepsis
    a. space
    a. sphincter
    a. stenosis
    a. surgery
    a. syphilis
    a. varix
anorectic, anoretic
    a. drug
anorectitis
anorectocolonic
anorectoplasty
    Laird-McMahon a.
    posterior sagittal a.
anorectum
anoretic (*var. of* anorectic)
anorexia
    a. nervosa (AN)
    a. nervosa and associated disorders (ANAD)
anorexia-cachexia syndrome
anorexiant
anorexic
anorexigenic
anorgasmia
anoscope
    Bacon a.
    Boehm a.
    Brinkerhoff a.
    Buie-Hirschman a.
    Ferguson a.
    Hirschmann a.
    Otis a.
    Pratt a.
    Pruitt a.
    Sims a.
    slotted a.
anoscopic
anoscopy
anosigmoidoscopy
anospinal center
anovaginal fistula
anovesical
anoxia
    chemical a.
    gastric a.

ANP
  atrial natriuretic peptide
  ANP receptor
ANS
  autonomic nervous system
Ansaid Oral
ansa pancreaticus
Anson-McVay femoral herniorrhaphy
antacid
  liquid a.
  Remegel Soft Chewable A.
  Trial A.
AntaGel Liquid
antagonist
  alpha-adrenergic a.
  alpha-1-adrenoceptor a.
  alpha-receptor a.
  beta-adrenergic a.
  BQ123 receptor a.
  calcium channel a. (CCA)
  CCK a.
  cholecystokinin a.
  cytokine a.
  dopamine a.
  endothelin a.
  EtA a.
  EtB a.
  histamine H2 a.
  histamine-2 receptor a. (H2RA)
  hormone a.
  H2 receptor a. (H2RA)
  5-HT$_3$, 5-HT$_4$ a.
  5HTM3 receptor a.
  interleukin-1 receptor a.
  intravenous H2 receptor a. (IVH2RA)
  KSG-504 CCK a.
  L-364,781 CCK a.
  L-365,260 CCK a.
  luteinizing hormone-releasing hormone a.
  opiate a.
  opioid a.
  PIVKA-II a.
  platelet glycoprotein 2b3a receptor a.
  potassium-canrenoate a.
  serotonin receptor a.
  TxA2 receptor a.
  type 3 serotonin receptor a.
antagonistic drug

antagonist-II
  prothrombin induced by vitamin K absence or a.-II (PIVKA-II)
antecedent pancreatic injury
antecolic
  a. anastomosis
  a. gastrectomy
  a. long-loop isoperistaltic gastrojejunostomy
antecubital arteriovenous fistula
anteflexed uterus
antegrade
  a. amnesia
  a. approach
  a. colonic enema (ACE)
  a. continence enema (ACE)
  a. continence enema procedure
  a. continence enema, in situ appendix
  a. contrast study
  a. cystography
  a. ejaculation
  a. endopyelotomy
  a. nephroscopy
  a. peristalsis
  a. pyelogram
  a. pyelography
  a. pyeloureterography
  a. scrotal sclerotherapy
  a. stent replacement
  a. ureteral drainage
  a. ureteroscopic manipulation
  a. urography
Antegren
antepartum constipation
anterior
  a. abdominal wall
  a. abdominal wall syndrome
  arteria caecalis a.
  arteria pancreaticoduodenalis superior a.
  a. axillary line (AAL)
  a. band of colon
  a. cecal artery
  a. cord syndrome
  a. duodenal ulcer
  a. esophageal sensor (AES)
  a. extremity
  a. fecal incontinence
  a. fissure
  a. fistula
  a. hemiblock

NOTES

anterior *(continued)*
- a. horn
- a. hypospadias
- a. innominate osteotomy
- a. nephrectomy
- a. oblique position
- a. pelvic exenteration
- a. perineum
- a. and posterior (A&P)
- a. rectopexy
- a. rectus fascia
- a. rectus sheath
- a. renal fascia
- a. resection
- a. rib impingement syndrome
- a. scrotal nerve
- a. spinal artery syndrome
- a. transabdominal approach
- a. urethra
- a. urethral valve
- a. vaginal wall sling (AVWS)
- a. wall antral ulcer

anterolateral thoracotomy incision
anteroposterior
anteroposterior cystoresectoscope
anterosuperior
- a. pancreaticoduodenal (ASPD)
- a. pancreaticoduodenal artery

anteverted uterus
antevesical hernia
anthelmintic
anthelone E, U
Anthos ht II automatic photometer
anthracene glycoside
anthracene-type laxative
anthraquinone laxative
anthrax
   intestinal a.
anthrone
- a. colorimetric technique
- a. method
- Rhein a.

anthropometric
- a. analysis
- a. calculation
- a. marker
- a. measurement

anthropometry
anthropomorphic parameter
anti-40 kDa colonic antigen
anti-ABO antibody
antiactin antibody
antiadhesive agent
anti-alpha fetoprotein
   ^{99m}Tc-labeled a.-a. f.
antiandrogenic activity
antiandrogen withdrawal syndrome
antibacterial personal catheter
antibasement membrane antibody

antibiotic
- a. absorption
- beta-lactam a.
- broad-spectrum a.
- a. enterocolitis
- a. group
- long-term a.
- macrolide a.
- a. management
- perioperative a.
- preoperative a.
- prophylactic a.
- a. prophylaxis
- a. therapy
- topical a.

antibiotic-associated
- a.-a. colitis (AAC)
- a.-a. diarrhea (AAD)
- a.-a. pseudomembranous colitis (AAPC, AAPMC)

antibiotic-coated stent
antibiotic-induced
- a.-i. diarrhea
- a.-i. enterocolitis

antibody
   Amerlex-M second a.
   anti-ABO a.
   antiactin a.
   antibasement membrane a.
   antibrush border a.
   anticardiolipin a. (ACA, ACLA)
   anticentromere a.
   anticolonic a.
   anticytokeratin monoclonal a.
   anti-DCP monoclonal a.
   antidelta IgM a.
   antidesmin monoclonal a.
   antiendomysial a. (anti-EMA)
   antiendomysium a.
   antiendothelial a.
   antienterocyte a.
   antiepithelial membrane antigen a.
   antiextractable nuclear a. (anti-ENA)
   anti-GBM a.
   antigliadin a. (AGA)
   antiglomerular basement membrane a.
   anti-HA a.
   anti-HAV IgM a.
   anti-HB a.
   anti-HBc IgM a.
   anti-HBs a.
   anti-HCV core a.
   anti-HD a.
   anti-HGF a.
   antihuman leukocyte antigen a.
   antiidiotype a.

anti-interleukin-2 receptor alpha monoclonal a.
antilymphocyte a.
antimicrosomal a.
antimitochondrial a. (AMA)
antineuronal nuclear a. (ANNA)
antineutrophil cytoplasmic a. (ANCA)
antineutrophil cytoplasmic IgG a.
antinuclear a. (ANA)
anti-PCNA/cyclin monoclonal a.
antiphospholipid a. (APA)
antiphospholipid-anticardiolipin a.
anti-RAP a.
anti-RAP-GST a.
antireticulin a.
anti-RNA polymerase a.
antirotavirus a.
anti-*Saccharomyces cerevisiae* a. (ASCA)
antismooth muscle a.
antisomatostatin a.
antisperm a.
anti-TBM a.
anti-Thy-1 a.
antithyroglobulin a. (ATA)
anti-TNF-alpha a.
antivimentin a.
assay for neutrophil a.'s
ATGAM polyclonal a.
basal cell-specific anticytokeratin a.
bladder a.
4B4 monoclonal a.
19B7 monoclonal a.
B72.3 murine monoclonal a.
a. to bromodeoxyuridine
cagA a.
CD14 monoclonal a.
celiac disease-specific EMA a.
CM1 polyclonal a.
a. to core peptide 9 (anti-CP9)
a. to core peptide 10 (anti-CP10)
a. to c100 protein
cytophilic a.
cytotoxic a.
eluted a.
a. to EMA
endomysial a. (EMA)
endomysium a.
endotoxin a.
enzyme-conjugated anti-IgA a.
fibronectin monoclonal a.
Flex Sure anti-H. pylori IgG a.
fluorescein isothiocyanate-conjugated a.
fluorescein isothiocyanate-labeled monoclonal a.
fluorescent antinuclear a. (FANA)
Fx1A a.
a. to GOR (anti-GOR)
a. to GOR epitope
HBe a.
HBeAb a.
HCV a.
a. to hepatis Be antigen
a. to hepatitis-associated antigen (anti-HAA)
a. to hepatitis A virus (anti-HAV)
hepatitis B core a. (HBcAb)
hepatitis Be a. (HBeAb, HbeAb)
a. to hepatitis Be antigen
hepatitis B surface a. (HBsAb)
a. to hepatitis B surface antigen
a. to hepatitis C virus (anti-HCV)
a. to hepatitis D virus (anti-HDV)
heterologous anti-GBM a.
Heymann a.
HMB-45 monoclonal a.
a. to HTLV-I (anti-HTLV-I)
humanized anti-CD3 monoclonal a.
humanized monoclonal a.
hybridoma-derived monoclonal a.
IgG2a a.
IgG alpha-gliadin a.
IgG reticulin a.
IgM anti-HAV a.
IgM anti-HBc a.
IgM-HA a.
immune rabbit a.
immunoglobulin A endomysial a.
immunoglobulin A transglutaminase a.
immunoglobulin G2a a.
immunoglobulin G antigliadin a.
indium-111 murine anti-CEA monoclonal a.
infectious mononucleosis heterophil a.
IOT29, clone K20 monoclonal a.
islet cell a. (ICA)
4KB5 monoclonal a.
a. to keratin
LDP-02 a.
a. to Leu M1

NOTES

antibody *(continued)*
    liver-kidney microsomal a.
    lymphocytotoxic a.
    M a.
    microsome a. (MCHA)
    milk protein a.
    mitochondrial a.
    monoclonal a. (MAb, mAb, MoAb)
    monoclonal anti-DNA a.
    MU-3 monoclonal a.
    mycelial a.
    mycobacterial a.
    OKT3 anti-T-cell a.
    OKT3 monoclonal a.
    p53 a.
    PAb 1801 monoclonal a.
    panel-reactive a. (PRA)
    para-ANC a.
    PBC-associated a.
    PC10 monoclonal a.
    perinuclear antineutrophil cytoplasmic a. (p-ANCA)
    phosphotyrosine a.
    polyclonal epidermal growth factor a.
    protein a. (PAb)
    recipient-derived anti-HLA a.
    serum virus a.
    smooth muscle a. (SMA)
    suitable rabbit polyclonal a.
    thyroglobulin a. (TGHA)
    thyroid microsomal a.
    a. to B72.3
    a. to c100 (anti-c100)
    a. to C22-3
    UCHL-1 monoclonal a.
    xenoreactive a.
    90Y-CYT-356 monoclonal a.
    ZCE 025 a.
antibody-dependent
    a.-d. cell-mediated cytotoxicity (ADCC)
    a.-d. cellular cytotoxicity (ADCC)
antibody-directed cytotoxic response
antibody-independent complement activation
antibody-mediated protection
antibrush border antibody
anti-c100
    antibody to c100
anticardiolipin
    a. antibody (ACA, ACLA)
    a. antibody syndrome
anti-CD3
    SMART a.
anti-CD45
anticentromere
    a. antibody
    a. autoantibody (ACA)

anticholinergic
    a. agent
    a. drug
    a. medication
    a. medicine therapy
anticholinesterase
    parasympathomimetic a.
antichymotrypsin
    prostate-specific antigen bound to alpha-1 a. (PSA-ACT)
anti-class II MAb
anti-claudin-7
anti-CMV antiserum
anticoagulant
    lupus a. (LA)
anticoagulant-induced hematuria
anticoagulation therapy
anticodon
anticolonic antibody
anticonvulsant agent hepatotoxicity
anti-CP9
    antibody to core peptide 9
anti-CP10
    antibody to core peptide 10
anticytokeratin monoclonal antibody
anticytokine
anti-DCP monoclonal antibody
antidelta IgM antibody
antidepressant
    a. drug hepatotoxicity
    tricyclic a.
antidesmin monoclonal antibody
antidiabetic agent hepatotoxicity
antidiarrheal (A-D)
    a. agent
    opioid a.
antidiuretic
    a. arginine vasopressin V2 receptor (AVPR2)
    a. hormone (ADH)
    a. hormonelike agent
anti-DNA
    a.-D. binding
    a.-D. immunological study
antidopaminergic
antidysenteric
anti-E2
    envelope 2 antigen
antielastase
anti-EMA
    antiendomysial antibody
antiemetic drug
anti-ENA
    antiextractable nuclear antibody
    anti-ENA immunological study
antiendomysial
    a. antibody (anti-EMA)
    a. antibody test
antiendomysium antibody

antiendothelial antibody
antiendotoxin measure
antienterocyte antibody
antiepileptic drug hypersensitivity
antiepithelial membrane antigen antibody
antiestrogen
antiextractable nuclear antibody (anti-ENA)
antifilarial
antifol
    Baker a.
antifolate
    multitargeted a.
antifungal
    a. agent
    a. esophageal infection
antifungal-resistant opportunistic infection
anti-GBM
    a.-GBM antibody
    a.-GBM disease
    a.-GBM glomerulonephritis
antigen (A/G)
    A a.
    adenoma-associated a.
    amebic lectin a.
    antibody to hepatitis-associated a. (anti-HAA)
    antibody to hepatitis Be a.
    antibody to hepatitis B surface a.
    anti-40 kDa colonic a.
    antineutrophil cytoplasmic a.
    antismooth muscle a. (ASMA)
    antiviral capsid a. (VCA)
    Australian a.
    B a.
    basement membrane a.
    bladder tumor a. (BTA)
    blood group a.
    C100-3 a.
    C22-3 a.
    Ca50 a.
    cancer a. 125 (CA-125)
    cancer-associated sialyl-Lea a.
    carbohydrate a. 19-9 (CA19-9)
    carcinoembryonic a. (CEA)
    CD25 a.
    cell membrane epithelial a.
    circulating tumor-associated a.
    class I, II a.
    a. DD23
    DD23 a.
    delta a.
    endogenous renal a.
    endomysium a.
    enterobacterial common a. (ECA)
    envelope 2 a. (anti-E2)
    epithelial membrane a.
    ethylchlorformate polymerized a.
    extracted nuclear a. (ENA)
    extrarenal a.
    factor VIII a.
    fetal sulfoglycoprotein a. (FSA)
    free prostate-specific a.
    free-to-total prostate-specific a. (FTPSA, F:T PSA)
    gastrointestinal cancer-associated a. (GICA)
    HBeAg a.
    hepatitis-associated a. (HAA)
    hepatitis B a. (HBAg)
    hepatitis B core a. (HBcAg)
    hepatitis Be a.
    hepatitis B early a. (HBeAg, HbeAg)
    hepatitis B surface a. (HBsAg)
    hepatitis B virus-encoded a.
    hepatitis D a. (HDAg)
    hidden a.
    histocompatibility a.
    HIV P24 a.
    HLA-DR a.
    human leukocyte a. (HLA)
    immunobead-reacting a.
    jejunum a.
    K a.
    40-kDa colonic a.
    leukocyte common a.
    Lewis A blood group a.
    Lewis B, X, Y a.
    liver membrane a.
    liver-specific a.
    M344 a.
    a. M344
    a. marker
    MHC class I, II a.
    monoclonal a.
    nephritogenic a.
    nuclear protein cyclin proliferating cell nuclear a.
    O a.
    P24 a.
    486p 3/12 a.

NOTES

antigen *(continued)*
  pancreatic oncofetal a. (POA)
  pHCV31 a.
  pHCV34 a.
  polysaccharide a.
  a. positive
  proliferating cell nuclear a. (PCNA)
  proliferating nuclear cell a. (PNCA)
  prostate gland prostate-specific membrane a.
  prostate-specific a. (PSA)
  prostate-specific membrane a. (PSMA)
  recombinant hepatitis C a.
  reticulin a.
  sialosyl-Tn a.
  sialyl Lewis A a.
  sialyl-Tn a.
  solubilized human leukocyte a.
  soluble egg a. (SEA)
  soluble liver a. (SLA)
  a. specific
  squamous cell carcinoma a.
  stage-specific embryonic a.
  a. stimulation
  a. stool detection test
  T a.
  T138 a.
  Thomsen-Friedenreich a.
  tissue polypeptide a.
  transplantation a.
  tumor-associated a. (TAA)
  tumor-rejection a.
  Ulex europeus I a.
  voiding dysfunctionrole of prostate stem cell a.
antigen-antibody system
antigen-dependent pathway
antigenemia
  PP65 a.
antigenic
  a. determinant
  a. modulation
  a. phenotype
antigen-independent
  a.-i. adhesion
  a.-i. pathway
antigen-presenting cell
antigen-specific
  nucleocapsid a.-s.
antigliadin
  a. antibody (AGA)
  luminal a.
antiglobulin (A/G)
antiglomerular
  a. basement membrane
  a. basement membrane antibody
  a. basement membrane antibody nephritis
  a. basement membrane disease
  a. basement membrane glomerulonephritis
  a. basement membrane-negative crescentric glomerular nephritis
anti-GOR
  antibody to GOR
anti-gp330 immunoglobulin G
anti-HAA
  antibody to hepatitis-associated antigen
anti-HA antibody
anti-HAV
  antibody to hepatitis A virus
    IgM anti-HAV
    anti-HAV IgM antibody
anti-HAV-positive
  IgG a.-HAV-p.
anti-HB antibody
anti-HBc
  a.-HBc IgM antibody
  monoclonal a.-HBc
anti-HBe
anti-HBs
  a.-HBs antibody
  Elecsys PreciControl a.-HBs
anti-HCV
  antibody to hepatitis C virus
    a.-HCV antibody third generation
    a.-HCV core antibody
anti-HD antibody
anti-HDV
  antibody to hepatitis D virus
anti-*Helicobacter*
  a.-*H.* pylori IgM
  a.-*H.* pylori treatment
antihepatitis A-IgM immunological study
anti-HGF antibody
antihistamine
anti-HSV IgM Ab titer
anti-HTLV-I
  antibody to HTLV-I
antihuman leukocyte antigen antibody
anti-Hu test
antihydropic
antihypertensive
  a. agent
  A. and Lipid-Lowering Treatment to Prevent Heart Attack Trial (ALLHAT)
  a. treatment
antiicteric
antiidiotype antibody
antiincontinence procedure
antiinfective biomaterial
antiinflammatory cytokine
antiinhibin

anti-interleukin-2 receptor alpha
 monoclonal antibody
antilipemic drug
antilithic
antiliver microsomal antibody detection
antilymphocyte
   a. antibody
   a. globulin
   a. heteroconjugate
   a. therapy
anti-M2 antimitochondrial antibody level
antimajor histocompatibility complex
antimegalin antiserum
antimesenteric
   a. border
   a. border of distal ileum
   a. enterotomy
   a. fat pad
   a. surface
antimesocolic side of cecum
antimicrobial
   a. agent
   macrolide a.
   a. prophylaxis
   a. resistance
   a. therapy
antimicrosomal antibody
Antiminth
antimitochondrial antibody (AMA)
antimony
   a. monocrystalline electrode
   a. pH electrode
   a. sodium tartrate
   a. trioxide
antimotility
   a. agent
   a. drug
antimüllerian derivative syndrome
antimuscarinic
   a. agent
   a. drug
antimycobacterial drug
antinatriuresis
antinauseant
antineoplastic drug hepatotoxicity
antineuronal
   a. enteric antibody test
   a. nuclear antibody (ANNA)
antineutrophil
   a. cytoplasmic antibody (ANCA)
   a. cytoplasmic antibody titer

   a. cytoplasmic antigen
   a. cytoplasmic autoantibody
   a. cytoplasmic IgG antibody
antineutrophilic cytoplasmic
 autoantibody-small vessel vasculitis
 (ANCA-SVV)
antinociceptive effect
antinuclear
   a. antibody (ANA)
   a. antibody immunological study
antioncogene therapy
antioxidant
   endogenous lipophilic a.
   A. Polyp Prevention Trial
anti-PCNA/cyclin monoclonal antibody
antiperistalsis
antiperistaltic
   a. anastomosis
   a. reflux
   a. technique
antiphospholipid
   a. antibody (APA)
   a. syndrome
antiphospholipid-anticardiolipin antibody
antiplasmin
   alpha-21 a.
antiporter
   Na+/H+ a.
antiproliferative
   a. activity
   a. effect
   a. immunosuppressant
antiproteinuric effect
antiprotozoal
antipsychotic drug hepatotoxicity
antipyrine clearance
anti-RAP antibody
anti-RAP-GST antibody
antireflux
   a. double-J stent
   a. flap-valve mechanism
   a. nipple
   a. operation
   a. procedure
   a. prosthesis
   a. regimen
   a. surgery
   a. therapy
   a. ureteral implantation technique
   a. valve
   a. wrap

NOTES

antirefluxing
    a. colonic conduit
    a. nipple
antireticulin antibody
anti-RNA polymerase antibody
antirotavirus antibody
antiruminant
anti-*Saccharomyces cerevisia* antibody (ASCA)
antisarcoma chemotherapy
anti-Schiff stain
antischistosomal
antisecretory
    a. agent
    a. drug
    a. opioid
    a. therapy
antisense
    a. DNA inhibition
    a. oligonucleotide
    a. RNA probe
    a. strategy
antiseptic
    Avagard Instant Hand A.
    a. dressing
antiseptic-impregnated central venous catheter
antiserum, pl. **antisera**
    anti-CMV a.
    antimegalin a.
    galanin a.
    nephrotoxic a.
    VIP a.
anti-SLA test
antismooth
    a. muscle antibody
    a. muscle antigen (ASMA)
antisomatostatin antibody
Antispas
antispasmodic
    a. agent
    a. drug
antisperm antibody
anti-SSA immunological study
anti-SSB immunological study
antistreptolysin-O titer
anti-Tamm-Horsfall protein
anti-TBM antibody
antithrombin III deficiency
anti-Thy-1
    a.-T.-1 antibody
    a.-T.-1 nephritis
antithymocyte
    a. antibody-induced glomerulonephritis
    a. gammaglobulin (ATGAM)
    a. globulin (ATG)
antithyroglobulin antibody (ATA)
antithyroid
    a. autoantibody
    a. drug hepatotoxicity
anti-TNF-alpha antibody
antitopoisomerase-I autoantibody
antitoxin
    dysentery a.
anti-TrkC antibody
antitubular basement membrane
antiulcer
Antivert
antivimentin antibody
antiviral
    a. capsid antigen (VCA)
    a. chemotherapy
Antizol for injection
Antopol-Goldman lesion
antra (*pl.* of antrum)
antral
    a. atrophic gastritis (AAG)
    a. biopsy
    a. cancer
    a. D, EC cell
    a. diverticulum of colon (ADC)
    a. edema
    a. gastric cell
    a. gastrin
    a. gastrin cell hyperfunction
    a. G-cell hyperplasia
    a. manometry
    a. membrane
    a. mucosa
    a. nodularity
    a. peptide
    a. peristalsis
    a. polyp
    a. pressure transducer
    a. resection
    a. scintigraphy
    a. somatostatin
    a. stasis
    a. stenosis
    a. stricture
    a. ulcer
    a. vascular ectasia
    a. web
antralization
antral-predominant gastritis
antral-type mucosa
antrectomy
    Roux-en-Y biliary bypass with a.
Antrenyl
Antrocol
antroduodenal
    a. manometry
    a. ulcer
antroduodenectomy
antroduodenojejunal manometry
antrofundal mucosa

antropyloric
antropyloroduodenal
    a. common chamber (APDCC)
    a. motility
    a. region
antrostomy, antrotomy
antrum, pl. **antra**
    cardiac a.
    duodenal a.
    gastric a.
    a. gastritis
    prepyloric a.
    a. pyloricum
    retained a.
    a. of stomach
    a. of Willis
anucleate fragment
anulus (var. of annulus), pl. **anuli**
anum
    per a.
anuresis
anuretic
anuria
    angioneurotic a.
    calculous a.
    compression a.
    flash pulmonary edema with a.
    obstructive a.
    postrenal a.
    prerenal a.
    renal a.
    suppressive a.
anuric
anus, pl. **ani**
    arcus tendineus musculi levatoris ani
    artificial a.
    atresia ani
    ectopic a.
    imperforate a.
    levator ani
    a. malformation
    patulous a.
    preternatural a.
    pruritus ani
    rosette appearance of a.
    Rusconi a.
    a. vesicalis
    a. vestibularis
    vulvovaginal a.
anusitis
Anusol HC, HC-1

anvil portion of EEA stapler
Anxanil
anxiety-related diarrhea
anxiolytic sedative
Anzemet
AOCLD
    acute on chronic liver disease
AOM
    azoxymethane
aorta
    abdominal a.
    supraceliac a.
aortic
    a. aneurysm
    a. dissection
    a. graft
    a. hiatus
    a. patch
    a. punch
    a. superior mesenteric artery bypass
    a. valvular stenosis
aortica
    dysphagia a.
aortoduodenal fistula (ADF)
aortoenteric
    a. fistula
    a. graft
aortoesophageal fistula
aortogastric fistula
aortograft duodenal fistula
aortography
    abdominal a.
    biplanar a.
aortohepatic arterial graft
aortoiliac anatomy
aortoostial lesion
aortorenal
    a. bypass
    a. bypass graft
    a. reimplantation
aortosigmoid fistula
aortotomy
AOSC
    acute obstructive suppurative cholangitis
AP
    adenomatous polyp
    alkaline phosphatase
        AP marker enzyme
A&P
    anterior and posterior
APA
    antiphospholipid antibody

NOTES

APAAP
  alkaline phosphatase-antialkaline phosphatase
APACHE
  acute physiology, age and chronic health evaluation
APACHE-II
  A.-II point
  A.-II score
  A.-II scoring system
APACHE-III scoring system
apancreatic
apatite
  a. calculus
  carbonate a.
APBD
  anomalous pancreaticobiliary duct
APBDJ
  anomalous pancreatobiliary duct junction
APBDU
  anomalous pancreaticobiliary ductal union
APBU
  anomalous pancreaticobiliary union
APC
  adenomatous polyp of colon
  adenomatous polyposis coli
  all-purpose capsule
  argon plasma coagulation
  argon plasma coagulator
    APC 300
    APC stool test
    APC tumor suppressor gene
APCR
  activated protein C resistance
APD
  automated peritoneal dialysis
APDCC
  antropyloroduodenal common chamber
apellous
apenteric
apepsia
  achlorhydria a.
apepsinia
aperistalsis
aperistaltic esophagus
Apert syndrome
aperture
  stomal a.
apex, pl. **apices**
  a. of duodenal bulb
  a. of external ring
aphallia
aphasia
apheresis
Aphrodyne
aphtha, pl. **aphthae**

aphthoid
  a. proctocolitis
  a. ulcer
aphthosa
  cachexia a.
aphthous
  a. erosion
  a. gastropathy
  a. stomatitis
  a. ulcer
aphthous-type lesion
API
  alkaline protease inhibitor
  transcription factor AP1
apical
  a. biopsy status
  a. canaliculus
  a. duodenal ulcer
  a. membrane
  a. polar nephrectomy
  a. sound
  a. thickening
apices (*pl. of* apex)
APKD
  adult polycystic kidney disease
aplasia
  bone marrow a.
  kidney a.
  pure red cell a. (PRCA)
  seminal vesicle a.
aplastic bone disease
APLD
  adult polycystic liver disease
apnea
  obstructive sleep a.
apo, Apo
  apolipoprotein
  apo A-I
  apo A-IV
  apo B
  apo B-48
Apo-Amitriptyline
Apo-Amoxi
APOB **gene**
Apo-Chlorax
Apo-Chlordiazepoxide
Apo-Cimetidine
Apo-Erythro
Apo-Erythro-ES
apoferritin
Apo-Hydroxyzine
apolipoprotein (apo, Apo)
  a. B-48
  a. B-containing lipoprotein
  a. B gene
  a. CII-CIII ratio
  a. synthesis

APOLT
    auxiliary partial orthotopic liver transplantation
Apo-Metronidazole
apomorphine
aponeurosis
    buccopharyngeal a.
    external oblique a.
    a. of external oblique
    a. of internal oblique
    ischiorectal a.
    superficial perineal a.
apoplexy
    abdominal a.
    mesenteric a.
    urethral a.
apoprotein
apoptosis
    a. in cell line
    crypt cell a.
    detachment-induced a.
    enterocyte a.
apoptotic
    a. cell death
    a. index
    a. response
Apo-Ranitidine
Apo-Sulfatrim
Apo-Tetra
Apo-Tolbutamide
Apo-Trimip
apparatus, pl. **apparatus**
    alimentary a.
    biliary a.
    contractile a.
    digestive a.
    GIA autosuture a.
    Golgi a.
    juxtaglomerular a.
    Manifold II slot-blot a.
    von Petz suturing a.
    Wangensteen suction a.
apparent
    a. digestive energy (ADE)
    a. mineral corticoid excess syndrome
appearance
    beaklike a.
    bird-beak a.
    bull's eye a.
    cloverleaf a.
    cobblestone a.
    coiled spring a.
    corkscrew a.
    ground-glass a.
    lead-pipe a.
    leafless tree a.
    mushroom-and-stem a.
    a. of normal colon vasculature
    normalized protein nitrogen a. (nPNA)
    picket fence a.
    pinwheel a.
    pseudo-Billroth I a.
    pseudotumor a.
    sausagelike a.
    sawtoothed a.
    soap sudsy a.
    spiculated a.
    spiderweb a.
    stack-of-coins a.
    string-of-beads a.
    tadpolelike a.
    target a.
    through-and-through a.
    tigroid a.
    toxic a.
    wind-sock a.
Appedrine
appendage
    cecal a.
    epiploic a.
    torsion of a.
    vermicular a.
appendagitis
appendectomy, appendicectomy (appy)
    colonoscopic a.
    emergency a.
    emergent a.
    incidental a.
    interval a.
    inversion a.
    inversion-ligation a.
    laparoscopic a.
    a. tape
    uncomplicated a.
appendiceal, appendical
    a. abscess
    a. adenocarcinoma
    a. intussusception
    a. Kaposi sarcoma
    a. mass
    a. mucocele
    a. opening

NOTES

appendiceal · application

appendiceal *(continued)*
    a. orifice
    a. perforation
    a. stump
appendicectasis
appendicectomy *(var. of* appendectomy*)*
appendices *(pl. of* appendix*)*
appendicism
appendicitis
    actinomycotic a.
    acute a.
    amebic a.
    bilharzial a.
    chronic a.
    a. by contiguity
    foreign body a.
    fulminating a.
    gangrenous a.
    a. granulosa
    helminthic a.
    left-sided a.
    lumbar a.
    myxoglobulosis a.
    necropurulent a.
    nonperforated a.
    a. obliterans
    obstructive a.
    pelvic a.
    perforated a.
    purulent a.
    recurrent a.
    relapsing a.
    retrocecal a.
    retroileal a.
    segmental a.
    skip a.
    stercoraceous a.
    subperitoneal a.
    suppurative a.
    traumatic a.
    verminous a.
appendicocecostomy
appendicocele
appendicocystostomy
    continent cutaneous a.
    dismembered reimplanted a.
    nonplicated a.
    orthotopic a.
    plicated a.
    reversed reimplanted a.
appendicoenterostomy
appendicolith
appendicolithiasis, appendilothiasis, appendolithiasis
appendicolysis
appendicopathy
appendicostomy
    Malone continent a.
appendicoumbilical stoma

appendicovesicostomy
    Mitrofanoff a.
appendicular
    a. artery
    a. colic
    a. dyspepsia
appendicularis
    arteria a.
appendilothiasis *(var. of* appendicolithiasis*)*
appendix, pl. **appendices**
    antegrade continence enema, in situ a.
    base of a.
    cecal a.
    divided a.
    a. dyspepsia
    a. epididymidis
    epiploic a.
    a. fibrosa
    gangrenous a.
    hot a.
    indurated a.
    inflamed a.
    Morgagni a.
    nonperforated a.
    normal a.
    paracecal a.
    perforated a.
    retrocecal a.
    retroileal a.
    ruptured a.
    simultaneous Malone antegrade continent enema and Mitrofanoff procedure using divided a.
    subcecal a.
    suppurative a.
    a. testis
    a. testis torsion
    vermiform a.
    xiphoid a.
appendolithiasis *(var. of* appendicolithiasis*)*
appetite
    a. disorder
    perverted a.
    voracious a.
apple
    cashew a.
apple-core lesion
apple-peel bowel syndrome
appliance
    external cooling a.
    Gentle Touch colostomy a.
    Karaya ring ileostomy a.
    ostomy a.
application
    laparoscopic clip a.
    research a.

ultrathin needle brachytherapy-style delivery renal a.

applicator
Betadine PrepStick Plus a.
Mick TP-200 a.
microwave a.
Multifire clip a.
multiload occlusive clip a.
resorbable thread clip a.
Stabiliplan orthovolt a.

Applied Biosystems 340A nucleic acid extractor

applier
Advanced surgical suture a.
clip a.
cotton-tipped a.
Endoclip a.
multiloaded clip a.
Stone clamp a.

Appolito suture

approach
Alken a.
anatomical a.
antegrade a.
anterior transabdominal a.
Bianchi a.
case-by-case a.
choledochofiberscopic a.
consortial a.
detailed stepwise a.
extrasphincteric a.
fascial sling a.
flank a.
Framingham risk-factor a.
gasless laparoscopic a.
Henry a.
invasive transvaginal a.
Kraske parasacral a.
laparoscopic-assisted a.
microbial a.
minilaparatomy a.
minimally invasive a.
percutaneous transhepatic a.
perineal a.
peroral a.
posterior lumbar a.
preperitoneal a.
Redman a.
retrograde a.
retroperitoneal a.
supraduodenal a.
surgical a.
thoracoabdominal extrapleural a.
thoracoabdominal intrapleural a.
transduodenal a.
transmural a.
transpapillary a.
transvesical laparoscopic a.
ureteroscopic a.
vaginal wall a.
ventral transperitoneal laparoscopic a.
wait-and-see a.

Appropriate Use of Gastrointestinal Endoscopy guidelines

approximation
a. suture
tissue a.
wound a.

approximator clamp

appy
appendectomy

APR
abdominoperineal resection

apraxia
constructional a.
swallow a.

APRE
acute-phase response element

aprepitant

Apresoline

aprindine

aproctia

apron
abdominal a.
fatty omental a.
a. skin incision

aprotinin

APRT
adenine phosphoribosyltransferase
APRT deficiency

APS
arterioportal vein shunting

APS-1
autoimmune polyglandular syndrome type 1

APSGN
acute poststreptococcal glomerulonephritis

APT-Downey alkali denaturation test

Aptosyn

aPTT
activated partial thromboplastin time

NOTES

APUD
    amine precursor uptake and decarboxylation
    APUD cell
apudoma
Aquachloral
AquaMEPHYTON
aquaporin-1
aquaporin water channel
AquaSens FMS 1000 fluid monitoring system
aquaticus
    Thermus a.
Aquazide-H
aqueous
    A. Charcodote
    a. phenol
AR
    aldose reductase
    AR mRNA
arabinotarda
    Shigella a. type A, B
arachidonic
    a. acid
    a. acid metabolite
    a. acid oxidation
arachis oil
arachnoid fibrosis
Aralen
Aramine
Arandel cell harvester
Aranesp
Arantius ligament
ARB
    angiotensin receptor blocker
arbaprostil
arbitrary unit (AU)
arborization of ducts
ARC
    AIDS-related complex
arc
    sacral reflex a.
    a. shadow
    tendinous a.
arcade
    gastroepiploic a.
ARCD
    acquired renal cystic disease
arch
    arterial a.
    cortical a.
    fallopian a.
    pubic a.
    Treitz a.
archaea
    methanogenic a.
architecture
    crypt a.
    distorted crypt a.
    hepatic a.
    intestinal villous a.
    lobular a.
arcuate
    a. artery
    a. line
    a. vein
arcus
    a. tendineus fasciae pelvis
    a. tendineus musculi levatoris ani
ARD
    acid-related disorder
    anorectal dressing
ardor urinae
ARDS
    adult respiratory distress syndrome
area, pl. **areae**
    cell surface a.
    choledochoduodenal a.
    a. gastrica
    areae gastricae
    gastrohepatic bare a.
    high-echoic a.
    intermicrovillar a.
    Killian-Jamieson a.
    medial preoptic a.
    midepigastric a.
    midrectal a.
    mycophenolate a.
    a. nuda hepatis
    Paget disease of perianal a.
    perianal a.
    pericolostomy a.
    peripancreatic a.
    periportal a.
    peristomal a.
    postcricoid a.
    a. postrema
    punctate a.
    retroperitoneal a.
    skip a.
    subhepatic a.
    target a.
    watershed a.
areflexia
    detrusor a.
areflexic bladder
Arena hemodialysis device
ARF
    acute renal failure
    mercuric chloride-induced ARF
argentaffin
    a. cell
    a. reaction test
    a. stain
Arginaid dietary supplement
arginase deficiency

arginine
  a. analog
  a. vasopressin (AVP)
arginosuccinate
argon
  a. beam coagulator
  A. Beamer 2 device
  a. beam plasma coagulation
  a. ion laser
  a. ion plasma coagulation
  a. laser therapy
  a. plasma coagulation (APC)
  a. plasma coagulator (APC)
  a. pumped dye laser
Argyle
  A. chest tube
  A. Ingram trocar catheter
  A. Medicut R catheter
Argyle-Salem sump tube
argyrophilia
  cytoplasmic a.
argyrophilic
  a. and argyrophobic neurons
  a. cell
ARI
  acute renal insufficiency
Arias syndrome
Aristocort
Aristospan
ARKD
  autosomal-recessive kidney disease
arm
  cell-mediated a.
  humoral a.
  Leonard A.
armamentarium
  contemporary urologic a.
Armanni-Ebstein lesion
Armanni-Ehrlich degeneration
ARMS-PCR
  amplification refractory mutation system-polymerase chain reaction
Army-Navy retractor
Arndorfer
  A. capillary perfusion system
  A. pneumohydraulic capillary infusion system
aromatase inhibitor
aromatic
  a. amine
  a. amino acid (AAA)
Aronson esophageal retractor

aroylhydrazone chelator
ARP
  acute recurrent pancreatitis
array
  DNA a.
arrest
  spermatogenic a.
Arrestin
arrhythmic frequency range
arrhythmogenicity
Arrow
  A. Raulerson syringe
  A. UserGard injection cap system
ARROWgard Blue hemodialysis catheter
arrowhead sign
ARS
  amylase-resistant starch
arsenical polyneuropathy
Artane
artefacta
  dermatitis a.
arteria, pl. arteriae
  a. appendicularis
  a. caecalis anterior
  a. caecalis posterior
  a. caudae pancreatis
  a. colica dextra
  a. colica media
  a. epigastrica inferior
  a. epigastrica superficialis
  a. epigastrica superior
  a. gastrica dextra
  arteriae gastricae breves
  a. gastrica posterior
  a. gastrica sinistra
  a. gastroomentalis dextra
  a. gastroomentalis sinistra
  a. hepatica communis
  a. hepatica propria
  arteriae ilei
  a. ileocolica
  arteriae intestinales
  arteriae jejunales
  a. lienalis
  a. lusoria
  a. mesenterica inferior
  a. mesenterica superior
  a. pancreatica dorsalis
  a. pancreatica inferior
  a. pancreatica magna
  arteriae pancreaticoduodenales inferiores

NOTES

arteria *(continued)*
    a. pancreaticoduodenalis superior anterior
    a. pancreaticoduodenalis superior posterior
    a. rectalis inferior
    a. rectalis media
    a. rectalis superior
    arteriae sigmoideae
    a. splenica
arteriae *(pl. of* arteria*)*
arterial
    a. ammonia
    a. aneurysm
    a. arch
    a. blood gas (ABG)
    a. blood sample
    a. circulation
    a. embolization
    a. line
    a. oxygen desaturation
    a. portography
    a. priapism
    a. saturation
    a. spider
    a. steal
    a. stimulation venous sampling (ASVS)
    a. thrombosis
    a. underfilling
    a. wall necrosis
arterial-enteric fistula
arterialization of portal vein
arteriogenic impotence
arteriogram
    hepatic a.
    superior mesenteric a.
arteriographic embolization
arteriography
    celiac a.
    celiomesenteric a.
    gastric a.
    hepatic a.
    mesenteric a.
    pancreaticoduodenal a.
    penile a.
    renal a.
    selective left gastric a.
    superselective a.
    visceral a.
arteriohepatic dysplasia
arteriolar
    a. hyalinosis
    a. nephrosclerosis
arteriole
    afferent glomerular a.
    efferent glomerular a.
    glomerular a.
    Isaacs-Ludwig a.
    juxtamedullary a.
    postglomerular a.
    preglomerular a.
    renal a.
arteriolopathy
    cyclosporine a.
arterioportal
    a. fistula
    a. vein shunting (APS)
    a. venous shunt
arterioportographical examination
arterioportography
arteriosclerosis obliterans
arteriosclerotic
    a. aneurysm
    a. renal artery disease (ASO-RAD)
arteriotomy
    end-to-side a.
arteriovenous (AV)
    a. access
    a. catheter
    a. fistula (AVF)
    a. hemofiltration
    a. malformation (AVM)
    a. shunt
arteritis
    radiation-induced obliterative a.
    Takayasu a.
    villous a.
artery
    abnormality of hepatic a.
    accessory obturator a.
    accessory superior colic a.
    adjacent hepatic a.
    adrenal a.
    anterior cecal a.
    anterosuperior pancreaticoduodenal a.
    appendicular a.
    arcuate a.
    ascending ileocolic a.
    ASPD a.
    atherosclerotic renal a.
    bladder a.
    bulbar a.
    bulbourethral a.
    caliber-persistent a.
    capsular a.
    carotid a.
    caudal pancreatic a.
    cavernosal a.
    colic a.
    common hepatic a. (CHA)
    common iliac a.
    common penile a.
    cremasteric a.
    cystic a.
    deep a.
    deferential a.

dorsal pancreatic a.
dorsal penile a.
a. of Drummond
epigastric a.
external iliac a.
femoral a.
gastric a.
gastroduodenal a. (GDA)
gastroepiploic a. (GEA, GEPA)
gluteal a.
gonadal a.
great pancreatic a.
helicine a.
hepatic a.
high transection of inferior mesenteric a.
hypogastric a.
ileal a.
ileocolic a.
iliac a.
inferior hemorrhoidal a.
inferior mesenteric a. (IMA)
inferior pancreatic a.
inferior pancreaticoduodenal a.
inferior phrenic a.
interlobar renal a.
internal iliac a.
internal pudendal a.
left gastroomental a.
lienal a.
lumbar a.
lusorian a.
mesenteric a.
middle adrenal a.
middle colic a. (MCA)
middle hemorrhoidal a.
obturator a.
ovarian a.
pancreatica magna a.
penile a.
phrenic a.
piriformis a.
polar a.
posterorsuperior pancreaticoduodenal a.
preureteral iliac a.
proper hepatic a.
prostatic a.
proximal superior mesenteric a.
pudendal a.
rectal a.
renal a. (RA)
retroduodenal a.
retrograde vascularization of superior mesenteric a.
right gastroomental a.
sacral a.
scrotal-perineal a.
spermatic a.
splenic a.
submucosal a.
superior hemorrhoidal a.
superior mesenteric a. (SMA)
superior vesical a.
testicular a.
umbilical a.
urethral a.
uterine a.
vesical a.
vesiculodeferential a.
a. weld strength

arthralgia
arthritic dose (A/D)
arthritis, pl. **arthritides**
    colitic a.
    dysenteric a.
    enteropathic reactive a.
    peripheral a.
    reactive a.
    rheumatoid a.
    temporomandibular a.
    urethral a.
    villous a.

arthropathy
    psoriatic a.

arthroplasty
arthrosia
    exanthesis a.

Articulator injection needle
artifact
    barium a.
    mirror-image a.
    pellet a.
    reverberation a.

artificial
    a. anus
    a. bezoar
    a. Carlsbad salt
    a. cystine stone
    a. erection
    a. erection test
    a. genitourinary sphincter
    a. genitourinary sphincter implantation

NOTES

artificial (continued)
    a. gut
    a. hepatic support
    a. insemination donor (AID)
    a. insemination husband (AIH)
    a. kidney
    a. Kissingen salt
    a. organ
    a. urethral sphincter (AUS)
    a. urinary sphincter (AUS)
    a. urinary sphincter implantation
    a. urinary sphincter pressure-regulating balloon
    a. Vichy salt
aryepiglottic
    a. fold
    a. muscle
arylamine
arytenoid
    a. adduction
    a. cartilage
AS
    anal sphincter
AS-800
    AS-800 artificial sphincter
    AS-800 balloon
    AS-800 cuff
    AS-800 male bulbous urethra
    AS-800 pump
ASA
    acetylsalicylic acid
4-ASA
    4-aminosalicylic acid
5-ASA
    5-aminosalicylic acid
    5-ASA agent
    5-ASA enema
Asacol delayed-release tablet
ASA-induced gastric ulceration
ASAP
    atypical small acinar proliferation of prostate
    ASAP channel-cut automated biopsy needle
    ASAP prostate biopsy needle
    ASAP Stacker automated multisample biopsy system
ASC
    acute suppurative cholangitis
ASCA
    anti-*Saccharomyces cerevisiae* antibody
ascariasis, ascaridiasis, ascaridosis, ascariosis
    biliary a.
    endobiliary a.
    intrahepatic a.
    pancreatic a.
ascaricidal
ascaricide

ascarid
ascaridiasis (*var. of* ascariasis)
ascaridosis (*var. of* ascariasis)
ascariosis (*var. of* ascariasis)
ascaris, pl. **ascarides**
    A. infestation
    A. lumbricoides
    A. suum
ascendens
    colon a.
ascending
    a. cholangitis
    a. colon
    a. ileocolic artery
    a. limb
    a. pyelography
    a. pyelonephritis
    a. urethrogram
ascent
    kidney a.
ascite
ascites
    a. adiposus
    bile a.
    biliary a.
    blood-tinged a.
    bloody a.
    chyliform a.
    a. chylosus
    chylous a.
    cirrhotic a.
    cloudy a.
    culture-negative neutrocytic a. (CNNA)
    demeclocycline-induced a.
    dialysis-related a.
    a. drainage tube
    eosinophilic a.
    a. euglobulin lysis time (AELT)
    exudative a.
    fatty a.
    gelatinous a.
    hemodialysis-associated a.
    hemorrhagic a.
    hydremic a.
    idiopathic a.
    malignant a.
    milky a.
    myxedema a.
    narrow albumin gradient a.
    nephrogenic a.
    nephrogenous dialysis a.
    neutrocytic a.
    nonchylous a.
    pancreatic a.
    pseudochylous a.
    refractory a.
    resistant a.
    straw-colored a.

tense a.
transudative a.
urinary a.
urine a.
wide albumin gradient a.
ascitic
    a. amylase
    a. fluid total protein (AFTP)
    a. tumor fluid (ATF)
ascitogenous
ascorbic acid
Ascriptin A/D
ASCUS
    atypical squamous cells of undetermined significance
asecretory
Aselli pancreas
aseptic
    a. anastomosis
    a. intermittent catheterization
    a. technique
    a. wound
Asepti-steryl disinfectant
Asepto irrigation syringe
ASGB
    adjustable silicone gastric banding
ASGE
    American Society for Gastrointestinal Endoscopy
Asherson syndrome
Ashkenazi Jewish community
ASHN
    acute sclerosing hyaline necrosis
Ashton
    A. brief
    A. pants
ASI
    A. prostatic stent
    A. Titan stent
asialia
asialoglycoprotein receptor
Asiatic
    A. cholera
    A. schistosomiasis
ASID Bonz PP infusion pump
asitia
Ask-Upmark
    A.-U. kidney
    A.-U. renal segment
ASLC
    acute self-limited colitis

ASMA
    antismooth muscle antigen
Asopa
    A. hypospadias repair
    A. procedure
ASO-RAD
    arteriosclerotic renal artery disease
asparaginase
asparagine
aspartate
    a. aminotransferase (AST)
    a. transferase
aspartyl protease-mediated cleavage
A-Spas
ASPD
    anterosuperior pancreaticoduodenal
    ASPD artery
aspect
    paraspinous a.
    spinous a.
    urological a.
aspergillosis esophagitis
Aspergillus
    A. bezoar
    A. *flavus*
    A. *fumigatus*
    A. infection
Aspergum
aspermatism
aspermatogenesis
aspermatogenic sterility
aspermia
asphyxiating thoracic dystrophy
aspidium
aspirate
    gastric a.
    heme-positive NG a.
    nasogastric a.
aspirated sample
aspirating needle
aspiration
    a. biopsy
    a. biopsy cytology
    a. catheter
    corporeal a.
    CT-guided fine-needle a.
    diagnostic a.
    a. and dissection tube
    endoscopic transesophageal fine-needle a.
    endoscopic ultrasound-guided fine-needle a. (EUS-FNA)

NOTES

aspiration *(continued)*
- epididymal sperm a. (ESA)
- EUS-guided fine-needle a.
- fetal bladder a.
- fine-needle a. (FNA)
- gastric a.
- Iglesias method of a.
- Levin tube a.
- lymphocele a.
- microepididymal sperm a. (MESA)
- microscopic epididymal sperm a.
- microsurgical epididymal sperm a. (MESA)
- a. mucosectomy
- percutaneous balloon a.
- percutaneous CT-guided a.
- percutaneous epididymal sperm a.
- percutaneous needle a.
- peritoneal a.
- a. pneumonia
- pulmonary a.
- real-time endoscopic ultrasound-guided fine-needle a.
- real-time fine-needle a. (RTFNA)
- seminal vesicle a.
- silent a.
- sonography-guided a.
- sperm a.
- suprapubic a.
- a. syringe
- tracheobronchial a.

aspirator
- Cavitron Ultrasonic Surgical A. (CUSA)
- Thorek gallbladder a.

aspirin
- enteric-coated a.

aspirin-induced gastritis
Aspisafe nasogastric tube
asplenia syndrome
Assam fever
assay
- Abbott IMx PSA a.
- acrosome reaction a.
- activity a.
- adherence a.
- amidolytic a.
- Aura-Tek FDP a.
- Ausab EIA a.
- Behring OPUS Plus immunofluorescence a.
- Bioclot protein S a.
- Bio-Rad protein a.
- BioWhittaker a.
- bladder tumor a.
- calprotectin a.
- ^{14}C glucose uptake a.
- Ciba-Corning ACS PSA a.
- *Clostridium difficile* toxin a.
- competition-binding a.
- competitive protein-binding a.
- cytotoxin a.
- disaccharidase a.
- electroimmunodiffusion a.
- electrophoretic mobility shift a.
- ELISA-like a.
- enhanced reverse transcriptase polymerase chain reaction a.
- enzyme-linked immunosorbent a. (ELISA)
- enzyme-linked immunosorbent a. I (ELISA-I)
- enzyme-linked immunosorbent a. II (ELISA-II)
- erythrocyte lysis a.
- estrogen receptor a. (ERA)
- fibroblast ECM adhesion a.
- fibroblast PMN adhesion a.
- Galacto-Light a.
- gastric-juice ammonia a.
- *Helicobacter pylori* stool a.
- heme-porphyrin a.
- hemizona a.
- HemoQuant a.
- HPLC fluorescence a.
- Hybritech Tandem prostate-pecific antigen a.
- Hybritech Tandem-R PSA a.
- IgA tTG a.
- IMMULITE 2000 free PSA a.
- IMMULITE 2000 third-generation PSA a.
- immunobead a.
- immunoradiometric a. (IRMA)
- IMx Hg a.
- indirect immunofluorescence a.
- inhibition a.
- Inno-LiPA a.
- intact hormone a.
- latex agglutination a.
- limiting dilution a.
- liquid chromatographic a.
- a. for neutrophil antibodies
- p53 a.
- PMN chemotaxis a.
- PP65 antigenemia a.
- Prometheus First Step inflammatory bowel disease screening a.
- Pros-Check PSA a.
- protein-protein a.
- PTH-rP by immunoradiometric a.
- Pyrilinks-D urinary a.
- qualitative microculture a.
- radioenzymatic a.
- radioimmunoinhibition a.
- radioimmunoprecipitation a.
- recombinant immunoblot a. (RIBA)

recombinant tissue transglutaminase radioligand a.
recombinant tTG radioligand a.
renal vein renin a. (RVRA)
representative electrophoretic mobility shift a.
Roche Elecsys free prostate-specific antigen a.
second-generation recombinant immunoblot a.
solution hybridization RNAse protection a.
sperm penetration a. (SPA)
stool antigen a.
stool toxin a.
Tandem-E-PSA immunoenzymetric a.
Tandem-ERA PSA immuenzymetric a.
Tandem-R PSA a.
tissue culture a.
TNF-alpha a.
Tosoh a.
toxin a.
transcriptase polymerase chain reaction a.
tumor necrosis factor-alpha a.
urine-based enzyme-linked immunosorbent a.
UroVysion a.
VERSANT HCV RNA qualitative a.
Vysis UroVysion DNA probe a.
Yang polyclonal a.
Yang Pros-Check PSA a.

assay-2
    recombinant immunoblot a.-2

assembly
    Dentsleeve extruded silastic perfused manometric a.
    dilating catheter-gastrostomy tube a.
    eight-lumen catheter a.
    Konigsberg five-channel solid-state catheter a.
    multiple sidehole manometric a.
    purpose-built silicone rubber multilumen manometric a.
    standard silicone manometric a.

assessment
    angiographic a.
    blood flow a.
    a. of bowel preparation quality
    endoscopic color Doppler a.
    extrapyramidal function a.
    integrated a.
    nutritional a.
    outcome and process a.
    penile vascular function a.
    Sepsis-Related Organ Failure A. (SOFA)
    urodynamic a.

ASSI
    Accurate Surgical and Scientific Instruments
        ASSI laparoscopic electrode
        ASSI METE-5168 end-to-end vasoepididymostomy
        ASSI METS-3668 Microspike approximator clamp
        ASSI MKCV-2040 Microspike approximator clamp
        ASSI MSPK-3678 Microspike approximator clamp

assistance
    Doppler a.

assistant
    gastrointestinal a. (GIA)

assisted
    a. reproduction
    a. reproductive technique

association
    American Anorexia/Bulimia A.
    American Diabetes A. (ADA)
    American Gastroenterological A. (AGA)
    American Urological A. (AUA)
    Internal Ostomy A. (IOA)
    megacystis-megaureter a.
    MURCS a.
    strong a.
    United Ostomy A. (UOA)

assumption of homogeneity

Assura
    A. closed minipouch
    A. convex drainable pouch
    A. convex urostomy pouch
    A. deluxe irrigation set
    A. economy irrigation set
    A. irrigation accessory
    A. irrigation sleeve
    A. pediatric pouch
    A. pediatric skin barrier flange
    A. standard drainable pouch

NOTES

Assura *(continued)*
    A. stoma cap
    A. stomy belt

AST
    acid suppression therapy
    aspartate aminotransferase
        AST test

AST/ALT ratio
asterixis
asteroid body
asthenospermia
asthenospermic
asthenoteratospermia
asthenozoospermia
Astler-Coller
    A.-C. classification A, B1, B2, C1, C2
    A.-C. modification of Dukes classification

ASTRA
    ASTRA profile
    ASTRA profile test

Astra/Merck Group
Astramorph
AstraZeneca Pharmaceuticals LP
astrovirus
    a. gastroenteritis
    human A. (HAstV)

Astwood-Coller staging system for carcinoma

ASVS
    arterial stimulation venous sampling

asymmetrical
asymmetric pupils
asymmetry
asymptomatic
    a. bacterium
    a. bacteriuria
    a. calculus
    a. gallstone
    a. hemodialysis patient
    a. hypocalcemia
    a. mass
    a. proteinuria
    a. pyelonephritis
    a. urinary tract infection (AUTI)
    a. urolithiasis

asystole
    lavage-induced cardiac a.

AT
    abdominal tympany
    adaptive thermogenesis

ATA
    antithyroglobulin antibody

Atabrine
Atarax
ataxia
    cerebellar a.
    late-onset a.

ATF
    ascitic tumor fluid

ATG
    antithymocyte giobulin

ATGAM
    antithymocyte gammaglobulin
        ATGAM polyclonal antibody

atheroembolic renal disease (AERD)
atheroembolism
atheroembolus
atherogenesis
atheromatous
atherosclerosis
    graft a.
    ostial artery a.

atherosclerosis-induced cavernosal ischemia

atherosclerotic
    a. abnormality
    a. plaque
    a. renal artery
    a. renal artery stenosis
    a. renovascular disease

Ativan
Atkins diet
Atkinson
    A. introducer
    A. prosthesis
    A. scoring system for dysphagia
    A. silicone rubber tube

Atlantic ileostomy catheter

ATN
    acute tubular necrosis
    atrasentan

atomic absorbance spectrophotometer

atonic
    a. bladder
    a. constipation
    a. dyspepsia
    a. esophagus

atony
    chronic intestinal a.
    gastric a.
    intestinal a.
    sphincter a.
    ureteral a.

atopic
    a. dermatitis
    a. eczema

atorvastatin
atovaquone
ATP
    adenosine triphosphate

***ATP7A* gene**
ATPase
    adenosine triphosphatase
    ATPase activity
    ATPase inhibitor

atracurium
atrasentan (ATN)
atrasentan HCl
atraumatic
    a. clamp
    a. grasper
    a. locking/grasping forceps
    a. suture
    a. tip
atresia
    anal a.
    a. ani
    anorectal a.
    bile duct a.
    biliary a.
    congenital biliary a.
    congenital duodenal a.
    duodenal a.
    esophageal a.
    extrahepatic bile duct a. (EHBDA)
    extrahepatic biliary a. (EBA)
    follicular a.
    gastric a.
    ileal a.
    intestinal a.
    intrahepatic a. (IHA)
    jejunoileal a.
    Kasai classification for extrahepatic bile duct a.
    meatal a.
    prepyloric a.
    pyloric a.
    suprapubic cystotomy tract urethral a.
    urethral a.
    vaginal a.
atretogastria
atrial
    a. liver pulse
    a. natriuretic factor (ANF)
    a. natriuretic peptide (ANP)
Atrigel
Atrocholin
atrophia (*var. of* atrophy)
atrophic
    a. cirrhosis
    a. gastritis
    a. pangastritis
    a. urethritis
    a. vagina
atrophicus
    lichen sclerosus et a.

atrophied
atrophy, atrophia
    acute yellow a.
    adrenal gland a.
    crypt a.
    familial microvillus a.
    fundic gland a.
    gastric mucosal a.
    healed yellow a.
    intestinal a.
    lobar a.
    mucosal a.
    multiple-system a.
    muscle a.
    parenchymal a.
    partial villous a. (PVA)
    proliferative inflammatory a.
    sclerotic a.
    seminal vesicle a.
    skin a.
    splenic a.
    subtotal villous a. (SVA)
    Sudeck a.
    tubular a.
    villous a.
    white a.
atropine
    a. derivative
    a. infusion
    a. methylnitrate
    a. sulfate
ATS
    autotransfusion
    ATS canister
attachment
    crystal a.
    mesenteric a.
    peritoneal a.
attack
    anginal a.
    Gowers a.
Attain tube feeding formula
attapulgite
attenuated adenomatous polyposis coli
attenuation
attic adhesion
atubular glomerulus
atypia
    cellular a.
    hepatocellular a.
atypical
    a. adenomatous hyperplasia (AAH)

NOTES

atypical *(continued)*
    a. distribution of disease
    a. ductular cell
    a. gallbladder disease
    a. glandular cells of unknown significance (AGUS)
    a. small acinar proliferation of prostate (ASAP)
    a. squamous cells of undetermined significance (ASCUS)
ATZ
    anal transitional zone
AU
    arbitrary unit
^{198}Au
    gold-198
AUA
    American Urological Association
    AUA Symptom Index
Aub-Dubois
    A.-D. standard
    A.-D. table
Auerbach
    A. and Meissner plexus
    A. mesenteric plexus
augmentation
    bladder a.
    a. cystoplasty
    a. enterocystoplasty
    gastroileac a.
    hemi-T a.
    ileocecocystoplasty bladder a.
    Mainz pouch a.
    orthotopic bladder a.
    a. plaque
    rectal a.
    ureteral bladder a.
    urothelial a.
augmented
    a. anastomotic urethroplasty
    a. biofeedback
    a. bladder
    a. valved rectum
Augmentin
AUR
    acute urinary retention
auranofin
Aura-Tek
    A.-T. FDP assay
    A.-T. FDP test
aureus
    methicillin-resistant *Staphylococcus a.* (MRSA)
    Staphylococcus a.
Auriculin
AUS
    artificial urethral sphincter
    artificial urinary sphincter
Ausab EIA assay

auscultation of bowel sounds
auscultatory
    a. sign
    a. sound
Ausonics OPUS-1
Australian antigen
australis
    Pseudo-nitzschia a.
autacoid
autemesia
Authority
    United Kingdom Transplant Support Service A. (UKTSSA)
AUTI
    asymptomatic urinary tract infection
Auto
    A. Suture Multifire Endo GIA 30 stapler
    A. Suture Premium CEEA stapler
autoanalyzer
    Beckman 2 a.
    Coulter automated a.
    Hitachi 737 a.
autoantibody
    anticentromere a. (ACA)
    antineutrophil cytoplasmic a.
    antithyroid a.
    antitopoisomerase-I a.
    circulating a.
    a. production
    ScI-70 a.
autoaugmentation
    bladder a.
    a. cystoplasty
    laparoscopic laser-assisted a.
autocholecystectomy
autoclave
    heat-sterilized by a.
    steam a.
    a. sterilized
autoclaved India ink
autoclaving
autocoid
autocrine
    a. motility factor (AMF)
    a. regulation
    a. reinforcing loop
autocystoplasty
autodigestion
autoerotic rectal trauma
autofluorescent endsocopic system
autogenous
    a. spermatocele
    a. tunica vaginalis graft
autografting
autoimmune
    a. cholangitis
    a. cirrhosis
    a. connective tissue disorder

a. deficiency syndrome
a. hemolytic anemia
a. hepatitis (AIH)
a. immunoglobulin mediation
a. interstitial nephritis
a. metaplastic atrophic gastritis (AMAG)
a. polyglandular syndrome type 1 (APS-1)
a. sensorineural hearing loss
a. thyroid disease
a. thyroiditis

autoimmunity
thyroid a.

autointoxicant
autointoxication
autolavage
autologous
a. chondrocyte
a. fat
a. HBcAg-specific CD4+
a. liver cell
a. rectus fascia
a. rectus fascia sling
a. transfusion

autolymphocyte-based treatment for renal cell carcinoma (ALT-RCC)
autolymphocyte therapy
automated
a. counter Technicon H.3 RTX
a. endoscopic system for optimal positioning (AESOP)
a. peritoneal dialysis (APD)

automatic
a. chemical analyzer
a. endoscopic reprocessor (AER)
a. needle driver
a. titration system

automatically sequenced
autonephrectomy
silent a.

autonomic
a. dysfunction
a. dysreflexia
a. hyperreflexia
a. nerve fiber
a. nerve-preserving three-space dissection
a. nervous system (ANS)
a. neurogenic bladder
a. neuropathy
a. seizure

autopepsia
autophosphorylation
autoplasty
peritoneal a.

autopoisonous
autoradiogram
autoradiography
autoreactivity
liver-directed a.

autoregressive
autoregulation
renal a.

autosomal-dominant
a.-d. disorder
a.-d. kidney disease
a.-d. polycystic kidney disease (ADPKD)

autosomally
a. inherited form of nephrolithiasis
a. recessive inherited disease

autosomal-recessive
a.-r. Alport syndrome
a.-r. mode
a.-r. polycystic kidney disease (ARPKD)

autosplenectomy
autostapling device
autosuture technique
Autotome rotatable sphincterotome
autotoxic
autotoxicosis
autotoxin
autotransfusion (ATS)
autotransplantation
colostomy pyloric a.
posttraumatic a.
pyloric a.
renal a.
a. of splenic fragment

auxiliary
a. heterotopic liver transplantation (AHLT)
a. partial orthotopic liver transplantation (APOLT)
a. partial orthotopic living donor transplantation
a. procedure
a. transplant

AV
arteriovenous
AV fistula
AV shunt

NOTES

Avagard Instant Hand Antiseptic
avascular
    a. cuff technique
    a. necrosis
    a. stricture
Avastin IV infusion
avenolith
Aventyl
average flow rate
AVF
    arteriovenous fistula
AVF-induced renal ischemia
AVH
    acute viral hepatitis
avian myeloblastosis virus reverse transcriptase
avidin-biotin complex (ABC)
avidin-biotin-peroxidase
    a.-b.-p. complex
    a.-b.-p. complex method
Avihepadnavirus
Avitene
avium
    Mycobacterium a.
avium-intracellulare
    Mycobacterium a.-i. (MAI)
AVM
    arteriovenous malformation
avoidance maneuver
AVP
    arginine vasopressin
AVPR2
    antidiuretic arginine vasopressin V2 receptor
avulsion
    splenic a.
AVWS
    anterior vaginal wall sling
AW
    actual weight
axes (*pl. of* axis)
axial
    a. flap
    a. hiatal hernia
    a. image
Axid
axillary adenopathy
Axiom double sump tube
axis, pl. **axes**
    bowel a.
    brain-gut a.
    cardiopyloric a.
    celiac a.
    crypt-villus a.
    a. deviation
    enteroinsular a.
    hypertension resistance a.
    hypothalamic-pituitary a. (HPA)
    hypothalamic-pituitary-testicular-penile a.
    macrophage-TGF-beta a.
    neurohumoral-immune a.
    pituitary-gonadal a.
    renin-angiotensin-aldosterone a.
    reproductive a.
axoaxonic synapse
Axokine
axonopathy
axon reflex
axoplasmic
AxSYM free PSA test
Aylett operation
Ayre brush
Azactam
azamethonium
azan stain
azapetine
Aza-Pred therapy
azar
    kala a.
azasteroid inhibitor
azathioprine
azide
    sodium a.
azidothymidine (AZT)
azithromycin
Azlin
azlocillin
Azo
    A. Gantanol
    A. Gantrisin
azole
    a. antifungal agent
    a. therapy
azoospermia, azoospermatism
    excretory a.
    occlusive a.
    steroid-induced a.
    unreconstructable obstructive a.
Azo-Standard
azotemia
    extrarenal a.
    prerenal a.
azotemic osteodystrophy
azoturia
azoturic
azoxymethane (AOM)
AZQ
    diaziquone
AZT
    azidothymidine
Aztec two-step
aztreonam
Azulfidine EN-tabs

azygos
    a. blood flow

coronary a.
a. vein

NOTES

B
    B antigen
    B bile
    B cellular phenotype
    B lymphocyte
    B & O No. 15A, 16A C-II suppository
    B ring
    B ring of esophagus

B-48
    apo B-48
    apolipoprotein B-48
    plasma apo B-48

B72.3
    antibody to B72.3

B_6
    vitamin B_6

1b
    HCV genotype 1b

B-1
    Dukes B-1

B2
    bromobenzene
    B2 glycoprotein I

B_{12}
    B_{12} anemia
    vitamin B_{12}

B12 immunological study
B1, B2 integrin
b558 membrane-bound cytochrome
B5 tumor marker
BA
    bile acid

Ba
    barium

Babcock
    B. clamp
    B. intestinal forceps

Babinski
    B. reflex
    B. sign

baby, pl. **babies**
    b. Balfour retractor
    Clinical Risk Index for Babies (CRIB)
    b. scope
    b. soft diet (BSD)

BabyBIG powder for IV infusion
BAC
    benzalkonium chloride

bacampicillin

bacillary
    b. dysentery
    b. peliosis

bacille Calmette-Guérin (BCG, bCG)
bacillus, pl. **bacilli**
    acid-fast b. (AFB)
    Calmette-Gúerin b.
    B. cereus
    B. cerreus
    coliform b.
    curved b.
    dysentery b.
    Friedländer b.
    Schmitz b.
    Shiga b.
    Sonne-Duval b.
    Stanley b.
    Whipple b.

bacitracin zinc
backflow
    pyelolymphatic b.
    pyelorenal b.
    pyelosinus b.
    pyelotubular b.
    pyelovenous b.

background
    experimental b.
    mucosal b.

Backhaus
    B. dilator
    B. towel clamp
    B. towel forceps

backleak
    acute tubular necrosis b.

backwash ileitis
baclofen
Bacon anoscope
Bacon-Babcock rectovaginal fistula operation
bacterascites
    monomicrobial nonneutrocytic b. (MNB)
    polymicrobial b.

bacteremia
    incidence of b.
    percentage frequency of b.
    risk of b.
    Streptococcus bovis b.

bacteria (*pl. of* bacterium)
bacterial
    b. adherence
    b. adhesin
    b. adhesion
    b. biofilm
    b. biofilm formation

bacterial *(continued)*
    b. cast
    b. cholangitis
    b. cirrhosis
    b. cleavage
    b. colitis
    b. complication
    b. culture
    b. cystitis
    b. endotoxin
    b. enterocolitis
    b. esophagitis
    b. flora
    b. food poisoning
    b. host interaction
    b. infection
    b. interference
    b. metabolism in intestine
    b. mucosal infiltration
    b. nephritis
    b. overgrowth
    b. overgrowth syndrome
    b. pathogenesis
    b. peritonitis
    b. prostatitis
    b. toxigenic diarrhea
    b. vaginosis
    b. vector
    b. virulence factor

bactericholia, bacteriocholia
bactericidal
    b. function of phagocyte
    b. stomach environment
bactericide
bacteriocholia *(var. of* bactericholia*)*
bacteriology
bacteriospermia
bacteriostatically
bacteriostatic barrier
bacterium, pl. **bacteria**
    asymptomatic b.
    Chauveau b.
    coliform b.
    colonic b.
    gram-negative b.
    gram-positive b.
    human gut b.
    intestinal b.
    mesophilic b.
    pathogenic b.
    planktonic b.
    pyogenic b.
    spiral b.
    toxigenic b.
    urease-producing b.
    urinalysis sediment microscopy b.
    uropathogenic b.

bacteriuria
    asymptomatic b.
    catheter-associated b.
Bacteroidaceae
Bacteroides
    B. distasonis
    B. eggerthii
    B. fragilis
    B. melaninogenicus
    B. ovatus
    B. praeacutus
    B. putredinis
    B. splanchnicus
    B. thetaiotaomicron
    B. uniformis
    B. ureolyticus
    B. vulgatus
bactibilia
Bactocill
Bactrim DS
baculovirus
baculum
BAD
    benign anorectal disease
BA-EDTA solution
Baehr-Lohlein lesion
Baermann
    B. stool filter
    B. stool test
bag
    Acme One Time enteral feeding b.
    Belly b.
    bile b.
    biohazard b.
    Bogota b.
    bowel b.
    breath b.
    Coloplast b.
    colostomy b.
    Davol feeding b.
    DeRoyal Surgical grab b.
    Dobbhoff enteral feeding b.
    endo catch b.
    EndoMate grab b.
    Entri-Pak enteral feeding b.
    eXtract specimen b.
    1090 Gavage b.
    Hollister urostomy b.
    ileostomy b.
    intestinal b.
    Keofeed enteral feeding b.
    Lahey liver transplant b.
    Le B.
    Mikulicz b.
    Mosher b.
    nylon tissue biopsy b.
    ostomy b.
    perfusate b.
    Perry b.

Petersen b.
Plummer b.
pneumatic b.
Polar enteral feeding b.
Rutzen ileostomy b.
stomal b.
Top-Fill enteral feeding b.
Vacutainer b.
Whitmore b.
BAGF
brachioaxillary bridge graft fistula
Bagley helical basket
BAIBF
bile acid-independent bile formation
Bainbridge
B. intestinal clamp
B. intestinal forceps
Bakamjian flap
Baker
B. antifol
B. intestinal decompression tube
B. jejunostomy tube
Bakes
B. common duct dilator
B. probe
BAL
blood alcohol level
balance
acid-base b.
chloride b.
electrolyte b.
equal fluid b.
glomerulotubular b.
metabolic b.
negative nitrogen b.
nitrogen b.
positive nitrogen b.
potassium b.
sodium b.
vagosympathetic b.
water b.
balanced
b. diet
b. electrolyte solution
b. salt solution (BSS)
b. voiding dysfunction
Balance lavage solution
balanic, balanitic
b. epispadias
b. hypospadias
balanitis
b. circinata

circinate b.
b. circumscripta plasmacellularis
b. diabetica
Follmann b.
b. gangraenosa
gangrenous b.
keratotic pseudoepitheliomatous b.
plasma cell b.
trichomonal b.
b. xerotica
b. xerotica obliterans (BXO)
yeast b.
b. of Zoon
balanoblennorrhea
balanocele
balanoplasty
balanoposthitis chronica circumscripta plasma cellularis
balanoposthomycosis
balanopreputial
balanorrhagia
balanorrhea
balantidial
b. colitis
b. dysentery
balantidiasis, balantidosis
Balantidium
B. coli
B. coli colitis
balanus
Balch 1 broth medium
bald gastric fundus
Baldwin perineum needle
Baldy-Webster operation
Balfour
B. abdominal retractor
B. gastroenterostomy
B. self-retaining retractor
Balkan
B. nephrectomy
B. nephritis
B. nephropathy
ball
b. electrode
food b.
fungal b.
gastrointestinal fungal b.
hair b.
b. myoma
B. operation
B. procedure
ureteropelvic fungus b.

NOTES

ball *(continued)*
  B. valve
  wool b.
Ballance sign
Ballenger forceps
Ballobes gastric balloon
balloon
  Acucise b.
  air-filled b.
  anchoring b.
  angioplasty b.
  artificial urinary sphincter pressure-regulating b.
  AS-800 b.
  Ballobes gastric b.
  banana-shaped b.
  barostat b.
  barostatic b.
  Brandt cytology b.
  b. catheter-assisted endoscopic snare papillectomy
  b. catheter and basket retrieval technique
  centering b.
  b. cholangiogram
  cylindrical b.
  b. cystoscope
  b. cytology
  DASH extraction b.
  b. decompression
  b. defecation
  b. dilating catheter
  b. dilation
  b. dilation of papilla
  b. dilator
  dissecting b.
  doughnut-shaped b.
  esophageal single b.
  b. expulsion test
  extraction b.
  Extractor XL triple-lumen retrieval b.
  fluid-filled b.
  Fogarty b.
  French Swan-Ganz b.
  Garren b.
  Garren-Edwards b.
  gastric b.
  Gau gastric b.
  Grüntzig b.
  Helmstein b.
  high-compliance latex b.
  hot wire b.
  hydrostatic b.
  intragastric b.
  Kaye nephrostomy tamponade b.
  b. kymography
  b. laser
  latex b.
  low-compliance b.
  mercury-containing b.
  Microvasive retrieval b.
  Microvasive Rigiflex through-the-scope b.
  occlusion b.
  b. occlusion cholangiography
  Percival gastric b.
  b. percutaneous transluminal angioplasty
  b. photodynamic therapy
  preperitoneal distention b. (PDB)
  b. proctogram
  Provocative sensitivity b.
  Quantum TTC biliary b.
  rectal b.
  b. reflex manometry
  retrieval b.
  Riepe-Bard gastric b.
  Rigiflex achalasia b.
  Rigiflex TTS b.
  scintigraphic b.
  Sengstaken-Blakemore esophageal b.
  silicone b.
  stone retrieval b.
  b. tamponade prosthesis
  Taylor gastric b.
  through-the-scope b.
  b. topogram
  treatment b.
  b. tube tamponade
  b. ureteral occlusion
  water displacing b.
  Wilson-Cook dilating b.
  Wilson-Cook esophageal b.
  Wilson-Cook gastric b.
  windowed esophageal b.
  wire-guided hydrostatic b.
ballooned hepatocyte
ballooning
  b. of cell
  b. degeneration
  b. degeneration of hepatocyte
  eosinophilic b.
  b. esophagoscope
  hepatocellular b.
  b. of papilla
balloon-occluded retrograde transvenous obliteration (B-RTO)
ballottable liver
ballottement
  abdominal b.
  kidney b.
  b. tenderness
balm
Balneol
BALP
  bone-specific alkaline phosphatase
balsalazide disodium

Balser fatty necrosis
BALT
    bronchus-associated lymphoepithelial tissue
Balthazar grading system
Baltimore Longitudinal Study of Aging (BLSA)
BAM
    bile acid malabsorption
Bamberger hematogenic albuminuria
bamboo jointlike appearance of gastric body
Bamethan
banana
    b. peel effect
    b. plug dipolar generator
    b.'s, rice, cereal, applesauce, tea, and toast (BRATT)
    b.'s, rice, cereal, applesauce, and toast (BRAT)
banana-shaped balloon
bancrofti
    Wuchereria b.
band
    adhesive b.
    anorectal b.
    cholecystoduodenal b.
    dysgenetic fibrous b.
    b. form
    free b. of colon
    genitomesenteric b.
    Harris b.
    Henle b.
    hymenal b.
    Ladd b.
    Lane b.
    b. ligation
    Lyon ring-constrictive b.
    Marlex b.
    mesocolic b.
    omental b.
    pecten b.
    peritoneal b.
    b. placement
    b. 3 protein
    retention b.
    silicone elastomer b.
    snap gauge b.
    b. and snare technique
    Swedish Adjustable Gastric B. (SAGB)
    WBC b.

bandage
    Sureseal pressure b.
    suspensory b.
    T b.
banded gastroplasty with divided pouch
banding
    adjustable silicone gastric b. (ASGB)
    b. cylinder
    esophageal b.
    hemorrhoidal b.
    laparoscopic adjustable gastric b.
    Lap-Band adjustable gastric b. (LAGB)
    laser adjustable silicone gastric b. (LASGB)
    mucosal b.
    suction b.
    variceal b.
Bandito single-band ligator
band-ligator device
band-snare technique
Banff classification
banjo-string adhesion
Bannayan-Zonana syndrome
Banocide
Banthine
Banti
    B. disease
    B. splenic anemia
    B. syndrome
BAO
    basal acid output
BAP
    bone alkaline phosphatase
BAR
    biofragmentable anastomotic ring
        Valtrac BAR
bar
    cricopharyngeal b.
    intersymphyseal b.
    leading b.
    Mercier b.
    symphyseal b.
barbed snare
barber pole sign
Barbidonna No. 2
Barbita
barbital-acetate buffer
barbotage

NOTES

Barcat
- B. procedure
- B. technique

Barcat-Redman hypospadias repair

Barcoo
- B. vomit
- B. vomitus

Bard
- B. alligator cup
- B. automatic reprocessor
- B. Biopty gun
- B. Biopty instrument
- B. BladderScan
- B. BladderScan bladder volume instrument
- B. BTA test
- B. button
- B. closed-end adhesive pouch
- B. Companion papillotome
- B. Director guidewire
- B. drainage adhesive pouch
- B. EndoCinch endoscopic suture system
- B. EndoCinch endoscopic suturing system
- B. endoscope transesophageal endoscopic plication
- B. Extra Ileo B pouch
- B. gastrostomy catheter
- B. gastrostomy feeding tube
- B. irrigation sleeve
- B. Memotherm colorectal stent
- B. oval cup
- B. PEG
- B. PEG tube
- B. Precisor direct bite forceps
- B. protective barrier
- B. protective barrier film
- B. security pouch
- B. Urolase
- B. Urolase fiber laser system
- B. Visilex mesh

Bardet-Biedl syndrome
Bardex-Foley catheter
Bard-Parker
- B.-P. blade
- B.-P. knife

BardPort implanted port
Bard-Stiegmann-Goff variceal ligation kit
bare area of liver
bariatric
- b. operation
- b. surgery

bariatrics
Baricon contrast medium
barium (Ba)
- b. artifact
- b. bezoar
- b. burger
- b. contrast radiography
- double tracking of b.
- b. enema (BE)
- b. enema reduction
- b. enema with air contrast
- b. esophagram
- b. granuloma
- b. meal
- b. paste
- b. peritonitis
- residual b.
- retained b.
- b. retention
- b. sediment in urine
- b. study
- b. sulfate
- b. sulfate solution
- b. sulfate for suspension
- b. swallow

barium-coated marshmallow
barium-impregnated marshmallow
Barnes common duct dilator
Barnett pouch
Baro-CAT
Baroflave contrast medium
barogenic perforation
Barophen
baroreceptor
- high-pressure arterial b.
- low-pressure cardiopulmonary b.
- renal b.
- sinoaortic b.

baroreceptor-mediated mesenteric arterial vasoconstriction
baroreflex
- cardiopulmonary b.

Barosperse contrast medium
barostat
- b. balloon
- electronic b.
- b. method
- rectal b.
- Synectics visceral stimulator electronic b.

barostatic balloon
barotrauma
Barr
- B. fistula hook
- B. fistula probe
- B. rectal retractor
- B. rectal speculum

barrel
- b. chest
- Opti-Vue plastic b.

Barrett
- B. carcinoma
- B. disease
- B. dysplasia

B. epithelium
B. esophagitis
B. esophagus (BE)
B. intestinal forceps
B. metaplasia
B. segment
B. syndrome
B. ulcer
Barrett-Clagett esophagogastrostomy
Barrett-Donovan-Mayo artificial bladder
Barrett-Murphy intestinal thumb forceps
barrier
ABO b.
bacteriostatic b.
Bard protective b.
bioabsorbable adhesion b.
blood-epididymis b.
blood-liquor b.
blood-testis b.
blood-urine b.
Colly-Seal wafer-type skin b.
Coloplast skin b.
Comfeel skin b.
Dansac skin b.
b. drape
filtration b.
gastric mucosal b.
high-pressure antireflux b.
Hollister Guardian F skin b.
INTERCEED absorbable adhesion b.
Nu-Hope Adhesive waterproof skin b.
pectin-base skin b.
Premium B.
ReliaSeal skin b.
seminiferous tubule blood-testis b.
Sween-A-Peel skin b.
United XL 14 skin b.
Barrington third reflex
Barron
B. ligation
B. rubber band ligator
Barr-Shuford rectal speculum
Barsony-Polgar syndrome
Bartel cytotoxicity
Barth hernia
Bartholin
B. cyst
B. gland
Bartonella henselae
Bartter syndrome

bar-type esophageal varix
baruria
BAS-300 transurethral thermotherapy device
basal
b. acid output (BAO)
b. acid secretion
b. anal canal pressure
b. anal sphincter pressure
b. androstenedione
b. carbohydrate oxidation rate
b. cell carcinoma
b. cell nevus syndrome
b. cell-specific anticytokeratin antibody
b. diet
b. ganglia
b. granular cell
b. interferon-gamma
b. lamina
b. metabolic rate (BMR, BRM)
b. metabolism (BM)
b. release of motilin
b. renal excretion
b. renal vascular resistance
b. secretory flow rate (BSFR)
b. secretory flow rate test
b. testosterone
Basaljel
basaloid squamous cell carcinoma (BSCC)
bascule
cecal b.
base
adhesive b.
b. of appendix
compressive b.
crypt b.
erythromycin b.
b. excess
Interstitial Cystitis Data B. (ICDB)
b. of renal pyramid
ulcer b.
baseball stitch
baseline
delta over b. (DOB)
b. recovered control
b. tenting
b. troponin T
basement
b. membrane

NOTES

basement *(continued)*
    b. membrane antigen
    b. membrane protein
bas-fond
basic
    b. diet
    b. dye
    b. fibroblast growth factor (bFGF)
    b. fibroblastic growth factor
    b. gastrin (BG)
basidiobolomycosis
Basidiobolus ranarum
basiliximab
basket
    Bagley helical b.
    DASH tipless extraction b.
    Dormia stone b.
    Eliminator stone extraction b.
    Ellik kidney stone b.
    b. extraction
    3.2F Cook N-Circle tipless stone b.
    b. forceps
    Gemini paired wire helical b.
    Glassman b.
    Helical b.
    laser lithotriptor b.
    minihelical b.
    nitinol b.
    Olympus stone retrieval b.
    Positrap miniretrieval b.
    b. procedure
    Pursuer CBD helical stone b.
    Pursuer minihelical stone b.
    retrieval b.
    Segura b.
    Segura-Dretler laser b.
    six-wire spiral-tip Segura b.
    sphincterotomy b.
    spiral b.
    stone retrieval b.
    trapped b.
basketing
    ureteral scoping b.
basket-type crushing forceps
baso
    basophil
basolateral membrane (BLM)
basophil (baso)
    WBC b.
Bassen-Kornzweig
    B.-K. disease
    B.-K. syndrome
Bassini
    B. inguinal hernia repair
    B. inguinal herniorrhaphy
    B. needle
    B. operation
Bates-corrected beta
Bates operation
bath
    alcohol cooling b.
    sitz b.
bathroom privilege
battery
    button b.
    b. ingestion
battery-powered endoscope
Battle
    B. incision
    B. operation
    B. sign
Battle-Jalaguier-Kammerer incision
bat-wing catheter
Bauhin
    valve of B.
    B. valve
Baumgarten
    B. cirrhosis
    B. syndrome
Baumrucker urinary incontinence clamp
Baveno portal hypertensive gastropathy grading system
Baxter
    B. CA-210 filter
    1550 B. hemodialyzer
    B. Interline IV system
Bayer
    B. Plus
    B. Versant HCV RNA 2.0 assay test kit
BayGam IM injection
Bay K 8644 channel agonist
Baylor bleeding score
bayonet stylet
bayonet-tip electrode
bayonet-type forceps
Bazex syndrome
BBDS
    benign bile duct stricture
BBM
    brush-border membrane
BBMV
    brush-border membrane vesicle
BBS
    brown bowel syndrome
BC
    biliary colic
    BC Cold Powder
BCA-1 protein assay kit
BCAA
    branched-chain amino acid
BCAA/AAA plasma ratio
BCAD 2 powder
B-cell
    B-c. antigen CD20
    B-c. cell differentiation factor
    B-c. cell epitope

B-c. cell line
B-c. cell PHSL
BCG, bCG
   bacille Calmette-Guérin
      BCG immunotherapy
      intravesical BCG
      BCG live
      BCG live intravesical injection
      Mycobacterium bovis BCG
      BCG vaccine
bcl-2
BCLA-4
   bladder cancer-specific nuclear matrix protein
BCM
   body cell mass
BCNU, bCNU
   carmustine
BCO
   biliary cholesterol output
BCR
   bulbocavernosus reflex
BDA
   bile duct adenoma
BDL
   bile duct ligation
bDNA
   branched-chain DNA
BDNF
   brain-derived neurotrophic factor
BDP
   beclomethasone dipropionate
B-D Safety-Gard needle
BE
   barium enema
   Barrett esophagus
Beacon surgical line
bead-chain
      b.-c. cystography
      Percoll b.-c.
      PMMA b.-c.
      Septopal b.-c.
      b.-c. study
beaded hepatic duct
beading sign
beaker cell
beaklike appearance
Beale
   sacculi of B.
beam
   x-ray b.

Beamer
   B. injection stent
   B. injection stent system
bear claw ulcer
Beardsley
   B. cecostomy trocar
   B. esophageal retractor
   B. intestinal clamp
   B. intestinal forceps
Bearn-Kunkel-Slater syndrome
Beasley-Babcock forceps
beaver
   B. blade
   B. dissector
   B. fever
BEB
   blind esophageal brushing
BEC
   biliary epithelial cell
Beck
   B. abdominal scoop
   B. aorta forceps
   B. Depression Inventory
   B. gastrostomy
   B. method
Beck-Jianu gastrostomy
Beckman
   B. airfuge
   B. 2 autoanalyzer
   B. ion-selective analyzer
   B. 39042 pH probe
Beckwith-Wiedemann syndrome
Béclard hernia
beclomethasone dipropionate (BDP)
BED
   binge-eating disorder
bed
      Advanta b.
      gallbladder b.
      graft b.
      hepatic b.
      liver b.
      nail b.
      b. pad
      portal vascular b.
      raw surface of liver b.
      stomach b.
      suburothelial vascular b.
      ulcer b.

NOTES

Bedge
    B. antireflux mattress
    B. pillow
bedside drainage (BSD)
bed-wetting alarm
Beebe hemostatic forceps
beef tapeworm
Beelith
Beer nephroureterectomy
BEF
    bronchoesophageal fistula
befacizumab
B.E. Glass abdominal retractor
behavior
    binge-purge b.
behavioral treatment
Behçet
    B. colitis
    B. disease
    B. syndrome
Behrend cystic duct forceps
Behring OPUS Plus immunofluorescence assay
beigelli
    Trichosporon b.
belch
    silent b.
belching
Belfield operation
Bell
    B. law
    B. muscle
    B. suture
Belladenal
belladonna
    tincture of b.
Bellafoline
Bellalphen
bell-clapper deformity
Bellergal-S
belli
    Isospora b.
Bellini
    B. duct
    B. duct carcinoma
    B. ligament
    B. tubule
bellow response
bell-shaped orifice
belly
    B. Bag
    Crix b.
    wooden b.
bellyache
BELS
    bioartificial extracorporeal liver support system
Belsey
    B. 270-degree fundoplication
    B. Mark IV antireflux operation
    B. Mark IV 240-degree fundoplication
    B. Mark IV procedure
    B. Mark IV repair
    B. Mark V operation
    B. partial fundoplication
    B. two-thirds wrap fundoplication
belt
    abdominal compression b.
    Assura stomy b.
    Coloplast ostomy b.
    B. technique
    b. test
Belt-Fuqua hypospadias repair
Belzer
    B. machine
    B. UW liver preservation solution
Benadryl
benazepril HCl
Bence
    B. Jones albumin
    B. Jones albumosuria
    B. Jones cylinder
    B. Jones globulin
    B. Jones protein
    B. Jones protein method
    B. Jones proteinuria
    B. Jones urine
bench
    b. surgery
    b. surgical technique
Benchekroun
    B. hydraulic ileal valve
    B. pouch
bend
    cautery b.
    iliac b.
bendroflumethiazide
Benedict
    B. and Franke method
    B. gastroscope
Benedict-Talbot body surface area method
benefit
    b. for the patient
    significant b.
Benelux Multicentre Trial Study Group
Benemid
Bengt-Johanson procedure
benign
    b. adenomatous polyp
    b. anorectal disease (BAD)
    b. bile duct stricture (BBDS)
    b. biliary stricture
    b. cystic mesothelioma
    b. cystic teratoma
    b. duodenocolic fistula
    b. familial hematuria

b. familial icterus
b. familial pemphigus
b. gastric ulcer
b. gastrocolonic-pancreatic fistula
b. hyperplastic gastropathy
b. lymphoma
b. lymphoma of rectum
b. mesenchymoma
b. mesothelioma of genital tract
b. mucous membrane pemphigoid (BMMP)
b. neoplastic precursor
b. nephrosclerosis
b. papillary stenosis
b. paroxysmal peritonitis
b. pneumatic colonoscopy complication
b. pneumoperitoneum
b. postoperative cholestasis
b. postoperative jaundice
b. prostatic enlargement (BPE)
b. prostatic hyperplasia (BPH)
b. prostatic hyperplasia transurethral vaporization
b. prostatic hypertrophy (BPH)
b. prostatic obstruction (BPO)
b. recurrent intrahepatic cholestasia
b. tumor
Béniqué sound
Bennett operation
benoxaprofen
benserazide
Benson pylorus separator
bentiromide test
Bentle button
bent nail syndrome
bentonite flocculation test
Bentson floppy-tipped guidewire
Bentson-type Glidewire guidewire
Bentyl
Bentylol
Benzacot Injection
benzaldehyde dehydrogenase
benzalkonium chloride (BAC)
benzamide prokinetic agent
benzathine penicillin
benzethonium chloride 0.025%
benzidine
benzimidazole
    substituted b.
benzoate
benzocaine

benzodiazepine conscious sedation
benzodiazepine-induced hypoventilation
benzoic acid
benzoin
    tincture of b.
benzoyl-tyrosyl-paraaminobenzoic acid (BT-PABA)
benzphetamine
benzquinamide
benzthiazide
benztropine
benzydamine
benzyl chloride
benzylpenicillin
BEP
    bleomycin, etoposide, cisplatin
Beppu score
bepridil
Berci-Shore
    B.-S. choledochoscope
    B.-S. choledochoscopy
Berens esophageal retractor
Bergenhem operation
Berger
    B. disease
    B. nephropathy
Bergkvist grading system
Bergman sign
Beriplast fibrin sealant
Berkeley-Bonney retractor
Berlin
    B. blue
    B. blue staining
Bernard
    B. canal
    B. duct
    B. glandular layer
Bernard-Sergent syndrome
Bernard-Soulier syndrome
Bernstein
    B. acid perfusion test
    B. gastroscope
berry aneurysm
Bertiella
    B. mucronata
    B. satyri
    B. studeri
Bertin
    hypertrophy of column of B.
Bertrand method
berylliosis
Besnier-Boeck-Schaumann disease

NOTES

BESP
Bipolar EndoStasis probe
Bessauds-Hilmand-Augier syndrome
Bessey-Lowry unit for alkaline phosphatase
Best
B. bite block
B. gallstone forceps
B. operation
B. right-angle colon clamp
bestatin
bestiarum
Aeromonas b.
besylate
amlodipine b.
beta
b. adrenergic blocker
b. aminoisobutyricaciduria
b. aminopropionitrile
Bates-corrected b.
b. blocker
b. chain
7-b.-epimer of chenodeoxycholic acid
epoetin b.
estrogen receptor b. (ER beta)
b. fetoprotein
b. galactosidase
b. galactosidase activity
growth factor b.
b. inhibin
interferon b.
b. interferon
b. microseminoprotein
b. sitosterolemia
transforming growth factor b. (TGF-beta)
beta-1
b.-1 chain
b.-1 chain integrin
transforming growth factor b.-1 (TGF-beta-1)
beta-2
b.-2 agonist
b.-2 microglobulin control
b.-2 test
transforming growth factor b.-2 (TGF-beta-2)
beta-3
b.-3 agonist
transforming growth factor b.-3 (TGF-beta-3)
beta-actin
b.-a. cDNA probe
b.-a. mRNA
b.-a. mRNA signal
beta-adrenergic
b.-a. agonist
b.-a. antagonist
b.-a. blockade
b.-a. receptor
beta-blocker therapy
Beta-Cap
B.-C. catheter closure
B.-C. II closure
Betadine
B. gel
B. PrepStick Plus applicator
B. scrub
17-beta-diol
5-alpha-androstane-3-alpha 17-b.-d.
5-alpha-androstane-3-beta 17-b.-d.
beta-endorphin
b.-e. peptide YY
beta-fibroblastic growth factor
beta-galactose
Betagan
beta-HCG, beta-hCG
b.-HCG autocrine motility factor
beta-hemolytic streptococcus
beta-hydroxyacyl-coenzyme A dehydrogenase
betahydroxylase
dopamine b.
3-beta-hydroxysteroid
3-b.-h. dehydrogenase
3-b.-h. dehydrogenase deficiency
betaine anhydrous solution
beta-lactam antibiotic
beta-lactamase-resistant penicillin
beta-lactam-associated diarrhea
betamethasone
topical b.
beta-2-microglobulin
beta-oxidation
mitochondrial fatty acid b.-o.
b.-o. pathway
beta-pleated sheet formation
BetaSorb device
beta-subunit
transmembrane b.-s.
beta-sympathomimetic tocolytic agent
beta-thromboglobulin
betaxolol
betazole stimulation test
bethanechol
b. chloride
b. hydrochloride
b. test
bethanidine
Bethesda System for cervicovaginal sample
Bethune shears
BetterMAN
bevacizumab
Bevan
B. abdominal incision
B. gallbladder forceps

B. operation
B. orchiopexy
bevel
    Menghini-type coring b.
beveled speculum
beverage
    Resource Fruit B.
bezafibrate
bezoar
    artificial b.
    Aspergillus b.
    barium b.
    fungal b.
    gastric b.
    medication b.
    orange b.
    percutaneous removal of b.
    persimmon b.
BF
    bile flow
bFGF
    basic fibroblast growth factor
BFR
    blood flow rate
BG
    basic gastrin
    bicolor guaiac
B2 glycoprotein I
BGP
    brain-type glycogen phosphorylase
BGV
    bleeding gastric varix
BHD
    Birt-Hogg-Dube
    BHD syndrome
BHDS
    Birt-Hogg-Dube syndrome
Bi
    bismuth
BIA
    bioelectrical impedance analysis
Biafine wound dressing emulsion
Bianchi approach
Biaxin
BIB
    biliointestinal bypass
bibasilar
bicalutamide
    b. monotherapy
    b. withdrawal phenomenon
BICAP
    Bipolar Circumactive Probe
    BICAP bipolar diathermy
    BICAP bipolar hemostasis probe
    BICAP coagulation
    BICAP electrocoagulation probe
    BICAP electrode probe
    BICAP endoscopic probe
    BICAP hemostatic system
    BICAP II cautery
    BICAP monopolar
    BICAP silver ACE
Bicarbolyte
bicarbonate (HCO^{3-})
    b. buffer system
    b. dialysate
    b. electrolyte
    potassium b.
    saliva b.
    serum b.
    sodium b.
    urinary b.
    b. wastage renal tubular acidosis
bicarotid trunk
BiCart dialysis fluid
biceps femoris musculocutaneous unit
bicho
Bicitra
BiCNU
bicolor guaiac (BG)
bicornuate uterus
bicoudate catheter
bicurved needle
bidigital rectal examination
bidirectional ligation
Biebl loop
bieneusi
    Enterocytozoon b.
Biermer disease
Biesiadecki fossa
bifid
    b. branches
    b. clitoris
    b. penis
    b. renal pelvis
    b. scrotum
    b. tongue
    b. ureter
bifida
    adolescent spina b.
    spina b.
Bifidobacterium
    B. bifidum
    B. brevis

NOTES

Bifidobacterium (continued)
    B. infantis
    B. longum
bifidum
    Bifidobacterium b.
bifidus
    Lactobacillus b.
bifocal multiplane rectal transducer
bifurcation
    b. of common bile duct
    hepatic b.
    tracheal b.
    b. tumor
Bigelow
    B. litholapaxy
    B. operation
bigeminy
biglycan
    proteoglycan b.
biguanides
Bihrle
    B. dorsal clamp
    B. dorsal clamp-T-C needle holder
BII
    BPH impact index
bikunin
bilabe
Bilagog
bilaminar embryonic disk
Bilarcil
bilateral
    b. anorchia
    b. cryptorchidism
    b. hydronephrosis
    b. lithotomy
    b. nephrectomy
    b. nephroureterectomy
    b. pheochromocytoma
    b. pudendal artery embolization
    b. renal tumor
    b. renal vein thrombosis
    b. subcostal incision
    b. transabdominal incision
    b. ureteral obstruction (BUO)
    b. ureterostomy takedown
    b. vagotomy
    b. Wilms tumor
bilayer
    lipid b.
    phospholipid b.
Bilbao-Dotter tube
bile
    A b.
    b. acid (BA)
    b. acid binder
    b. acid breath test
    b. acid diarrhea type 1, 2
    b. acid-EDTA solution
    b. acid-independent bile formation (BAIBF)
    b. acid malabsorption (BAM)
    b. acid pool
    b. acid sequestrant
    b. acid therapy
    b. acid tolerance test
    b. ascites
    B b.
    b. bag
    C b.
    canalicular b.
    b. capillary
    clear b.
    cloudy b.
    b. concretion
    cystic b.
    b. duct
    b. duct abscess
    b. duct adenoma (BDA)
    b. duct atresia
    b. duct brushing
    b. duct canaliculus
    b. duct cancer
    b. duct cannulation
    b. duct carcinoma
    b. duct cyst
    b. duct dyskinesia
    b. duct epithelial cell
    b. duct hypoplasia
    b. duct ligation (BDL)
    b. duct lumen
    b. duct paucity
    b. duct pressure
    b. duct proliferation
    b. duct stenosis
    b. duct stone
    b. duct stricture
    b. duct trauma
    b. duct-type cytokeratin
    b. ductular cholestasis
    extravasated b.
    b. flow (BF)
    b. infarct
    inspissated b.
    b. lake
    limy b.
    lithogenic b.
    milk-of-calcium b.
    b. papilla
    b. peritonitis
    b. phospholipid concentration (BPC)
    b. phospholipid output (BPO)
    b. pleuritis
    b. plug
    b. pulmonary embolism
    b. reflux
    b. reflux gastritis
    b. salt (BS)

b. salt aggregation
b. salt-binding resin
b. salt concentrate (BSC)
b. salt deficiency
b. salt diarrhea
b. salt export pump (BSEP)
b. salt injury
b. salt-losing enteropathy
b. salt metabolism (BSM)
b. salt output (BSO)
b. salt-phospholipid ratio
b. salt-stimulated lipase (BSSL)
b. secretory failure
SI of b.
b. solubility test
stagnant b.
b. stasis
supersaturated b.
thick b.
b. thrombus
turbid b.
viscid b.
viscous b.
white b.
bile-laden macrophage
bile-stained
    b.-s. fluid
    b.-s. vomitus
bile-tinged fluid
bilharzial
    b. appendicitis
    b. bladder cancer syndrome
    b. dysentery
    b. worm
bilharzial-related cancer
bilharziasis
bilharzioma
bili
    bilirubin
    bili light
    Bili mask
biliaris
    collum vesicae b.
    corpus vesicae b.
    ductus b.
    fossa vesicae b.
    fundus vesicae b.
    vesica b.
biliary
    b. abscess
    b. actinomycosis
    b. air

b. angiography
b. apparatus
b. ascariasis
b. ascites
b. atresia
b. balloon catheter
b. balloon dilator
b. balloon probe
b. calculus
b. canaliculus
b. cannulation
b. carcinoma
b. cholangitis
b. cholesterol output (BCO)
b. cholesterol secretion
b. cirrhosis
b. cirrhotic liver
b. clonorchiasis
b. colic (BC)
b. cryptosporidiosis
b. cycle
b. cyst
b. cystadenocarcinoma
b. cystadenoma
b. decompression
b. dilation
b. dilator catheter
b. diverticulum
b. drainage
b. duct
b. ductules
b. dyskinesia
b. dyspepsia
b. dyssynergia
b. echinococcosis
b. endoprosthesis
b. endoprosthesis insertion
b. endoscopic sphincterotomy
b. epithelia hyperplasia
b. epithelial cell (BEC)
b. excretion
b. fibroadenomatosis
b. fibrosis
b. fistula
b. gland
b. hypercholesterolemia xanthomatosis
b. immunoglobulin
b. infestation
b. instrumentation
b. leakage
b. lipid

NOTES

biliary *(continued)*
- b. lithotripsy
- b. manometry
- b. microhamartoma
- b. mud
- b. orifice
- b. pancreatitis
- b. papillomatosis
- b. passage
- b. piecemeal necrosis
- b. plexus
- b. prosthesis
- b. radicle
- b. reconstruction
- b. saturation index
- b. scintiscan
- b. sclerosis
- b. sepsis
- b. sludge
- b. sphincter
- B. Spiral Z stent
- b. stasis
- b. steatorrhea
- b. stenting
- b. stent patency
- b. structure
- B. Symptoms Questionnaire (BSQ)
- b. tract
- b. tract disease
- b. tract obstruction
- b. tract pain (BTP)
- b. tract pressure
- b. tract stone
- b. tract stricture
- b. tract torsion
- b. tract tumor
- b. tree
- b. tree duplication

biliary-bronchial fistula
biliary-cutaneous fistula
biliary-duodenal pressure gradient
biliation
Bilibed
BiliBlanket Phototherapy System
BiliBottoms
BiliCheck
- B. breath analyzer device
- B. test

bilicyanin
bilifaction, bilification
bilifer
- canaliculus b.

biliferi
- ductuli b.
- ductus b.

biliferous
bilification *(var. of* bilifaction*)*
biliflavin
bilifulvin

bilifuscin
biligenesis
biligenetic
biligenic
Biligrafin contrast medium
bilihumin
bilin
bilioduodenal
- b. fistula
- b. prosthesis

bilioenteric
- b. anastomosis
- b. bypass
- b. fistula

biliointestinal bypass (BIB)
biliopancreatic
- b. bypass (BPB)
- b. diversion
- b. diversion with duodenal stent
- b. fistula
- b. obesity surgery
- b. shunt

bilious
- b. cholera
- b. colic
- b. diarrhea
- b. emesis
- b. flux
- b. leakage
- b. remittent fever
- b. remittent malaria
- b. stool
- b. vomit
- b. vomiting

biliousness
biliprasin
biliptysis
bilirachia
bilirubin (bili)
- conjugated b.
- delta b.
- direct b.
- b. encephalopathy
- b. ester conjugate
- fat-soluble b.
- fractionation of b.
- indirect b.
- b. infarct
- b. pigment gallstone
- b. protein conjugate
- serum b.
- b. test
- total b.
- unconjugated b. (UCB)
- urinary b.
- urine b.
- water-soluble b.

bilirubinate stone
bilirubinemia

bilirubinoid
bilirubinometer
    direct-reading b.
bilirubinuria
bilis
    Helicobacter b.
    vesicula b.
Biliscopin contrast medium
Bilitec
    fiberoptic spectrophotometer B. 2000
    B. 2000 intraluminal fiberoptic probe
bilitherapy
biliuria
biliverdin
Bilivist contrast medium
Billingham-Bookwalter rectal fenestrated blade
Billroth
    B. cord
    B. forceps
    B. gastroduodenoscopy
    B. gastroenterostomy type I, II
    B. gastrojejunostomy type I, II
    B. hypertrophy
    B. I gastroduodenostomy
    B. II anastomotic scar
    B. II anatomy
    B. I, II anastomosis
    B. I, II gastrectomy
    B. I, II operation
    B. I, II reconstruction
    B. strand
    B. venae cavernosae
bilobar
    b. hyperplasia
    b. hypertrophy
bilobate false aneurysm
bilobed
    b. gallbladder
    b. polypoid lesion
bilocular stomach
biloma
Bilopaque contrast medium
Biloptin contrast medium
Biltricide
Bimexes
bimucosa
    fistula b.
binary factor

binder
    bile acid b.
    Dale abdominal b.
    T b.
    b. test
binding
    anti-DNA b.
    crystal b.
    phosphotyrosine-SH2 b.
    ryanodine b.
    soluble CD44 b.
    sperm-immunobead b.
    vasoactive intestinal polypeptide b.
binge
binge-eating disorder (BED)
bingeing and purging
binge-purge behavior
binucleate renal tubule epithelial cell
bioabsorbable adhesion barrier
bioactive antimicrobial coated solid alloplast
bioartificial
    b. extracorporeal liver support system (BELS)
    b. liver support device
bioassay
    mink cell b.
bioavailability
Biocef
biochanin A
biochemical
    b. characterization
    b. marker
Bioclot protein S assay
biocompatibility
biocompatible
    b. material
    b. membrane
Biodan Prostathermer
biodegradable microsphere
biodistribution of N-isopropyl-p-iodoamphetamine
bioeffect
bioelectrical impedance analysis (BIA)
Bio-Enzabead test
biofeedback
    augmented b.
    bladder b.
    cystometric b.
    sensory b.
    b. therapy
    voiding b.

NOTES

biofilm
  bacterial b.
  b. formation
  microbial b.
  polymicrobial b.
  resistance monomicrobial b.
biofilm-related encrustation
BioFIT Herbgels
Biofix stent
biofragmentable anastomotic ring (BAR)
Bio-Gel HTP
Biogenex antigen retrieval method
biogenic amine
Bio-Gen urine test strip
Bioglass
biohazard bag
bioincompatible membrane
Biolab
  Malakit *Helicobacter pylori* B.
biologic
  b. collagen-based tissue-matrix graft
  b. marker
  b. response modifier (BRM)
  b. response modifier therapy
biological predictors for treatment outcome of transurethral microwave thermotherapy
BioLogic-DTPF system
BioLogic-DT system
biomarker
  intermediate b.
biomaterial
  alloplastic b.
  antiinfective b.
  Emerge b.
  encrustation of b.
  MycroMesh b.
  b. surface
  technical b.
  b. type
biomaterial-associated infection
biomedical
  B. Instruments and Products (BIP)
  b. research
  b. science
biomembrane
BIO 101 MERmaid DNAkit
biomodulation
Biomox
biooclusive dressing
Bioplastique
biopsy
  adrenal cortex fine-needle b.
  alcohol-fixed gastric b.
  antral b.
  aspiration b.
  bite b.
  bladder b.
  blind percutaneous liver b.
  bone marrow b.
  borderline b.
  brush b.
  b. channel
  cholangioscopic forceps b.
  CLO b.
  cold cup b.
  colonic b.
  colonoscopic b.
  colorectal b.
  cone b.
  contralateral testicular b.
  core needle b.
  corporal b.
  corpus cavernosum b.
  Crosby-Kugler capsule for b.
  CT-guided liver b.
  CT-guided needle-aspiration b.
  cup bladder b.
  cytologic b.
  diathermic loop b.
  digitally guided b.
  direct-vision liver b.
  double-bite b.
  duodenal b.
  endoluminal ultrasonography-guided fine-needle aspiration b.
  endoscopic small bowel b.
  endoscopic strip b.
  endoscopic transbronchial real-time ultrasound-guided b.
  endoscopic transpapillary b.
  endourologic b.
  ERCP-guided b.
  esophageal b.
  EUS-guided Tru-Cut needle b.
  fine-needle aspiration b. (FNAB)
  fine-needle capillary b.
  b. forceps
  four-quadrant jumbo b.
  freehand b.
  full-thickness b.
  fundic b.
  b. of gastric mucosa
  grasp b.
  guided transcutaneous b.
  guillotine needle b.
  b. gun
  hot b.
  ileal b.
  incisional b.
  b. instrument
  intestinal b.
  jejunal drainage and b.
  jumbo b.
  laparoscopic b.
  large forceps b.
  large-particle b.
  laser-guided b.

lift-and-cut b.
liver b.
Menghini technique for percutaneous liver b.
morphological study of renal b.
mucosal b.
multiple b.'s
native renal b.
needle aspiration b. (NABX)
needle core b. (NCB)
open b.
paracollicular b.
percutaneous fine-needle pancreatic b.
percutaneous liver b. (PLB)
percutaneous native renal b.
percutaneous pancreas b.
peritoneal b.
peroral jejunal b.
pinch b.
plugged liver b.
pouch b.
prostate gland b.
protocol b.
PTC-guided b.
punch b.
b. punch
random bladder b.
rectal b.
renal b.
saucerized b.
scan-directed b.
sextant transrectal ultrasound-guided b.
shave b.
skinny-needle b.
small bowel b.
snap-frozen b.
snare excision b.
snare loop b.
sonoguided b.
strip b.
suction b.
systematic sextant b.
tangential b.
targeted b.
testicular b.
transcutaneous b.
transfemoral liver b.
transgastric fine-needle aspiration b.
transitional zone b.
transjugular liver b.
transpapillary b.
transperineal ultrasound-guided template b.
transrectal ultrasonography-guided b.
transrectal ultrasound-guided sextant b.
transvenous liver b.
trephine b.
Tru-Cut needle b.
ultrasound-guided anterior subcostal liver b.
ultrasound-guided systematic sextant b.
b. urease test
vaginal cone b.
Vim-Silverman technique for liver b.
Watson capsule b.

biopsy-verified chronic glomerulonephritis

Biopty
    B. cut needle
    B. gun

Bio-Rad protein assay
bioresorbable stent
Biosafe PSA4 screen
biosampler
    Accellon Combi cervical b.

Biosearch 7000 enteral feeding pump
BioSling bioabsorbable urethral sling
BioSorb resorbable urology stent
Biostent biliary stent
biosynthesis
biota
    gastrointestinal b.

Biotel home screening test
biothesiometry
    penile b.

biotin
    b. deficiency
    endogenous b.

biotinylated DNA probe
Bio-Tract proprietary strain
biotransformation
BioWhittaker
    B. assay
    B. assay test

BIP
    Biomedical Instruments and Products
    BIP biopsy instrument
    BIP high-speed multibiopsy needle

biperiden

NOTES

biphasic diurnal rhythm
4,5-biphosphate
    phosphatidylinositol 4,5-b.
biplanar aortography
biplane sector probe
bipolar
    b. bleeding
    b. cautery probe BP-7350A
    B. Circumactive Probe (BICAP)
    B. Circumactive Probe coagulation
    b. coagulating forceps
    b. electrocautery
    b. electrocoagulation (BPEC)
    B. EndoStasis probe (BESP)
    b. esophageal recording
    b. glass electrode
    b. hemostasis probe
    b. neuron
    b. sphincterotome
    b. TURP
    b. urological loop
Birbeck granule
bird-beak
    b.-b. appearance
    b.-b. configuration
    b.-b. narrowing
birefringence
Birt-Hogg-Dube (BHD)
    B.-H.-D. syndrome (BHDS)
birth trauma
Bisac-Evac
bisacodyl
    Fleet B.
    b. tannex
bisantrene
Bisco-Lax
Bishop-Koop ileostomy
Biskra button
bismuth (Bi)
    B. benign bile duct stricture classification
    b. classification, types I-IV
    b. compound
    b., metronidazole, tetracycline (BMT)
    b. nephropathy
    b. salt
    b. sclerotherapy
    b. subsalicylate (BSS)
    b. triple monocapsule
    b. triple regimen
    b. triple therapy
    b. tumor
bismuthate
bismuth-free triple therapy
Bisodol
bisoprolol
bisphosphonate
bistable

bistriazole
bitartrate
    cysteamine b.
bite
    b. biopsy
    b. biopsy forceps
bithionol
Bitome
    B. bipolar sphincterotome
    B. bipolar system
    B. catheter
Bittorf reaction
bivalve mollusc
bizarre leiomyoma
black
    B. Beauty ureteral stent
    b. clot
    b. cohosh
    b. esophagus
    b. faceted stone
    b. hairy tongue
    b. jaundice
    b. liver disease
    b. pigment gallstone
    b. pigment stone
    b. sickness
    b. silk suture (BSS)
    b. tarry stool
    b. urine
    b. vomit
    b. vomitus
Black-Draught Lax-Senna
bladder
    b. acontractility
    acute phase of neurogenic b.
    b. agenesis
    alloplastic prostatic b.
    amebiasis of b.
    amyloidosis of b.
    b. angiosarcoma
    b. antibody
    areflexic b.
    b. artery
    atonic b.
    b. augmentation
    augmented b.
    b. autoaugmentation
    autonomic neurogenic b.
    Barrett-Donovan-Mayo artificial b.
    b. biofeedback
    b. biopsy
    b. calculus
    b. cancer
    b. cancer angiogenic factor
    b. cancer-specific nuclear matrix protein (BCLA-4)
    b. *Candida* infection
    b. capacity
    b. carcinoma in situ

b. carcinosarcoma
b. chimney procedure
b. chondrosarcoma
b. choriocarcinoma
color Doppler imaging of ureteral jet into b.
b. compliance
compliance of b.
congenital bifid b.
b. congenital diverticulum
b. congenital megacystis
b. cooling reflex
cord b.
b. cuff
b. decompensation
b. decompression
defunctionalized b.
b. denervation
b. descensus
distended b.
b. diverticulectomy
dome of b.
double b.
dropped b.
b. duplication
b. dysplasia
b. ear
embryonal transitory b.
b. emptying
encysted b.
b. enlargement
b. epithelium
b. erosion
b. examination
b. excision
b. exstrophy
fasciculated b.
b. filling
b. fistula
gastric b.
Gilchrist ileocecal b.
b. granular cell myoblastoma
b. hernia
high-riding b.
b. histology
b. hydrodistention
hyperreflexic b.
hypertonic b.
b. hypoplasia
hypotonic b.
ileal b.
ileocecal b.

ileocolonic b.
b. imaging
b. incontinence
b. infusion
b. inhibition
b. injury
b. innervation
b. intravesical pressure
inversion of b.
b. inverted papilloma
b. involuntary contraction
b. irrigation
irritable b.
kidneys, ureters, b. (KUB)
b. leiomyosarcoma
b. leukoplakia
b. liposarcoma
low-compliance b.
b. lymphohemangioma
b. lymphoma
b. malacoplakia
b. malignant melanoma
b. mapping
b. mast cell
Mayo b.
b. mesonephric adenocarcinoma
b. mucosal graft
b. muscarinic receptor
b. neck
b. neck closure (BNC)
b. neck contracture
b. neck detrusor muscle
b. neck dysfunction
b. neck hypermobility
b. neck obstruction
b. neck-preserving technique
b. neck reconstruction
b. neck sphincteric function
b. neck support pessary
b. neck support prosthesis
b. neck suspension (BNS)
b. neck-to-urethra anastomosis
b. neck transurethral resection
b. neck tubularization
b. neck Y-V plasty
b. neoplasm
b. nephrogenic adenoma
nephroureterectomy with en bloc removal of cuff of b.
nervous b.
b. neurofibroma
neurogenic b.

NOTES

bladder *(continued)*
neuropathic b.
b. neurosis
b. nonepithelial tumor
nonneurogenic neurogenic b.
orthotopic b.
b. osteosarcoma
b. outflow obstruction
b. outlet
b. outlet closure
b. outlet kinesiologic study
b. outlet obstruction (BOO)
b. outlet reconstruction
overactive b.
b. overdistention
b. pain
b. palpation
pancreatic b.
b. patch
b. perforation
b. pheochromocytoma
b. pillar block
pine cone appearance of b.
b. plasmacytoma
b. plate
poorly compliant b.
b. postcystourethropexy instability
b. preservation
b. pressure (BP)
b. pressure sensor
b. prolapse
prosthetic b.
pseudoneurogenic b.
b. pseudosarcoma
psychologic nonneuropathic b.
reflex neurogenic b.
reflex neuropathic b.
b. regeneration
b. replacement
b. replacement urinary pouch
b. retraction
b. rhabdomyosarcoma
ruga of urinary b.
b. rupture
sacculated b.
b. sarcoma
b. schistosomiasis
b. sensation
b. small cell carcinoma
b. smooth muscle
b. spasm
spinning top deformity of b.
b. squamous cell carcinoma
b. squamous metaplasia
stammering b.
b. stone
b. storage function
strangulation of b.
b. stress relaxation
b. substitution
summit of b.
b. support
suprapubic aspiration of b.
teardrop b.
thimble b.
b. thimble
tic douloureux of b.
trabeculated b.
b. training
b. transection
transitional cell carcinoma of b. (TCCB)
b. transitional cell carcinoma
b. trauma
b. trigone
b. tuberculosis
tuberculosis of kidney and b.
b. tumor (BT)
b. tumor antigen (BTA)
b. tumor antigen test
b. tumor assay
b. ulcer
b. ultrasonography
uninhibited neurogenic b.
uninhibited overactive b.
unstable b.
ureteral jet into b.
urinary b.
uvula of b.
valve b.
vascular malformation of b.
b. vein
vertex of urinary b.
b. viscoelasticity
b. volume
b. washing
b. worm
b. xanthoma
b. yolk sac tumor

BladderChek
NMP22 B.

BladderManager portable ultrasonic device

BladderScan
Bard B.
B. BVI2500 ultrasound scanner
B. ultrasound

blade
Bard-Parker b.
Beaver b.
Billingham-Bookwalter rectal fenestrated b.
Bookwalter-Cook anal anorectal b.
Bookwalter malleable retractor b.
Bookwalter-Mayo b.
Bookwalter-Parks anal sphincter b.
Bovie b.
Deaver-type b.

knife b.
malleable b.
razor b.
scalpel b.
Blair silicone drain
Blaivas
    B. classification of urinary incontinence
    B. urinary incontinence classification
Blake gallstone forceps
Blakemore-Sengstaken tube
Blakemore tube
Blalock pulmonary artery forceps
Blanchard hemorrhoid forceps
blanching
    b. of lesion
    b. of mucosa
bland
    b. diet
    b. food
    b. pulmonary hemorrhage
    b. thrombosis
Bland-Altman analysis
blanket
    Gaymar water-circulating b.
blast
    b. cell
    b. injury
    refractory anemia with excess b.'s (RAEB)
    white blood cell b.
blastema
    renal b.
blastocyst hatching
Blastocystis hominis
blastoid transformation
blastomere
Blastomyces dermatitidis
blastomycosis
    peritoneal b.
Blatin
    B. sign
    B. syndrome
bleb
bleed
    gastrointestinal b.
    GI b.
    herald b.
    postgastrectomy b.
    postpolypectomy b.
bleeder

bleeding
    b. acid-peptic disease
    active source of b.
    acute variceal b.
    b. angioma
    bipolar b.
    b. colonic angiodysplasia
    colorectal variceal b.
    contact b.
    b. control
    diverticular b.
    b. diverticulosis
    b. diverticulum
    duodenal b.
    dysfunctional b.
    esophageal variceal b.
    esophagogastric variceal b.
    excessive b.
    first variceal b.
    functional b.
    gastric varix b.
    b. gastric varix (BGV)
    b. gastritis
    gastrointestinal b. (GIB)
    GI b.
    b. hemorrhoid
    b. jejunal metastasis
    jetlike b.
    b. lesion
    lower gastrointestinal b. (LGIB)
    lower GI b.
    massive colonic diverticular b.
    minute b.
    mucosal b.
    obscure gastrointestinal b.
    occult gastrointestinal b.
    painless rectal b.
    pancreatitis-related b.
    peptic ulcer b.
    per anum b.
    b. per rectum
    b. pile
    b. point
    b. polyp
    prevention of first b.
    b. proctitis
    rectal b.
    recurrent b.
    severe variceal b.
    b. site
    b. site localization
    b. time

NOTES

bleeding (continued)
    b. tumor
    b. ulcer
    upper gastrointestinal b. (UGIB)
    vaginal b.
    variceal b.

blend
    b. waveform
    b. waveform desiccation

blended
    b. current
    b. cut
    b. electrocautery

blenderized diet
blennemesis
blennorrhagica
    keratoderma b.
    keratosis b.

blennuria
bleomycin
    carboplatin, etoposide, b. (CEB)
    b., etoposide, cisplatin (BEP)
    platinum, etoposide, b. (PEB)
    platinum, Velban, b. (PVB)
    b. sulfate
    b. toxicity
    Velban, actinomycin D, b. (VAB)
    vinblastine, actinomycin D, b. (mini-VAB)

bleomycin-associated adult respiratory distress syndrome
blepharitis
blepharospasm
blind
    b. cautery
    b. enema
    b. esophageal brushing (BEB)
    b. fistula
    b. intestine
    b. limb
    b. lithotripsy
    b. loop
    b. loop syndrome (BLS)
    b. percutaneous liver biopsy
    b. stump
    b. subtotal colectomy
    b. technique
    b. upper esophageal pouch

blindgut
blindness
    river b.

blink
    acoustic b.

blinking reflex
BLL
    blood lead level

BLM
    basolateral membrane

bloat

bloc
    harvesting en b.

Blocadren
Bloch-Paul-Mikulicz operation
block
    abdominal ganglion b.
    Best bite b.
    bladder pillar b.
    caudal b.
    celiac plexus b.
    collision b.
    endoscopic ultrasound-guided celiac plexus b.
    Marcaine b.
    nerve b.
    neurolytic celiac plexus b.
    OB-10 Comfort bite b.
    periprostatic b.
    portal b.
    prostatic b.
    transitory b.

Block-Ace solution
blockade
    adjuvant alpha b.
    alpha sympathetic b.
    androgen b.
    beta-adrenergic b.
    cavernosal alpha b.
    combined androgen b. (CAB)
    differential neuroaxial b.
    lipoxygenase b.
    maximal androgen b. (MAB)
    muscarinic b.
    reversible b.

blockage
    complete hormonal b.

blocked aerogastria
blocker
    alpha-1 b.
    angiotensin receptor b. (ARB)
    beta adrenergic b.
    calcium channel b.
    calcium entry b.
    H2 b.
    histamine b. (HB)
    nicotinic receptor b.
    proton pump b.
    RAS b.
    renin-angiotensin system b.
    starch b.

blocking
    electrical b.
    thermal b.

Blocksom vesicostomy
Blom-Singer
    B.-S. esophagoscope
    B.-S. tracheoesophageal fistula

blood
    b. admixed with stool

b. agar plate
b. alcohol level (BAL)
b. ammonia
bright red b.
b. calculus
b. cast
b. clot
clotted b.
b. coagulation
b. coagulation disorder
b. collection
crossmatched b.
b. culture
dark burgundy b.
b. flow
b. flow assessment
b. flow rate (BFR)
frank b.
b. gas on oxygen
b. gas on room air
b. group antigen
b. lead level (BLL)
maroon b.
nonhemolyzed b.
nostril b.
occult b.
b. on surface of stool
oozing b.
b. passed with stool
b. per rectum (BPR)
b. pH
b. pressue change
b. pressure (BP)
b. sample
spurting b.
b. in stool
stool for occult b.
b. transfusion
b. type
typed b.
b. urea concentration
b. urea level
b. urea nitrogen (BUN)
b. vessel
whole b.

bloodborne
b. non-A non-B hepatitis
b. pathogen
b. transmission

blood-contactin catheter
blood-epididymis barrier

Bloodgood
B. operation
B. procedure

blood-liquor barrier
blood-streaked stool
bloodstream infection (BSI)
blood-testis barrier
blood-testis-epididymis
blood-tinged ascites
blood-type diet
blood-urine barrier
blood-water clearance

bloody
b. ascites
b. diarrhea
b. discharge
b. peritoneal fluid
b. stool
b. vomitus

blooming effect
blot
Southern b.
Western b.

blotting
ECL Western b.
enhanced chemiluminescence Western b.
Western b.

Blount disease
blow-hole
b.-h. cecostomy
b.-h. ileostomy

blown pupil
BLQ
both lower quadrants

BLS
blind loop syndrome

BLSA
Baltimore Longitudinal Study of Aging

BLT
bright light therapy

blue
Alcian b.
Berlin b.
carmine b.
b. diaper syndrome
b. dot sign
eosin-methylene b. (EMB)
Evans b.
B. Max balloon catheter
methylene b.
b. navel

NOTES

blue *(continued)*
    periodic acid-Schiff-Alcian b. (PAS-AB)
    b. rubber bleb nevus syndrome
    b. toe syndrome
    toluidine b.
    Urolene B.
    b. varix

Bluemle pump

Blumberg
    inguinal ligament of B.
    B. sign

Blumer rectal shelf

blunt
    b. abdominal trauma
    b. liver trauma
    b. needle
    b. pancreatic trauma
    b. probe
    b. and sharp dissection

blunting
    costophrenic b.
    haustral b.
    b. of valve

blunt-tipped obturator

blush
    delayed b.
    immediate b.

B-lymphocyte
    B-l. activation
    B-l. system

BM
    basal metabolism
    bowel movement

BMD
    bone mineral densitometry
    bone mineral density

BMI
    body mass index

BMMP
    benign mucous membrane pemphigoid

B-mode
    B-m. imaging
    B-m. ultrasonography
    B-m. ultrasound image

BMR
    basal metabolic rate

BMS
    burning mouth syndrome

BMT
    bismuth, metronidazole, tetracycline
    bone marrow transplantation

BNC
    bladder neck closure

BNO
    bowels not open

BNP
    brain natriuretic peptide

BNS
    bladder neck suspension

boardlike
    b. rigidity
    b. rigidity of abdomen

Boari
    B. bladder flap
    B. bladder flap procedure
    B. operation
    B. ureteral flap repair

Boari-Ockerblad
    B.-O. flap
    B.-O. principle

Boas
    B. algesimeter
    B. point
    B. sign
    B. test meal

boat-shaped abdomen

Bochdalek
    foramen of B.
    B. hernia

Bodansky unit

Boden-Gibb tumor staging

Bodenhammer rectal speculum

body
    acidophilic b.
    anal foreign b.
    angularis b.
    anorectal foreign b.
    asteroid b.
    bamboo jointlike appearance of gastric b.
    Call-Exner b.
    b. cell mass (BCM)
    CMV inclusion b.
    cobblestone appearance of gastric b.
    coccidian b.
    colonic foreign b.
    b. composition analysis
    compressible cavernous b.
    corneal foreign b.
    Councilman b.
    Cowdry type A inclusion b.
    crescentic b.
    Cyanobacterium-like b.
    Donovan b.
    duodenal foreign b.
    embryoid b.
    b. of epididymis
    epithelial inclusion b.
    esophageal foreign b.
    esophageal Lewy b.
    falciform b.
    b. fluid osmolality
    foreign b.
    B. Fortress Natural Amino tablet
    gastric foreign b.

b. habitus
Highmore b.
Howell-Jolly b.
inclusion b.
ingested foreign b.
intracytoplasmic CMV inclusion b.
intraepithelial b.
intranuclear CMV inclusion b.
Jaworski b.
juxtaglomerular b.
ketone b. (KB)
Lafora b.
lower GI tract foreign b.
Mallory hyaline b.
malpighian b.
b. mass index (BMI)
Michaelis-Gutmann b.
oval fat b.
penile b.
perineal b.
polar b.
b. position
b. of pubis
rectal foreign b.
renal tumorlike pyonephrosis with foreign b.
retained foreign b. (RFB)
Savage perineal b.
Schaumann b.
Schiller-Duval b.
S-shaped b.
string-of-pearls appearance of gastric b.
b. substance isolation (BSI)
Symington b.
upper GI tract foreign b.
vaginal foreign b.
vermiform b.
viral inclusion b.
b. water
b. weight (BW)
zebra b.'s

Boeck sarcoma
Boehm
B. anoscope
B. proctoscope
B. rectal diagnostic and treatment set
B. sigmoidoscope
Boehringer kit

Boerema
B. anterior gastropexy
B. hernia repair
Boerhaave syndrome
Boettcher crystal
boggy prostate
Bogota bag
Bogros space
Bohr effect
bol
Bolande tumor
Boley vascular ectasia
bolster suture
bolus
alimentary b.
b. challenge test
b. dressing
b. extraction
b. feeding
food b.
heparin b.
b. hold-up
marshmallow b.
b. transport
bombesin receptor
bone
adynamic b.
b. alkaline phosphatase (BAP)
b. disease
b. formation
innominate b.
b. marrow aplasia
b. marrow biopsy
b. marrow-derived B cell
b. marrow stem cell
b. marrow transplantation (BMT)
b. marrow transplantation-related problem
b. metastasis
b. mineral densitometry (BMD)
b. mineral density (BMD)
b. morphogenic protein
b. scan
b. turnover marker
bone-specific alkaline phosphatase (BALP)
Bonine
Bonney test
bony
b. defect
b. dysraphism
b. landmark

NOTES

bony *(continued)*
  b. pelvis
  b. spicule
  b. tenderness
BOO
  bladder outlet obstruction
Bookler swivel-ball laparoscope holder
Bookwalter
  B. malleable retractor blade
  B. retractor system
  B. ring retractor
Bookwalter-Cook anal anorectal blade
Bookwalter-Goulet retractor
Bookwalter-Hill-Ferguson rectal retractor
Bookwalter-Mayo blade
Bookwalter-Parks anal sphincter blade
Bookwalter-St. Mark deep pelvic retractor
Boost Nutritional Energy Drink
BOR
  bowels open regularly
  branchio-otorenal
borborygmus, pl. **borborygmi**
Borchardt triad
border
  antimesenteric b.
  brush b.
  b. cell
  fundopyloric mucosal b.
  intestinal brush b. (IBB)
  lobulated b.
  mucosal b.
  scalloped antimesenteric b.
  b. zone
borderline biopsy
bore
  magnetic b.
Borge clamp
boring pain
Boros esophagoscope
Borreliosis classification for advanced gastric cancer
Borrmann
  B. gastric cancer
  B. gastric cancer classification
  B. gastric cancer typing system type I–IV
  B. gastric carcinoma types I–IV
  B. scirrhous carcinoma
Bors ice water test
Bosniak
  B. classification
  B. criteria
  B. lesion category I–IV
bosselated surface
both
  b. lower quadrants (BLQ)
  b. upper quadrants (BUQ)
Botkin disease

Botox
botryoid
  interlabial sarcoma b.
  b. sarcoma
botryoides
  sarcoma b.
botryomycosis
  cecal b.
Bottini operation
bottle
  McGaw plastic b.
  Nu-Hope urine collection b.
  b. operation
  Vacutainer b.
botulinum
  Clostridium b.
  b. toxin (BTX)
  b. toxin injection
botulism immune globuln intravenous
Bouchard
  B. disease
  B. index
bougie
  acorn-tipped b.
  b. à boule
  bulbous b.
  Celestin dilator b.
  b. dilator
  Eder-Puestow b.
  elastic b.
  elbowed b.
  EndoLumina b.
  filiform b.
  following b.
  French b.
  Hegar intrarectal b.
  Hurst mercury b.
  Hurst-type b.
  Jackson esophageal b.
  Klebanoff common duct b.
  large-diameter b.
  Maloney b.
  mercury-weighted rubber b.
  polyvinyl b.
  Savary b.
  Savary-Gilliard Silastic flexible b.
  Savary-Gilliard wire-guided b.
  tapered rubber b.
  through-the-scope b.
  Trousseau esophageal b.
  Wales rectal b.
  wax-tipped b.
  wire-guided polyvinyl b.
bougienage
  esophageal b.
  Hurst b.
  peroral b.
  transgastric esophageal b.
bouillon

Bouin fixative solution
boulardii
    Saccharomyces b.
boule
    bougie à b.
bouquet fever
Bourne test
Bourneville disease
bouton en chemise
Bouveret
    B. syndrome
    B. ulcer
Bouveret-Duguet ulcer
Bovie
    B. blade
    B. cautery
    B. coagulation
    B. electrocautery
    B. electrocoagulation unit
    B. holder
bovied
bovine
    b. dermal collagen
    b. graft
    b. serum albumin (BSA)
    b. thrombin
    b. trypsin
bovis
    Cysticercus b.
    Moraxella b.
    Mycobacterium b.
    Streptococcus b.
bowed sternum
bowel
    b. adherent to omentum
    aganglionic b.
    b. axis
    b. bag
    b. bypass
    b. bypass syndrome
    competent b.
    b. content
    b. continuity
    dead b.
    detubularized small b.
    dilated loops of b.
    b. dilation
    b. disease
    B. Disease Questionnaire
    b. displacement
    entrapment of b.
    fixed segment of b.
    fluid-filled small b.
    b. forceps
    b. function
    gangrenous b.
    b. gas
    b. grasper
    greedy b.
    b. habit
    incarcerated b.
    b. incontinence
    infarcted b.
    b. injury
    b. intussusception
    b. irrigation
    ischemic b.
    kink in b.
    Ladd correction of malrotation of b.
    large b.
    b. loop
    b. lumen
    b. movement (BM)
    b. necrosis
    necrotizing vasculitis of b.
    Noble surgical plication of b.
    b.'s not open (BNO)
    b. obstruction
    b.'s open regularly (BOR)
    b. perforation
    b. plate
    pleating of small b.
    b. preparation
    b. preparation complication
    prolapsed b.
    b. pseudoobstruction
    b. refashioning procedure
    b. resection
    b. rest (BR)
    small b.
    b. sounds normal (BSN)
    b. sounds normal and active (BSNA)
    b. stoma
    strangulated b.
    b. tone
    toxic dilatation of b.
    b. wall
    b. wall induration
bowel-emptying regimen
Bowen
    B. disease

NOTES

Bowen *(continued)*
   B. papule
   B. patch
bowenoid papulosis
Bower PEG tube
bowler hat sign
Bowman
   B. capsule
   B. space
   B. space cyst
Boyarsky
   B. BPH symptom score
   B. symptom scoring system
Boyce
   longitudinal nephrotomy of B.
   B. modification of Sengstaken-Blakemore tube
   B. sign
Boyce-Vest procedure
Boyden
   B. sphincter
   B. test
   B. test meal
boydii
   Pseudallescheria b.
   Shigella b.
Boyle and Goldstein saline test
Bozeman
   B. forceps
   B. operation
Bozeman-Fritsch catheter
Bozicevich test
BP
   bladder pressure
   blood pressure
BP-7350A
   bipolar cautery probe BP-7350A
BPB
   biliopancreatic bypass
BPC
   bile phospholipid concentration
BPE
   benign prostatic enlargement
BPEC
   bipolar electrocoagulation
BPH
   benign prostatic hyperplasia
   benign prostatic hypertrophy
   BPH impact index (BII)
BPO
   benign prostatic obstruction
   bile phospholipid output
BPR
   blood per rectum
BQ123 receptor antagonist
BR
   bowel rest
BR96
   monoclonal antibody BR96

Braasch
   B. bulb
   B. catheter
   B. direct catheterization cystoscope
Braasch-Kaplan direct-vision cystoscope
brachial pressure index
brachioaxillary bridge graft fistula (BAGF)
brachioradialis
brachiosubclavian bridge graft fistula (BSGF)
brachyesophagus
BrachySeed
   B. brachytherapy seed
   B. Pd-103 implant
   B. prostate cancer treatment
BrachyTherapy
   Varian B.
brachytherapy
   interstitial b.
   intracavitary application b.
   PharmaSeed I-125 b.
   salvage b.
   transperineal interstitial permanent prostate b. (TIPPB)
Brackin
   B. ureterointestinal anastomosis
   B. ureterointestinal anastomosis technique
Bradley
   B. classification of voiding dysfunction
   B. disease
   B. loop
bradyarrhythmia
bradycardia
   reflex b.
   sinus b.
bradygastria
bradykinin
bradypepsia
bradyphagia
bradyspermatism
bradystalsis
bradytrophia
bradytrophic
bradyuria
brain
   b. metastasis
   b. myoinositol content
   b. natriuretic peptide (BNP)
   b. stem-sacral loop
   b. tumor
brain-derived neurotrophic factor (BDNF)
Brainerd diarrhea
brain-gut
   b.-g. axis
   b.-g. peptide

brain-heart
    b.-h. infusion agar
    b.-h. infusion plate
brain-type glycogen phosphorylase (BGP)
brake
    duodenal b.
    ileal b.
bran
branch
    bifid b.'s
    b. duct-type tumor
    lateral b.
    b. pancreatic duct
    b. renal artery disease
    side b.
branched
    b. crypt
    b. renal calculus
    b. stone
    b. vascular graft
branched-chain
    b.-c. alpha-ketoacid dehydrogenase
    b.-c. amino acid (BCAA)
    b.-c. DNA (bDNA)
brancher
    b. deficiency
    b. deficiency glycogenosis
    b. enzyme
    b. glycogen storage disease
branching
    b. complex staghorn calculus
    b. tubule formation
branchiogenous cyst
branchio-otorenal (BOR)
    b.-o. syndrome
Brandel cell harvester
Brandt cytology balloon
brash
    sour b.
    water b.
    weaning b.
brasiliensis
    Nippostrongylus b.
    Paracoccidioides b.
BRAT
    bananas, rice, cereal, applesauce, and toast
    BRAT diet

BRATT
    bananas, rice, cereal, applesauce, tea, and toast
    BRATT diet
Braun
    B. anastomosis
    B. enteroenterostomy
    B. stent
Braune
    B. muscle
    B. valve
Braun-Jaboulay gastroenterostomy
Bravo
    B. Catheter-Free pH testing system
    B. pH Monitor
BRBPR
    bright red blood per rectum
BrDu, BrdU, BrdUrd
    bromodeoxyuridine
    BrDu staining
break
    b. cluster homology gene
    mucosal b.
breakage
    intracorporeal needle b.
breakbone fever
breakfast
    Ewald b.
    test b.
Breakstone lithotriptor
breakthrough
    b. dose
    nocturnal acid b. (NAB)
breast
    b. cancer
    b. cancer-associated protein pS2 expression
breath
    b. alkane
    b. alkane testing
    b. bag
    b. ethane level
    b. hydrogen excretion test
    b. isotope bacterial urease detection
    liver b.
    b. odor
    b. pentane test
    b. sound
    uremic b.
breath-hold MR cholangiography
breathing
    deep b.

NOTES

breathing *(continued)*
    diaphragmatic b.
    intermittent positive-pressure b. (IPPB)
    Kussmaul b.
    mouth b.
    sleep-disordered b. (SDB)
Breisky-Navratil straight retractor
Brennemann syndrome
Brenner tumor
brequinar sodium
Brescia-Cimino
    B.-C. fistula
    B.-C. shunt
Breslow-Day test
Brethine
Bretschneider histidine tryptophan solution
bretylium
breve
    Gymnodinium b.
breves
    arteriae gastricae b.
Brevibloc
brevis
    Bifidobacterium b.
Brewer
    B. infarct
    B. point
BRIC
    benign recurrent intrahepatic cholestasis
Bricanyl
Bricker
    B. ileal conduit
    B. operation
    B. pouch
    B. technique
    B. ureteroileostomy
    B. urinary diversion
bridge
    agar b.
    Albarran reflecting b.
    B. Assurant biliary stent delivery system
    colostomy b.
    B. deep surgery forceps
    loop ostomy b.
    mucosal b.
    suture b.
    B. X3 renal stent system
bridging
    b. fibrosis
    b. hepatic necrosis
    mucosal b.
    portal-to-portal b.
    b. therapy
bridle
    control b.

brief
    Ashton b.
    Holyoke b.
    Kim Care contour b.
    B. Male Sexual Function Inventory for Urology
    Suretys incontinence b.
Brigham sling
bright
    B. disease
    b. light therapy (BLT)
    b. red blood
    b. red blood per rectum (BRBPR)
    b. red vomitus
brim
    pelvic b.
Brinkerhoff
    B. anoscope
    B. rectal speculum
Brinton disease
Bristol
    B. female lower urinary tract symptom
    B. nomogram for uroflowmetry
BRM
    basal metabolic rate
    biologic response modifier
broad-based
    b.-b. gait
    b.-b. polyp
broadening
    spectral b.
broad-spectrum
    b.-s. antibiotic
    b.-s. therapy
Brödel line
Broder index
Brodie sign
Broesike fossa
broken stent retrieval device
bromelain
bromfenac
bromide
    cetyldimethylethyl ammonium b.
    clidinium b.
    emepronium b.
    ethidium b.
    hexamethonium b.
    mepenzolate b.
    methantheline b.
    methscopolamine b.
    propantheline b.
    valethamate b.
bromine-75
bromobenzene (B2)
bromocriptine dopaminergic medication
bromodeoxyuridine (BrDu, BrdU, BrdUrd)

antibody to b.
b. cell kinetics
5-bromodeoxyuridine
bromodiphenhydramine
Bromo Seltzer
brompheniramine
bromsulfophthalein (BSP)
bromsulphalein (BSP)
b. clearance
bronchial
b. carcinoid
b. obstruction
b. sound
bronchium, pl. **bronchia**
bronchobiliary fistula
Broncho-Cath double-lumen endotracheal tube
bronchoesophageal fistula (BEF)
bronchoesophagology
bronchoesophagoscopy
bronchopancreatic fistula
bronchophony
bronchopulmonary
b. dysplasia
b. foregut malformation
bronchoscope
Fujinon EB-410S b.
Savary b.
bronchospasm
bronchovisceral fistulectomy
bronchus
bronchus-associated lymphoepithelial tissue (BALT)
Bronkosol
Brooke ileostomy
bropirimine
broth
cysteine *Brucella* b.
tryptic soy b.
brown
b. bowel syndrome (BBS)
B. dietary method for colon preparation
b. pigment gallstone
b. pigment stone
b. stool
B. and Wickham pressure profile method
Brown-Buerger cystoscope
Browne operation
brownian motion

Browning and Parks continence grading system category A, B, C, D
Brown-McHardy
B.-M. pneumatic dilator
B.-M. pneumatic mercury bougie dilation
Brown-Mueller
B.-M. T-bar fastener
B.-M. T fastener
Broyle
B. esophagoscope
B. retrograde cystoscope
B-RTO
balloon-occluded retrograde transvenous obliteration
Brucella melitensis
brucellosis
Brudzinski sign
Bruel-Kjaer
B.-K. axial transducer
B.-K. scanner
B.-K. 1846 ultrasound system
Bruening esophagoscope
Brugia
B. lymphatic obstruction
B. malayi
B. timori
bruisability
easy b.
bruit
abdominal b.
carotid b.
femoral b.
vascular b.
Brunn epithelial nest
Brunner
B. gland
B. gland adenoma
B. gland of duodenum
B. gland hamartoma
B. gland hyperplasia
B. intestinal forceps
B. ligature set
B. tissue forceps
brunneroma of duodenum
Brunschwig operation
brush
Ayre b.
b. biopsy
b. border
b. catheter

NOTES

brush *(continued)*
    Combo Cath wire-guided cytology b.
    Cragg thrombolytic b.
    b. cytology
    cytology b.
    Cytolong b.
    Endovations disposable cytology b.
    Glassman b.
    Olympus cytology b.
    scraping b.
    sheathed cytology b.
    Suction oral b.

brush-border
    b.-b. digestion
    b.-b. disaccharidase specific activity
    b.-b. enzyme activity
    b.-b. hydrolase activity
    b.-b. hydrolysis
    b.-b. marker enzyme
    b.-b. membrane (BBM)
    b.-b. membrane vesicle (BBMV)

brushing
    bile duct b.
    blind esophageal b. (BEB)
    cytologic b.
    b. urea breath test

brushite
Bruton disease
Bruton-type agammaglobulinemia
Bryan-Leishman stain
BS
    bile salt
BSA
    bovine serum albumin
BSA-induced overload proteinuria
BSC
    bile salt concentrate
B-scanner
BSCC
    basaloid squamous cell carcinoma
BSD
    baby soft diet
    bedside drainage
BSD-300 device
BSEP
    bile salt export pump
BSFR
    basal secretory flow rate
        BSFR test
BSGF
    brachiosubclavian bridge graft fistula
BSI
    bloodstream infection
    body substance isolation
BSM
    bile salt metabolism
BSN
    bowel sounds normal

BSNA
    bowel sounds normal and active
BSO
    bile salt output
BSP
    bromsulfophthalein
    bromsulphalein
        BSP retention
        BSP test
BSQ
    Biliary Symptoms Questionnaire
BSS
    balanced salt solution
    bismuth subsalicylate
    black silk suture
BSSL
    bile salt-stimulated lipase
BT
    bladder tumor
BTA
    bladder tumor antigen
        BTA stat test
        BTA TRAK test
BTP
    biliary tract pain
BT-PABA
    benzoyl-tyrosyl-paraaminobenzoic acid
        BT-PABA test
BTX
    botulinum toxin
        BTX injection
bubble
    cavitation b.
    collapse of cavitation b.
    Garren-Edwards gastric b.
    Garren gastric b.
    gastric air b.
    GEG b.
    intragastric b.
    intraluminal gas b.
    plasma b.
    b. therapy
bubo
    chancroidal b.
    gonorrheal b.
    indolent b.
    nonvenereal b.
    strumous b.
    venereal b.
bubonocele
buccal
    b. mucosa
    b. mucosal patch graft
    b. mucosal substitution urethroplasty
    b. mucosal urethral replacement
    b. smear
buccopharyngeal aponeurosis
bucket-handle incision
Buck fascia

buckling test
Bucladin-S
buclizine
bucrylate sclerosant
bud
    dorsal b.
    ureteral b.
    ureteric b.
    ventral b.
Budd
    B. cirrhosis
    B. disease
    B. jaundice
    B. syndrome
Budd-Chiari
    B.-C. disease
    B.-C. syndrome
BUD drainage catheter
budesonide capsule
Buerhenne stone basket technique
buetschlii
    Iodamoeba b.
Buffaprin caplet
buffer
    barbital-acetate b.
    cacodylate b.
    guanidinium thiocyanate b.
    HEPES b.
    ice-cold sucrose b.
    Krebs-Henseleit bicarbonate b. (KHB)
    Krebs-Ringer bicarbonate b.
    PBS-Tween b.
    Rapid-hyb b.
    b. solution
    b. system
buffered
    b. formalin
    b. saline
Bufferin Arthritis Strength caplet
buffering
    intracellular b.
Bugbee
    B. electrocautery
    B. electrode
Buie
    B. biopsy forceps
    B. fistula probe
    B. fulguration electrode
    B. pile clamp
    B. pile forceps
    B. position
    B. rectal injection cannula
    B. rectal scissors
    B. rectal suction tip
    B. rectal suction tube
    B. sigmoidoscope
Buie-Hirschman anoscope
Buie-Smith retractor
Build Up enteral feeding
bulb
    apex of duodenal b.
    Braasch b.
    b. of corpus cavernosum
    b. deformity
    duodenal b.
    genital end b.
    b. suction
bulbar
    b. artery
    b. colliculus
    b. peptic ulcer
    b. urethra
bulbi (*pl. of* **bulbus**)
bulbocavernosus
    b. fat pad
    b. reflex (BCR)
bulbocavernous reflex latency measurement
bulbomembranous
    b. stricture
    b. urethra
    b. urethral squamous cell carcinoma
bulboprostatic repair
bulbospongiosus muscle
bulbourethral
    b. artery
    b. carcinoma
    b. gland
    b. stricture
bulbourethralis
    ductus glandulae b.
bulbous
    b. bougie
    b. urethral cuff implantation
bulb-tip
    b.-t. retrograde study
    b.-t. retrograde ureterogram
bulbus, pl. **bulbi**
    b. penis
    b. urethrae
bulgaricus
    Lactobacillus b.

NOTES

bulge
  inguinal b.
  luminal b.
bulging
  anal b.
  b. flank
  b. papilla
  b. of perineum
bulimia nervosa
bulimorexia
bulk
  b. agent
  b. laxative
bulkage
bulking
  b. agent
  b. technique
bulk-producing laxative
bulky
  b. colonic pouch
  b. dressing
  b. malignancy
  b. stool
bulla, pl. **bullae**
Bullard intubating laryngoscope
bulldog
  b. clamp
  b. forceps
bullet probe
bullet-tip
  b.-t. catheter
  b.-t. dilator
bullosa
  epidermolysis b. (EB)
  Herlitz junctional epidermolysis b.
bullous
  b. edema
  b. edema vesicae
  b. pemphigoid
bull's
  b. eye appearance
  b. eye lesion
bumetanide
Bumex
bumper
  Cloverleaf internal b.
  dome-shaped internal b.
  gastrostomy b.
  PEG b.
BUN
  blood urea nitrogen
bunching
  accordion-like b.
  b. maneuver
bundle
  coherent b.
  conjoined fiber b.
  fiber b.
  fiberoptic b.
  b. of His
  image guide b.
  intermediate filament b.
  light guide b.
  master IG b.
  microfilament b.
  neovascular b.
  vasa recta b.
BUN-to-creatinine ratio
BUO
  bilateral ureteral obstruction
bupivacaine hydrochloride
buprenorphine narcotic analgesic therapy
bupropion
BUQ
  both upper quadrants
bur
  ultrasonic oscillating b.
Burch
  B. iliopectineal ligament urethrovesical suspension
  B. procedure
  B. retropubic colposuspension
Burch-Cooper ligament sling
burden
  stone b.
Burdwan fever
burger
  barium b.
Bürger-Grütz syndrome
Burhenne steerable catheter
buried
  b. bumper syndrome
  b. penis
  b. suture
  b. vaginal island
Burkitt lymphoma
burn
  genital b.
  thermal b.
  transmural b.
burned-out
  b.-o. mucosa
  b.-o. testis cancer
  b.-o. tumor
burnetii
  Coxiella b.
Burnett syndrome
burning
  b. drops sign
  b. feet syndrome
  b. mouth syndrome (BMS)
  b. pain
  b. sensation
Burnishine disinfectant
Burow vein
burp
burrowing incision

Burrow solution
bursa, pl. **bursae**
    b. of Fabricius
bursitis
    omental b.
bursoscopy
    supragastric b.
burst
    oxidative b.
    phagocyte respiratory b.
    respiratory b.
bursula
Buschke-Löwenstein tumor
Busch umbilical scissors
Buselmeier shunt
buserelin acetate
bush tea
buski
    Fasciolopsis b.
Busodium
BuSpar
buspirone hydrochloride
busulfan
butabarbital sodium
Butalan
butalbital
1-butanol
Butibel
Butisol Sodium
butorphanol
butter
    b. meal
    b. stool
Butterfield cystoscope
butterfly, pl. **butterflies**
    b. endoluminal gastroplasty procedure
    b. hematoma
    b. needle
    b. rash
    butterflies in stomach
buttock
button
    Bard b.
    b. battery
    b. battery ingestion
    Bentle b.
    Biskra b.
    compression b.
    b. drainage
    b. of duodenum
    b. electrode
    b. gastrostomy
    gastrostomy b.
    Jaboulay b.
    Murphy b.
    Olympus One-Step B.
    One-Step gastric b.
    B. One-Step gastrostomy device
    peritoneal b.
    Surgitek b.
    b. suture
buttonhole
    b. incision
    b. preputial transposition
    b. puncture technique
button-type G tube
buttress
    fascia lata b.
butyl aminobenzoate
butylbromide
    hyoscine b.
butyl-silane extraction column
butyrate
butyricum
    Clostridium b.
Butyrovibrio
butzleri
    Acrobacter b.
BW
    body weight
BXO
    balanitis xerotica obliterans
Byars flap
Byclomine
Byler
    B. disease
    B. syndrome
bypass
    Alden loop gastric b.
    aortic superior mesenteric artery b.
    aortorenal b.
    bilioenteric b.
    biliointestinal b. (BIB)
    biliopancreatic b. (BPB)
    bowel b.
    cardiopulmonary b.
    duodenoileal b. (DIB)
    gastric b. (GBP)
    gastroduodenal-to-renal artery b.
    b. graft
    Greenville gastric b.
    Griffen Roux-en-Y b.
    Hallberg biliointestinal b.

NOTES

bypass *(continued)*
    hepatic-to-renal artery saphenous vein b.
    hepatorenal b.
    ileorenal b.
    intestinal b.
    jejunal b.
    jejunoileal b. (JIB)
    laparoscopic gastric b.
    long-limb surgical b.
    mesenterorenal b.
    partial ileal b.
    Payne-DeWind jejunoileal b.
    percutaneous biliary b.
    b. procedure
    Roux-en-Y gastric b.
    Scopinaro pancreaticobiliary b.
    Scott jejunoileal b.
    splenorenal b.
    superior mesenterorenal b.
    thoracic aortorenal b.
    venovenous b.
    b. wire

bystander effect

Bywaters syndrome

C
- C bile
- C graft
- C of Hosmer-Lemeshow ratio test
- C loop of duodenum

C3
- C3 convertase
- C3 deposit
- C3 immunological study
- seminal plasma C3

C4
- leukotriene C_4

C100-3
- C100-3 antigen
- C100-3 hepatitis C marker

C-11
- carbon-11

^{14}C
- ^{14}C glucose uptake assay
- ^{14}C UBT
- ^{14}C urea breath test

C3a
- plasma-activated complement 3
- C3a complement

C4a
- plasma-activated complement 4

C5a
- plasma-activated complement 5

c100
- antibody to c. (anti-c100)

C18 Sep-Pack column
C-1 esterase inhibitor
C1q nephropathy
C3b, C4b receptor
CA
- carbonic anhydrase
- cholic acid
  - CA cellulose acetate membrane hollow-fiber dialyzer
  - CA 1-18 tumor marker
  - CA 72-4 tumor marker

CA19-9
- carbohydrate antigen 19-9
  - CA19-9 test

Ca2+
- inositol 1,4,5-triphosphate Ca2+

CA110 dialyzer
CA-125
- cancer antigen 125

Ca50 antigen
CAA
- coloanal anastomosis

Ca^{2+}-activated K+
CAB
- combined androgen blockade

cable
- fiberoptic light c.
- internal fiberoptic c.
- leakage bypass c.
- light c.

Cabot-Nesbit orchiopexy
Cacchi-Ricci
- C.-R. disease
- C.-R. syndrome

cachectic
- c. diarrhea
- c. edema
- c. fever
- c. pallor

cachectin
cachexia
- c. aphthosa
- Grawitz c.
- malignant c.
- tumor c.
- urinary c.
- vascular c.

CaCo2 cell
$CaCO_3$ crystal
cacodylate buffer
cadaver
- c. kidney
- c. renal preservation

cadaveric
- c. intestinal transplant
- c. pericardial graft
- c. renal transplant
- c. renal transplantation
- c. segmental graft

cadaveris
- *Clostridium c.*

caddy stool
cadmium-induced nephrotoxicity
cadmium nephropathy
caecalis
- fossa c.

caecus minor ventriculi
cafe
- c. coronary
- c. coronary syndrome

Cafergot
caffeine
- c., alcohol, pepper, spicy foods (CAPS)
- c. clearance
- c. gut

caffeinism
CAG
- cholangiogram

CAG *(continued)*
    cholangiography
    chronic atrophic gastritis
cagA
    cytotoxin-associated gene A
        cagA antibody
        cagA gene
        cagA protein
cagA-negative *Helicobacter pylori*
cagA-positive *Helicobacter pylori*
CAGEIN
    catheter-guided endoscopic intubation
cag PAI gene
CAH
    chronic active hepatitis
    chronic aggressive hepatitis
    congenital adrenal hyperplasia
CAI
    carbonic anhydrase inhibitor
    Clinical Activity Index
Cajal
    interstitial cells of C. (ICC)
cake kidney
Cal
    C. Carb 600 with Vitamin D antacid tablet
    C. Carb 600 with Vitamin D dietary supplement tablet
    C. Power calorie supplement
Calan
calbindin
    subserosal c.
calbindin-D9k
    vitamin D-dependent c.-D9k
calcaneal ultrasound bone densitometry
calcareous
    c. pancreatitis
    c. renal calculus
Calcibind
Calcidrine syrup
calcific
    c. flocculate
    c. flocculus
    c. pancreatitis
calcification
    carbonate apatite c.
    dystrophic c.
    kidney c.
    laminated c.
    pancreatic c.
    retroperitoneal c.
    scrotal c.
    scrotum c.
    tram-line c.
    ureteric c.
calcified
    c. enterolith
    c. gallstone
    c. zone

calciform cell
calcifying pancreatitis
Calcijex
calcineurin
    c. inhibitor
    c. inhibitor-free immunosuppressive regimen
    c. inhibitor toxicity
calcinosis
    c. cutis, Raynaud phenomenon, esophageal motility disorder, sclerodactyly, and telangiectasia (CREST)
    c. cutis, Raynaud phenomenon, sclerodactyly, and telangiectasia (CRST)
    tumoral c.
calciphylaxis
calcite
calcitonin
    c. gene-related peptide (CGRP)
    serum c.
Cal-Citrate
calcitriol trial
calcium
    c. acetate
    c. ATPase pump
    c. bilirubinate stone
    c. carbonate
    c. carbonate and simethicone
    c. channel
    c. channel antagonist (CCA)
    c. channel blocker
    c. chloride
    c. concentration
    cytosolic c.
    c. deficiency
    dietary c.
    c. electrolyte
    c. entry blocker
    c. excretion
    exogenous c.
    extracellular c.
    c. gluconate
    c. homeostasis
    c. hydrogen phosphate
    c. infusion test
    intracytoplasmic c.
    c. ionophore
    c. metabolism
    c. oxalate
    c. oxalate calculus
    c. oxalate crystallization
    c. oxalate dihydrate
    c. oxalate dihydrate stone
    c. oxalate monohydrate crystal
    c. oxalate monohydrate stone
    c. oxalate nephrolithiasis
    c. oxalate stone former

c. oxalate urolithiasis
c. oxaluria
c. phosphate calculus
c. phosphate nephrocalcinosis
c. phosphate urolithiasis
plasma ionized c.
renal absorption of c.
renal excretion of c.
serum c.
c. supplementation
UFT/leucovorin c.
urinary c.
calcium-activated potassium channel
calcium-binding protein
calcium-calmodulin complex
calcium-creatinine ratio
calcium-free dialysate
calcium-phosphate homeostasis
calcium-regulated protein
calcium-rich, gluten-free diet
calcium-specific binding protein
Calciviridae
calcivirus
human enteric c. (HuCV)
calcoaceticus
Acinetobacter c.
calculation
anthropometric c.
c. of renal ammonium excretion
calculi (*pl. of* calculus)
calculosis
calculous
c. anuria
c. cholecystitis
c. cirrhosis
c. formation
c. gallbladder disease
c. pyelitis
calculus, pl. **calculi**
alternating c.
alvine c.
ammonium acid urate c.
apatite c.
asymptomatic c.
biliary c.
bladder c.
blood c.
branched renal c.
branching complex staghorn c.
calcareous renal c.
calcium oxalate c.
calcium phosphate c.

caliceal diverticular c.
carbonate apatite c.
cat's eye c.
cholesterol c.
combination c.
common duct c.
coral c.
c. culture
cystine c.
decubitus c.
dendritic c.
diagnosing ureteral c.
2,8-dihydroxyadenine c.
c. disease
encysted c.
fibrin c.
fusible c.
gallbladder c.
gastric c.
gonecystic c.
hemp seed c.
hepatic c.
impacted c.
indigo c.
indinavir c.
infection c.
intestinal c.
intrarenal c.
jackstone c.
lower ureteric c.
male predominance of urinary tract c.
matrix c.
metabolic c.
midureteral c.
c. migration
mulberry c.
nephritic c.
noncalcareous renal c.
nonstruvite c.
oxalate c.
pancreatic c.
pocketed c.
preputial c.
primary renal c.
prostatic c.
proximal ureteral c.
c. radiography
recurrent urinary c.
renal pelvis c.
salivary c.
secondary renal c.

NOTES

calculus *(continued)*
    seminal vesicle c.
    silicate c.
    small solitary renal c.
    solitary lower pole c.
    spermatic c.
    spurious c.
    staghorn c.
    stomach c.
    struvite c.
    submucosal c.
    treatment of renal c.
    triamterene c.
    unilateral ureteral c.
    upper urinary tract c.
    urate c.
    ureteric c.
    urethral c.
    uric acid c.
    urinary c.
    urostealith c.
    vesical c.
    vesicoprostatic c.
    Volkmann spoon for pancreatic c.
    weddellite c.
    whewellite c.
    xanthic c.
    xanthine c.
Calcutript
    C. electrohydraulic lithotriptor
    Karl Storz C.
CALD
    chronic active liver disease
caldesmon
Caldwell needle/cannula Quick-Tap paracentesis system
Calglycine
Calgocide disinfectant
caliber
    loop c.
    c. probe
caliber-persistent
    c.-p. artery
    c.-p. artery of stomach
    c.-p. vessel
calibrate
calibration of cardia
calibrator
    c. serum
    Vitros Immunodiagnostic Products HBsAg Reagent Pack and C.
caliceal, calyceal
    c. diverticular calculus
    c. diverticulum
    c. drainage
    c. extension
    c. filling time
    c. fistula
    c. fornix
    c. infundibulum
    c. puncture
calicectasis, caliectasis, calycectasis, calyectasis *(var. of* calycectasis*)*
calicectomy, caliectomy, calycectomy
calices *(pl. of* calix*)*
calicine
Caliciviridae virus family
Calicivirus **gastroenteritis**
calicoplasty, calycoplasty, calyoplasty
calicotomy, calycotomy, calyotomy
Calicylic
caliectasis *(var. of* calicectasis*)*
caliectomy *(var. of* calicectomy*)*
calioplasty
caliorrhaphy, calyorrhaphy
caliotomy
calipers
    Lange skinfold c.
calix, pl. calices
    anomalous c.
    c. clubbing
    c. elongation
    c. enlargement
    extrarenal c.
    kidney c.
    minor c.
    multiple calices
    c. obstruction
    c. orchid
    c. puncture
Cal-Lac
Callaway formula
Call-Exner body
Calmette-Guérin
    bacille C.-G. (BCG, bCG)
    Calmette-Gúerin bacillus
    intravesical bacillus C.-G.
calmodulin
Calmoseptine ointment
Calogen LCT emulsion
caloric
    c. intake
    c. supplement
calorie
    high c.
calorimeter
Calot
    C. operation
    C. triangle
calpain in acute tubular necrosis
calponin
calprotectin
    c. assay
    fecal c.
calretinin
Caluso PEG gastrostomy tube
calyceal *(var. of* caliceal*)*

calycectasis, calicectasis (*var. of* calicectasis)
calycectomy (*var. of* calicectomy)
calycoplasty (*var. of* calicoplasty)
calycotomy (*var. of* calicotomy)
calyectasis (*var. of* calicectasis)
Calymmatobacterium granulomatis
calyoplasty (*var. of* calicoplasty)
calyorrhaphy (*var. of* caliorrhaphy)
calyotomy (*var. of* calicotomy)
calyx, pl. **calyces**
CAM
    complementary and alternative medicine
Camalox
Cambridge pancreatitis classification I–IV
camera
    c. adapter
    Anger scintillation c.
    charge-coupled device monochrome c.
    Circon-ACMI MicroDigital-I c.
    endoscopic c.
    field-of-view c.
    Fujinon FG-series endoscopic c.
    gamma scintillation c.
    Gammatone II gamma c.
    instant c.
    motion picture c.
    Olympus OM-1 reflex c.
    Olympus OM-series endoscopic c.
    Olympus OM-2 c. with SM-45 enlarging adapter
    Olympus OTV-S-series miniature c.
    Olympus SCA-series endoscopic c.
    Pen-F half-frame c.
    Pentax endoscopic c.
    Polaroid c.
    positron c.
    single-lens reflex c.
    still c.
    television c.
Cameron
    C. electrosurgical unit
    C. erosion
    C. lesion
    C. omniangle gastroscope
    C. ulcer
Cameron-Miller
    C.-M. electrocoagulation unit
    C.-M. electrode
    C.-M. monopolar probe
    C.-M. suction-coagulator
Camey
    C. enterocystoplasty
    C. enterocystoplasty urinary diversion
    C. I, II operation
    C. ileocystoplasty
    C. I orthotopic urinary diversion
    C. neobladder
    C. procedure
    C. reservoir
    C. urinary pouch
cAMP
    cyclic adenosine monophosphate
    5′-cyclic adenosine monophosphate
    vasopressin-induced cAMP
Campbell
    C. procedure
    C. sound
    C. technique
    C. trocar
camper
    C. angle
    C. chiasm
    fascia of C.
    C. fascia
    C. ligament
    C. plane
Camptosar injection
camptothecin
Campy-BAP culture medium
Campylobacter
    C. cinaedi
    C. coli
    C. doylei
    C. fetus
    C. fetus colitis
    C. fetus enteritis
    C. hyointestinalis
    C. jejuni
    C. lari
    C. pylori
    C. pyloridis gastritis
    C. test
    C. upsaliensis
Campylobacter-**like**
    C.-l. organism (CLO)
    C.-l. organism test (CLOtest)
Camwrap plastic covering

NOTES

Canada-Cronkhite syndrome
Canadian Urology Oncology Group (CUOG)
canal
  abdominal c.
  Alcock c.
  alimentary c.
  anal c.
  Bernard c.
  femoral c.
  c. of Hering
  histologic anal c.
  inguinal c.
  c. of Nuck
  pancreatobiliary c.
  pecten of anal c.
  pleuroperitoneal c.
  portal c.
  pudendal c.
  pyloric c.
  Santorini c.
  c. stenosis
  ventricular c.
  vesicourethral c.
  c. of Wirsung
canalicular
  c. bile
  c. bile plug
  c. cholestasis
  c. cryptorchidism
canaliculus, pl. **canaliculi**
  apical c.
  bile duct c.
  biliary c.
  c. bilifer
  pili torti et c.
  pseudobile c.
  secretory c.
Canasa suppository
cancelling A's test
cancer
  American Joint Committee on C. (AJCC)
  American Joint Committee on Cancer/International Union Against C. (AJCC/UICC)
  Amsterdam criteria for hereditary nonpolyposis colorectal c.
  androgen-independent prostate c.
  c. antigen 125 (CA-125)
  antral c.
  bile duct c.
  bilharzial-related c.
  bladder c.
  Borreliosis classification for advanced gastric c.
  Borrmann gastric c.
  breast c.
  burned-out testis c.
  c. cell growth
  c. cell heterogeneity
  clear cell renal c.
  colon c.
  colorectal c. (CRC)
  columnar cuff c.
  cryoablation for prostate c.
  de novo liver c.
  depressed c.
  depressed-type colorectal c.
  diagnosis of bladder c.
  disseminated c.
  c. doubling time
  c. drug resistance
  duodenal c.
  early gastric c. (EGC)
  endocrine c.
  esophageal c.
  esophagogastric junction c.
  European Organization for Research and Treatment of C. (EORTC)
  exenterative surgery for pelvic c.
  extragonadal germ cell c.
  extrahepatic bile duct c.
  familial colon c.
  c. family syndrome
  gastric c.
  gastrointestinal c.
  GI c.
  hereditary nonpolyposis colon c. (HNPCC)
  hereditary nonpolyposis colorectal c.
  hereditary papillary renal c. (HPRC)
  high-grade synchronous colon c.
  hypoechoic c.
  hypopharyngeal c.
  incurable c.
  intraepithelial c.
  intramucosal c.
  Japanese classification of c.
  large bowel c.
  liver c.
  low-lying rectal c.
  lung c.
  markers for c.
  Matritech NMP22 test for bladder c.
  metachronous colon c.
  metastatic c.
  Mostofi-grade prostate c.
  mucin-producing c.
  new chemotherapy combinations for advanced bladder c.
  nonfixed c.
  nonpolyposis colorectal c.
  obstructing c.
  ovarian c.
  pancreatic c. (PC)

pancreatoduodenal c.
papillary renal c.
polypoid c.
postgastrectomy c.
primary colorectal c. (PCRC)
prostate c. (PCa)
C. of the Prostate Strategic Urologic Research Endeavor
rectal c.
rectosigmoid c.
recurrent colorectal c. (RCRC)
restaging of c.
c. screening
squamous cell c.
staging of c.
stenotic c.
suburothelial infiltrative c.
superficial bladder c.
superficial depressed c.
teratoma testicular c.
testis c.
transplanted c.
treatment of bladder c.
urethral c.
urologic system c.
urothelial c.
Whitmore classification of prostate c.

cancer-associated sialyl-Lea antigen
cancerous erosion
Candela
    C. MDA-200 Lasertripter
    C. MiniScope
    C. Model MDL 2000 laser
    C. 405-nm pulsed-dye laser
candesartan
    luminal c.
Candida
    C. albicans
    C. esophagitis
    C. glabrata
    C. immitis
    C. immunological study
    C. infection
    C. krusei
    C. neoformans
    C. peritonitis
    C. symptom
    systemic *C.*
    C. treatment
    C. tropicalis

    ureteral *C.*
    vaginal *C.*
candidal
    c. cellulitis
    c. cystitis
    c. esophagitis
    c. infection
    c. intertrigo
    c. overgrowth
candidemia
candidiasis, candidosis
    esophageal c. (EC)
    vulvovaginal c.
candidum
    Geotrichum c.
canine sphincter
caninum
    Dipylidium c.
canis
    Toxocara c.
canister
    ATS c.
canker sore
Cannon
    C. point
    C. ring
cannula, pl. cannulas, cannulae
    Buie rectal injection c.
    contour ERCP c.
    double-lumen irrigation c.
    ERCP c.
    Flexicath silicone subclavian c.
    Fluoro Tip ERCP c.
    Franklin-Silverman biopsy c.
    Hasson open laparoscopy c.
    Intraducer peritoneal c.
    Jetco-Spray C.
    LaparoSAC single-use obturator and c.
    laparoscopic c.
    large-bore c.
    Makler c.
    Mayo-Ochsner suction trocar c.
    Medicut c.
    Olympus monopolar c.
    perfusion c.
    polyethylene c.
    portal c.
    Ramirez Silastic c.
    Tandem XL triple-lumen ERCP c.
    Teflon ERCP c.
    Veress c.

NOTES

cannula *(continued)*
    washout c.
    c. with preloaded guidewire
cannulation, cannulization
    bile duct c.
    biliary c.
    c. of biliary tree
    c. catheter
    deep c.
    duct c.
    endoscopic retrograde c.
    endoscopic transpapillary c.
    ERCP c.
    ex vivo c.
    freehand c.
    postsphincterotomy ERCP c.
    retrograde c.
    selective ductal c.
    stricture c.
    transpapillary c.
cannulatome
    Cotton c.
Can-Opt
    C.-O. dual-lumen ERCP system
    C.-O. stand-alone dual-lumen ERCP catheter
C-ANP
    C-type atrial natriuretic peptide
C22-3 antigen
    antibody to C22-3 a.
Cantil
Cantlie line
Cantor tube
Cantwell-Ransley
    C.-R. cavernocavernostomy
    C.-R. epispadias repair
    C.-R. technique
    C.-R. urethroplasty
CAP
    carcinoma of prostate
    chronic alcoholic pancreatitis
cap
    Assura stoma c.
    Coloplast stoma c.
    continent anal c.
    ConvaTec Active Life stoma c.
    duodenal c. (DC)
    c. method
    phrygian c.
    c. polyposis
    pyloric c.
    stoma c.
    Sur-Fit Natura flange c.
    Sur-Fit stoma c.
    ZE c.
capacitive coupling
capacity
    acid-neutralizing c. (ANC)
    bladder c.
    cystometric bladder c.
    fluid absorptive c.
    functional bladder c.
    galactose elimination c. (GEC)
    gastric c.
    iron-binding c. (IBC)
    maximum bladder c.
    maximum cystometric c.
    peritoneal membrane solute transport c.
    PMN oxidative burst c.
    pressure-specific bladder c.
    rectal c.
    total iron-binding c. (TIBC)
    unbound iron-binding c. (UIBC)
capacity-limited kinetics
cap-assisted resection
CAPD
    chronic ambulatory peritoneal dialysis
    continuous ambulatory peritoneal dialysis
capecitabine
Capener gouge
Cape Town technique
cap-fitted
    c.-f. endoscope
    c.-f. gastroscopy
    c.-f. panendoscope
capillarectasia
Capillaria philippinensis
capillariasis
    intestinal c.
capillaritis
    pulmonary c.
capillaropathy
capillary
    bile c.
    c. dilation
    c. endothelial cell
    glomerular c.
    c. hemangioma
    c. hyperfiltration
    c. network
    peritubular c.
    c. permeability
    c. refill
    C. System slide holder
    c. wall
capillary-leak phenomenon
capillary-lymphatic invasion
capillata
    Absidia c.
capistration
capita (*pl. of* caput)
capitatum
    Trichosporon c.
capitonnage
caplet
    Buffaprin c.
    Bufferin Arthritis Strength c.

Renax film-coated c.
Strovite Advance c.
Vanquish Analgesic C.'s
Capmul 8210
capnography
capnometry
capotement
Capoten
Capozide
CAPPP
    Captopril Prevention Project
capreomycin
CAPS
    caffeine, alcohol, pepper, spicy foods
capsaicin
    intravesical c.
CAPS-free diet
capsid-encoding region
capsula
    c. adiposa renis
    c. fibrosa
    c. fibrosa hepatitis
    c. fibrosa perivascularis
    c. fibrosa renis
    c. glomeruli
    c. pancreatitis
capsular
    c. artery
    c. blood vessel
    c. cirrhosis of liver
    c. flap pyeloplasty
    c. nephritis
    c. penetration
    c. tear
capsulatum
    Histoplasma c.
capsule
    acidophilus c.
    all-purpose c. (APC)
    Bowman c.
    budesonide c.
    Carey c.
    Cenogen-OB c.
    Crosby c.
    Detrol LA c.
    dutasteride c.
    c. endoscopy
    enteric-coated c.
    c. enteroscopy
    Entero-Test c.
    Entocort EC oral c.
    fascial c.

c. flap technique
Gerota c.
Given imaging capsule/M2A c.
Glisson c.
hepatic c.
hepatobiliary c.
L-carnitine c.
liver c.
M2A capsule/Given imaging c.
M2A Swallowable Imaging C.
Max-EPA c.
müllerian c.
mycophenolate mofetil c.
Orfadin c.
c. of pancreas
pH-sensitive radiotelemetry c.
polysaccharide c.
prostatic c.
radioisotope c.
radiotelemetering c.
Rebetol c.
renal c.
ribavirin 200 mg c.
Sitzmarks radiopaque marker in gelatin c.
splenic c.
Synalgos-DC C.'s
tolterodine tartrate c.
Watson c.
capsules/tablets
    Disalcid c./t.
capsulitis
    hepatic c.
capsuloma
capsuloplasty
capsulotomy
    renal c.
CapSure continence shield
Captiflex polypectomy snare
Captivator polypectomy snare
captivus
    penis c.
captopril
    c. plasma renin activity test
    C. Prevention Project (CAPPP)
    c. renogram
    c. renography
captopril-DTPA
    c.-DTPA scanning
captopril-enhanced renography
caput, pl. **capita**
    c. epididymidis

NOTES

caput *(continued)*
    c. gallinaginis
    c. medusae
    c. pancreatis
Carafate
CaraKlenz skin cleanser
carbachol
carbamazepine hepatotoxicity
carbamoyl phosphate synthetase deficiency
carbamylated hemoglobin
carbamylation
carbamylcholine
carbenicillin
carbenoxolone
Carbicarb
carbidopa dopaminergic medication
CarboFlex odor-control dressing
carbohydrate
    c. antigen 19-9 (CA19-9)
    c. antigen 19-9 immunohistochemical expression
carbohydrate-free
    Ross c.-f. (RCF)
carbohydrate-induced hyperlipidemia
carbohydraturia
carbolfuchsin stain
carbon
    c. dioxide acidosis
    c. dioxide insufflator
    c. dioxide laser
    c. dioxide laser plaque ablation
    c. dioxide trapping agent
    c. tetrachloride
    c. tetrachloride-induced liver regeneration
    c. tetrachloride nephropathy
carbon-11 (C-11)
carbon-14
    c. urea breath test
    c. urinary excretion test
carbon-13 urea breath test (^{13}C-UBT)
carbonate
    aluminum c.
    c. apatite
    c. apatite calcification
    c. apatite calculus
    c. apatite stone
    calcium c.
    dihydroxyaluminum sodium c.
    lanthanum c.
    magnesium c.
carbonic
    c. anhydrase (CA)
    c. anhydrase II
    c. anhydrase inhibitor (CAI)
carbonuria
carboplatin, etoposide, bleomycin (CEB)
carboprost tromethamine
Carbowax
carboxamide
    dimethyltriazenoimidazole c. (DTIC)
carboxyamidotriazole
carboxykinase
    phosphoenolpyruvate c. (PEPCK)
carboxylic ester hydrolase (CEH)
carboxyl-terminal amidation
carboxymethylcellulose jelly
carboxypeptidase
    c. B-like enzyme
    porcine c. B
carboxyterminal
    c. noncollagenous domain
    c. PTH
carbuncle
    kidney c.
    renal c.
carbunculoid
carbuterol
Carcassonne perineal ligament
carcinoembryonic antigen (CEA)
carcinogenesis
    chemical c.
    colorectal c.
    oncogene-induced c.
carcinogenicity
carcinogenic nitrosamine
carcinoid
    bronchial c.
    duodenal c.
    c. flush
    gastric c.
    gastroduodenal c.
    hindgut c.
    c. secretory granule
    seminal vesicle c.
    c. syndrome
    testis c.
    c. tumor
carcinoma, *pl.* **carcinomas, carcinomata**
    acinar cell c.
    acinar hepatocellular c.
    adenoid cystic c.
    adenosquamous cell c.
    adrenal cortex c.
    ameboma mimicking c.
    ampullary c.
    ampullopancreatic c.
    anal epidermoid c.
    anorectal c.
    Astwood-Coller staging system for c.
    autolymphocyte-based treatment for renal cell c. (ALT-RCC)
    Barrett c.
    basal cell c.
    basaloid squamous cell c. (BSCC)
    Bellini duct c.

bile duct c.
biliary c.
bladder small cell c.
bladder squamous cell c.
bladder transitional cell c.
Borrmann gastric c. types I–IV
Borrmann scirrhous c.
bulbomembranous urethral squamous cell c.
bulbourethral c.
cervical c.
cholangiocellular c. (CCC)
cholangitis c.
clear cell hepatocellular c.
clear cell nonpapillary c.
collecting duct c.
colon c.
colorectal c. (CRC)
cystic renal cell c. (CRCC)
deleted in colorectal c. (DCC)
diffuse hepatocellular c.
downstaging of advanced esophageal c.
Dukes classification of c.
Edmondson grading system for hepatocellular c.
embryonal cell c.
embryonal testicular c.
encapsulated renal cell c.
encephaloid gastric c.
endometrial c.
epidermoid c.
esophageal squamous cell c.
excavated gastric c.
c. ex pleomorphic adenoma
fibrolamellar hepatocellular c. (FL-HCC)
flat c.
flat-type c.
focal c.
gallbladder c.
gastric c.
genitourinary c.
germ cell c.
hepatocellular c. (HCC)
hereditary nonpolyposis colorectal c.
hilar c.
increased risk of penile c.
intramucosal c.
invasive c.
islet cell c.
Jass staging for rectal c.

Jewett classification of bladder c.
kidney c.
large bowel c.
laryngeal c.
linitis plastica c.
liver cell c.
medullary thyroid c.
metastatic prostatic c.
metastatic renal cell c. (MRCC)
microtrabecular hepatocellular c.
monofocal papillary c.
mucin-hypersecreting c.
mucinous c.
mucoepidermoid c.
mutated colorectal c. (MCC)
nodular transitional cell c.
nongerm cell c.
nonseminomatous testicular c.
nonsmall cell lung c.
oat cell c.
obstructing rectosigmoidal c.
oropharyngeal c.
ovarian c.
pancreatic c. (PCA)
pancreatic acinar cell c.
pancreatic islet cell c.
papillary gastric c.
papillary renal cell c.
papillary transitional cell c.
pediatric c.
penile c.
perforated c.
periampullary c.
peritoneal c.
PIVKA-II EIA kit for hepatocellular c.
polypoid c.
primary lung c.
primary transitional cell c.
c. of prostate (CAP)
prostate gland small cell c.
prostatic urethral transitional cell c.
protuberant c.
rectal linitis plastica colorectal c.
renal cell c. (RCC)
renipelvic transitional cell c.
renomedullary c.
RLP colorectal c.
sarcomatoid squamous cell c.
scirrhous c.
sclerosing hepatic c. (SHC)
secondary metastatic c.

NOTES

carcinoma *(continued)*
    sessile nodular c.
    sigmoid colon c.
    signet-ring cell c.
    signet-ring pattern of gastric c.
    c. in situ (CIS)
    c. in situ of glans penis
    splenic flexure c.
    sporadic nonfamilial clear cell c.
    squamous cell c. (SCC)
    stage B, C c.
    superficial esophageal c. (SEC)
    superficial gastric c.
    superficially spreading c.
    supraglottic squamous cell c.
    testicular c.
    TNM classification of c.
    Tp53-mutated c.
    transitional cell c.
    transthoracic resection of esophageal c.
    tubular c.
    ulcerating c.
    unresectable hepatocellular c.
    ureteral c.
    urethral c.
    urothelial c.
    verrucous c.
    vulvar c.
    yolk sac c.
carcinomatosis
    peritoneal c.
    c. peritonei
carcinosarcoma
    bladder c.
    gastric c.
    kidney c.
    polypoid exophytic nonulcerating c.
    renal c.
card
    Hemoccult II c.
cardia
    achalasia c.
    calibration of c.
    crescent gastric c.
    gastric c.
    c. intestinal metaplasia (CIM)
    patulous c.
    c. of stomach
cardiac
    c. antrum
    c. beta-adrenoreceptor hyporesponsiveness
    c. beta receptor
    c. cirrhosis
    c. decompression
    c. glycoside
    c. impression on liver
    c. output
    c. output/cardiac index (CO/CI)
    c. proteinuria
    c. sphincter
    c. stomach
    c. stomach mucosa
    c. sympathovagal tone
cardiac-type
    c.-t. gland
    c.-t. mucosa
cardialgia
cardiectomy
cardinal
    c. ligament
    c. suture
    c. vein
cardiochalasia
cardiodiosis
cardioesophageal (CE)
    c. junction (CEJ)
    c. mucosal junction
    c. reflex
    c. relaxation
    c. sphincter
cardiofundic gastropathy
cardiohepatic
    c. angle
    c. triangle
cardiohepatomegaly
cardiomegaly
cardiomyopathy
    uremic c.
cardiomyotomy
    Heller c.
cardiopexy
    ligamentum teres c.
cardioplasty
cardiopulmonary
    c. baroreflex
    c. baroreflex dysfunction
    c. baroreflex function
    c. bypass
    c. complication
cardiopyloric axis
cardiorespiratory complication
cardiospasm
cardiotomy
cardiotoxicity
    ipecac-induced c.
cardiovascular
    c. complication
    c. disease
    c. disorder
    c. drug hepatotoxicity
    c. mortality
carditis
    gastric c.
Cardizem
CARD15 polymorphism
Cardura

care
  Advanced-RF Natal C.
  cost-effective c.
  c. pathway
  surgical c.
caretaker gene
Carey capsule
Carey-Coons biliary endoprosthesis kit
Ca-Rezz moisture barrier cream
caribi
Carignan syndrome
carina, pl. **carinae**
carinate abdomen
carinii
  Pneumocystis c.
carious teeth
Carle analytic gas chromatograph
Carlesta
C-arm
  C-a. fluoroscope
  C-a. fluoroscopy
Carmalt
  C. clamp
  C. forceps
  C. hemostat
Carman-Kirklin
  C.-K. meniscus complex
  C.-K. meniscus sign
Carman sign
Carmel clamp
carminative
carmine
  c. blue
  contrast chromoscopy using indigo c. (CCIC)
  indigo c.
carmustine (BCNU, bCNU)
Carnett sign
Carney
  C. complex
  C. syndrome
carnitine
Carnitor
carnosinuria
Carnot
  C. function
  C. test
Caroid
Caroli
  C. disease
  C. syndrome
Caroli-Sarles classification

carotene
  serum c.
carotenemia
carotid
  c. artery
  c. bruit
Carpenter syndrome
carphenazine
Carrel
  C. aortic patch
  C. aortic patch anastomosis
carrier
  c. of allele
  Deschamps ligature c.
  Endo-Assist disposable ligature c.
  gene c.
  Goldwasser suture c.
  hepatitis c.
  nongene c.
  Pereyra ligature c.
  Raz double-prong ligature c.
  Semb ligature c.
Carr-Locke injection needle
Carson
  C. internal/external endopyelotomy stent
  C. Zero Tip balloon dilation catheter
cart
  Fujinon videoendoscopy c.
carteolol
Carter-Horsley-Hughes syndrome
Carter-Thomason
  C.-T. port closure device
  C.-T. suture passer
cartilage
  arytenoid c.
cartridge
  Clark hemoperfusion c.
  Dimension RxL PSA Flex reagent c.
Cartrol Oral
cartwheel configuration
caruncle
  Morgagni c.
  urethral c.
carvedilol
Cary-Blair medium
Casale
  C. vasectomy
  C. vesicostomy

NOTES

cascade
    clotting c.
    fibrogenic c.
    intrarenal matrix-degrading enzyme c.
    MAP kinase signaling c.
    metastatic c.
    signaling c.
    c. stomach
cascara
    c. sagrada
    c. sagrada and aloe
case
    poor surgical risk c.
    primary c.
    secondary c.
caseating
    c. granuloma
    c. necrosis
caseation
case-by-case approach
Casec calcium supplement
casei
    Lactobacillus c.
casein refeeding
caseosa
    nephritis c.
caseous nephritis
Case Power protein supplement
cashew apple
CAS 200 image cytometer
CaSki cell line
Casodex
Casola cecostomy
Casoni skin test
cast
    bacterial c.
    blood c.
    coarse granular c.
    erythrocyte c.
    esophageal c.
    fat c.
    fatty c.
    fine granular c.
    granular c. (GC)
    hematin c.
    hyaline c.
    c. nephropathy
    proteinaceous c.
    red blood cell c.
    c. syndrome
    urinalysis sediment microscopy c.
    urinary sediment c.
    white blood cell c.
Castellani paint
Castleman
    C. disease
    C. tumor
castlike tube

Castoria
    Fletcher's C.
castor oil
castrate
castration
    functional c.
    medical c.
    radiologic c.
catabolism
catalase
Catapres
catarrhal
    c. cholangitis
    c. cystitis
    c. dysentery
    c. dyspepsia
    c. gastritis
    c. jaundice
    c. nephritis
catastrophic complication
catatonic trypsinogen DNA screening
catecholamine
    adrenal c.
    c. excess state
    plasma c.
    c. synthetic enzyme
    urinary c.
catecholaminergic
category
    NIH Classification C. I–IV
category-specific isolation
cat-eye syndrome
catgut
    chromic c.
catharsis
cathartic
    c. colitis
    c. colon
    osmotic c.
Cathelin segregator
catheter
    Ablaser laser delivery c.
    Abscession biliary drainage c.
    Accurate c.
    Achiever balloon dilation c.
    acorn-tipped c.
    Acucise balloon c.
    Acucise endopyelotomy c.
    Allis c.
    Amplatz c.
    Angiocath PRN c.
    angiographic end-hole c.
    angiography c.
    AngioJet Xpeedior c.
    angioplasty balloon c.
    antibacterial personal c.
    antiseptic-impregnated central venous c.
    Argyle Ingram trocar c.

catheter · catheter

Argyle Medicut R c.
ARROWgard Blue hemodialysis c.
arteriovenous c.
aspiration c.
Atlantic ileostomy c.
c. bacterial interference
balloon dilating c.
Bardex-Foley c.
Bard gastrostomy c.
bat-wing c.
bicoudate c.
biliary balloon c.
biliary dilator c.
Bitome c.
blood-contactin c.
Blue Max balloon c.
Bozeman-Fritsch c.
Braasch c.
brush c.
BUD drainage c.
bullet-tip c.
Burhenne steerable c.
cannulation c.
Can-Opt stand-alone dual-lumen ERCP c.
Carson Zero Tip balloon dilation c.
central venous c.
Chemo-Port c.
Cholangiocath c.
c. cholangiogram
cholangiographic c.
Clay-Adams PE-10, PE-50 c.
coaxial c.
cobra c.
coil c.
Coil-Cath c.
c. coiling sign
colon motility c.
combination biliary brush c.
Comfort Cath I, II c.
Conceptus Soft Seal cervical c.
Conceptus Soft Torque uterine c.
Conceptus VS c.
condom c.
cone-tip c.
conical c.
Cook TPN c.
Cooled ThermoCath treatment c.
Cope loop nephrostomy c.
Corflo percutaneous access c.
coudé c.

Councill c.
CRE balloon c.
Curl Cath c.
DASH ERCP c.
decompression c.
c. á demeure
Dentsleeve single multilumen extrusion c.
de Pezzer c.
dilating c.
dilation c. (DC)
Dormia stone basket c.
Dotter c.
double-J c.
double-lumen balloon c.
double-lumen injection c.
Dow-Corning ileal pouch c.
Dowd II prostatic balloon dilatation c.
drainage c.
dual-lumen c. (DLC)
Duo-Flow c.
DURAglide 3 stone balloon c.
eight-lumen esophageal manometry c.
elbowed c.
Eliminator balloon c.
end-hole ureteral c.
endoscopic retrograde cholangiopancreatography c.
EndoSound endoscopic ultrasound c.
epidural c.
ERCP c.
esophageal motility perfused c.
esophageal perfusion c.
exdwelling ureteral occlusion balloon c.
exit site of c.
external ureteral c.
Extractor three-lumen retrieval balloon c.
5F c.
female c.
femoral hemodialysis c.
fenestrated c.
fiberoptic c.
Flexima ureteral c.
Flexxicon Blue dialysis c.
Flexxicon II PC internal jugular c.
Fogarty balloon biliary c.
Fogarty irrigation c.

NOTES

catheter *(continued)*
Foley c.
four-lumen polyvinyl manometric c.
French Cope loop nephrostomy c.
French mushroom-tip c.
French pigtail nephrostomy c.
French Teflon pyeloureteral c.
Gauder Silicon PEG c.
Glidex coated Percuflex c.
Glo-tip biliary c.
G91-9215 monocrystant antimony pH c.
Gold Probe Direct bipolar hemostasis c.
Gold Probe electrohemostasis c.
Gore-Tex c.
Gouley c.
Graham c.
Greenfield caval c.
Grüntzig balloon c.
c. guide
guiding c.
Handi-Cath c. kit
Hemoject injection c.
HemoSplit c.
hooked c.
Howmedica slit c.
Hurwitz dialysis c.
Hydromer grafted c.
hydrostatic balloon c.
ILUS c.
indwelling urinary c.
injection c.
intraarterial chemotherapy c.
intracholedochal manometric c.
intraductal imaging c.
intrathecal c.
intravascular ultrasound c.
c. irrigation
IVUS c.
Jackson-Pratt c.
Jelco c.
Kaye tamponade balloon c.
Kendall Foley c.
kidney internal splint/stent c.
Kish urethral illuminate c.
KISS c.
Konigsberg c.
Kumpe c.
Lane gastroenterostomy c.
large-bore c.
LeVeen c.
LifeJet c.
Lifemed c.
long-term indwelling c.
lumen-seeking c.
Mahurkar c.
male c.
Malecot reentry c.
Malecot suprapubic c.
Mallinckrodt c.
manometry c.
Mark IV Moss decompression-feeding c.
MaxForce TTS biliary balloon dilatation c.
MaxForce TTS high-performance balloon dilatation c.
measuring-mounting c.
Medicut c.
Medina ileostomy c.
Medi-Tech bipolar c.
Medi-Tech steerable c.
Memokath c.
Mentor nonhydrophilic PVC c.
Mentor straight c.
metal ball-tip c.
metallic-tip c.
Mewissen infusion c.
microtip sensor c.
microtip transducer c.
Microvasive balloon c.
Millar urodynamic c.
MiniBard c.
Missouri c.
Mistifier spray c.
MM c.
modified aspirating c.
MS Classique balloon dilatation c.
multifiber c.
multilumen manometric c.
mushroom c.
nasobiliary drainage c.
nasocystic c.
nasopancreatic c.
nasovesicular c.
needle-tip c.
Nélaton c.
nephrostomy c.
10 o'clock selector c.
olive-tipped c.
Olympus PW-1L wash c.
Olympus PW-5V spray c.
On-Command c.
open-ended ureteral c.
oral suction c.
over-the-wire balloon c.
Passage biliary dilatation c.
Passport Balloon-on-a-Wire dilatation c.
PE-MV balloon dilatation c.
Percuflex c.
percutaneous femoral vein c.
percutaneous nephrostomy Malecot c.
percutaneous transhepatic biliary drainage c.
percutaneous transhepatic pigtail c.

peritoneal dialysis c. (PDC)
PermCath dual-lumen c.
Pezzer c.
Phantom 5 Plus ST balloon dilatation c.
Phillips c.
pigtail c.
Pollack ureteral c.
polyethylene c.
polyurethane nasoenteric c.
polyvinyl chloride c.
Porges c.
Port-A-Cath c.
portal c.
postprostatectomy hemostatic c.
Pourchez XpressO hemodialysis c.
c. probe
c. probe-assisted endoluminal ultrasonography (CP-EUS)
c. probe ultrasound
prostatic c.
PTHC c.
pulse spray c.
pusher c.
PVC c.
pyeloureteral c.
Quinton c.
Quinton-Mahurkar dual-lumen peritoneal c.
radiopaque ERCP c.
Ranfac cholangiographic c.
Reddick cystic duct cholangiogram c.
red rubber Robinson c.
Release-NF c.
retrograde occlusion balloon c.
Rigiflex ABD balloon dilatation c.
Rigiflex biliary balloon dilatation c.
Rigiflex esophageal TTS balloon c.
Rigiflex OTW balloon dilatation c.
Rigiflex TTS balloon dilatation c.
Ring biliary drainage c.
Robinson c.
ruler c.
Sacks QuickStick c.
Sacks Single-Step c.
SchonCath chronic dialysis c.
self-drainage c.
self-retaining c.
shepherd's hook c.
shepherd's hook-shaped angiographic c.

Siegel-Cohen dilating c.
Silastic c.
silicone rubber Dacron cuffed c.
silver c.
SIM 2 c.
Simmons c.
Simplastic c.
single-lumen Broviac silicone c.
SmartCath esophageal balloon c.
Soehendra graduated dilating c.
solid-state esophageal manometry c.
Sonicath endoluminal ultrasound c.
c. sonography
Spectrum silicone Foley c.
spiral-tip c.
Stamey-Malecot c.
Stamey open-tip ureteral c.
standard ERCP c.
stenting c.
Stretta c.
subclavian c.
Suction Buster c.
Supra-Foley c.
surgically implanted hemodialysis c. (SIHC)
Surgitek c.
Swan-Ganz pulmonary artery c.
Swan-Ganz thermodilution c.
swan-neck Missouri c.
swan-neck pediatric Coil-Cath c.
SynchroMed infusion system intraspinal c.
synthetic five-channel water-perfused motility c.
Tandem thin-shaft transureteroscopic balloon dilatation c.
tapered-tip hydrophilic-coated push c.
Taut cystic duct c.
Teflon guiding c.
Tenckhoff peritoneal dialysis c.
Tenckhoff two-cuff c.
Texas-style two-piece c.
three-way irrigating c.
toposcopic c.
Toronto-Western c.
torque c.
Trabucco double balloon c.
Trach-Eze closed suction c.
Tracker c.
transanal c.
transducer c.

NOTES

catheter *(continued)*
- translumbar inferior vena cava c.
- transurethral c.
- Tratner c.
- trial without c. (TWOC)
- Trilogy low-profile balloon dilatation c.
- triple-lumen manometry c.
- c. tunnel infection
- Tyshak c.
- Uldall subclavian hemodialysis c.
- ureteral occlusion balloon c.
- Urocath external c.
- urodynamic c.
- UroMax II high-pressure balloon c.
- Uro-San Plus external c.
- Van Andel dilating c.
- van Sonnenberg gallbladder c.
- Vaxcel dialysis c.
- VTC biliary c.
- Vygon Nutricath S c.
- washing c.
- water-infusion esophageal manometry c.
- water-perfused c.
- whistle-tip ureteral c.
- Willscher c.
- Wilson-Cook fine-needle aspiration c.
- Wilson-Cook Quantum TTC esophageal balloon dilatation c.
- winged c.
- Witzel enterostomy c.
- Xpeedior c.
- Z-Med c.

catheter-associated bacteriuria
catheter-based ultrasound probe
catheter-guided endoscopic intubation (CAGEIN)
catheterization
- aseptic intermittent c.
- clean intermittent c. (CIC)
- clean intermittent bladder c.
- cystic duct c.
- hepatic vein c.
- in-and-out c.
- intermittent c.
- c. pouch
- c. pouch rupture
- retrourethral c.
- Seldinger cystic duct c.
- selective c.
- subclavian vein c.
- c. test
- transhepatic c.
- transnasal bile duct c.
- transpapillary c.
- umbilical vein c.
- ureteral c.
- urethral c. (UC)
- urinary c.

catheterize
catheter-related bloodstream infection (CR-BSI)
Cath-Secure
- C.-S. catheter holder
- C.-S. tape

cation
- cosecreted c.
- c. exchange
- c. exchanger
- c. exchange resin
- c. transport

cationic
- c. colloidal gold (CCG)
- c. dye

cationized ferritin
cat's eye calculus
Cattell T tube
cauda
- c. epididymis
- c. equina
- c. equina lesion
- c. equina syndrome

caudal
- c. block
- c. mesonephros
- c. pancreatic artery
- c. pancreaticojejunostomy
- c. pole
- c. regression syndrome
- c. traction

caudate
- c. eminence of liver
- c. lobe
- c. lobe of liver

caustic
- c. acid
- c. alkali
- c. colitis
- c. esophagitis
- c. ingestion
- c. stricture
- c. substance

cauterization
- colon c.

cauterize
cautery
- c. bend
- BICAP II c.
- blind c.
- Bovie c.
- endoscopic laser c.
- c. knife
- looped c.
- c. pencil
- snare c.

cava (*pl. of* cavum)

caval-atrial shunt
caveola
caveolated cell
caveolin-1
Caverject
CaverMap
    C. procedure
    C. surgical device
cavernitis, cavernositis
    fibrous c.
cavernocavernostomy
    Cantwell-Ransley c.
cavernosa (*pl. of* cavernosum)
cavernosae
    Billroth venae c.
cavernosal
    c. abscess
    c. alpha blockade
    c. alpha blockade technique
    c. artery
    c. nerve
    c. nerve-sparing radical prostatectomy
    c. systolic pressure
    c. vein
cavernositis (*var. of* cavernitis)
cavernosogram
cavernosography
cavernosometry
    dynamic infusion c.
    gravity c.
cavernosonography
    dynamic infusion cavernosometry and c.
cavernosorum
    tunica albuginea corporum c.
cavernospongiosum shunt
cavernostomy
cavernosum, pl. cavernosa
    bulb of corpus c.
    fibrotic corpus c.
Cavernotome
cavernous
    c. artery blood flow
    c. artery blood flow acceleration
    c. artery dilation
    c. artery disease
    c. artery injury
    c. artery occlusion pressure
    c. autonomic nerve dysfunction
    c. fibrosis
    c. hemangioma
    c. nerve
    c. nerve mapping
    c. transformation of portal vein (CTPV)
cavernovenous leakage
CAVH
    chronic active viral hepatitis
    continuous arteriovenous hemofiltration
CAVH-B
    chronic active viral hepatitis, type B
CAVHD
    continuous arteriovenous hemodialysis
CAVHDF
    continuous arteriovenous hemodiafiltration
CAVH-NAB
    chronic active viral hepatitis non-A non-B
caviae
    Aeromonas c.
Cavilon diabetes foot care kit
cavitas peritonealis
cavitating tuberculoma
cavitation
    c. bubble
    c. bubble activity
    pulmonary c.
Cavitron Ultrasonic Surgical Aspirator (CUSA)
cavity
    abdominal c.
    abdominopelvic c.
    Cutinova C.
    intraperitoneal c.
    nephrotomic c.
    peritoneal c.
    retroperitoneal c.
    tension-free closure of abdominal c.
cavography
    synchronous inferior c.
    synchronous superior c.
    vena c.
cavotomy
CAVU
    continuous arteriovenous ultrafiltration
cavum, pl. cava
    inferior vena cava (IVC)
    infrahepatic vena cava
    c. pelvis
    retrohepatic vena cava
    c. retzii

NOTES

cavum *(continued)*
    suprahepatic vena cava
    vena cava
    c. vesicouterinum
cayetanensis
    Cyclospora c.
CBAVD
    congenital bilateral absence of vas deferens
CBC
    complete blood count
CBD
    common bile duct
        CBD 2 choledochoscope
        CBD stone
CBDE
    common bile duct exploration
CBDM
    common bile duct microlithiasis
CBDS
    common bile duct stone
C-beta gene
CBH
    chronic benign hepatitis
CBI
    continuous bladder irrigation
^{13}C-bicarbonate breath test
CBP
    chronic bacterial prostatitis
    copper-binding protein
        CBP test
C^{13} breath test
CBS
    colloidal bismuth subcitrate
CC, Crcl
    Adalat CC
CCA
    calcium channel antagonist
CCC
    cholangiocellular carcinoma
    chronic calculous cholecystitis
    cylindrical confronting cisterna
CCD
    charge-coupled device
    cortical collecting duct
        CCD endoscope
        CCD perfusion
CCE
    cholesterol crystal embolization
CCFA
    Crohn and Colitis Foundation of America
CCG
    cationic colloidal gold
C-cholylglycine breath excretion test
CCIC
    contrast chromoscopy using indigo carmine

CCK
    cholecystokinin
        CCK antagonist
CCK-8
    cholecystokinin octapeptide
CCK-LI
    cholecystokinin-like immunoreactivity
CCKNOW
    Crohn and Colitis Knowledge
        CCKNOW score
CCK-OP
    cholecystokinin octapeptide
CCK-PZ
    cholecystokinin-pancreozymin
CCL-64 cell
CCL-277 colon cancer cell
CCl4-induced cirrhosis
CCNU
    cyclohexylchloroethylnitrosurea
        methyl CCNU
CCP
    chronic calcifying pancreatitis
    colitis cystica profunda
CCPD
    continuous cycling peritoneal dialysis
CCUP
    colpocystourethropexy
CD
    Clostridium difficile
    collecting duct
    common duct
    Crohn disease
    cystic duct
        CD activity index
CD3+ T cell
CD4+
    autologous HBcAg-specific CD4+
    CD4+ cell
    CD4+ T-cell count
CD4
    CD4 lymphocyte count
    CD4 molecule
    CD4 phenotype
    CD4 protein
    CD4 T cell
CD8+
    CD8+ cell
    CD8+ T lymphocyte
CD8
    CD8 lymphocyte
    CD8 lymphocyte count
    CD8 molecule
    CD8 phenotype
    CD8 protein
CD117
    c-kit protooncogene
CD20
    B-cell antigen CD20

C&D
    cystoscopy and dilation
CD2-positive cell
CD3-T-cell receptor complex
CD4+–CD8+ T-cell ratio
CD14 monoclonal antibody
CD23 enterocyte
CD25 antigen
CD2-associated protein
CD3 protein
CD45RO-positive memory T cell
CDA
    chenodeoxycholic acid
CDAD
    Clostridium difficile-associated diarrhea
CDAI
    Crohn Disease Activity Index
CDC
    Centers for Disease Control and Prevention
    choledochocholedochostomy
    complement-dependent cytotoxicity
    Crohn disease of colon
CDC42 protein
CDCA
    chenodeoxycholic acid
CDE
    common duct exploration
    cystine dimethylester
CDEIS
    Crohn Disease Endoscopic Index of Severity
CDJ
    choledochojejunostomy
CDK
    cyclin-dependent kinase
cDNA
    complementary deoxyribonucleic acid
        HSP-70 cDNA
        cDNA probe
CDNF
    ciliary-derived neurotrophic factor receptor
CDP
    computerized dynamic posturography
CD45RO lymphocyte
CDS
    commercial dialysis solution
CD3+ T cell
CDY
    cystoduodenostomy

CE
    cardioesophageal
    conjugated estrogen
CEA
    carcinoembryonic antigen
        CEA test
CE-AD gastric lesion staging by endoscopy
CEA-Scan
CeaVac
CEB
    carboplatin, etoposide, bleomycin
ceca (*pl. of* cecum)
cecal
    c. appendage
    c. appendix
    c. bascule
    c. botryomycosis
    c. colonoscopy
    c. cystoplasty
    c. dilation
    c. diverticulitis
    c. diverticulum
    c. fissure
    c. fold
    c. gangrene
    c. haustrum
    c. hernia
    c. homogenate
    c. imbrication procedure
    c. mucosal nodule
    c. necrosis
    c. perforation
    c. sacculation
    c. serosa
    c. ulcer
    c. vascular ectasia
    c. volvulus
cecectomy
Cecil
    C. operation
    C. procedure
    C. repair
    C. urethral stricture syndrome
    C. urethroplasty
cecitis
Ceclor
cecocolic intussusception
cecocolon
cecocolopexy
cecocolostomy
cecocystoplasty

NOTES

cecofixation
cecoileal reflux
cecoileostomy
cecopexy
cecoplication
cecoproctostomy
cecoptosis
cecorrhaphy
cecosigmoidostomy
cecostomy
 blow-hole c.
 Casola c.
 Chait percutaneous c.
 ileal Malone c.
 Malone c.
 percutaneous catheter c.
 percutaneous endoscopic c.
 tube c.
cecotomy
cecoureterocele
cecum, pl. ceca
 antimesocolic side of c.
 coned c.
 cone-shaped c.
 conical c.
 watermelon c.
Cedax
CEEA
 curved end-to-end anastomosis
 CEEA stapler
CE-EUS
 contrast-enhanced endoscopic ultrasonography
cefaclor
cefadroxil monohydrate
Cefadyl
cefamandole
CE-FAST
 contrast-enhanced fast sequence
cefazolin sodium
cefdinir
cefditoren pivoxil
cefepime
cefixime
cefmenoxine
cefmetazole
Cefobid
cefonicid
cefoperazone
ceforanide
Cefotan
cefotaxime
cefotetan disodium
cefotiam
cefoxitin
cefpirome
cefpodoxime proxetil
cefprozil
cefsulodin

ceftazidime
ceftibuten
Ceftin Oral
ceftizoxime
ceftriaxone
 c. pseudolithiasis
 c. sodium
cefuroxime
C-EGD
 conventional upper esophagogastroduodenoscopy
cEGF
 concentration epidermal growth factor
CEH
 carboxylic ester hydrolase
CEJ
 cardioesophageal junction
celandine
 greater c.
Celebrex
Celecoxib Long-Term Arthritis Safety Study (CLASS)
Celestin
 C. dilator bougie
 C. endoprosthesis
 C. esophageal tube
 C. graduated dilator
 C. latex rubber tube
 C. prosthesis
Celestone
celiac, coeliac, coeliac
 c. angiogram
 c. angiography
 c. arteriography
 c. axis
 c. axis compression
 c. dimple
 c. disease-specific EMA antibody
 c. flux
 c. lymph node
 c. plexus
 c. plexus block
 c. plexus neurolysis (CPN)
 c. plexus reflex
 c. plexus sectioning
 c. rickets
 c. sprue
 c. sprue disease
 c. syndrome
 c. trunk
 c. tumor
celiacography
celiac-superior mesenteric ganglia
celiacus
 truncus c.
celiagra
celiectomy
celiocentesis
celioenterotomy

celiogastrostomy
celiogastrotomy
celiomesenteric arteriography
celiomyalgia
celiomyomotomy
celioparacentesis
celiopathy
celiorrhaphy
celioscope
celioscopy, coelioscopy (*var. of* coelioscopy)
celiotomy
    exploratory c.
    c. incision
    vaginal c.
    ventral c.
celitis
cell
    absorptive c.
    acid c.
    acinar c.
    acinic c.
    acinous c.
    adelomorphous c.
    algoid c.
    amine precursor uptake and decarboxylation c.
    c. analysis system
    C. Analysis System 200 image cytometer
    aneuploid c.
    antigen-presenting c.
    antral D, EC c.
    antral gastric c.
    APUD c.
    argentaffin c.
    argyrophilic c.
    atypical ductular c.
    autologous liver c.
    ballooning of c.
    basal granular c.
    beaker c.
    bile duct epithelial c.
    biliary epithelial c. (BEC)
    binucleate renal tubule epithelial c.
    bladder mast c.
    blast c.
    bone marrow-derived B c.
    bone marrow stem c.
    border c.
    CaCo2 c.
    calciform c.

capillary endothelial c.
caveolated c.
CCL-64 c.
CCL-277 colon cancer c.
CD4+ c.
CD8+ c.
CD2-positive c.
CD45RO-positive memory T c.
CD3+ T c.
CD4 T c.
central c.
centroacinar c.
chalice c.
chief c.
chromaffin c.
chromogranin A immunoreactive c.
COLO 320 colon cancer c.
columnar-cuboidal adenocarcinoma c.
connective tissue-type mast c. (CTMC)
c. count
crypt c.
c. culture transwell
c. cycle marker
cytotoxic T c.
Davidoff c.
delomorphous c.
dendritic reticular c.
diploid c.
DNA haploid c.
donor dendritic c.
Dukes signet c. A, B, C
dysmorphic red blood c.
dysplastic c.
EC c.
ECL c.
effector c.
endocrine c.
endodermic c.
endothelial c.
enteric ganglion c.
enterochromaffin c.
enterochromaffin-like c.
enteroendocrine c.
epithelial c. (EC)
epithelial endocrine c.
eumorphic red blood c.
exfoliative epithelial colonic c.
F9 c.
fat c.
fat-storing liver c.

NOTES

cell (continued)
- fatty liver c. (FLC)
- fetal liver-derived B c.
- flare c.
- flattened epithelial microfold c.
- flexura hepatica c.
- foam c.
- gastric pacemaker c.
- gastrin c.
- gastrin-secreting c.
- Gaucher c.
- giant c.
- GI pacemaker c.
- glitter c.
- glomerular contractile c.
- glomerular epithelial c.
- gluconeogenic-competent human proximal tubule c.
- goblet c.
- graft parenchymal c.
- Grimelius-positive c.
- ground-glass c.
- GTL-16 gastric carcinoma c.
- haploid c.
- HBV-specific T c.
- Heidenhain c.
- HeLa c.
- helper T c.
- hematopoietic c.
- hepatic stellate c. (HSC)
- hepG2 c.
- HGF-stimulated renal epithelial c.
- histamine-producing mast c.
- HLF c.
- hobnailed c.
- HT-29 c.
- human cytotoxic T c.
- human intestinal epithelial Coco-2 c.
- human umbilical vein endothelial c. (HUVEC)
- hypochromic red c.
- IEC-6 c.
- IEL T c.
- IgA-producing c.
- IgG-producing c.
- infiltrating inflammatory c.
- infiltrating T c.
- intercalated c.
- interstitial immunocompetent c.
- interstitial mononuclear c.
- intestinal absorptive c.
- intestinal endocrine c.
- intestinal epithelial c.
- intestinal mucosal mast c. (IMMC)
- intraglomerular mesangial c.
- IPEC-J2 c.
- islet c.
- Ito c.
- JR-St c.
- KATO-III c.
- killer T c.
- Kulchitsky c.
- Kupffer c. (KC)
- L c.
- LAK c.
- lamina propria lymphoid c.
- Langerhans c.
- Langhans c.
- LE c.
- Leydig c.
- LIM 2537 c.
- c. line
- lipid-laden clear c.
- littoral c.
- liver-deprived epithelial clonic c.
- LLC-PK1-FBPase+ c.
- LLC-PK renal tubular c.
- lymphocyte-target c.
- lymphokine-activated killer c.
- lymphomononuclear c.
- M c.
- macula densa c.
- mast c.
- MDCK epithelial c.
- c. membrane
- c. membrane epithelial antigen
- memory T c.
- mesangial c. (MC)
- mesenchyma c.
- microfold c.
- MN c.
- mucous neck c.
- mucus-secreting c.
- multinucleated giant c.
- murine B16 c.
- murine lymphoid c.
- murine mesangial c. (MMC)
- murine proximal tubule c.
- myeloid dentritic c.
- myenteric ganglion c.
- myointimal c.
- natural killer c.
- c. necrosis
- neuroendocrine c.
- NK c.
- nonalpha nonbeta pancreatic islet c.
- nonantigen-expressing target c.
- noncleaved B c.
- nonrosetted c.
- nuclear-tagged c.
- oat c.
- OK c.
- OKT4 c.
- OKT8 c.
- osteoclast-like giant c. (OCLG)
- oxyntic c.
- P c.

pacemaker c.
packed red blood c.'s
pale c.
pancreatic acinar c.
pancreatic islet c.
Paneth c.
PAP-HT25 c.
paracrine c.
parietal c.
peptic c.
percentage of hypochromic red c.'s (%HYPO)
peripheral blood mononuclear c. (PBMC)
peripheral T c.
perisinusoidal c.
peritoneal mesothelial c.
peritubular myoid c.
phagocytic stellate c.
phenotypes of mast c.'s
Pick c.
pigment-laden Kupffer c.
pit c.
plasma c.
PLC-PRF 5 c.
PMN c.
Pockel c.
polymorphonuclear c.
postreceptor signaling of parietal c.
PP-immunoreactive c.
primed c.
principal c. (PC)
proliferating tubular c.
c. proliferation
prostate gland stromal c.
proximal tubular c.
ptyocrinous c.
pulpar c.
purified T c.
Q c.
C. Recovery System (CRS)
rectal epithelial c.
red blood c.'s (RBC)
renal collecting duct c.
renal proximal tubular c.
renal tubule epithelial c.
renocortical tubule c.
renomedullary interstitial c. (RMIC)
S c.
C. Saver
Schwann c.
schwannian spindle c.

secretory c.
semen round c.
seminiferous tubule Sertoli c.
senescent c.
c. separation technique
serotonin c.
Sertoli c.
Sertoli-Leydig c.
signet-ring c.
silver c.
sinusoidal endothelial c. (SEC)
sinusoid lining c.
small granule c.
C. Soft 2000 semen analyzer
C. Soft system
somatostatin c.
spillage of tumor c.'s
spindle c.
squamous c.
stellate c.
stem c.
c. substratum
suppressor T c.
c. surface area
c. surface receptor
SW 480 c.
c. swelling
T84 c.
target c.
T effector c.
tetraploid c.
thymus-derived c.
tolerogenic dendritic c.
transblotting c.
c. transfected
transitional c.
triploid c.
Trypan blue-stained c.
tubular epithelial c.
tumor c.
c. type
undifferentiated c.
unit of packed red blood c.'s (UPRBC)
upregulation of monocyte chemoattractant protein-1 genecytoplasm of c.
ureteral muscle c.
urinalysis sediment microscopy c.
urine glitter c.
vascular permeation of tumor c.
vascular smooth muscle c. (VSMC)

NOTES

cell *(continued)*
    villous-tip c.
    villus c.
    von Hansemann c.
    von Kupffer c.
    white blood c.'s (WBC)
    xanthoma c.
    XL1-Blue c.
    zymogenic c.
cell-adhesion molecule
cell-cell
    c.-c. adhesion
    c.-c. contact
    c.-c. interaction
CellCept
cell-mediated
    c.-m. arm
    c.-m. cytotoxicity
    c.-m. hepatic injury
    c.-m. immunity
    c.-m. immunohistological response
    c.-m. mechanism
    c.-m. suppression
cell-positive margin
cell-surface sialylation
Cell-Track
cellular
    c. atypia
    c. differentiation
    c. electrophysiology
    c. enzyme
    c. immune response
    c. immunity
    c. infiltration
    c. peptide
    c. proliferation
    c. tumor suppressor
cellularis
    balanoposthitis chronica circumscripta plasma c.
cellule
cellulitis
    candidal c.
    vaginal cuff c.
cellulosae
    Cysticercus c.
cellulose
    c. diacetate membrane
    c. phosphate
cellulose-based membrane
celomic epithelium
celoscope
celoscopy
celotomy
Celsius thermometer
cement
    latex-base skin c.
    Torbot c.
    Wacker Sil-Gel 604 silicone c.

CE-M gastric lesion staging by endoscopy
C-EMR
    cutting endoscopic mucosal resection
Cenogen-OB capsule
center
    anospinal c.
    C.'s for Disease Control and Prevention (CDC)
    freestanding ambulatory surgical c.
    organized germinal c.
    pontine micturition c. (PMC)
    rectovesical c.
    swallowing c.
    vomiting c.
centering balloon
centigrade thermometer
centigray
centimeter
    joules per c. (J/cm)
centipoise
central
    c. adrenergic agent
    c. cell
    c. cystocele
    c. echogenicity
    c. hyaline sclerosis
    c. hyperalimentation
    c. lacteal
    c. necrosis
    c. nervous system (CNS)
    c. spot
    c. vagal nerve stimulation
    c. venous alimentation
    c. venous catheter
    c. venous pressure (CVP)
    c. venous pressure line
centrifugal pump
centrifugation
    density gradient c.
    Ficoll-Hypaque gradient c.
    Polyprep c.
centrifuge
    Ficoll-Hypaque density gradient c.
centrifuged
centrilobular
    c. acidophilic necrosis
    c. cholestasis
    c. pancreatitis
    c. region of liver
centrizonal necrosis
centroacinar cell
Century bicarbonate dialysis control unit
Ceo-Two laxative
cephalad traction
cephalexin
cephalin-cholesterol flocculation test
cephalocyst

cephalosporin
    prophylactic c.
    second-generation c.
    third-generation c.
cephalothin
cephalotrigonal technique
cephapirin sodium
cephradine
Cephulac
Ceplene
CERA
    continuous erythropoiesis receptor activator
Ceralas PDT 633 diode laser system
ceramic element
ceramidase deficiency
ceramide lactoside lipidosis
c-ErbB-2/Neu oncoprotein
cercaria
cercaricidal
cerclage
    McDonald c.
    Shirodkar cervical c.
cerebellar ataxia
cerebelloretinal hemangioblastomatosis
cerebral
    c. edema
    c. fluid shunt
    c. hemangioblastoma
    c. palsy
    c. perfusion pressure (CPP)
cerebral-brain stem circuit
cerebral-sacral loop
cerebrohepatorenal syndrome (CHRS)
cerebrooculofacial syndrome
cerebrospinal
    c. fluid (CSF)
    ventricular c.
cerebrotendinous xanthomatosis
cerebrovascular
    c. complication
    c. disease
Cerespan
Ceretec
cereus
    Bacillus c.
cerevisiae
    Saccharomyces c.
Cerezyme
cerivastatin
ceroid-laden macrophage

certainty
    varying degrees of c.
cerulein
    exogenous cholecystokinin or c.
ceruloplasmin
    serum c.
cerumen obstruction
cervical
    c. carcinoma
    c. discharge
    c. erosion
    c. esophagogastric anastomosis
    c. esophagus
    c. friability
    c. gastroesophagostomy
    c. inflammation
    c. intraepithelial neoplasia (CIN)
    c. irregularity
    c. lymphadenopathy
    c. motion tenderness
    c. mucus-sperm interaction
    c. neuroblastoma
    c. polyp
    c. position
    c. spasm
    c. ulcer
    c. wart
cervicitis
    mucopurulent c.
    schistosomal c.
cervicocolpitis
cervicovaginitis
CESD
    cholesterol ester storage disease
cesium
cesium-137 wire
CE-SM gastric lesion staging by endoscopy
Cestoda **tapeworm**
cestode
cestodiasis
Cetacaine topical anesthetic
cetirizine
CETP
    cholesterol ester transfer protein
Cetuximab (IMC-C225)
cetyldimethylethyl ammonium bromide
Ceylon sore mouth
CF
    cystic fibrosis
        CF epithelium
CF-200Z Olympus colonoscope

NOTES

CF-HM
    C.-H. endoscope
    C.-H. fiberscope
    C.-H. magnifying colonoscope
CF-LB3R colonoscope
C-Flex
    C-F. Amsterdam stent
    C-F. ureteral stent
c-fos
    c-fos induction
    c-fos protooncogene
CF100TL
    Olympus CF100TL
CFTR
    cystic fibrosis transmembrane conductance regulator
        CFTR gene analysis
CFU
    colony-forming unit
CF-UHM colonoscope
CF-UM3 echocolonoscope
CG
    chronic glomerulonephritis
^{14}C-glycocholate breath test
C-glycocholic acid breath test
CGM
    coffee-grounds material
cGMP
    cyclic guanosine monophosphate
    5'-cyclic guanosine monophosphate
cGMP-mediated relaxant
CGN
    chronic glomerulonephritis
CGRP
    calcitonin gene-related peptide
CGS
    computer graphic simulation
c-GVHD
    chronic graft-versus-host disease
CGY
    cystogastrostomy
cGy radiation measure
CH
    chronic hepatitis
CH-40 activated charcoal
CHA
    common hepatic artery
Chaffin-Pratt drain
Chagas-Cruz disease
Chagas disease
chagasi
    Leishmania donovani c.
Chagasic megaesophagus
chain
    alpha-3, -4, -5 c.
    alpha-4 c.
    alpha-5 c.
    beta c.
    beta-1 c.
    c. cystogram
    c. cystourethrography
    food c.
    gamma light c.
    J c.
    kappa light c.
    monoclonal light c.
    obturator lymphatic c.
    c. suture
    sympathetic c.
chain-of-lakes
    c.-o.-l. deformity
    c.-o.-l. filling defect
    c.-o.-l. sign
chain-terminating inhibitor
chair
    Hausted all-purpose c.
    Vess c.
Chait percutaneous cecostomy
chalasia
chalazion
chalice cell
challenge
    c. diet
    fluid c.
    food c.
    gluten c.
    jejunal gluten c.
    rectal gluten c.
    solid bolus c.
challenging patient population
chamaedrys
    Teucrium c.
chamber
    antropyloroduodenal common c. (APDCC)
    deglutitive pharyngeal c.
    hyperbaric oxygen c.
    Makler counting c.
    Microcell c.
    10 Pa Amicon c.
    Sigma 34 monoplace hyperbaric c.
    Ussing c.
chancre
    hunterian c.
    Nisbet c.
chancroid
chancroidal bubo
chancrous
change
    blood pressue c.
    degenerative c.
    ductal c.
    enzyme c.
    erosive prepyloric c.
    fibrocystic c.
    fractional weight c.
    large cell c. (LCC)
    mesangiolytic c.

mesenchymal c.
morphologic c.
morphological c.
obstructive c.
orthostatic c.
pancreatic ductal morphological c.
phlegmonous c.
polyneuropathy, organomegaly, endocrinopathy, monoclonal protein, and skin c.'s (POEMS)
postsurgical c.
segmental c.
sensorium c.
spatial c.
trophic c.
ultrastructural basket-weave c.

channel
aquaporin water c.
biopsy c.
calcium c.
calcium-activated potassium c.
chloride c.
common c.
detrusor muscle potassium c.
epithelial sodium c. (ENaC)
gastric c.
ion c.
ligand-gated c.
lymph c.
lymphatic c.
Malone antegrade continent enema c.
Mitrofanoff catheterizable c.
pancreatic duct-choledochus c.
pancreaticobiliary common c.
potassium c.
preputial transverse island flap and glans c.
pyloric c.
Sonotrode c.
stomalike c.
stretch-sensitive ion c.
suction c.
thin-walled vascular c.
treatment c.
urea c.
voltage-dependent anion c.
voltage-gated c.
water c.

chaparral leaf
chaperone
retinoid c.

characteristic
anatomical c.
client-patient c.
performance c.
receiver-operating c. (ROC)

characterization
biochemical c.

***c*-Ha-ras gene**
CharcoAid
charcoal
activated c. (AC)
CH-40 activated c.
c. filter
c. hemoperfusion
hemoperfusion with c.
mitomycin adsorbed onto activated c. (M-CH)
C. Plus
c. suspension

CharcoCaps
Charcodote
Aqueous C.

Charcot
C. cirrhosis
C. intermittent fever
C. syndrome
C. triad
C. triangle

Charcot-Boettcher crystals and filaments
Charcot-Leyden crystal
Chardonna-2
CHARGE
coloboma, heart disease, atresia choanae, retarded growth, genital hypoplasia, and ear abnormalities
CHARGE abnormalities
CHARGE syndrome

charge
c. selectivity
urine net c. (UNC)

charge-coupled
c.-c. device (CCD)
c.-c. device endoscope
c.-c. device monochrome camera

Charrière scale
Chassard-Lapiné projection
chasteberry
ChAT
choline acetyltransferase

Chatillon
C. Digital Force gauge
C. dolorimeter

NOTES

Chauffard point
Chauveau bacterium
Cheatle
    C. salt
    C. slit
Cheatle-Henry
    C.-H. hernia
    C.-H. incision
checklist
    Hopkins symptom c.
Checklist-90R
    Symptom C.
Cheek-Perry syndrome
cheesy
    c. necrosis
    c. nephritis
Cheetah radiopaque contrast medium
cheilitis
    granulomatous c.
cheilosis
chelate
    gadolinium c.
chelator
    aroylhydrazone c.
Chelidonium majus
Chelsea-Eaton anal speculum
Chemet
chemical
    c. anoxia
    c. carcinogenesis
    c. cholecystitis
    c. cystitis
    cystogenic c.
    c. gastritis
    c. gastropathy
    c. litholysis
    c. peritonitis
    c. prostatitis
    c. splanchnicectomy
    c. urinalysis
chemical-induced esophagitis
chemically defined diet
chemiluminescence
    enhanced c. (ECL)
    luminol-enhanced c.
chemise
    bouton en c.
chemistry
    phosphoramidite c.
chemoattractant
chemodissolution
chemoembolization
    transarterial c. (TACE)
    transcatheter arterial c. (TACE)
chemoimmunotherapy
chemokine-orchestrated chemotaxis
chemokine receptor
chemolysis
    intrarenal c.

Chemo-Port catheter
chemoprevention of aging
chemoprophylaxis
    long-term low-dose maintenance c.
    traveler's c.
chemoradiation
    neoadjuvant c.
    c. therapy (CRT)
chemoradiotherapy
chemoreceptor
chemosensitivity
chemosis
chemotactic
    c. factor
    c. peptide
chemotaxis
    chemokine-orchestrated c.
    c. of polymorphonuclear leukocyte
chemotherapeutic
    c. agent
    c. agent hepatotoxicity
chemotherapy
    adjuvant hepatic arterial infusion c.
    antisarcoma c.
    antiviral c.
    continuous infusion c.
    cytotoxic c.
    c. gonadotoxicity
    hepatic arterial infusion c.
    high-dose c. (HDC)
    intraarterial c.
    intraperitoneal hyperthermic c. (IPHC)
    intrathecal c.
    intravesical c.
    IP c.
    neoadjuvant c.
    platinum-based consolidation c.
    polyantibiotic c.
    c. of primary tumor
    response rate to c.
chemotherapy-induced
    c.-i. nausea
    c.-i. nausea and emesis (CINE)
    c.-i. sterility
    c.-i. vomiting
Chemstrip
    C. bG reagent
    C. LN dipstick
ChemTrak
    C. AccuMeter
    C. AccuMeter screen
Chenix Tablet
chenodeoxycholate
chenodeoxycholic acid (CDA, CDCA)
chenodiol
Cherchevski disease
Cherney incision

cherry
    c. angiomas
    c. red spot (CRS)
    c. sponge
Cherry-Crandall method for testing serum lipase
chest
    barrel c.
    flail c.
    c. pain
    c. physiotherapy
    c. tube
    c. tube scar
Chester-Winter procedure
Chevalier
    C. Jackson esophagoscope
    C. Jackson gastroscope
chevron incision
chew-and-spit test
chewing gum diarrhea
CHF
    congenital hepatic fibrosis
CHI
    creatinine height index
Chiari
    C. disease
    C. malformation
chiasm
    Camper c.
Chiba
    C. needle
    C. percutaneous cholangiogram
Chibroxin
chief cell
Chilaiditi
    C. sign
    C. syndrome
child
    C. class A–C
    C. class A–C patient
    C. classification of hepatic risk criteria A–C
    cystinuric c.'s
    C. esophageal varix classification
    c. esophagoscope
    C. hepatic dysfunction classification
    C. intestinal forceps
    C. liver criteria
    C. liver disease classification
    C. operation
    C. pancreaticoduodenostomy

childhood
    extraordinary urinary frequency syndrome of c.
    papular acrodermatitis of c.
    urolithiasis in c.
    c. visceral myopathy (CVM)
Child-Phillips bowel plication
Child-Pugh
    C.-P. class A–C
    C.-P. classification
    C.-P. criteria
    C.-P. score
children
    c. coma scale
    C.'s Hospital intestinal forceps
Childs-Phillips intestinal plication needle
Child-Turcotte classification (CTC)
Child-Turcotte-Pugh (CTP)
    C.-T.-P. classification
chili-bean pseudopolyp
Chilomastix mesnili
chimney
    Roux-Y c.
China ink
Chinese restaurant syndrome (CRS)
chip
    prostatic c.
Chiron
    C. RIBA HCV test
    C. RIBA HCV test system second generation
chiufa
chlamydia
    C. psittaci
    C. trachomatis
    C. trachomatis infection
    c. urethritis
chloracetic
chloral hydrate
chlorambucil
chloramphenicol
chlorazepate
chlordiazepoxide
chlorhydria
chloride
    adrenalin c.
    ambenonium c.
    c. balance
    benzalkonium c. (BAC)
    benzethonium c. 0.025%
    benzyl c.
    bethanechol c.

NOTES

chloride *(continued)*
- calcium c.
- c. channel
- choline c.
- c. concentration
- CYT-356 radiolabeled with 111 indium c.
- c. electrolyte
- endrophonium c.
- mercury c. (HgCl2)
- mivacurium c.
- oxybutynin c.
- polyvinyl c. (PVC)
- potassium c. (KCl)
- c. secretion
- serum c.
- c. shunt
- sodium c.
- strontium-89 c.
- tetramethyl ammonium c. (TEMAC)
- titanous c.
- tridihexethyl c.
- urinary c.

chloride-to-phosphate ratio
chloridorrhea
- familial c.

chlorisondamine
chlormadinone acetate
chloroazotemic nephritis
chlorodontia
chloroform toxicity
chlorohydrate
- linsidomine c.

chloroma
- gastric c.

Chloromycetin
chloroplast
chloroprocaine
chloroquine-induced damage
chloroquine phosphate
chlorothiazide
chlorotrianisene
chlorozotocin
chlorpheniramine
chlorphenoxamine
chlorpromazine
chlorpromazine-induced cholestasis
chlorprothixene
chlorthalidone
chlorzoxazone toxicity
choana, pl. **choanae**
chocolate agar medium
CHOD-PAP cholesterol reagent
Cho/Dyonics two-portal endoscope
choice
- Medi-Jector C.

Choice2 test
choking
Cholac

cholagogic
cholagogue
cholaneresis
cholangeitis
cholangiectasis
cholangioadenoma
cholangiocarcinoma
- hilar c.
- metastatic c.
- perihilar c.
- peripheral c. (PCC)
- peripheral intrahepatic c.
- type III c.

Cholangiocath catheter
cholangiocatheter
- cystic duct c.
- saline-filled c.

cholangiocellular carcinoma (CCC)
cholangiocholecystocholedochectomy
cholangiodrainage
- endosonography-guided c.
- EUS-guided c.
- percutaneous transhepatic c. (PTCD)

cholangiodysplastic pseudocirrhosis
cholangioenterostomy
- intrahepatic c.

cholangiofibroma
cholangiofibromatosis
cholangiogastrostomy
cholangiogram (CAG)
- balloon c.
- catheter c.
- Chiba percutaneous c.
- common duct c.
- contrast selective c.
- cystic duct c.
- endoscopic retrograde c.
- fine-needle percutaneous c.
- fine-needle transhepatic c.
- intraoperative c.
- intravenous c. (IVC)
- occlusion c.
- operative c.
- percutaneous transhepatic c. (PTC, PTHC)
- pernasal c.
- retrograde c.
- serial c.'s
- thin-needle percutaneous c.
- transgastric c.
- transhepatic c.
- T-tube c. (TTC)

cholangiographic
- c. catheter
- c. findings

cholangiography (CAG)
- balloon occlusion c.
- breath-hold MR c.
- cystic duct c.

delayed operative c.
direct percutaneous transhepatic c.
drip infusion c. (DIC)
endoscopic retrograde c. (ERC)
fine-needle transhepatic c. (FNTC, FNTHC)
intraoperative c. (IOC)
intravenous c. (IVC)
magnetic resonance c. (MRC)
nasobiliary drain c.
non-breath-hold MR c.
operative c.
percutaneous hepatobiliary c.
percutaneous transhepatic c. (PTC, PTHC)
postoperative c.
retrograde c.
transabdominal c.
transhepatic c. (TC, THC)
T-tube c.

cholangiograsper
Storz c.

cholangiohepatitis
Oriental c.
recurrent pyogenic c. (RPC)

cholangiohepatoma
cholangiojejunostomy
intrahepatic c.

cholangiolar
cholangiole
cholangiolitic
c. cirrhosis
c. hepatitis

cholangiolitis
cholangioma
cholangiopancreatography
endoscopic retrograde c. (ERCP)
endoscopic ultrasound retrograde c.
magnetic resonance c. (MRCP)

cholangiopancreatoscopy
peroral c. (PCPS)

cholangiopathy
destructive c.
eosinophilic c.

cholangiophytiasis
cholangioscope
Olympus CHF-Q10 c.
prototype c.

cholangioscopic forceps biopsy
cholangioscopy
intraductal c.

percutaneous transhepatic c. (PTCS)
peroral c. (PCS)

cholangiostomy
cholangiotomy
cholangiovenous
c. communication
c. reflux

cholangitic
c. abscess
c. biliary cirrhosis

cholangitis
acute obstructive suppurative c. (AOSC)
acute suppurative c. (ASC)
ascending c.
autoimmune c.
bacterial c.
biliary c.
c. carcinoma
catarrhal c.
chronic nonsuppurative destructive c.
destructive c.
fibrous obliterative c.
granulomatous c.
idiopathic autoimmune c.
intrahepatic sclerosing c.
c. lenta
lymphoid c.
nonsuppurative destructive c.
obstructive c.
pleomorphic destructive c.
postendoscopic c.
posttransplantation c.
primary sclerosing c. (PSC)
progressive suppurative c.
pyogenic c.
rejection c.
sclerosing c.
secondary sclerosing c.
septic c.
small-duct primary sclerosing c.
suppurative c.
transient c.
viral c.

cholanopoiesis
cholanopoietic
cholascos
cholate
cholebilirubin
Cholebrine contrast medium
cholechromopoiesis

NOTES

cholecyanin
cholecystagogic
cholecystagogue
cholecystalgia
cholecystatony
cholecystectasia
cholecystectomy
    endoscopic laser c.
    laparoscopic c. (LC)
    laparoscopic laser c. (LLC)
    minilaparoscope c.
    prophylactic c.
    three-trocar technique for laparoscopic c.
    c. treatment
    videolaseroscopy c.
cholecystendysis
cholecystenteric fistula
cholecystenteroanastomosis
cholecystenterostomy
cholecystenterotomy
cholecystic
cholecystis
cholecystitis
    acalculous c.
    acute c. (AC)
    acute acalculous c.
    calculous c.
    chemical c.
    chronic calculous c. (CCC)
    c. cystica
    c. emphysematosa
    emphysematous c.
    erythromycin-induced c.
    follicular c.
    gangrenous c.
    gaseous c.
    c. glandularis proliferans
    perforated c.
    c. with cholelithiasis
    xanthogranulomatous c.
cholecystobiliary fistula
cholecystocele
cholecystocholangiography
cholecystocholedochal fistula
cholecystocholedocholithiasis
cholecystocolonic fistula
cholecystocolostomy
cholecystocolotomy
cholecystoduodenal
    c. band
    c. fistula
    c. ligament
cholecystoduodenocolic
    c. fistula
    c. fold
cholecystoduodenostomy
cholecystoendoprosthesis
    endoscopic retrograde c. (ERCCE)

cholecystoenterostomy
cholecystoenterotomy
cholecystogastric
cholecystogastrostomy
cholecystogram
    oral c. (OCG)
cholecystography
    drip infusion c.
    intravenous c.
    oral c.
    post-fatty meal c.
cholecystoileostomy
cholecystointestinal
cholecystojejunostomy
cholecystokinetic food
cholecystokinin (CCK)
    c. antagonist
    c. cholescintigraphy
    c. octapeptide (CCK-8, CCK-OP)
    c. test
cholecystokinin-like immunoreactivity (CCK-LI)
cholecystokinin-pancreozymin (CCK-PZ)
cholecystolithiasis
cholecystolithotomy
    percutaneous c. (PCCL)
    percutaneous transhepatic c. (PCTCL)
cholecystolithotripsy
cholecystomy
cholecystonephrostomy
cholecystoparesis
    diabetic c.
cholecystopathy
cholecystopexy
cholecystoptosis
cholecystopyelostomy
cholecystorrhaphy
cholecystoscopy
    percutaneous transhepatic c. (PTCC)
cholecystosis
    hyperplastic c.
cholecystostomy
    laparoscopy-guided subhepatic c.
    percutaneous transhepatic c.
cholecystotomy
    transpapillary endoscopic c. (TEC)
choledochal
    c. basal pressure
    c. cyst grades I, II, III, IV, IVa
    c. region
    c. sphincter
    c. sphincterotomy
choledochectomy
choledochendysis
choledochiarctia
choledochitis
choledochocele
choledochocholedochostomy (CDC)

choledochocolonic fistula
choledochocyst
choledochocystostomy
choledochodochorrhaphy
choledochoduodenal
    c. area
    c. fistula
    c. fistulotomy
    c. junction
    c. junctional stenosis
choledochoduodenostomy
choledochoenteric fistula
choledochoenterostomy
choledochofiberoscopy
    T-tube tract c.
choledochofiberscope
    Olympus URF-P2
    translaparoscopic c.
choledochofiberscopic approach
choledochogram
choledochography
choledochohepatostomy
choledochoileostomy
choledochojejunostomy (CDJ)
    end-to-side c.
    loop c.
    retrocolic end-to-side c.
    Roux-en-Y c.
choledocholith
choledocholithiasis
    Glasgow classification of c.
    rendezvous technique for treatment of c.
choledocholithotomy
choledocholithotripsy
choledochopancreatic ductal junction
choledochoplasty
choledochorrhaphy
choledochoscope
    Berci-Shore c.
    CBD 2 c.
    flexible fiberoptic c.
    Hopkins rod-lens system for rigid c.
    Machida c.
    Olympus CHF-P20 c.
    Olympus XCHF-37 c.
    URF-P2 c.
choledochoscopic guidance
choledochoscopy
    Berci-Shore c.
    cystic duct c.
    jejunostomy tract c.
    operative c.
    percutaneous c.
    postoperative c.
    T-tube tract c.
choledochostomy
choledochotomy
    c. incision
    longitudinal c.
choledochus
    ductus c.
choleglobin
cholehepatic shunt pathway
choleic acid
cholelith, chololith
cholelithiasis, chololithiasis
    cholecystitis with c.
    cholesterol c.
    intrahepatic c.
    c. prevalence
cholelithic, chololithic
cholelithic dyspepsia
cholelitholysis
cholelithoptysis
cholelithotomy
cholelithotripsy
cholemesis
cholemia
    familial c.
    Gilbert c.
cholemic nephrosis
cholepathia spastica
choleperitoneum
choleperitonitis
cholepoiesis, cholopoiesis
cholepoietic
choleprasin
cholera
    Asiatic c.
    bilious c.
    c. infantum
    c. morbus
    c. nostras
    pancreatic c.
    c. sicca
    summer c.
    c. toxin
    c. toxin-induced diarrhea
cholerae
    Vibrio c.
choleraesuis
    Salmonella c.

NOTES

choleraic diarrhea
choleresis
choleretic
    c. effect
    c. enteropathy
cholerheic
choleriform enteritis
cholerigenic, cholerigenous
cholerine
choleroid
cholerrhagia
cholerrhagic
cholescintigram
cholescintigraphy
    cholecystokinin c.
    hepatobiliary c.
    morphine c.
    radionuclide c.
CholestaGel
cholestasis, cholestasia
    acute drug-induced c.
    benign postoperative c.
    benign recurrent intrahepatic c. (BRIC)
    bile ductular c.
    canalicular c.
    centrilobular c.
    chlorpromazine-induced c.
    contraceptive pill-induced c.
    drug-induced c.
    estrogen-induced c.
    extrahepatic c.
    familial c.
    hepatocanalicular c.
    hepatocellular c.
    high-grade c.
    intrahepatic c.
    methyltestosterone-induced c.
    neonatal c.
    Norwegian c.
    c. patient
    pericentral c.
    c. of pregnancy
    progressive familial intrahepatic c. (PFIC)
    pure c.
    recurrent c.
    tolbutamide-induced c.
cholestatic
    c. hepatosis icterus gravidarum
    c. hypersensitivity
    c. jaundice
    c. liver disease
    c. reaction
    c. syndrome
    c. viral hepatitis
cholesteatoma
cholesterol
    c. calculus
    c. cholelithiasis
    c. crystal embolization (CCE)
    dietary c.
    c. embolism
    c. emboli syndrome
    c. embolus
    c. ester
    c. ester storage disease (CESD)
    c. ester transfer protein (CETP)
    high-density lipoprotein c. (HDLC)
    low-density lipoprotein c. (LDLC)
    c. monohydrate crystal
    c. polyp
    radioactive c.
    c. saturation index (CSI)
    seminal plasma c.
    serum c.
    c. solitaire
    c. stone
    very low density lipoprotein c.
    VLDL c.
cholesterol-cholesteroloxidase-phenol 4-aminophenazone method
cholesterol-containing gallstone
cholesteroleresis
cholesterosis, cholesterolosis
    acalculous c.
    c. of gallbladder
    c. of mucosal surface
cholesteryl ester
cholestyramine
    C. Light
    c. therapy
Choletec
choletelin
choletherapy
choleverdin
cholic
    c. acid (CA)
    c. acid clearance
cholicele
choline
    c. acetyltransferase (ChAT)
    c. chloride
    c. deficiency liver disease
    seminal plasma c.
cholinergic
    c. agonist
    c. innervation
    c. neuron
    c. receptor
    c. syndrome
cholochrome
chologenetic
Cholografin contrast medium
chololith (*var. of* cholelith)
chololithiasis (*var. of* cholelithiasis)
chololithic (*var. of* cholelithic)
cholopoiesis (*var. of* cholepoiesis)

cholorrhea
choloscopy
Cholybar
cholyl-^{14}C-glycine
chondrocyte
    autologous c.
chondrocyte-alginate gel
chondrodysplasia
    Jansen-type metaphyseal c.
Chondrogel
chondrogenic differentiation
chondroitin
chondroitinuria
chondrosarcoma
    bladder c.
Chooz
chorda
    c. gubernaculum
    c. spermatica
chordee
    acquired c.
    congenital c.
    c. correction
    fibrous c.
    lateral c.
    residual c.
chordeic penis
choreoathetosis
choriocarcinoma
    bladder c.
chorioepithelioma
chorionic
chorista
choristoma
choroid plexus cyst (CPC)
Christie gallbladder retractor
Christmas
    C. tree appearance of pancreas
    C. tree sign
Christopher-Williams overtube
chromaffin
    c. cell
    c. tissue
chromaffinoma
chromagranin
chromatofocusing pH range
chromatograph
    Carle analytic gas c.
    QuinTron Microlyzer 12 c.
chromatography
    column c.
    denaturing high-performance liquid c. (dHPLC)
    gas c.
    gel filtration c.
    high-performance liquid c. (HPLC)
    high-pressure liquid c. (HPLC)
    ion c.
    solid-phase extraction c.
    stool c.
    thin-layer c. (TLC)
    Varian model 3600 gas c.
chromatopectic (var. of chromopectic)
chromatopexis (var. of chromopexy)
chromic
    c. catgut
    c. catgut suture
    c. gut suture
chromium
    c. deficiency
    c. sesquioxide
51-chromium-labeled ethylenediaminetetraacetate (^{51}Cr-EDTA)
chromocystoscopy
chromoendoscope
chromoendoscopy
    Lugol c.
    magnification c.
    methylene blue c.
    phenol red c.
chromogen
chromogranin
    c. A immunoreactive cell
    c. stain
chromopectic, chromatopectic, chromopexic
chromopexy, chromatopexis
chromophobe
    c. adenoma
    c. cell tumor
chromophore-enhanced laser welding
chromoscopy
    gastric c.
chromosomal
    c. abnormality
    c. marker
chromosome
    c. deletion
    human c. 6
    c. insertion
    c. instability
    c. inversion

NOTES

chromosome *(continued)*
   c. karyotype
   c. marker
   marker c.
   c. morphology
   Philadelphia c.
   c. ploidy
   X, Y c.
chromoureteroscopy
chronic
   c. abacterial prostatitis
   c. active gastritis
   c. active hepatitis (CAH)
   c. active liver disease (CALD)
   c. active pouchitis
   c. active viral hepatitis (CAVH)
   c. active viral hepatitis non-A non-B (CAVH-NAB)
   c. active viral hepatitis, type B (CAVH-B)
   c. aggressive hepatitis (CAH)
   c. alcoholic cirrhosis
   c. alcoholic pancreatitis (CAP)
   c. alcohol-induced pancreatitis
   c. allograft nephropathy
   c. allograft rejection
   c. ambulatory peritoneal dialysis (CAPD)
   c. anoplasty treatment
   c. appendicitis
   c. atrophic duodenitis
   c. atrophic gastritis (CAG)
   c. autoimmune hepatitis
   c. bacterial enteropathy
   c. bacterial prostatitis (CBP)
   c. bacterial pyelonephritis
   c. benign hepatitis (CBH)
   c. calcifying pancreatitis (CCP)
   c. calculous cholecystitis (CCC)
   c. cholestatic liver disease
   c. cicatrizing enteritis
   c. cystic gastritis
   c. diarrhea
   c. diverticulitis
   c. erosion
   c. erosive gastritis
   c. fibrosing hepatitis
   c. fibrosing pancreatitis
   c. follicular gastritis
   c. functional constipation
   c. functional gastrointestinal symptom
   c. functional symptomatology
   c. gastrointestinal blood loss
   c. GI blood loss
   c. glomerular disease
   c. glomerulonephritis (CG, CGN)
   c. graft dysfunction
   c. graft-versus-host disease (c-GVHD)
   c. granulomatous disease
   c. hepatitis (CH)
   c. hepatitis A, B, C, D, E, F
   c. hypokalemic nephropathy
   c. idiopathic constipation
   c. idiopathic intestinal pseudoobstruction (CIIP)
   c. idiopathic jaundice
   c. inflammatory bowel disease (CIBD)
   c. inflammatory cell infiltrate
   c. interstitial gastritis
   c. interstitial hepatitis
   c. intestinal atony
   c. intestinal dysmotility (CID)
   c. intestinal ischemic syndrome
   c. intestinal pseudoobstruction (CIP, CIPO)
   c. intestinal pseudoobstruction syndrome
   c. intravenous supplementation
   c. ischemic colonic lesion caused by phlebosclerosis (CICLP)
   c. lead poisoning
   c. liver disease (CLD)
   C. Liver Disease Questionnaire (CLDQ)
   c. lobular hepatitis (CLH)
   c. low-frequency electrical stimulation
   c. membranous glomerulonephritis (CMGN)
   c. mercury poisoning
   c. metabolic acidosis
   c. nonbacterial prostatitis (CNP)
   c. nonimmune gastritis
   c. nonsuppurative destructive cholangitis
   c. obstructive pulmonary disease (COPD)
   c. obstructive uropathy
   c. pancreatitis (CP)
   c. pancreatitis of Kasugai
   c. parenchymal liver disease
   c. pelvic pain syndrome (CPPS)
   c. peptic esophagitis
   c. periesophagitis
   c. persistent hepatitis (CPH)
   c. progressive hepatitis
   c. progressive tubulointerstitial disease
   c. prostate pain syndrome (CPPS)
   c. prostatitis-like symptom
   c. prostatitis/pelvic pain syndrome (CPPS)
   c. pyelonephritis (CP, CPN)
   c. radiation proctitis

chronic · Ciba-Corning

c. regurgitation
c. rejection after renal transplantation
c. relapsing pancreatitis
c. renal failure (CRF)
c. renal failure glomerulonephritis
c. renal insufficiency (CRI)
c. sacral neuromodulation
c. sacral-spinal nerve stimulation
c. sclerosing hyaline fibrosis
c. superficial gastritis (CSG)
c. transplant rejection
c. tubular damage
c. type B hepatitis
c. ulcer
c. ulcerative colitis (CUC)
c. ulcerative proctitis
c. urate nephropathy
c. urethral syndrome
c. urinary retention (CUR)
c. viral hepatitis

chronica
enteritis cystica c.
gastrorrhea continua c.
ileocolitis ulcerosa c.

chronically inflamed gallbladder
chronic-continuous type
chronicus
lichen simplex c.

chronobiological parameter
chronotropism
Chronulac
CHRP
coagulation and hemostatic resection of prostate

CHRPE
congenital hypertrophy of retinal pigment epithelium

CHRS
cerebrohepatorenal syndrome

CHUK
conserved helix-loop-helix ubiquitous kinase

Church deep surgery scissors
Churg-Strauss syndrome
Chwalla membrane
chylangioma
chylaqueous
chylectasia
chyle cyst

chyli
cisterna c.
receptaculum c.

chylifaction
chylifactive
chyliferous vessel
chylification
chyliform ascites
chylocele
parasitic c.

chyloderma
chylomediastinum
chylomicron
c. core
c. production
c. retention disease
c. secretion

chyloperitoneum
chylophoric
chylopoiesis
chylopoietic disease
chylorrhea
chylosa
diarrhea c.

chylosis
chylothorax
chylous
c. ascites
c. ascitic fluid
c. fistula
c. leukemia
c. peritonitis
c. urine

chyluria
chylus
chyme
c. discharge
c. transport

Chymex
chymification
chymobilia
iatrogenic c.

chymopoiesis
chymorrhea
chymotrypsin
CI
confidence interval

CIA
congenital intestinal aganglionosis

Cialis
Ciba-Corning ACS PSA assay

NOTES

cibalis
    fistula c.
CIBD
    chronic inflammatory bowel disease
cibenzoline
cibi
    fastidium c.
CIC
    clean intermittent catheterization
cicatricial
    c. stricture
    c. tissue
cicatrix, pl. **cicatrices**
cicatrization
CICLP
    chronic ischemic colonic lesion caused by phlebosclerosis
CID
    chronic intestinal dysmotility
Cidecin
Cidex
    C. activated dialdehyde solution
    C. Plus solution
cidofovir
cIEL
    crypt intraepithelial lymphocyte
CIFN
    consensus interferon
    CIFN therapy
cigarette drain
cigar-shaped hyperchromatic nucleus
ciguatera fish poisoning
C-III
    Testred C-III
CIIP
    chronic idiopathic intestinal pseudoobstruction
Cilaidit syndrome
cilastin
ciliary-derived neurotrophic factor receptor (CDNF)
ciliary dysentery
ciliate dysentery
Cillium
CIM
    cardia intestinal metaplasia
cimetidine
Cimicifuga heracleifolia
CIN
    cervical intraepithelial neoplasia
cinacalcet
cinaedi
    Campylobacter c.
    Helicobacter c.
CINE
    chemotherapy-induced nausea and emesis
cinedefecogram
cinedefecography
cine-esophagogram
cine-esophagoscope
cine-esophagoscopy
cinefluorographic study
cinefluorography
cinefluoroscopic method
cinegastroscopy
cineloop memory function
cineradiographic analysis
cineurography
cinnamic acid
Cinobac Pulvules
cinoxacin
CIP
    chronic intestinal pseudoobstruction
CIPO
    chronic intestinal pseudoobstruction
ciprofloxacin hydrochloride
Cipro XR
circadian
    c. gastric acidity
    c. periodicity
    c. rhythm
    c. rhythmicity
    c. testosterone pattern
circadian-shaped infusion
Circe device
circinata
    balanitis c.
circinate balanitis
circle
    c. of death
    c. needle
    Pagenstecher c.
Circon-ACMI
    C.-ACMI lithotriptor
    C.-ACMI MicroDigital-I camera
    C.-ACMI miniscope
    C.-ACMI MR-6, MR-9 ureteroscope
    C.-ACMI USL-2000 rigid device
circuit
    cerebral-brain stem c.
    enteric neuronal c.
    enteric secretomotor c.
    extracorporeal cardiopulmonary c.
circuitous
circular
    c. anal dilator
    c. dichroism
    c. folds of Kerckring
    c. muscle
    c. muscle fiber
    c. myotomy
    c. stapled anastomosis
    c. stapler
    c. stapler donut
    c. stapling device
    c. suture
    c. tape
    c. vesicomyotomy (CVM)

circulares
    plicae c.
circulating
    c. autoantibody
    c. enzyme
    c. immunocomplex immunological study
    c. tumor-associated antigen
circulation
    arterial c.
    collateral abdominal c.
    cutaneous collateral c.
    enterohepatic c. (EHC)
    hepatic c.
    hyperdynamic c.
    mesenteric c.
    portal c.
    portal-collateral c.
    venous c.
circulatory embarrassment
circumanal
circumcaval ureter
circumcise
circumcised
circumcision
    c. complication
    contraindication to c.
    meatal stenosis after c.
    Plastibell c.
    routine neonatal c.
    sleeve-type c.
    trapped penis after c.
circumductive
circumference
    abdominal c. (AC)
circumferential
    c. fundoplication
    c. margin
    c. mucosal dissection
    c. transanal sleeve advancement flap
circumflex vein
circumintestinal
circumlocution
circumumbilical incision
cirrhogenous, cirrhogenic
cirrhosis
    acholangic biliary c.
    acute juvenile c.
    alcoholic c. (AC)
    atrophic c.
    autoimmune c.
    bacterial c.
    Baumgarten c.
    biliary c.
    Budd c.
    calculous c.
    cardiac c.
    CCl4-induced c.
    Charcot c.
    cholangiolitic c.
    cholangitic biliary c.
    chronic alcoholic c.
    compensated c.
    congestive c.
    CPH-CAH c.
    Cruveilhier-Baumgarten c.
    cryptogenic c.
    decompensated alcoholic c.
    decompensated liver c.
    drug-induced c.
    end-stage c.
    fatty c.
    focal biliary c.
    frank c.
    glabrous c.
    Glisson c.
    Hanot c.
    hemochromatotic c.
    hepatic c.
    hepatitis C antiviral long-term treatment to prevent c. (HALT-C)
    histologic c.
    hypertrophic c.
    hypochlorhydric c.
    incomplete c.
    juvenile c.
    Laënnec c.
    liver c. (LC)
    macronodular c.
    Maixner c.
    Mayo Clinic system for primary biliary c.
    micronodular c.
    mixed c.
    multilobular c.
    necrotic c.
    nonazotemic c.
    nutritional c.
    obstructive biliary c.
    periportal c.
    pigmentary c.
    pipestem c.
    portal c.

NOTES

cirrhosis *(continued)*
    posthepatic c.
    postnecrotic c.
    primary biliary c. (PBC)
    progressive familial c.
    secondary biliary c.
    stasis c.
    c. of stomach
    syndrome of primary biliary c.
    Todd c.
    toxic c.
    type C c.
    unilobular c.
    vascular c.
cirrhotic
    c. ascites
    c. gastritis
    c. hydrothorax
    c. liver
cirsocele
cirsoid aneurysm
cirsomphalos
CIS
    carcinoma in situ
cisapride
    rectal c.
cisapride-assisted lavage
cisapride-functional dyspepsia trial
CISCA
    cisplatin, cyclophosphamide, Adriamycin
    CISCA protocol
cis-diaminedichloroplatinum
cisplatin
    bleomycin, etoposide, c. (BEP)
    c., cyclophosphamide, Adriamycin (CISCA)
    c. doxorubicin, cyclophosphamide
    etoposide, ifosfamide, c.
    methotrexate, c. (MC)
    c., methotrexate, Velban (CMV)
    c., methotrexate, vinblastine (CMV)
    methotrexate, vinblastine, Adriamycin, c. (MVAC, M-VAC)
    methotrexate, vinblastine, epirubicin, c. (M-VEC)
    c. nephropathy (CPN)
cisplatin-Lipiodol-Spongel (CLS)
cisterna, pl. **cisternae**
    c. chyli
    cylindrical confronting c. (CCC)
CIT
    cold ischemia time
Citra Forte
citrate
    clomiphene c.
    c. infusion
    lead c.
    c. of magnesia
    magnesium c.
    c. metabolism
    piperazine c.
    potassium c.
    ranitidine bismuth c. (RBC)
    c. replacement fluid
    seminal plasma c.
    sildenafil c.
    sodium c.
    c. supplementation
    c. synthase
    c. test
    urinary c.
citric
    c. acid
    c. acid bladder mixture
citrinum
    Penicillium c.
Citrobacter
    C. amalonaticus
    C. diversus
    C. freundii
    C. intermedius
Citrocarbonate
Citroma
Citro-Mag
Citro-Nesia
Citrotein liquid feeding
Citrucel Sugar-Free
citrulline
citrullinemia
Civiale operation
CIXU
    constant infusion excretory urogram
c-jun
    c-jun oncogene
    c-jun protooncogene
***c-kit* protooncogene (CD117)**
CK-MB
    muscle-brain isoenzyme of creatine kinase
CKPT
    combined kidney and pancreas transplant
CLA
    conjugated linoleic acid
    CLA echoendoscope
^{13}C-labeled cholesteryl octanoate breath test
C-lactose test
Clado ligament
cladribine
Claforan
Clagett-Barrett
    C.-B. esophagogastroscopy
    C.-B. esophagogastrostomy
Clagett esophagogastrostomy
clam
    c. enterocystoplasty
    c. ileocystoplasty

clamp
Abadie enterostomy c.
Adson c.
Allen anastomosis c.
Allen intestinal c.
Allen-Kocher c.
Allis c.
anastomosis c.
approximator c.
ASSI METS-3668 Microspike approximator c.
ASSI MKCV-2040 Microspike approximator c.
ASSI MSPK-3678 Microspike approximator c.
atraumatic c.
Babcock c.
Backhaus towel c.
Bainbridge intestinal c.
Baumrucker urinary incontinence c.
Beardsley intestinal c.
Best right-angle colon c.
Bihrle dorsal c.
Borge c.
Buie pile c.
bulldog c.
Carmalt c.
Carmel c.
Collins umbilical c.
Cope crushing c.
Cope modification of Martel intestinal c.
Crawford c.
Crile appendix c.
Crile hemostatic c.
Cunningham urinary incontinence c.
curved Mayo c.
Daniel colostomy c.
Dardik c.
DeBakey c.
DeMartel appendix c.
DeMartel-Wolfson anastomosis c.
Dennis c.
Dixon-Thomas-Smith c.
Doyen intestinal c.
Earle hemorrhoid c.
Edna towel c.
Fehland intestinal c.
Fogarty c.
Foss anterior resection c.
Foss intestinal c.
Furniss anastomosis c.
Furniss-Clute duodenal c.
Gant c.
Glassman noncrushing gastrointestinal c.
Goldblatt c.
Goldstein Microspike approximator c.
Gomco umbilical c.
Haberer intestinal c.
Harvey Stone c.
Hayes anterior resection c.
Hayes colon c.
Heaney c.
hemorrhoidal c.
hemostatic c.
Hendren c.
Herrick kidney c.
hilar c.
Hirschmann pile c.
Hunt colostomy c.
Hurwitz esophageal c.
Hurwitz intestinal c.
intestinal c.
Jarvis hemorrhoid c.
Jarvis pile c.
Kane umbilical c.
Kapp-Beck colon c.
Kelly c.
Kelsey pile c.
kidney pedicle c.
Kleinschmidt appendectomy c.
Kocher c.
Lane gastroenterostomy c.
Lane intestinal c.
laparoscopic Allis c.
Linnartz intestinal c.
Linton tourniquet c.
Madden intestinal c.
Martel c.
Masters intestinal c.
Masters-Schwartz liver c.
Mayo abdominal c.
Mayo-Robson intestinal c.
McCleery-Miller intestinal c.
McDougal prostatectomy c.
McLean pile c.
Meeker gallbladder c.
metal wing c.
Microspike approximator c.
microvascular c.
Mikulicz c.
Millin T c.

NOTES

clamp *(continued)*
    Mixter c.
    Mogen c.
    Moreno gastroenterostomy c.
    mosquito hemostatic c.
    Moynihan c.
    Myles hemorrhoidal c.
    noncrushing bowel c.
    Nussbaum intestinal c.
    occlusive c.
    Ochsner c.
    O'Hanlon intestinal c.
    Olsen cholangiogram c.
    Parker-Kerr intestinal c.
    partialocclusion c.
    Payr pyloric c.
    Péan c.
    pedicle c.
    Pemberton sigmoid c.
    penile c.
    Pennington c.
    Petz c.
    Phillips rectal c.
    Rankin c.
    Redo intestinal c.
    right-angle c.
    Roosevelt c.
    rubber-sheathed c.
    rubber-shod c.
    Satinsky c.
    Schwartz c.
    Scudder intestinal c.
    self-retraction c.
    serrefine c.
    Shoemaker intestinal c.
    Singley intestinal ring c.
    slotted nerve c.
    Stetten intestinal c.
    Stille c.
    Stone-Holcombe intestinal c.
    Stone intestinal c.
    straight mosquito c.
    Strelinger colon c.
    T c.
    tonsil c.
    tubing c.
    vascular c.
    von Petz c.
    Wangensteen anastomosis c.
    Wirthlin splenorenal c.
    Wolfson intestinal c.
    Wylie hypogastric c.
    Zachary Cope-DeMartel c.
    Zeppelin c.
    Zipser penile c.
clamping
    hyperglycemic c.
clamshell technique
clandestine intake

clapotage, clapotement
clarithromycin
    lansoprazole, amoxicillin, c.
    omeprazole, amoxicillin, c. (OAC)
    omeprazole, metronidazole, c. (OMC)
    ranitidine bismuth citrate, amoxicillin, c. (RAC)
    c. triple therapy
Clark
    C. common duct dilator
    C. hemoperfusion cartridge
    C. operation
    C. sign
Clarke-Hadfield syndrome
Clarke-Reich knot pusher
CLASS
    Celecoxib Long-Term Arthritis Safety Study
class
    Child c. A–C
    Child-Pugh c. A–C
    GR drug c.
    c. I, II antigen
    c. I, II MHC molecule
Classen-Demling papillotome
classic
    c. achalasia
    c. high-pressure low-flow voiding
    c. triad of Rigler
classical transactivator
classification
    AJCC TNM tumor c.
    Anderson c.
    Ann Arbor c.
    Astler-Coller c. A, B1, B2, C1, C2
    Astler-Coller modification of Dukes c.
    Banff c.
    Bismuth benign bile duct stricture c.
    Blaivas urinary incontinence c.
    Borrmann gastric cancer c.
    Bosniak c.
    Cambridge pancreatitis c. I–IV
    Caroli-Sarles c.
    Child esophageal varix c.
    Child hepatic dysfunction c.
    Child liver disease c.
    Child-Pugh c.
    Child-Turcotte c. (CTC)
    Child-Turcotte-Pugh c.
    Correa c.
    Cotton c.
    Couinaud c.
    CTP c.
    Dagradi esophageal variceal c.
    Dubin-Amelar varicocele c.

classification · clearance

Dukes c.
Forrest c.
Fredrickson c.
gastric mucosal pattern c.
Hald-Bradley c.
Hetzel-Dent c.
IGCCCG c.
International Continence Society voiding function c.
International Germ Cell Cancer Collaborative Group c.
Japanese cancer c.
Jewett bladder carcinoma c.
Kasugai c.
Kelami c.
LA c.
Lapides c.
Lauren gastric carcinoma c.
Los Angeles c.
Lukes-Collins c.
Marseille pancreatitis c.
Marsh c.
McNeer c.
megaureter c.
Ming gastric carcinoma c.
modified Bismuth-Corlete c.
Mt. Sinai c.
Musshoff modification of Ann Arbor c.
NIH-CPSI prostatitis c.
Pugh c.
Ranson acute pancreatitis c.
Rappaport c.
reflux esophagitis c. I–IV
Santiani-Stone c.
Siurala c.
Solcia c.
Sonnenberg c.
Stamey c.
Sumikoshi c.
Sydney system gastritis c.
c. system
TNM carcinoma c.
UICC tumor c.
Visick dysphagia c.
voiding dysfunction c.
Whitehead c.
WHO gastric carcinoma c.
clathrin-coated pit
claudication
claudin-2-positive zone
CLAVE needleless system

clavulanate
clavulanic acid
Clavulin
claw forceps
Clay-Adams PE-10, PE-50 catheter
Claybrook sign
clay-colored stool
CLD
  chronic liver disease
  NBNC CLD
  non-B, non-C CLD
CLDQ
  Chronic Liver Disease Questionnaire
CLE
  columnar-lined esophagus
  long-segment CLE
  short-segment CLE
clean
  c. intermittent bladder catheterization
  c. intermittent catheterization (CIC)
clean-catch urine specimen
cleaner
  Endozime AW bacteriostatic enzyme c.
cleaning
  diathermic c.
cleanser
  CaraKlenz skin c.
  Rediwash skin c.
  UltraKlenz skin c.
cleansing hypertonic phosphate enema
clean-voided specimen (CVS)
clear
  c. bile
  c. cell adenocarcinoma
  c. cell carcinoma of kidney
  c. cell hepatocellular carcinoma
  c. cell nonpapillary carcinoma
  c. cell renal cancer
  c. cell sarcoma
  c. discharge
  enemas until c.
  c. liquid diet
clearance
  aminopyrine c.
  antipyrine c.
  blood-water c.
  bromsulphalein c.
  caffeine c.
  cholic acid c.
  complete stone c.

NOTES

clearance *(continued)*
    creatinine c. (Crcl)
    ^{51}Cr-labeled albumin c.
    dextran c.
    equivalent residual renal urea c. (eKru)
    esophageal acid c.
    fractional c.
    hepatic c.
    24-hour creatinine c.
    hydrogen gas c.
    ICG c.
    I-125 iothalamate c.
    immunoglobulin G c.
    increased peritoneal c.
    indocyanine green c.
    instantaneous c.
    integrated c.
    inulin c.
    iodoantipyrine c.
    iothalamate c.
    kidney c.
    lithium c. (CLi)
    lowest c.
    luminal acid c.
    mucociliary c.
    osmolar c.
    PAH c.
    paraaminohippurate c.
    plasma c.
    prescribed c.
    renal c.
    retinyl ester c.
    stone c.
    theophylline c.
    urea c.
    in vitro c.
    in vivo c.
    whole-blood c.
clearing
    esophageal c.
cleavage
    aspartyl protease-mediated c.
    bacterial c.
    embryonic c.
    c. plane
cleaved extracellular domain
cleft palate
Cleocin
Cleveland
    C. Clinic Incontinence Score
    C. Clinic weighted scale of endoscopic procedures
CLH
    chronic lobular hepatitis
CLi
    lithium clearance

click
    intermittent c.
    systolic c.
clidinium bromide
client-patient characteristic
CLIM computer program
clindamycin
Clindex
clinic
    hospital-based c.
    urology c.
clinical
    c. activity
    C. Activity Index (CAI)
    c. determinant
    c. findings
    c. hypergastrinemia
    c. implication
    c. improvement
    c. indication
    c. investigation
    c. monitoring
    c. parameter
    c. problem
    c. protocol
    c. rejection
    C. Risk Index for Babies (CRIB)
    c. sequela
    c. trial
    c. trial for kidney disease
clinically
    c. insignificant
    c. stable human renal allograft
clinicobiological criteria
clinicopathological
clinicopathologic staging
Clinifeed Iso enteral feeding
Clinitest-negative stool
Clinitest-positive stool
Clinitest stool test
Clinoril
Clinoxide
clip
    absorbable c.
    c. applier
    Heifitz c.
    Hulka c.
    laparoscopic tie c.
    Lapra-Ty c.
    metal c.
    Michel c.
    silver c.
    titanium c.
    towel c.
    von Petz suture c.
    Weck c.
Clipoxide
clipping
    endoluminal c.

endoscopic c.
laser c.
Clirans T-series dialyzer
clitoral
    c. index
    c. recession
clitoridis
    preputium c.
clitoris, pl. **clitorides**
    bifid c.
clitoroplasty
clitorovaginoplasty
CLO
    Campylobacter-like organism
    CLO biopsy
cloaca, pl. *cloacae*
    congenital c.
    Enterobacter cloacae
    persistent c.
    c. septation
cloacal
    c. exstrophy
    c. exstrophy one-stage repair
    c. exstrophy two-stage repair
    c. malformation
    c. membrane
    c. plate
    c. remnant
    c. septum
cloacogenic polyp
clodronate
clofazimine
clofibrate
Clomid
clomiphene
    c. citrate
    c. test
clomipramine
clonal
    c. anergy
    c. deletion
    c. dilution
clonality
clonazepam
clone
    gliadin-specific T-cell c.
clonic contraction
clonidine suppression test
cloning
    molecular c.
clonogenic repopulation

clonorchiasis, clonorchiosis
    biliary c.
    hepatic c.
Clonorchis sinensis
clonus
    left-sided c.
    right-sided c.
C-loop
Cloquet
    C. hernia
    node of C.
clorazepate dipotassium
clortermine
closed
    c. afferent loop
    c. colon
    c. continuous lavage
    c. drainage
    c. duodenum
    c. efferent loop
    c. esophagus
    c. eyes sign
    c. hemorrhoidectomy
    c. injury
    c. morphology
    c. pylorus
    c. tubule fixation technique
closed-end ostomy pouch
closed-loop intestinal obstruction
closed-suction
    c.-s. drain
    c.-s. drainage system
closing pressure
Clostoban
clostridial nephritis
Clostridium
    C. algidicarnis
    C. botulinum
    C. butyricum
    C. cadaveris
    C. coccoides
    C. difficile (CD)
    C. difficile-associated diarrhea (CDAD)
    C. difficile enteritis
    C. difficile enterotoxin
    C. difficile toxin assay
    C. fallax
    C. leptum
    C. perfringens
    C. ramosum
    C. tertium

NOTES

Clostridium *(continued)*
    C. tetani
    C. welchii
closure
    Beta-Cap catheter c.
    Beta-Cap II c.
    bladder neck c. (BNC)
    bladder outlet c.
    delayed primary c. (DPC)
    exstrophy c.
    Graham c.
    ileostomy c.
    muscularis tunnel c.
    primary c.
    pyelotomy c.
    secondary c.
    Smead-Jones c.
    stapled c.
    Sur-Fit Natura irrigation sleeve tail c.
    sutureless colostomy c.
    Tom Jones c.
    Witzel c.
    wound c.
clot
    adherent c.
    black c.
    blood c.
    c.'s and debris
    fresh c.
    fundic c.
    hematuria with c.'s
    intraluminal c.
    nonadherent c.
    overlying c.
    sentinel c.
CLOtest
    Campylobacter-like organism test
clot-induced urinary tract obstruction
clotrimazole
clotted blood
clotting
    c. abnormality
    c. cascade
    c. factor
    c. parameter
    c. time
cloud
    c. phenomenon
    plasma c.
cloudy
    c. ascites
    c. bile
    c. fluid
cloverleaf
    c. appearance
    c. deformity
    c. excision of hemorrhoid
    C. internal bumper

cloxacillin-induced cholestatic jaundice
Cloxapen
CLS
    cisplatin-Lipiodol-Spongel
club
    American Endosonography C. (AEC)
clubbed
    c. common bile duct
    c. finger
    c. penis
clubbing
    calix c.
    finger c.
    c. of fingers and toes
clustered
    c. jejunal waves
    c. waves (CW)
cluster of grapelike cysts
clusterin mRNA
CLVP
    contact laser vaporization of prostate
clysis
clysma
Clysodrast
clyster
CM1 polyclonal antibody
CMA
    cow's milk allergy
c-met
    c-met oncogene
    c-met protein
    c-met receptor
CMG
    cystometrogram
CMGN
    chronic membranous glomerulonephritis
C-mount adapter
CMSE
    cow's milk-sensitive enteropathy
CMV
    cisplatin, methotrexate, Velban
    cisplatin, methotrexate, vinblastine
    cytomegalovirus
        CMV colitis
        CMV esophagitis
        CMV inclusion body
        CMV inclusion cyst
        CMV infection
        CMV ulcerative disease
CMV-associated ulceration
CMV-induced esophageal ulceration
CMV-related ulcer
c-myc
    c-myc oncogene
    c-myc protooncogene
CNDI
    congenital nephrogenic diabetes insipidus

CNNA
    culture-negative neutrocytic ascites
CNP
    chronic nonbacterial prostatitis
    C-type natriuretic peptide
CNS
    central nervous system
    congenital nephrotic syndrome
CO_2
    CO_2 breath test
    CO_2 electrolyte
    CO_2 laser
    CO_2 laser probe
Co
    coenzyme
CoA
    coenzyme A
coagulase
    c. waveform
    c. waveform desiccation
coagulase-negative *Staphylococcus*
coagulating
    c. current
    c. electrode
    c. forceps
coagulation
    argon beam plasma c.
    argon ion plasma c.
    argon plasma c. (APC)
    BICAP c.
    Bipolar Circumactive Probe c.
    blood c.
    Bovie c.
    coaptive c.
    disseminated intravascular c. (DIC)
    EHT c.
    electrohydrothermal c.
    endoscopic microwave c.
    free-beam c.
    heater probe c.
    c. and hemostatic resection of prostate (CHRP)
    hot biopsy monopolar c.
    infrared c.
    interstitial laser c. (ILC)
    laser c.
    microwave c.
    monopolar c.
    multipolar c.
    c. necrosis
    c. probe
    semen c.
    c. time
    tissue c.
coagulative
    c. laser therapy
    c. necrosis
coagulator
    argon beam c.
    argon plasma c. (APC)
    ERBE Unit argon plasma c.
    infrared c.
    microwave tissue c.
    Redfield infrared c.
Coaguloop resection electrode
coagulopathy
    iatrogenic c.
    c. pancreatitis
coagulum pyelolithotomy
coalesce
coalescence
coalescent ulcer
coalition
    Digestive Disease National C. (DDNC)
coaptation
coaptive coagulation
coarctation
coarse
    c. granular cast
    c. material
    c. nodularity
coarsely granular kidney
coat
    fibromuscular c.
    hydrated gelatinous c.
    muscular c.
Coat-A-Count Free PSA IRMA test
coated biopsy forceps
coaxial
    c. catheter
    c. snare
cobalamin deficiency
cobalophilin
cobalt-60
Coban
    C. dressing
    C. tape
Cobb collar
cobbler's stitch
cobblestone
    c. appearance
    c. appearance of gastric body
    c. filling defect

NOTES

cobblestone *(continued)*
    c. mucosa
    c. pattern
    c. pattern of hepatocyte
cobblestonelike monolayer
cobblestoning
    c. of colon
    c. of mucosa
    mucosal c.
    c. sign
Cobe Centrysystem dialyzer 400 HG
COBED tube
^{57}Co B$_{12}$ excretion
cobra
    c. catheter
    c. venom factor (CVF)
cobra-head
    c.-h. deformity
    c.-h. sign
cocaine
    c. hepatotoxicity
    c. package ingestion
cocarcinogen
cocarcinogenic
    c. FBA
    c. fecal bile acid
coccidian
    c. body
    c. *Cyclospora*
    c. sporulation
    unsporulated c.
coccidian-like
coccidioidal
    c. cystitis
    c. endometritis
    c. peritonitis
Coccidioides immitis peritonitis
coccidioidomycosis
coccidiosis
coccidium
coccoides
    Clostridium c.
coccoid form of *Helicobacter pylori*
coccygeal
    c. fistula
    c. pelvis
coccygeus muscle
Cochin China diarrhea
Cochran-Mantel-Haenszel test
CO/CI
    cardiac output/cardiac index
Cockcroft-Gault
    C.-G. equation
    C.-G. formula
Cock operation
Cockroft method
cocktail
    GI c.
    lytic c.

CO_2-CO_2 abundance ratio
^{13}C-octanoic acid gastric emptying breath test
coculture system
CODAS software
code
    genetic c.
Coding Systems for a Thesaurus of Adverse Reaction Terms (COSTART)
codominant phenotype
codon
    premature stop c.
coefficient
    glomerular ultrafiltration c.
    inbreeding c.
    mass transfer area c. (MTAC)
    prostatic pressure c. (PPC)
    sieving c. (SC)
    ultrafiltration c.
    c. of variation
coeliac (*var. of* celiac)
coeliac (*var. of* celiac)
coelioscopy, celioscopy (*var. of* celioscopy)
coenzyme (Co)
coenzyme A (CoA)
coerulea
    Absidia c.
coeundi
    impotentia c.
coexpress
coffee-grounds
    c.-g. emesis
    c.-g. material (CGM)
    c.-g. vomit
    c.-g. vomitus
Coffey
    C. technique
    C. ureterointestinal anastomosis
Cogentin
cognition
cognitive function
Cohen
    C. antireflux procedure
    C. cross-trigonal reimplantation
    C. cross-trigonal technique
    C. syndrome
    C. test
    C. ureteroneocystostomy
coherent
    c. bundle
    C. model 90-K laser
cohosh
    black c.
coil
    c. catheter
    endoanal c.
    endoesophageal MRI c.
    endoprostatic c.

endorectal-pelvic phased-array c.
Gianturco c.
helical c.
Helmholtz double-surface c.
interlocking detachable c.'s
intraurethral c.
MRCP using HASTE with phased-array c.
pelvic phased-array c. (PPA)
secretory c.
spring-wire c.
c. stent
Stylet internal esophageal MRI c.

Coil-Cath catheter
coiled
    c. spring appearance
    c. spring sign
coiled-coil motif
coimmunoprecipitated
coincubation
    sperm immunobead c.
coinfection
coit
***COL4A3* gene**
***COL4A4* gene**
***COL4A5* gene**
Colace
Colapinto needle
Colaris
    C. genetic susceptibility test
    C. molecular diagnostic test
Colax-C
Colazal
Colazide
colchicine
cold
    c. biopsy forceps
    c. cup biopsy
    c. cup resection
    c. defect
    c. flushing
    c. forceps ablation
    c. ischemia time (CIT)
    c. knife
    c. knife endoureterotomy
    c. knife hook
    c. knife incision
    c. scissors
    c. snare ablation
    c. snare excision
    C. Spor disinfectant
    c. spot

    c. storage
    c. stress test
Cole
    C. duodenal retractor
    C. sign
colectasia
colectomy
    abdominal c.
    blind subtotal c.
    laparoscopic c.
    segmental c.
    subtotal c.
    total abdominal c. (TAC)
    transverse c.
    c. ulcerative colitis
coleoptosis
Colestid
colestipol hydrochloride
Coley toxin
coli
    adenomatous polyposis c. (APC)
    adherent invasive *Escherichia c.*
    attenuated adenomatous polyposis c.
    Balantidium c.
    Campylobacter c.
    diffuse adherent *Escherichia c.* (DAEC)
    enteroadherent *Escherichia c.* (EAEC)
    enteroaggregative *Escherichia c.* (EAEC, EaggEC)
    enterohemorrhagic *Escherichia c.* (EHEC)
    enteroinvasive *Escherichia c.* (EIEC)
    enteropathogenic *Escherichia c.* (EPEC)
    enterotoxigenic *Escherichia c.* (ETEC)
    Escherichia c.
    familial adenomatous polyposis c.
    familial polyposis c. (FPC)
    flexura lienalis c.
    haustra c.
    juvenile polyposis c.
    labium inferius valvulae c.
    labium superius valvulae c.
    melanosis c.
    nonpathogenic *Escherichia c.*
    pneumatosis cystoides c. (PCC)
    polyposis c.

NOTES

coli *(continued)*
    Shiga toxin-producing
       Escherichia c. (STEC)
    Taeniae c.
colibacillosis
colic, colica
    acute ureteric c.
    appendicular c.
    c. artery
    biliary c. (BC)
    bilious c.
    copper c.
    crapulent c.
    Devonshire c.
    endemic c.
    episodic c.
    esophageal c.
    flatulent c.
    gallstone c.
    gastric c.
    hepatic c.
    c. impression
    c. impression on liver
    infantile c.
    intestinal c.
    lead c.
    mucous c.
    multiple recurrent renal c.
    c. myoneurosis
    c. omentum
    painter's c.
    pancreatic c.
    c. patch
    c. patch esophagoplasty
    pseudoesophageal c.
    pseudomembranous c.
    renal c.
    saburral c.
    c. sacculation
    saturnine c.
    stercoraceous c.
    ureteral c.
    uterine c.
    vermicular c.
    verminous c.
    wind c.
    worm c.
    zinc c.
colicky abdominal pain
colicoplegia
colicystopyelitis
coliform
    c. bacillus
    c. bacterium
    c. urinary infection
colipase
colipase-dependent lipase
coliplication
colipuncture

Colirest
colistimethate
colistin
colitic
    c. arthritis
    c. mucosa
colitis, pl. **colitides**
    acute infectious c.
    acute self-limited c. (ASLC)
    adaptic c.
    adenovirus c.
    allergic c.
    amebic c.
    antibiotic-associated c. (AAC)
    antibiotic-associated
       pseudomembranous c. (AAPC, AAPMC)
    bacterial c.
    balantidial c.
    Balantidium coli c.
    Behçet c.
    Campylobacter fetus c.
    cathartic c.
    caustic c.
    chronic ulcerative c. (CUC)
    CMV c.
    colectomy ulcerative c.
    collagenous c.
    Crohn c.
    c. cystica profunda (CCP)
    c. cystica superficialis
    cytomegalovirus c.
    diabetic c.
    distal c.
    diversion c.
    drug-induced c.
    eosinophilic c.
    familial ulcerative c.
    focal c.
    fulminant toxic c.
    fulminating ulcerative c.
    gangrenous ischemic c.
    granulomatous transmural c.
    c. gravis
    hemorrhagic c.
    iatrogenic c.
    idiopathic c.
    indeterminate c. (IC)
    infectious c.
    inflammatory c.
    intractable ulcerative c.
    ischemic c.
    left-sided c.
    lymphocytic c.
    microscopic c.
    milk-sensitive c.
    mucosal ulcerative c. (MUC)
    mucous c.
    myxomembranous c.

necrotic hemorrhagic c.
neutropenic c.
nonantibiotic c.
nonspecific c.
pantothenic acid deficiency-induced c.
patchy c.
c. perineal complication
peroxynitrite-induced c.
c. polyposa
progesterone-associated c.
pseudomembranous c. (PMC)
radiation-induced c.
regional c.
Salmonella c.
segmental ischemic c.
sexually transmitted c.
Shigella c.
single-stripe c. (SSC)
toxic c.
transmural c.
tuberculous c.
ulcerative c. (UC)
uremic c.
viral c.
Yersinia enterocolitica c.

colla (*pl. of* collum)
Collaborative Transplant Study (CTS)
collagen
alpha-2-beta-1 integrin cell-surface c.
bovine dermal c.
Contigen glutaraldehyde cross-linked c.
degradation of c.
c. deposition
glutaraldehyde cross-linked c. (GAX)
c. injection
c. maturation
pressure-injected bovine c.
c. synthesis
c. synthesis inhibitor
c. types I–XIII
c. vascular disease

collagenase
interstitial c.

collagenofibrotic glomerulopathy
collagenous
c. colitis
c. sprue

collapse
c. of cavitation bubble
parenchymal c.
collapsed ileum
collapsing
c. FSGS
c. glomerulopathy
collar
Cobb c.
polyglycolic acid c.
preputial c.
ulcer c.
collar-button
c.-b. appearance in colon
c.-b. ulceration
collar-buttonlike ulcer
collateral
c. abdominal circulation
portal azygous c.
vasodilation of portasystemic c.
collecting
c. duct (CD)
c. duct carcinoma
c. system
c. tube
c. tubule
c. venule
collection
American type culture c.
blood c.
duodenal fluid c.
encysted intraabdominal c.
fluid c.
24-hour urine c.
pancreatic fluid c. (PFC)
perinephric fluid c.
peripancreatic fluid c.
pus c.
quantitative stool c.
semen c.
collector
Grass force displacement fluid c.
Misstique female external urinary c.
Colles fascia
colli
cystitis c.
colliculectomy
colliculitis
colliculus, pl. **colliculi**
bulbar c.

NOTES

colliculus *(continued)*
   seminal c.
   c. seminalis
collimator
   high-sensitivity c.
Collin
   C. abdominal retractor
   C. intestinal forceps
   C. intestinal retractor
   C. knife
   C. mesher
   C. tissue forceps
   C. tongue forceps
Collin-Duval intestinal thumb forceps
Collings
   C. electrode
   C. electrosurgery knife
Collins
   C. indigo carmine solution
   C. intracellular electrolyte solution
   C. umbilical clamp
colliquative
   c. diarrhea
   c. necrosis
   c. proteinuria
Collis
   C. antireflux operation
   C. gastroplasty
   C. repair
collision block
Collis-Nissen
   C.-N. fundoplication
   C.-N. gastroplasty
colloid
   c. osmotic pressure
   c. shift on liver-spleen scan
   c. solution
   sulfur c. (SC)
   ^{99m}Tc albumin c.
   ^{99m}Tc sulfur c. (^{99m}Tc SC)
   ^{99m}Tc tin c.
   technetium-99m tin c.
colloidal
   c. bismuth subcitrate (CBS)
   c. bismuth suspension
   c. oatmeal
   c. thorium
colloid-producing adenocarcinoma
collum, pl. **colla**
   c. glandis penis
   c. vesicae biliaris
   c. vesicae felleae
Colly-Seal wafer-type skin barrier
coloanal anastomosis (CAA)
coloboma, heart disease, atresia choanae, retarded growth, genital hypoplasia, and ear abnormalities (CHARGE)
colobronchial fistula
colocalization
colocalized
ColoCARE fecal occult blood test
colocecostomy
colocentesis
colocholecystic fistula
colocholecystostomy
coloclysis
colocolic intussusception
COLO 320 colon cancer cell
colocolonic
   c. anastomosis
   c. fistula
colocolostomy
colocolponeopoiesis
Colocort
colocutaneous fistula
colocystoplasty
   seromuscular c.
colodyspepsia
coloenteric fistula
coloenteritis
colofixation
cologastrocutaneous fistula
Cologel
colography
   computed tomography c.
   CT c.
   magnetic resonance c.
colohepatopexy
coloileal fistula
cololysis
colometrometer
colon
   adenomatous polyp of c. (APC)
   aganglionic segment of c.
   anterior band of c.
   antral diverticulum of c. (ADC)
   c. ascendens
   ascending c.
   c. cancer
   c. cancer resection
   c. cancer screening
   c. carcinoma
   cathartic c.
   c. cauterization
   closed c.
   cobblestoning of c.
   collar-button appearance in c.
   coned-down appearance of c.
   Crohn disease of c. (CDC)
   c. cutoff sign
   c. descendens
   descending c. (DC)
   distal c.
   diverticula of c.
   diverticular disease of c. (DDC)
   endometriosis of c.
   fascia of c.

foreshortening of c.
free band of c.
frenum of valve of c.
gangrenous c.
giant c.
haustra of c.
hepatic flexure of c.
hypoganglionosis of c.
iliac c.
c. impression
c. incarceration
institutional c.
inverted diverticulum of c.
irritable c. (IC)
knuckle of c.
lateral reflection of c.
c. lavage cytology
lead-pipe c.
left c.
longitudinal band of c.
longitudinal fasciculi of c.
loop of redundant c.
c. medial reflection
mesenteric attachments of c.
mesosigmoid c.
midsigmoid c.
c. motility catheter
pelvic c.
perforation of c.
perisigmoid c.
c. procedure
rectosigmoid c.
right c.
saccular c.
sacculation of c.
c. schistosomiasis
sigmoid c.
c. sigmoideum
c. single-stripe sign
spastic c.
spiculation on c.
spike burst on electromyogram of c.
c. splenic flexure
thrifty c.
toxic dilation of c.
c. transit marker study
transverse c.
c. transversum
c. tumor cell lysis
unstable c.
c. urinary conduit

valve of c.
varix of c.
volvulus of c.
watermelon c.

colonalgia
colonic
c. adenocarcinoma
c. adenoma
c. arterial spider
c. bacterium
c. biopsy
c. circular muscle
c. dilation
c. distention
c. diverticulosis
c. diverticulum
c. duplication
c. electromyogram
c. epithelial proliferation
c. explosion
c. fistula
c. flora
c. food
c. foreign body
c. gas
c. hamartoma
c. hemorrhage
c. hyperalgesia
c. ileus
c. inertia
c. infiltration
c. insufflation
c. interposition
c. ischemia
c. J pouch
c. J-pouch reservoir
40-kDa c. antigen
c. lavage
c. lavage solution
c. leiomyoma
c. lesion identification
c. lipoma
c. loop
c. lymphoid nodule
c. manometry
c. mass
c. metaplasia
c. metastasis
c. microflora
c. motility
c. mucosal line
c. mucosal pattern

NOTES

colonic *(continued)*
    c. mucosal surface
    c. myenteric plexus
    c. necrosis
    c. neoplasia
    c. nodular lymphoid hyperplasia
    c. obstruction
    c. obstruction technique
    c. patch
    c. perforation
    c. permeability
    c. pit
    c. pitting
    c. polyp
    c. polyposis
    c. polyposis syndrome
    c. propulsion
    c. prostaglandin
    c. pseudoobstruction
    c. pseudoobstruction syndrome
    c. purge preparation
    c. schistosomiasis
    c. solitary ulcer syndrome
    c. stent
    c. tattoo
    c. transabdominal sonography (CTAS)
    c. transit study
    c. transit test
    c. transit time
    c. trauma
    c. tuberculosis
    c. ulcer
    c. varix
    c. vascular lesion
    c. villus
    c. volvulus
    c. wall
    c. Z stent
colonization
    gut c.
    intestinal c.
    jejunal c.
    stool c.
Colonlite bowel preparation
colonofiberscope
    Olympus CG-P-series c.
colonography
    CT c.
    endoluminal CT c.
    magnetic resonance c. (MRC)
colonopathy, colopathy
    fibrosing c.
colonorrhagia
colonorrhea
colonoscope, coloscope
    ACMI fiberoptic c.
    CF-HM magnifying c.
    CF-LB3R c.
    CF-UHM c.
    CF-200Z Olympus c.
    double-channel c.
    FCS-ML II c.
    fiberoptic c.
    Fujinon EC-130LT c.
    Fujinon EC-200LT c.
    Fujinon EC-410MP c.
    Fujinon EC-300MS c.
    Fujinon FE-100LR c.
    Innoflex variable-stiffness c.
    Machida FCS-ML II magnifying c.
    magnifying c.
    Olympus CF-HM-series magnifying c.
    Olympus CF-MB/LB c.
    Olympus CF-MB-M c.
    Olympus CF-MB-series c.
    Olympus CF24OZI c.
    Olympus CF-PL-series c.
    Olympus CF-P20S fiberoptic c.
    Olympus CF-1T100L c.
    Olympus CF-T-series c.
    Olympus CF-TVL-series c.
    Olympus CF-UHM-series c.
    Olympus CF-UM3 c.
    Olympus CF-VL-series c.
    Olympus CF-200Z c.
    Olympus CV-series c.
    Olympus PCF-100 pediatric c.
    Olympus PCF-130 pediatric c.
    Olympus PCF-series pediatric c.
    Olympus SIF-M magnifying c.
    PCF-140L pediatric c.
    pediatric c.
    Pentax FC-series c.
    Pentax VSB-P2900 pediatric c.
    single-channel c.
    standard c.
    Toshiba TCE-M-series c.
colonoscopic
    c. appendectomy
    c. biopsy
    c. decompression
    c. diagnosis
    c. disimpaction
    c. endoluminal ultrasound
    c. findings
    c. polypectomy
    c. removal
    c. sclerotherapy
    c. study
    c. tattoo
    c. view of adenoma
colonoscopist
colonoscopy, coloscopy
    cecal c.
    c. complication
    diagnostic c.

colonoscopy · colorectostomy

emergency c.
high-magnification c.
magnifying c.
pediatric c.
c. screening
splenic flexure c.
surveillance c.
tandem c. (TC)
c. technique with external straightener
therapeutic c.
total c.
upper endoscopy and c.
urgent c.
Virtual Vision audiovisual system for EGD and c.

colonoscopy-induced hyponatremic encephalopathy
colonoscopy-related
    c.-r. emphysema
    c.-r. incarceration
colonostomy
colony count
colony-forming unit (CFU)
colony-stimulating
    c.-s. factor (CSF)
    c.-s. factor-1 (CSF-1)
colopathy (*var. of* colonopathy)
coloperineal fistula
colopexostomy
colopexotomy
colopexy
Coloplast
    C. bag
    C. closed pouch
    C. conseal plug
    C. drainable pouch
    C. flange minicap
    C. flange pouch
    C. irrigation faceplate
    C. irrigation kit
    C. minipouch
    C. ostomy belt
    C. ostomy irrigation set
    C. skin barrier
    C. skin barrier paste
    C. skin barrier ring
    C. stoma cap
    C. stoma cone
    C. transparent irrigation sleeve
coloplasty pouch
coloplication

coloproctectomy
coloproctia
coloproctitis
coloproctology
coloproctostomy
coloptosis, coloptosia
colopuncture
color
    c. Doppler imaging of ureteral jet into bladder
    c. Doppler ultrasonography
    c. flow Doppler
    c. flow Doppler imaging
    stool c.
    urinalysis c.
    urine c.
color-coded
    c.-c. Doppler sonography
    c.-c. duplex sonography
colorectal
    c. adenocarcinoma
    c. anastomosis
    c. biopsy
    c. cancer (CRC)
    c. cancer screening
    c. cancer syndrome
    c. carcinogenesis
    c. carcinoma (CRC)
    c. disease
    c. endoluminal ultrasound
    c. endometriosis
    c. lymphoma
    c. mass
    c. motility
    c. mucosa
    c. neoplasm
    c. physiologic dysfunction
    c. physiologic study
    c. polyp
    c. resection
    c. snare
    c. stricture
    c. surgeon
    c. surgery (CRS)
    c. trauma
    c. tumor
    c. tumorigenesis
    c. ulcer
    c. variceal bleeding
    c. villous adenoma
colorectal/ovarian (CR/OV)
colorectostomy

NOTES

colorectum
colorimetric detection
Colormate TLc BiliTest System
colorrhagia
colorrhaphy
colorrhea
coloscope (*var. of* colonoscope)
coloscopy (*var. of* colonoscopy)
Coloscreen
    C. Self-test
    C. VPI
Coloshield
colosigmoidostomy
colosigmoid resection
colostomy
    c. bag
    c. bridge
    continent c.
    decompression c.
    descending loop c.
    Devine c.
    diverting loop c.
    divided-stoma c.
    double-barrel c.
    dry c.
    end c.
    end-loop c.
    end-sigmoid c.
    end-to-side ileotransverse c.
    exteriorization c.
    Hartmann c.
    ileoascending c.
    ileosigmoid c.
    ileotransverse c.
    irrigation of c.
    longitudinal c.
    loop transverse c.
    Mikulicz c.
    nonirrigating descending c.
    permanent end c.
    c. pyloric autotransplantation
    resective c.
    c. rod
    sigmoid-end c.
    sigmoid-loop rod c.
    c. soiling
    takedown of c.
    temporary end c.
    terminal c.
    transverse c.
    transverse-loop rod c.
    Turnbull c.
    Wangensteen c.
    wet c.
colosuspension
    Stamey c.
colotomy
    Allingham c.
coloureteral fistula

Colour-Quad-System imaging system
colouterine fistula
colovaginal fistula
colovenous fistula
colovesical fistula
colpocleisis
    Latzko partial c.
colpocystocele
colpocystotomy
colpocystoureterotomy
colpocystourethropexy (CCUP)
colpogram
colpoperineoplasty
colpopexy
    transvaginal sacrospinous c.
colporectopexy
colporrhaphy
colposuspension
    Burch retropubic c.
    laparoscopic needle c.
    laparoscopic retropubic c.
    retropubic c.
colpoureterotomy
column
    anal c.
    butyl-silane extraction c.
    c. chromatography
    C18 Sep-Pack c.
    hemicrypt c.
    c. of Morgagni
    rectal c.
    Sepharose 4B-coupled-protein-A c.
    variceal c.
columna, pl. columnae
    columnae anales
    columnae rectales
    columnae renales
columnar
    c. cuff
    c. cuff cancer
    c. epithelium
    c. metaplasia
    c. mucosa
columnar-cuboidal adenocarcinoma cell
columnar-lined esophagus (CLE)
Coly-Mycin M, S
colypeptic
CoLyte bowel preparation
coma
    acute hepatic c.
    ammoniagenic c.
    electrolyte imbalance c.
    hepatic c.
comatose
CombiDERM nonadhesive absorbant dressing
Combidex
combination
    c. biliary brush catheter

c. calculus
prednisone-colchicine c.
synergistic c.
combined
    c. androgen blockade (CAB)
    c. antegrade and retrograde dilation
    c. chemoradiation therapy
    c. endoscopic sandwich technique
    c. fat- and carbohydrate-induced hyperlipidemia
    c. hemorrhoids
    c. hiatal hernia
    c. intracavernous injection and stimulation test
    c. kidney and pancreas transplant (CKPT)
    c. percutaneous-endoscopic management of perforated esophagus
    c. ureterolysis
comblike redness sign
Combo Cath wire-guided cytology brush
comet sign
Comfeel
    C. Purilon
    C. skin adhesive
    C. skin barrier
Comfort Cath I, II catheter
comfrey
Comhaire grading system
co-mitogen
commensal flora
commercial dialysis solution (CDS)
comminution
    stone c.
common
    c. bile duct (CBD)
    c. bile duct compression
    c. bile duct exploration (CBDE)
    c. bile duct microlithiasis (CBDM)
    c. bile duct obstruction
    c. bile duct stent
    c. bile duct stone (CBDS)
    c. bile duct varix
    c. cavity phenomenon
    c. channel
    c. duct (CD)
    c. duct calculus
    c. duct cholangiogram
    c. duct exploration (CDE)
    c. duct sound
    c. hepatic artery (CHA)
    c. hepatic duct
    c. iliac artery
    c. iliac vein
    c. penile artery
    c. pH electrode
    c. variable immunodeficiency (CVI)
communicating hydrocele
communication
    anomalous pancreaticobiliary c.
    cholangiovenous c.
    horseshoe c.
    pseudocyst c.
communis
    arteria hepatica c.
    ductus hepaticus c.
community
    Ashkenazi Jewish c.
comorbid condition
comorbidity
companion
    C. 2
    C. feeding pump
comparison
    c. of depth of tissue injury
    prospective c.
    c. of rates of appropriate EGD long-term management of patients
compartment
    infracolic c.
    inframesocolic c.
    posterior pararenal c.
    supracolic c.
Compat 199205 enteral feeding pump
compatibility
    in vitro c.
Compazine
Compeed Skinprotector dressing
compendium
    urologic drug c.
compensated
    c. cirrhosis
    c. dysphagia for solid food
compensatory testicular hypertrophy
competent
    c. bowel
    c. ileocecal valve
competition-binding assay
competitive protein-binding assay
Compleat-B liquid feeding
complement
    c. activation

NOTES

complement *(continued)*
    C3a c.
    c. fixation test
    c. hemolytic activity
    c. level
    plasma-activated c. 3 (C3a)
    plasma-activated c. 4 (C4a)
    plasma-activated c. 5 (C5a)
    prostate gland C3 c.
    c. receptor type 1 (CR1)
    c. regulatory protein
    total hemolytic c.
complementary
    c. and alternative medicine (CAM)
    c. deoxyribonucleic acid (cDNA)
    c. DNA
    c. single-stranded antisense riboprobe
complement-dependent cytotoxicity (CDC)
complement-independent autologous phase
complement-mediated
    c.-m. experimental glomerulonephritis
    c.-m. immune glomerular disease
complete
    c. anatomical recovery
    c. blood count (CBC)
    c. blood count test
    c. bowel obstruction
    c. duplication
    c. hormonal blockage
    c. male epispadias
    c. PEG pull
    c. PEG push
    Pepcid C.
    c. repair of bladder exstrophy
    c. replacement PEG
    c. Savary
    c. stone clearance
    c. stone fragmentation
    c. surgical exploration (CSE)
    c. ureteral stricture
    c. urological imaging
completion gastrectomy
complex
    adenylate cyclase c.
    AIDS-related c. (ARC)
    anisoylated plasminogen-streptokinase activator c.
    c. anorectal fistula
    antimajor histocompatibility c.
    avidin-biotin c. (ABC)
    avidin-biotin-peroxidase c.
    calcium-calmodulin c.
    c. calyceal pattern
    Carman-Kirklin meniscus c.
    Carney c.
    CD3-T-cell receptor c.
    c. class II expression
    dorsal vagal c.
    dorsal vein c. (DVC)
    c. enterocele
    epispadias-exstrophy c.
    exstrophy-epispadias c.
    gastroduodenal artery c.
    Golgi c.
    Heymann nephritis antigenic c. (HNAC)
    histocompatibility c.
    c. hypospadias
    IGF-BP3 c.
    inflammatory polyp-fold c. (IPFC)
    interdigestive migrating motor c.
    interdigestive myoelectric c.
    lactase-ceramidase c.
    major histocompatibility c. (MHC)
    membrane-attack c.
    membrane-bound multicomponent enzyme c.
    Meyenburg c.
    migrating motor c. (MMC)
    migrating myoelectric c.
    mitochondrial c.
    muscle-alginate c.
    Mycobacterium avium c.
    nephroblastomatosis c. (NBC)
    OEIS c.
    oligohydramnios c.
    oligometric c.
    c. papillary infolding
    penoscrotal transposition c.
    phagocytic respiratory burst oxidase c.
    polysaccharide-iron c.
    c. reconstructive surgery
    rectal motor c.
    refined carbohydrate c.
    c. renal procedure
    sling-ring c.
    c. stone
    surface membrane actin cytoskeleton c.
    T-cell antigen receptor/CD3 c.
    thrombin-antithrombin III c.
    tuberous sclerosis c. (TSC)
    urobilin c.
    von Meyenburg c. (VMC)
compliance
    bladder c.
    c. of bladder
    detrusor c.
    rectal c.
    vesical c.
complication
    anastomotic c.
    bacterial c.

c. of benign gastric ulcer
benign pneumatic colonoscopy c.
bowel preparation c.
cardiopulmonary c.
cardiorespiratory c.
cardiovascular c.
catastrophic c.
cerebrovascular c.
circumcision c.
colitis perineal c.
colonoscopy c.
cystolitholapaxy experienced c.
endoscopy c.
extraintestinal c.
feeding c.
gastrointestinal c.
hematologic c.
infectious c.
intraoperative c.
laparoscopy c.
metabolic c.
metastatic c.
neurologic c.
opportunistic c.
postbiopsy vascular c.
postoperative c.
potential c.
pouch-specific c.
pulmonary c.
relatively minimal c.
renal c.
sclerotherapy c.
significant reported c.
stent-related c.
urethral reconstruction c.
vascular access c.

component
Knodell c.
lymphoid c.
secretory c. (SC)
serum amyloid P c.
shock wave lithotripsy cavitation c.
suburethral c.
tachykinin c.

composite prosthesis
composition
adrenal gland c.
cystine c.
stone c.
urinary c.
urine c.

compound
bismuth c.
c. cyst
gold c.
guanidino c.
NGD-95-1 antiobesity c.
nitroso c.
tetrapyrrol c.

Compound-65 Pulvules
Darvon C.-65 P.

comprehensive review
compressible cavernous body
compression
abdominal c. (AC)
c. anuria
c. button
c. button gastrojejunostomy
celiac axis c.
common bile duct c.
duodenal c.
esophageal c.
extramural common bile duct c.
extrinsic biliary c.
extrinsic pancreatic c.
gastric c.
mechanical variceal c.
renal venous outflow c.
spinal cord c.
c. syndrome
c. ultrasound (CUS)

compressive base
compressor urethra
compromise
vascular c.

Compro suppository
computed
c. tomodensitometry
c. tomographic angiography (CTA)
c. tomography (CT)
c. tomography arterial portography
c. tomography colography
c. tomography during arterial portography (CTAP, CT-AP)
c. tomography technology

computer-aided
c.-a. ambulatory gastrojejunal manometry
c.-a. diagnostic system

computer-controlled sedation infusion system
computer graphic simulation (CGS)
computerization

NOTES

computerized
    c. dynamic posturography (CDP)
    c. electronic endoscopy
    c. image analysis system
    c. phonoenterography
    c. tomographic hepatic angiography (CTHA)
    c. tomography (CT)
Compu-void
comutagenic
Comvax
ConA, con A
con A/anti-con A perfusion
concealed
    c. hemorrhage
    c. hypospadias
    c. penis
    c. umbilical stoma
    c. vomiting
Concentraid Nasal
concentrate
    bile salt c. (BSC)
    human thrombin c.
    Maalox Therapeutic C.
    therapeutic c. (TC)
concentrated urine
concentration
    albumin plasma c.
    aminothiol c.
    amylase c.
    bile phospholipid c. (BPC)
    blood urea c.
    calcium c.
    chloride c.
    dialysate glucose c.
    endothelin-1 c.
    endothelin-3 c.
    c. epidermal growth factor (cEGF)
    expiratory breath ethanol c.
    extrapolated plasma caffeine c.
    fasting plasma caffeine c.
    fluoroquinolone seminal plasma c.
    hepatic iron c. (HIC)
    hyaluronic acid c.
    hydrogen ion c. (pH)
    mean corpuscular hemoglobin c. (MCHC)
    millimolar c.
    minimal inhibitory c. (MIC)
    phospholipid-bound choline c.
    plasma caffeine c.
    plasma-free choline c.
    plasma gastrin c.
    plasma norepinephrine c.
    plasma renin c.
    plasma urea c.
    predialysis plasma phosphate c.
    renal vein renin c. (RVRC)
    retinol c.
    saturation riboprobe c.
    semen sperm c.
    serum calcium c.
    serum ferritin c.
    sodium butyrate c.
    spermatozoon c.
    subsaturation riboprobe c.
    testosterone plasma c.
    thyroid hormone serum c.
    timed average urea c. (TACurea)
    total homocysteine plasma c.
    total protein c.
    urinary c.
    urine c.
concentric
    c. hyaline inclusion
    c. needle
    c. needle electrode
concept
    evolving c.
    exudate-transudate c.
    Valsalva leak-point pressure c.
conceptus
    c. dose
    C. Robust guidewire
    C. Soft Seal cervical catheter
    C. Soft Torque uterine catheter
    C. VS catheter
concern
    Rating Form of Inflammatory Bowel Disease Patient C.'s (RFIPC)
concomitant
    c. antireflux surgery
    c. disease
    c. hypertension
    c. medication effect
    c. prolapse
concrement
concretion
    bile c.
    fecal c.
    intestinal c.
concurrent hepatic laceration
concussion
    hydraulic abdominal c.
condition
    acid-peptic c.
    comorbid c.
    c.'s of impaired sodium transport
    intersex c.
    pathological hypersecretory c.
    pathophysiology of c.
    physiological c.
    urologic c.
conditioning
    c. film
    c. film deposition
    interceptive c.

conditioning · congenital

semantic c.
c. therapy
condom
   c. catheter
   c. catheter endoscopic ultrasound
   female c.
   c. urinal
conductance
   potassium c.
   selective paracellular c.
   urethral electrical c.
conducted current
conduction defect
conductivity
   electrical c.
conduit
   antirefluxing colonic c.
   Bricker ileal c.
   colon urinary c.
   cutaneous appendiceal c.
   ileal urinary c.
   jejunal urinary c.
   Malone c.
   Mitrofanoff c.
   nonrefluxing colon c.
   sigmoid c.
   urinary c.
   Yang-Monti c.
condyloma, pl. **condylomata**
   c. acuminatum
   anal c.
   flat c.
   c. latum
   perianal c.
   pointed c.
condylomatosis
Condylox
cone
   c. biopsy
   Coloplast stoma c.
   hard sonolucent plastic c.
   Stone C.
   vaginal c.
coned cecum
coned-down appearance of colon
cone-shaped cecum
cone-tip catheter
confidence
   c. interval (CI)
   c. ring
configuration
   bird-beak c.
   cartwheel c.
   golf-hole c.
   horseshoe c.
   laparoscopy trocar c.
   pouch c.
   rat-tail c.
   W-pouch c.
confluence
confluent hepatic necrosis
confocal laser scanning microscopy
conformal radiation therapy
congenital
   c. adrenal hyperplasia (CAH)
   c. bifid bladder
   c. bilateral absence of vas deferens (CBAVD)
   c. biliary atresia
   c. biliary cyst
   c. bladder diverticulum
   c. chloride diarrhea
   c. chordee
   c. cloaca
   c. cystic disease
   c. cystosis
   c. diaphragm
   c. diaphragmatic hernia
   c. diverticulosis
   c. double kidney
   c. duodenal atresia
   c. enterocele
   c. enterocyte heparan sulphate deficiency
   c. epispadias
   c. esophageal stenosis
   c. hepatic fibrosis (CHF)
   c. hydrocele
   c. hyperbilirubinemia
   c. hypertrophic pyloric stenosis
   c. hypertrophy of retinal pigment epithelium (CHRPE)
   c. hypoplasia
   c. intestinal aganglionosis (CIA)
   c. lactic acidosis
   c. malrotation of gut
   c. megacolon
   c. mesoblastic nephroma
   c. nephrogenic diabetes insipidus (CNDI)
   c. nephrosis
   c. nephrotic syndrome (CNS)
   c. penile curvature
   c. penile deviation (CPD)

NOTES

congenital (continued)
- c. polycystic disease (CPD)
- c. portacaval shunt
- c. pyloric membrane
- c. pyloric stenosis
- c. pylorospasm
- c. renal artery aneurysm
- c. renal lymphangiectasia
- c. renal mass
- c. sodium diarrhea (CSD)
- c. splenic cyst
- c. splenomegaly
- c. ureteral stricture
- c. ureteropelvic junction obstruction
- c. urethral stricture
- c. urethroperineal fistula
- c. urethrorectal fistula
- c. urologic abnormality
- c. uropathy

congenitally altered anatomy

congenitum
- megacolon c.

congested
- c. kidney
- c. mucosa

congestion
- active c.
- hepatic c.
- passive c.
- renal c.

congestive
- c. cirrhosis
- c. heart failure
- c. hepatomegaly
- c. hypertensive gastropathy
- c. splenomegaly

Congo
- C. red dye
- C. red stain

congolense
- *Trypanosoma c.*

congophilic material

congruent grade A study

conical
- c. catheter
- c. cecum
- c. centrifuge tube
- c. glans
- c. trocar

conical-tip electrode

conjoined
- c. fiber bundle
- c. tendon

conjugate
- bilirubin ester c.
- bilirubin protein c.
- goat antirabbit HRP c.
- xenobiotic glutathione c.

conjugated
- c. bile acid
- c. bilirubin
- c. estrogen (CE)
- c. hyperbilirubinemia
- c. linoleic acid (CLA)

conjunctival
- c. erythema
- c. icterus

connecting tubule

connective
- c. tissue
- c. tissue disease
- c. tissue disorder
- c. tissue-type mast cell (CTMC)

connector
- Luer-Lok c.
- T c.
- Tuohy-Borst c.
- wire loop c.
- Y-port c.

Connell
- C. incision
- C. stitch
- C. suture

connexin 43

conniventes
- valvulae c.

Conn syndrome

conorii
- *Rickettsia c.*

Conradi line

Conray 60, 70, 280 contrast material

conscious sedation

Conseal
- C. one-piece continent colostomy system
- C. ostomy irrigation set

consecutive asymptomatic patients

consensual reflex

consensus interferon (CIFN)

consequence
- metabolic c.'s

conservation
- VP4 protein c.

conservatively
- managed c.

conservative management

conserved helix-loop-helix ubiquitous kinase (CHUK)

consideration
- transplant c.

consistency
- doughy c.

consortial approach

consortium
- Pediatric Peritoneal Dialysis Study c.

constant
    c. infusion excretory urogram (CIXU)
    Michaelis c. (Km)
Constene
constipated
constipation
    antepartum c.
    atonic c.
    chronic functional c.
    chronic idiopathic c.
    drug-induced c.
    functional c.
    gastrojejunal c.
    geriatric c.
    idiopathic c.
    intractable c.
    outlet obstruction c.
    postpartum c.
    psychogenic c.
    slow-transit c. (STC)
    spastic c.
constipation-predominant irritable bowel syndrome
constitutional
    c. hepatic dysfunction
    c. hyperbilirubinemia
constricting pain
constriction
    mesenteric artery c.
    c. ring
constrictive pericarditis
construction
    Abbe-McIndoe vaginal c.
    ileal reservoir c.
    Lich ureteral implantation for neobladder c.
    neovagina c.
    pelvic ileal reservoir c.
    phallic c.
    sphincteric c.
    U-pouch c.
    vaginal c.
constructional apraxia
consult
    prompt GI c.
consumption
    alcohol c.
    EtOH c.
    salt c.
    whole-cell oxygen c.

contact
    c. bleeding
    cell-cell c.
    c. dermatitis
    c. dissolution
    c. laser vaporization
    c. laser vaporization of prostate (CLVP)
    c. laxative
    c. lithotripsy
    c. probe
contact-tip laser system
contagiosum
    giant molluscum c.
    molluscum c.
container
    Safe-T-Flex enteral feeding c.
contamination
    fecal c.
    c. of food
    postautoclave c.
    c. of water
contemporary urologic armamentarium
content
    abdominal c.'s
    bowel c.
    brain myoinositol c.
    gastric c.
    hepatic malondialdehyde c.
    intestinal c.
    luminal c.
    mucosal hexosamine c.
    renocortical malondialdehyde c.
    reticulocyte hemoglobin c.
    total glutathione c.
contexture analysis
Contigen
    C. Bard collagen implant
    C. glutaraldehyde cross-linked collagen
contiguity
    appendicitis by c.
contiguous loop
Contimed II pelvic floor muscle monitor
continence
    diurnal c.
    fecal c.
    c. nipple
    c. ring
    satisfactory c.
    urinary c.

NOTES

continence-preserving resection
continent
   c. abdominal wall stoma
   c. anal cap
   c. cateterizable appendicovesicostomy using Mitrofanoff principle
   c. catheterizable urinary diversion
   c. colostomy
   c. cutaneous appendicocystostomy
   c. cutaneous diversion
   c. cutaneous reservoir
   c. ileal reservoir
   c. ileal reservoir catheterization pouch
   c. ileostomy
   c. ileovesicostomy
   c. of stool
   c. supravesical bowel urinary diversion
   c. valve
   c. vesicostomy
continuity
   bowel c.
   small bowel c.
   urinary c.
continuous
   c. ambulatory infusion
   c. ambulatory peritoneal dialysis (CAPD)
   c. arteriovenous hemodiafiltration (CAVHDF)
   c. arteriovenous hemodialysis (CAVHD)
   c. arteriovenous hemofiltration (CAVH)
   c. arteriovenous hemofiltration with dialysis
   c. arteriovenous ultrafiltration (CAVU)
   c. bladder drainage
   c. bladder irrigation (CBI)
   c. catheter drainage
   c. cycler-assisted peritoneal dialysis
   c. cycling peritoneal dialysis (CCPD)
   c. drip feeding
   c. erythropoiesis receptor activator (CERA)
   c. hypothermic pulsatile perfusion
   c. incontinence
   c. infusion chemotherapy
   c. murmur
   c. NG suction
   c. prophylaxis
   c. pullthrough technique
   c. renal replacement therapy (CRRT)
   c. suction drainage
   c. suture
   c. venovenous hemodiafiltration (CVVHDF)
   c. venovenous hemodialysis (CVVHD)
   c. venovenous hemofiltration (CVVH)
continuous-flow
   c.-f. fluorometer
   c.-f. resectoscope
continuously perfused probe
ContiRing
contour
   c. ERCP cannula
   isodose c.
   sawtooth irregularity of bowel c.
contraception
contraceptive
   c. device
   c. pill-induced cholestasis
contractile
   c. apparatus
   c. ring dysphagia
   c. stricture
contractility
   normal detrusor c.
   ureter c.
contraction
   alcohol-induced extracellular volume c.
   anal sphincter c.
   bladder involuntary c.
   clonic c.
   crural c.
   detrusor c.
   fat-induced gallbladder c.
   gallbladder c.
   giant migrating c. (GMC)
   high-amplitude c. (HAPC)
   hourglass c.
   hunger c.'s
   isotonic c.
   paradoxical puborectalis c.
   peristaltic c.
   phase II c.
   phasic c.
   primary c.
   propagated antroduodenal c.
   propagation of c.
   reflex detrusor c.
   ringlike c.
   secondary c.
   sliding filament model of c.
   slow phasic c.
   sustained detrusor c.
   tertiary c.
   tonic c.
   voluntary sphincter c.
contraction-relaxation cycle

Contractubex gel
contracture
    bladder neck c.
    Dupuytren c.
    postinflammatory c.
    severe recurrent bladder neck c.
contradictory result
contraindication
    c. to circumcision
    laparoscopy c.
Contrajet ERCP contrast delivery system
contralateral
    c. reflux
    c. testicular biopsy
contrast
    c. agent
    barium enema with air c.
    c. chromoscopy using indigo carmine (CCIC)
    Cysto Conray c.
    dilute iodinated c.
    double c.
    dynamic c.
    c. enema
    c. enhancement
    c. esophagography
    c. esophagram
    c. filling
    c. fluid
    c. medium
    c. selective cholangiogram
    Solutrast 300 c.
    water-soluble c.
contrast-associated renal failure
contrast-enhanced
    c.-e. computed tomography
    c.-e. endoscopic ultrasonography (CE-EUS)
    c.-e. fast sequence (CE-FAST)
contrast-induced renal failure
control
    androgen gonadotropin feedback c.
    baseline recovered c.
    beta-2 microglobulin c.
    bleeding c.
    c. bridle
    electronic pain c.
    endoscopic c.
    fluoroscopic c.
    foot pedal suction c.
    gender-matched c.
    c. glucose
    hemorrhage c.
    c. level
    neural c.
    pain c.
    symptom c.
controlled
    c. expansion (CX)
    c. radial expansion (CRE)
controller
    Actis venous flow c. (VFC)
conus medullaris
ConvaTec
    C. Active Life stoma cap
    C. colostomy pouch
    C. Durahesive Wafer ostomy
    C. Little One Sur-Fit pouch
    C. Sur-Fit two-piece pouch
convection
convective transport
conventional
    c. concentric electromyography
    c. cystoscopy
    c. hemodialysis
    c. static scanner
    c. stent
    c. treatment
    c. upper esophagogastroduodenoscopy (C-EGD)
Converspaz
convertase
    C3 c.
convexity
convex margin
convolution
    entire distal c.
ConXn
COOH-terminal SH2 domain
Cook
    C. biopsy gun
    18F C. Enforcer
    3.2F C. N-Circle tipless stone basket
    C. plastic Luer Lok adapter
    C. rectal speculum
    C. stent
    C. tissue morcellator
    C. TPN catheter
    C. urological trocar
Cooke-Apert-Gallais syndrome
coolant

NOTES

cooled
- c. antenna zone
- c. catheter transurethral microwave thermotherapy
- c. catheter TUMT
- C. ThermoCath treatment catheter

cooler

cooling
- external c.
- homogenous c.
- ice c.
- immersion c.
- nerve c.
- perfusion c.
- surface c.
- transarterial perfusion c.
- urethral c.
- whole body c.

cool-temperature hemodialysis
Coomassie brilliant blue technique
Coombs test
Coons/Carey endoprosthesis
Coons guide
Cooper
- C. hernia
- C. herniotome
- C. irritable testis
- C. ligament
- C. ligament hernioplasty
- C. ligament sling

cooperi
- fascia propria c.

coordination
- R-wave c.

COPD
- chronic obstructive pulmonary disease

Cope
- C. crushing clamp
- C. loop nephrostomy catheter
- C. loop nephrostomy tube
- C. modification of Martel intestinal clamp
- C. sign
- C. viscerotomy anchor
- C. wire

Copegus
copious irrigation
copolymerized substrate
copper
- c. colic
- c. deficiency
- c. nephropathy

copper-binding
- c.-b. protein (CBP)
- c.-b. protein test

copper-deficiency anemia
copracrasia
copremesis
Coprinus **mushroom**

coproantibody
Coprococcus
coprolith
coproma
coproplanesia
coproporphyria
- erythropoietic c.
- hereditary c. (HCP)
- variegate c.

coproporphyrin
coprostasis
coracidium
coral calculus
Corbus disease
cord
- Billroth c.
- c. bladder
- genital c.
- gubernacular c.
- hepatic c.
- hepatocytic c.
- c. hydrocele
- inguinal c.
- lipoma of c.
- microsurgical denervation of spermatic c.
- nephrogenic c.
- palpable c.
- S c.
- spermatic c.
- c. structure
- tethered spinal c.
- tunic of spermatic c.
- umbilical c.
- vocal c.

Cordis-Hakim shunt
corditis
Cordonnier
- C. technique ureterocolonic anastomosis
- C. ureteroileal loop

cordotomy
core
- chylomicron c.
- c. needle biopsy
- c. temperature
- c. of tumor

core-cut system
CoreTherm high-energy device
core-through optical urethrotomy
Corflo
- C. enteral feeding tube
- C. PEG tube
- C. percutaneous access catheter

Corgard
Cori
- C. cycle
- C. disease

coring
    c. out
    uterine c.
coring-out procedure
Corinthian stent
corkscrew
    c. appearance
    c. esophagus
Corlopam
corneae
    Vittaforma c.
corneal
    c. foreign body
    c. reflex
    c. ulcer
Cornelia de Lange syndrome
corner
    c. suture
    C. tampon
cornerstone immunosuppressant
cornflake esophageal motility test
cornstarch-rich diet
cornucopia
    sinusoidal endothelium c.
corona, pl. **coronae**
    c. glandis penis
    c. radiata
coronal
    c. adhesion
    c. epispadias
    c. hypospadias
    c. slice
    c. sulcus
coronary
    c. artery disease
    c. azygos
    cafe c.
    c. ligament
    c. sinus
coronavirus
Coronavirus **gastroenteritis**
Corpak
    C. feeding tube
    C. weighted-tip self-lubricating tube
corpora (*pl. of* corpus)
corporal
    c. biopsy
    c. plication procedure
    c. rotation procedure
corporeal
    c. aspiration
    c. fibrosis

    Nesbit c.
    c. reconstruction
    c. sinusoid
    c. venoocclusive dysfunction
corporoplasty
    incisional c.
    modified Essed-Schroeder c.
corporotomy
corpus, pl. **corpora**
    corpora amylacea
    c. callosum agenesis
    c. cavernosum biopsy
    c. cavernosum dilation
    c. cavernosum muscarinic receptor
    c. cavernosum papaverine injection
    c. cavernosum penile electromyography
    c. cavernosum tunica covering
    c. epididymidis
    c. gastricum
    c. gastritis
    Highmore c.
    c. Highmori
    c. pancreatis
    c. spongiosum
    c. spongiosum fibrosis
    c. spongiosum hypoplasia
    c. spongiosum penis
    c. ventriculare
    c. ventriculi
    c. vesicae biliaris
    c. vesicae felleae
    c. wolffi
corpuscle
    Jaworski c.'s
    juxtamedullary renal c.
    malpighian c.'s
    pacinian c.
    renal c.'s
Correa classification
correction
    chordee c.
    Yates c.
Correctol
correlation
    Pearson product c.
    significant c.
    Spearman rank c.
Corrigan pulse
corrosive
    c. esophageal stricture

NOTES

corrosive *(continued)*
    c. esophagitis
    c. gastritis
Corson
    C. needle
    C. needle electrosurgical probe
Cortef
Cortenema retention enema
cortex, pl. **cortices**
    aberrant suprarenal c.
    adrenal c.
    fetal adrenal c.
    c. glandulae suprarenalis
    kidney c.
    renal c.
    total measured renal c.
Corticaine
cortical
    c. abscess
    c. adenoma
    c. arch
    c. collecting duct (CCD)
    c. collecting tubule
    c. interstitial volume fraction
    c. labyrinth
    c. loss
cortices (*pl. of* cortex)
corticoadenoma
    adrenal c.
corticoadrenal
    renal c.
corticomedullary
    c. demarcation
    c. differentiation
    c. junction
corticosteroid
    c. regulation of amiloride-sensitive sodium channel subunit
    c. therapy
    c. treatment
corticotropin
corticotropin-releasing hormone (CRH)
Cortifoam
cortisol
    c. hypersecretion
    c. metabolism
    plasma c.
    urinary c.
cortisone acetate
Cortisporin
Cortone Acetate
Cortrophin-Zinc
Cortrosyn stimulation test
corymbifera
    Absidia c.
    Mucor c.
Corynebacterium
    C. minutissimum
    C. parvum
    C. tenuis
cosecreted cation
cosine curve
cosinor analysis
cosinor rhythmometry
Cosmegen
cosmesis
cost
    c. effective
    c. of therapy
costal margin
COSTART
    Coding Systems for a Thesaurus of Adverse Reaction Terms
        COSTART system
cost-conscious healthcare system
cost-effective care
Costello
    C. laser ablation of prostate
    C. protocol
costive
costiveness
costochondral
    c. junction
    c. tenderness
costocolic fold
costophrenic blunting
costovertebral
    c. angle tenderness (CVAT)
    c. ligament
    c. sulcus
cosyntropin stimulation test
Cotazym-S
cotransporter
    c. mRNA
    NA+-glucose c.
    taurine c. (TCT)
Cotrim
cotrimoxazole
cotton
    C. cannulatome
    C. classification
    Oxycel c.
    C. sphincterotome
    c. suture
    c. swab test
Cotton-Huibregtse double pigtail stent
Cotton-Leung biliary stent
cottonseed oil
cotton-tipped applier
cotton-wool spot (CWS)
coudé catheter
cough stress test
Couinaud classification
Coulter automated autoanalyzer
Coumadin
coumarin
    c. dye laser

c. flashlamp-pumped pulsed-dye laser
c. green tunable dye laser lithotripsy
coumestrol
Councill catheter
Councilman
  C. body
  C. lesion
Council-tip tube
count
  Addis c.
  CD4 lymphocyte c.
  CD8 lymphocyte c.
  CD4+ T-cell c.
  cell c.
  colony c.
  complete blood c. (CBC)
  granulocyte c.
  hemolysis, elevated liver enzymes, and low platelet c. (HELLP)
  instrument c.
  lymphocyte c.
  mitosis c.
  needle c.
  peripheral leukocyte c.
  c.'s per minute (cpm, CPM)
  platelet c.
  red blood cell c.
  sponge c.
  too numerous to c. (TNTC)
  white blood cell c. (WBC)
  whole crypt mitotic c.
counter
  LKB-Wallac scintillation c.
  RackBeta scintillation c.
countercurrent
  c. exchange
  c. mechanism
  c. multiplication
  c. multiplier
  c. multiplier principle
counterirritation
counterstaining
  sequential c.
countertransporter
  sodium-lithium c. (SLC)
coup de sabre
coupling
  capacitive c.
  electromechanical c.
  excitation-contraction c.

pharmacomechanical c.
slow wave c.
c. stoichiometry
Courtney
  deep postanal space of C.
  C. space
Courvoisier
  C. gallbladder
  C. gastroenterostomy
  C. law
  C. sign
Courvoisier-Terrier syndrome
couvade syndrome
Couvelaire ileourethral anastomosis
cover
  Foxy Pouch c.
  laparotomy pad c.
  Nu-Hope pouch c.
  pad c.
  Sur-Fit Pouch c.
covered
  c. biliary metal stent
  c. self-expanding prosthesis
covering
  Camwrap plastic c.
  corpus cavernosum tunica c.
  Permalume c.
Cowan 1 strain
Cowden
  C. disease
  C. syndrome
Cowdry type A inclusion body
Cowen sign
Cowper
  C. cyst
  C. gland
  C. syringocele
cow's
  c. milk allergy (CMA)
  c. milk protein allergy
  c. milk-sensitive enteropathy (CMSE)
COX
  cyclooxygenase
  COX enzyme system
  COX mRNA
COX-1, -2
  cyclooxygenase-1
  COX-1, -2 enzyme
  COX-1, -2 inhibition
COX-2
  cyclooxygenase-2

NOTES

COX-2 *(continued)*
    COX-2 inhibitor
    COX-2 selective nonsteroidal antiinflammatory drug
Coxiella burnetii
Cox-Mantel test
Cox regression model
coxsackievirus infection A, B
CP
    chronic pancreatitis
    chronic pyelonephritis
        CP test
CPA
    cyproterone acetate
CPC
    choroid plexus cyst
CPD
    congenital penile deviation
    congenital polycystic disease
CP-EUS
    catheter probe-assisted endoluminal ultrasonography
CPH
    chronic persistent hepatitis
CPH-CAH cirrhosis
CPK
    creatine phosphokinase
C-plasty
cpm, CPM
    counts per minute
CPN
    celiac plexus neurolysis
    chronic pyelonephritis
    cisplatin nephropathy
        EUS CPN
CPP
    cerebral perfusion pressure
CPPS
    chronic pelvic pain syndrome
    chronic prostate pain syndrome
    chronic prostatitis/pelvic pain syndrome
CR1
    complement receptor type 1
CR103
    OncoScint CR103
CR49
    RIGScan CR49
cracker test
cradle
    acoustically transparent c.
Crafoord thoracic scissors
Cragg
    C. Endopro System I stent
    C. thrombolytic brush
cramp
crampy abdominal pain
cranial
    c. mesonephros
    c. pole

craniocaudal
Cranley phleborrheograph
crapulent colic
crapulous diarrhea
crassi
    folliculi lymphatici solitarii intestini c.
crater
    ulcer c.
Crawford clamp
CR Bard Urolase
CR-BSI
    catheter-related bloodstream infection
CRC
    colorectal cancer
    colorectal carcinoma
CRCC
    cystic renal cell carcinoma
Crcl *(var. of* CC*)*
    creatinine clearance
CRE
    controlled radial expansion
        CRE balloon catheter
C-reactive protein (CRP)
cream
    Analpram-HC anorectal c.
    Ca-Rezz moisture barrier c.
    Dermovate c.
    lidocaine-prilocaine c.
    Prudoxin c.
    rectal c.
    Sween C.
    Topicort C.
    triamcinolone c.
crease
    inguinal c.
    midline abdominal c.
    skin c.
    torso c.
creatine phosphokinase (CPK)
creatinine
    c. clearance (Crcl)
    c. height index (CHI)
    plasma c.
    pretreatment serum c.
    c. production
    serum c. (SCr)
    c. test
    urinary albumin to c. (UA/C)
creation
    diverting stoma c.
    Politano-Leadbetter tunnel c.
    tunnel c.
creatorrhea
Credé maneuver
^{51}Cr-EDTA
    51-chromium-labeled ethylenediaminetetraacetate
        ^{51}Cr-EDTA excretion

creep
    ureter c.
creeping of mesenteric fat
Creevy evacuator
CREG
    crossreactive group
cremaster
    Henle internal c.
    c. muscle
cremasteric
    c. artery
    c. fascia
    c. fiber
    c. muscle
    c. reflex
    c. vessel
Cremer-Ikeda papillotome
cremnocele
crenate margin
Creon 10, 20
crepitus
crescendo-decrescendo
crescendoing bowel sounds
crescent
    c. fold
    c. gastric cardia
    glomerular c.
    c. snare
crescentic
    c. body
    c. fold disease
    c. glomerulonephritis
    c. nephritis
C-resistance
Crespo operation
CREST
    calcinosis cutis, Raynaud phenomenon, esophageal motility disorder, sclerodactyly, and telangiectasia
    CREST syndrome
crest
    cupula of ampullary c.
    c. factor
    haustral c.
    iliac c.
    jejunal c.
    urethral c.
Creutzfeldt-Jakob disease
crevicular fluid
CRF
    chronic renal failure

CRH
    corticotropin-releasing hormone
CRI
    chronic renal insufficiency
CRIB
    Clinical Risk Index for Babies
cricoid
    c. aneurysm
    c. myotomy
cricomyotomy
cricopharyngeal
    c. achalasia
    c. bar
    c. diverticulum
    c. myotomy
    c. spasm
    c. sphincter
cricopharyngeus muscle
cri du chat syndrome
Crigler-Najjar
    C.-N. disease
    C.-N. jaundice
    C.-N. syndrome type I, II
Crile
    C. angle retractor
    C. appendix clamp
    C. bile duct forceps
    C. gall duct forceps
    C. hemostat
    C. hemostatic clamp
    C. malleable retractor
    C. nerve hook
Crile-Wood needle holder
criminal nerve
crinogenic
crisis, pl. **crises**
    abdominal c.
    Addison c.
    adrenal c.
    Dietl c.
    gastric c.
    scleroderma renal c.
crista
    c. urethralis
    c. urethralis masculinae
    c. urethralis virilis
cristate margin
criteria
criterion
    Amsterdam c.'s
    Bosniak c.'s

NOTES

criterion *(continued)*
- Child classification of hepatic risk c.'s A–C
- Child liver c.'s
- Child-Pugh c.'s
- clinicobiological c.'s
- DeMeester c.'s
- evidence-based c.'s
- Foley c.'s
- Forrest c.
- Ganau c.
- c. for grading of clinical studies and recommendations
- Harvey and Bradshaw c.
- histopathologic c.
- Hogan/Geenen c.
- King's College ALF c.
- Lown c.
- Manning c.
- manometric c.
- morphometric c.
- Munich inclusion c.
- O'Duffy c.
- Pugh modification of Child c.
- Ranson c.
- Rome c. I, II
- Savary-Miller c.
- variceal size inclusion c.
- well-defined anatomical entry c.

critical diarrhea
Criticare HN elemental liquid feeding
CRIT-LINE instrument
Crix belly
Crixivan lithiasis
^{51}Cr-labeled
- ^{51}Cr-l. albumin clearance
- ^{51}Cr-l. EDTA

crochet knot
Crohn
- C. colitis
- C. and Colitis Foundation of America (CCFA)
- C. and Colitis Knowledge (CCKNOW)
- C. disease (CD)
- C. Disease Activity Index (CDAI)
- C. disease of colon (CDC)
- C. Disease Endoscopic Index of Severity (CDEIS)
- C. duodenal ulcer
- C. duodenitis
- C. ileitis
- C. ileocolitis
- C. regional enteritis
- C. small intestine

cromakalim
cromoglycate
- disodium c.
- sodium c.

cromolyn sodium
Cronkhite-Canada syndrome
Crosby capsule
Crosby-Kugler capsule for biopsy
cross
- gastrointestinal c.
- Maltese c.
- c. vasovasotomy

crossbar
- c. deformity
- inner c.
- outer c.
- c. symptom of Frankel

crossbridge
- c. cycle
- dephosphorylated myosin c.
- myosin c.

cross-clamped, crossclamped
Crosseal fibrin sealant
crossed
- c. renal ectopia
- c. testicular ectopia

cross-folding
crosshatch mark
crossmatch
- flow cytometry c. (FCXM)
- T-cell c.

crossmatched blood
crossover
- c. design
- c. vasectomy

cross-phosphorylation
crossreactive group (CREG)
crossreactivity
- direct c.

cross-sectional
cross-section of collecting duct
crosstalk
- receptor c.

cross-trigonal repair
Crotalaria
Croton lechleri
- *Croton lechleri* tree

croupous
- c. cystitis
- c. membrane
- c. nephritis

CR/OV
- colorectal/ovarian
- OncoScint CR/OV
  - OncoScint CR/OV Bcarcinoma localization scintigraphy
  - OncoScint CR/OV carcinoma localization scintigraphy

crowding
- variable nuclear c.

crow's foot pattern
CRP
- C-reactive protein

CRRT
    continuous renal replacement therapy
CRS
    Cell Recovery System
    cherry red spot
    Chinese restaurant syndrome
    colorectal surgery
CRST
    calcinosis cutis, Raynaud phenomenon, sclerodactyly, and telangiectasia
        CRST syndrome
CRT
    chemoradiation therapy
cruciate incision
cruciferous vegetable
crude
    c. cost analysis
    c. drug
    c. incidence rate
    c. urine
cruentes
    vomitus c.
crunch
    mediastinal c.
    c. stick anastomosis
crural
    c. contraction
    c. fold
    c. fossa
    c. vein
    c. venous leakage
crus, pl. **crura**
    c. of diaphragm
    penile c.
    c. penis
    tinea cruris
crush
    c. kidney
    c. syndrome
crusher
crutched
    c. stick-type biliary duct stent
    c. stick-type polyurethane endoprosthesis
Cruveilhier
    C. disease
    C. sign
    C. ulcer
Cruveilhier-Baumgarten
    C.-B. anomaly
    C.-B. cirrhosis
    C.-B. murmur
    C.-B. sign
    C.-B. syndrome
Cruz-Chagas disease
cruzi
    Trypanosoma c.
cryaerophilus
cryoablation
    Endocare renal c.
    c. for prostate cancer
    renal c.
    salvage c.
cryofibrinogenemia
cryogenic ablation
cryoglobulinemia
    essential mixed c.
    mixed essential c.
    type II c.
CryoNeedle
    SeedNet gold ultrathin C.
    C. technology
cryoprecipitate
cryoprecipitated plasma
cryopreservation
    sperm c.
    spermatozoon c.
Cryoprobe
cryoprostatectomy
cryospray
cryostat
    c. tissue
    Tissue Tek-II c.
cryosurgery
cryosurgical
    c. ablation
    c. ablation of prostate (CSAP)
cryotherapy
    endoscopic spray c.
crypt
    c. abscess
    anal c.
    c. architectural distortion
    c. architecture
    c. atrophy
    c. base
    branched c.
    c. cell
    c. cell apoptosis
    c. defensin
    c. epithelium
    forked c.
    c. of Haller
    c. hook

NOTES

crypt *(continued)*
    c. hyperplasia
    c. hypertrophy
    ileal c.
    c. intraepithelial lymphocyte (cIEL)
    Lieberkühn c.
    c. of Littré
    Luschka c.
    Morgagni c.
    mucous c.
    multilocular c.
crypta, pl. **cryptae**
    cryptae mucosae duodeni
Cryptaz
cryptdin
cryptectomy
cryptitis
    neutrophilic c.
cryptococcal pyelonephritis
cryptococcosis
    adrenal c.
    genital c.
    prostatic c.
    renal c.
Cryptococcus neoformans
cryptogenic
    c. chronic hepatitis
    c. cirrhosis
    c. hypertransaminasemia
    c. liver disease
cryptoglandular
cryptolith
cryptorchidectomy
cryptorchidism, cryptorchism
    abdominal c.
    bilateral c.
    canalicular c.
    ectopic c.
    femoral c.
    inguinal c.
    nonpalpable c.
    c. torsion
cryptorchidopexy
Cryptosporidia-**induced diarrhea**
cryptosporidial infection
cryptosporidiosis
    biliary c.
Cryptosporidium
    C. muris
    C. oocyst
    C. parvum
    C. species
crypt-villus
    c.-v. axis
    c.-v. site
    c.-v. unit
crystal
    c. attachment
    c. binding
    Boettcher c.
    $CaCO_3$ c.
    calcium oxalate monohydrate c.
    Charcot-Leyden c.
    cholesterol monohydrate c.
    cystine c.
    c. morphology
    oxalate c.
    phosphate c.
    piezoelectric c.
    quick-dissolving c.
    Reinke c.
    c. retention
    thymol c.
    triple-phosphate c.
    urate c.
    uric acid c.
    urinalysis sediment microscopy c.
    urinary c.
crystal-cell interaction
crystallization
    c. abnormality
    calcium oxalate c.
crystallography
    optical c.
    x-ray c.
crystalloid
    hypertonic c.
    c. solution
crystalluria
crystalluridrosis
crystal-phospholipid interaction
C&S, C+S
    culture and sensitivity
        C&S test
CSAP
    cryosurgical ablation of prostate
CS-5 cryosurgical system
CSD
    congenital sodium diarrhea
CS-9000 densitometer
CSE
    complete surgical exploration
CSF
    cerebrospinal fluid
    colony-stimulating factor
        CSF glucose
        CSF glutamine
        CSF glutamine test
        CSF protein
CSF-1
    colony-stimulating factor-1
CSG
    chronic superficial gastritis
CSI
    cholesterol saturation index
CSM Stretta system
CT
    computed tomography

computerized tomography
   CT colography
   CT colonography
   CT during arterial portography (CTAP, CT-AP)
   helical CT
   renal helical CT (RHCT)
   CT scan
   CT scan with contrast enhancement
   spiral CT
   CT Twin scanner
   unenhanced helical CT

CTA
   computed tomographic angiography

CTAP, CT-AP
   computed tomography during arterial portography
   CT during arterial portography

CTAS
   colonic transabdominal sonography

CTC
   Child-Turcotte classification

Ctenochaetus strigosus

C-terminal propeptide of type I procollagen

CT-guided
   CT-g. abscess drainage
   CT-g. celiac plexus neurolysis
   CT-g. fine-needle aspiration
   CT-g. liver biopsy
   CT-g. needle-aspiration biopsy
   CT-g. PEG
   CT-g. percutaneous endoscopic gastrostomy
   CT-g. pseudocyst drainage

CTHA
   computerized tomographic hepatic angiography

CTL
   cytolytic T lymphocyte
   cytotoxic T lymphocyte

CTL-mediated lysis

CTMC
   connective tissue-type mast cell

CTP
   Child-Turcotte-Pugh
   CTP classification

CTPV
   cavernous transformation of portal vein

C-Trak
   C-T. analyzer
   C-T. handheld gamma detector
   C-T. probe
   C-T. surgical guidance system

^{14}C-triolein breath test

CTS
   Collaborative Transplant Study

C-type
   C-t. atrial natriuretic peptide (C-ANP)
   C-t. natriuretic peptide (CNP)

cube
   Gelfoam c.

cubilin

cuboidal epithelium

Cub R-200 enteral feeding pump

^{13}C-UBT
   carbon-13 urea breath test

CUC
   chronic ulcerative colitis

Cucurbita pepo

cuff
   c. abscess
   AS-800 c.
   bladder c.
   columnar c.
   c. electrode
   rectal muscle c.
   suprahepatic caval c.
   vaginal c.

cuffed
   c. endotracheal tube
   c. esophageal endoprosthesis

cuffitis

cul-de-sac
   c.-d.-s. of Douglas
   c.-d.-s. fluid
   c.-d.-s. mass

culdocentesis

culdoplasty
   McCall c.

culdoscope

culdoscopy

Cullen sign

Culp
   C. spiral flap pyeloplasty
   C. ureteropelvioplasty

Culp-DeWeerd
   C.-D. spiral flap pyeloplasty
   C.-D. ureteropelvioplasty

culture
   aerobic c.
   allogeneic mixed leukocyte c.
   anaerobic c.

NOTES

culture *(continued)*
    bacterial c.
    c. of biopsy specimen
    blood c.
    calculus c.
    fluid c.
    glomerular cell c.
    hanging-drop c.
    c. medium
    mixed growth on c.
    mixed leukocyte c. (MLC)
    semiquantitative c.
    c. and sensitivity (C&S, C+S)
    c. and sensitivity test
    shell vial c.
    stool c.
    tissue c.
    urine c.
    viral c.
cultured rat mesangial
Culturelle
culture-negative neutrocytic ascites (CNNA)
cumulative damage hypothesis
cumulus
Cunningham-Cotton sleeve coaxial dilator
Cunninghamella
Cunningham urinary incontinence clamp
CUOG
    Canadian Urology Oncology Group
cup
    Bard alligator c.
    Bard oval c.
    c. bladder biopsy
    ileostomy c.
    stone c.
    vaginal fistula c.
cup-and-spill stomach
cup-patch technique
Cuprimine
cuprophane membrane
cupula, pl. **cupulae**
    c. of ampullary crest
    gas c.
CUR
    chronic urinary retention
curative tumor resection
curd
    alum c.
^{13}**C-urea**
    synthetic ^{13}C-u.
C-urea breath excretion
curette, curet
    Spratt c.
C-urinary excretion
Curl Cath catheter

curling
    esophageal c.
    1C. ulcer
Curran syndrome
currant jelly stool
Currarino triad
current
    c. algorithm
    blended c.
    coagulating c.
    conducted c.
    cutting c.
    c. density
    electrocoagulating c.
    electrosurgical c.
    high-frequency electrosurgical c.
    membrane c.
    Olympus PSD-10 electrosurgical blend c.
    pure cutting c.
    c. treatment modality
Curschmann disease
curtsy
    Vincent c.
curvatura
    c. gastrica major
    c. gastrica minor
    c. ventriculi major
    c. ventriculi minor
curvature
    congenital penile c.
    penile c.
    c. of stomach
curve
    angulus on lesser c.
    cosine c.
    disease-free survival c.
    gallbladder emptying-refilling c.
    Kaplan-Meier c.
    learning c.
    loss of sigmoid c.
    sigmoid c.
    c. of stream
    time-activity c.
    time-concentration c.
    triphasic cystometric c.
curved
    c. bacillus
    c. dissecting forceps
    c. end-to-end anastomosis (CEEA)
    c. flank position
    c. hemostat
    c. linear-array
    c. Maryland forceps
    c. Mayo clamp
    c. Mayo scissors
    c. transjugular needle
curved-array echoendoscope
curved-needle surgeon's knot

curvilinear scanning echoendoscope
Curvularia lunata
CUS
  compression ultrasound
CUSA
  Cavitron Ultrasonic Surgical Aspirator
  CUSA dissector
Cushing
  C. disease
  C. forceps
  C. medicamentosus syndrome
  C. suture
  C. ulcer
  C. vein retractor
cushingoid facies
Cushing-Rokitansky ulcer
cushion
  air c.
  GasBGon filter seat c.
  hemorrhoidal c.
  partial water bath and water c.
  Positron Plus c.
  c. sign
  tissue c.
Custom Ultrasonic automatic reprocessor
cut
  blended c.
  electrosurgical c.
  field c.
  c. surface of liver
  c. waveform
  c. waveform desiccation
cut-and-push method of PEG tube removal
cutaneobiliary fistula
cutaneous
  c. advancement flap
  c. appendiceal conduit
  c. collateral circulation
  c. dropsy
  c. EGG
  c. electrical field stimulation
  c. electrogastrogram
  c. hemangioma
  c. horn of penis
  c. hyperesthesia
  c. ileocystostomy
  c. lesion
  c. lichen amyloidosis
  c. loop ureterostomy
  c. metastasis

  c. pyelostomy
  c. recording
  c. reflex
  c. schistosomiasis japonica
  c. T-cell lymphoma
  c. urinary diversion
  c. vesicostomy
cutback
  c. anoplasty
  vaginal c.
cutback-type vaginoplasty
cutdown liver
cuticular flap
Cutinova
  C. Cavity
  C. foam
  C. Hydro
  C. Hydro Thin
cutis laxa
cutter
  Endopath endoscopic linear c.
  linear staple c.
  Nu-Hope hole c.
  Proximate linear c.
  rib c.
  suture c.
cutting
  c. current
  c. electrode
  c. endoscopic mucosal resection (C-EMR)
  c. LR needle
  c. wire
CV-1 videoscope
CVAT
  costovertebral angle tenderness
CVF
  cobra venom factor
CVI
  common variable immunodeficiency
CVM
  childhood visceral myopathy
  circular vesicomyotomy
CVP
  central venous pressure
CVS
  clean-voided specimen
  cyclic vomiting syndrome
CVVH
  continuous venovenous hemofiltration
CVVHD
  continuous venovenous hemodialysis

NOTES

CVVHDF
 continuous venovenous hemodiafiltration
CW
 clustered waves
CWS
 cotton-wool spot
CX
 controlled expansion
  CX Plus prosthesis
CXM prosthesis
C282Y
 C282Y hemochromatosis
 C282Y mutation
cyanate
 urea-derived c.
cyanide
 potassium c.
cyanoacrylate
 c. glue
 c. injection
 N-butyl c.
2-cyanoacrylate
 isobutyl 2-c.
***Cyanobacterium*-like body**
cyanocobalamin
 c. injection
 c. radioactive agent
cyanosis
 enterogenous c.
cyanotic kidney
cybernetic regulation of blood pressure
cyclamate
cyclase
 adenylate c. (AC)
 guanylate c.
 guanylyl c.
 ligand-triggered membrane guanylate c.
cycle
 biliary c.
 contraction-relaxation c.
 Cori c.
 crossbridge c.
 cyclin/PCNA during cell c.
 diurnal c.
 gastric c.
 glutathione redox c.
 Krebs c.
 liver-adipose tissue c.
 Schiff biliary c.
 tricarboxylic acid c.
 urea c.
cycler
 Perkin-Elmer 9600 thermal c.
cyclic
 c. adenosine monophosphate (cAMP)
 c. guanosine monophosphate (cGMP)
 c. proteinuria
 c. urinary disinfectant
 c. vomiting
 c. vomiting syndrome (CVS)
5'-cyclic
 5'-c. adenosine monophosphate (cAMP)
 5'-c. guanosine monophosphate (cGMP)
cyclical vomiting
cyclin
cyclin-dependent
 c.-d. kinase (CDK)
 c.-d. kinase inhibitor
cycling dialysis
cyclin/PCNA during cell cycle
cyclizine
cyclobenzaprine
cyclocytidine
Cyclogyl
cycloheximide
cyclohexylchloroethylnitrosurea (CCNU)
cyclooxygenase (COX)
 c. inhibition
 c. inhibitor
 c. messenger ribonucleoprotein acid
 c. metabolite
 c. mRNA
 c. pathway
cyclooxygenase-1 (COX-1, -2)
cyclooxygenase-2 (COX-2)
 c.-2 inhibitor
 c.-2 selective nonsteroidal antiinflammatory drug
cyclooxygenase-dependent mechanism
cyclopentamine
cyclophosphamide
 cisplatin, doxorubicin, c.
 escalated methotrexate, vinblastine, Adriamycin, cisplatin or c. (E-MVAC)
 5-fluorouracil, Adriamycin, c. (FAC)
 c., Velban, actinomycin D, bleomycin, platinum (VAB-VI)
 vincristine, Adriamycin, c. (VAC)
cycloserine
Cyclospora
 C. cayetanensis
 coccidian *C.*
cyclosporine
 c. A-induced hepatotoxicity
 c. arteriolopathy
 c. for microemulsion
 c. nephrotoxicity
 c. toxicity
 c. tubulopathy
 withdrawal of c.
cyclosporine-induced optic neuropathy

Cyclotrac-SP radioimmunoassay
cycrimine
cylinder
    AMA inflatable c.
    AMS 700CX penile prosthesis c.
    banding c.
    Bence Jones c.
    high-pressure inflatable prosthesis c.
    inflated rubber c.
    Mentor Bioflex c.
    suction c.
    Ultrex c.
cylindrical
    c. balloon
    c. confronting cisterna (CCC)
    c. diffuser
    c. mucosal resection
cylindruria
Cymed Micro Skin one-piece drainage pouch
CyPat treatment
cypionate
    c. ester
    testosterone c.
CYP isozyme
cyproheptadine
cyproterone acetate (CPA)
cyst
    adrenal gland c.
    adventitious c.
    air c.
    allantoic c.
    alveolar hydatid c.
    Bartholin c.
    bile duct c.
    biliary c.
    Bowman space c.
    branchiogenous c.
    choledochal c. grades I, II, III, IV, IVa
    choroid plexus c. (CPC)
    chyle c.
    cluster of grapelike c.'s
    CMV inclusion c.
    compound c.
    congenital biliary c.
    congenital splenic c.
    Cowper c.
    daughter c.
    dermoid c.
    duplication c.
    Echinococcus liver c.
    endoscopic management of choledochal c.
    Entamoeba coli c.
    enteric c.
    enterogenous c.
    epidermal c.
    epidermoid c.
    epididymal c.
    esophageal duplication c.
    extramucosal c.
    extraparenchymal renal c.
    false c.
    fatty c.
    c. fenestration
    Gartner duct c.
    gas c.
    gastric duplication c.
    glomerular c.
    granddaughter c.
    grapelike c.
    hepatic echinococcal c.
    hydatid c.
    ileal duplication c.
    inclusion c.
    intraluminal c.
    intratesticular c.
    isolated c.
    junctional c.
    kidney c.
    lucent c.
    macroscopic liver c.
    median raphe c.
    mesenteric c.
    mother c.
    müllerian duct c.
    multilocular c.
    multiloculated c.
    neoplastic c.
    noncommunicating biliary c.
    nonepithelial c.
    nonparasitic splenic c.
    omental c.
    ovarian dermoid c.
    pancreatic c.
    parapelvic c.
    parasitic c.
    paraurethral c.
    parovarian c.
    penile c.
    peripelvic c.
    pilonidal c.
    presacral c.

NOTES

cyst *(continued)*
    prosthetic utricle c.
    c. puncture device
    pyelocalyceal c.
    pyelogenic renal c.
    renal sinus c.
    retention c.
    retrorectal c.
    Rosen c.
    sacrococcygeal pilonidal c.
    scrotum c.
    sebaceous c.
    secondary c.
    seminal vesicle hydatid c.
    simple renal c.
    solitary hepatic c.
    sterile c.
    suburethral epithelial inclusion c.
    tailgut c. (TGC)
    Tarlov c.
    testicular c.
    tunic c.
    tunica albuginea c.
    unicameral c.
    unilocular ovarian c.
    urachal c.
    urethral c.
    urinary c.
    vitellointestinal c.
cystadenocarcinoma
    biliary c.
    pancreatic mucinous c.
    stage III papillary serous c.
cystadenoma
    biliary c.
    ductal c.
    ductectatic mucinous c.
    endoscopic ultrasound-guided ethanol lavage of pancreatic c.
    glycogen-rich c.
    hepatic c.
    mucinous c.
    ruptured appendiceal c.
Cystagon
cystalgia
cystamine
Cysta-Q
cystathionine gamma-lyase
cystatin C
cystatrophia
cystauchenitis
cystauchenotomy
cystauxe
cysteamine bitartrate
cysteamine-induced duodenal ulcer
cystectasia, cystectasy
cystectomy
    palliative c.
    partial c.
    pilonidal c.
    radical c.
    salvage c.
    simple c.
    subtrigonal c.
    supratrigonal c.
    total c.
cysteine
    c. *Brucella* broth
    c. sulfinic acid
cysteinyl leukotriene
cystelcosis
cystendesis
cystenterostome
    diathermic c.
cystenterostomy
    direct c.
    endoscopic c.
cysterethism
cystgastrostomy
    surgical c.
cysthypersarcosis
cystic
    c. artery
    c. bile
    c. cystitis
    c. degeneration
    c. dilation
    c. duct (CD)
    c. duct angiogram
    c. duct catheterization
    c. duct cholangiocatheter
    c. duct cholangiogram
    c. duct cholangiography
    c. duct choledochoscopy
    c. duct leakage
    c. duct lumen
    c. duct stenosis
    c. duct stone
    c. echinococcosis
    c. epithelial proliferation
    c. fibrosis (CF)
    c. fibrosis gene probe
    c. fibrosis transductance regulator
    c. fibrosis transmembrane conductance regulator (CFTR)
    c. hamartoma
    c. liver disease
    c. mass
    c. nephroma
    c. plexus
    c. puncture
    c. renal cell carcinoma (CRCC)
    c. Wilms tumor
cystica
    cholecystitis c.
    cystitis c.
    pyelitis c.
    pyeloureteritis c.

ureteritis c.
urethritis c.
cystic-choledochal junction
cysticercosis
cysticercus
    C. *bovis*
    C. *cellulosae*
    c. disease
cysticohepatic junction
cysticolithectomy
cysticolithotripsy
cysticorrhaphy
cysticotomy
cysticus
    ductus c.
    polypus c.
cystidolaparotomy, cystidoceliotomy
cystidotrachelotomy
cystine
    c. calculus
    c. composition
    c. crystal
    c. dimethylester (CDE)
    c. metabolism
    c. stone
    c. supersaturation
    c. urolithiasis
cystinosis
    neuropathic c.
cystinuria
cystinuric
    c. children
    c. patient
cystis fellea
Cystistat
cystistaxis, cystostaxis
cystitis
    acute hemorrhagic c. (AHC)
    allergic c.
    amicrobic c.
    bacterial c.
    candidal c.
    catarrhal c.
    chemical c.
    coccidioidal c.
    c. colli
    croupous c.
    cystic c.
    c. cystica
    diagnosing interstitial c.
    dimethyl sulfate c.
    diphtheritic c.
    DMSO c.
    c. emphysematosa
    emphysematous c.
    eosinophilic c.
    exfoliative c.
    follicular c.
    c. follicularis
    gangrenous c.
    glandular c.
    c. glandularis
    hemorrhagic c.
    honeymoon c.
    Hunner interstitial c.
    incrusted c.
    interstitial c.
    mechanical c.
    nonbacterial c. (NBC)
    nonulcerative interstitial c.
    panmural c.
    papillary c.
    radiation c.
    recurrent c.
    reservoir of underdiagnosed and misdiagnosed interstitial c.
    c. senilis feminarum
    subacute c.
    submucous c.
    sympathetic c.
    uncomplicated c.
    viral c.
    xanthogranulomatous c.
cystitis-causing strain
Cysto
    C. Conray contrast
    C. Flex stent
    Urovist C.
Cystocath
cystocele
    central c.
    grade 4 c.
    lateral c.
cystochrome
cystochromoscopy
cystocolostomy
cystocolpoproctography
    fluoroscopic c.
cystodiaphanoscopy
cystodiathermy
    flexible c.
cystodistention

NOTES

cystodiverticulum
cystoduodenostomy (CDY)
    endoscopic c.
cystodynia
cystoenterocele
cystoenterostomy
cystoepiplocele
cystoepithelioma
cystofiberscope
    Olympus CYF-3 OES c.
cystofibroma
cystogastric fistula
cystogastrostomy (CGY)
    endoscopic ultrasound-guided c.
cystogastrotome
cystogenic chemical
cystogram
    air c.
    chain c.
    excretory c. (XC)
    gravity c.
    micturating c.
    postvoiding c. (PVC)
    retrograde c. (RC)
    static c.
    stress c.
    surveillance c.
    voiding c. (VCG)
cystography
    antegrade c.
    bead-chain c.
    radionuclide c.
    retrograde c.
    suprapubic c.
    triple-voiding c.
cystohepatic triangle
Cysto-Hypaque
cystojejunostomy
    Roux-en-Y c.
cystolateral pancreatojejunostomy
cystolith
cystolithectomy
cystolithiasis
cystolithic
cystolitholapaxy experienced complication
cystolithotomy
cystometer
    Lewis c.
cystometric
    c. biofeedback
    c. bladder capacity
cystometrogram (CMG)
    filling c.
cystometrographic monitoring
cystometrography
    voiding c.
cystometry
    filling c.
    gas c.

    multichannel c.
    provoked c.
    saline c.
    screening c.
    simultaneous urethral c.
    spontaneous c.
    transballoon c.
    voiding c.
    water c.
cystonephrosis
cystoneuralgia
cystopancreatography
cystopanendoscopy
cystoparalysis
cystopericystectomy
cystoperitoneal shunt
cystopexy
cystophotography
cystophthisis
cystoplasty
    augmentation c.
    autoaugmentation c.
    cecal c.
    flap valve c.
    Gil-Vernet ileocecal c.
    human lyophilized dura c.
    laparoscopic c.
    nonsecretory sigmoid c.
    sigmoid c.
    urinary tract reconstruction augmentation c.
cystoplegia
cystoplelography (*var. of* cystopyelogram)
cystoproctostomy
cystoprostatectomy
    salvage c.
cystoprostatourethrectomy
cystoprostatovesiculectomy
cystoptosis, cystoptosia
cystopyelitis
cystopyelogram, cystoplelography
cystopyelonephritis
cystoradiography
cystorectocele
cystorectostomy
cystoresectoscope
    ALR c.
    anteroposterior c.
    Damon-Julian c.
    Julian c.
cystorrhagia
cystorrhaphy
cystorrhea
cystosarcoma phyllodes
cystoschisis
cystoscope
    Albarran laser c.
    balloon c.

Braasch direct catheterization c.
Braasch-Kaplan direct-vision c.
Brown-Buerger c.
Broyle retrograde c.
Butterfield c.
French c.
InjecTx c.
Judd c.
Kelly c.
Kidd c.
Laidley double-catheterizing c.
Lowsley-Peterson c.
McCarthy-Campbell miniature c.
McCarthy Foroblique panendoscope c.
McCrea c.
Miller c.
Morganstern continuous-flow operating c.
National general purpose c.
Nesbit c.
Olympus fiberoptic c.
Storz c.
Surgitek graduated c.
Young c.

cystoscopic
    c. electrohydraulic lithotripsy
    c. urography

cystoscopy
    conventional c.
    c. and dilation (C&D)
    percutaneous fetal c.
    steerable c.
    virtual c.

cystose, cystous

cystosis
    congenital c.

cystospasm
Cystospaz
Cystospaz-M
cystospermitis
cystostaxis (*var. of* cystistaxis)

cystostomy
    suprapubic c.
    trocar c.
    c. tube

cystotome
    Kelman air c.
    Kelman double-bladed c.
    Kelman knife c.
    Kelman knife-cannula c.
    McIntyre reverse c.
    Mendez ultrasonic c.
    reverse c.

cystotomy
    open c.
    suprapubic c.

cystotrachelotomy
cystoureteritis
cystoureterogram
cystoureterography
cystoureteropyelitis
cystoureteropyelonephritis

cystourethrectomy
    total c.

cystourethritis
cystourethrocele

cystourethrogram
    micturating c.
    micturition c.
    retrograde c.
    voiding c. (VCUG)

cystourethrography
    chain c.
    expression c.
    isotope voiding c. (IVCU)
    micturating c. (MCU)
    radionuclide voiding c.
    voiding c.

cystourethropexy
    laparoscopic c.
    Marshall-Marchetti-Krantz c.
    obturator shelf c.
    Pereyra-Raz c.

cystourethroplasty
    Kropp c.
    Leadbetter c.

cystourethroscope
    ACMI c.
    microlens c.
    O'Donoghue c.
    Wappler microlens c.

cystourethroscopy
    dynamic c.

cystous (*var. of* cystose)

CYT-356 radiolabeled with 111 indium chloride
Cytadren
cytarabine
Cytocare Prolase II
cytocentrifuge
    c. preparation
    c. set

cytochalasin B

NOTES

cytochrome
    b558 membrane-bound c.
    c. P450
    c. P450 enzyme
    c. P450 enzyme system
    c. P450 metabolite
cytochrome-*c* oxidase deficiency
cytodiagnosis
CytoGam
cytogenetic analysis
cytokeratin
    bile duct-type c.
    hepatocyte-type c.
    c. staining
cytokine
    c. antagonist
    antiinflammatory c.
    fibrogenic c.
    fibrosis-promoting c.
    c. gene expression
    GM-CSF c.
    c. profile
    proinflammatory c.
    c. therapy
    c. tumor necrosis factor-alpha
cytologic
    c. biopsy
    c. brushing
    c. diagnosis
    C. software
    c. specimen
cytology
    aspiration biopsy c.
    balloon c.
    brush c.
    c. brush
    colon lavage c.
    endoscopic brush c.
    endoscopic retrograde c.
    endoscopic transesophageal fine-needle aspiration c.
    c. examination
    exfoliative c.
    fine-needle aspiration c. (FNAC)
    gastric brush c.
    guided-needle aspiration c.
    lavage c.
    needle aspiration c.
    salvage c.
    touch c.
    urine c.
    voiding urine c. (VUC)
    wire-guided c.
Cytolong brush
cytolysis inhibitor
cytolytic
    c. action
    c. therapy
    c. T lymphocyte (CTL)

cytoma
cytomegalovirus (CMV)
    c. colitis
    c. enterocolitis
    c. esophagitis
    c. hepatitis
    c. immune globulin
    c. infection
cytometer
    CAS 200 image c.
    Cell Analysis System 200 image c.
    Dickinson FACS 400-series flow c.
    EPICS C-flow c.
    EPICS Elite flow c.
    EPICS 700-series flow c.
    EPICS V-flow c.
    FACScan flow c.
cytometric
    c. analysis
    c. pattern
cytometry
    deoxyribonucleic acid flow c.
    DNA flow c.
    flow c.
    fluorescence-activated flow c.
    image c.
    static image DNA c.
cytopenia
cytophilic antibody
cytophotometry
    static c.
cytoplasm
    eosinophilic c.
cytoplasmic
    c. adaptor protein
    c. argyrophilia
    perinuclear antineutrophil c. (p-ANC)
    c. staining
    c. urease
cytoprotective prostaglandin
cytoreduction
    ultrasonic c.
cytoreductive
    c. nephrectomy
    c. surgery
Cytosar
Cytoscreen
    C. Human Eotaxin immunoassay
    C. human interferon-gamma ELISA kit
cytosine
    5-methyl c.
cytoskeletal link
cytoskeleton
    prostate gland c.
cytoskeleton-altering toxin
cytosol

cytosolic
    c. calcium
    c. face
cytospin collection fluid
CytoTAb
Cytotec
cytotoxic
    c. agent
    c. antibody
    c. chemotherapy
    c. liver disease
    c. T cell
    c. T-cell response
    c. T lymphocyte (CTL)
cytotoxicity
    antibody-dependent cell-mediated c. (ADCC)
    antibody-dependent cellular c. (ADCC)
    Bartel c.
    cell-mediated c.
    complement-dependent c. (CDC)
    lymphocyte c.
cytotoxin
    c. assay
    c. necrotizing factor
    VacA c.
    vacuolating toxin gene A c.
cytotoxin-associated
    c.-a. gene A (cagA)
    c.-a. gene A protein
Cytoxan
Czerny
    C. rectal speculum
    C. suture
Czerny-Kocher-Perthes incision
Czerny-Lembert suture

NOTES

D
  D cell
  D cell density
  1,25-dihydroxyvitamin D
D3
  dihydroxyvitamin D3
  1,25-dihydroxyvitamin D3
    (1,25(OH)2 D3)
  25-hydroxyvitamin D3 (25(OH)D3)
  I-alpha-hydroxyvitamin D3
  1,25(OH)2 D3
    1,25-dihydroxyvitamin D3
3-D
  three-dimensional
  3-D gadolinium-enhanced MR angiography
  3-D linear endosonography
  3-D sonography
D_4
  leukotriene D_4
D16S283 marker
D16S291 marker
D16S84 marker
D4S231 marker
D4S414 marker
DAB
  diaminobenzidine
dacarbazine
  doxorubicin, bleomycin sulfate, vinblastine, d. (ABVD)
dacliximab
daclizumab
Dacogen
Dacomed
  D. Catalyst VCD
  D. snap gauge
Dacron
  D. interposition graft
  D. mesh
  D. prosthesis
  D. suture
Dacron-impregnated Silastic sheet
DAEC
  diffuse adherent *Escherichia coli*
DAF
  decay-accelerating factor
DAG
  diacylglycerol
  diffuse antral gastritis
  dimeric acidic glycoprotein
Dagradi esophageal variceal classification
DAH
  diffuse alveolar hemorrhage
daidzein

daily
  d. hemodialysis
  d. intermittent peritoneal dialysis (DIPD)
  d. protein intake (DPI)
Dairy Ease chewable tablets
d-ALA
  delta-aminolevulinic acid
Dalalone
  D. D.P.
  D. L.A.
Dale
  D. abdominal binder
  D. Foley catheter holder
DALM
  dysplasia-associated lesion or mass
Dalmane
dalteparin sodium
dam
  rubber d.
damage
  chloroquine-induced d.
  chronic tubular d.
  drug-induced esophageal d. (DIED)
  flucloxacillin-associated liver d.
  gastric mucosal d.
  Graham scale for drug-induced gastric d.
  histologic d.
  hypertensive end-organ d.
  indomethacin-induced mucosal d.
  ischemic tubular d.
  microsomal d.
  oropharyngeal d.
  parenchymal d.
  probable long-term kidney d.
  renal parenchymal d.
  renal structural d.
  results in tissue d.
  tubular d.
Damon-Julian cystoresectoscope
Danazol
Danbolt-Closs syndrome
Dance sign
dandy
  d. fever
  D. nerve hook
Dane particle
Daniel colostomy clamp
Dansac
  D. Karaya Seal one-piece drainage pouch
  D. ostomy irrigation set
  D. skin barrier
  D. Standard Ileo pouch

dansylcadaverine
Dantec
    D. 12-channel Urocolor Video system
    D. Etude uroflow transducer
    D. Menuet system
    D. rotating disk flowmeter
    D. Urodyn 1000 flowmeter
    D. Urodyn 1000 uroflowmeter
danthron
Dantrium
dantrolene sodium
Danubian endemic familial nephropathy
dapsone
daptomycin for injection
darbepoetin alfa
Darbid
Dardik clamp
D-arginine
    enantiomer D-a.
Daricon PB
Darier disease
darifenacin
dark
    d. adaptation study
    d. burgundy blood
    d. concentrated urine
    d. spot
    d. stool
darting incision
dartoic
dartoid
dartos
    d. fascia
    d. muscle
    d. pedicled flap
    d. pouch procedure
Darvocet-N 100
Darvon Compound-65
DASH
    dietary approach to stop hypertension
    DASH ERCP catheter
    DASH extraction balloon
    DASH sphincterotome
    DASH system
    DASH tipless extraction basket
DAT
    diet as tolerated
data
    long-term followup d.
    multiple testing of d.
    paucity of clinical d.
    perioperative d.
    questionnaire d.
    randomized clinical trial d.
    tolerability d.
    volumetric d.
date fever

daughter
    d. cyst
    d. endoscopic retrograde cholangiopancreatoscopy system
    d. nodule
daunorubicin
DaunoXome
Davidoff cell
David rectal speculum
da Vinci Surgical System
Davis
    D. interlocking sounds
    D. intubated ureterostomy
    D. intubated ureterotomy
    D. loop
    D. spatula
    D. technique
Davol
    D. colon tube
    D. feeding bag
    D. feeding tube
    D. sump drain
    D. tunneler
DAWG
    demucosalized augmentation with gastric segment
    DAWG procedure
daycare diarrhea
daytime incontinence
DAZ **gene**
DBCP
    dibromochloropropane
DBP
    vitamin D-binding protein
DBSQ
    Diabetes Bowel Symptom Questionnaire
DBW
    desirable body weight
DC
    descending colon
    dilation catheter
    duodenal cap
    DC locus allelic
DCBE
    double-contrast barium enema
DCC
    deleted in colorectal carcinoma
DCC **gene**
DCGI
    double-contrast barium examination of upper gastrointestinal tract
DCP
    des-gamma-carboxy prothrombin
3-DCRT
    three-dimensional conformal radiation therapy
DCT
    distal convoluted tubule

3-DCTP
three-dimensional CT pancreatography
DD
digestive disease
DD23
DD23 antigen
antigen DD23
DDAVP
deamino-D-arginine-vasopressin
desmopressin
DDAVP nasal spray
DDC
diverticular disease of colon
ddC, ddc
dideoxycytidine
ddI, ddi
didanosine
D-dimer
DDNC
Digestive Disease National Coalition
DDS
Denys-Drash syndrome
DDS-Acidophilus
DDV ligator
DE
duodenal exclusion
de
de novo
de novo autoimmune hepatitis
de novo liver cancer
de novo malignancy
de novo needle-knife technique
de novo renal disease
de Pezzer catheter
de Toni-Debré-Fanconi syndrome
de Toni-Fanconi-Debré syndrome
dead
d. bowel
d. space
DEAE
diethylaminoethyl
deafferentation
deafness
lentigines, electrocardiographic conduction abnormalities, ocular hypertelorism, pulmonary stenosis, abnormal genitalia, retardation of growth, and d. (LEOPARD)
de-air

deaminase
adenosine d.
porphobilinogen d. (PBG-D)
deamino-D-arginine-vasopressin (DDAVP)
Dean
D. stage
D. stage I, II radiation proctitis
death
apoptotic cell d.
circle of d.
hepatocellular d.
ischemic tubular cell d.
liver d.
Deaver
D. incision
D. operating scissors
D. retractor
window of D.
Deaver-type blade
deazaaminopterin
DeBakey
D. clamp
D. forceps
DeBakey-Cooley retractor
Debioclip single-dose delivery system
Debove membrane
debrancher
d. deficiency
d. enzyme
d. glycogen storage disease
Debré-de Toni-Fanconi syndrome
debridement
debris
clots and d.
degenerating cellular d.
purulent d.
stonelike d.
debrisoquin
debulking
percutaneous d.
d. therapy
tumor d.
DEC
diethylcarbamazine
Decadron
decanoate
nandrolone d.
decapacitation factor
Decapeptyl
decapsulation of kidney
decarboxylase
histidine d. (HDC)

NOTES

decarboxylase *(continued)*
    ornithine d. (ODC)
    uroporphyrinogen d. (UROD)
decarboxylation
    amine precursor uptake and d. (APUD)
decay-accelerating factor (DAF)
decerebrate posturing
Decholin
decidualis
    periappendicitis d.
Declomycin
decompensated
    d. alcoholic cirrhosis
    d. liver cirrhosis
    d. neobladder
decompensation
    bladder d.
    detrusor muscle d.
decompression
    abdominal d.
    balloon d.
    biliary d.
    bladder d.
    cardiac d.
    d. catheter
    colonoscopic d.
    d. colostomy
    ductal d.
    endoscopic biliary d.
    gastric d.
    hydrostatic d.
    intestinal d.
    long intestinal tube d.
    nasogastric d.
    operative d.
    palliative d.
    PEG-assisted d.
    percutaneous transhepatic d.
    pericardial d.
    portal d.
    surgical d.
    transduodenal endoscopic d.
    d. tube
    tube d.
    variceal d.
decongestant
decontamination
    selective intestinal d. (SID)
decorin
    proteoglycan d.
decorticate posturing
decortication
    renal cyst d.
decreased
    d. peristalsis
    d. postprandial-to-fasting power ratio
decrescendo

decubitus
    d. calculus
    lateral d.
    d. position
    d. ulcer
dedifferentiate
deep
    d. abdominal ring
    d. artery
    d. breathing
    d. cannulation
    d. cervical fascia
    d. dorsal vein
    d. interloop abscess
    d. jaundice
    d. muscular plexus
    d. pain
    d. perineal space
    d. postanal anorectal space
    d. postanal space of Courtney
    d. tendon reflex
    d. trigone
    d. venous thrombosis
deepithelialization
deepithelialized flap
deep-seated fungal infection
defecate
    urge to d.
defecating proctogram
defecation
    balloon d.
    fragmentary d.
    infrequent d.
    obstructive d.
    painful d.
    d. syncope
defecatory
    d. difficulty
    d. dyschezia
    d. straining
    d. urgency
defecogram
defecography
    FECOM artificial stool for d.
defecometry
defect
    acidemia d.
    acidification d.
    acinar d.
    acquired neutrophil chemotaxis d.
    amorphous filling d.
    bony d.
    chain-of-lakes filling d.
    cobblestone filling d.
    cold d.
    conduction d.
    fascial d.
    fetal alcohol syndrome ureter d.
    filling d.

frondlike filling d.
hernial d.
hot d.
inherited d.
interventricular d.
intraluminal filling d.
intrapelvic filling d.
isolation d.
lobulated filling d.
mesenteric d.
plaquelike linear d.
polypoid filling d.
portal perfusion d.
renal concentrating d.
tailing d.
uterine lateral fusion d.

defensin
crypt d.

deferens
ampulla of vas d.
congenital bilateral absence of vas d. (CBAVD)
ductus d.
ectopic vas d.
vas d.

deferentectomy
deferential artery
deferentis
ampulla ductus d.
diverticula ampullae ductus d.

deferentitis
deferoxamine mesylate infusion test
defervescence
deficiency
acquired lactose d.
adenine phosphoribosyltransferase d.
adult lactase d.
aldosterone d.
alpha-1-antitrypsin d.
17-alpha-hydroxylase d.
amylo-1,6-glucosidase d.
androgen d.
d. anemia
antithrombin III d.
APRT d.
arginase d.
aucrose-isomaltase d.
11-beta-hydroxylase d.
3-beta-hydroxysteroid dehydrogenase d.
bile salt d.
biotin d.

brancher d.
calcium d.
carbamoyl phosphate synthetase d.
ceramidase d.
chromium d.
cobalamin d.
congenital enterocyte heparan sulphate d.
copper d.
cytochrome-*c* oxidase d.
debrancher d.
20,22-desmolase d.
dietary d.
disaccharidase d.
d. disease
enteropeptidase d.
essential fatty acid d. (EFAD)
estrogen d.
familial high-density lipoprotein d.
folate d.
follicle-stimulating hormone d.
fructose aldolase d.
fructose diphosphatase d.
fumarylacetoacetate hydrolase d.
glucose-6-phosphatase d.
glucuronyl transferase d.
gonadotropin-releasing hormone d.
growth hormone d.
hepatic phosphorylase d.
hypoxanthine-guanine phosphoribosyltransferase d.
IgA d.
immune d.
intestinal lactase d.
intrinsic sphincter d. (ISD)
iron d.
lactase d.
long-chain acyl-CoA dehydrogenase d.
magnesium d.
medium-chain acyl-CoA dehydrogenase d.
niacin d.
nutritional d.
ornithine carbamoyl transferase d.
pancreatic lipase d.
PiZZ alpha-1-antitrypsin d.
potassium d.
protein C, S d.
pyridoxal 5′-phosphate d.
riboflavin d.
S-adenosylmethionine d.

NOTES

deficiency *(continued)*
    sodium d.
    sucrose-isomaltase d. (SID)
    testosterone d.
    thiamine d.
    triglyceride enzyme d.
    UDPGT d.
    uridine diphosphate glucuronosyltransferase d.
    vaginal estrogen d.
    vitamin A, D d.
    zinc d.
deficiens
    ejaculatio d.
deficit
    lateralizing sensory d.
    neurologic d.
defined-formula diet
defloration pyelitis
Deflux
    D. injectable gel
    D. injectable implant
    D. system implant
deformability
    hepatic d.
deformans
    peritonitis d.
deformity
    Akerlund d.
    bell-clapper d.
    bulb d.
    chain-of-lakes d.
    cloverleaf d.
    cobra-head d.
    crossbar d.
    duodenal bulb d.
    gross d.
    hourglass d.
    keyhole d.
    limb d.
    nasal d.
    penile d.
    phrygian cap d.
    swan-neck d.
    trefoil d.
    ureterocele cobra-head d.
    Whitehead d.
    Z-type d.
defunctionalization
defunctionalized bladder
defunctioning efficiency
Defyne urethral assist device
degassed water
degenerating cellular debris
degeneration
    acidophilic d.
    acute hepatocellular d.
    Armanni-Ehrlich d.
    ballooning d.
    cystic d.
    feathery d.
    fistulous d.
    hepatocerebral d.
    hepatolenticular d.
    macular d.
degenerative
    d. change
    d. nephritis
degloving
    penile shaft d.
deglutible
deglutition
    d. disorder
    d. mechanism
    d. reflex
deglutitive
    d. inhibition
    d. pharyngeal chamber
deglutitory
Degos
    D. disease
    D. syndrome
degradation
    d. of collagen
    gastric mucosal d.
    haptocorrin d.
    proteolytic d.
degradative enzyme
degranulation
    mast cell d.
degree
    50-d. Foroblique optic laparoscope
    0-d. forward optic laparoscope
    d. of hyperreflexia
    120-d. lens
    d. of objectivity
    10-d. operating laparoscope
dehisced
dehiscence
    abdominal incision d.
    d. of cystic stump
    Killian d.
    staple line d.
    suture line d.
    wound d.
DEHOP
    diethylhomospermine
dehydrated ethanol
dehydration
    absolute d.
    d. fever
    hyperosmotic nonketotic d.
dehydrocholaneresis
dehydroemetine
dehydroepiandrosterone (DHA)
    d. sulfate (DHAS)
dehydrogenase
    alcohol d. (ADH)

aldehyde d. (ALDH)
alpha-ketoacid d.
benzaldehyde d.
beta-hydroxyacyl-coenzyme A d.
3-beta-hydroxysteroid d.
branched-chain alpha-ketoacid d.
glutamate d. (GLDH)
glyceraldehyde phosphate d. (GAPD, GAPDH)
glyceraldehyde-3-phosphate d. (GAPDH, G3PDH)
ketoglutarate d. (KGDH)
lactate d. (LDH)
lactic acid d. (LDH)
long-chain 3-hydroxyacyl coenzyme A d. (LCHAD)
medium-chain acyl-CoA d. (MCAD)
pyruvate d. (PDH)
sorbitol d. (SDH)
succinate d.
xanthine d. (XDH)

deionized formamide
Deisting technique
dejecta
dejection
Dejerine-Sottas syndrome
Delatestryl
delavirdine
delay
excretory d.
gastric emptying d.
outlet d.

delayed
d. anastomosis
d. blush
d. capillary refill
d. colonic transit
d. gallbladder emptying
d. graft function (DGF)
d. hyperacute transplant rejection
d. liquid gastric emptying
d. nephrogram
d. operative cholangiography
d. primary closure (DPC)
d. primary intention
d. primary intention healing
d. upstroke
d. ureteral anastomotic stenosis
d. vesicoureteral reflux

delayed-release tablet
delayed-type hypersensitivity (DTH)

del Castillo syndrome
deleted
d. in colon carcinoma gene
d. in colorectal carcinoma (DCC)

deletion
chromosome d.
clonal d.
d. mutation
d. and mutation detection enhancement gel
d. polymorphism
somatic allelic d.

Delflex peritoneal dialysis solution
delivery
energy d.
PlasmaKinetic radiofrequency energy d.
vectorial d.

delomorphous cell
Delorme
D. operation for rectal prolapse
D. procedure
D. rectal prolapse operation
D. transrectal excision

delta
d. agent hepatitis
d. antigen
d. bilirubin
d. hepatitis superinfection
d. over baseline (DOB)
d.'s per mil
d. virus

delta-aminolevulinic acid (d-ALA)
Delta-Cortef
delta-5-pregnenolone
Deltasone
Deltatrac Metabolic Monitor
delusional
Demadex
demand
increased clinical d.

demarcate
demarcation
corticomedullary d.

DeMartel
D. appendix clamp
D. appendix forceps

DeMartel-Wolfson
D.-W. anastomosis clamp
D.-W. clamp holder

demasculinization
demeclocycline-induced ascites

NOTES

DeMeester
  D. acid score
  D. criteria
dementia
  dialysis d.
Demerol
demethylchlortetracycline
Deming operation
Demling-Classen sphincterotome
demonstrated hypertensive rate
demucosalized augmentation with gastric segment (DAWG)
denaturation
denaturing high-performance liquid chromatography (dHPLC)
Denck esophagoscope
dendritic
  d. calculus
  d. cell therapy
  d. reticular cell
dendriticum
  Diphyllobothrium d.
denervated sphincter of Oddi
denervation
  bladder d.
  detrusor d.
  partial bladder d.
  peripheral bladder d.
  sinoaortic d. (SAD)
dengue
  hemorrhagic d.
  d. hemorrhagic fever
  d. hemorrhagic fever infection
  d. shock syndrome
  d. virus
Denhardt solution
Denis
  D. Browne abdominal retractor
  D. Browne operation
  D. Browne pouch
  D. Browne urethroplasty technique
Dennis
  D. clamp
  D. colorectal tube
  D. intestinal forceps
  D. intestinal tube
Dennis-Brooke ileostomy
Dennis-Varco pancreaticoduodenostomy
Denonvilliers fascia
densa
  lamina d.
  macula d.
  nascent macula d.
dense
  d. adhesion
  d. polyposis
densitometer
  CS-9000 d.
  Hoefer GS 300 laser d.
  Hologic d.
densitometric unit
densitometry
  bone mineral d. (BMD)
  calcaneal ultrasound bone d.
  double x-ray d.
density
  bone mineral d. (BMD)
  current d.
  D cell d.
  electrosurgical current d.
  fat d.
  filtration slit-length d.
  gastrin mRNA:G-cell d.
  d. gradient centrifugation
  grain d.
  intramural microvessel d.
  lumbar spine bone mineral d. (LSBM)
  prostate-specific antigen d. (PSAD)
  radiopaque d.
  slit pore length d.
Dent
  D. disease
  D. supplement
dentate
  d. line
  d. margin
denticulatum
  pentastomum d.
Dentsleeve
  D. device
  D. extruded silastic perfused manometric assembly
  D. pneumohydraulic perfusion system
  D. single multilumen extrusion catheter
  D. sleeve sensor
denuded mucosa
denutrition
Denver
  D. peritoneovenous shunt
  D. pleuroperitoneal shunt
Denys-Drash syndrome (DDS)
deodorized tincture of opium (DTO)
deoxycholate
  sodium d.
deoxycholic acid
deoxycorticosterone
deoxycytidine
  fluoromethylene d.
deoxydoxorubicin
deoxyepinephrine
5′-deoxy-5-fluorouridine (5′-DFUR)
1-deoxy-galactonojirimicin (DGJ)
deoxyribonucleic
  d. acid (DNA)

d. acid flow cytometry
d. acid synthesizer
deoxyspergualin (DSP)
15-deoxyspergualin
DePage-Janeway gastrostomy
Depakene
deparaffinization
Depen
dependent rubor
dephosphorylated myosin crossbridge
depleted lysate
depletion
    mucous d.
    nephropathy of potassium d.
    plasma volume d.
    potassium d.
    protein d.
    syndrome of chloride d.
deployment
    stent d.
depMedalone
depolarization
Depo-Predate
Depo-Provera
deposit
    C3 d.
    electron-dense mesangial d.
    fatty d.
    hemosiderin d.
    liver d.
    mesangial d.
    peritoneal d.
    seminal vesicle amyloid d.
    subendothelial d.
    subepithelial d.
deposition
    collagen d.
    conditioning film d.
    encrustation d.
    heavy chain d.
    ion beam-assisted d.
    matrix d.
    microdroplet fat d.
    perisinusoidal fibrin d.
Depostat
depot
    d. injection
    Lupron D.
    Sandostatin LAR d.
    Trelstar D.
Depo-Testosterone

depressed
    d. adenoma
    d. cancer
    d. tumor
depressed-type colorectal cancer
depression
    orbital d.
    pterygoid d.
    respiratory d.
    spermatogenesis d.
    d. surface
deprivation
    androgen d.
    neoadjuvant hormonal d.
deranged hemostatic mechanism
derangement
    metabolic d.
derivative
    atropine d.
    ergot d.
    fibrate d.
    hematoporphyrin d. (HpD)
    isoxazole d.
    Photofrin d.
    Photoscan-3 hematoporphyrin d.
    photosensitizing hemoporphyrin d.
    pivalate d.
    sialylated d.
    sphingolipid d.
derma
dermal
    d. island-flap anoplasty
    d. suture
Dermalene suture
Dermalon suture
dermatan sulfate
dermatitidis
    Blastomyces d.
dermatitis, pl. dermatitides
    allergic d.
    d. artefacta
    atopic d.
    contact d.
    factitial d.
    d. herpetiformis (DH)
    irritant d.
    seborrheic d.
    Toxicodendron d.
dermatofibroma
dermatological tumor
dermatolymphatic invasion

NOTES

dermatomyositis
    paraneoplastic d.
dermatopathic enteropathy
dermatophyte infection
dermatosis, pl. **dermatoses**
    acute febrile neutrophilic d.
    d. of hemodialysis
    neutrophilic d.
    reactive inflammatory vascular d.
dermoid cyst
Dermovate cream
DeRoyal Surgical grab bag
DES
    diethylstilbestrol
    diffuse esophageal spasm
desaturation
    arterial oxygen d.
    oxygen d.
descendens
    colon d.
descending
    d. colon (DC)
    d. diaphragm
    d. duodenum
    d. inhibitory reflex
    d. loop colostomy
    d. perineum syndrome
    d. urography
descensus
    d. aberrans testis
    bladder d.
    d. paradoxus testis
    rectal d.
    renal d.
    d. uteri
    d. ventriculi
descent
    open renal d.
    pelvic floor d.
    perineal d.
    testicular d.
    total d.
    vaginal d.
Deschamps ligature carrier
DESD
    detrusor external sphincter dyssynergia
deserpidine
Desferal Mesylate challenge for hemochromatosis
desferrioxamine
des-gamma-carboxy
    d.-g.-c. prothrombin (DCP)
    d.-g.-c. prothrombin level
desiccation
    blend waveform d.
    coagulase waveform d.
    cut waveform d.
    electrosurgical d.

design
    crossover d.
    microwave antenna d.
desipramine hydrochloride
desirable body weight (DBW)
Desjardins
    D. gallbladder forceps
    D. gallbladder probe
    D. gallbladder scoop
    D. gall duct probe
    D. gallstone forceps
    D. gallstone probe
    D. gallstone scoop
    D. point
Desmarres paracentesis knife
desmin
desmoid tumor
desmolase
    20,22-d. deficiency
desmoplastic
    d. reaction
    d. response
desmopressin (DDAVP)
    d. acetate
    d. response
desmosomal junction
desmosome
desoximetasone
desquamated epithelium
desquamation
    tubular cell d.
dessusception
destruction
    fibroproliferative d.
    d. of laminin
    long-term graft d.
destructive
    d. cholangiopathy
    d. cholangitis
destruens
    adenoma d.
Desyrel
detachable miniloop ligation
detachment
    mucosal d.
    transvesical laparoscopic d.
detachment-induced apoptosis
Detachol adhesive remover
detail
    outstanding anatomical d.
detailed stepwise approach
detection
    antiliver microsomal antibody d.
    breath isotope bacterial urease d.
    colorimetric d.
    fluorescent d.
    gastroenteropathy d.
    hepatitis B DNA d.
    hepatitis C virus RNA d.

immunohistochemical d.
d. of malignancy
radioactive d.
d. rate
RIGScan CR49 test for colorectal cancer d.

detector
C-Trak handheld gamma d.
Early D.

deterioration
d. of graft function
marked d.
renal d.

determinant
antigenic d.
clinical d.
MAb IOT2-recognizing monomorphic DR d.

determination
IHA d.
indirect hemagglutination d.

detorsion

Detrol
D. LA
D. LA capsule

detrusodetrusor facilitative reflex

detrusor
acontractile d.
d. acontractility
d. activity index
d. areflexia
d. compliance
d. contraction
d. contraction strength
d. denervation
d. external sphincter dyssynergia (DESD)
d. hyperactivity
d. hyperreflexia
hypocontractile d.
d. hypocontractility
d. instability (DI)
d. muscle decompensation
d. muscle flap
d. muscle inhibition
d. muscle instability
d. muscle leak-point pressure
d. muscle myosin
d. muscle overactivity
d. muscle potassium channel
d. muscle pressure-flow micturition study

d. muscle protrusion junction
d. muscle stability
d. muscle trabeculation
d. muscle underactivity
d. myectomy
d. recovery
d. sphincter dyssynergia (DSD)
d. urethral dyssynergia
d. urinae

detrusorectomy
detrusorrhaphy
detrusosphincteric inhibitory reflex
detrusourethral inhibitory reflex
detubularization principle
detubularized
d. right colon reservoir
d. small bowel

detumescence
deuterium oxide
devascularization
paraesophagogastric d.
Sugiura paraesophagogastric d.

devastated urethra
devazepide
developer
Hemoccult Sensa d.

developing high-grade dysplasia
development
dynamic d.
embryologic d.

deviation
axis d.
congenital penile d. (CPD)
tongue d.
tracheal d.
ulnar d.
uvular d.

device
Accutorr oscillometric d.
ACMI ulcer measuring d.
Acucise balloon cutting d.
AcuSnare polypectomy d.
AcuTrainer handheld electronic d.
Aerochamber pediatric spacer d.
angled delivery d. (ADD)
Arena hemodialysis d.
Argon Beamer 2 d.
autostapling d.
band-ligator d.
BAS-300 transurethral thermotherapy d.
BetaSorb d.

NOTES

device *(continued)*
BiliCheck breath analyzer d.
bioartificial liver support d.
BladderManager portable ultrasonic d.
broken stent retrieval d.
BSD-300 d.
Button One-Step gastrostomy d.
Carter-Thomason port closure d.
CaverMap surgical d.
charge-coupled d. (CCD)
Circe d.
Circon-ACMI USL-2000 rigid d.
circular stapling d.
contraceptive d.
CoreTherm high-energy d.
cyst puncture d.
Defyne urethral assist d.
Dentsleeve d.
Digiflator digital inflation d.
Digitrapper MK III ambulatory d.
Dilamezinsert d.
double-headed P190 stapling d.
EEA stapling d.
endoscopically deliverable tissue-transfixing d.
endoscopic hemoclip d.
endoscopic mucosal resection with ligating d.
ErecAid vacuum erection d.
Erlangen magnetic colostomy d.
external urethral barrier d.
extracorporeal liver assist d. (ELAD)
extracorporeal organ bioartificial liver d.
fingerstick d.
flexible delivery d.
flexible endoscopic suturing d.
flexible Olympus GF-eUM3 d.
Flexible Sew-Right d.
Flexible Ti-Knot d.
fog reduction elimination d. (FRED)
gastroesophageal antireflux d. (GARD)
Gastro-Port II feeding d.
GIA autosuture d.
Gould polygraph gastric motility measuring d.
head-mounted d.
hemoclipping application d.
Hepatix d.
HX-5/6-1 endoscopic clipping d.
implantable penile venous compression d.
indwelling stomal d.
infection-prevention d.
Insuflon insulin delivery d.
InterStim d.
IntraSonix TULIP laser d.
ISOBAR barostat distension d.
ligation d.
linear stapling d.
Macroplastique implantation d.
Makler insemination d.
Makler sperm-counting d.
Menuet Compact urodynamic testing d.
Microgyn II urinary incontinence d.
Microvasive Gold probe bipolar electrocautery d.
miniature ultrasound suction d.
Mission vacuum constriction d.
Mission vacuum erection d.
multiband ligating d.
Multifire Endo GIA stapling d.
Nachlas-Linton esophagogastric balloon tamponade d.
needlescope d.
Nottingham KeyMed introducing d.
NovolinPen d.
Olympus clip-fixing d.
Olympus LUS-1 rigid d.
Olympus LUS-2 ultrasonic energy rigid d.
Olympus UES-series snare cautery d.
OraSure salivary collection d.
OSB gastrostomy d.
PC Polygraf HR d.
pneumatic compression d. (PCD)
PortSaver PercLoop d.
Pos-T-Vac vacuum erection d.
ProCon incontinence d.
prophylactic d.
Prostathermer d.
Prostatron transurethral thermotherapy d.
ProTack tacking d.
pyxigraphic d.
Q-Maxx side-firing laser d.
Quantum inflation d. (QID)
Relia-Flow d.
Richard Wolf model 2271.004 ultrasonic energy rigid d.
Rigiflator handheld inflation/deflation d.
RigiScan d.
ring-type rigidity measuring d.
robotic-automated assist d.
roticulator stapling d.
silicone pressure sensor d.
Soehendra stent retrieval d.
SofTouch vacuum erection d.
Sonoblate ablation d.
Sony Promavica still capture d.

Stone Cone nitinol stone retrieval d.
Swiss Lithoclast Master d.
Synergist vacuum erection d.
targeted cryoablation d.
TA stapling d.
Techstar percutaneous closure d.
temporary endoprosthetic d.
testicular hypothermia d.
TherMatric hyperthermia d.
TherMatrx TMx-2000 d.
Thermex-II transurethral prostate heating d.
thread-locking d.
transparent elastic band ligating d.
TriClip endoscopic clipping d.
Trimedyne Optilase 1000 d.
Turapy d.
UV-Flash ultraviolet germicidal exchange d.
vacuum constriction d. (VCD)
vacuum entrapment d.
vacuum erection d. (VED)
vacuum extraction d.
vacuum tumescence d.
variceal pressure measuring d.
Visiport d.
VTU-1 vacuum erection d.
Wallstent delivery d.
Wedge electrosurgical resection d.
wire-guided metal spiral retrieval d.
Wolf Piezolith 2300 lithotripsy d.

device-related urinary tract infection

Devine
D. colostomy
D. exclusion
D. hypospadias repair

Devine-Devine procedure

Devine-Horton flip-flap for hypospadias repair

devitalization

devolvulization
endoscopic d.

Devonshire colic

Dew sign

DEX
dexloxiglumide

DEXA
dual-energy x-ray absorptiometry
DEXA absorption

dexamethasone
d. sodium phosphate

d. suppression test
vincristine, doxorubicin, d. (VAD)

Dexatrim
dexbrompheniramine
Dexedrine
dexfenfluramine
dexloxiglumide (DEX)
Dexol 300
Dexon
D. polyglycolic acid mesh
D. suture

dexpanthenol
dexter
ductus hepaticus d.
ductus lobi caudati d.

dextra
arteria colica d.
arteria gastrica d.
arteria gastroomentalis d.
flexura coli d.

dextran
d. 40, 70, 75
d. clearance
iron d.
d. sieving
d. sodium sulfate (DSS)

dextrin
dextrinizing time
dextrinosis
limit d.

dextroamphetamine
dextrogastria
dextropropoxyphene
dextrose
DF
discriminant function

DFT
Doppler flow test

5'-DFUR
5'-deoxy-5-fluorouridine

d-galactosamine
DGER
duodenal gastroesophageal reflux
duodenogastroesophageal reflux

DGF
delayed graft function

DGHAL
Doppler-guided hemorrhoidal artery ligation

DGJ
1-deoxy-galactonojirimicin

NOTES

DGR
    duodenogastric reflux
DH
    dermatitis herpetiformis
    diaphragmatic hernia
DHA
    dehydroepiandrosterone
DHA-paclitaxel
    Taxoprexin DHA-p.
DHAS
    dehydroepiandrosterone sulfate
DHD
    donor hepatic duct
DHFK
    Dow Hollow Fiber kidney
DHPG
    dihydroxypropoxymethyl guanine
dHPLC
    denaturing high-performance liquid chromatography
DHSI
    Digestive Health Status Instrument
DHT
    dihydrotestosterone
DI
    detrusor instability
    distal intestine
DiaBeta
diabetes
    alimentary d.
    D.'s Bowel Symptom Questionnaire (DBSQ)
    fibrocalculous pancreatic d. (FCPD)
    gestational d.
    d. home screening test
    d. insipidus
    insulin-dependent d.
    d. mellitus
    pancreatic d.
diabetic
    d. autonomic neuropathy
    d. cholecystoparesis
    d. colitis
    d. diarrhea
    d. diet
    d. enteropathy
    d. gastroparesis
    d. gastropathy
    d. impotence
    insulin-treated d.
    d. ketoacidosis
    d. microangiopathy
    d. nephropathy
    d. patient
    Resource D.
    d. urine
diabetica
    balanitis d.

diabeticorum
    gastroparesis d.
DiabetiSweet
DiabetiTrim
Diabinese
diabrosis
diacetate
    $2',7'$-dichlorofluoresin d.
diachorema
diachoresis
Diacol
diacylglycerol (DAG)
Diacyte DNA ploidy analysis
Diagnex
    D. Blue test
    D. Blue test for gastric acid
diagnosing
    d. interstitial cystitis
    d. ureteral calculus
diagnosis, pl. **diagnoses**
    algorithm of d.
    d. of bacterial prostatitis
    d. of bladder cancer
    colonoscopic d.
    cytologic d.
    differential d.
    endoscopic ultrasonographic d.
    endoscopic ultrasound d.
    enteroscopy d.
    histologic d.
    missed d.
    needle biopsy d.
    noninvasive d.
    pancreatic tumor d.
    pathological d.
    photodynamic d. (PPD)
    prenatal d.
    scintigraphic d.
    serologic d.
    d. of testicular tumor
    ultrasonic d.
    wastebasket d.
diagnostic
    d. angiography
    d. aspiration
    d. colonoscopy
    d. duodenoscope
    d. fiberoptic stomatoscopy
    d. imaging evaluation
    d. laparoscope
    d. laparoscopy
    d. paracentesis
    d. surgery
    d. technique
    d. upper endoscopy
    d. uroradiology
    d. yield
diagram
    schematic d.

diagraph
Dialose
Dialume
Dialyflex dialysis fluid
dialysance
dialysate
    bicarbonate d.
    calcium-free d.
    ethanol and phosphate-enriched d.
    d. glucose concentration
    high-calcium d.
    low-calcium d.
    peritoneal d.
dialysate-to-plasma ratio
dialysis
    d. access infection
    d. access surgery
    d. adequacy
    automated peritoneal d. (APD)
    chronic ambulatory peritoneal d. (CAPD)
    continuous ambulatory peritoneal d. (CAPD)
    continuous arteriovenous hemofiltration with d.
    continuous cycler-assisted peritoneal d.
    continuous cycling peritoneal d. (CCPD)
    cycling d.
    daily intermittent peritoneal d. (DIPD)
    d. dementia
    d. disequilibrium syndrome
    d. encephalopathy syndrome
    d. equilibrium syndrome
    extended daily d. (EDD)
    extracorporeal d.
    high-efficiency d.
    high-flux d.
    home d.
    d. modality
    nightly intermittent peritoneal d. (NIPD)
    d. osteomalacia
    D. Outcomes Quality Initiative (DOQI)
    peritoneal d. (PD)
    d. to plasma
    profiled d.
    renal d.
    short daily d.
    d. shunt
    slow low-efficiency d. (SLED)
    sustained low-efficiency d. (SLED)
    terminal anuria vesical d.
    title peritoneal d. (TPD)
dialysis-associated hypotension
dialysis-related ascites
dialytic
    d. treatment
    d. ultrafiltration (DU)
dialyzer
    AN69 membrane d.
    CA110 d.
    CA cellulose acetate membrane hollow-fiber d.
    Clirans T-series d.
    double d.
    Fresenius AG d.
    Gambro d.
    high-flux d.
    hollow-fiber d.
    d. membrane
    parallel plate d.
    760 polysulfone d.
    Renaflo hollow-fiber d.
    Renalin d.
    Renatron d.
    Terumo d.
diameter
    distal bile duct d.
    inner d. (ID)
    lower infundibula d.
    luminal d.
    maximum d.
    outer d. (OD)
    renal artery d.
    unequal calf d.
diaminedichloroplatinum
diamine oxidase
diaminobenzidine (DAB)
    3′,3-d. tetrahydrochloride
diamond
    d. flap
    D. stent
    D. tube
diamond-jaw needle holder
diamorphine
Dianeal K-141
diaphoresis
diaphoretic
diaphragm
    accessory d.

NOTES

diaphragm *(continued)*
- congenital d.
- crus of d.
- descending d.
- d. disease
- duodenal d.
- endoscopic ablation of antral d.
- leaves of d.
- mucosal ileal d.
- pelvic d.
- prepyloric antral d.
- slit d.
- urogenital d.

diaphragmatic
- d. abscess
- d. breathing
- d. hernia (DH)
- d. hernia trauma
- d. hiatus
- d. hump
- d. injury
- d. muscle
- d. pinch
- d. pinchcock
- d. surface of liver

diaphragmatocele

diaphragmlike
- d. stenosis
- d. stricture

diarrhea
- acute infectious d.
- *Aeromonas* d.
- alcoholic d.
- antibiotic-associated d. (AAD)
- antibiotic-induced d.
- anxiety-related d.
- bacterial toxigenic d.
- beta-lactam-associated d.
- bile acid d. type 1, 2
- bile salt d.
- bilious d.
- bloody d.
- Brainerd d.
- cachectic d.
- chewing gum d.
- choleraic d.
- cholera toxin-induced d.
- chronic d.
- d. chylosa
- *Clostridium difficile*-associated d. (CDAD)
- Cochin China d.
- colliquative d.
- congenital chloride d.
- congenital sodium d. (CSD)
- crapulous d.
- critical d.
- *Cryptosporidia*-induced d.
- daycare d.
- diabetic d.
- dientamoeba d.
- dysenteric d.
- elixir d.
- endemic d.
- enteral d.
- enterotoxin d.
- explosive d.
- factitious d.
- familial chloride d.
- fatty acid d.
- fermentative d.
- flagellate d.
- fructose d.
- functional d.
- gastrogenic d.
- gastrogenous d.
- gluten-sensitive d.
- hemorrhagic d.
- hill d.
- ileostomy d.
- infantile d.
- infectious nosocomial d.
- infectious viral d.
- inflammatory d.
- intermittent d.
- intractable d.
- irritative d.
- lactose-associated d.
- lienteric d.
- liquid d.
- magnesium-induced d.
- malabsorptive d.
- maldigestive d.
- mechanical d.
- morning d.
- mucous d.
- nausea, vomiting, d. (NVD)
- neurogenic secretory d.
- nocturnal d.
- osmotic d.
- d. pancreatica
- pancreatogenous d.
- paradoxical d.
- parenteral d.
- postvagotomy d.
- putrefactive d.
- raw milk-associated d.
- rotavirus d.
- rotavirus-associated d.
- runner's d.
- secretory d.
- serous d.
- severe secretory d.
- sodium anion d.
- sorbitol d.
- stercoraceous d.
- d. stool
- summer d.

diarrhea · diencephalic

toddler's d.
toxic d.
toxigenic d.
traveler's d.
tropical d.
tubercular d.
unrelenting d.
viral d.
virulent d.
d. and vomiting (D&V)
watery d.
white d.
diarrheagenic (*var. of* diarrheogenic)
diarrheal, diarrheic
diarrhea-predominant irritable bowel syndrome
diarrheogenic, diarrheagenic
diary
    voiding d.
DiaScreen 10 Reagent Strip
Diasonics
    D. DRF ultrasound unit
    D. Therasonic lithotriptor
Diasorb
diastase
    d. digestion
    pancreatic d.
    d. predigestion
diastasis
    palpable rib d.
    pubic d.
    rectus d.
    d. rectus abdominis
    wide pubic d.
diastatic serosal tear
Diastat vascular access graft
diastematomyelia
diathermal snare
diathermic
    d. cleaning
    d. cystenterostome
    d. fistulotomy
    d. loop
    d. loop biopsy
    d. precut needle
    d. puncture
    d. resection
diathermocoagulation
diathermy
    BICAP bipolar d.
    d. hemorrhoidectomy
    d. scissors

    d. technique
    d. wire
diathesis, pl. **diatheses**
diatrizoate
    meglumine d.
    postdilation meglumine d.
    d. sodium enema
    sodium methylglucamine d.
diatrizoic acid
diazepam emulsified injection
diaziquone (AZQ)
diazoxide
DIB
    duodenoileal bypass
dibasic
    d. aminoacidopathy
    d. amino acid residue
Dibent Injection
Dibenzyline
dibromochloropropane (DBCP)
dibucaine
DIC
    disseminated intravascular coagulation
    drip infusion cholangiography
    DIC parameter
dichlorofluorescein
dichlorofluoresin
    2',7'-d. diacetate
dichotomization
dichroism
    circular d.
Dickinson FACS 400-series flow cytometer
Dickson osteotomy
diclofenac
    d. analgesic therapy
    d. sodium
dicloxacillin
dicyclomine
didactic teaching session
didanosine (ddI, ddi)
didelphys
    uterus d.
dideoxycytidine (ddC, ddc)
Didrex
Didronel
didymalgia
didymitis
DIED
    drug-induced esophageal damage
diencephalic syndrome

NOTES

dientamoeba
    d. diarrhea
    D. fragilis

diet
    absolute d.
    acid-ash d.
    ADA d.
    advance to regular d.
    alkaline-ash d.
    Andresen d.
    d. as tolerated (DAT)
    Atkins d.
    baby soft d. (BSD)
    balanced d.
    basal d.
    basic d.
    bland d.
    blenderized d.
    blood-type d.
    BRAT d.
    BRATT d.
    calcium-rich, gluten-free d.
    CAPS-free d.
    challenge d.
    chemically defined d.
    clear liquid d.
    cornstarch-rich d.
    defined-formula d.
    diabetic d.
    disease-specific d.
    Ebstein d.
    elemental d.
    elimination d.
    exclusion d.
    fasting d.
    fen-phen d.
    fiber-deficient d.
    fractionated d.
    fructose-free d.
    full liquid d.
    galactose-free d.
    gastric d.
    Giordano-Giovannetti d.
    gluten-free d. (GFD)
    gluten-rich d.
    grapefruit d.
    high-bulk, low-fat d.
    high-calorie d.
    high-carbohydrate d.
    high-fat d.
    high-fiber d.
    high-protein d.
    high-roughage d.
    high-starch d.
    hypercaloric d.
    hyperprotidic d.
    immune-enhancing d. (IED)
    K d.
    K+2 d.
    lactose-free d. (LFD)
    liquid d.
    liver d.
    low available carbohydrate d.
    low-calorie d.
    low-fat d. (LFD)
    low-fiber d.
    low-lactose d.
    low-oxalate d.
    low-residue d.
    low-roughage d.
    low-sodium d.
    low-tyrosine, low-phenylalanine d.
    Meulengracht d.
    milk d.
    modified liver d.
    Moro-Heisler d.
    Paleolithic d.
    phen-fen d.
    Portagen d.
    progressive d.
    reducing d.
    regular d.
    rice-fruit d.
    Schmidt d.
    semielemental d.
    Sippy d.
    smooth d.
    soft bland d.
    steroid-dependent d.
    steroid-refractory d.
    d. therapy
    Travasorb Hepatic D.
    Travasorb Renal D.
    vegetarian d.
    Weight Watchers d.
    Western d.

dietary
    d. approach to stop hypertension (DASH)
    d. calcium
    d. cholesterol
    d. deficiency
    d. energy intake
    d. fat
    d. fiber
    d. gluten
    d. habit
    d. L-arginine supplementation
    d. nitrite
    d. oxalate
    d. phosphate
    d. phosphorus
    d. potassium
    d. protein
    d. protein intolerance
    d. protein restriction
    d. purine
    d. sodium

dietetic regimen
dietetics
diethylaminoethyl (DEAE)
diethylcarbamazine (DEC)
diethylenetriamine
    d. pentaacetic acid (DTPA)
    d. pentaacetic acid renal scan
    d. pentaacetic acid renography
diethylenetriamine-pentaacetic acid-galactosyl-human serum albumin
diethylhomospermine (DEHOP)
diethylpropion
diethylstilbestrol (DES)
dieting plateau
dietitian
Dietl crisis
Dieulafoy
    D. anomaly
    D. cirsoid aneurysm
    D. disease
    D. gastric erosion
    D. gastric lesion
    D. theory
    D. triad
    D. ulcer
    D. vascular malformation
difference
    potential d. (PD)
    substantial regional d.
    transmembrane electrical potential d.
    transmucosal potential d. (TMPD)
different
    d. osmolarity
    d. thermotherapy
differential
    d. diagnosis
    d. loading
    d. neuroaxial blockade
    d. renal function test
    d. ureteral catheterization test
    WBC d.
    white blood count d.
differentiated teratoma
differentiation
    cellular d.
    chondrogenic d.
    corticomedullary d.
    endothelial cell d.
    genital d.
    gonadal d.
    impaired cell d.
    osteogenic d.
    rhabdomyoblastic d.
    sexual d.
DiffGAM
difficile
    Clostridium d. (CD)
difficult nephrectomy
difficulty
    defecatory d.
Diff-Quik stain
diffractometry
    x-ray d.
Diffu-K
diffuse
    d. adherent *Escherichia coli* (DAEC)
    d. alveolar hemorrhage (DAH)
    d. alveolar hemorrhage syndrome
    d. angiodysplasia
    d. angiokeratoma
    d. antral gastritis (DAG)
    d. diabetic glomerulosclerosis
    d. esophageal spasm (DES)
    d. hepatocellular carcinoma
    d. hyperplastic polyposis
    d. irregular narrowing of pancreatic duct
    d. liver disease
    d. lobular fibrosis
    d. malignant mesothelioma (DMM)
    d. mesangial proliferation
    d. mesangial sclerosis (DMS)
    d. metastasis
    d. mucosal polyposis
    d. nodular hyperplasia (DNH)
    d. pain
    d. pancreatitis
    d. patchy nephrogram
    d. proliferative glomerulonephritis
    d. redness (DR)
    d. suppurative nephritis
    d. tenderness
    d. varioliform gastritis
    d. vasculitis of polyarteritis nodosa type
diffusely tender abdomen
diffuser
    cylindrical d.
diffusion
    disk d.
    interstitial d.

NOTES

diffusion *(continued)*
    pericapillary d.
    transcapillary d.
diffusive transport
diffusum
    angiokeratoma corporis d.
Diflucan
diflunisal
difluoromethylornithine
DIF-test
  direct immunofluorescence test
digastric
    d. anterior muscle
    d. impression
    d. posterior muscle
    d. triangle
Di-Gel
DiGeorge
    D. anomaly
    D. syndrome
Digepepsin
digestant
digestion
    brush-border d.
    diastase d.
    duodenal d.
    proteolytic d.
    RNAse d.
    solid food d.
digestive
    d. apparatus
    d. disease (DD)
    D. Disease National Coalition (DDNC)
    d. enzyme
    d. fever
    d. gastrosuccorrhea
    d. glycosuria
    D. Health Status Instrument (DHSI)
    D. Health Status Instrument survey
    d. system
    d. tract
    d. tube
digestive-respiratory
    d.-r. fistula (DRF)
    d.-r. fistula stent
digestorius
    apparatus d.
    tubus d.
Digibar 190
Digiflator digital inflation device
digit
    sausage d.
digital
    d. manipulation of pubic hair
    d. rectal evacuation
    d. rectal examination (DRE)
    d. stream segment
    d. venous subtraction angiography (DSA)
digitalis
digitally guided biopsy
digitonin
Digitrapper
    D. Gold MK III solid-state data logger
    D. Mark II pH monitoring system
    D. MK III
    D. MK III ambulatory device
    D. MK III portable digital recorder
    Synthetics dual-channel solid-state D.
diglycoaldehyde
Dignity incontinence pants
digoxin
dihydrate
    calcium oxalate d.
    octahedral-shaped d.
dihydrochloride
    histamine d.
    nolatrexed d.
dihydroergotoxine
dihydropyridine
dihydrotestosterone (DHT)
    d. gel
    d. synthesis
dihydroxyadenine
    2,8-d. calculus
    d. urolithiasis
dihydroxyaluminum
    d. aminoacetate
    d. sodium carbonate
dihydroxyeicosatrienoic acid
dihydroxyphenylalanine (DDC, DOPA)
dihydroxypropoxymethyl guanine (DHPG)
dihydroxy salt
1,25-dihydroxyvitamin
    1,25-d. D
    1,25-d. D3 (1,25(OH)2 D3)
dihydroxyvitamin D3
diiodohydroxyquin
diisopropyliminodiacetic
    d. acid (DISDA, DISIDA)
    d. acid enterogastroesophageal reflux study
Dilamezinsert (DMI)
    D. device
    D. penile prosthesis
    D. urologic instrument
Dilantin
dilatation *(var. of* dilation)
dilated
    d. bile duct
    d. gallbladder
    d. loops of bowel

dilated · dilator

    d. pupil
    d. vein
dilating
    d. catheter
    d. catheter-gastrostomy tube assembly
    d. set
dilation, dilatation
    achalasia balloon d.
    anal d.
    aneurysmal d.
    balloon d.
    biliary d.
    bowel d.
    Brown-McHardy pneumatic mercury bougie d.
    capillary d.
    d. catheter (DC)
    cavernous artery d.
    cecal d.
    colonic d.
    combined antegrade and retrograde d.
    corpus cavernosum d.
    cystic d.
    cystoscopy and d. (C&D)
    ductal d.
    Eder-Puestow d.
    endoscopic balloon d. (EBD)
    endoscopic balloon sphincter d. (EBSD)
    endoscopic papillary balloon d. (EPBD, EPD)
    esophageal d.
    d. of esophagus
    extrahepatic biliary cystic d.
    gastric d.
    Grüntzig balloon d.
    d. of hemorrhoid
    hepatic web d.
    hydrostatic balloon d.
    inadequate d.
    intrahepatic biliary cystic d.
    intrahepatic ductal d.
    Lord d.
    Maloney d.
    mechanical ureteral d.
    medical d.
    mucosal vascular d.
    percutaneous balloon d.
    periportal sinusoidal d.
    peroral esophageal d.

    pneumatic bag esophageal d.
    pneumatic balloon catheter d.
    pneumostatic d.
    prostate gland transurethral balloon d.
    pyloric d.
    d. range
    rectal d.
    d. of stomach
    submucosal vascular d.
    d. therapy
    through-the-scope balloon d.
    tract d.
    transurethral balloon d.
    TTS balloon d.
    upper tract d.
    urethral d.
    Uromat d.
    Wirsung d.
dilator
    achalasia d.
    Achiever balloon d.
    American Dilation System d.
    American Endoscopy d.
    Amplatz fascial d.
    anal d.
    Backhaus d.
    Bakes common duct d.
    balloon d.
    Barnes common duct d.
    biliary balloon d.
    bougie d.
    Brown-McHardy pneumatic d.
    bullet-tip d.
    Celestin graduated d.
    circular anal d.
    Clark common duct d.
    Cunningham-Cotton sleeve coaxial d.
    Dotter d.
    Eder-Puestow metal olive d.
    Einhorn d.
    Eliminator PET biliary balloon d.
    ERCP d.
    esophageal balloon d.
    Ferris biliary duct d.
    fluoroscopy-guided balloon d.
    French d.
    Garrett d.
    Grüntzig d.
    Hegar rectal d.
    high-diameter d.

NOTES

dilator *(continued)*
    Hurst bullet-tip d.
    Hurst mercury-filled d.
    Hurst-Tucker pneumatic d.
    hydrostatic d.
    KeyMed advanced d.
    Kollmann d.
    Kron bile duct d.
    Kron gall duct d.
    Maloney-Hurst d.
    Maloney mercury-filled esophageal d.
    Maloney tapered-tip d.
    mercury-filled d.
    mercury-weighted d.
    metal olive d.
    Microvasive CRE esophageal d.
    Microvasive Rigiflex balloon d.
    modified polyethylene d.
    Mosher d.
    Murphy common duct d.
    Nottingham One-Step tapered d.
    Nottingham ureteral d.
    Olbert balloon d.
    olive-tipped plastic d.
    Optilume prostate balloon d.
    over-the-endoscope Witzel d.
    d. placement
    d. placement failure
    Plummer d.
    pneumatic balloon d.
    polyethylene balloon d.
    polyvinyl d.
    probe d.
    prostate balloon d.
    Quantum TTC balloon d.
    Ramstedt pyloric stenosis d.
    rectal d.
    Rider-Moeller d.
    Rigiflex achalasia d.
    Rigiflex TTS balloon d.
    Russell peel-away sheath d.
    Savary-Gilliard over-the-wire d.
    Savary tapered thermoplastic d.
    Sippy esophageal d.
    Soehendra catheter d.
    Starck d.
    Stucker bile duct d.
    tapered-tip d.
    through-the-scope d.
    TTS d.
    Tucker spindle-shaped d.
    vessel d.
    Walther d.
    Witzel pneumatic d.
Dilaudid
dilaurate
    fluorescein d. (FDL)
dildo, dildoe

dilemma of distal ureter
dilevalol
dilinoleoylphosphatidylcholine (DLPC)
Dilomine
diltiazem therapy
dilute
    d. iodinated contrast
    d. Russell viper venom test (DRVVT)
dilution
    agar d.
    clonal d.
    serial d.
dilutional hyponatremia
dimenhydrinate
dimension
    D. Free prostate-specific antigen Flex reagent cartridge test
    D. RxL PSA Flex reagent cartridge
dimercaptosuccinic
    d. acid (DMSA)
    d. acid renal scan
    d. acid scintigraphy
dimeric
    d. acidic glycoprotein (DAG)
    d. IgA
dimerization
dimethyl
    d. iminodiacetic acid scan
    d. sulfate cystitis
    d. sulfoxide (DMSO)
dimethylester
    cystine d. (CDE)
1,2-dimethylhydrazine
dimethyl-4-phenylpiperazinium (DMPP)
dimethylpolysiloxane (DMPS)
dimethylsulfoxide
dimethyltriazenoimidazole carboxamide (DTIC)
diminished
    d. bowel sounds
    d. branching abnormality
    d. gag reflex
diminuta
    Hymenolepis d.
diminutive
    d. adenomatous polyp
    d. colonic polyp
    d. hyperplastic polyp
dimorphic
dimple
    celiac d.
dimpling
    focal d.
    postanal d.
    skin d.
Dinamap Plus monitor

dinitrate
    isosorbide d.
    d. and mononitrate ester
dinitrochlorobenzene (DNCB)
Dinitrophenol
dinner
    d. pad
    test d.
Dinophysis
    D. acuminata
    D. fortii
dinucleotide
    flavin adenine d.
    nicotinamide adenine d. (NADH)
Diocto-C, -K
diode
    interstitial d.
    d. laser
Diodrast
Dioeze
Diogenes syndrome
Diomed laser
DIONEX 2000 system
Diosuccin
dioxide
    thorium d.
DiPAS-positive granule
DIPD
    daily intermittent peritoneal dialysis
Dipentum
dipeptidase
    N-acetylated alpha-linked d.
dipeptide
diphallia
diphallus
diphemanil methylsulfate
Diphenatol
diphenhydramine
diphenoxylate
diphenylthiazole
diphosphatase
    adenosine d. (ADPase)
diphosphate (DP)
    adenosine d. (ADP)
    d. buffer solution
5′-diphosphate
    uridine 5′-d. (UDP)
diphosphonate
    ^{99m}Tc-labeled stannous methylene d.
diphtheria

diphtheritic
    d. cystitis
    d. enteritis
diphyllobothriasis
Diphyllobothrium
    D. alascence
    D. dendriticum
    D. latum
    D. nihonkaiense
    D. pacificum
    D. parvum
    D. taenioides
    D. ursi
dipivoxil
    adefoir d.
diploid
    d. cell
    d. tumor
diploidy
dipole
dipotassium
    clorazepate d.
dipropionate (DP)
    beclomethasone d. (BDP)
Diprospan
dipslide
    Uricult d.
dipstick
    Chemstrip LN d.
    d. protein
    urinalysis d.
    urine d.
Dipylidium caninum
dipyridamole
direct
    d. bilirubin
    d. cautery puncture
    d. crossreactivity
    d. cystenterostomy
    d. extension
    d. fragmentation technique
    d. immunobead test
    d. immunofluorescence test (DIF-test)
    d. inguinal hernia
    d. laryngoscopy
    d. manipulation
    d. nerve stimulation graciloplasty
    d. percutaneous jejunostomy (DPJ)
    d. percutaneous jejunostomy tube
    d. percutaneous transhepatic cholangiography

NOTES

direct *(continued)*
    d. repeat
    d. tubular toxicity
    d. vesicoureteral scintigraphy (DVS)
    d. vision
direct-beam coupler for TURP
direct-current
    d.-c. electrocoagulation
    d.-c. electrotherapy trial
direction
    isoperistaltic d.
director
    grooved d.
    D. Guidewire system
    Larry rectal d.
    probe and groove d.
direct-reading bilirubinometer
direct-vision
    d.-v. internal urethrotomy (DVIU)
    d.-v. liver biopsy
Direx Tripter X-1 lithotriptor
dirithromycin
Disa
    D. electromyography
    D. needle electrode
    D. 5500 urograph
disaccharidase
    d. assay
    d. deficiency
    d. enzyme activity
disaccharide
    d. intolerance
    d. lactose
    nonabsorbable d.
    d. tripeptide
disaggregation
Disalcid capsules/tablets
disappearing phenomenon
disassembly
    technique of penile d.
disc *(var. of* disk*)*
discharge
    anal d.
    bloody d.
    cervical d.
    chyme d.
    clear d.
    nasal d.
    nipple d.
    purulent d.
    urethral d. (UD)
    vaginal d.
discoid
    d. lupus erythematosus
    d. rash
discoloration
discomfort
    epigastric d.
    postligation d.
    posttreatment d.
    preexisting d.
disconnection
    ureteroendoscopic d.
discontinuation
    transient d.
discontinuity
    pelvic d.
discrete
    d. bleeding source
    d. mass
    d. narrowing
    d. nodule
    d. organ enlargement
discriminant function (DF)
discriminator
    EMI APED amplifier d.
    model 500A gamma camera d.
DISDA
    diisopropyliminodiacetic acid
disease
    acalculous gallbladder d.
    acid-peptic d.
    acquired cystic kidney d. (ACKD)
    acquired renal cystic d. (ARCD)
    actinomycotic esophageal d.
    acute abdominal vascular d.
    acute graft-versus-host d.
    acute idiopathic inflammatory bowel d.
    acute on chronic liver d. (AOCLD)
    acute polycystic d.
    Addison d.
    adrenal d.
    adult celiac d. (ACD)
    adult familial hyaline membrane d.
    adult polycystic kidney d. (APKD)
    adult polycystic liver d. (APLD)
    adynamic bone d. (ABD)
    African-American Study of Kidney D.
    Ajmalin liver d.
    Albarran d.
    alcoholic liver d. (ALD)
    alpha-1-antitrypsin d. (AATD)
    alpha-1-antitrypsin deficiency d.
    alpha-chain d.
    alpha heavy-chain d.
    Alstrom d.
    alveolar hydatid d.
    American Association for the Study of Liver D.'s (AASLD)
    Andersen d.
    anorectal d.
    anti-GBM d.
    antiglomerular basement membrane d.
    aplastic bone d.

arteriosclerotic renal artery d. (ASO-RAD)
atheroembolic renal d. (AERD)
atherosclerotic renovascular d.
atypical distribution of d.
atypical gallbladder d.
autoimmune thyroid d.
autosomal-dominant polycystic kidney d. (ADPKD)
autosomally recessive inherited d.
autosomal-recessive kidney d. (ARKD)
autosomal-recessive polycystic kidney d.
Banti d.
Barrett d.
Bassen-Kornzweig d.
Behçet d.
benign anorectal d. (BAD)
Berger d.
Besnier-Boeck-Schaumann d.
Biermer d.
biliary tract d.
black liver d.
bleeding acid-peptic d.
Blount d.
bone d.
Botkin d.
Bouchard d.
Bourneville d.
bowel d.
Bowen d.
Bradley d.
brancher glycogen storage d.
branch renal artery d.
Bright d.
Brinton d.
Bruton d.
Budd d.
Budd-Chiari d.
Byler d.
Cacchi-Ricci d.
calculous gallbladder d.
calculus d.
cardiovascular d.
Caroli d.
Castleman d.
cavernous artery d.
celiac sprue d.
cerebrovascular d.
Chagas d.
Chagas-Cruz d.

Cherchevski d.
Chiari d.
cholestatic liver d.
cholesterol ester storage d. (CESD)
choline deficiency liver d.
chronic active liver d. (CALD)
chronic cholestatic liver d.
chronic glomerular d.
chronic graft-versus-host d. (c-GVHD)
chronic granulomatous d.
chronic inflammatory bowel d. (CIBD)
chronic liver d. (CLD)
chronic obstructive pulmonary d. (COPD)
chronic parenchymal liver d.
chronic progressive tubulointerstitial d.
chylomicron retention d.
chylopoietic d.
clinical trial for kidney d.
CMV ulcerative d.
collagen vascular d.
colorectal d.
complement-mediated immune glomerular d.
concomitant d.
congenital cystic d.
congenital polycystic d. (CPD)
connective tissue d.
Corbus d.
Cori d.
coronary artery d.
Cowden d.
crescentic fold d.
Creutzfeldt-Jakob d.
Crigler-Najjar d.
Crohn d. (CD)
Cruveilhier d.
Cruz-Chagas d.
cryptogenic liver d.
Curschmann d.
Cushing d.
cysticercus d.
cystic liver d.
cytotoxic liver d.
Darier d.
debrancher glycogen storage d.
deficiency d.
Degos d.
de novo renal d.

NOTES

disease *(continued)*
Dent d.
diaphragm d.
Dieulafoy d.
diffuse liver d.
digestive d. (DD)
diverticular d.
drug-related liver d.
Dubin-Sprinz d.
Ducrey d.
duodenal ulcer d.
Dupuytren d.
Durand-Nicholas-Favre d.
early-onset graft-versus-host d.
Ebstein d.
echinococcal cyst d.
endoscopy-negative reflux d. (ENRD)
end-stage liver d. (ESLD)
end-stage renal d. (ESRD)
Epstein d.
estrogen-induced liver d.
extensive pelvic d.
extraabdominal d.
extracapsular d.
extraintestinal d.
extramammary Paget d. (EMPD)
Fabry d.
familial Crohn d.
fatty liver d.
Fenwick d.
fibroobliterative d.
fibropolycystic liver d.
fistulizing Crohn d.
fistulous Crohn d.
Forbes d.
Fournier d.
fulminant Crohn d.
functional bowel d.
gamma heavy chain d.
Gamna d.
gastric mucosal d.
gastritis-associated peptic ulcer d.
gastroduodenal Crohn d.
gastroesophageal reflux d. (GERD)
Gaucher d.
Gee d.
Gee-Herter d.
Gee-Herter-Heubner d.
Gee-Thaysen d.
Gierke d.
Gilbert d.
glomerular basement membrane d.
glomerulocystic kidney d.
glycogen storage d.
Goldstein d.
gonococcal perihepatis pelvic inflammatory d.
Goodpasture d.
Gordon d.
G protein d.
graft-versus-host d. (GVHD)
granulomatous bowel d.
Graves d.
Grey Turner d.
Gross d.
H d.
Hailey-Hailey d.
halothane-induced d.
Hanot d.
Harley d.
Hartnup d.
HBsAg-negative anti-HCV-negative chronic liver d.
heavy chain deposition d.
Hebra d.
hemorrhage in inflammatory bowel d.
hepatic cystic d.
hepatic Hodgkin d.
hepatic metastatic d.
hepatic venoocclusive d.
hepatic venous web d.
hepatitis C virus-associated venoocclusive d.
hepatobiliary fibropolycystic d.
hepatobiliary tract d.
hepatocellular d.
hepatolenticular d.
herring-worm d.
Hers d.
Herter d.
Herter-Heubner d.
Heubner-Herter d.
Hirschsprung d.
Hodgkin d.
homologous protein overload d.
hookworm d.
Hutinel d.
hydatid cyst d.
hyperacute graft-versus-host d.
hypertensive autosomal-dominant polycystic kidney d.
hypoplastic glomerulocystic d.
idiopathic inflammatory bowel d. (IIBD)
ileocolic d.
ileocolonic Crohn d.
immunodeficiency d.
immunoproliferative small intestinal d. (IPSID)
inactive Crohn d.
infantile celiac d.
infantile polycystic d. (IPCD)
infiltrative d.
inflammatory bowel d. (IBD)
intramural atheromatous d.
iron storage d.

ischemic bowel d.
Johne d.
juvenile nephronophthisis-medullary cystic d.
Kashin-Beck d.
Katayama d.
Kennedy d.
Keshan d.
kidney glomerulocystic d.
Kimmelstiel-Wilson d.
Kimura d.
Kinnier Wilson d.
Klebs d.
Klemperer d.
Kohlmeier-Degos d.
Kyasanur Forest d.
Kyrle d.
Lane d.
Larrey-Weil d.
Leigh d.
Leiner d.
Leyden d.
Lhermitte-Duclos d.
Liddle d.
light-chain deposition d. (LCDD)
Lignac d.
Lignac-Fanconi d.
liver hydatid d.
Löwe d.
luminal Crohn d.
lung d.
Lyell d.
Lyme d.
lysosomal storage d. (LSD)
Mackenzie d.
macrovascular d.
malabsorption d.
malignant biliary obstructive d.
Manson d.
maple-syrup urine d. (MSUD)
Marchiafava-Micheli d.
Marie-Strumpell d.
Marion d.
medullary cystic d.
Ménétrier d.
Ménière d.
Menkes d.
mesenteric inflammatory venoocclusive d. (MIVOD)
mesenteric vascular d.
metabolic liver d.
metabolic stone d.

metastatic Crohn d. (MCD)
microcystic d. of renal medulla
microvillus inclusion d.
Milroy d.
minimal change d.
mixed connective tissue d. (MCTD)
Model for End-Stage Liver D. (MELD)
modification of diet in renal d. (MDRD)
mucosal lesion of acid peptic d.
multicystic kidney d.
Munk d.
muscle layer d.
mycobacterial d.
myeloproliferative d.
National Institute of Diabetes, Digestive and Kidney D. (NIDDK)
neoplastic d.
neurogenic bladder d.
neurohumoral d.
Niemann-Pick d.
nil d.
Nisbet d.
non-A–G chronic liver d.
nonalcoholic fatty liver d. (NAFLD)
non-B non-C chronic liver d. (NBNC CLD)
noncalculous d.
noncommunicating polycystic d.
nondiabetic proteinuric renal d.
nonerosive gastroesophageal reflux d.
nonerosive reflux d. (NERD)
nonobstructive hepatic parenchymal d.
nonorgan confined d.
oasthouse urine d.
obstructive gastroduodenal Crohn d.
Ohara d.
oral d.
organic neurologic d.
Ormond d.
Osler-Weber-Rendu d.
ovarian d.
Paget extramammary d.
Paget perianal d.
panacinar d.
pancreatic d.

NOTES

disease (continued)
  pancreaticobiliary d.
  parasitic liver d.
  parathyroid d.
  parenchymal liver d.
  Parkinson d.
  paroxysmal motor d.
  patella d.
  Payr d.
  pediatric end-stage liver d. (PELD)
  pediatric stone d.
  pelvic inflammatory d. (PID)
  peptic reflux d.
  peptic ulcer d. (PUD)
  perforated ulcer d.
  perianal Crohn d.
  perineal Crohn d.
  Peyronie d.
  pilonidal sinus d.
  polycystic kidney d.
  polycystic liver d. (PCLD, PLD)
  Pompe d.
  post jejunoileal bypass hepatic d.
  Potter d.
  predominant hyperparathyroid bone d. (PHBD)
  preeclamptic liver d.
  preexisting d.
  primary glomerular d.
  protozoan d.
  pseudoalcoholic liver d.
  pseudo-Whipple d.
  radiation-induced d.
  Rayer d.
  reactive airway d. (RAD)
  recessive polycystic kidney d.
  rectal d.
  recurrent episodes of *Clostridium difficile* d. (RCCD)
  reflux d.
  Reichmann d.
  Reiter d.
  renal arterial occlusive d.
  renal bone d.
  renal cystic d.
  renal fibromuscular d.
  renal hydatid d.
  Rendu-Osler-Weber d.
  renovascular d.
  rheumatic d.
  Rokitansky d.
  Rossbach d.
  Ruysch d.
  Saunders d.
  Schilder d.
  Schindler d.
  schistosomal liver d.
  Schönlein-Henoch d.
  Schultz d.
  scleroderma bowel d.
  sexually related intestinal d.
  sexually transmitted d. (STD)
  sickle cell d.
  sigmoid d.
  skeletal muscle d.
  skin d.
  small intestinal Crohn d.
  space-occupying d.
  Spencer d.
  steely-hair d.
  Steinert d.
  steroid-dependent Crohn d.
  steroid-refractory Crohn d.
  Stokvis d.
  stone d.
  Strachan d.
  stress-related mucosal d. (SRMD)
  Stühmer d.
  subacute liver d.
  subserosal d.
  suprahilar d.
  systemic mast cell d.
  Takayasu d.
  Tangier d.
  terminal ileal d.
  testicular Hodgkin d.
  Thaysen d.
  thin basement membrane d. (TBMD)
  thin glomerular basement membrane d.
  thromboembolic d.
  thyroid d.
  Tis d.
  transfusion-related chronic liver d.
  transmittable d.
  tubulointerstitial d.
  tufting d.
  tunnel d.
  unilocular hydatid d.
  upper tract d.
  uremic medullary cystic d.
  urinary tract d.
  urologic d.
  valvular heart d.
  Van Bogaert d.
  van Buren d.
  van den Bergh d.
  vascular d.
  venereal d.
  venoocclusive liver d.
  venous outflow obstructive d.
  venous web d.
  von Gierke d.
  von Hippel-Lindau d.
  von Recklinghausen d.
  von Rokitansky d.
  von Willebrand d.

disease · disorder

Wassilieff d.
Weber-Christian d.
Weil d.
Werdnig-Hoffman d.
Westphal-Strümpell d.
Whipple d. (WD)
Wilkie d.
Wilson d. (WD)
Wolman d.
X-linked chronic granulomatous d. (X-CGD)

diseased organileal pouch-anal anastomosis
disease-free survival curve
disease-specific
d.-s. diet
d.-s. isolation

dish
Side-Fire reflecting d.

disialosyl Lea
DISIDA
diisopropyliminodiacetic acid
DISIDA enterogastroesophageal reflux study
DISIDA scan

disimpaction
colonoscopic d.

disinfectant
Abocide d.
Actril d.
Asepti-steryl d.
Burnishine d.
Calgocide d.
Cold Spor d.
cyclic urinary d.
Endospore d.
Enzol d.
Metricide d.
Omnicide d.
ProCide d.
Sporacidin d.
Vespore d.
Wavicide d.

disinfection
high-level d. (HLD)

disintegration
endoscopic stone d.

DisIntek reagent strip
disjoined pyeloplasty
disk, disc
anal d.
bilaminar embryonic d.

d. diffusion
d. kidney
laser d.
d. margin
Marlen double-faced adhesive d.
Molnar d.

dislodgement
electrode d.

dislodger
stone d.

dismembered
d. anastomosis
d. pyeloplasty
d. reimplanted appendicocystostomy

dismutase
superoxide d. (SOD)

disobliteration
disodium
balsalazide d.
cefotetan d.
d. cromoglycate
d. edetate

Disolan
Disonate
disopyramide phosphate (DP)
disorder
absence of comorbid d.'s
acid-base d.
acid-related d. (ARD)
acid secretory d.
anorexia nervosa and associated d.'s (ANAD)
appetite d.
autoimmune connective tissue d.
autosomal-dominant d.
binge-eating d. (BED)
blood coagulation d.
cardiovascular d.
connective tissue d.
deglutition d.
esophageal motility d. (EMD)
esophageal motor d.
evacuation d.
fat storage d.
feeding d.
functional bowel d. (FBD)
functional gastrointestinal d. (FGID)
gastric motility d.
Hartnup d.
humoral immunodeficiency d.
intestinal motility d.
iron overload d.

NOTES

disorder *(continued)*
- lower motor neuron bladder d.
- lymphoproliferative d.
- metabolic d.
- mixed connective tissue d.
- motility d.
- myeloproliferative d.
- National Association of Anorexia Nervosa and Associated D.'s
- neurodegenerative d.
- neurogenic d.
- neurologic d.
- nonspecific esophageal motility d. (NEMD)
- papulosquamous d.
- pelvic floor d.
- posttransplant lymphoproliferative d. (PTLD)
- psychological d.
- psychosomatic d.
- pulmonary d.
- rectal evacuatory d. (RED)
- seizure d.
- spastic motor d.
- urachal d.
- vasomotor d.
- vesiculobullous d.
- wound healing d.

disordered
- d. acrosome reaction of spermatozoon
- d. motility

Di-Sosul

dispar
- *Entamoeba d.*

Di-Spaz

Dispenstirs

displacement
- bowel d.
- fiber lock d.
- fish-hook d.
- gallbladder d.
- tumor d.

display
- high-definition video d. (HDVD)

disposable
- d. forceps
- d. pudendal nerve electrode
- d. sheathed flexible sigmoidoscope
- d. trocar

disposable-sheath flexible gastroscope

disrupted peristalsis

disruption
- pancreatic duct d.

disruptor
- endocrine d.

Disse
- space of D.

dissecting
- d. abdominal aneurysm
- d. balloon
- d. renal artery aneurysm

dissection
- aortic d.
- autonomic nerve-preserving three-space d.
- blunt and sharp d.
- circumferential mucosal d.
- electrosurgical d.
- en bloc d.
- extended obturator node and iliopsoas node d.
- extraperitoneal endoscopic pelvic lymph node d. (EEPLND)
- finger fracture d.
- flap d.
- intersphincteric rectal d.
- intracapsular d.
- intramural air d.
- laparoscopic pelvic lymph node d. (LPLND)
- lateral node d.
- limited obturator node d.
- lymph node d.
- d. margin
- meticulous d.
- minilaparotomy pelvic lymph node d.
- nerve-sparing lymph node d.
- node d.
- partial zonal d. (PZD)
- pelvic d.
- per anum intersphincteric rectal d.
- plane of d.
- rectal d.
- renal hilar d.
- retroperitoneal lymph node d. (RPLD)
- scissors d.
- d. scissors
- sharp d.
- spontaneous d.
- submucosal d.
- suprahilar lymph node d.
- three-field d.
- three-space d.
- ultrasonic d.
- ureteral d.

dissector
- Beaver d.
- CUSA d.
- Kittner d.
- McDonald stone d.
- Mixter d.
- peanut d.
- Spacemaker balloon d.

sponge d.
ultrasonic aspirator and d.
disseminated
    d. cancer
    d. CMV infection
    d. histoplasmosis
    d. intravascular coagulation (DIC)
    d. lupus erythematosus (DLE)
    d. metastasis
    d. peritoneal adenomucinosis
    d. strongyloidiasis
dissemination
    metastatic d.
dissimilatory sulfate reduction
dissociated medium
dissolution
    contact d.
    d. of gallstone
    MTBE gallstone d.
distal
    d. bile duct
    d. bile duct diameter
    d. blind stomach
    d. colitis
    d. colon
    d. convoluted tubule (DCT)
    d. duodenum
    d. esophageal ring
    d. esophageal stenosis
    d. esophageal stricture
    d. esophagus
    d. gastrectomy
    d. ileitis
    d. intestine (DI)
    d. neoplasia
    d. nephron segment
    d. pancreatectomy
    d. pouch leak
    d. renal tubular acidosis (dRTA)
    d. renal tubular necrosis
    d. shave section
    d. splenorenal shunt (DSRS)
    d. tubular acting agent
    d. tubule (DT)
    d. ureter
    d. ureteral anatomy
    d. ureterectomy
    d. venous plexus
distance
    peritoneal-anal d.
distant
    d. abscess

    d. heart sounds
    d. metastasis
    d. pH probe location
distasonis
    Bacteroides d.
distended
    d. abdomen
    d. bladder
distensibility
distention
    abdominal d.
    colonic d.
    esophageal balloon d.
    gaseous d.
    gastric d.
    intestinal d.
    intraesophageal balloon d. (IEBD)
    intraluminal d.
    isobaric gastric d.
    postprandial d.
    rectal d.
    d. ulcer
    visible abdominal d.
distomiasis
    intestinal d.
distorted crypt architecture
distortion
    crypt architectural d.
distress
    epigastric d.
    functional bowel d. (FBD)
    mild d.
    moderate d.
    respiratory d.
distribution
    folate d.
    geographic d.
    hit-skip d.
    intrarenal d.
    liver d.
    node d.
    d. ratio (DR)
    vasoactive intestinal peptide d.
    volume of d. (Vd)
disturbance
    acid-base d.
    gait d.
    phytoestrogen-induced menstrual cycle d.
disulfide cross linked fibril
disulfiram

NOTES

disulfiram-like effect
dithiothreitol (DTT)
Ditropan XL
Dittel
    D. operation
    D. sound
Diucardin
Diupres
diuresis
    alcohol d.
    osmotic d.
    postobstructive d.
    solute d.
    tubular d.
    water d.
diuretic
    high-ceiling d.
    hydragogue d.
    kaliuretic d.
    loop d.
    d. nuclear renography
    osmotic d.
    potassium-sparing d.
    refrigerant d.
    d. renal quantitative camera study
    d. renal scintigraphy
    thiazide d.
diuretic-induced hypokalemia
diuria
Diurigen
diurnal
    d. continence
    d. cycle
    d. enuresis
    d. incontinence
    d. urine osmolality
    d. variation
Diutensen-R
diutinum
    erythema elevatum d.
divalent mineral
diversion
    acidosis after urinary intestinal d.
    biliopancreatic d.
    Bricker urinary d.
    Camey enterocystoplasty urinary d.
    Camey I orthotopic urinary d.
    d. colitis
    continent catheterizable urinary d.
    continent cutaneous d.
    continent supravesical bowel urinary d.
    cutaneous urinary d.
    double-T pouch urinary d.
    Duke pouch cutaneous urinary d.
    external biliary d.
    fecal d.
    Gil-Vernet ileocecal cystoplasty urinary d.
    Gil-Vernet orthotopic urinary d.
    Hammock technique urinary d.
    hemi-Kock urinary d.
    heterotopic d.
    ileal conduit urinary d.
    ileal neobladder urinary d.
    ileocecal cutaneous d.
    ileocolic urinary d.
    ileocolonic pouch urinary d.
    Indiana continent reservoir urinary d.
    initial proximal d.
    jejunal cutaneous urinary d.
    Kock pouch cutaneous urinary d.
    Leadbetter ileal loop d.
    Le Bag urinary d.
    LeDuc technique urinary d.
    Mainz pouch cutaneous urinary d.
    orthotopic urinary d.
    partial external biliary d.
    primary urinary d.
    d. proctitis
    rectal bladder urinary d.
    split-nipple technique urinary d.
    stone in urinary d.
    Studer reservoir urinary d.
    subcutaneous urinary d.
    supravesical urinary d.
    tunneled technique urinary d.
    urinary intestinal d.
    Wallace technique urinary d.
diversionary ileostomy
diversus
    Citrobacter d.
diverticula (*pl.* of diverticulum)
diverticular
    d. abscess
    d. bleeding
    d. disease
    d. disease of colon (DDC)
    d. hemorrhage
    d. phlegmon
diverticulectomy
    bladder d.
    endocavitary bladder d.
    Harrington esophageal d.
    pharyngoesophageal d.
    urethral d.
    vesical d.
diverticulitis
    acute d.
    cecal d.
    chronic d.
    duodenal d.
    d. evaluation
    Meckel d.
    perforating d.
    sigmoid d.
diverticulogram

diverticuloma
diverticulopexy
diverticuloscope
    soft d.
diverticulosis
    acquired d.
    bleeding d.
    colonic d.
    congenital d.
    esophageal intramural d.
    gastric d.
    giant d.
    jejunal d.
diverticulostomy
    endoscopic stapling d.
diverticulotomy
    endoscopic d.
    endoscopic clip-and-cut d.
diverticulum, pl. **diverticula**
    d. of Akerlund
    diverticula ampullae ductus deferentis
    angioarchitecture of arterial supply of d.
    biliary d.
    bladder congenital d.
    bleeding d.
    caliceal d.
    cecal d.
    diverticula of colon
    colonic d.
    congenital bladder d.
    cricopharyngeal d.
    Dohlman endoscopic repair of Zenker d.
    duodenal d.
    epiphrenic d.
    esophageal d.
    false d.
    fluid-filled d.
    d. fulguration
    Ganser d.
    giant colonic d. (GCD)
    Graser d.
    Heister d.
    hepatic d.
    Hutch d.
    hypopharyngeal d.
    d. ilei verum
    inflamed d.
    intestinal d.
    intraluminal duodenal d. (IDD)
    intramural d.
    inverted sigmoid d.
    juxtapapillary duodenal d.
    Kirchner d.
    long-neck d.
    Meckel d.
    midesophageal d.
    mucosal d.
    noncommunicating d.
    d. of Nuck
    pancreatic d.
    perforated d.
    periampullary duodenal d.
    peripapillary d.
    Pertik d.
    pharyngeal d.
    pharyngoesophageal d.
    pressure d.
    Rokitansky d.
    ruptured sigmoid d.
    sigmoid d.
    solitary d.
    supradiaphragmatic d.
    thin-walled d.
    traction d.
    unroofing of d.
    urachal d.
    ureteric d.
    urethral d.
    vesical d.
    vesicourachal d.
    volvulated Meckel d.
    Zenker d.
diverting
    d. loop colostomy
    d. loop ileostomy
    d. stoma
    d. stoma creation
divided appendix
divided pancreas
divided-stoma colostomy
division
    urethral plate d.
divisum
    incomplete pancreas d. (IPD)
    pancreas d. (PD)
Dixon-Thomas-Smith clamp
Dizac
DJJ
    duodenojejunal junction
DLC
    dual-lumen catheter

NOTES

DLE
 disseminated lupus erythematosus
DLPC
 dilinoleoylphosphatidylcholine
DM
 duodenal mucosa
DMEM
 Dulbecco modified Eagle medium
DMI
 Dilamezinsert
  DMI urologic instrument
DMM
 diffuse malignant mesothelioma
DMPP
 dimethyl-4-phenylpiperazinium
DMPS
 dimethylpolysiloxane
DMS
 diffuse mesangial sclerosis
DMSA
 dimercaptosuccinic acid
  DMSA scan
  DMSA scintigraphy
  ^{99m}Tc DMSA
DMSO
 dimethyl sulfoxide
  DMSO cystitis
DNA
 deoxyribonucleic acid
  DNA aneuploidy
  DNA array
  complementary DNA
  DNA flow cytometry
  genomic DNA
  DNA haploid cell
  HBV genomic DNA
  hepatitis B-like DNA
  DNA hypomethylation
  DNA immunization
  DNA labeling kit
  DNA laddering
  DNA microarray technology
  DNA ploidy analysis
  DNA ploidy pattern
  DNA polymerase
  DNA polymorphism
  DNA proliferation
  DNA Sequencing System
  single-parameter DNA
  DNA stemline
  DNA synthesis
DNCB
 dinitrochlorobenzene
  DNCB immunological study
DNH
 diffuse nodular hyperplasia
DOB
 delta over baseline

Dobbhoff
 D. biofeedback monitor
 D. bipolar coagulation probe
 D. enteral feeding bag
 D. gastrectomy feeding tube
 D. gastric decompression tube
 D. PEG tube
dobutamine
docetaxel
Dock test meal
Docucal-P
docusate sodium
dodecadactylitis
dodecadactylon
dog-ear of anastomosis
Dogiel type I, II morphology
DO2-haplotype
Dohlman
 D. endoscopic repair of Zenker diverticulum
 D. esophagoscope
dolasetron
dolichocolon with pseudoobstruction
DoLi S extracorporeal shock wave lithotriptor
Dolobid
dolorimeter
 Chatillon d.
dolorosa
 nephritis d.
dolphin grasping forceps
dolphin-type atraumatic forceps
domain
 alternative cell attachment d.
 carboxyterminal noncollagenous d.
 cleaved extracellular d.
 COOH-terminal SH2 d.
 effector d.
 Kringle d.
 membrane-spanning d. (MDS)
 NH2-terminal SH2 d.
 nucleotide-binding d. (NBD)
 SH2-binding d.
 src-homology 2 d.
 trefoil d.
dome
 d. of bladder
 gallbladder d.
 d. of liver
 trabeculation of bladder d.
Domeboro solution
dome-shaped internal bumper
dome-tip electrode
domiciliary urinary tract infection
dominant inheritance model
Domino transplant
domperidone
domperidone-functional dyspepsia trial

donation
  live renal d.
  organ d.
Donnagel
Donnagel-PG
Donnamar
Donna-Sed
Donnatal No. 2
Donnazyme
donor
  d. age-dependent effect
  artificial insemination d. (AID)
  d. dendritic cell
  four-antigen matched d.
  d. hematopoietic cell microchimerism
  d. hepatectomy
  d. hepatic duct (DHD)
  d. kidney
  kidney d.
  living d. (LD)
  living adult-to-adult d.
  living related d.
  living unrelated d. (LURD)
  marginal kidney d.
  d. nephrectomy
  nitric oxide d.
  d. of nitric oxide
  related living d. (RLD)
  sulfhydryl d.
donor/recipient race matching
donor-specific
  d.-s. alloantibody
  d.-s. transfusion (DST)
donor-type microchimerism
Donovan body
donovani
  Leishmania donovani d.
donovanosis
Donphen
donut
  circular stapler d.
doom
  triangle of d.
DOPA
  dihydroxyphenylalanine
dopamine
  d. agonist
  d. antagonist
  d. betahydroxylase

dopaminergic
  d. agonist
  d. medication
Dopar
dopexamine
Doppler
  D. assistance
  color flow D.
  D. color flow imaging
  D. effect
  endoscopic color D.
  D. flow test (DFT)
  D. operation
  penile D.
  D. perfusion index (DPI)
  D. probe
  pulsed D.
  D. QAD-1
  D. Quantum color flow system
  D. sonography of SMA
  D. ultrasonography
  D. ultrasonography angiography
  D. ultrasound (DUS)
  D. ultrasound intestinal blood flow measurement
Doppler-guided hemorrhoidal artery ligation (DGHAL)
DOQI
  Dialysis Outcomes Quality Initiative
d'orange
  peau d.
Dor fundoplication
Dormia
  D. noose
  D. stone basket
  D. stone basket catheter
Dornier
  D. compact lithotriptor
  D. extracorporeal shock wave lithotripsy
  D. gallstone lithotriptor
  D. HM3, HM4 electrohydraulic lithotriptor
  D. MFL 5000 urological workstation
  D. MPL 9000 electrohydraulic lithotriptor ultrasound focusing system
  D. MPL 9000 gallstone lithotripsy
  D. MPL 5000 lithotriptor
  D. Urotract cystoscopy table

NOTES

dorsal
    d. bud
    d. curve plication
    d. lithotomy
    d. lithotomy position
    d. lumbotomy
    d. lumbotomy incision
    d. mesogastrium
    d. nerve conduction velocity
    d. nerve of penis
    d. pancreatic artery
    d. pancreatic duct
    d. penile artery
    d. point
    d. rhizotomy
    d. root ganglion
    d. slit
    d. tunical tuck
    d. vagal complex
    d. vein
    d. vein complex (DVC)
    d. vein patch graft
dorsalis
    arteria pancreatica d.
    tabes d.
dorsocranial
dorsosacral position
dorsum
    d. of penis
    d. of testis
dosage
    radiation d.
    sclerosant d.
dose
    arthritic d. (A/D)
    breakthrough d.
    conceptus d.
    d. optimized therapy (DOT)
    d. response
dosepak
    Hytrin D.
dosimeter
    single-channel in vivo light d.
Dostent
DOT
    dose optimized therapy
    TherMatrx DOT
dot-blot hybridization
dot-plotted probe
Dotter
    D. catheter
    D. dilator
Doubilet
    D. sphincterotome
    D. sphincterotomy
double
    d. accessory channel therapeutic endoscope
    d. balloon method of enteroscopy
    d. balloon technique
    d. bladder
    d. bubble duodenal sign
    d. contrast
    d. dialyzer
    d. duct sign
    d. enterostomy
    d. gallbladder
    d. gracilis wrap
    d. halo sign
    d. incontinence
    d. intussusception
    d. J-shaped reservoir
    d. penis
    d. pyloroplasty
    d. pylorus
    d. reverse alpha-sigmoid loop
    d. stapling technique (DST)
    d. strength (DS)
    d. tracking of barium
    d. uterus
    d. x-ray densitometry
double-antibody sandwich system
double-barrel
    d.-b. colostomy
    d.-b. ileostomy
    d.-b. reservoir
double-bite biopsy
double-blind randomized study
double-chamber hemodiafiltration
double-channel
    d.-c. colonoscope
    d.-c. endoscope
    d.-c. esophagogram
    d.-c. fistulotome
    d.-c. sphincterotome
    d.-c. videoendoscope
double-contrast
    d.-c. barium enema (DCBE)
    d.-c. barium enema examination
    d.-c. barium examination of upper gastrointestinal tract (DCGI)
    d.-c. barium meal
    d.-c. esophagram
    d.-c. radiography
    d.-c. roentgenography
double-cuff urinary sphincter
double-dose IV Timentin
double-faced island flap for hypospadias repair
double-folded cup-patch technique
double-headed
    d.-h. P190 stapler
    d.-h. P190 stapling device
double-head spermatozoon
double-J
    d.-J. catheter
    d.-J. indwelling catheter stent
    d.-J. silicone stent

d.-J. Surgitek catheter stent
d.-J. ureteral stent
double-loop
d.-l. pouch
d.-l. tourniquet
double-lumen
d.-l. balloon catheter
d.-l. endoprosthesis
d.-l. gastric laryngeal mask airway
d.-l. injection catheter
d.-l. irrigation cannula
d.-l. tapered-tip papillotome
d.-l. tube
double-peaked wave
double-pigtail
d.-p. endoprosthesis
d.-p. prosthesis
d.-p. stent
double-puncture laparoscopy
double-spoon forceps
double-stapled
d.-s. ileal pouch-anal anastomosis
d.-s. ileal reservoir
double-staple technique
DoubleStent
D. biliary endoprosthesis
D. biliary endoprosthesis stent
double-tail spermatozoon
double-T pouch urinary diversion
double-wing shape
doubling time
doubly ligated
doughnut
d. lesion
stapler d.
doughnut-shaped balloon
doughy
d. abdomen
d. consistency
Douglas
D. abscess
cul-de-sac of D.
D. fold
line of D.
D. pouch
D. rectal snare
rectouterine pouch of D.
semicircular line of D.
doula
Dow-Corning ileal pouch catheter

Dowd II prostatic balloon dilatation catheter
Dow Hollow Fiber kidney (DHFK)
down
D. syndrome
tacked d.
downhill esophageal varix
downregulation after furosemide treatment
downscatter
downstage
downstaging
d. of advanced esophageal carcinoma
hormonal d.
downstream
d. signaling protein
d. signal transduction
downward retraction
doxacurium
doxazosin mesylate
doxepin
doxercalciferol injection
Doxinate
doxorubicin
d., bleomycin sulfate, vinblastine (ABV)
d., bleomycin sulfate, vinblastine, dacarbazine (ABVD)
doxycycline-metronidazole-bismuth subcitrate triple therapy
doxycycline monohydrate
Doyen
D. abdominal retractor
D. abdominal scissors
D. gallbladder forceps
D. intestinal clamp
D. intestinal forceps
D. operation
D. raspatory
D. rib elevator
doylei
Campylobacter d.
DP
diphosphate
dipropionate
disopyramide phosphate
D.P.
Dalalone D.P.
DP-1 lithotriptor
DPC
delayed primary closure

NOTES

DPEG
    dual percutaneous endoscopic gastrostomy
D-penicillamine
DPI
    daily protein intake
    Doppler perfusion index
DPJ
    direct percutaneous jejunostomy
    DPJ tube
D-P urea ratio
DQ2 haplotype
DR
    diffuse redness
    distribution ratio
    HLA DR
DR2
    DR2 1501 HLA-DRB tissue type
    DR2 1502 HLA-DRB tissue type
    DR2 1601 HLA-DRB tissue type
    DR2 1602 HLA-DRB tissue type
DR7
    DR7 haplotype
    DR7 HLA-DRB tissue type
DR1 HLA-DRB tissue type
DR3
    HLA DR3
    DR3 HLA-DRB tissue type
DR4
    HLA DR4
    DR4 HLA-DRB tissue type
DR5
    heterozygous DR5
DR9 HLA-DRB tissue type
drag
    solvent d.
dragon pyelogram
drain
    Blair silicone d.
    Chaffin-Pratt d.
    cigarette d.
    closed-suction d.
    Davol sump d.
    ERCP nasobiliary d.
    fluted J-Vac d.
    four-wing Malecot d.
    Hemovac Suction Standard d.
    Hollister irrigator d.
    Jackson-Pratt d.
    J-Vac d.
    Mikulicz d.
    nasobiliary d. (NBD)
    nasocystic d.
    Nélaton rubber tube d.
    Penrose sump d.
    perineal d.
    Pezzer d.
    Quad-Lumen d.
    Redivac suction d.
    Redon d.
    Relia-Vac d.
    Snyder d.
    stab-wound d.
    suction d.
    sump d.
    surgical d.
    T d.
    Teflon nasobiliary d.
    transnasal pancreaticobiliary d.
    transpapillary d.
    T-tube d.
    two-wing Malecot d.
    van Sonnenberg sump d.
    d. volume
    Wangensteen d.
drainable ostomy pouch
drainage
    antegrade ureteral d.
    bedside d. (BSD)
    biliary d.
    button d.
    caliceal d.
    d. catheter
    closed d.
    continuous bladder d.
    continuous catheter d.
    continuous suction d.
    CT-guided abscess d.
    CT-guided pseudocyst d.
    duodenal d.
    endoscopic biliary d.
    endoscopic nasobiliary d. (ENBD)
    endoscopic nasobiliary catheter d.
    endoscopic pancreatic d.
    endoscopic retrograde biliary d. (ERBD)
    endoscopic transgastric d.
    endoscopic transpapillary cyst d. (ETCD)
    external d.
    gravity-dependent d.
    guided percutaneous d.
    incision and d. (I&D)
    internal biliary d.
    J-Vac closed wound d.
    lymphocele internal d.
    lymphocele percutaneous d.
    nasobiliary d.
    nasogastric d.
    nasopancreatic d.
    open d.
    pancreaticoduodenal venous d.
    passive chest d.
    percutaneous abscess d.
    percutaneous antegrade biliary d.
    percutaneous biliary d. (PBD)
    percutaneous transhepatic d. (PTD)

percutaneous transhepatic biliary d. (PTBD)
postoperative irrigation-suction d.
Pyridium test of vaginal d.
sanguineous d.
serosanguineous d.
suction d.
suprapubic cystomy d.
tidal d.
transduodenal d.
transgastric d.
transhepatic biliary d.
transluminal pseudocyst d.
transmural d. (TMD)
transpapillary d.
T-tube d.
d. tube
Wangensteen d.
wound d.

drainage-resistant pseudocyst
draining sinus
drain-trap stomach
Drake uroflowmeter
Drake-Willock
    D.-W. delivery system
    D.-W. peritoneal dialysis system
Dramamine
Drapanas shunt
drape
    barrier d.
    fenestrated d.
    Lingeman 3-in-1 procedure d.
    Lingeman TUR d.
    O'Connor d.
    surgical d.
Drash syndrome
DRB **gene**
DRE
    digital rectal examination
Dreiling tube
Dremel Moto-Tool
dressing
    Acticoat composite d.
    Acticoat foam d.
    Adaptic d.
    adhesive d.
    anorectal d. (ARD)
    antiseptic d.
    bioocclusive d.
    bolus d.
    bulky d.
    CarboFlex odor-control d.
    Coban d.
    CombiDERM nonadhesive absorbant d.
    Compeed Skinprotector d.
    dry sterile d.
    Elastoplast d.
    d. forceps
    gauze d.
    Kling d.
    LYOfoam d.
    Montgomery strap d.
    nonadhesive d.
    occlusive collodion d.
    Op-Site d.
    pressure d.
    SaliCept freeze-dried d.
    Signa Dress Hydrocolloid d.
    sterile d.
    Tegaderm d.
    Telfa d.
    Tielle Plus hydropolymer d.
    tie-over d.
DRF
    digestive-respiratory fistula
dribble
    postmicturition d.
    postvoid d.
dribbling
    urinary d.
drift
    pronator d.
drilling tract
drink
    Boost Nutritional Energy D.
    HeartBar Orange D.
drinking
    d. habit
    psychogenic water d.
    voluntarily stopping eating and d. (VSED)
drip
    alkaline milk d.
    d. infusion cholangiography (DIC)
    d. infusion cholecystography
    intragastric d.
    intravenous d.
    Murphy d.
    postnasal d.
driver
    automatic needle d.
    Haney needle d.
    laparoscopic needle d.

NOTES

driver *(continued)*
    long vascular needle d.
    needle d.
    Szabo-Berci needle d.
dromedary hump
dronabinol
drooling
droop
    flank d.
drooping lily sign
droperidol
dropped bladder
dropsical
    d. nephritis
    d. nephropathy
dropsy
    abdominal d.
    cutaneous d.
    nutritional d.
    peritoneal d.
Drosophila melanogaster
dRTA
    distal renal tubular acidosis
drug
    aminobiphosphonate gastrotoxic d.
    anorectic d.
    antagonistic d.
    anticholinergic d.
    antiemetic d.
    antilipemic d.
    antimotility d.
    antimuscarinic d.
    antimycobacterial d.
    antisecretory d.
    antispasmodic d.
    d. carrier system
    COX-2 selective nonsteroidal antiinflammatory d.
    crude d.
    cyclooxygenase-2 selective nonsteroidal antiinflammatory d.
    d. hepatotoxicity
    H2 receptor-blocking d.
    hydrocholeretic d.
    immunoregulatory d.
    immunosuppressive d.
    d. intoxication
    lipid-lowering d.
    d. metabolism
    neurolytic d.
    neuropsychotropic d.
    nitric oxide-releasing nonsteroidal antiinflammatory d.'s (NO-NSAIDs)
    nonnephrotoxic d.
    nonsteroidal antiinflammatory d. (NSAID)
    parasympatholytic d.
    parasympathomimetic d.
    portal hypotensive d.
    prokinetic d.
    psychotropic d.
    d. reaction
    recreational d.
    d. resistance
    second-line d.
    serotonergic d.
    d. therapy
    vasoactive d.
drug-induced
    d.-i. acute hepatic injury
    d.-i. acute pancreatitis
    d.-i. acute tubular necrosis
    d.-i. cholestasis
    d.-i. cirrhosis
    d.-i. colitis
    d.-i. constipation
    d.-i. erection
    d.-i. esophageal damage (DIED)
    d.-i. esophagitis
    d.-i. gastritis
    d.-i. hepatitis
    d.-i. pain
    d.-i. priapism
    d.-i. renal failure
    d.-i. steatosis
    d.-i. ulcer
drug-related liver disease
Drummond
    artery of D.
    marginal artery of D.
DRVVT
    dilute Russell viper venom test
DRw8 HLA-DRB tissue type
DRw10 HLA-DRB tissue type
DRw11 HLA-DRB tissue type
DRw12 HLA-DRB tissue type
DRw13 HLA-DRB tissue type
DRw14 HLA-DRB tissue type
dry
    d. colostomy
    d. ejaculation
    d. heaves
    d. mucous membrane
    d. skin
    d. sterile dressing
    d. swallow
    d. swallow on esophageal manometry
    d. vomiting
    d. weight
DS
    double strength
    Bactrim DS
    Septra DS
    Sulfatrim DS
    trimethoprim-sulfamethoxazole DS

DSA
  digital venous subtraction angiography
DSD
  detrusor sphincter dyssynergia
DSP
  deoxyspergualin
DSRS
  distal splenorenal shunt
DSS
  dextran sodium sulfate
DST
  donor-specific transfusion
  double stapling technique
  duodenal secretin test
DT
  distal tubule
DTH
  delayed-type hypersensitivity
DTIC
  dimethyltriazenoimidazole carboxamide
DTO
  deodorized tincture of opium
DTPA
  diethylenetriamine pentaacetic acid
    indium-111 DTPA
    DTPA renal scan
    DTPA renography
DTT
  dithiothreitol
DU
  dialytic ultrafiltration
  duodenal ulcer
Dua antireflux stent
dual
  d. percutaneous endoscopic gastrostomy (DPEG)
  d. percutaneous gastrostomy tube
dual-axis confocal microscope
dual-endoscope technique
dual-energy
  d.-e. CT scan
  d.-e. x-ray absorptiometry (DEXA, DXA)
  d.-e. x-ray absorption
dual-lumen
  d.-l. catheter (DLC)
  d.-l. papillotome
DualMesh hernia repair
dual-phase helical computed tomography
dual-photon absorptiometry
dual-plane catheter-based ultrasound
Dual-Port system

dual-pulse lithotripter
Dubin-Amelar varicocele classification
Dubin-Johnson syndrome
Dubin-Sprinz
  D.-S. disease
  D.-S. syndrome
Dubowitz syndrome
Duchenne-type muscular dystrophy
duck-bill forceps
Duckett
  D. meatal advancement
  D. procedure
Ducrey disease
ducreyi
  Haemophilus d.
duct
  absence of diluted d.
  accessory pancreatic d.
  anomalous junction of pancreaticobiliary d.'s (AJPBD)
  anomalous pancreaticobiliary d. (APBD)
  arborization of d.'s
  beaded hepatic d.
  Bellini d.
  Bernard d.
  bifurcation of common bile d.
  bile d.
  biliary d.
  branch pancreatic d.
  d. cannulation
  clubbed common bile d.
  collecting d. (CD)
  common d. (CD)
  common bile d. (CBD)
  common hepatic d.
  cortical collecting d. (CCD)
  cross-section of collecting d.
  cystic d. (CD)
  diffuse irregular narrowing of pancreatic d.
  dilated bile d.
  distal bile d.
  donor hepatic d. (DHD)
  dorsal pancreatic d.
  ductal d.
  ejaculatory d.
  epididymis lymphatic d.
  excretory d.
  extrahepatic bile d.
  fusiform widening of d.
  gall d.

NOTES

duct *(continued)*
    Gartner d.
    genu of pancreatic d.
    hepatic d.
    horseshoe anomaly of pancreatic d.
    impacted cystic d.
    infected bile d.
    infundibulum of bile d.
    inner medullary collecting d. (IMCD)
    interlobular bile d.
    intrahepatic bile d.
    intrapancreatic bile d.
    irregular d.
    left hepatic d. (LHD)
    Leydig d.
    d. lumen
    Luschka d.
    main pancreatic d. (MPD)
    medullary collecting d.
    mesonephric d.
    middle extrahepatic bile d.
    müllerian d.
    narrow-caliber d.
    nontransected pancreatic d.
    normal-caliber d.
    outer medullary collecting d.
    pancreatic d.
    papillomatosis of intrahepatic bile d.
    perilobular d.
    peripheral bile d.
    preampullary portion of bile d.
    prepapillary bile d.
    proximal bile d.
    Rathke d.
    right hepatic d.
    d. of Santorini
    serpiginous microcystic d.
    Skene d.
    spiral fold of cystic d.
    Stensen d.
    subvesical d.
    tapered common bile d.
    tear d.
    terminal bile d.
    terminal inner medullary collecting d.
    thoracic d.
    upstream pancreatic d.
    vitelline d.
    vitellointestinal d. (VID)
    Wharton d.
    d. of Wirsung
    d. of Wolff
    wolffian d.
ductal
    d. adenocarcinoma of prostate
    d. change
    d. cystadenoma
    d. decompression
    d. dilation
    d. duct
    d. epithelial hyperplasia
    d. epithelium
    d. hypertension
    d. obstruction
    d. stricture
    d. system
    d. system perforation
ductectatic
    d. mucinous cystadenoma
    d. tumor
ductogram
    pancreatic d.
ductography
    peroral retrograde pancreaticobiliary d.
    postsphincterotomy d.
ductopenia
    idiopathic adulthood d.
    mild idiopathic adulthood biliary d. (MIAD)
ductopenic rejection
ductular structure
ductule
    biliary d.'s
    inferior aberrant d.
    superior aberrant d.
ductulus, pl. **ductuli**
    d. aberrans superior
    ductuli aberrantes
    ductuli biliferi
    ductuli efferentes
    ductuli interlobulares
    ductuli prostatica
ductus
    d. biliaris
    d. biliferi
    d. choledochus
    d. cysticus
    d. deferens
    d. ejaculatorius
    d. epididymidis
    d. excretorius vesiculae seminalis
    d. glandulae bulbourethralis
    d. hepaticus communis
    d. hepaticus dexter
    d. hepaticus sinister
    d. lobi caudati dexter
    d. lobi caudati sinister
    d. mesonephricus
    d. muelleri
    d. pancreaticus
    d. pancreaticus accessorius
    d. paraurethrales urethrae femininae
    d. prostatici
    d. Wolffi

Duette double-lumen ERCP instrument
Duffield deep surgery scissors
Dufourmentel technique
DUG
 dynamic urinary graciloplasty
Duhamel
 D. laparoscopic pullthrough anastomosis
 D. operation
 D. pullthrough procedure
Duke
 D. pouch
 D. pouch cutaneous urinary diversion
Dukes
 D. B-1
 D. classification
 D. classification of carcinoma
 D. signet cell A, B, C
 D. stage
 D. staging system
Dul45 cell line
Dulbecco modified Eagle medium (DMEM)
Dulcolax bowel preparation
dull
 d. pain
 d. to percussion abdomen
dullness
 hepatic d.
 liver d.
 d. to percussion
 shifting d.
 splenic d.
 tympanitic d.
dumbbell-shaped
 d.-s. caliceal extension
 d.-s. shadow
Dumdum fever
dumerili
 Seriola d.
Dumon-Gilliard
 D.-G. endoprosthesis system
 D.-G. prosthesis introducer
 D.-G. prosthesis pushing tube
dumping
 late d.
 d. stomach
 d. syndrome
dump kidney
duocrinin

duodenal
 d. acidification
 d. adenocarcinoma
 d. adenoma
 d. ampulla
 d. antrum
 d. atresia
 d. biopsy
 d. bleeding
 d. brake
 d. bulb
 d. bulb deformity
 d. cancer
 d. cap (DC)
 d. carcinoid
 d. C loop
 d. cluster unit
 d. compression
 d. diaphragm
 d. digestion
 d. diverticulitis
 d. diverticulum
 d. drainage
 d. effect
 d. endoscopic polypectomy
 d. erosion
 d. exclusion (DE)
 d. fistula
 d. fluid collection
 d. fold
 d. foreign body
 d. fossa
 d. gastrinoma
 d. gastroesophageal reflux (DGER)
 d. hemangiomatosis
 d. hematoma
 d. histoplasmosis
 d. impression
 d. impression on liver
 d. injury
 d. juice
 d. leiomyoma
 d. lesion
 d. loop
 d. lumen
 d. lymphoma
 d. lymphonodular hyperplasia
 d. mass
 d. metastasis
 d. mucosa (DM)
 d. neurofibroma
 d. obstruction

NOTES

duodenal *(continued)*
  d. orifice
  d. papilla
  d. polyp
  d. polyposis
  d. pressure wave
  d. secretin test (DST)
  d. seromyectomy
  d. smear
  d. stenosis
  d. stump
  d. sweep
  d. switch
  d. telangiectasia
  d. terminus
  d. trauma
  d. tube
  d. tuberculosis
  d. tumor
  d. ulcer (DU)
  d. ulceration
  d. ulcer disease
  d. ulceroinflammatory ulcer
  d. ulcer perforation (DUP)
  d. varix
  d. villus
  d. wall hamartoma
  d. web
duodenale
  Ancylostoma d.
duodenalis
  Giardia d.
duodenectomy
duodeni
  cryptae mucosae d.
duodenitis
  chronic atrophic d.
  Crohn d.
  erosive d.
duodenobiliary
  d. pressure gradient
  d. reflux
duodenocaval fistula
duodenocholangeitis
duodenocholecystostomy
duodenocholedochotomy
duodenocolic fistula
duodenocystostomy
duodenoduodenostomy
duodenoenterocutaneous fistula
duodenoenterostomy
duodenogastric reflux (DGR)
duodenogastroesophageal reflux (DGER)
duodenogastroscopy
  retrograde d. (RDG)
duodenogastrostomy
  end-to-side d.
duodenogram

duodenography
  hypotonic d.
duodenohepatic
duodenoileal bypass (DIB)
duodenoileostomy
duodenojejunal
  d. angle
  d. flexure
  d. fold
  d. fossa
  d. hernia
  d. junction (DJJ)
  d. recess
  d. sphincter
duodenojejunalis
  flexura d.
duodenojejunostomy
  suprapapillary Roux-en-Y d.
duodenolysis
duodenomesocolic fold
duodenopancreatic reflux
duodenorrhaphy
duodenoscope
  diagnostic d.
  endoscopic ultrasound d.
  Fujinon DUO-XT d.
  Fujinon ED7-XT d.
  Fujinon ED-200XU d.
  Fujinon ED-310XU d.
  Fujinon ED-410XU d.
  Fujinon EVD-XT d.
  Fujinon FD-100XU d.
  JF-200 d.
  JF-IT20 d.
  large-channel therapeutic d.
  master d.
  Olympus EW-series fiberoptic d.
  Olympus JF1T10 fiberoptic d.
  Olympus PJF-series pediatric d.
  Olympus TJF-10, -100, -200 d.
  Pentax d.
  side-viewing fiberoptic d.
  standard d.
  therapeutic side-viewing d.
  TJF-100, -130 large-channel d.
duodenostomy
  Witzel d.
duodenotomy
  transverse d.
duodenovideoscope
  small-caliber d.
duodenum
  Brunner gland of d.
  brunneroma of d.
  button of d.
  C loop of d.
  closed d.
  d. deformed by scarring
  descending d.

distal d.
gastric metaplasia of d.
mucous crypt of d.
obstruction d.
scarified d.
ulcer d.

duodenum-preserving pancreatic head resection
Duodopa
Duo-Flow catheter
Duosol
Duo-Tube feeding tube
DUP
duodenal ulcer perforation
DUPAN 2 tumor marker
Duphalac
Duplay operation
duplex
d. Doppler endosonography
d. ileum
d. sonography
duplicated gallbladder
duplicate uterus
duplication
alimentary tract d.
d. anomaly
biliary tree d.
bladder d.
colonic d.
complete d.
d. cyst
gastric cystic d.
incomplete d.
renal d.
tubular colonic d.
urethra d.
Dupuytren
D. contracture
D. disease
D. hydrocele
D. suture
D. tourniquet
durability
long-term d.
durable healing
Duracep biopsy forceps
DURAglide 3 stone balloon catheter
Dura-II positionable penile prosthesis
Duralone
dural patch reconstruction
Duramorph
Durand-Nicholas-Favre disease

Duraphase inflatable penile prosthesis
Durasphere injectable bulking agent
duration
esophageal body contraction d.
mean treatment d.
phasic wave d.
d. time
Duricef
Duroziez sign
Durrani dorsal vein complex ligation needle
DUS
Doppler ultrasound
duskiness
stomal d.
dusky stoma
dutasteride capsule
Duval
D. distal pancreaticojejunostomy
D. procedure
Duverney foramen
Duvoid
D&V
diarrhea and vomiting
DVC
dorsal vein complex
DVIU
direct-vision internal urethrotomy
DVS
direct vesicoureteral scintigraphy
dwarf kidney
dwell period
DXA
dual-energy x-ray absorptiometry
D-xylose
D-x. absorption test
D-x. malabsorption
dyad
mother-infant d.
dyadic relationship
Dyazide
Dyclone
dye
Alcian blue d.
basic d.
cationic d.
Congo red d.
Evans blue d.
indigo carmine d.
indocyanine green d. (ICG)
iodine d.
Kiton red d.

NOTES

dye *(continued)*
    d. laser
    metachromatic d.
    methylene blue d.
    orthochromatic d.
    radiopaque d.
    rapid emptying of d.
    rhodamine 6G d.
    d. scattering method
    d. sham intrarenal lesion
    d. spraying
dye-exclusion test
dye-injection endoscopic retrograde pancreatography
Dynabac
DynaCirc
Dynaflex
    D. penile implant
    D. penile prosthesis
Dynalink 0.035 biliary self-expanding stent system
dynamic
    d. closure pressure
    d. contrast
    d. cystourethroscopy
    d. development
    d. fluorescein angiography
    d. fluorescence videoendoscopy
    d. ileus
    d. infusion cavernosometry
    d. infusion cavernosometry and cavernosonography
    d. proctography
    d. urethral profile study
    d. urinary graciloplasty (DUG)
dynamoscopy
dynograph
dynorphin
dyphylline
Dyrenium
dysarthric
dysautonomia
    familial d.
    Riley-Day syndrome of familial d.
dysbiosis
dyschezia
    defecatory d.
dyscoordinate hyoid movement
dysdiadochokinesia
dysenteriae
    Shigella d.
dysenteric
    d. algid malaria
    d. arthritis
    d. diarrhea
dysentery
    amebic d.
    d. antitoxin
    bacillary d.
    d. bacillus
    balantidial d.
    bilharzial d.
    catarrhal d.
    ciliary d.
    ciliate d.
    epidemic d.
    flagellate d.
    Flexner d.
    fulminant d.
    fulminating d.
    giardiasis d.
    helminthic d.
    institutional d.
    Japanese d.
    malarial d.
    malignant d.
    protozoan d.
    schistosomal d.
    scorbutic d.
    Shiga d.
    Shigella d.
    Sonne d.
    spirillar d.
    spirochetal d.
    sporadic d.
    viral d.
dysesthesia
dysfunction
    anal sphincter d.
    anorectal sensorimotor d.
    autonomic d.
    balanced voiding d.
    bladder neck d.
    Bradley classification of voiding d.
    cardiopulmonary baroreflex d.
    cavernous autonomic nerve d.
    chronic graft d.
    colorectal physiologic d.
    constitutional hepatic d.
    corporeal venoocclusive d.
    ejaculatory d.
    erectile d.
    esophageal body motor d.
    evidence-based review of sphincter of Oddi d.
    gastric d.
    geriatric voiding d.
    hereditary spastic paraplegia voiding d.
    hindgut d.
    International Continence Society classification of voiding d.
    intracorporeal therapy of erectile d.
    intraurethral therapy of erectile d.
    intrinsic sphincter d. (ISD)
    Lapides classification of voiding d.
    late graft d.
    lower urinary tract d. (LUTD)

dysfunction · dyspepsia

low-pressure, low-flow voiding d.
mechanoreceptor d.
multiple organ system d. (MOSD)
neurogenic erectile d.
neuroimmune d.
neuropathic voiding d.
neutrophil d.
nondiabetic neurogenic erectile d.
nonneurogenic voiding d.
oral therapy of erectile d.
outlet d.
pancreatic exocrine d.
pediatric voiding d.
pelvic floor d.
platelet d.
postgastrectomy d.
postparacentesis circulatory d. (PCD)
posttransplant renal d.
progressive renal d.
psychogenic erectile d.
psychologic d.
puborectalis d.
reflex voiding d.
sensory voiding d.
sphincter d.
sphincter of Oddi d. (SOD)
transfer d.
traumatic corporeal venoocclusive d.
tubular cell d.
urodynamic d.
venoocclusive d.
visceral d.

dysfunctional
d. bleeding
d. voiding

dysgenesis
anorectal d.
gonadal d.
mixed gonadal d.

dysgenetic
d. fibrous band
d. gonad

dysgenitalism
dysgerminoma
dysgeusia
dysgonesis
dyskeratosis follicularis
dyskinesia
bile duct d.
biliary d.
primary ciliary d.

dyskinetic
d. cilia syndrome
d. puborectalis

dyslipidemia
dyslipidosis
dysmetabolic syndrome
dysmorphic
d. erythrocyte
d. red blood cell
d. vessel

dysmorphy
extrarenal d.

dysmotility
chronic intestinal d. (CID)
d. dyspepsia
esophageal d.
gallbladder d.

dysmotility-like dyspepsia
dysnatremia
dysorexia
dyspareunia
dyspepsia
acid d.
adhesion d.
appendicular d.
appendix d.
atonic d.
biliary d.
catarrhal d.
cholelithic d.
dysmotility d.
dysmotility-like d.
fermentative d.
flatulent d.
functional d.
gastric d.
gastroduodenal d.
mononuclear d.
nervous d.
nonorganic d.
nonulcer d. (NUD)
Optimal Regimen Cures *Helicobacter*-Induced D. (ORCHID)
postcholecystectomy flatulent d.
Quality of Life in Reflux and D. (QOLRD)
reflex d.
reflux d.
refluxlike d.
ulcer d.
ulcerlike d.

NOTES

dyspeptic
    d. symptom
    d. urine
dyspeptica
    angina d.
dysperistalsis
dysphagia, dysphagy
    d. after antireflux surgery
    d. aortica
    Atkinson scoring system for d.
    contractile ring d.
    esophageal d.
    d. inflammatoria
    liquid food d.
    d. lusoria
    malignant d.
    d. nervosa
    neurogenic d.
    onset of d.
    oropharyngeal d.
    d. paralytica
    postvagotomy d.
    preesophageal d.
    progressive d.
    sideropenic d.
    soft food d.
    solid food d.
    d. spastica
    transfer d.
    vallecular d.
    d. valsalviana
dysphagic
dysphasia
    panostotic fibrous d.
    polyostotic fibrous d.
dysphonia
dysphoria
dysplasia
    acrocephalopolydactylous d.
    anal squamous d.
    anal transitional zone d.
    arteriohepatic d.
    Barrett d.
    bladder d.
    bronchopulmonary d.
    developing high-grade d.
    epithelial d.
    fibromuscular d. (FMD)
    fibrous d.
    flat d.
    genital d.
    high-grade d. (HGD)
    kidney d.
    liver cell d.
    low-grade d. (LGD)
    lung d.
    malignant d.
    mucosal d.
    multicystic renal d.
    neuroectodermal d.
    nonulcer d.
    polypoid d.
    renal segmental renal d.
    urothelial d.
    vesicourethral reflux and renal d. (VURD)
dysplasia-associated lesion or mass (DALM)
dysplasia-to-carcinoma sequence
dysplastic
    d. cell
    d. focus
    d. kidney
    d. mucosa
dyspnea
Dysport
dyspragia
    d. angiosclerotica
    d. intermittens
    d. intermittens angiosclerotica intestinalis
dysraphic malformation
dysraphism
    bony d.
    neurospinal d.
    occult spinal d.
    spinal d.
    spine d.
dysreflexia
    autonomic d.
dysregulated immune response
dysrhythmia
    ESWL-related d.
    gastric electrical d.
    glucagon-evoked gastric d.
dysspermatogenic sterility
dyssynergia
    biliary d.
    detrusor external sphincter d. (DESD)
    detrusor sphincter d. (DSD)
    detrusor urethral d.
    pelvic floor d.
    rectoanal d.
    rectosphincteric d.
    vesical external sphincter d. (VSD)
    vesicosphincteric d.
dystonia
dystonic phenomenon
dystopia
    d. transversa externa testis
    d. transversa interna testis
dystopic kidney
dystrophic
    d. calcification
    d. penis
dystrophica
    epidermolysis bullosa d.

dystrophy
- adiposogenital d.
- asphyxiating thoracic d.
- Duchenne-type muscular d.
- hyperplastic d.
- Jeune asphyxiating thoracic d.
- muscular d.
- myotonic muscular d.
- oculocerebrorenal d.
- oculopharyngeal muscular d.
- reflex sympathetic d.
- Steinert myotonic d.

dystrypsia
dysuresia
dysuria
- psychic d.

dysuria-pyuria syndrome
dysuric
dyszoospermia

NOTES

E
    erythrocyte
        E rosetted
        E sign
        E test
E1
    prostaglandin E1
E2
    prostaglandin E2 (PGE2)
E-1023
    enzyme immunoassay E-1023
E1, E2, E6 protein
e10 electrosurgery system
EABV
    effective arterial blood volume
Eadie-Hofstee
    E.-H. plot
    E.-H. transformation
EAEC
    enteroadherent *Escherichia coli*
    enteroaggregative *Escherichia coli*
EaggEC
    enteroaggregative *Escherichia coli*
Eagle-Barrett syndrome
Eagle minimal essential medium (EMEM)
EAL
    endoscopic aspiration lumpectomy
EAM
    endoscopic aspiration mucosectomy
EAP
    etoposide, Adriamycin, Platinol
ear
    bladder e.
Earle
    E. hemorrhoid clamp
    E. medium
    E. rectal probe
    E. sign
    E. solution
early
    E. Detector
    e. dumping syndrome
    e. gastric cancer (EGC)
    e. growth response factor-alpha
    e. preimplantation cell screening (EPICS)
    e. satiety
    e. signs of dilutional hyponatremia
early-onset graft-versus-host disease
earth eating
EAS
    external anal sphincter
Easi-Lav lavage
easily reducible hernia

EasiVac evacuator
Easprin
EAST1
    enteroaggregative *Escherichia coli* heat-stable enterotoxin 1
Eastern Cooperative Oncology Group (ECOG)
Eastman cystic duct forceps
easy bruisability
EATCL
    enteropathy-associated T-cell lymphoma
eater
    liver e.
eating
    earth e.
EAUS
    endoanal ultrasound
EB
    epidermolysis bullosa
EBA
    extrahepatic biliary atresia
E-Base
Ebbehoj procedure
EBCT
    electron-beam computerized tomography
EBD
    endoscopic balloon dilation
EBL
    endoscopic band ligation
    estimated blood loss
Ebola hemorrhagic fever
E1b protein
ebrotidine
EBRT
    external-beam radiation therapy
EBS
    estrogen binding site
EBSD
    endoscopic balloon sphincter dilation
Ebstein
    E. diet
    E. disease
    E. lesion
EBV
    Epstein-Barr virus
EC
    epithelial cell
    esophageal candidiasis
    EC cell
    Entocort EC
    thymic EC
ECA
    enterobacterial common antigen
Ecabet Sodium (ES)
E-cadherin

EC cell
ECF
  extracellular fluid
ECGF
  endothelial cell growth factor
Echinacea purpura
echinococcal
  e. cyst disease
  e. liver abscess
echinococcosis, echinococciasis
  biliary e.
  cystic e.
  hepatic e.
  hepatic-alveolar e.
Echinococcus
  E. granulosus
  life cycle of *E.*
  E. liver cyst
  E. multilocularis
echinostomiasis
echo
  gradient e.
  magnetization prepared-rapid gradient e. (MP-RAGE)
  e. pattern
  e. sign
echocolonoscope
  CF-UM3 e.
  Olympus CF-UM3 flexible e.
echo-Doppler
echoduodenoscope
echoduodenoscopy
echoendoscope
  CLA e.
  curved-array e.
  curvilinear scanning e.
  electronic radial-array e.
  FG-36 UA curved linear-array e.
  GF-UM30P linear-oriented radial scanning e.
  large-channel video curvilinear e.
  linear-array e.
  oblique viewing e.
  Olympus CF-UM-series e.
  Olympus EUM-20 e.
  Olympus GF-UC30P e.
  Olympus GF-UCT30P linear-array e.
  Olympus GF-UM30P e.
  Olympus GF-UM29 radial scanner e.
  Olympus GIF20 e.
  Olympus GIF-EUM2 e.
  Olympus GIF-series e.
  Olympus GIF-1T10 e.
  Olympus JF-UM20 e.
  Olympus linear-array e.
  Olympus UM-20 radial e.
  Olympus VU-M2 e.
  Olympus XIF-UM3 e.
  Pentax FG-36-UX linear-array e.
  Pentax linear-array e.
  radial-sector scanning e.
echoendoscopy
echogastroscope
echogenic
  e. cardiac focus
  e. duct margin
  e. liver
echogenicity
  central e.
echographic
echolucent
echomorphologic
echo-poor
  e.-p. layer
  e.-p. lesion
echoprobe
  Olympus XMP-U2 catheter e.
echorich
EchoSeed radioactive iodine-125 brachytherapy seed
echotexture
EchoTip Ultra endoscopic needle
echovirus infection
ECI automatic reprocessor
Eck fistula
Eckhout vertical gastroplasty
ECL
  enhanced chemiluminescence
  enterochromaffin-like
    ECL cell
    ECL cell hyperplasia
    ECL hypertrophy and hyperplasia
    ECL Western blotting
ECLoma
  enterochromaffin-like gastric carcinoid tumor
ECLP
  extracorporeal liver perfusion
ECM
  extracellular matrix
  extracolonic malignancy
ECOG
  Eastern Cooperative Oncology Group
  ECOG performance status scale
ecology
  microbial e.
Ecotrin
ECP
  eosinophil cationic protein
ECPL
  endocavitary pelvic lymphadenectomy
ectacolia
ectasia
  antral vascular e.
  Boley vascular e.
  cecal vascular e.

gastric antral vascular e. (GAVE)
gastric vascular e. (GVE)
mucinous ductal e. (MDE)
precaliceal canalicular e.
tortuous venous e.
vascular e.
venous e.
ectatic
e. vascular lesion
e. vessel
ecthyma gangrenosum
ectocolon
ectoderm
ectodermal
ectoperitoneal
ectoperitonitis
ectopia, ectopy
acquired gastric e.
crossed renal e.
crossed testicular e.
gastric mucosal e.
intraabdominal transverse testicular e.
renal e.
transverse testicular e.
ureteral e.
e. vesicae
ectopic
e. adrenal rest
e. anus
e. cryptorchidism
e. gastric mucosa
e. gestation
e. kidney
e. pancreas
e. pheochromocytoma
e. schistosomiasis
e. scrotum
e. sigmoid pregnancy
e. testis
e. ureter
e. ureterocele
e. varix
e. vas deferens
ectoscopy
ECU
extracorporeal ultrafiltration
ECV
esophageal collateral vein
extracellular fluid volume
eczema
atopic e.

ED1
monoclonal antibody ED1
EDA+
extradomain A positive
EDAP LT.01 lithotriptor
EDD
extended daily dialysis
Edebohls
E. operation
E. position
edema
acute idiopathic scrotal e.
alimentary e.
angioneurotic e.
antral e.
bullous e.
cachectic e.
cerebral e.
focal e.
idiopathic e.
laryngeal e.
nephritic e.
nephrotic e.
pedal e.
penile e.
perianal e.
pericholecystic e.
peripheral extremity e.
pitting e.
pulmonary e.
sacral e.
edematous
e. gallbladder
e. hyperemic mucosa
e. pancreatitis
e. tag
edentulous
Eder-Bernstein gastroscope
Eder-Chamberlin gastroscope
Eder gastroscope
Eder-Hufford
E.-H. gastroscope
E.-H. rigid esophagoscope
Eder-Palmer
E.-P. semiflexible fiberoptic endoscope
E.-P. semiflexible gastroscope
Eder-Puestow
E.-P. bougie
E.-P. dilation
E.-P. dilator shaft
E.-P. guidewire

NOTES

Eder-Puestow *(continued)*
- E.-P. metal olive dilator
- E.-P. olive

edetate
- disodium e.

Edex

edge
- e. enhancement
- heaped-up e.
- hepatic e.
- ligament reflecting e.
- liver e.
- Poupart ligament shelving e.
- ulcer with heaped-up e.

EdGr
- Edmondson grading
- EdGr system

edible vaccine

Edlich gastric lavage tube

Edmondson
- E. grading (EdGr)
- E. grading system
- E. grading system for hepatocellular carcinoma

Edmondson-Steiner histologic grading of hepatocellular carcinoma I, II, III, IVa

Edna towel clamp

EDNO
- endothelium-derived nitric oxide

EDP
- endoscopic digital pancreatography

EDRF
- endothelium-derived relaxing factor

edrophonium
- e. provocation
- e. test

ED-Spaz

EDTA
- ethylenediaminetetraacetic acid
- ^{51}Cr-labeled EDTA

Edwardsiella tarda

Edwards syndrome

ED7-XU2

EEA
- end-to-end anastomosis
   - EEA stapler gun
   - EEA stapling device
   - EEA stapling of varices

EEG
- electroencephalography

EEGF
- esophageal epidermal growth factor

EEJ
- electroejaculation

EEPLND
- extraperitoneal endoscopic pelvic lymph node dissection

EES
- expandable esophageal stent

EET
- epoxyeicosatrienoic acid

EFA
- essential fatty acid

EFAD
- essential fatty acid deficiency

effacement
- villous e.

effect
- analgesic e.
- antinociceptive e.
- antiproliferative e.
- antiproteinuric e.
- banana peel e.
- blooming e.
- Bohr e.
- bystander e.
- choleretic e.
- concomitant medication e.
- disulfiram-like e.
- donor age-dependent e.
- Doppler e.
- duodenal e.
- esophageal e.
- first-pass e.
- gastric e.
- gender e.
- gene-inductive e.
- Haldane e.
- halo e.
- hypothermic e.
- e. of inhibition
- inhibitory e.
- intracellular flush e.
- irradiation e.
- J-curve e.
- kidney shock wave e.
- local alcohol instillation e.
- long-term renal functional e.
- membrane e.
- metabolic e.
- mitogenic e.
- mutagenic e.
- normothermic e.
- octreotide e.
- physiological trophic e.
- pinchcock e.
- placebo e.
- preservation times e.
- proapoptotic e.
- prokinetic e.
- sieving e.
- snowstorm e.
- soar-crash e.
- systemic e.
- topic e.
- tubulotoxic e.

effective
    e. arterial blood volume (EABV)
    cost e.
    e. dose equivalent radiation
    e. lithotriptor
    e. renal plasma flow (ERPF)

effector
    e. cell
    e. domain
    locally acting paracrine e.
    e. response

EFFERdose
    Zantac E.

efferent
    e. glomerular arteriole
    e. limb
    e. loop
    e. loop syndrome
    e. renal sympathetic nerve activity (ERSNA)

efferentes
    ductuli e.

Effer-Syllium

efficacious noninvasive anesthesia-independent first-line method

efficacy
    e. of neuromodulation
    poor long-term e.

efficiency
    defunctioning e.

effluent
    anal e.
    ileal e.
    ileostomy e.
    peritoneal dialysis e. (PDE)
    transverse colostomy e.

efflux

effort rupture of esophagus

effusion fluid

E2F protein

EG
    eosinophilic gastroenteritis
    esophagogastrectomy
    esophagogastric

EGBT
    esophagogastric balloon tamponade

EGC
    early gastric cancer

EGD
    esophagogastroduodenoscopy

EGE
    eosinophilic gastroenteritis

egesta

EGF
    epidermal growth factor
    ^{125}I-h-EGF
    intragastric EGF
    luminal EGF
    subcutaneous EGF

EGFR
    epidermal growth factor receptor

EGG
    electrogastrogram
    electrogastrography
    cutaneous EGG

eggerthii
    Bacteroides e.

egg yolk-cobalamin absorption test (EYCAT)

EGM
    extraglomerular mesangium

egophony

EGS
    electrogalvanic stimulation
    EGS Model 100 electrogalvanic stimulator

EGTA
    esophageal gastric tube airway
    ethyleneglycoltetraacetic acid

Egyptian splenomegaly

EHBDA
    extrahepatic bile duct atresia

EHC
    enterohepatic circulation

EHEC
    enterohemorrhagic *Escherichia coli*

EHL
    electrohydraulic lithotripsy
    endoscopic hemorrhoid ligation
    EHL probe

Ehlers-Danlos syndrome

EHM
    extrahepatic metastasis

EHPVO
    extrahepatic portal vein obstruction

Ehrlich
    E. abdominoplasty
    E. diazo reaction
    E. reagent

Ehrmann alcohol test meal

EHT
    electrohydrothermal
    EHT coagulation
    EHT electrode

NOTES

EIA
    enzyme immunoassay
        HCV EIA II
        Helicobacter pylori stool antigen EIA
        EIA kit

EIA-2
    second-generation enzyme immunoassay

eicosanoid synthesis

eicosapentaenoic acid (EPA)

EIEC
    enteroinvasive *Escherichia coli*

eight-channel cross-sectional anal sphincter probe

eight-lumen
    e.-l. catheter assembly
    e.-l. esophageal manometry catheter

Einhorn
    E. dilator
    E. string test

EIS
    endoscopic injection sclerotherapy

Eisenberger technique

Eitest MONO P-II test

ejaculatio
    e. deficiens
    e. praecox
    e. retardata

ejaculation
    antegrade e.
    dry e.
    electrostimulation-induced e.
    e. failure
    premature e.
    retrograde e.

ejaculatorius
    ductus e.

ejaculatory
    e. duct
    e. duct obstruction
    e. duct reflux
    e. duct transurethral resection
    e. duct ultrasonography
    e. dysfunction
    e. impotence

ejaculum

ejecta

ejection

EJP
    excitatory junction potential

ekiri

eKru
    equivalent residual renal urea clearance

Ektachem slide test

EL2-LS2 flexible video laparoscope

ELAD
    extracorporeal liver assist device

ELAM-1
    endothelial leukocyte adhesion molecule-1
    ligand for ELAM-1

Elastalloy
    E. esophageal endoprosthesis
    E. esophageal stent

elastase
    neutrophil e.
    serum e. 1

elastic
    e. band ligation
    e. bougie
    e. ligature
    e. O ring
    e. scattering spectroscopy
    e. silicone membrane

elastica interna

elasticum
    pseudoxanthoma e.

elastin stain

elastolysis
    generalized e.

Elastoplast dressing

Elavil

ELBF
    estimated liver blood flow

ELBNS
    extraperitoneal laparoscopic bladder neck suspension

elbowed
    e. bougie
    e. catheter

Elecsys
    E. anti-HBs immunoassay
    E. 1010 and 2010 immunoanalyzer
    E. PreciControl anti-HBs

elective resection

electric
    e. tissue morcellator
    e. zone

electrical
    e. blocking
    e. conductivity
    e. waveform

electroacupuncture

electroblotting

electrocautery
    bipolar e.
    blended e.
    Bovie e.
    Bugbee e.
    e. knife
    light e.
    monopolar e.
    multipolar e.
    needle-knife e. (NKE)
    Neomed e.

electrocautery · electrofulguration

    e. pencil
    e. resection
electrocholecystectomy
electrocholecystocausis
electrocoagulating
    e. biopsy forceps
    e. current
electrocoagulation
    bipolar e. (BPEC)
    direct-current e.
    endoscopic e.
    Gold Probe e.
    monopolar e.
    multipolar e. (MPEC)
    e. necrosis
    snare e.
    transendoscopic e.
electrocystography
electrode
    abdominal patch e.
    ACMI monopolar e.
    antimony monocrystalline e.
    antimony pH e.
    ASSI laparoscopic e.
    ball e.
    bayonet-tip e.
    bipolar glass e.
    Bugbee e.
    Buie fulguration e.
    button e.
    Cameron-Miller e.
    coagulating e.
    Coaguloop resection e.
    Collings e.
    common pH e.
    concentric needle e.
    conical-tip e.
    cuff e.
    cutting e.
    Disa needle e.
    e. dislodgement
    disposable pudendal nerve e.
    dome-tip e.
    EHT e.
    electrohydrothermal e.
    e. electrolyte
    Eppendorf needle e.
    flat spatula e.
    foramen e.
    glass pH e.
    Greenwald Control Tip cystoscopic e.
    Gyrus bipolar e.
    hook-tip laparoscopic e.
    indifferent e.
    intraluminal reference e.
    ion-specific e.
    e. jelly
    J-hook tip laparoscopic e.
    knife e.
    loop-tipped e.
    McCarthy e.
    Medtronic thin flexible antimony e.
    Microelectrode MI-506 small-caliber pH e.
    Microglass pH e.
    midgastric e.
    e. migration
    model 440 M1.5, M4 e.
    modified thermal nitinol e.
    needle e.
    needle-tip laparoscopic e.
    Neil-Moore e.
    pencil-tipped e.
    e. placement
    e. probe
    renal sympathetic nerve activity recording e.
    reusable laparoscopic e.
    right-angle e.
    rollerball e.
    single-fiber EMG e.
    Smith e.
    spatula-tip laparoscopic e.
    spoon-tip laparoscopic e.
    St. Mark pudendal e.
    surface e.
    three-quarter circle e.
    unipolar glass e.
    VaporTrode e.
    wire e.
electrodiathermy
electroejaculation (EEJ)
    rectal probe e.
electroejaculator
    G&S E.
electroencephalography (EEG)
electroendosmosis
electroevaporation
electrofulguration

NOTES

electrogalvanic
  e. stimulation (EGS)
  e. stimulator
electrogastrogram (EGG)
  cutaneous e.
electrogastrograph
electrogastrography (EGG)
electrohemostasis
electrohydraulic
  e. generator
  e. lithotripsy (EHL)
  e. lithotripsy probe
  e. lithotriptor
  percutaneous transhepatic choledochoscopic e.
  e. shock wave lithotripsy (ESWL)
electrohydrothermal (EHT)
  e. coagulation
  e. electrode
electroimmunodiffusion assay
electroincision
electrolithotrity
electrolyte
  e. abnormality
  e. balance
  bicarbonate e.
  calcium e.
  chloride e.
  CO_2 e.
  electrode e.
  e. excretion
  e. flush solution
  e. imbalance coma
  e. loss
  potassium e.
  e. preparation
  sodium e.
  stool e.
electrolyte-polyethylene glycol lavage solution
electromagnetic
  e. flow transducer
  e. lithotriptor
electromechanical
  e. coupling
  e. impactor (EMI)
electromicroscopy
electromyogram (EMG)
  colonic e.
electromyography
  conventional concentric e.
  corpus cavernosum penile e.
  Disa e.
  intraanal e.
  needle electrode e.
  noninvasive intraanal e.
  pelvic floor e.
  e. of penile corpus cavernosum muscle
  rhabdosphincter e.
  single-fiber needle e.
  surface pelvic floor e.
  ureteral e.
  video pressure flow e.
electron
  e. immunoperoxidase observation
  e. microscopy
electron-beam computerized tomography (EBCT)
electron-dense mesangial deposit
electronic
  e. barostat
  e. pain control
  e. radial-array echoendoscope
  e. radial-array endoscope
electron-microscopic evidence
electrophoresis
  agarose gel e.
  horizontal e.
  e. immunoblot analysis
  immunofixation e. (IFE)
  polyacrylamide gel e. (PAGE)
  pulsed-field gel e. (PFGE)
  serum protein e. (SPEP)
  sodium dodecyl sulfate polyacrylamide gel e. (SDS-PAGE)
  urine protein e. (UPEP)
electrophoretic
  e. mobility
  e. mobility shift assay
electrophysiology
  cellular e.
  e. of gastric musculature
  GI e.
electropneumatic endoscopic lithotriptor
electroresection
electrosensitivity
  mucosal e. (MES)
electrostimulation
electrostimulation-induced ejaculation
electrosurgery
  EUS probe-guided e.
electrosurgical
  e. current
  e. current density
  e. curved scissors
  e. cut
  e. cutting knife
  e. desiccation
  e. dissection
  e. fulguration
  e. generator
  e. monopolar spatula probe
  e. needle
  e. snare
  e. snare polypectomy

e. spatula
e. unit (ESU)
electrotherapy
electrovaporization
    prostate gland e.
    transurethral e.
Elema-Siemens AB pressure transducer
element
    acute-phase response e. (APRE)
    androgen receptor e.
    ceramic e.
    estrogen response e. (ERE)
    glucocorticoid response e. (GRE)
    hepatic subcellular e.
    interferon-stimulated regulatory e. (ISRE)
    thyroid hormone response e. (TRE)
elemental
    e. diet
    e. phosphate
elephantiasis
    genital e.
    e. scroti
elevated WBC
elevation
    mucosal e.
elevator
    Alexander e.
    Doyen rib e.
    Ellik kidney stone e.
    Freer e.
    Stille e.
eleventh
    e. rib flank incision
    e. rib transperitoneal incision
ELF
    etoposide, leucovorin, 5-fluorouracil
    ELF chemotherapy protocol
Eligard sustained-release subcu injection
elimination
    e. diet
    pyelography by e.
    spontaneous partial e.
    stool e.
eliminator
    E. balloon catheter
    E. biliary stent
    Fecal Odor E. (FOE)
    E. nasobiliary catheter set
    E. pancreatic stent
    E. PET biliary balloon dilator
    E. stone extraction basket

ELISA
    enzyme-linked immunosorbent assay
    first-generation ELISA
    gliadin ELISA
    Heprofile ELISA
    ELISA Kit Alfa-gliatest
    sensitive and specific ELISA
    TG ELISA
    tissue transglutaminase ELISA
    ELISA titer
ELISA-I
    enzyme-linked immunosorbent assay I
ELISA-II
    enzyme-linked immunosorbent assay II
ELISA-I, -II, -III test
ELISA-like assay
elixir
    e. diarrhea
    Hemocyte-F e.
    Susano E.
Ellik
    E. evacuator
    E. kidney stone basket
    E. kidney stone elevator
Elliot position
Elliott gallbladder forceps
ellipsoid method
elliptical incision
Ellis types 1, 2 glomerulonephritis
Ellis-van Creveld syndrome
Ellsner gastroscope
Elmiron
ELMISKOP 101 electron microscope
elongated pseudostratified nucleus
elongation
    calix e.
Eloxatin
ELP
    enterocolic lymphocytic phlebitis
Elspar
ELT
    endoscopic laser therapy
eltor
    Vibrio e.
    Vibrio cholerae biotype *e.*
eluate
    acetonitrile e.
elucidation
EluHair
ELUS
    endoluminal rectal ultrasonography

NOTES

elusive
    e. polyp
    e. ulcer
eluted antibody
elutriation
    T-cell depletion by e.
El-Zimaity triple stain
EM
    erythema multiforme
    esophageal manometry
EMA
    endomysial antibody
        antibody to EMA
        IgA EMA
emaciation
EMAG
    environmental metaplastic atrophic gastritis
emasculation
EMB
    eosin-methylene blue
        EMB agar
embarrassment
    circulatory e.
    respiratory e.
embolectomy
    renal artery e.
emboli (*pl. of* embolus)
embolic
    e. agent
    e. nephritis
embolism
    air e.
    bile pulmonary e.
    cholesterol e.
    hemodialysis air e.
    mesenteric arterial e.
    postoperative cholesterol e.
    pulmonary e.
    renal artery e.
embolization
    e. of aneurysm
    angiographic variceal e.
    arterial e.
    arteriographic e.
    bilateral pudendal artery e.
    cholesterol crystal e. (CCE)
    Gelfoam e.
    hyperselective e.
    iliac artery e.
    percutaneous transhepatic liver biopsy with tract e. (PBTE)
    portal e. (PE)
    renal artery cholesterol e.
    splenic arterial e.
    superselective transcatheter e.
    transarterial catheter e. (TACE)
    transcatheter arterial e. (TAE)
    transcatheter hepatic arterial e.
    transcatheter splenic arterial e. (TSAE)
    transcatheter variceal e.
    transhepatic e. (THE)
    varicocele e.
embolotherapy
    transcatheter e.
embolus, pl. **emboli**
    cholesterol e.
    metallic e.
    pulmonary e.
    renal cholesterol e.
    talc e.
EMBP
    estramustine-binding protein
embryoid body
embryologic development
embryology
embryoma of kidney
embryonal
    e. adenoma
    e. adenomyosarcoma
    e. adenosarcoma
    e. cell carcinoma
    e. nephroma
    e. testicular carcinoma
    e. transitory bladder
    e. tumor
embryonic cleavage
Emcyt
EMD
    esophageal motility disorder
EMDA
    intravesical electromotive drug administration
EMEM
    Eagle minimal essential medium
emepronium bromide
Emerge biomaterial
emergency
    e. appendectomy
    e. colonoscopy
    e. laparotomy
emergency-to-elective workload
emergent appendectomy
emerging profile
emesis
    bilious e.
    chemotherapy-induced nausea and e. (CINE)
    coffee-grounds e.
emetatrophia
Emete-Con
emetic reflex
emetine
emetocathartic
emetogenic injury
Emetrol
EMF oral liquid

EMG
  electromyogram
    MyoTrac EMG
    sphincter EMG
EMI
  electromechanical impactor
    EMI APED amplifier discriminator
    EMI 9813B photomultiplier
eminence
  hypothenar e.
  thenar e.
emissary vein of penis
emission
  gamma e.
  nocturnal e.
Emitasol nasal therapy
Emitrip
emitter
  light e.
EMLA
  eutectic mixture of local anesthetics
    EMLA anesthetic
emollient laxative
Emory score
EMPD
  extramammary Paget disease
emperipolesis
emphysema
  alpha-1-antitrypsin disease-related e.
  colonoscopy-related e.
  endoscopy-related e.
  intestinal e.
  panacinar e.
  panlobular e.
  subcutaneous e.
  unilateral periorbital e.
emphysematosa
  cholecystitis e.
  cystitis e.
emphysematous
  e. cholecystitis
  e. cystitis
  e. gastritis
  e. pyelonephritis
empty
  e. intestine
  e. sella syndrome
emptying
  bladder e.
  delayed gallbladder e.
  delayed liquid gastric e.
  e. delta volume

  gastric e. (GE)
  liquid e.
  neorectal e.
  rapid gastric e.
  rectal e.
  Roux limb e.
  solid e.
  T-1/2 time of gastric e.
empyema of gallbladder
empyocele
EMR
  endoscopic magnetic resonance
  endoscopic mucosal resection
EMRC
  endoscopic mucosal resection, cap method
EMRL
  endoscopic mucosal resection with ligation
EMRT
  endoscopic mucosal resection, tube method
EMS
  esophageal manometric sequence
emtricitabine
emulsion
  Biafine wound dressing e.
  Calogen LCT e.
  intralipid fat e.
  intravenous lipid e.
  lipid e.
  e. proteinuria
Emulsoil bowel preparation
E-MVAC
  escalated methotrexate, vinblastine, Adriamycin, cisplatin or cyclophosphamide
E-Mycin
EN
  enema
  enteral nutrition
en
  en bloc dissection
  en bloc distal pancreatectomy
  en bloc endoscopic resection
  en bloc kidney transplantation
  en bloc technique
  en bloc ureter
  en bloc vein resection
  en coup de sabre
  en face
  en face view

NOTES

ENA
    extracted nuclear antigen
        ENA screen
ENaC
    epithelial sodium channel
enalapril
enalaprilat
enalkiren
enamel pellicle formation
ENANB
    enterically transmitted non-A non-B
        ENANB hepatitis
enanthate
        e. ester
        testosterone e.
enantiomer D-arginine
ENBD
    endoscopic nasobiliary drainage
encapsulated
        e. carcinoid tumor
        e. plasmodium
        e. renal cell carcinoma
encapsulation
    peritoneal e.
    tumor e.
Encare tube feeding formula
encasement
        pancreatic duct e.
        ureteral e.
encelialgia
encelitis
Encephalitozoon intestinalis
encephaloid gastric carcinoma
encephalomyopathy
    mitochondrial
        neurogastrointestinal e. (MNGIE)
encephalopathy
    bilirubin e.
    colonoscopy-induced
      hyponatremic e.
    hepatic e. (HE)
    myoclonic e.
    portosystemic e. (PSE)
    postshunt e.
    subclinical hepatic e. (SHE)
    uremic e.
    Wernicke e.
encephalotrigeminal syndrome
encircle
encirclement
    anal e.
encoding virulence
encopresis
encroachment
    scrotal e.
encrustation
    e. analysis
    biofilm-related e.
    e. of biomaterial
    e. deposition
    e. of stent
encrusted
    e. pyelitis
    e. ureteral stent
encystation
encysted
    e. bladder
    e. calculus
    e. hydrocele
    e. intraabdominal collection
end
    advanced glycation e. (AGE)
    e. colostomy
    esophageal Z stent with fully
      coated flange e.'s
    e. ileostomy
    e. stoma
endarterectomy
    e. knife
    renal e.
    transaortic e.
endeavor
    Cancer of the Prostate Strategic Urologic Research E.
endemic
    e. colic
    e. deep mycosis
    e. diarrhea
    e. hematuria
    e. nonbacterial infantile gastroenteritis
end-end stapler
Endep
end-expiratory intragastric pressure
end-filling pressure
end-fire transrectal probe
end-hole ureteral catheter
end-labeling
    nick e.-l.
end-loop
    e.-l. colostomy
    e.-l. ileocolostomy
    e.-l. ileostomy
    e.-l. stoma
endo
    e. catch bag
    E. GIA 30, 60 stapler
    E. GIA suture stapler
    E. Hernia stapler
    E. pants
endoabdominal fascia
endoanal
    e. coil
    e. magnetic resonance imaging
    e. mucosectomy
    e. probe
    e. ultrasound (EAUS)
    e. ultrasound scan

EndoAnchor
endoappendicitis
Endo-Assist
    E.-A. disposable atraumatic grasping forceps
    E.-A. disposable hemostat
    E.-A. disposable ligature carrier
    E.-A. disposable needle holder
    E.-A. reusable knot pusher
endoauscultation
Endo-Avitene
    E.-A. MCH
    E.-A. microfibrillar collagen hemostat
Endo-Babcock stapler
endobag
endobiliary ascariasis
EndoBlade
    LaserSonics E.
endobrachyesophagus
endobronchial
    e. fistula
    e. stent
Endocam
endocamera
    Polaroid e. EC-3
endocarditis
    enterococcal e.
    high risk for e.
    infective e.
    marantic e.
    native valve bacterial e.
    Streptococcus bovis e.
Endocare renal cryoablation
endocast
    three-dimensional pelvicaliceal e.
endocavitary
    e. bladder diverticulectomy
    e. pelvic lymphadenectomy (ECPL)
    e. radiation
endocholedochal
EndoCinch suturing system
Endoclip applier
EndoCoil
    E. biliary stent
    E. esophageal stent
endocolitis
endocrine
    e. cancer
    e. cell
    e. disruptor
    e. mimic
    e. screening
    e. system
    e. therapy
endocrinopathy
Endocut
endocutter
    Long45 e.
endocystitis
endocytosis
    fluid-phase e.
endocytotic vesicle
endodermal
endodermic cell
Endo-Dop transendoscopic Doppler catheter probe system
Endodynamics suction polyp trap
endoenteritis
endoesophageal MRI coil
endoesophagitis
endogastric
endogastritis
Endo-Gauge
endogenous
    e. biotin
    e. lipophilic antioxidant
    e. mutation
    e. obesity
    e. opioid
    e. peroxidase
    e. peroxidase activity
    e. pyrogen
    e. renal antigen
endograsper
endoherniorrhaphy
Endolav
    E. lavage pump
    Meditron EL-100 E.
endoligature
Endoloop suture
EndoLumina bougie
endoluminal
    e. clipping
    e. CT colonography
    e. endoscopy
    e. gastroplication
    e. rectal ultrasonography (ELUS)
    e. ultrasonography-guided fine-needle aspiration biopsy
    e. ureteral ultrasound
EndoMate grab bag
endometrial carcinoma
endometrioid

NOTES

endometrioma
    ovarian e.
endometriosis
    e. of colon
    colorectal e.
    e. vesicae
endometritis
    coccidioidal e.
endometrium
endomorph
endomorphic
endomorphy
endomysial
    e. antibody (EMA)
    e. antibody test
    e. IgA
endomysium
    e. antibody
    e. antigen
EndoNet
    Pentax E.
endonuclease
    restriction e.
Endopath
    E. EMS hernia stapler
    E. endoscopic linear cutter
    E. Optiview laparoscopic obturator
    E. 30, 60 stapler
endopeptidase
    neutral e.
    pancreatic e.
endoperitoneal
endoperitonitis
endoperoxide
    PGG2 e.
    PGH2 e.
endophlebitis hepatica obliterans
endophotography
endophytic
endoplasmic
    e. reticulum
    e. reticulum-bound polysome
Endo-P-Probe
endoprobe
    rotating e.
endoprostatic coil
endoprosthesis
    biliary e.
    Celestin e.
    Coons/Carey e.
    crutched stick-type polyurethane e.
    cuffed esophageal e.
    double-lumen e.
    double-pigtail e.
    DoubleStent biliary e.
    Elastalloy esophageal e.
    endoscopic biliary e.
    esophageal e.
    exchange of e.
    expandable biliary e.
    expandable metal mesh e.
    IntraStent DoubleStrut biliary e.
    KeyMed Atkinson e.
    large-bore biliary e.
    Medoc-Celestin e.
    pancreatic e.
    peroral e.
    pigtail e.
    3/4-pigtail plastic e.
    plastic e.
    polyethylene e.
    Proctor-Livingston e.
    self-expandable stainless steel braided e.
    straight e.
    Titan e.
    transpapillary endoscopic e.
    UroLume e.
    VIABIL biliary e.
    Wallstent e.
    Wilson-Cook e.
endopyeloplasty
    percutaneous e.
endopyelotomy
    Acucise e.
    antegrade e.
    e. failure
    e. incision
    retrograde e.
    e. stent
    ureteroscopic e.
endopyeloureterotomy
    percutaneous e.
endoradiosonde
endorectal
    e. advancement flap
    e. coil magnetic resonance imaging
    e. ileal pouch
    e. ileal pullthrough
    e. probe
    e. pullthrough procedure
    e. surface coil MRI
    e. ultrasound (ERUS)
endorectal-pelvic phased-array coil
endosac
endoscissors
    rotating e.
endoscope
    AccuSharp e.
    ACMI e.
    activated capsule e.
    battery-powered e.
    cap-fitted e.
    CCD e.
    CF-HM e.
    charge-coupled device e.
    Cho/Dyonics two-portal e.

endoscope · endoscope

double accessory channel therapeutic e.
double-channel e.
Eder-Palmer semiflexible fiberoptic e.
electronic radial-array e.
end-viewing e.
EVIS 140 Q series e.
EVIS 140 S wide-screen e.
FCS two-channel ultra high-magnification e.
FG-series two-channel e.
FGS-ML-series two-channel e.
FGS-series two-channel e.
FGS-SML-series two-channel e.
fiberoptic e.
flexible fiberoptic e.
forward-viewing e.
Fujinon EG-FP-series e.
Fujinon EVE-series e.
Fujinon EVG-CT e.
Fujinon EVG-FP-series e.
Fujinon EVG-F-series e.
Fujinon FP-series e.
GIF N30 fiberoptic pediatric e.
GIF-Q240 upper digestive tract e.
GIF XP20 e.
GIF XQ10 upper e.
Hirschowitz e.
e. impaction
intraductal e.
JFB III e.
JF-20 side-viewing fiberoptic e.
J-shaped e.
Karl Storz e.
Kussmaul e.
large-channel e.
lateral-viewing e.
looping of e.
magnifying e.
Messerklinger e.
mother-daughter e.
Navigator flexible e.
near-infrared electronic e.
oblique viewing e.
Olympus Aloka GF-EU-series e.
Olympus CF 2301 e.
Olympus CF-UM20 ultrasonic e.
Olympus CF-UM20 ultrasound e.
Olympus CF-200Z e.
Olympus CV-series e.
Olympus DES-series e.
Olympus EUM-20 e.
Olympus EUS-series e.
Olympus EVIS Q-series e.
Olympus GF-UM30P e.
Olympus GF-UM20 radial scanning e.
Olympus GF-UM3 ultrasonic e.
Olympus GF-UM20 ultrasound e.
Olympus GIF-D2 e.
Olympus GIF-HM-series e.
Olympus GIF-J-series e.
Olympus GIF-P e.
Olympus GIF-Q200 e.
Olympus GIF-2T10 e.
Olympus GIF-2T200 e.
Olympus GIF-T-series e.
Olympus GIF-XP-series e.
Olympus GIF-XQ240 e.
Olympus GIF-XV-series e.
Olympus JF1T e.
Olympus JF-T-series e.
Olympus JF-TV-series e.
Olympus JF-V-series e.
Olympus PJF e.
Olympus PJF-series pediatric e.
Olympus P-series e.
Olympus SIF-SW fiberoptic e.
Olympus SIF-100 video push e.
Olympus 2T100 e.
Olympus TJF-100 e.
Olympus UM-series e.
Olympus V-series e.
Olympus XCF-XK-series e.
Olympus XGF-UCT30 e.
Olympus XP-series e.
Olympus XQ-200, XQ-230 video e.
Olympus Zoom e.
pediatric e.
Pentax EG-2901, -2940, -3800 e.
Pentax ESI-2000 fiberoptic e.
Pentax FG-38X e.
Pentax VSB-2000 fiberoptic e.
rigid e.
semiflexible e.
semirigid e.
side-viewing e.
Simpson e.
Surgenomic e.
therapeutic e.
transcutaneous sonogram e.
two-channel e.

NOTES

endoscope *(continued)*
  UGI e.
  ultrasonic e.
  ultrasound e.
  ultrathin e.
  upper GI e.
  variable stiffness e.
  Visicath e.
  Weerda e.
  wireless capsule e.
endoscope-body position relationship
endoscopic
  e. ablation of antral diaphragm
  e. access
  e. adrenalectomy
  e. alligator forceps
  e. aspiration lumpectomy (EAL)
  e. aspiration mucosectomy (EAM)
  e. atrophic gastritis
  e. balloon dilation (EBD)
  e. balloon sphincter dilation (EBSD)
  e. band ligation (EBL)
  e. band ligation of varix
  e. band ligator
  e. BICAP probe
  e. biliary decompression
  e. biliary drainage
  e. biliary endoprosthesis
  e. biliary sphincterotomy
  e. biliary stent
  e. biliary stent placement
  e. biopsy forceps
  e. biopsy site
  e. botulinum toxin injection
  e. brush cytology
  e. camera
  e. clip-and-cut diverticulotomy
  e. clipping
  e. color Doppler
  e. color Doppler assessment
  e. color Doppler ultrasonography
  e. control
  e. cystenterostomy
  e. cystoduodenostomy
  e. data acquisition
  e. detachable miniloop ligation
  e. devolvulization
  e. digital pancreatography (EDP)
  e. diverticulotomy
  e. Doppler probe
  e. Doppler ultrasound-guided injection therapy
  e. electrocoagulation
  e. electrohydraulic lithotripsy
  e. enterogastric reflux gastritis
  e. enucleation
  e. epinephrine injection
  e. erythematous/exudative gastritis
  e. esophageal mucosal resection tube technique
  e. esophagitis
  e. esophagogastric variceal ligation
  e. examination
  e. extirpation cicatricial obliteration
  e. extraction pancreatic duct stone
  e. findings
  e. fine-needle puncture
  e. fistulotomy
  e. flowprobe
  e. four-quadrant tattoo
  e. fulguration
  e. gastroenteric anastomosis with magnets
  e. gastrostomy tube
  e. grasping forceps
  e. guidance
  e. heater probe thermocoagulation
  e. heat probe
  e. hemoclip device
  e. hemoclipping
  e. hemoclip therapy
  e. hemorrhagic gastritis
  e. hemorrhoid ligation (EHL)
  e. hemostasis
  e. hemostatic therapy
  e. Ho:YAG lithotripsy
  e. incision
  e. India ink injection
  e. injection sclerosis
  e. injection sclerotherapy (EIS)
  e. injection therapy
  e. intervention
  e. jejunostomy
  e. laser cautery
  e. laser cholecystectomy
  e. laser recanalization
  e. laser therapy (ELT)
  e. light source
  e. magnet-assisted nonsurgical technique
  e. magnetic extractor
  e. magnetic resonance (EMR)
  e. magnetic resonance scanning
  e. management
  e. management of choledochal cyst
  e. manometry
  e. metallic stent lithotripsy
  e. microwave
  e. microwave coagulation
  e. monitoring
  e. mucosal resection (EMR)
  e. mucosal resection, cap method (EMRC)
  e. mucosal resection, tube method (EMRT)
  e. mucosal resection with ligating device

endoscopic · endoscopic

e. mucosal resection with ligation (EMRL)
e. nasobiliary catheter drainage
e. nasobiliary drainage (ENBD)
e. oblique aspiration mucosectomy
e. optical coherence tomography
e. optical urethrotomy
e. pancreatic drainage
e. pancreatic duct sphincterotomy
e. pancreatic sphincterotomy (EPS)
e. pancreatic stenting (EPS)
e. pancreatic therapy
e. papillary balloon dilation (EPBD, EPD)
e. papillotomy (EPT)
e. papillotomy and stenting
e. patchiness
e. photography
e. pulsed-dye laser
e. pulsed-dye laser lithotripsy
e. raised erosive gastritis
e. reflectance
e. reflectance spectrophotometry
e. removal of fragment
e. resection of antral web
e. retroflexion
e. retrograde biliary drainage (ERBD)
e. retrograde biliary stenting
e. retrograde cannulation
e. retrograde cholangiogram
e. retrograde cholangiography (ERC)
e. retrograde cholangiopancreatography (ERCP)
e. retrograde cholangiopancreatography catheter
e. retrograde cholecystoendoprosthesis (ERCCE)
e. retrograde cytology
e. retrograde ileography
e. retrograde pancreatography (ERP)
e. retrograde parenchymography (ERP)
e. retrograde parenchymography of pancreas (ERPP)
e. retrograde sclerotherapy
e. rugal hyperplastic gastritis
e. scissors
e. sclerotherapy (ES)
e. sessile polypectomy
e. sewing machine
e. sewing machine technology
e. sigmoidopexy
e. small bowel biopsy
e. snare
e. snare ampullectomy
e. snare resection
e. sphincterectomy
e. sphincter of Oddi manometry
e. sphincterotomy (ES)
e. sphincterotomy-induced duodenal perforation
e. sphincterotomy-induced pancreatitis
e. spray cryotherapy
e. stapling diverticulostomy
e. stent exchange
e. stigma
e. stigmata of hemorrhage
e. stone disintegration
e. stone manipulation
e. stone removal
e. strictureplasty
e. stricturotomy
e. strip biopsy
e. surveillance
e. suture-cutting forceps
e. system
e. thermal ablation
e. thermodisinfector
e. transbronchial real-time ultrasound-guided biopsy
e. transesophageal fine-needle aspiration
e. transesophageal fine-needle aspiration cytology
e. transgastric drainage
e. transpancreatic ampullary septotomy
e. transpapillary biopsy
e. transpapillary cannulation
e. transpapillary catheterization of gallbladder (ETCG)
e. transpapillary cyst drainage (ETCD)
e. transpapillary drainage of pancreatic abscess
e. treatment
e. ultrasonographic diagnosis
e. ultrasonographic imaging
e. ultrasonography (EUS)
e. ultrasound (EUS)
e. ultrasound-assisted band ligation

NOTES

endoscopic *(continued)*
- e. ultrasound diagnosis
- e. ultrasound duodenoscope
- e. ultrasound evaluation
- e. ultrasound-guided celiac plexus block
- e. ultrasound-guided celiac plexus neurolysis
- e. ultrasound-guided cystogastrostomy
- e. ultrasound-guided ethanol lavage of pancreatic cystadenoma
- e. ultrasound-guided fine-needle aspiration (EUS-FNA)
- e. ultrasound-guided fine-needle injection
- e. ultrasound-guided pancreatic gastrostomy
- e. ultrasound probe
- e. ultrasound retrograde cholangiopancreatography
- e. variceal band ligation
- e. variceal ligation (EVL)
- e. variceal sclerotherapy
- e. washing pipe
- e. Waterpik

endoscopically
- e. deliverable tissue-transfixing device
- e. guided segmental gut lavage
- e. normal patient

endoscopic-controlled lithotripsy
endoscopist
endoscopy
- advanced therapeutic e.
- American Society for Gastrointestinal E. (ASGE)
- 5-aminolevulinic acid-induced fluorescence e.
- anal e.
- capsule e.
- CE-AD gastric lesion staging by e.
- CE-M gastric lesion staging by e.
- CE-SM gastric lesion staging by e.
- e. complication
- computerized electronic e.
- diagnostic upper e.
- endoluminal e.
- enhanced magnification e.
- Erlanger active stimulator for interventional e.
- fiberoptic e.
- flexible e.
- fluorescein electronic e.
- fluorescent electronic e.
- gastrointestinal e.
- high-altitude e.
- high-magnification e.
- high-resolution e.
- infrared e.
- intestinal e.
- intraoperative biliary e.
- light-induced fluorescence e. (LIFE)
- open-access e. (OAE)
- outpatient e.
- pancreaticobiliary e.
- pediatric e.
- peripartum e.
- peroral e.
- postsurgical e.
- primary diagnostic e.
- e. procedure
- rapid exchange technique for therapeutic e.
- screening e.
- e. suite
- surveillance e.
- TEM transanal e.
- therapeutic pancreaticobiliary e.
- therapeutic upper e.
- transcolonic e.
- transesophageal e.
- transmural e.
- UGI e.
- ultrahigh-magnification e.
- ultrathin e.
- upper alimentary e.
- upper gastrointestinal e. (UGIE)
- videocapsule e.
- virtual e.
- wireless capsule e. (WCE)
- e. with iodine staining

endoscopy-negative reflux disease (ENRD)
endoscopy-related emphysema
Endoshears
EndoSheath
- Vision System E.

endosnare
endosonographer
endosonographically targeted injection
endosonographic staging
endosonography
- anal e. (AES)
- anorectal e.
- 3-D linear e.
- duplex Doppler e.
- high-frequency e.
- e. instrument
- rectal e.
- three-dimensional linear e.

endosonography-guided
- e.-g. celiac plexus neurolysis
- e.-g. cholangiodrainage
- e.-g. drainage of pancreatic pseudocyst

EndoSound
  E. endoscopic ultrasound catheter
  E. ultrasound probe
Endospore disinfectant
Endostapler
Endostat II bipolar/monopolar electrosurgical generator
endostethoscope
Endotek machine
endothelia (*pl. of* endothelium)
endothelial
  e. cell
  e. cell differentiation
  e. cell growth factor (ECGF)
  e. leukocyte adhesion molecule-1 (ELAM-1)
  e. tube
endothelial-dependent relaxation
endothelialis
  hepatic e.
endothelin (ET)
  e. A (EtA)
  e. antagonist
  e. A receptor
  e. B (EtB)
  renal e.
  selective e. A
endothelin-1 (ET-1)
  e.-1 concentration
endothelin-3 (ET-3)
  e.-3 concentration
endothelioma
endotheliosis
  glomerular e.
endothelium, pl. **endothelia**
  gastrointestinal e.
  sinusoidal e.
endothelium-dependent
  e.-d. fibrinolysis
  e.-d. vasodilation
endothelium-derived
  e.-d. nitric oxide (EDNO)
  e.-d. relaxing factor (EDRF)
  e.-d. relaxing hormone
EndoTherapy
Endotorque
  Greenen E.
endotoxemia
  systemic e.
endotoxin
  e. antibody
  bacterial e.

endotracheal
  e. intubation
  e. tube (ET)
  e. tube placement
ENDO-Tube nasojejunal feeding tube
endoureteral ultrasound sonography
endoureterotomy
  cold knife e.
endourologic
  e. biopsy
  e. management
endourological
  e. cold-knife incision
  e. failure
  e. procedure
  e. training
endourology
  reconstructive e.
  therapeutic e.
endovascular
  e. stent grafting
  e. stenting
  e. treatment
Endovations disposable cytology brush
endovenous
Endozime
  E. AW bacteriostatic enzyme cleaner
  E. sponge
endplate
  motor e.
end-point dilution titer
Endrate
endrophonium chloride
end-sigmoid colostomy
end-stage
  e.-s. cirrhosis
  e.-s. liver disease (ESLD)
  e.-s. renal disease (ESRD)
  e.-s. renal failure
end-to-end
  e.-t.-e. anastomosis (EEA)
  e.-t.-e. anastomotic repair
  e.-t.-e. branch reanastomosis
  e.-t.-e. enterostomy
end-to-side
  e.-t.-s. anastomosis
  e.-t.-s. arteriotomy
  e.-t.-s. choledochojejunostomy
  e.-t.-s. duodenogastrostomy
  e.-t.-s. ileotransverse colostomy
  e.-t.-s. portacaval shunt

NOTES

end-to-side *(continued)*
    e.-t.-s. reimplantation
    e.-t.-s. vasoepididymostomy technique

Enduron

Enduronyl

end-viewing
    e.-v. endoscope
    e.-v. gastroscope

Enecat CT concentrated rectal suspension

enema (EN)
    air-contrast barium e. (ACBE)
    5-aminosalicylic acid e.
    analeptic e.
    antegrade colonic e. (ACE)
    antegrade continence e. (ACE)
    5-ASA e.
    barium e. (BE)
    blind e.
    cleansing hypertonic phosphate e.
    contrast e.
    Cortenema retention e.
    diatrizoate sodium e.
    double-contrast barium e. (DCBE)
    flatus e.
    Fleet Babylax e.
    flexible barium e.
    flocculation on barium e.
    full-column barium e.
    Gastrografin e.
    glycerin e.
    high e.
    hydrocortisone e.
    hydrogen peroxide e.
    Hypaque e.
    Kayexalate e.
    lactulose e.
    Malone antegrade colonic e.
    Malone antegrade continence e.
    Malone antegrade continent e. (MACE)
    meglumine diatrizoate e.
    mesalamine e.
    methylene blue e.
    nuclear e.
    NuLYTELY e.
    nutrient e.
    oil retention e.
    pancreatic e.
    phosphate e.
    Phospho-Soda e.
    povidone-iodine e.
    prednisolone e.
    puddling on barium e.
    retention e.
    retrograde flow on barium e.
    Rowasa e.
    saline cleansing e.
    single-contrast barium e.
    small bowel e.
    soapsuds e. (SSE)
    sorbitol e.
    steroid foam e.
    sucralfate retention e.
    sulfasalazine e.
    tap water e.
    theophylline olamine e.
    tranexamic acid e.
    turpentine e.
    e.'s until clear
    water-soluble contrast e.

enemator

energy
    apparent digestive e. (ADE)
    e. delivery
    e. dispersive x-ray analysis
    mean e.

Enfamil
    E. LIPIL formula
    E. Low Iron liquid
    E. with iron formula

enflurane

Enforcer
    18F Cook E.

Engerix-B
    HBV E.-B

engorgement
    liver e.
    venous e.

engraftment

enhanced
    e. chemiluminescence (ECL)
    e. chemiluminescence Western blotting
    enhance visualization
    e. magnification endoscopy
    e. reverse transcriptase polymerase chain reaction assay
    e. technical feasibility
    e. virulence

enhancement
    contrast e.
    CT scan with contrast e.
    edge e.
    hybrid rapid acquisition with relaxation e. (HRARE)

enlarged
    e. prostate
    e. uterus

enlargement
    benign prostatic e. (BPE)
    bladder e.
    calix e.
    discrete organ e.
    ovarian e.
    parotid gland e.
    penile e.

salivary gland e.
tonsillar e.
tube e.
uterine e.

enolase
neuron-specific e. (NSE)

Enovil
enoxacin
enoxaparin
e. sodium
e. sodium injection

ENRD
endoscopy-negative reflux disease

Enrich
E. feeding
E. protein and calorie supplement

ENS
enteric nervous system

ensheathing trocar
ensnarement
Ensure
E. HIN tube feeding formula
E. Plus
E. Plus formula
E. Plus liquid feeding
E. pudding

entactin
entamebiasis
entamebic abscess
Entamoeba
E. coli cyst
E. dispar
E. histolytica
E. histolytica abscess

entecavir
enteradenitis
EnteraFlo feeding tube
enteral
e. absorption
e. alimentation
e. diarrhea
e. feeding
e. nutrition (EN)

enteralgia
enterdynia
enterectasis
enterectomy
enterelcosis
enteric
e. adenovirus
e. cyst
e. excitatory motoneuron
e. fever
e. fistula
e. ganglion
e. ganglion cell
e. hormone
e. hyperoxaluria
e. immunogen
e. infection
e. inhibitory motoneuron
e. interneuron
e. nervous system (ENS)
e. neuronal circuit
e. neuronal reflex
e. oxaluria
e. pathogen
e. secretomotor circuit
e. vasodilator neuron

enterically
e. transmitted non-A non-B (ENANB)
e. transmitted non-A non-B hepatitis (ET-NANBH)

enteric-coated
e.-c. aspirin
e.-c. capsule

entericus
liquor e.
succus e.

enteritidis
Salmonella e.

enteritis
e. anaphylactica
Campylobacter fetus e.
choleriform e.
chronic cicatrizing e.
Clostridium difficile e.
Crohn regional e.
e. cystica chronica
diphtheritic e.
eosinophilic e.
granulomatous e.
e. gravis
hemorrhagic e.
idiopathic diffuse ulcerative nongranulomatous e.
leishmanial e.
mucomembranous e.
mucous e.
myxomembranous e.
e. necroticans
pellicular e.
phlegmonous e.

NOTES

enteritis *(continued)*
    e. polyposa
    protozoan e.
    pseudomembranous e.
    radiation e.
    regional e. (RE)
    segmental e.
    Streptococcus e.
    tuberculous e.
    ulcerative e.
    viral e.
    Yersinia e.
enteroadherent *Escherichia coli* (EAEC)
enteroaggregative
    e. *Escherichia coli* (EAEC, EaggEC)
    e. *Escherichia coli* heat-stable enterotoxin 1 (EAST1)
enteroanastomosis
enteroanthelone
enteroapocleisis
Enterobacter
    E. aerogenes
    E. cloacae
    E. hafniae
    E. liquefaciens
Enterobacteriaceae
enterobacterial common antigen (ECA)
enterobiliary
Enterobius vermicularis
enterobrosis, enterobrosia
enterocele
    complex e.
    congenital e.
    iatrogenic e.
    partial e.
    e. pulsion
    rectocele, cystocele, e.
    e. sac
    secondary e.
    simple e.
    e. traction
enterocele-like central hernia
enterocentesis
enteroceptive
enterocholecystostomy
enterocholecystotomy
enterochromaffin cell
enterochromaffin-like (ECL)
    e.-l. cell
    e.-l. gastric carcinoid tumor (ECLoma)
enterocinesia
enterocinetic
enterocleisis
    omental e.
enteroclysis
    small bowel e.
    e. tube

enterococcal
    e. endocarditis
    e. sepsis
enterococcus, pl. **enterococci**
    vancomycin-resistant e. (VRE)
enterocolectomy
enterocolic
    e. fistula
    e. lymphocytic phlebitis (ELP)
enterocolitica
    Yersinia e.
enterocolitis
    Aeromonas-associated e.
    antibiotic e.
    antibiotic-induced e.
    bacterial e.
    cytomegalovirus e.
    gangrenous ischemic e.
    granulomatous e.
    hemorrhagic e.
    Hirschsprung-associated e. (HAEC)
    necrotizing e. (NEC)
    nontuberculous mycobacteria-associated e.
    pericrypt eosinophilic e.
    pseudomembranous e.
    radiation e.
    regional e.
    Salmonella typhimurium e.
enterocolostomy
enterocutaneous
    e. fistula
    e. intubation
enterocyst
enterocystocele
enterocystoma
enterocystoplasty
    augmentation e.
    Camey e.
    clam e.
    sigmoid e.
enterocyte
    e. apoptosis
    CD23 e.
    intestinal e.
    small intestinal e.
Enterocytozoon bieneusi
enterodiol
enterodynia
enteroendocrine cell
enteroenteral fistula
enteroenteric
    e. anastomosis
    e. fistula
enteroenterostomy
    Braun e.
    Parker-Kerr closed method of end-to-end e.
    two-layer e.

enterogastric reflex
enterogastritis
enterogastrone
enterogenic proteinuria
enterogenous
　　e. cyanosis
　　e. cyst
enteroglucagon
enterogram
enterograph
enterography
enterohemorrhagic *Escherichia coli* (EHEC)
enterohepatic circulation (EHC)
enterohepatitis
enterohepatocele
enteroidea
enteroinsular axis
enterointestinal
enteroinvasive *Escherichia coli* (EIEC)
enterokinase
enterokinesia
enterokinetic
enterolactone
enterolith
　　calcified e.
enterolithiasis
enterolithotomy
enterology
enterolysis
enteromegaly, enteromegalia
enteromenia
enteromesenteric occlusion
enterometer
enteromycodermitis
enteromycosis
enteromyiasis
enteron
enteronitis
　　polytropous e.
Enteron Pharmaceuticals, Inc.
enteroparesis
enteropathic
　　e. organism
　　e. reactive arthritis
enteropathica
　　acrodermatitis e.
enteropathogen
enteropathogenic *Escherichia coli* (EPEC)
enteropathy
　　allergic e.

　　bile salt-losing e.
　　choleretic e.
　　chronic bacterial e.
　　cow's milk-sensitive e. (CMSE)
　　dermatopathic e.
　　diabetic e.
　　food-sensitive e.
　　gluten e.
　　gluten-sensitive e. (GSE)
　　HIV-1 e.
　　idiopathic e.
　　protein-losing e.
　　radiation e.
　　soya-induced e.
enteropathy-associated T-cell lymphoma (EATCL)
enteropeptidase deficiency
enteroperitoneal abscess
enteropexy
enteroplasty
enteroplegia
Enteroport feeding pump
enteroproctia
enteroptosis
enteroptychia, enteroptychy
enterorrhagia
enterorrhaphy
enterorrhea
enterorrhexis
enteroscope
　　magnifying e.
　　Olympus 215-cm e.
　　Olympus SIF-10 e.
　　Olympus SIF-M-series video e.
　　Olympus SIF-Q240 e.
　　Olympus SIF-SW-series video e.
　　Olympus SIF-100 video push e.
　　Pentax VSB-P-series e.
　　push e.
　　Sonde e.
　　temporary e.
　　tube e.
　　variable stiffness e.
　　video push e.
enteroscopy
　　capsule e.
　　e. diagnosis
　　double balloon method of e.
　　intraoperative e. (IOE)
　　push e.
　　push-type e.
　　Roux-en-Y limb e.

NOTES

enteroscopy *(continued)*
    small bowel e. (SBE)
    Sonde e.
    total peroral intraoperative e.
    transgastrostomic e. (TGE)
    video small bowel e.
    virtual e.
enterosepsis
enterosorption
enterospasm
enterostasis
enterostaxis
enterostenosis
enterostomal therapy (ET)
enterostomy
    double e.
    end-to-end e.
    gun-barrel e.
    tube e.
    Witzel e.
Entero-Test capsule
enterotome
enterotomy
    antimesenteric e.
    inadvertent e.
    e. incision
    longitudinal e.
enterotoxemia
enterotoxication
enterotoxigenic *Escherichia coli* **(ETEC)**
enterotoxin
    Clostridium difficile e.
    e. diarrhea
    enteroaggregative *Escherichia coli* heat-stable e. 1 (EAST1)
    heat-labile e.
    heat-stable e. (ST)
enterotoxism
enterotropic
enterourethral fistula
enterourethrostomy
enterourinary fistula
enterovaginal fistula
enterovenous
enterovesical fistula
enterovesical/urethral fistulae
enterovirus
enterozoon, pl. **enterozoa**
Enterra
    E. gastrointestinal pacemaker
    E. Therapy
    E. Therapy implantable neurostimulation system
Enteryx
    E. GERD procedure kit
    E. implant
    E. implantation
    intentional injection of E.
    E. procedure
    E. technology for GERD
Entery-X-Procedure
enthesis
enthetic
entire distal convolution
entocele
Entocort
    E. EC
    E. EC oral capsule
entoderm
Entolase
Entralife HN tube feeding formula
entrapment
    e. of bowel
    e. sac
    e. sack introducer
Entri-Pak
    E.-P. enteral feeding bag
    E.-P. tube feeding formula
EntriStar
    E. feeding tube
    E. polyurethane PEG tube
Entrition
    E. Entri-Pak feeding
    E. tube feeding formula
EntroEase
    E. Dry powder for oral suspension
    E. oral radiopaque contrast medium suspension
entropion
    eversion e.
entry site
enucleation
    endoscopic e.
enucleator
    Young e.
Enulose
enuresis
    adult-onset nocturnal e.
    e. alarm
    e. alarm technique
    diurnal e.
    learned e.
    monosymptomatic nocturnal e. (MNE)
    nocturnal e.
    psychologic e.
    sleep e.
enuretic absence
envelope 2 antigen (anti-E2)
environment
    acidic e.
    bactericidal stomach e.
environmental metaplastic atrophic gastritis (EMAG)
enzimoimmunoassay MEIA Abbott
Enzol disinfectant
Enzygnost anti-HIV 1+2 test

enzymatic, enzymic
  e. fat necrosis
  e. protein
  e. spectrophotometric analysis
enzyme
  angiotensin-converting e. (ACE)
  AP marker e.
  brancher e.
  brush-border marker e.
  carboxypeptidase B-like e.
  catecholamine synthetic e.
  cellular e.
  e. change
  circulating e.
  COX-1, -2 e.
  cytochrome P450 e.
  debrancher e.
  degradative e.
  digestive e.
  gluconeogenesis-associated e.
  glycolytic e.
  glycosaminoglycan-degrading e.
  HK e.
  e. immunoassay (EIA)
  e. immunoassay E-1023
  immunoreactive trypsin e.
  insulin-degrading e. (IDE)
  Ku-Zyme HP pancreatic e.
  lactase e.
  LDH e.
  lipase e.
  lipolytic e.
  liver e.
  lysosomal e.
  NAG lysosomal marker e.
  pancreatic isoamylase e.
  plasma e.
  proteinase e.
  proteolytic e.
  e. replacement therapy
  restriction e.
  SDH e.
  zinc-requiring e.
enzyme-conjugated anti-IgA antibody
enzyme-linked
  e.-l. immunosorbent assay (ELISA)
  e.-l. immunosorbent assay I (ELISA-I)
  e.-l. immunosorbent assay II (ELISA-II)
enzymic (*var. of* enzymatic)
enzymology

Enzymun test
EOA
  esophageal obturator airway
EOB-DTPA contrast agent
  gadolinium EOB-DTPA c. a. (Gd-EOB-DTPA)
EOG
  eosinophilic gastroenteritis
EORTC
  European Organization for Research and Treatment of Cancer
eosin
  hematoxylin and e. (H&E)
  e. stain
eosin-methylene
  e.-m. blue (EMB)
  e.-m. blue agar
eosinophil
  e. cationic protein (ECP)
  e. protein X (EPX)
eosinophilia
eosinophilic
  e. ascites
  e. ballooning
  e. cholangiopathy
  e. colitis
  e. cystitis
  e. cytoplasm
  e. enteritis
  e. esophagitis
  e. gastritis
  e. gastroenteritis (EG, EGE, EOG)
  e. gastroenteritis syndrome
  e. gastroenteropathy
  e. granuloma
  e. ileal perforation
  e. major basic protein
eosinophiluria
Eovist
EP2-EP3 protein
EPA
  eicosapentaenoic acid
EPBD
  endoscopic papillary balloon dilation
EPC
EPD
  endoscopic papillary balloon dilation
EPEC
  enteropathogenic *Escherichia coli*
ephedrine sulfate
EpHM
  intraesophageal pH monitoring

NOTES

EPI
    exocrine pancreatic insufficiency
epicardia
epicardial
epicritic pain
EPICS
    early preimplantation cell screening
        EPICS C-flow cytometer
        EPICS Elite flow cytometer
        EPICS 700-series flow cytometer
        EPICS V-flow cytometer
epicystitis
epicystotomy
epidemic
    e. dysentery
    e. gangrenous proctitis
    e. hemorrhagic fever
    e. hepatitis
    e. hypochlorhydria
    e. nausea
    e. nephritis
    e. nephropathy
    e. nonbacterial gastroenteritis
    e. vomiting
epidemica
    nephropathia e.
epidemiologic
epidemiological
epidemiology
epidermal
    e. cyst
    e. growth factor (EGF)
    e. growth factor receptor (EGFR)
    e. stria
epidermidis
    Staphylococcus e.
epidermoid
    e. carcinoma
    e. cyst
epidermolysis
    e. bullosa (EB)
    e. bullosa acquisita
    e. bullosa dystrophica
Epidermophyton floccosum
epididymal
    e. abscess
    e. cyst
    e. infection
    e. sarcoidosis
    e. sperm aspiration (ESA)
    e. tubule
    e. tunic
epididymectomy
epididymidis
    appendix e.
    caput e.
    corpus e.
    ductus e.
    globus major e.
    globus minor e.
    vas e.
epididymis, pl. **epididymides**
    body of e.
    cauda e.
    e. epithelium
    e. filariasis
    e. lymphatic duct
    e. marsupialization
    e. micropuncture
    microsurgical extraction of sperm from e. (MASE)
    e. obstruction
    e. percutaneous puncture
    e. secretion
epididymisoplasty
epididymitis
    acute e.
    mumps e.
    spermatogenic e.
epididymodeferentectomy
epididymodeferential
epididymography
epididymoorchitis
    pediatric cryptococcal e.
epididymoplasty
epididymotomy
epididymovasectomy
epididymovasostomy
    microsurgical e. (MSEV)
epididymovesiculography
epidural
    e. catheter
    e. space
epifluorescence microscopy
epigastralgia
epigastric
    e. angle
    e. artery
    e. discomfort
    e. distress
    e. fold
    e. fossa
    e. hernia
    e. incision
    e. pain
    e. puncture
    e. reflex
    e. spot
    e. zone
epigastrica
    plica e.
epigastrium
    palpation in e.
epigastrocele
epigastrography
    impedance e.
epigenetic

epiglottis
    omega-shaped e.
epiillumination
EpiLeukin
Epimorph
epinephrectomy
epinephrine
epinephritis
epinephroma
epinephros
epiphenomenon
epiphrenic diverticulum
epiplocele
epiploectomy
epiploenterocele
epiploic
    e. abscess
    e. appendage
    e. appendix
    e. foramen
epiploicum
    foramen e.
epiploitis
epiploon
    great e.
    lesser e.
epiplopexy
epiploplasty
epiplorrhaphy
epipodophyllotoxin
epirubicin
episcleritis
episiotomy scar
episode
    mitochondrial encephalomyopathy, lactic acidosis and strokelike e.'s
    multiple acute rejection e.'s
    e. of pouchitis
    reduced rejection e.
    subsequent rejection e.
    urinary incontinence e.
episodic
    e. colic
    e. vomiting
epispadia (*var. of* epispadias)
epispadiac
    e. opening
    e. orifice
epispadial
epispadias, epispadia
    balanic e.
    complete male e.
    congenital e.
    coronal e.
    female e.
    incontinent e.
    male e.
    penile e.
    penopubic e.
    e. repair
    subsymphyseal e.
epispadias-exstrophy complex
epistaxis
    Gull renal e.
    renal e.
epitaxial nucleation
epithelia (*pl. of* epithelium)
epithelial
    e. cell (EC)
    e. dysplasia
    e. endocrine cell
    e. growth factor
    e. inclusion body
    e. membrane antigen
    e. regenerative process
    e. restitution and renewal
    e. sodium channel (ENaC)
    e. tumor
epitheliitis
epithelioid
    e. granuloma
    e. leiomyoma
epithelium, pl. epithelia
    adenomatous e.
    airway e.
    Barrett e.
    bladder e.
    celomic e.
    CF e.
    columnar e.
    congenital hypertrophy of retinal pigment e. (CHRPE)
    crypt e.
    cuboidal e.
    desquamated e.
    ductal e.
    epididymis e.
    flattening of ileal e.
    follicle-associated e.
    gastric foveolar e.
    gastric-type surface e.
    germinal e.
    heterotopic cylindric ciliated e.
    hyperplastic foveolar e.

NOTES

epithelium *(continued)*
    metaplastic e.
    nonkeratinizing squamous e.
    nontumorous e.
    oviduct e.
    parietal e.
    proliferation of gastric e.
    renal tubular e.
    seminiferous tubule e.
    short-segment Barrett e.
    specialized columnar e. (SCE)
    squamous e.
    surface e.
    transitional e.
    tumorous e.
    villous e.
epithelium-lined tubule
epitope
    antibody to GOR e.
    B-cell e.
    Goodpasture e.
    HLA class II-restricted T-cell e.
    immunodominant T-cell e.
    Lewis Y carbohydrate e.
    nephritogenic e.
    T-cell e.
epitrochlear
epityphlitis
epityphlon
Epivir-HBV
EPL
    extracorporeal piezoelectric lithotripsy
    Piezolith EPL
EPO, Epo
    erythropoietin
        glycosylation of EPO
Epodyl
epoetin
    e. alfa
    e. beta
Epogen
Epon 812 resin
epoöphoron
epoprostenol sodium
epoxyeicosatrienoic acid (EET)
EPP
    erythropoietic proporphyria
Eppendorf
    E. needle electrode
    E. tube
Epping jaundice
EPS
    endoscopic pancreatic sphincterotomy
    endoscopic pancreatic stenting
EPS-21
    PerryMeter anal electromyographic sensor EPS-21
epsilon-aminocaproic acid

EPSP
    excitatory postsynaptic potential
Epstein
    E. disease
    E. nephrosis
    E. syndrome
Epstein-Barr
    E.-B. viral infection
    E.-B. virus (EBV)
EPT
    endoscopic papillotomy
EPX
    eosinophil protein X
Equagesic
Equalactin
equal fluid balance
equation
    Cockcroft-Gault e.
    Harris-Benedict energy requirement e.
    Henderson-Hasselbalch e.
    Nernst e.
    Portsmouth predictor e.
Equilet
equilibrium
    acid-base e.
    Gibbs-Donnan e.
    solute e.
equina
    cauda e.
equivalent
    meconium ileus e. (MIE)
    e. residual renal urea clearance (eKru)
equivocal
equol
ER
    estrogen receptor
ERA
    estrogen receptor assay
eradication therapy
ER alpha
    estrogen receptor alpha
ERBD
    endoscopic retrograde biliary drainage
ERBE
    ERBE electrical coagulation instrument
    ERBE electrical cutting instrument
    ERBE electrocautery unit
    ERBE Unit argon plasma coagulator
ER beta
    estrogen receptor beta
Erbitux
erbium:YAG laser
Erbotom F2 electrocoagulation unit
ERC
    endoscopic retrograde cholangiography

ERCCE
    endoscopic retrograde cholecystoendoprosthesis
ERCP
    endoscopic retrograde cholangiopancreatography
        ERCP balloon extractor
        ERCP cannula
        ERCP cannulation
        ERCP catheter
        ERCP conventional prosthesis
        ERCP dilator
        ERCP guidewire
        ERCP manometry
        ERCP nasobiliary drain
        ERCP sphincterotome
ERCP-guided biopsy
ERCP-induced splenic rupture
ERE
    estrogen response element
ErecAid
    E. vacuum erection device
    E. vacuum system
erectile
    e. dysfunction
    e. potency
    e. sinusoid
erection
    artificial e.
    artificial e. test
    drug-induced e.
    e. hemodynamics
    intraoperative penile e.
    Medicated Urethral System for E. (MUSE)
    medication-associated e.
    nocturnal e.
    nonbuckling e.
    penile e.
    pharmacologically induced e.
    psychogenic e.
    reflex e.
    reflexogenic e.
    vacuum constriction e.
ERF
    esophagorespiratory fistula
Ergamisol
ergonovine test
ergot
    e. alkaloid
    e. derivative
ergotamine

erigendi
    impotentia e.
erigentes
    nervi e.
ERK
    extracellular signal-regulated protein kinase
Erlangen
    E. magnetic colostomy device
    E. papillotome
    E. pull-type precut papillotomy
    E. pull-type sphincterotomy
Erlanger active stimulator for interventional endoscopy
erlotinib (OSI-774)
eroded polyp
erosion
    aphthous e.
    bladder e.
    Cameron e.
    cancerous e.
    cervical e.
    chronic e.
    Dieulafoy gastric e.
    duodenal e.
    gastric antral e.
    gastric mucosal e.
    gravity-induced e.
    idiopathic chronic e.
    implant e.
    limiting plate e.
    linear e.
    mucosal e.
    salt-and-pepper duodenal e.
    small bowel e.
    stress e.
erosive
    e. duodenitis
    e. esophagitis
    e. gastritis
    e. gastropathy
    e. prepyloric change
erosive-hemorrhagic gastritis
erotic vomiting
ERP
    endoscopic retrograde pancreatography
    endoscopic retrograde parenchymography
ERPF
    effective renal plasma flow
ERPP
    endoscopic retrograde parenchymography of pancreas

NOTES

ERSNA
  efferent renal sympathetic nerve activity
ERT
  estrogen replacement therapy
ertapenem sodium
eructation
  nervous e.
ERUS
  endorectal ultrasound
ERxin multicomponent penile injection
Eryc
EryPed
erysipelas
Ery-Tab
erythema
  conjunctival e.
  e. elevatum diutinum
  joint e.
  e. multiforme (EM)
  necrolytic migratory e.
  e. nodosum
  palmar e.
  e. toxicum
  urethromeatal e.
erythematosus
  discoid lupus e.
  disseminated lupus e. (DLE)
  lupus e.
  procainamide-induced systemic lupus e.
  systemic lupus e. (SLE)
erythematous
  e. gastropathy
  e. streak
erythrasma
Erythrocin
erythrocyte (E)
  e. aggregation
  e. cast
  dysmorphic e.
  eumorphic e.
  e. lysis assay
  neuraminidase-treated sheep e.
  e. sedimentation rate (ESR)
  e. sedimentation rate test
  e. sickling
erythrocytosis
  absolute e.
  stress e.
erythrocyturia
erythroid
  e. colony formation
  e. hypoplasia
erythromycin
  e. base
  e. estolate hepatotoxicity
  e. ethylsuccinate
  e. gluceptate
  e. lactobionate

erythromycin-induced cholecystitis
erythroplasia
  Queyrat e.
  Zoon e.
erythropoiesis
  ineffective e.
erythropoietic
  e. coproporphyria
  e. proporphyria (EPP)
  e. protoporphyria
erythropoietin (EPO, Epo)
  human recombinant e.
  e. hyporesponsiveness
  recombinant human e. (rh-EPO)
  e. therapy
ES
  Ecabet Sodium
  endoscopic sclerotherapy
  endoscopic sphincterotomy
ESA
  epididymal sperm aspiration
Esbach method
escalated methotrexate, vinblastine, Adriamycin, cisplatin or cyclophosphamide (E-MVAC)
Escherichia
  E. coli
  E. faecalis
escutcheon
  female e.
  male e.
E-selectin expression
Esidrix
ESI fiberoptic sigmoidoscope
Esimil
ESLD
  end-stage liver disease
esmolol
esogastritis
esomeprazole magnesium
EsophaCoil
  E. prosthesis
  E. self-expanding esophageal stent
esophagalgia
esophageal
  e. A, B ring
  e. achalasia
  e. acid clearance
  e. acid infusion test
  e. acid sensitivity
  e. adenocarcinoma
  e. atresia
  e. balloon dilator
  e. balloon distention
  e. balloon tamponade
  e. banding
  e. banding technique
  e. band ligation
  e. biopsy

esophageal · esophageal

- e. biopsy specimen
- e. body contraction amplitude
- e. body contraction duration
- e. body motor dysfunction
- e. bougienage
- e. cancer
- e. candidiasis (EC)
- e. cast
- e. clearing
- e. colic
- e. collateral vein (ECV)
- e. compression
- e. condyloma acuminatum
- e. condyloma virus
- e. contractile ring
- e. curling
- e. dilation
- e. dilation treatment
- e. diverticulum
- e. duplication cyst
- e. dysmotility
- e. dysphagia
- e. ectopic sebaceous gland
- e. effect
- e. endoprosthesis
- e. epidermal growth factor (EEGF)
- e. extirpation
- e. fistula
- e. foreign body
- e. function test
- e. fungal infection
- e. gastric tube airway (EGTA)
- e. globus
- e. globus sensation
- e. groove
- e. hyperkeratosis
- e. hyperkinsis
- e. hypomotility
- e. impression
- e. inlet
- e. intramural diverticulosis
- e. intramural hematoma
- e. intramural pseudodiverticulosis
- e. intubation
- e. I stent
- e. leiomyoma
- e. Lewy body
- e. lumen
- e. malignancy
- e. manometric sequence (EMS)
- e. manometry (EM)
- e. mass
- e. motility
- e. motility disorder (EMD)
- e. motility perfused catheter
- e. motor disorder
- e. mucosa
- e. mucosal gland
- e. mucosal ring
- e. muscular ring
- e. myotomy
- e. obstruction
- e. obturator airway (EOA)
- e. osteophyte
- e. paralysis
- e. perforation
- e. perfusate
- e. perfusion catheter
- e. peristalsis
- e. peristaltic pressure
- e. pH monitoring
- e. photodynamic therapy
- e. plexus
- e. polyp
- e. prosthesis
- e. reflux
- e. resection
- e. rupture
- e. scleroderma
- e. shunt
- e. single balloon
- e. sling procedure
- e. sound
- e. spasm
- e. sphincter
- e. sphincter relaxation
- e. squamous cell carcinoma
- e. squamous papilloma
- e. stenosis
- e. stethoscope
- e. Strecker stent
- e. stricture
- e. tear
- e. transection
- e. transit scan
- e. transit time
- e. trauma
- e. tube
- e. tuberculosis
- e. tumor
- e. ulcer
- e. ulceration
- e. valve (ESV)
- e. variceal bleeding

NOTES

esophageal *(continued)*
- e. variceal hemorrhage (EVH)
- e. variceal sclerosant
- e. variceal sclerosis
- e. variceal sclerotherapy (EVS)
- e. varix
- e. wall
- e. wall thickness (EWT)
- e. web
- e. Z stent with anchors
- e. Z stent with Dua antireflux stent
- e. Z Stent with Dua antireflux valve
- e. Z stent with fully coated flange ends

esophagectasia, esophagectasis

esophagectomy
- Ivor Lewis two-stage subtotal e.
- transhiatal blunt e.
- transhiatal radical e.
- transhiatal simple e.
- transthoracic e.
- e. with thoracotomy

esophagi (*pl. of* esophagus)

esophagism
- hiatal e.

esophagismus

esophagitis
- acid-pepsin reflux e.
- acid-peptic e.
- acute corrosive e.
- acute necrotizing e.
- alkaline reflux e.
- aspergillosis e.
- bacterial e.
- Barrett e.
- *Candida* e.
- candidal e.
- caustic e.
- chemical-induced e.
- chronic peptic e.
- CMV e.
- corrosive e.
- cytomegalovirus e.
- e. dissecans superficialis
- drug-induced e.
- endoscopic e.
- eosinophilic e.
- erosive e.
- herpes simplex e.
- herpetic e.
- herpetiform e.
- histological e.
- infectious e.
- *Leishmania* e.
- Los Angeles Classification grade A, B, C, D e.
- *Monilia* e.
- monilial e.
- mucormycosis e.
- nonerosive e.
- nonreflux e.
- nonspecific e.
- peptic e.
- pill e.
- pill-induced e.
- polycystic chronic e.
- radiation e.
- reflux e. (RE)
- refractory e.
- retention e.
- Savary-Gilliard e. grade I, II
- Savary-Miller grade I-III erosive e.
- Savary-Miller grade I-III reflux e.
- severe erosive e.
- severe reflux e.
- stasis e.
- streptococcal e.
- tetracycline-induced spongiotic e.
- thrush e.
- tuberculous infectious e.
- ulcerative reflux e.

esophagobronchial fistula

esophagocardial malignancy

esophagocardiomyotomy

esophagocardioplasty

esophagocele

esophagocolic anastomosis

esophagocologastrostomy

esophagocoloplasty

esophagoduodenostomy

esophagodynia

esophagoenterostomy

esophagoesophagostomy

esophagofiberscope

esophagofundopexy

esophagogastrectomy (EG)
- Ivor Lewis e.
- thoracoabdominal e.

esophagogastric (EG)
- e. balloon tamponade (EGBT)
- e. fat pad
- e. intubation
- e. junction
- e. junction cancer
- e. pH-metry
- e. variceal bleeding
- e. varix

esophagogastroanastomosis

esophagogastroduodenoscopy (EGD)
- conventional upper e. (C-EGD)
- pediatric e.
- small-caliber e.

esophagogastromyotomy

esophagogastropexy
- intercostal pedicle e.

esophagogastroplasty
    Grondahl-Finney e.
esophagogastroscopy
    Abbott e.
    Clagett-Barrett e.
    intrathoracic e.
    Johnson e.
    Thal e.
    Woodward e.
esophagogastrostomy
    Abbott e.
    Barrett-Clagett e.
    Clagett e.
    Clagett-Barrett e.
    intrathoracic e.
    Johnson e.
    Thal e.
    Woodward e.
esophagogram
    double-channel e.
    solid-column e.
    tube e.
esophagography
    contrast e.
esophagojejunal anastomosis
esophagojejunoplasty
esophagojejunostomy
    loop e.
    Roux-en-Y e.
esophagolaryngectomy
esophagology
esophagomalacia
esophagomediastinal fistula
esophagometer
esophagomycosis
esophagomyotomy
    Heller e.
esophagopharynx
esophagoplasty
    colic patch e.
esophagopleural fistula
esophagoplication
esophagoprobe
    Olympus ultrasonic e.
esophagoproximal gastrectomy
esophagoptosis
esophagopulmonary fistula
esophagorespiratory fistula (ERF)
esophagosalivary reflex
esophagosalivation
esophagoscope
    ACMI fiberoptic e.
    ballooning e.
    Blom-Singer e.
    Boros e.
    Broyle e.
    Bruening e.
    Chevalier Jackson e.
    child e.
    Denck e.
    Dohlman e.
    Eder-Hufford rigid e.
    fiberoptic e.
    Foregger rigid e.
    Foroblique fiberoptic e.
    full-lumen e.
    Haslinger e.
    Holinger e.
    infant e.
    Jackson e.
    Jesberg e.
    J-scope e.
    large-bore rigid e.
    LoPresti fiberoptic e.
    Moersch e.
    Mosher e.
    Moure e.
    Negus rigid e.
    Olympus EF-series e.
    optical e.
    oval e.
    oval-open e.
    Roberts folding e.
    Roberts oval e.
    Sam Roberts e.
    Schindler e.
    Storz e.
    Tesberg e.
    Tucker e.
    Universal e.
    Yankauer e.
esophagoscopy
    flexible e.
    prospective blinded study of diagnostic e.
    rigid e.
esophagospasm
esophagostenosis
esophagostoma
esophagostomy
esophagotome
esophagotomy
esophagotracheal fistula

NOTES

esophagram
    barium e.
    contrast e.
    double-contrast e.
esophagus, pl. **esophagi**
    abdominal part of e.
    achalasia-like e.
    aperistaltic e.
    A ring of e.
    atonic e.
    Barrett e. (BE)
    black e.
    B ring of e.
    cervical e.
    closed e.
    columnar-lined e. (CLE)
    combined percutaneous-endoscopic management of perforated e.
    corkscrew e.
    dilation of e.
    distal e.
    effort rupture of e.
    external coat of e.
    Heller-Belsey correction of achalasia of e.
    Heller-Nissen correction of achalasia of e.
    hypersensitive e.
    introitus esophagi
    long-segment Barrett e. (LSBE)
    nutcracker e.
    pneumatic bag dilation of e.
    primary malignant melanoma of e. (PMME)
    pseudosarcoma of e.
    pseudowatermelon e.
    scleroderma of e.
    short-segment Barrett e. (SSBE)
    spastic e.
    strictured e.
    thoracic e.
    tortuous e.
    variceal sclerotherapy in e.
esorubicin
ESPGHAN
    European Society of Pediatric Gastroenterology, Hepatology, and Nutrition
esprolol plus Viagra
ESR
    erythrocyte sedimentation rate
        ESR immunological study immunological study
ESRD
    end-stage renal disease
Essed
    E. plication method
    E. surgical procedure

essential
    e. amino acid
    e. fatty acid (EFA)
    e. fatty acid deficiency (EFAD)
    e. hematuria
    e. mixed cryoglobulinemia
estazolam
Esteem advanced vacuum therapy for impotence
ester
    cholesterol e.
    cholesteryl e.
    cypionate e.
    dinitrate and mononitrate e.
    enanthate e.
    injectable e.
    N^G-nitro-L-arginine methyl e. (L-NAME)
esterase
    leukocyte e.
    e. stain
    urinary leukocyte e.
esterification
esterified fecal acid
esthesioneuroblastoma
estimate
    significant parameter e.
    ultrasonography e.
estimated
    e. blood loss (EBL)
    e. liver blood flow (ELBF)
estimation
    Kaplan-Meier e.
Estracyt
estradiol-releasing silicone vaginal ring
estradiol transdermal patch
estramustine
    e. phosphate
    e. phosphate sodium
estramustine-binding protein (EMBP)
Estring estradiol vaginal ring
estrogen
    e. binding site (EBS)
    conjugated e. (CE)
    e. deficiency
    e. receptor (ER)
    e. receptor alpha (ER alpha)
    e. receptor assay (ERA)
    e. receptor beta (ER beta)
    e. replacement therapy (ERT)
    e. response element (ERE)
    e. testicular secretion
estrogen-induced
    e.-i. cholestasis
    e.-i. liver disease
estrone
Estroven
ESU
    electrosurgical unit

ESV
　esophageal valve
ESWL
　electrohydraulic shock wave lithotripsy
　　Modulith SL 20 device for ESWL
ESWL-related dysrhythmia
ET
　endothelin
　endotracheal tube
　enterostomal therapy
ET-1
　endothelin-1
ET-3
　endothelin-3
EtA
　endothelin A
　　EtA antagonist
　　EtA receptor
etanercept
EtB
　endothelin B
　　EtB antagonist
　　EtB receptor
ETCD
　endoscopic transpapillary cyst drainage
ETCG
　endoscopic transpapillary catheterization of gallbladder
ETEC
　enterotoxigenic *Escherichia coli*
ethacrynic acid
ethambutol
Ethamolin
ethanol (EtOH, ETOH)
　　e. abuse
　　dehydrated e.
　　e. enriched
　　gastric first-pass metabolism of e. (GFPM)
　　hydrolyzed in e.
　　e. injection
　　e. injection therapy
　　e. and phosphate-enriched dialysate
　　e. sclerotherapy
ethanolamine oleate sclerosant
ethanol-induced tumor necrosis (ETN)
ethanolism
ethanol-specific impairment
Ethaquin
ethaverine
ethchlorvynol

ether
　methyl-*tert*-butyl e. (MTBE)
　trimethylsilyl e.
Ethezyme debriding ointment
Ethibond suture
Ethicon
　E. CDH29 stapler
　E. TLH30 stapler
　E. trocar
ethidium
　e. bromide
　e. bromide staining
Ethiflex suture
Ethilon suture
ethinylestradiol
ethiofos
ethionamide
ethmoid
ethoglucid
ethopropazine
ethosuximide
Ethox feeding tube
ethoxysclerol
Ethril
ethyl alcohol
ethylcellulose
ethylchlorformate polymerized antigen
ethylene
　ethyleneglycoltetraacetic acid (EGTA)
　e. glycol
　e. oxide
　e. oxide gas (ETO)
ethylenediamine
　theophylline e.
ethylenediaminetetraacetate
　51-chromium-labeled e. (^{51}Cr-EDTA)
ethylenediaminetetraacetic acid (EDTA)
ethyleneglycoltetraacetic acid (EGTA)
ethylsuccinate
　erythromycin e.
5-ethynyluracil
Ethyol
etidronate
etiology
etiopathogenesis
ETN
　ethanol-induced tumor necrosis
ET-NANBH
　enterically transmitted non-A non-B hepatitis

NOTES

ETO
  ethylene oxide gas
  ETO sterilization
etodolac
EtOH, ETOH
  ethanol
  EtOH consumption
etomidate
etoposide
  e., Adriamycin, Platinol (EAP)
  e., ifosfamide, cisplatin
  e. injection
  e., leucovorin, 5-fluorouracil (ELF)
  platinum, e. (PE)
EU
  excretory urography
eubacterial strain
Eubacterium
  E. lentum
  E. limosum
  E. rectale
Eucestoda
euchlorhydria
eucholia
euchylia
euglycemic hyperinsulinemia
Eulexin plus LHRH-A chemotherapy/radiation therapy protocol
eumorphic
  e. erythrocyte
  e. red blood cell
eupancreatism
eupepsia, eupepsy
eupeptic
euperistalsis
Euphorbia resinifera
Euro-Collins
  E.-C. fluid
  E.-C. solution
European
  E. Organization for Research and Treatment of Cancer (EORTC)
  E. primary sclerosing cholangitis patient
  E. retrospective study
  E. Society of Pediatric Gastroenterology, Hepatology, and Nutrition (ESPGHAN)
Eurotransplant kidney allocation
EUS
  endoscopic ultrasonography
  endoscopic ultrasound
    EUS CPN
    evaluation of pancreatic cystic lesions with EUS
    EUS probe-guided electrosurgery
EUS-AD gastric lesion staging by endoscopic ultrasonography
EUS-FNA
  endoscopic ultrasound-guided fine-needle aspiration
EUS-guided
  EUS-g. celiac plexus neurolysis
  EUS-g. cholangiodrainage
  EUS-g. fine-needle aspiration
  EUS-g. FNA
  EUS-g. Tru-Cut needle biopsy
EUS-M gastric lesion staging by endoscopic ultrasonography
EUSN-1 EchoTip needle
EUS-SM gastric lesion staging by endoscopic ultrasonography
eutectic
  e. mixture
  e. mixture of local anesthetics (EMLA)
Eutonyl
euvolemic hyponatremia
Evac-Q-Kwik bowel preparation
evacuation
  digital rectal e.
  e. disorder
  hematobilia e.
  ileal reservoir e.
  e. pouchography
  e. proctography
  rectal e.
  stool e.
evacuator
  Creevy e.
  EasiVac e.
  Ellik e.
  McCarthy e.
  Toomey e.
  Urovac bladder e.
Evac-U-Gen
Evac-U-Lax
evagination
Evalose
evaluation
  acute physiology, age and chronic health e. (APACHE)
  adolescent urologic e.
  diagnostic imaging e.
  diverticulitis e.
  endoscopic ultrasound e.
  followup e.
  geriatric incontinence e.
  Heart Outcomes Prevention E. (HOPE)
  manometric e.
  medical e.
  metabolic e.
  e. of pancreatic cystic lesions with EUS
  percutaneous nerve e. (PNE)
  peripheral nerve e. (PNE)

evaluation · examination

postoperative e.
presurgical medical e.
pretransplant e.
prospective e.
risk e.
serum metabolic e.
sexual e.
status e.
e. of symptomatic hydronephrosis
urinary tract four-glass e.
urodynamic e.
videourodynamic e.
evanescent
Evans
    E. blue
    E. blue dye
EVE Fujinon videocolonoscope
event
    thromboembolic e.
eventration
Everett pile forceps
Everett-TeLinde operation
ever-expanding armamentarium of therapeutic modalities
ever-increasing knowledge
everolimus pharmacokinetics
eversion
    e. entropion
    e. normal
    e. operation
    e. orchiopexy
    vaginal e.
everted umbilicus
everting suture
EVH
    esophageal variceal hemorrhage
evidence
    electron-microscopic e.
    e. of inflammation
    solid e.
evidence-based
    e.-b. criteria
    e.-b. dietary/fluid modification
    e.-b. position statement
    e.-b. review of sphincter of Oddi dysfunction
eviration
EVIS
    EVIS EXERA
    EVIS EXERA Video System
    EVIS 140 Q series endoscope
    EVIS 140 S wide-screen endoscope

evisceration
    pelvic e.
    total abdominal e. (TAE)
EVL
    endoscopic variceal ligation
evoked potential
evolving concept
EVS
    esophageal variceal sclerotherapy
Ewald
    E. breakfast
    E. gastroscope
    E. node
    E. test meal
    E. tube
Ewing sarcoma
EWT
    esophageal wall thickness
ex
    e. vivo
    e. vivo cannulation
    e. vivo liver-directed gene therapy
    e. vivo perfusion
exacerbation of pain
examination
    abdominal tomodensitometric e.
    adolescent genitourinary e.
    anorectal e.
    arterioportographical e.
    bidigital rectal e.
    bladder e.
    cytology e.
    digital rectal e. (DRE)
    double-contrast barium enema e.
    endoscopic e.
    fistula in ano endoscopic e.
    followup e.
    merthiolate fresh stool e.
    microscopic urine e.
    motor e.
    nonrehydrated guaiac e.
    parasite e.
    peroral pneumocolon e.
    physical e.
    prostate gland color flow Doppler e.
    radial e.
    rectal e.
    reflux small bowel e.
    retrograde small bowel e.
    tomodensitometric e.
    vertical strip-pattern breast e.

NOTES

exanthematicus
  ichthyismus e.
exanthesis arthrosia
excavated gastric carcinoma
excavatio, pl. **excavationes**
  e. rectouterina
  e. rectovesicalis
  e. vesicouterina
excavation
  ischiorectal e.
  rectoischiadic e.
excavatum
  pectus e.
Excel disposable biopsy forceps
excess
  base e.
  e. mucus
  severe aldosterone e.
excessive
  e. bleeding
  e. straining
exchange
  anion e.
  cation e.
  countercurrent e.
  e. of endoprosthesis
  endoscopic stent e.
  extensive plasma e.
  guidewire e.
  plasma e.
  rapid e. (RX)
  short-dwell hypertonic e.
  sodium e.
  stent e.
  wire-guided balloon-assisted
    endoscopic biliary stent e.
exchanger
  cation e.
  heat e.
  thymocyte NA+/H+ e.
excision
  abdominoperineal e.
  adrenal gland laparoscopic e.
  Allingham rectum e.
  bladder e.
  cold snare e.
  Delorme transrectal e.
  full-thickness local e. (FTLE)
  Gibson e.
  laparoscopic abdominoperineal e.
  laser hemorrhoid e.
  mesorectal e.
  pouch e.
  sinus e.
  total mesorectal e. (TME)
  transanal e.
excitation-contraction coupling

excitatory
  e. junction potential (EJP)
  e. postsynaptic potential (EPSP)
excitotoxic food poisoning
exclusion
  Devine e.
  e. diet
  duodenal e. (DE)
  subtotal gastric e.
excoriation
excrement
excrementitious
excrescence
  polypoid e.
excreta
excrete
excretion
  basal renal e.
  biliary e.
  calcium e.
  calculation of renal ammonium e.
  ^{57}Co B$_{12}$ e.
  ^{51}Cr-EDTA e.
  C-urea breath e.
  C-urinary e.
  electrolyte e.
  fecal fat e. (FFE)
  glucose e.
  24-hour fecal fat e.
  net acid e. (NAE)
  pulmonary methane e.
  e. pyelography
  quantified protein e.
  renal acid e.
  renal ammonium e.
  renal phosphate e.
  renal sodium e.
  urate renal e.
  urinary chloride e.
  urinary glycosaminoglycan e.
  urinary kallikrein e.
  urinary oxalate e.
  urinary protein e.
  urinary sodium e. (UNaV)
  urinary urea nitrogen e. (UUN)
  waste nitrogen e.
  water e.
  whole-kidney fractional e.
excretor
  methane (CH4) e.
  non-CH4 e.
excretory
  e. azoospermia
  e. cystogram (XC)
  e. delay
  e. duct
  e. function
  e. urogram (XU)
  e. urography (EU, EXU)

excursion
  respiratory e.
excystation
exdwelling ureteral occlusion balloon catheter
exendin
exenteration
  anterior pelvic e.
  pelvic e.
  posterior pelvic e.
  supralevator pelvic e.
  total pelvic e.
exenterative surgery for pelvic cancer
exenteritis
EXERA
  EVIS EXERA
exercise
  Kegel pelvic muscle e.
  pelvic floor e. (PFE)
  pelvic floor muscle e.
  vaginal cone for pelvic floor e.
exercise-associated acute renal failure
exercise-induced hematuria
exeresis
  palliative e.
exertional rhabdomyolysis
exertion-induced pain
exfoliative
  e. cystitis
  e. cytology
  e. epithelial colonic cell
  e. gastritis
exisulind
exit
  e. site
  e. site of catheter
  e. site infection
Ex-Lax
Exna
exocolitis
exocrine
  e. function
  e. pancreas
  e. pancreatic hypoplasia
  e. pancreatic insufficiency (EPI)
exocytosis
  granulocyte e.
exoenzyme-S
exogastric
exogastritis
exogenous
  e. androgen

e. calcium
e. cholecystokinin or cerulein
e. hyperglyceridemia
e. IGF-1
e. obesity
e. PGE2
e. thiol
exomphalos
exon
  e. 1–5
  e. skipping
exopeptidase
  pancreatic e.
exophytic
  e. adenocarcinoma
  e. lesion
  e. mass
  e. wart
exotoxin
  Pseudomonas e. A
expandable
  e. biliary endoprosthesis
  e. esophageal stent (EES)
  e. intrahepatic portacaval shunt stent
  e. metallic stent
  e. metal mesh endoprosthesis
  e. olive
expander
  rectal e.
expanding retroperitoneal hematoma
expansile abdominal mass
expansion
  controlled e. (CX)
  controlled radial e. (CRE)
  intravascular volume e.
  mesangial matrix e.
  plasma volume e.
  sudden e.
  volume e.
expenditure
  resting energy e. (REE)
experience
  initial clinical e.
  personal e.
experiment
  Nussbaum e.
experimental
  e. background
  e. glomerulonephritis
  e. maneuver
expertise

NOTES

expiratory breath ethanol concentration
explant
exploration
- common bile duct e. (CBDE)
- common duct e. (CDE)
- complete surgical e. (CSE)
- laparoscopically guided transcystic e.
- laparoscopic transcystic duct e.
- prior negative inguinal e.
- renal e.
- repeat e.
- transcystic duct/common bile duct e. (TCD/CBDE)

exploratory
- e. celiotomy
- e. laparotomy

explosion
- colonic e.

explosive
- e. diarrhea
- e. doubling time
- e. vomiting

exponential rate
exposure
- occupational toxin e.
- postural quantitative analysis of acid e.
- radiation e.
- tobacco dose e.
- toxin e.

expression
- breast cancer-associated protein pS2 e.
- carbohydrate antigen 19-9 immunohistochemical e.
- complex class II e.
- e. cystourethrography
- cytokine gene e.
- E-selectin e.
- fibronectin e.
- e. of hemin receptor
- p53 e.
- renal tissue kallikrein e.
- tissue-specific gene e.

exquisite
- e. pain
- e. tenderness

exquisitely tender abdomen
exsanguinating hemorrhage
exsanguination
exsiccation fever
exstrophic bladder plate
exstrophy
- bladder e.
- cloacal e.
- e. closure
- complete repair of bladder e.
- vesical e.

exstrophy-epispadias complex
extended
- e. daily dialysis (EDD)
- e. left subcostal incision
- e. obturator node and iliopsoas node dissection
- e. pelvic lymphadenectomy
- e. pyelolithotomy
- e. pyelotomy
- e. release (XL, XR)
- e. right hepatectomy

extensibility
- penile e.

extension
- caliceal e.
- direct e.
- dumbbell-shaped caliceal e.
- e. fiber
- full e.
- superficial e.

extensive
- e. fibrosis
- e. pelvic disease
- e. plasma exchange

exteriorization colostomy
exteriorize
externa
- fascia spermatica e.
- lamina rara e. (LRE)
- muscularis e.

external
- e. abdominal ring
- e. anal sphincter (EAS)
- e. anal sphincter muscle
- e. anorectal mucosal prolapse
- e. biliary diversion
- e. biliary fistula
- e. biliary lavage
- e. coat of esophagus
- e. cooling
- e. cooling appliance
- e. drainage
- e. hemorrhoid
- e. iliac artery
- e. inguinal ring
- e. ligament
- e. oblique
- e. oblique aponeurosis
- e. oblique fascia
- e. oblique muscle
- e. pressure transducer
- e. proctotomy
- e. receiving
- e. recording
- e. rectal sphincter
- e. rotation
- e. shock wave lithotripsy
- e. skin tag
- e. spermatic fascia

e. spermatic vein
e. sphincter ani profundus muscle
e. sphincterotomy
e. stimulus
e. straightener
e. striated urinary sphincter
e. swelling
e. trauma
e. ureteral catheter
e. urethral barrier device
e. urethral sphincter
e. urethrotomy
e. vacuum therapy
external-beam
    e.-b. irradiation
    e.-b. radiation therapy (EBRT)
externally releasable knot
externi
    urethritis orificii e.
extirpation
    esophageal e.
    surgical e.
extra
    e. heart sounds
    E. Stiff Amplatz wire
extraabdominal disease
extraanatomical renal revascularization technique
extracapillary crescent formation
extracapsular
    e. disease
    e. tumor
extracellular
    e. calcium
    e. fluid (ECF)
    e. fluid volume (ECV)
    e. hyperosmolarity
    e. lipid
    e. matrix (ECM)
    e. matrix molecule
    e. potassium
    e. signal-regulated protein kinase (ERK)
    e. superoxide
extracellulary
extracolonic malignancy (ECM)
extracorporeal
    e. anastomosis
    e. cardiopulmonary circuit
    e. dialysis
    e. liver assist device (ELAD)
    e. liver perfusion (ECLP)

e. organ bioartificial liver device
e. partial nephrectomy
e. piezoelectric lithotripsy (EPL)
e. piezoelectric lithotriptor
e. piezoelectric shock wave lithotripsy
e. renal preservation
e. repair
e. shock
e. shock wave
e. shock wave lithotriptor
e. surgery
e. ultrafiltration (ECU)
e. whole-organ perfusion
extract
    lipidosterol e.
    Mycobacterium phlei cellular e.
    numerous plant e.'s
    pollen e.
    Pygeum e.
    Serenoa repens e.
extracted
    e. ductal sperm
    e. nuclear antigen (ENA)
extraction
    e. balloon
    e. balloon technique
    basket e.
    e. bile duct stone
    bolus e.
    foreign body e.
    harpoon e.
    e. pancreatic stone
    stone e.
    testicular sperm e. (TESE)
    ultrasound basket e.
extractor
    Applied Biosystems 340A nucleic acid e.
    endoscopic magnetic e.
    ERCP balloon e.
    Glassman stone e.
    Soehendra stent e.
    E. three-lumen retrieval balloon catheter
    E. XL triple-lumen retrieval balloon
eXtract specimen bag
extractum senna
extradomain A positive (EDA+)
extradural electrical stimulation
extraesophageal symptom

NOTES

extraglandular endocrine cell
　proliferation
extraglomerular mesangium (EGM)
extragonadal
　　e. germ cell cancer
　　e. germ cell neoplasm
extrahepatic
　　e. bile duct
　　e. bile duct atresia (EHBDA)
　　e. bile duct cancer
　　e. bile duct obstruction
　　e. biliary atresia (EBA)
　　e. biliary cystic dilation
　　e. biliary obstruction
　　e. biliary stricture
　　e. cholestasis
　　e. manifestation
　　e. metastasis (EHM)
　　e. portal vein
　　e. portal vein obstruction (EHPVO)
　　e. portal venous hypertension
　　e. shunt
extraintestinal
　　e. complication
　　e. disease
extralymphatic metastasis
extramammary Paget disease (EMPD)
extramedullary
　　e. hematopoiesis
　　e. plasmacytoma
extramucosal
　　e. cyst
　　e. mass
extramural
　　e. common bile duct compression
　　e. lesion
　　e. pseudocyst
Extraneal 7.5% peritoneal dialysis
　solution
extraordinary urinary frequency
　syndrome of childhood
extrapancreatic
　　e. nerve plexus
　　e. pseudocyst
extraparenchymal renal cyst
extraperitoneal
　　e. endoscopic pelvic lymph node
　　　dissection (EEPLND)
　　e. excision of lower one-third of
　　　ureter
　　e. fascia
　　e. laparoscopic bladder neck
　　　suspension (ELBNS)
　　e. laparoscopic nephrectomy
　　e. laparoscopy
　　e. rupture
　　e. supracostal live-donor
　　　nephrectomy
　　e. tissue
　　totally e. (TEP)
extrapolated plasma caffeine
　concentration
extraprostatitis
extrapudendal pelvic nerve
extrapulmonary *Pneumocystis carinii*
　infection
extrapyramidal function assessment
extrarenal
　　e. antigen
　　e. azotemia
　　e. calix
　　e. dysmorphy
　　e. mass
　　e. renal pelvis
　　e. uremia
　　e. vasculitis
extrasphincteric
　　e. anal fistula
　　e. approach
extraurethral incontinence
extravaginal torsion
extravasated
　　e. bile
　　e. iodinated contrast material
extravasation
　　e. of contrast medium
　　peripelvic e.
　　pyelosinus e.
　　red blood cell e.
　　urinary e.
　　urine e.
extravascular space
extraversion
　　urinary e.
extravesical
　　e. anastomosis
　　e. pathology
　　e. reimplantation
　　e. seromuscular tunnel
　　e. ureteral reimplantation technique
　　e. ureterolysis
extravisceral aneurysm
extremitas, pl. extremitates
extremity
　　anterior e.
　　inferior e.
　　posterior e.
　　superior e.
　　e. weakness
extrinsic
　　e. biliary compression
　　e. mass
　　e. pancreatic compression
　　e. ureteral obstruction
　　e. ureteropelvic junction obstruction
extrude
extruding mucus

extubate
extussusception
EXU
    excretory urography
exuberant granulation tissue
exudate
    fibrinopurulent e.
    mucopurulent e.
    pharyngeal e.
    whitish e.
exudate-transudate concept
exudative
    e. ascites
    e. nephritis
    e. peritonitis
exulceratio simplex
EYCAT
    egg yolk-cobalamin absorption test
eyelet
EZ
    EZ Detect colorectal screening test kit
    EZ vascular 35 linear stapler
EZH2 protein
Ez-HBT
E-Z Paque

NOTES

F-18, ^{18}F
   fluorine-18
      F-18 fluorodeoxyglucose positron emission tomography
F2 focal point
F60S polysulfone
F9 cell
Faber
   F. anemia
   F. syndrome
fabianii
   Hansenula f.
FABP
   fatty acid-binding protein
Fabricius
   bursa of F.
Fabry disease
FAC
   5-fluorouracil, Adriamycin, cyclophosphamide
face
   cytosolic f.
   en f.
   linear streaks en f.
   stable f.
faceplate
   Coloplast irrigation f.
   Marlen Neoprene All-Flexible f.
   Torbot f.
   United Surgical Hypalon f.
faceted gallstone
facies
   f. abdominalis
   f. anterior pancreatis
   cushingoid f.
   f. diaphragmatica hepatis
   f. hepatica
   f. inferior hepatis
   f. inferior pancreatis
   moon f.
   f. posterior hepatis
   f. posterior pancreatis
   Potter f.
   f. superior hepatis
   f. visceralis hepatis
facile working knowledge
faciodigital syndrome
FACS
   fluorescence-activated cell sorter
FACScan
   fluorescence-activated cell sorter scan
      FACScan flow cytometer
F-actin filament

factitial
   f. dermatitis
   f. proctitis
factitious diarrhea
Factive
factor
   acidic fibroblast growth f.
   acid-inhibitory f.
   adverse prognostic f.
   alcoholic prognostic f.
   analysis of virulence f.
   angiogenic f.
   atrial natriuretic f. (ANF)
   autocrine motility f. (AMF)
   bacterial virulence f.
   basic fibroblast growth f. (bFGF)
   basic fibroblastic growth f.
   B-cell differentiation f.
   beta-fibroblastic growth f.
   beta-HCG autocrine motility f.
   binary f.
   bladder cancer angiogenic f.
   brain-derived neurotrophic f. (BDNF)
   chemotactic f.
   clotting f.
   cobra venom f. (CVF)
   colony-stimulating f. (CSF)
   concentration epidermal growth f. (cEGF)
   crest f.
   cytotoxin necrotizing f.
   decapacitation f.
   decay-accelerating f. (DAF)
   endothelial cell growth f. (ECGF)
   endothelium-derived relaxing f. (EDRF)
   epidermal growth f. (EGF)
   epithelial growth f.
   esophageal epidermal growth f. (EEGF)
   fibroblast-derived f.
   fibroblast growth f. (FGF)
   gastric inhibitor f.
   glial cell line-derived neurotrophic f. (GDNF)
   glial-derived neurotrophic f. (GDNF)
   glycosylation-inhibiting f. (GIF)
   glycyrrhetinic acidlike f. (GALF)
   granulocyte colony-stimulating f. (G-CSF)
   granulocyte-macrophage colony-stimulating f. (GM-CSF)
   growth f.

factor *(continued)*
    guanine nucleotide-releasing f. (GNRF)
    f. H
    heat-labile f. (HLF)
    heparin-binding epidermal growth f. (HB-EGF)
    hepatocyte growth f. (HGF)
    histamine-releasing f. (HRF)
    host f.
    human epidermal growth f. (h-EGF)
    human growth f. (HGF)
    important risk f.
    independent positive predictive f.
    independent risk f.
    f.'s influencing colonic involvement in patients
    insulinlike growth f. (IGF)
    intrinsic f. (IF)
    keratinocyte growth f. (KGF)
    Kruppel-like f. 6 (KLF6)
    luminal CCK-releasing f.
    luteinizing hormone-follicle-stimulating hormone-releasing f.
    macrophage colony-stimulating f. (M-CSF)
    maternal age as risk f.
    migration inhibition f. (MIF)
    mineralocorticoid-independent f.
    müllerian inhibiting f.
    negative anatomical f.
    nerve growth f. (NGF)
    neurohumoral f.
    new differentiation f. (NDF)
    nonimmune f.
    nuclear roundness f.
    osteoclast-activating f.
    oxidase cytosolic f.
    paracrine f.
    pathogenetic f.
    patient f.
    platelet f. 4
    platelet-activating f. (PAF)
    platelet-derived growth f. (PDGF)
    P-Mod-S f.
    polypeptide growth f.
    prognostic f.
    progression f.
    prostatic antibacterial f.
    psychological f.
    review f.
    salivary epidermal growth f. (sEGF)
    scatter f.
    serum blocking f.
    somatotropin release-inhibiting f. (SRIF)
    sperm motility-inhibiting f.
    sperm survival f.
    testis-determining f.
    thrombotic risk f.
    transcription f.
    transfer f.
    transforming growth f. (TGF)
    trefoil f.
    tumor necrosis f. (TNF)
    urethral resistance f. (URA)
    vascular endothelial growth f. (VEGF)
    vascular permeability f. (VPF)
    f. VIII antigen
    virulence f.
    von Willebrand f.
    washout f.
    well-known virulence f.
    Wyanoids Relief F.
    f. Xa
    f. XIa
    f. XIIa
factor-1
    colony-stimulating f.-1 (CSF-1)
    heparin-binding growth f.-1
    insulinlike growth f.-1 (IGF-1)
    salivary epidermal growth f.-1
factor-2
    insulinlike growth f.-2 (IGF-2)
factor-alpha
    cytokine tumor necrosis f.-a.
    early growth response f.-a.
factor-beta-1, -2, -3
Fader Tip ureteral stent
faecalis
    Enterococcus f.
    Escherichia f.
    Streptococcus f.
FAG
    fundic atrophic gastritis
Fahrenheit thermometer
failed
    f. adaptation
    f. antireflux surgery
    f. nipple valve
    f. recovery of potency
    f. transplant
failure
    acute hepatic f.
    acute intrinsic renal f.
    acute liver f. (ALF)
    acute renal f. (ARF)
    anatomic fundoplication f.
    anemia of chronic renal f.
    bile secretory f.
    chronic renal f. (CRF)
    congestive heart f.
    contrast-associated renal f.
    contrast-induced renal f.
    dilator placement f.

drug-induced renal f.
ejaculation f.
endopyelotomy f.
endourological f.
end-stage renal f.
exercise-associated acute renal f.
fulminant hepatic f. (FHF)
fulminant hepatocellular f.
fulminant liver f.
hyperacute liver f. (HALF)
intubation f.
irradiation f.
kidney f.
late-onset hepatic f.
liver f.
multiorgan system f.
multiple organ f. (MOF)
multiple organ system f. (MOSF)
multiple-system organ f. (MSOF)
multisystem organ f. (MSOF)
nephrotoxic acute renal f.
nonoliguric acute renal f.
oliguric renal f.
paracetamol acute liver f.
parenchymatous acute renal f.
postischemic acute renal f.
pouch f.
radiocontrast-induced acute renal f.
renal f.
respiratory f.
shock wave lithotripsy f.
sling f.
subacute liver f. (SALF)
subfulminant liver f.
surgical f.
f. to thrive
treatment f.
vascular access f.

Fairley
F. bladder washout localization technique
F. bladder washout test

falciform
f. body
f. ligament

falciparum
f. fever
f. malaria
Plasmodium f.

Falk appendectomy spoon
fallax
Clostridium f.

fallopian
f. arch
f. tube
Fallot tetralogy
F2-alpha
prostaglandin F2-a. (PGF2-alpha)
false
f. aneurysm
f. channel formation
f. colonic obstruction
f. cyst
f. diverticulum
f. membrane
f. negative (FN)
f. negative rate in high-risk patient
f. positive (FP)
f. positive scintiscan
f. tympanites
FAM
5-fluorouracil, Adriamycin, mitomycin C
famciclovir
FAMe
fluorouracil, Adriamycin, mitomycin C
familial
f. adenomatous polyposis (FAP)
f. adenomatous polyposis coli
f. aggregation
f. amyloid polyneuropathy (FAP)
f. atypical multiple-mole melanoma (FAMM)
f. atypical multiple-mole melanoma syndrome
f. benign hematuria
f. chloride diarrhea
f. chloridorrhea
f. cholemia
f. cholestasis
f. chronic idiopathic jaundice
f. chylomicronemia syndrome
f. colon cancer
f. colonic varix
f. colorectal polyposis
f. combined hyperlipidemia
f. Crohn disease
f. dysautonomia
f. fat-induced hyperlipidemia
f. gastrointestinal polyposis
f. hamartomatous polyposis
f. hepatitis
f. high-density lipoprotein deficiency
f. hyperaldosteronism

NOTES

familial *(continued)*
- f. hyperbetalipoproteinemia and hyperprebetalipoproteinemia
- f. hypercholesteremic xanthomatosis
- f. hypercholesterolemia
- f. hypercholesterolemia with hyperlipidemia
- f. hyperchylomicronemia
- f. hyperchylomicronemia with hyperprebetalipoproteinemia
- f. hyperlipoproteinemia type II
- f. hypertriglyceridemia
- f. hypocalciuric hypercalcemia (FHH)
- f. hypocalciuric hypocalcemia
- f. intestinal neurofibromatosis
- f. intestinal polyposis
- f. intestinal pseudoobstruction
- f. juvenile nephronophthisis
- f. juvenile polyposis (FJP)
- f. lipoprotein lipase inhibitor
- f. Mediterranean fever (FMF)
- f. microvillus atrophy
- f. nephritis serum
- f. nephrosis
- f. nonhemolytic jaundice
- f. pancreatitis
- f. paroxysmal polyserositis (FPP)
- f. pheochromocytoma
- f. polyposis coli (FPC)
- f. polyposis syndrome
- f. predisposition
- f. pseudohyperkalemia
- f. recurrent polyserositis
- f. ulcerative colitis
- f. unconjugated hyperbilirubinemia
- f. visceral myopathy (FVM)
- f. visceral neuropathy (FVN)

family
- Caliciviridae virus f.
- inter-alpha inhibitor f.
- secretin-glucagon-vasoactive intestinal peptide f.
- S100 super f.
- tachykinin-bombesin f.
- trefoil factor f. (TFF)

FAMM
familial atypical multiple-mole melanoma
FAMM syndrome

famotidine
- f. maintenance treatment
- f. pharmacokinetics

FAMTX
fluorouracil, Adriamycin, methotrexate with leucovorin rescue

FANA
fluorescent antinuclear antibody

Fanconi-de Toni-Debré syndrome
Fanconi syndrome

fan elevator retractor
fan-shaped biopsy technique
fan-type laparoscopic retractor
FAP
familial adenomatous polyposis
familial amyloid polyneuropathy
5-fluorouracil, Adriamycin, Platinol

Farabeuf retractor
farmer's lung
Fas
- *Fas* gene
- Fas immunostaining

fascia, pl. **fasciae**
- anal f.
- anterior rectus f.
- anterior renal f.
- autologous rectus f.
- Buck f.
- Camper f.
- f. of Camper
- Colles f.
- f. of colon
- cremasteric f.
- dartos f.
- deep cervical f.
- Denonvilliers f.
- f. diaphragmatis pelvis inferior
- f. diaphragmatis pelvis superior
- endoabdominal f.
- external oblique f.
- external spermatic f.
- extraperitoneal f.
- fusion f.
- Gerota f.
- inferior f.
- internal abdominal f.
- internal oblique f.
- internal spermatic f.
- investing f.
- ischiorectal f.
- kidney Gerota f.
- f. lata
- f. lata buttress
- f. lata suburethral sling
- lateral oblique f.
- levator f.
- lumbodorsal f.
- lumbosacral f.
- paracolonal f.
- pelvic f.
- f. pelvis
- f. pelvis visceralis
- f. penis profunda
- f. penis superficialis
- perineal f.
- perirenal f.
- posterior renal f.
- prevertebral f.
- f. propria cooperi

prostatic f.
psoas f.
pubocervical f.
pubovesicocervical f.
rectal f.
rectosacral f.
rectovesical f.
rectus f.
renal f.
f. renalis
rim of f.
Scarpa f.
spermatic f.
f. spermatica externa
f. spermatica interna
subperitoneal f.
subserous f.
superficial f.
transversalis f.
umbilicovesical f.
f. of urogenital trigone
vesicopelvic f.
Waldeyer f.

fasciae (*pl. of* fascia)
fascial
f. capsule
f. defect
f. layer
f. sling approach
f. stranding
fasciculata
zona f.
fasciculated bladder
fasciculation
fasciitis
necrotizing f.
fasciocutaneous flap
Fasciola
F. gigantica
F. hepatica
F. hepatica infestation
fascioliasis
hepatic f.
Fascioloides magna
fasciolopsiasis
Fasciolopsis buski
fashion
Heineke-Mikulicz f.
helical f.
LeDuc f.
retrograde f.

fast
f. cholinergic input
f. spin-echo acquisition MRI
fasted-to-fed pattern
fastener
Brown-Mueller T f.
Brown-Mueller T-bar f.
ROC XS suture f.
T f.
fastidium cibi
fasting
f. C-peptide level
f. diet
intermediate f.
f. motor pattern
partial f.
f. plasma caffeine concentration
f. serum gastrin
f. serum gastrin level
total f.
FastPack system
FasTrac hydrophilic coated guidewire
FasTracker 325 coaxial microcatheter
fast-twitch striated muscle fiber
fat
abdominal f.
autologous f.
f. cast
f. cell
creeping of mesenteric f.
f. density
dietary f.
fecal f.
herniated preperitoneal f.
f. indigestion
f. infiltration
ischiorectal f.
macrovesicular f.
microvesicular f.
f. pad
paratesticular f.
pericolic f.
perinephric f.
peripelvic f.
perirectal f.
perirenal f.
perivesical f.
preperitoneal f.
properitoneal f.
protruding f.
retroperitoneal f.
serosal creeping f.

NOTES

fat (continued)
    f. storage disorder
    subcutaneous f.
    submucosal f.
    f. wrapping
fat-free supper (FFS)
fatigue
    structural f.
    suture f.
fat-induced gallbladder contraction
fat-soluble
    f.-s. bilirubin
    f.-s. vitamin
fat-storing liver cell
fat-suppressed spin-echo (FSSE)
fatty
    f. acid
    f. acid-binding protein (FABP)
    f. acid diarrhea
    f. acid-free bovine serum albumin
    f. ascites
    f. cast
    f. cirrhosis
    f. cyst
    f. deposit
    f. food
    f. food intolerance
    f. infiltration of liver
    f. kidney
    f. liver (FL)
    f. liver cell (FLC)
    f. liver disease
    f. liver hepatitis
    f. liver and kidney syndrome (FLKS)
    f. liver of pregnancy
    f. meal
    f. meal sonogram (FMS)
    f. metamorphosis
    f. necrosis
    f. omental apron
    f. stool
    f. tissue
favorable outcome
favored gait
FB-25K jumbo biopsy forceps
FBA
    fecal bile acid
    cocarcinogenic FBA
FBD
    functional bowel disorder
    functional bowel distress
FBDSI
    Functional Bowel Disorder Severity Index
FBI
    food-borne illness
FBV
    fiber bundle volume

FCC-COCA1 **gene**
F circle
FCIS
    Flint Colon Injury Scale
FCPD
    fibrocalculous pancreatic diabetes
FCS
    fluorescence correlation spectroscopy
        FCS two-channel ultra high-magnification endoscope
FCS-ML
    fluorescence correlation spectroscopy magnifying light
        FCS-ML II colonoscope
        FCS-ML II fiberscope
        FCS-ML II gastroscope
FCXM
    flow cytometry crossmatch
FDI
    frequency-duration index
FDL
    fluorescein dilaurate
        FDL test
FDP
    fibrin/fibrinogen degradation product
Fe
    iron
        Slow Fe
feasibility
    enhanced technical f.
feathery degeneration
feature
    manometric f.
    pathognomonic f.
    unique esophageal f.
febrile
    f. agglutinins
    f. morbidity
    f. pleomorphic anemia
    f. proteinuria
    f. urine
fecal
    f. abscess
    f. alpha-1-antitrypsin test
    f. analysis
    f. bile acid (FBA)
    f. calprotectin
    f. concretion
    f. contamination
    f. contamination of food
    f. contamination of water
    f. continence
    f. diversion
    f. fat
    f. fat excretion (FFE)
    f. fat test
    f. fistula
    f. flora
    f. fluid

    f. frequency (FF)
    f. homogenate
    f. impaction
    f. incontinence
    f. leukocyte
    f. leukocyte count test
    f. marker
    f. material
    f. obstruction
    f. occult blood test (FOBT)
    f. occult blood testing
    F. Odor Eliminator (FOE)
    f. paradoxical puborectalis spasm
    f. peritonitis
    f. PMN-elastase
    f. reservoir
    f. residue
    f. seepage
    f. soiling
    f. spillage
    f. stasis
    f. tagging
    f. transmission
    f. tumor
    f. urobilinogen
    f. vomiting
fecalith
fecaloid
fecaloma
fecal-oral
    f.-o. route
    f.-o. transmission
fecaluria
Fecatest
feces
    impacted f.
    inspissated f.
    retained f.
Fechtner syndrome
FECOM artificial stool for defecography
feculence
feculent vomitus
fecundity
fed
    f. motor pattern
    f. response
Federici sign
fedotozine
feedback
    tubuloglomerular f. (TGF)

feeding
    Amin-Aid powdered f.
    bolus f.
    Build Up enteral f.
    Citrotein liquid f.
    Clinifeed Iso enteral f.
    Compleat-B liquid f.
    f. complication
    continuous drip f.
    Criticare HN elemental liquid f.
    f. disorder
    Enrich f.
    Ensure Plus liquid f.
    enteral f.
    Entrition Entri-Pak f.
    Finkelstein f.
    Flexical enteral f.
    forced f., forcible f.
    Fortison enteral f.
    gastric f.
    gastrostomy f.
    f. gastrostomy
    f. gastrostomy tube
    gavage f.
    half-strength f.
    Hepatic-Aid powdered f.
    HN f.
    hyperosmotic f.
    intermittent drip f.
    intravenous f.
    Isocal HCN liquid f.
    Isotein HN f.
    isotonic f.
    jejunostomy elemental diet f.
    jejunostomy tube f.
    lactose-free f.
    Lonalac f.
    low-residue f.
    Magnacal liquid f.
    Meritene liquid f.
    modified sham f.
    nasal f.
    nasoenteric f.
    nasojejunal f.
    Osmolite HN enteral f.
    parenteral f.
    Portagen f.
    postoperative regimen for oral early f. (PROEF)
    Precision Isotein HN powdered f.
    Precision Isotonic powdered f.
    Precision LR powdered f.

NOTES

feeding *(continued)*
    Renu enteral f.
    Resource enteral f.
    semielemental enteral f.
    sham f.
    Stresstein liquid f.
    Sustacal HC liquid f.
    Sustagen liquid f.
    thermic effect of f. (TEF)
    transitional f.
    transpyloric f.
    TraumaCal enteral f.
    Traum-Aid HBC enteral f.
    Travasorb HN powdered f.
    Travasorb MCT liquid f.
    Travasorb STD liquid f.
    tube f.
    f. tube placement
    f. vessel
    Vital HN f.
    Vitaneed f.
    Vivonex HN powdered f.
    Vivonex TEN f.
Feen-a-Mint
FEFEK
    fractional excretion of potassium
Fehland intestinal clamp
Feldene
FELI
    fractional excretion of lithium
Felig insulin pump
felineus
    Opisthorchis f.
felis
    Helicobacter f.
fellea
    cystis f.
    vesica f.
    vesicula f.
felleae
    collum vesicae f.
    corpus vesicae f.
    fossa cystidis f.
    fundus vesicae f.
felodipine
Felty syndrome
female
    f. catheter
    f. condom
    f. epispadias
    f. escutcheon
    f. hypospadias
    f. pelvis
    f. perineum
    f. urethral syndrome
feminae
    hydrocele f.
    ostium urethrae externum f.
    tunica spongiosa urethrae f.

feminarum
    cystitis senilis f.
Femina vaginal weight
feminina
    urethra f.
femininae
    ductus paraurethrales urethrae f.
feminizing
    f. genitoplasty
    f. surgery
femoral
    f. artery
    f. bruit
    f. canal
    f. cryptorchidism
    f. hemodialysis catheter
    f. hernia
    f. ligament
    f. nerve
    f. testis
    f. triangle
FemSoft insert
FENa
    fractional excretion of sodium
fenbufen
fencing reflex
fenestrated
    f. catheter
    f. cup biopsy forceps
    f. drape
    f. ellipsoid spiked open-span biopsy forceps
    f. spiked open-span jumbo biopsy forceps
fenestration
    cyst f.
fenfluramine
Fenger gallbladder probe
fennelliae
    Helicobacter f.
fenofibrate
fenoldopam
fenoprofen
fen-phen diet
fentanyl
Fenwick disease
Fenwick-Hunner ulcer
Feosol
Ferguson
    F. abdominal scissors
    F. anal retractor
    F. anoscope
    F. gallstone scoop
    F. hemorrhoidectomy
    F. needle
    F. technique
    F. tenaculum forceps
Ferguson-Moon rectal retractor
Feridex IV

fermentative
  f. diarrhea
  f. dyspepsia
Ferrein
  F. tube
  F. tubule
ferric hyaluronate gel
ferricytochrome-C
Ferris
  F. biliary duct dilator
  F. common duct scoop
ferritin
  anionic f.
  cationized f.
  serum f.
ferrofluid
ferromagnetic tamponade
ferrous
  f. salt poisoning
  f. sulfate
fertile eunuch syndrome
fertility status
fertilization
  in vitro f.
FertilMARQ home diagnostic screening test kit
ferumoxides injectable solution
ferumoxsil
Festalan
Festal II
fetal
  f. adrenal cortex
  f. adrenal gland hemorrhage
  f. alcohol syndrome ureter defect
  f. arginine vasopressin
  f. bladder aspiration
  f. calf serum
  f. liver-derived B cell
  f. macrosomia
  f. sulfoglycoprotein antigen (FSA)
fetalis
  nonimmune hydrops f. (NIHF)
fetid
fetoprotein
  alpha f. (AFP)
  anti-alpha f.
  beta f.
  fucosylation index of alpha f.
  gamma f.
fetor
  fetor f.

fetus
  Campylobacter f.
Feulgen
  F. reaction
  F. staining
fever
  Aden f.
  Assam f.
  beaver f.
  bilious remittent f.
  bouquet f.
  breakbone f.
  Burdwan f.
  cachectic f.
  Charcot intermittent f.
  dandy f.
  date f.
  dehydration f.
  dengue hemorrhagic f.
  digestive f.
  Dumdum f.
  Ebola hemorrhagic f.
  enteric f.
  epidemic hemorrhagic f.
  exsiccation f.
  falciparum f.
  familial Mediterranean f. (FMF)
  filarial f.
  food f.
  hemorrhagic f.
  hemorrhagic f. with renal syndrome
  hepatic intermittent f.
  inanition f.
  intermittent hepatic f.
  Katayama f.
  Kinkiang f.
  Korean hemorrhagic f.
  Lassa hemorrhagic f.
  low-grade f.
  Manchurian hemorrhagic f.
  Mediterranean f.
  polka f.
  Q f.
  solar f.
  spiking f.
  thirst f.
  typhoid f.
  urticarial f.
  viral hemorrhagic f.
  Yangtze Valley f.
fexofenadine

NOTES

FF
    fecal frequency
    follicular fluid
FFE
    fecal fat excretion
^{18}F-fluorodeoxyglucose
FFP
    fresh frozen plasma
FFS
    fat-free supper
FG-36 UA curved linear-array echoendoscope
FGF
    fibroblast growth factor
FGID
    functional gastrointestinal disorder
FG-series two-channel endoscope
FGS-ML II gastroscope
FGS-ML-series two-channel endoscope
FGS-series two-channel endoscope
FGS-SML-series two-channel endoscope
FG-32UA
    Pentax FG-32UA
    Pentax/Hitachi FG-32UA
FHF
    fulminant hepatic failure
FHH
    familial hypocalciuric hypercalcemia
FHVP
    free hepatic venous pressure
fialuridine
fiber
    afferent nerve f.
    autonomic nerve f.
    f. bundle
    f. bundle volume (FBV)
    circular muscle f.
    cremasteric f.
    dietary f.
    extension f.
    fast-twitch striated muscle f.
    GBM collagen f.
    hypogastric f.
    Indigo diffuse f.
    intrapelvic somatic f.
    f. lock displacement
    oblique gastric f.
    optical f.
    oxidative-glycolytic f.
    pain f.
    PediaSure with f.
    psyllium husk f.
    ragged-red f.
    sacral afferent f.
    sling muscle f.
    slow-twitch striated muscle f.
    SLT 7 laser f.
    splanchnic afferent f.
    Trimedyne Flex MAX f.
    UltraLine f.
    Urolase neodymium:YAG laser f.
    viscoelastic collagen f.
Fiberall
fibercolonoscope
    Olympus CF-20 f.
FiberCon
fiber-deficient diet
fiberduodenoscope
fiberendoscope
fibergastroscope
    fluorescence f.
fiberoptic
    f. bundle
    f. catheter
    f. colonoscope
    f. endoscope
    f. endoscopy
    f. esophagoscope
    f. gastroscope
    f. injection sclerotherapy (FIS)
    f. instrument technology
    f. light cable
    f. panendoscopy
    f. sensor
    f. sigmoidoscope
    f. sigmoidoscopy
    f. spectrophotometer Bilitec 2000
fiberoptics
fiberscope
    CF-HM f.
    FCS-ML II f.
    gastrointestinal f.
    GIF-HM f.
    Hirschowitz gastroduodenal f.
    Olympus Aloka EU-MI ultrasound gastrointestinal f.
    Olympus GF-EU1 gastrointestinal f.
    Olympus GIF-Q30 f.
    Olympus OES f.
    Olympus XK-series oblique-viewing flexible f.
    pediatric f.
    Pentax f.
    side-viewing f.
    ultrasound gastrointestinal f.
fibra
    f.'s obliquae ventriculi
    f.'s oblique gastricae
fibrate derivative
fibril
    disulfide cross linked f.
    twisted beta-pleated sheet f.
fibrillary glomerulonephritis
fibrin
    f. calculus
    f. glue
    f. injection
    f. score

f. seal
f. sealant
f. split product (FSP)
f. sponge
f. spraying
f. strand
f. tissue adhesive

fibrin/fibrinogen degradation product (FDP)

fibrinogen degradation product

fibrinoid necrosis

fibrinolysis
endothelium-dependent f.

fibrinolytic activity

fibrinopeptide-A

fibrinopurulent exudate

fibroadenoma

fibroadenomatosis
biliary f.

fibroadipose tissue

fibroblast
f. ECM adhesion assay
f. growth factor (FGF)
HE9 f.
human synovial f.
interstitial f.
perivascular f.
f. PMN adhesion assay
quiescent human f.
3T3 murine f.

fibroblast-derived factor

fibrocalculous pancreatic diabetes (FCPD)

fibrocollagenous tissue

fibrocongestive splenomegaly

fibrocystic
f. change
f. disease of pancreas

fibrodysplastic

fibroelastic
f. connective tissue stroma
f. tissue

fibroelastosis

fibrofatty
f. adventitia
f. infiltration of pancreas

fibrogenesis

fibrogenic
f. cascade
f. cytokine

fibroid
f. induration

f. polyp
uterine f.

fibrolamellar
f. hepatocarcinoma
f. hepatocellular carcinoma (FL-HCC)
f. hepatoma

fibrolipomatous nephritis

fibroma
kidney f.
ovarian f.
renal f.
testicular f.
f. of testis
ungual f.

fibromatogenic

fibromatoid

fibromatosis
aggressive f.
mesenteric f.
penile f.
f. ventriculi

fibromatous

fibromectomy

fibromuscular
f. coat
f. dysplasia (FMD)
f. hyperplasia

fibromyalgia

fibromyoma

fibromyxoma

fibronectin
f. expression
f. monoclonal antibody
plasma f.
urinary f.

fibronectin-binding protein

fibroobliterative disease

fibroplasia
adventitial f.
intimal f.
medial f.
perimedial f.
string-of-beads appearance of renal medial f.
subadventitial f.

fibroplastica
gastritis granulomatosa f.

fibropolycystic liver disease

fibroproliferative destruction

fibropurulent perisplenitis

NOTES

fibrosa
    appendix f.
    capsula f.
    tunica f.
fibrosarcoma
    kidney f.
fibrosing
    f. cholestatic hepatitis B
    f. colonopathy
    f. piecemeal necrosis
fibrosis
    acholangic biliary f.
    alcoholic f.
    anal f.
    arachnoid f.
    biliary f.
    bridging f.
    cavernous f.
    chronic sclerosing hyaline f.
    congenital hepatic f. (CHF)
    corporeal f.
    corpus spongiosum f.
    cystic f. (CF)
    diffuse lobular f.
    extensive f.
    hepatic f.
    idiopathic retroperitoneal f.
    interlobular f.
    interstitial f.
    intralobular f.
    liver f.
    mixed intralobular f.
    noncirrhotic portal f. (NCPF)
    pancreatic f.
    paravariceal f.
    penile f.
    pericentral f.
    periductal f.
    perilobular f.
    perinephretic f.
    peripancreatic f.
    periportal f.
    periportal-perisinusoidal f.
    perisinusoidal f.
    periureteral f.
    perivenular f.
    portal-to-portal f.
    portal tract f.
    postoperative retroperitoneal f.
    progressive perivenular alcoholic f. (PPAF)
    retroperitoneal f.
    f. score
    secondary biliary f.
    segmental bile duct f.
    sinusoidal f.
    stripe interstitial f.
    transmural f.
    tubulointerstitial f.
    vesical f.
fibrosis-promoting cytokine
fibrotic corpus cavernosum
fibrous
    f. adhesion
    f. appendage of liver
    f. capsule of liver
    f. cavernitis
    f. chordee
    f. dysplasia
    f. histiocytoma
    f. nephritis
    f. obliterative cholangitis
    f. septum
    f. sheath
    f. stroma
    f. tissue
    f. tunic
    f. tunic of liver
fibrovascular polyp
Ficoll-Hypaque
    F.-H. density gradient centrifuge
    F.-H. gradient centrifugation
    F.-H. gradient sedimentation
field cut
field-of-view camera
Fiessinger-Leroy-Reiter syndrome
figure-of-eight suture
filament
    actin f.
    Charcot-Boettcher crystals and f.'s
    F-actin f.
filamentous morphology
filarial
    f. abscess
    f. fever
    f. funiculoepididymitis
    f. hydrocele
    f. lymphedema
    f. orchitis
filariasis
    amicrofilaremic f.
    epididymis f.
    late-period f.
    occult f.
    prepatent-period f.
filiform
    f. bougie
    f. and follower
    f. polyp
    f. polyposis
    f. stricture
    f. tip
filling
    bladder f.
    contrast f.
    f. cystometrogram
    f. cystometry

f. defect
gallbladder f.
muscle f.
rectal f.

film
Bard protective barrier f.
conditioning f.
high abdominal plain f.
organic conditioning f.
plain f.
postevacuation f.
soft x-ray f.

filmy adhesion
filter
Amicon D-20 f.
Baermann stool f.
Baxter CA-210 f.
charcoal f.
fluorescence excitation f.
Fresenius F-40 f.
Gambro FH88H f.
Gene Screen nylon membrane f.
Greenfield f.
Hospal Biospal f.
interference barrier f.
Millex-GS pore-size f.
Millex-GV f.
Millipore f.
nitrocellulose f.
Percoll f.
Renal System HF250 f.
suprarenal Greenfield f.
Sur-Fit auto-lock closed-end pouch with f.
Sur-Fit Natura opaque closed-end pouch with f.
Zeta probe nylon f.

filtered
f. fraction
f. glucose

filtering
high-pass f.

filtrate
Folin f.

filtration
f. barrier
f. fraction
glomerular f.
kidney magnesium f.
f. slit-length density
f. slit membrane

f. slit pores
spontaneous ascites f.

fimbria, pl. **fimbriae**
final
f. motor neuron
f. position

finasteride
finding
anatomical f.'s
cholangiographic f.'s
clinical f.'s
colonoscopic f.'s
endoscopic f.'s
focal f.'s
intraoperative f.'s
manometric f.'s
physical examination f.'s
preliminary f.'s
relevant gastroduodenal f.'s
RNA-based f.'s
roentgen f.'s
sensory f.'s
spinal f.'s
ultrasonographic f.'s
unexplained f.'s

fine
f. gastric mucosal pattern
f. granular cast
f. needle
f. reticular pattern
f. tissue forceps

finely
f. fatty foamy liver
f. granular kidney

fine-needle
f.-n. aspiration (FNA)
f.-n. aspiration biopsy (FNAB)
f.-n. aspiration cytology (FNAC)
f.-n. capillary biopsy
f.-n. percutaneous cholangiogram
f.-n. transhepatic cholangiogram
f.-n. transhepatic cholangiography (FNTC, FNTHC)
f.-n. vasography

fine-toothed forceps
finger
clubbed f.
f. clubbing
f. fracture dissection
f. fracture technique
f. intrinsic

NOTES

finger *(continued)*
    f. ring
    zinc f.
fingerbreadth
fingerlike
    f. epithelial process
    f. villus
fingerprick latex agglutination test
fingerprinting
    peptide mass f.
fingerstick device
fingertip lesion
Finkelstein feeding
Finney
    F. Flexirod penile prosthesis
    F. gastroenterostomy
    F. operation
    F. pyloroplasty
    F. strictureplasty
Finochietto retractor
FIO$_2$
    fractional percentage of inspired oxygen
Fioricet
Fiorinal
Firlit-Kluge stent
First-Choice drainable pouch
first-degree relative
first-generation ELISA
first-line
    f.-l. screening technique
    f.-l. treatment
first-order kinetics
first-pass
    f.-p. effect
    f.-p. metabolism (FPM)
first-set phenomenon
first-stage repair
first variceal bleeding
FIS
    fiberoptic injection sclerotherapy
Fischer test meal
FISH
    fluorescence in situ hybridization
fish
    f. bone ingestion
    f. oil
    f. oil supplementation
    f. tapeworm
Fishberg method
Fisher
    F. Accumet pH meter
    F. Capillary System
    F. exact probability test
    F. two-tailed exact test
fish-hook displacement
Fishman-Doubilet test
fishmouth
    f. anastomosis
    f. incision

fish-scale gallbladder
fissura, pl. **fissurae**
    f. ligamenti teretis
    f. ligamenti venosi
fissural
fissure
    Allingham f.
    anal f.
    f. in ano
    anterior f.
    cecal f.
    f. of ligamentum teres
    f. of ligamentum venosum
    longitudinal f.
    portal f.
    posterior f.
    f. of round ligament
    transverse f.
    umbilical f.
fissurectomy
fissured tongue
fissurelike ulceration
fist fornication
fistula, pl. **fistulae, fistulas**
    abdominal f.
    airway-arterial f.
    amphibolic f., amphibolous f.
    anal f.
    f. in ano
    f. in ano endoscopic examination
    anorectal f.
    anovaginal f.
    antecubital arteriovenous f.
    anterior f.
    aortoduodenal f. (ADF)
    aortoenteric f.
    aortoesophageal f.
    aortogastric f.
    aortograft duodenal f.
    aortosigmoid f.
    arterial-enteric f.
    arterioportal f.
    arteriovenous f. (AVF)
    AV f.
    benign duodenocolic f.
    benign gastrocolonic-pancreatic f.
    biliary f.
    biliary-bronchial f.
    biliary-cutaneous f.
    bilioduodenal f.
    bilioenteric f.
    biliopancreatic fistula
    f. bimucosa
    bladder f.
    blind f.
    Blom-Singer tracheoesophageal f.
    brachioaxillary bridge graft f. (BAGF)

brachiosubclavian bridge graft f. (BSGF)
Brescia-Cimino f.
bronchobiliary f.
bronchoesophageal f. (BEF)
bronchopancreatic f.
caliceal f.
cholecystenteric f.
cholecystobiliary f.
cholecystocholedochal f.
cholecystocolonic f.
cholecystoduodenal f.
cholecystoduodenocolic f.
choledochocolonic f.
choledochoduodenal f.
choledochoenteric f.
chylous f.
f. cibalis
coccygeal f.
colobronchial f.
colocholecystic f.
colocolonic f.
colocutaneous f.
coloenteric f.
cologastrocutaneous f.
coloileal f.
colonic f.
coloperineal f.
coloureteral f.
colouterine f.
colovaginal f.
colovenous f.
colovesical f.
complex anorectal f.
congenital urethroperineal f.
congenital urethrorectal f.
cutaneobiliary f.
cystogastric f.
digestive-respiratory f. (DRF)
duodenal f.
duodenocaval f.
duodenocolic f.
duodenoenterocutaneous f.
Eck f.
endobronchial f.
enteric f.
enterocolic f.
enterocutaneous f.
enteroenteral f.
enteroenteric f.
enterourethral f.
enterourinary f.
enterovaginal f.
enterovesical f.
enterovesical/urethral fistulae
esophageal f.
esophagobronchial f.
esophagomediastinal f.
esophagopleural f.
esophagopulmonary f.
esophagorespiratory f. (ERF)
esophagotracheal f.
external biliary f.
extrasphincteric anal f.
fecal f.
forearm graft arteriovenous f.
f. formation
gastric f.
gastrocolic f.
gastrocutaneous f.
gastroduodenal f.
gastroenteric f.
gastrointestinal f.
gastrojejunocolic f.
genitourinary f.
graft-enteric f.
hepatic f.
hepaticopulmonary f.
hepatopleural f.
horseshoe f.
H-type f.
iatrogenic prostatourethral-rectal f.
iatrogenic rectourethral f.
ileosigmoid f.
ileovesical f.
intersphincteric anal f.
intestinal f.
intrahepatic AV f.
intrahepatic spontaneous arterioportal f.
ischiorectal f.
jejunocolic f.
kidney arteriovenous f.
low intersphincteric anal f.
malignant esophagopericardial f.
Mann-Bollman f.
mesenteric arteriovenous f.
mucous f.
pancreatic cutaneous f.
pancreaticopleural f.
pancreatic-portal vein f.
pararectal f.
parietal f.
pelvirectal f.

NOTES

fistula *(continued)*
    perianal f.
    perianal and enterourethral fistulae
    perineal urinary f.
    perirectal f.
    pleurobiliary f.
    postbiopsy f.
    postoperative pleurobiliary f.
    posttraumatic pancreatic-cutaneous f.
    pouch f.
    primary arteriovenous f.
    f. probe
    prostatourethral f.
    prostatourethral-rectal f.
    pseudocystobiliary f.
    psuedocystolonic f.
    radiation-induced vesicovaginal f.
    radiocephalic f.
    rectal f.
    rectolabial f.
    rectoneovaginal f.
    rectourethral f.
    rectourinary f.
    rectovaginal f.
    rectovesical f.
    rectovestibular f.
    rectovulvar f.
    renal arteriovenous f.
    renogastric f.
    residual rectoperineal f.
    respiratory-esophageal f.
    retroperitoneal f.
    seton treatment of high anal f.
    sigmoidovesical f.
    spermatic f.
    splanchnic AV f.
    splenic AV f.
    splenobronchial f.
    stercoraceous f.
    suprapapillary f.
    suprasphincteric f.
    sylvian f.
    thigh graft arteriovenous f.
    Thiry f.
    Thiry-Vella f. (TVF)
    thoracic f.
    tracheoesophageal f. (TEF)
    f. tract
    transsphincteric anal f.
    ulcerogenic f.
    umbilical f.
    urachal f.
    ureterocolic f.
    ureterocutaneous f.
    ureterouterine f.
    ureterovaginal f.
    urethral f.
    urethrocavernous f.
    urethrocutaneous f.
    urethrorectal f.
    urethrovaginal f.
    urinary umbilical f.
    urogenital f.
    vaginal f.
    vasocutaneous f.
    Vella f.
    vesical f.
    vesicocolic f.
    vesicocolonic f.
    vesicocutaneous f.
    vesicoenteric f.
    vesicointestinal f.
    vesicorectal f.
    vesicosalpingovaginal f.
    vesicoumbilical f.
    vesicouterine f.
    vesicovaginal f. (VVF)
    vesicovaginorectal f.
    vulvorectal f.
fistulation
    spreading f.
fistulectomy
    bronchovisceral f.
fistulization
fistulizing Crohn disease
fistuloenterostomy
fistulogram
fistulography
fistulotome
    double-channel f.
    needle-knife f.
fistulotomy
    choledochoduodenal f.
    diathermic f.
    endoscopic f.
    laying-open f.
    needle-knife f. (NKF)
    Parks method of anal f.
    Parks staged f.
    primary f.
fistulous
    f. Crohn disease
    f. degeneration
    f. orifice
    f. tract
FITC
    fluorescein isothiocyanate
Fite stain
Fitz
    F. law
    F. syndrome
Fitz-Hugh and Curtis syndrome
FIV-ASA suppository
five-port fan placement
fixation
    f. anomaly
    intestinal f.
    pubic f.

fixation · flap

sacrospinalis ligament vaginal f.
sacrospinous ligament vaginal f.
superior passive f.
tissue f.

fixative
Saccomanno f.
Zamboni f.

fixed
f. drain pipe urethra
f. drug reaction
f. and dynamic urethral compression treatment
f. ring retractor
f. segment of bowel

Fix and Perm permeabilizing kit

FJP
familial juvenile polyposis

FK506

FK-13K-1 jumbo biopsy forceps

FL
fatty liver
full liquids

flabby abdomen

flaccid penis

flagellate
f. diarrhea
f. dysentery

flagellum, pl. **flagella**
polar sheathed flagella

Flagyl

flail chest

flame photometry

flammeus
nevus f.

flange
Assura pediatric skin barrier f.

flank
f. approach
f. approach adrenalectomy
bulging f.
f. droop
f. incision
f. mass
f. nephrectomy
f. pain
f. position
f. roll positioning
f. surgery

flanking sequence

FLAP
fluorouracil, leucovorin rescue, Adriamycin, Platinol

flap
abdominal fasciocutaneous f.
advancement of rectal f.
advancement sleeve f.
axial f.
Bakamjian f.
Boari bladder f.
Boari-Ockerblad f.
Byars f.
circumferential transanal sleeve advancement f.
cutaneous advancement f.
cuticular f.
dartos pedicled f.
deepithelialized f.
detrusor muscle f.
diamond f.
f. dissection
endorectal advancement f.
fasciocutaneous f.
forearm f.
foreskin f.
Fortunoff f.
gracilis muscle f.
House sliding advancement f.
ischemia or sloughing of the f.
island groin f.
island pedicle f.
latissimus dorsi free f.
liver f.
Martius labial fat pad f.
Mathieu island onlay f.
microvascular f.
musculocutaneous f.
myocutaneous f.
Ockerblad-Boari f.
omental pedicle f.
onlay island f.
paraexstrophy skin f.
parameatal-based f.
pedicle island f.
pedicle muscle f.
penile island f.
random f.
rectus abdominis musculocutaneous f.
rectus femoris f.
renal capsular f.
Scardino f.
surgical f.
f. technique
tensor fascia lata f.

NOTES

flap *(continued)*
    tubed groin f.
    tubularized cecal f.
    upper arm f.
    U-shaped skin f.
    vaginal f.
    f. valve
    f. valve antireflux procedure
    f. valve cystoplasty
    f. valve principle
    vastus lateralis muscle f.
    ventrum penis f.
flapping tremor sign
flap-valve mechanism
flare
    f. cell
    pancreatic f.
flare-up
FLASH
    flat low-angle shot
    FLASH pulse sequence
flashlamp pumped-dye laser
flash pulmonary edema with anuria
flat
    f. adenoma
    f. carcinoma
    f. condyloma
    f. depressed lesion
    f. dysplasia
    f. elevated lesion
    f. hyperplasia
    f. low-angle shot (FLASH)
    f. plate of abdomen
    f. polycyclic ulceration
    f. rectal adenocarcinoma
    f. spatula electrode
    f. ulcer
flattened
    f. duodenal fold
    f. epithelial microfold cell
flattening
    histogram f.
    f. of ileal epithelium
flat-type carcinoma
flatulence
flatulent
    f. colic
    f. dyspepsia
Flatulex
flatus
    f. enema
    f. incontinence
    f. tube insertion
Flavimonas
flavin
    f. adenine dinucleotide
    f. mononucleotide
flavivirus
Flavobacterium meningosepticum
flavonol
flavoxate hydrochloride
flavus
    Aspergillus f.
FLC
    fatty liver cell
flea-bitten kidney
flecainide
Fleet
    F. Babylax enema
    F. Bisacodyl
    F. bowel preparation
    F. Enema Mineral Oil
    F. Flavored Castor Oil
    F. Phospho-soda
    F. Phospho-soda buffered saline laxative
fleroxacin
Fletcher's Castoria
flexed
Flexeril
flexible
    f. aspiration needle
    f. barium enema
    f. bronchoscopy simulator
    f. cystodiathermy
    f. delivery device
    f. dental suction
    f. endoscopic overtube
    f. endoscopic suturing device
    f. endoscopy
    f. esophagoscopy
    f. fiberoptic choledochoscope
    f. fiberoptic endoscope
    f. forward-viewing panendoscope
    7-8F f. scope
    f. gastroscope
    f. laparoscopy
    f. nephroscope
    f. nephroscopy
    f. Olympus GF-eUM3 device
    F. Sew-Right device
    f. sigmoidoscope
    f. sigmoidoscopy
    F. Ti-Knot device
    f. ureteropyeloscopy
    f. ureterorenoscopy
    f. ureteroscope
    f. videolaparoscope (FVL)
flexible-tip guidewire
Flexical enteral feeding
Flexicath silicone subclavian cannula
Flexi-Flate
    F.-F. I, II penile prosthesis
    F.-F. penile implant
Flexiflo
    F. Companion enteral feeding pump
    F. II enteral feeding pump

F. Inverta-PEG gastrostomy kit
F. Inverta-PEG tube
F. Lap J laparoscopic jejunostomy kit
F. over-the-guidewire gastrostomy kit
F. stoma-creator tube
F. Stomate low-profile gastrostomy tube
F. Top-Fill Enteral Nutrition System
F. tungsten weighted feeding tube
F. Versa-PEG tube

Flexima
F. biliary stent
F. ureteral catheter

Flexirod penile prosthesis
Flexi-Stent
Freeman pancreatic F.-S.

Flexner dysentery
flexneri
Shigella *f.*

FlexSure
F. anti-H. pylori IgG antibody
F. HP test
F. in-office rapid serology test kit
F. whole-blood test

flexura, pl. flexurae
f. coli dextra
f. coli sinistra
f. duodeni inferior
f. duodeni superior
f. duodenojejunalis
f. hepatica cell
f. lienalis coli
f. perinealis recti
f. sacralis recti

flexural rigidity
flexure
anorectal f.
colon splenic f.
duodenojejunal f.
hepatic f.
left colonic f.
perineal f.
right colonic f.
sigmoid f.
splenic f.

Flexxicon
F. Blue dialysis catheter
F. II PC internal jugular catheter

FLH
focal lymphoid hyperplasia
FL-HCC
fibrolamellar hepatocellular carcinoma
FLI
fluorescent light intensity
Flint Colon Injury Scale (FCIS)
flip-flap
Mathieu-Horton-Devine f.-f.
f.-f. procedure
f.-f. technique
flipped T wave
FLKS
fatty liver and kidney syndrome
floating
f. gallbladder
f. gallstone
f. stent
f. stool
f. table
Flocare 500 feeding pump
floccosum
Epidermophyton *f.*
flocculate
calcific f.
flocculation on barium enema
flocculus, pl. flocculi
calcific f.
Flo-Gard pump
Flolan
Flomax
Flood syndrome
floor
inguinal f.
f. of inguinal region
pelvic f.
floppy
f. Nissen fundic wrap
f. Nissen fundoplication
floppy-tipped guidewire
flora
bacterial f.
colonic f.
commensal f.
fecal f.
GI tract f.
gut f.
intestinal f.
normal f.
protective probiotic f.
proximal human colonic f.

NOTES

florid
    f. bile duct lesion
    f. polyposis
Florida
    F. pouch urinary reservoir
    F. urinary pouch
Floropryl
flosulide
flow
    azygos blood f.
    bile f. (BF)
    blood f.
    cavernous artery blood f.
    f. cytometric analysis
    f. cytometric study
    f. cytometry
    f. cytometry analysis
    f. cytometry crossmatch (FCXM)
    effective renal plasma f. (ERPF)
    estimated liver blood f. (ELBF)
    forearm blood f.
    gastric mucosal blood f.
    hepatic blood f.
    hepatofugal f.
    hepatopetal f.
    high-velocity f.
    light f.
    f. microsphere fluorescent immunoassay technique
    mucosal blood f.
    nephron plasma f.
    noninvasive assessment of urinary f.
    obstruction of bile f.
    outer cortical blood f. (OCBF)
    pancreatic blood f.
    peak f.
    plasma f.
    f. rate
    renal blood f. (RBF)
    renal plasma f. (RPF)
    splanchnic blood f.
    splenic venous blood f.
    tubular fluid f.
    turbulent f.
    urinary f.
    f. volume
flower
    passion f.
flowmeter
    Dantec rotating disk f.
    Dantec Urodyn 1000 f.
    laser Doppler f.
    Life-Tech f.
    model 500F electromagnetic f.
    Transonics laser-Doppler f.
flowprobe
    endoscopic f.
Flow-Thru feeding tube
Floxin
floxuridine
flucloxacillin
flucloxacillin-associated liver damage
flucloxacillin-induced delayed cholestatic hepatitis
fluconazole
fluctuance
fluctuant mass
fluctuation
    GB vol+ f.
    spontaneous f.
flucytosine
fludarabine phosphate
Fluhrer rectal probe
fluid
    f. absorptive capacity
    f. analysis
    ascitic tumor f. (ATF)
    BiCart dialysis f.
    bile-stained f.
    bile-tinged f.
    bloody peritoneal f.
    cerebrospinal f. (CSF)
    f. challenge
    chylous ascitic f.
    citrate replacement f.
    cloudy f.
    f. collection
    contrast f.
    crevicular f.
    cul-de-sac f.
    f. culture
    cytospin collection f.
    Dialyflex dialysis f.
    effusion f.
    Euro-Collins f.
    extracellular f. (ECF)
    fecal f.
    follicular f. (FF)
    forward motility protein of epididymal f.
    free f.
    f. intake postoperatively
    intracellular f. (ICF)
    intraglandular f.
    irrigating f.
    I.V. f.
    LDH level of ascitic f.
    LKB Optiphase 2 scintillation f.
    f. loss
    malodorous f.
    milky f.
    motor oil peritoneal f.
    Niflex PEG-based lavage f.
    nonmalodorous f.
    oviductal f.
    peripancreatic f.
    peritoneal f.

peritubular f.
f. phase marker
primary infection of ascetic f.
prune juice peritoneal f.
renal tubular f.
f. replacement therapy
f. restriction
f. resuscitation
sanguineous f.
seminal f.
f. sequestration
serosanguineous f.
f. shift
straw-colored f.
synovial f.
testicular interstitial f. (TIF)
f. transport
turbid peritoneal f.
University of Wisconsin preservation f.
f. wave

fluid-air interface
fluid-debris level
fluid-filled
f.-f. balloon
f.-f. diverticulum
f.-f. sac
f.-f. small bowel

fluidity
hepatocellular basolateral plasma membrane f.

fluidjet technology-assisted mucosal resection
fluid-phase
f.-p. endocytosis
f.-p. pinocytosis

fluid:ultrafiltrate
tubular f.:u. (TF/UF)

fluke
giant intestinal f.
liver f.

flulike syndrome
flumazenil
flumecinol
flunarizine
flunisolide
fluocinolone
fluorescein
f. dilaurate (FDL)
f. dilaurate test
f. electronic endoscopy
f. isothiocyanate (FITC)

f. isothiocyanate-conjugated antibody
f. isothiocyanate-labeled monoclonal antibody
linear f.
scattered f.
sodium f. (NaF)
f. string test
superficial f.

fluoresceinuria
fluorescence
f. angiography
f. correlation spectroscopy (FCS)
f. correlation spectroscopy magnifying light (FCS-ML)
f. excitation filter
f. fibergastroscope
f. intensity
pericentral pyridine nucleotide f.
periportal pyridine nucleotide f.
f. in situ hybridization (FISH)

fluorescence-activated
f.-a. cell sorter (FACS)
f.-a. cell sorter scan (FACScan)
f.-a. flow cytometry

fluorescent
f. antinuclear antibody (FANA)
f. detection
f. electronic endoscopy
f. gene scanning
f. image analysis
f. light intensity (FLI)
f. treponemal antibody absorption (FTA-ABS)
f. treponemal antibody absorption test

fluoride
phenyl-methane-sulfonyl f.

fluorine-18 (F-18, ^{18}F)
5-fluorocytosine
fluorodeoxyuridine (FUDR)
fluorodopan
fluorometer
continuous-flow f.

fluorometholone
fluoromethylene deoxycytidine
FluoroPlus Roadmapper
fluoroquinolone
f. seminal plasma concentration
f. therapy

fluoroscope
C-arm f.

NOTES

fluoroscopic
   f. control
   f. cystocolpoproctography
   f. guidance
   f. monitoring
fluoroscopy
   C-arm f.
   oblique f.
fluoroscopy-guided balloon dilator
Fluoro Tip ERCP cannula
Fluorotome double-lumen sphincterotome
fluorouracil
   f., Adriamycin, methotrexate with leucovorin rescue (FAMTX)
   f., Adriamycin, mitomycin C (FAMe)
   etoposide, leucovorin, 5-f. (ELF)
   f., leucovorin rescue, Adriamycin, Platinol (FLAP)
   MeCCNU, Oncovin, f. (MOF)
5-fluorouracil (5-FU)
   5-f., Adriamycin, cyclophosphamide (FAC)
   5-f., Adriamycin, mitomycin C (FAM)
   5-f., Adriamycin, Platinol (FAP)
   5-f., mitomycin C radiation (FUMIR)
fluorourodynamics
fluoxetine hydrochloride
fluoxymesterone
FLUP
   front-loading ultrasound probe
fluphenazine
flurbiprofen
flush
   carcinoid f.
   saline f.
   f. stoma
flushing
   cold f.
   f. syndrome
flush-tank sign
flutamide therapy
fluted J-Vac drain
fluvastatin
fluvialis
   Vibrio f.
fluvoxamine
flux
   bilious f.
   celiac f.
   lumen-to-bath sodium f.
   paracellular f.
   proton f.
   sodium f.
FMD
   fibromuscular dysplasia

FMF
   familial Mediterranean fever
fMLP, FMLP
   N-formyl-methionyl-leucyl-phenylalanine
     fMLP chemoattractant receptor
fMLP-stimulated O_2
fMRI
   functional magnetic resonance imaging
FMS
   fatty meal sonogram
FN
   false negative
FNA
   fine-needle aspiration
     EUS-guided FNA
FNAB
   fine-needle aspiration biopsy
FNAC
   fine-needle aspiration cytology
FNH
   focal nodular hyperplasia
FNTC, FNTHC
   fine-needle transhepatic cholangiography
foal adhesion kinase
foam
   f. cell
   Cutinova f.
   hydrocortisone f.
foamy
   f. liver
   f. stool
Fobi pouch
FOBT
   fecal occult blood test
     FOBT positive
focal
   f. accumulation of tracer
   f. bacterial nephritis
   f. biliary cirrhosis
   f. carcinoma
   f. colitis
   f. collagen synthesis
   f. colonic mucosal ulcer
   f. dimpling
   f. edema
   f. fatty infiltration
   f. fatty infiltration of liver
   f. findings
   f. hepatocellular necrosis
   f. ileus
   f. lymphoid hyperplasia (FLH)
   f. necrotizing glomerulonephritis
   f. nodular hyperplasia (FNH)
   f. nonfatty infiltration of liver
   f. pancreatitis
   f. proliferative glomerulonephritis
   f. sclerosis
   f. segmental glomerulosclerosis (FSGS)

    f. stricture
    f. tenderness
    f. tumor
focus, pl. **foci**
    aberrant crypt f. (ACF)
    dysplastic f.
    echogenic cardiac f.
    tumor f.
    f. of tumor
focused shock wave
FOE
    Fecal Odor Eliminator
Foerster
    F. abdominal ring retractor
    F. sponge forceps
Fogarty
    F. balloon
    F. balloon biliary catheter
    F. biliary probe
    F. clamp
    F. irrigation catheter
fog reduction elimination device (FRED)
folate
    f. anemia
    f. deficiency
    f. distribution
    f. malabsorption
    polyglutamate f.
    red blood cell f.
    serum f.
fold
    aryepiglottic f.
    cecal f.
    cholecystoduodenocolic f.
    costocolic f.
    crescent f.
    crural f.
    Douglas f.
    duodenal f.
    duodenojejunal f.
    duodenomesocolic f.
    epigastric f.
    flattened duodenal f.
    gastric f.
    gastropancreatic f.
    giant gastric f.
    gluteal f.
    haustral f.
    Heister f.
    Hensing f.
    hepatopancreatic f.
    ileocolic f.
    inferior duodenal f.
    inguinal f.
    interhaustral f.
    Jonnesco f.
    Kerckring f.
    left pancreaticogastric f.
    middle rectal f.
    mucosal f.
    Nélaton f.
    palatopharyngeal f.
    paraduodenal f.
    parietocolic f.
    f. pattern
    peritoneum lateral umbilical f.
    peritoneum medial f.
    peritoneum median f.
    rectal f.
    rugal f.
    semilunar-shaped f.
    sentinel f.
    sigmoid f.
    spiral f.
    superior duodenal f.
    Treves f.
    triradiate cecal f.
    vascular cecal f.
    vertical f.
folded fundus
Foley
    F. catheter
    F. criteria
    nitrofurazone F. (NF)
    F. operation
    F. Y-plasty
    F. Y-plasty pyeloplasty
    F. Y-type ureteropelvioplasty
    F. Y-V plasty
    F. Y-V pyeloplasty
    F. Y-V ureteropelvioplasty
Folgard
foliaceus
    pemphigus f.
foliate papillae
folic
    f. acid
    f. acid malabsorption
Folin
    F. filtrate
    F. gravimetric method
    F. phenol reagent
Folin-Benedict-Myers method

NOTES

Folin-Denis method
folinic acid
follicle
    ileal f.
    Lieberkühn f.
    lymphoid f.
    mucosal lymphoid f.
follicle-associated epithelium
follicle-stimulating
    f.-s. hormone (FSH)
    f.-s. hormone deficiency
    f.-s. hormone inhibin regulation
    f.-s. hormone secretion
follicular
    f. atresia
    f. cholecystitis
    f. cystitis
    f. fluid (FF)
    f. gastritis
    f. lymphoid hyperplasia
follicularis
    cystitis f.
    dyskeratosis f.
    keratosis f.
folliculitis
folliculus, pl. folliculi
    f. lymphatica
    folliculi lymphatici aggregati
    folliculi lymphatici gastrici
    folliculi lymphatici recti
    folliculi lymphatici solitarii
    folliculi lymphatici solitarii intestini crassi
    folliculi lymphatici solitarii intestini tenuis
    folliculi lymphatici splenici
follitropin alfa for injection
Follmann balanitis
follower
    filiform and f.
following bougie
followthrough
    small bowel f. (SBFT)
followup
    f. evaluation
    f. examination
    median f.
fomepizole
Fontana-Masson stain
food
    f. allergen
    f. allergy
    f. ball
    bland f.
    f. bolus
    f. bolus impaction
    f. bolus obstruction
    caffeine, alcohol, pepper, spicy f.'s (CAPS)
    f. chain
    f. challenge
    cholecystokinetic f.
    colonic f.
    compensated dysphagia for solid f.
    contamination of f.
    fatty f.
    fecal contamination of f.
    f. fever
    gas-producing f.
    Lactobacillus plantarum-fermented f.
    medical f.
    methionine-rich f.
    NutraPrep f.
    f. particle
    f. poisoning
    f. protein-induced enterocolitis syndrome (FPIES)
    f. residue
    sieving of solid f.
    solid f.
    f. supplement
food-borne illness (FBI)
FoodSCAN food allergy test
food-sensitive enteropathy
foot
    f. pedal suction control
    f. process (FP)
footprint
foramen, pl. foramina
    f. of Bochdalek
    f. of Bochdalek hernia
    Duverney f.
    f. electrode
    epiploic f.
    f. epiploicum
    greater sciatic f.
    f. of Morgagni
    omental f.
    f. omentale
    pleuroperitoneal f.
    f. of Winslow
Forbes disease
force
    isometric f.
forced
    f. alimentation
    f. feeding
forceps
    ACMI Martin endoscopy f.
    Adair-Allis f.
    Adson-Brown tissue f.
    Adson tissue f.
    Allen intestinal f.
    alligator jaws Olympus FG 6L grasping f.
    alligator-type grasping f.
    Allis f.
    angled dissecting f.

atraumatic locking/grasping f.
Babcock intestinal f.
Backhaus towel f.
Bainbridge intestinal f.
Ballenger f.
Bard Precisor direct bite f.
Barrett intestinal f.
Barrett-Murphy intestinal thumb f.
basket f.
basket-type crushing f.
bayonet-type f.
Beardsley intestinal f.
Beasley-Babcock f.
Beck aorta f.
Beebe hemostatic f.
Behrend cystic duct f.
Best gallstone f.
Bevan gallbladder f.
Billroth f.
biopsy f.
bipolar coagulating f.
bite biopsy f.
Blake gallstone f.
Blalock pulmonary artery f.
Blanchard hemorrhoid f.
bowel f.
Bozeman f.
Bridge deep surgery f.
Brunner intestinal f.
Brunner tissue f.
Buie biopsy f.
Buie pile f.
bulldog f.
Carmalt f.
Child intestinal f.
Children's Hospital intestinal f.
claw f.
coagulating f.
coated biopsy f.
cold biopsy f.
Collin-Duval intestinal thumb f.
Collin intestinal f.
Collin tissue f.
Collin tongue f.
Crile bile duct f.
Crile gall duct f.
curved dissecting f.
curved Maryland f.
Cushing f.
DeBakey f.
DeMartel appendix f.
Dennis intestinal f.

Desjardins gallbladder f.
Desjardins gallstone f.
disposable f.
dolphin grasping f.
dolphin-type atraumatic f.
double-spoon f.
Doyen gallbladder f.
Doyen intestinal f.
dressing f.
duck-bill f.
Duracep biopsy f.
Eastman cystic duct f.
electrocoagulating biopsy f.
Elliott gallbladder f.
Endo-Assist disposable atraumatic grasping f.
endoscopic alligator f.
endoscopic biopsy f.
endoscopic grasping f.
endoscopic suture-cutting f.
Everett pile f.
Excel disposable biopsy f.
FB-25K jumbo biopsy f.
fenestrated cup biopsy f.
fenestrated ellipsoid spiked open-span biopsy f.
fenestrated spiked open-span jumbo biopsy f.
Ferguson tenaculum f.
fine tissue f.
fine-toothed f.
FK-13K-1 jumbo biopsy f.
Foerster sponge f.
foreign body retrieving f.
Foss intestinal clamp f.
Fujinon biopsy f.
gallstone f.
Gavin-Miller intestinal f.
Gemini gall duct f.
Gerald f.
Gilbert cystic duct f.
Glassman-Allis intestinal f.
Glenn diverticulum f.
Gold deep surgery f.
grasping f.
grasp tripod f.
Gray cystic duct f.
Green cystic duct f.
Haberer intestinal f.
Halsted f.
Hamilton deep surgery f.
Harrington f.

NOTES

forceps *(continued)*
Hasson bullet-tip f.
Hasson needle-nose f.
Hasson ring f.
Hasson spike-tooth f.
Healy intestinal f.
high-frequency hemostatic f.
hook f.
hot biopsy f.
hot flexible f.
Jarvis hemorrhoid f.
jeweler's f.
Johns Hopkins gallbladder f.
Judd-Allis intestinal f.
Judd-DeMartel gallbladder f.
Julian splenorenal f.
jumbo biopsy f.
Keen Edge disposable biopsy f.
Kelly f.
Kelly-Murphy f.
Kent deep surgery f.
Kleppinger f.
Kocher f.
Koerte gallstone f.
Lahey-Babcock f.
Lahey gall duct f.
Lalonde hook f.
lancet-shaped biopsy f.
Lane intestinal f.
Laplace f.
Lawrence deep surgery f.
Leonard deep surgery f.
Lillie intestinal f.
Lockwood-Allis intestinal f.
long-jaw disposable f.
loop-type snare f.
loop-type stone-crushing f.
Lovelace f.
Lower gall duct f.
Luer hemorrhoid f.
Maxum reusable f.
Mayo-Blake gallstone f.
Mayo-Péan f.
Mayo-Robson intestinal f.
Mazzariello-Caprini f.
McGill f.
McGivney hemorrhoid f.
McNealey-Glassman-Mixter f.
Medicon-Jackson rectal f.
Michigan intestinal f.
Microvasive disposable alligator-shaped f.
Microvasive radial-jaw 3 biopsy f.
Microvasive radial-jaw 1597-20 large-capacity biopsy f.
Microvasive radial-jaw 31263-20 large-capacity biopsy f.
Mikulicz peritoneal f.
Miller rectal f.
Millin f.
Mill-Rose RiteBite biopsy f.
Mixter gallstone f.
mosquito f.
Moynihan artery f.
Moynihan gall duct f.
Muir hemorrhoid f.
Multibite biopsy f.
Nelson f.
Nissen gall duct f.
no-scalpel vasectomy fixator ring clamp f.
Nussbaum intestinal f.
Ochsner f.
O'Hara f.
Olympus alligator-jaw endoscopic f.
Olympus basket-type endoscopic f.
Olympus Endo-Therapy disposable biopsy f.
Olympus FB-20C endoscopic f.
Olympus FBK-13 f.
Olympus FB-25K endoscopic f.
Olympus FB-24U biopsy f.
Olympus FG-12U wide-mouth f.
Olympus FK-13-1 biopsy f.
Olympus FS-K-series endoscopic suture-cutting f.
Olympus grasping rat-tooth f.
Olympus hot biopsy f.
Olympus magnetic extractor f.
Olympus minisnare f.
Olympus pelican-type endoscopic f.
Olympus rat-tooth endoscopic f.
Olympus reusable oval-cup f.
Olympus rubber-tip endoscopic f.
Olympus shark-tooth endoscopic f.
Olympus tripod-type endoscopic f.
Olympus W-shaped endoscopic f.
Ombrédanne f.
Orr gall duct f.
packing f.
Payr pyloric f.
Péan f.
pelican biopsy f.
Pennington f.
Percy intestinal f.
perforating f.
pinch f.
Porter duodenal f.
Positrap three-prong nonretracting grasping f.
Potts f.
Potts-Smith f.
Precisor Direct Bite biopsy f.
Precisor disposable biopsy f.
Quire mechanical finger f.
Radial Jaw bladder biopsy f.
Radial Jaw hot biopsy f.

Radial Jaw III Max Capacity 1589 biopsy f.
Radial Jaw III Max Capacity with needle biopsy f.
Radial Jaw III single-use biopsy f.
Rampley sponge-holding f.
Randall stone f.
Ratliff-Blake gallstone f.
Ratliff-Mayo f.
rat-tooth Olympus FG 8L grasping f.
Reich-Nechtow f.
f. removal
ring f.
RiteBite biopsy f.
Robbers f.
Robson intestinal f.
Rochester-Carmalt f.
Rochester gallstone f.
Rochester-Mixter f.
Rochester-Ochsner f.
Rochester-Péan f.
Rudd Clinic hemorrhoidal f.
Russian tissue f.
Schindler peritoneal f.
Schnidt gall duct f.
Schnidt thoracic f.
Schoenberg intestinal f.
Scudder intestinal f.
Seitzinger tripolar cutting f.
Semken tissue f.
Shark disposable biopsy f.
shark-tooth f.
Singley intestinal f.
smooth tissue f.
spiral gallstone f.
sponge f.
sponge-holding f.
spoon f.
Steinmann intestinal f.
Stille-Barraya intestinal f.
Stille gallstone f.
stone-grasping f.
stone-holding basket f.
straight Maryland f.
SureBite biopsy f.
Therma Jaw disposable hot biopsy f.
Therma Jaw hot urologic f.
Thorek gallbladder f.
Thorek-Mixter gallbladder f.
three-armed basket f.

three-pronged grasping f.
tissue f.
tonsil f.
toothed tissue f.
traumatic grasping f.
tripod grasping f.
Troutman rectus f.
Turner-Warwick stone f.
Turrell-Wittner rectal f.
Varco gallbladder f.
Westphal gall duct f.
Williams intestinal f.
W-shaped f.
Yeoman rectal biopsy f.
Yeoman-Wittner rectal f.
Young intestinal f.

forcible feeding
Forder retractor
Fordyce
    angiokeratoma of F.
    F. granule
    F. spot
forearm
    f. blood flow
    f. flap
    f. graft arteriovenous fistula
Foregger rigid esophagoscope
foregut
foreign
    f. body
    f. body appendicitis
    f. body extraction
    f. body ingestion
    f. body management
    f. body reaction
    f. body removal
    f. body retrieving forceps
    f. body sensation
    f. body trauma
    f. object
foreshortening of colon
foreskin
    f. flap
    f. manual retraction
    f. restoration
Forest I, II lesion
forestomach
forgotten stent
fork
    stimulation f.
forked crypt

NOTES

form
- band f.
- trophozoite f.
- wave f.
- wax-matrix slow-release f.
- WBC immature f.'s

Formad kidney

formaldehyde
- gelatin resorcinol and f. (GRF)
- f. solution

formalin
- buffered f.
- intravesical f.

formalin-fixed tissue

formamide
- deionized f.

formate

formation
- abscess f.
- adhesion f.
- bacterial biofilm f.
- beta-pleated sheet f.
- bile acid-independent bile f. (BAIBF)
- biofilm f.
- bone f.
- branching tubule f.
- calculous f.
- enamel pellicle f.
- erythroid colony f.
- extracapillary crescent f.
- false channel f.
- fistula f.
- gallstone f.
- germinal center f.
- Gothic arch f.
- idiopathic calcium (renal) stone f. (ICSF)
- indicator of reactive oxygen species f.
- kerion f.
- median bar f.
- micelle f.
- nurse cell f.
- physicochemical basis of gallstone f.
- prostanoid f.
- prosthesis-related seroma f.
- pseudoaneurysm f.
- recurrent calcium stone f.
- renal stone f.
- scar tissue f.
- stone granuloma f.
- struvite crystal f.
- ultimate fistula f.

formatio reticularis

forme
- f. fruste
- f. tardive

formed
- angle f.
- f. stool

former
- calcium oxalate stone f.
- pouch f.
- stone f.

formigenes
- *Oxalobacter f.*

formin

formononetin

formula, pl. **formulas, formulae**
- Advance f.
- Attain tube feeding f.
- Callaway f.
- Cockcroft-Gault f.
- F. EM oral suspension
- Encare tube feeding f.
- Enfamil LIPIL f.
- Enfamil with iron f.
- Ensure HIN tube feeding f.
- Ensure Plus f.
- Entralife HN tube feeding f.
- Entri-Pak tube feeding f.
- Entrition tube feeding f.
- Formula 2 tube feeding f.
- heartburn relief f. (HRF)
- hydrolyzed whey f.
- Isomil SF f.
- I-Soyalac f.
- Jevity tube feeding f.
- Lofenalac f.
- Lonalac f.
- Natural stool f.
- Nursoy f.
- Nutramigen f.
- Portagen f.
- predigested protein f.
- Pregestimil f.
- ProSobee liquid f.
- RCF f.
- Reabilan HN tube feeding f.
- Similac PM 60/40 low-iron f.
- SMA f.
- Soyalac f.
- soy-based f.
- Van Slyke f.
- Vitaneed tube feeding f.

Formulex

formyl peptide receptor

fornication
- fist f.

fornix, pl. **fornices**
- caliceal f.
- gastric f.

Foroblique
- F. fiberoptic esophagoscope
- F. lens
- F. resectoscope

Forrest
    F. classification
    F. classification of gastroduodenal ulcer
    F. criteria
Forssell sinus
FortaPerm surgical sling
Fortaz
Forte
    Pamine F.
    Robinul F.
fortii
    Dinophysis f.
Fortison enteral feeding
fortuitum
    Mycobacterium f.
Fortuna syringe
Fortunoff flap
forward motility protein of epididymal fluid
forward-viewing
    f.-v. endoscope
    f.-v. position
    f.-v. telescope
    f.-v. videocolonoscope
foscarnet
    f. therapy
    f. treatment
fosfomycin tromethamine
fosinopril
Fosrenol
Foss
    F. anterior resection clamp
    F. bifid gallbladder retractor
    F. biliary duct retractor
    F. intestinal clamp
    F. intestinal clamp forceps
fossa, pl. **fossae**
    Biesiadecki f.
    Broesike f.
    f. caecalis
    crural f.
    f. cystidis felleae
    duodenal f.
    duodenojejunal f.
    epigastric f.
    Gruber-Landzert f.
    Hartmann f.
    hypochondriac f.
    iliac f.
    inferior digital f.
    intrabulbar f.
    ischiorectal f.
    Jonnesco f.
    Landzert f.
    lateral f.
    f. of male urethra
    f. of Morgagni
    f. navicularis
    f. navicularis urethrae
    f. ovalis
    paravesical f.
    piriform f.
    prostatic f.
    rectal f.
    retrocolic f.
    f. subinguinalis
    subsigmoid f.
    Treitz f.
    f. vesicae biliaris
fotemustine
Fothergill sign
Fouchet test
foul-smelling
    f.-s. odor
    f.-s. stool
foundation
    American Digestive Health F. (ADHF)
    American Liver F. (ALF)
four
    f. lines sign
    f. phases of swallowing
four-antigen matched donor
four-glass test
Fourier
    F. transform analysis
    F. transform infrared spectroscopy (FTIR)
four-lumen
    f.-l. polyvinyl manometric catheter
    f.-l. tube
Fournier
    F. disease
    F. gangrene
    F. sign
    F. syphiloma
four-port diamond placement
four-pronged polyp grasper
four-quadrant
    f.-q. incision
    f.-q. jumbo biopsy
    f.-q. tattooing
four-wing Malecot drain

NOTES

fovea
    Morgagni f.
foveola, pl. **foveolae**
    gastric f.
    foveolae gastricae
foveola-gland ratio
foveolar
    f. gastric mucosa
    f. hyperplasia
foveolate
Fowler position
Fowler-Stephens
    F.-S. maneuver
    F.-S. orchiopexy
    F.-S. procedure
    F.-S. test
Foxy Pouch cover
FP
    false positive
    foot process
FPC
    familial polyposis coli
FPIES
    food protein-induced enterocolitis syndrome
FPM
    first-pass metabolism
FPP
    familial paroxysmal polyserositis
fPSA
    free PSA
fraction
    alpha-gliadin f.
    anionic IgG 4 f.
    cortical interstitial volume f.
    filtered f.
    filtration f.
    gallbladder ejection f. (GBEF)
    globulin f.
    mesangial volume f.
    micronized flavonidic f.
    nonnuclear f.
    non-T-cell f.
    nuclear f.
    packing f.
    plasma protein f.
    recombination f.
fractional
    f. clearance
    f. excretion of lithium (FELI)
    f. excretion of potassium (FEFEK)
    f. excretion of sodium (FENa)
    f. percentage of inspired oxygen (FIO_2)
    f. proximal reabsorption
    f. weight change
fractionated
    f. diet
    f. voiding

fractionation of bilirubin
fracture
    micronized purified flavonoid f. (MPFF)
    pelvis f.
    penis f.
    trabecular bone f.
fragilis
    Bacteroides f.
    Dientamoeba f.
fragment
    anucleate f.
    autotransplantation of splenic f.
    endoscopic removal of f.
    N-terminal f.
    nuclear f.
    residual f.
fragmentary defecation
fragmentation
    complete stone f.
    laser-induced f.
    stone f.
    ultrasonic f.
Fragmin
Fraley
    F. sign
    F. syndrome
frame
    nitinol mesh-covered f.
    Stryker f.
frameshift
Framingham risk-factor approach
Francis test
Franco operation
frank
    f. blood
    f. blood in stool
    f. cirrhosis
    f. pus
Frankel
    crossbar symptom of F.
Frankfeldt rectal snare
Franklin-Silverman biopsy cannula
Franseen needle
Franz abdominal retractor
Fraser syndrome
Frazier
    F. suction tip
    F. suction tube
FreAmine amino acid solution
FRED
    fog reduction elimination device
FREDDY Nd:YAG laser
Frederick-Miller tube
frederiksenii
    Yersinia f.
Fredet-Ramstedt
    F.-R. operation
    F.-R. pyloromyotomy

Fredrickson classification
free
 f. acetate
 f. air
 f. band of colon
 f. fatty acid
 f. fecal bile acid
 f. fluid
 f. hepatic venous pressure (FHVP)
 f. jejunal graft
 f. prostate-specific antigen
 f. PSA (fPSA)
 f. radical
 f. radical scavenger
 f. reflux
 f. resection
 f. ribosome
 Ross carbohydrate f. (RCF)
 f. subphrenic gas
 f. testosterone
 f. thyroxine (FT4)
 f. tie
free-beam
 f.-b. coagulation
 f.-b. laser system
Freedom
 F. Clear long-seal male external catheter line
 F. Clear LS male external catheter line
 F. Clear sport-sheath male external catheter line
 F. Clear SS male external catheter line
free-floating testis
free-GEPA graft
freehand
 f. biopsy
 f. cannulation
freeing up of adhesion
Freeman pancreatic Flexi-Stent
Freer elevator
freestanding ambulatory surgical center
free-to-total
 free-to-total prostate-specific antigen (FTPSA, F:T PSA)
 f.-t.-t. PSA
 f.-t.-t. PSA ratio
freezing
 gastric f.
Freiburg biopsy set
fremitus

frena (*pl. of* frenum)
frenal
French
 F. bougie
 F. Cope loop nephrostomy catheter
 F. cystoscope
 F. dilator
 F. double-J ureteral stent
 F. eye needle
 F. introducer set
 F. mushroom-tip catheter
 F. Pharmacovigilance system
 F. pigtail nephrostomy catheter
 F. scale
 F. Swan-Ganz balloon
 F. Teflon pyeloureteral catheter
 F. T tube
frenectomy
frenoplasty
Frenta
 F. Mat feeding pump
 F. System II feeding pump
frenulum, pl. frenula
 f. of duodenal papilla
 f. of ileocolic valve
 f. of prepuce of penis
 f. preputii penis
 f. valvae ilealis
 f. valvae ileocaecalis
frenum, pl. frena
 f. of Morgagni
 f. of valve of colon
frequency
 fecal f. (FF)
 operating f.
 pulse repetition f. (PRF)
 f. of stool
 urinary f.
frequency-doubled-double pulse ND:YAG laser
frequency-duration index (FDI)
frequency-urgency-pain syndrome
frequent
 f. hemodialysis
 f. joint manifestation
Fresenius
 F. AG dialyzer
 F. F-40 filter
 F. 2008H hemodialysis machine
 F. volumetric dialysate balancing system

NOTES

fresh
   f. clot
   f. frozen plasma (FFP)
Freter theory
Freund adjuvant
freundii
   Citrobacter f.
Frey
   F. gastric pit
   F. hair
Freyer operation
friability
   cervical f.
friable mucosa
friction
   f. knot
   f. rub
friction-fit adapter
Friderichsen-Waterhouse syndrome
Friedländer bacillus
Friedman perineal retractor
Frimberger-Karpiel 12 o'clock papillotome
Fritsch retractor
Froehlich (*var. of* Fröhlich)
frogleg position
frog-spawnlike mucosa
Fröhlich, Froehlich
   F. syndrome
frondlike filling defect
frontal tenderness
front-loading ultrasound probe (FLUP)
Frostberg reversed-3 sign
frothy
frozen section
fructose
   f. aldolase
   f. aldolase deficiency
   f. diarrhea
   f. diphosphatase deficiency
   f. intolerance
   seminal plasma f.
fructose-1,6-bisphosphatase
fructose-free diet
fruity odor
fruste
   forme f.
Frykman-Goldberg
   F.-G. operation for rectal prolapse
   F.-G. procedure
FSA
   fetal sulfoglycoprotein antigen
FSGS
   focal segmental glomerulosclerosis
   collapsing FSGS
FSH
   follicle-stimulating hormone
FSP
   fibrin split product

FSSE
   fat-suppressed spin-echo
FT4
   free thyroxine
FTA-ABS
   fluorescent treponemal antibody absorption
   FTA-ABS test
FTIR
   Fourier transform infrared spectroscopy
FTLE
   full-thickness local excision
FTPSA, F:T PSA
   free-to-total prostate-specific antigen
5-FU
   5-fluorouracil
fucosidosis
fucosylation index of alpha fetoprotein
fucosyltransferase gene
FUDR
   fluorodeoxyuridine
fugax
   proctalgia f.
Fujinon
   F. biopsy forceps
   F. CEG-FP-series videoelectroscope
   F. DUO-XT duodenoscope
   F. EB-410S bronchoscope
   F. EC7-CM2 videocolonoscope
   F. EC-130LT colonoscope
   F. EC-200LT colonoscope
   F. EC-410MP colonoscope
   F. EC-300MS colonoscope
   F. ED7-XT duodenoscope
   F. ED-200XU duodenoscope
   F. ED-310XU duodenoscope
   F. ED-410XU duodenoscope
   F. ED7-XU2 videoduodenoscope
   F. EG-310D gastroscope
   F. EG-200FP gastroscope
   F. EG-FP-series endoscope
   F. EG-410HR gastroscope
   F. ES-200ER sigmoidoscope
   F. EVC-M videocolonoscope
   F. EVD-XL videoduodenoscope
   F. EVD-XT duodenoscope
   F. EVE-series endoscope
   F. EVG-CT endoscope
   F. EVG-FP-series endoscope
   F. EVG-F-series endoscope
   F. FD-100XU duodenoscope
   F. FE-100LR colonoscope
   F. FG-series endoscopic camera
   F. FP-series endoscope
   F. FS-100ER sigmoidoscope
   F. GF-100PE gastroscope
   F. PRO-PC flexible fiberoptic sigmoidoscope

F. 400-series super image videogastroscope
F. SIG-E2 fiberoptic sigmoidoscope
F. SIG-EK-series flexible fiberoptic sigmoidoscope
F. SIG-E-series flexible fiberoptic sigmoidoscope
F. SIG-ET-series flexible fiberoptic sigmoidoscope
F. SP-501 sonoprobe system
F. UGI-FP-series videoendoscope
F. videoendoscopy cart
F. videoendoscopy system
F. 310XU videoduodenoscope

FUL
functional urethral length

fulguration
diverticulum f.
electrosurgical f.
endoscopic f.

full
f. extension
f. liquid diet
f. liquids (FL)
f. Monti procedure
f. Monti technique
f. range of motion

full-bladder technique
full-column barium enema
Fuller
F. operation
F. rectal shield

full-length viral genome
full-lumen esophagoscope
fullness
abdominal f.
adnexal f.
postprandial f.
pyloric f.

full-surface micromesh teeth
full-thickness
f.-t. biopsy
f.-t. graft
f.-t. local excision (FTLE)

fulminant
f. Crohn disease
f. dysentery
f. hepatic failure (FHF)
f. hepatitis A–E
f. hepatocellular failure
f. liver failure

f. toxic colitis
f. viral hepatitis (FVH)

fulminating
f. appendicitis
f. dysentery
f. pancreatitis
f. ulcerative colitis

fumagillin
fumarylacetoacetate hydrolase deficiency
fumigatus
Aspergillus f.

FUMIR
5-fluorouracil, mitomycin C radiation

function
anal sphincter f.
bladder neck sphincteric f.
bladder storage f.
bowel f.
cardiopulmonary baroreflex f.
Carnot f.
cineloop memory f.
cognitive f.
delayed graft f. (DGF)
deterioration of graft f.
discriminant f. (DF)
excretory f.
exocrine f.
gallbladder f.
gastrin cell f.
graft f.
impaired colonic motor f.
International Index of Erectile F. (IIEF)
kidney f.
Leydig cell secretory f.
Maddrey discriminant f.
native kidney f.
neoanal f.
organ f.
P450 f.
pharyngoesophageal f.
preoperative f.
proximal tubule f.
PTEN suppressor gene f.
puborectalis muscle f.
pudendal nerve f.
rectoanal f.
rectosigmoid f.
renal f.
Sertoli cell secretory f.
sexual f.
sieving f.

NOTES

function (continued)
    sphincter f.
    splenic f.
    split renal f.

functional
    f. bladder capacity
    f. bleeding
    f. bowel disease
    f. bowel disorder (FBD)
    F. Bowel Disorder Severity Index (FBDSI)
    f. bowel distress (FBD)
    f. bowel syndrome
    f. castration
    f. constipation
    f. cystic duct obstruction
    f. diarrhea
    f. disorder stomach
    f. dyspepsia
    f. gastrointestinal disorder (FGID)
    f. hepatic volume
    f. impotence
    f. incontinence
    f. magnetic resonance imaging (fMRI)
    f. pain
    f. plasminogen
    f. profile length
    f. reconstruction
    f. trauma
    f. urethral length (FUL)

fundal
    f. gastritis
    f. plication
    f. pouch
    f. varix

fundectomy
fundi (*pl. of* fundus)
fundic
    f. atrophic gastritis (FAG)
    f. biopsy
    f. clot
    f. gland atrophy
    f. gland gastritis
    f. gland heterotopia
    f. gland polyp
    f. mucosa
    f. plexus
    f. varix

fundic-antral junction
fundiform ligament
fundoplasty
    Gomez f.
    Thal f.

fundoplication
    anatomically correct f.
    Belsey 270-degree f.
    Belsey Mark IV 240-degree f.
    Belsey partial f.
    Belsey two-thirds wrap f.
    circumferential f.
    Collis-Nissen f.
    Dor f.
    floppy Nissen f.
    Hill esophageal f.
    intrathoracic Nissen f.
    laparoscopic Nissen and Toupet f.
    Nissen 360-degree wrap f.
    Nissen laparoscopic f.
    partial f.
    Rossetti modification of Nissen f.
    slipped Nissen f.
    supraphysiological f.
    Toupet partial posterior f.

fundopyloric mucosal border
fundus, pl. **fundi**
    bald gastric f.
    folded f.
    gallbladder f.
    gastric f.
    f. gastricus
    f. rotation gastroplasty
    f. of stomach
    f. ventricularis
    f. ventriculi
    f. vesicae biliaris
    f. vesicae felleae
    f. vesicae urinariae

fundusectomy
fungal
    f. ball
    f. bezoar
    f. infection
    f. liver abscess
    f. peritonitis
    f. pyelonephritis
    f. spore

fungating growth
fungemia
fungi (*pl. of* fungus)
Fungi-Fluor
    F.-F. chitin stain
    F.-F. procedure

fungiform papilla
Fungizone
fungoides
    mycosis f.

fungosa
    gastrosia f.

funguria
fungus, pl. **fungi**
    ovoid f.
    f. testis

funicular
    f. hydrocele
    f. inguinal hernia
    f. stump

funiculi (*pl. of* funiculus)

funiculitis
funiculoepididymitis
    filarial f.
funiculopexy
funiculus, pl. **funiculi**
    hepatic f.
    f. spermaticus
funis
funisitis
funnel
    stent f.
funnel-neck prostate
Furacin
Furadantin
fura-2 pentapotassium salt
furazolidone
Furlow
    F. cylinder inserter
    F. introducer
Furlow-Fisher modification of Virag 1 operation
Furniss
    F. anastomosis clamp
    F. ureterointestinal anastomosis
Furniss-Clute duodenal clamp
furnissii
    Vibrio f.
furor medicus
furosemide washout renogram
Furoxone
furrier suture
furrow
    Liebermeister f.

furuncle
furunculosis
Fusarium solani
fused kidney
fusible calculus
fusiform
    f. renal artery aneurysm
    f. widening of duct
fusion
    f. fascia
    splenogonadal f.
    tissue f.
    urethrohymenal f.
    viral membrane f.
Fusobacterium
Futura resectoscope sheath
future
    f. role of target of rapamycin inhibitors in renal transplantation
    f. of stent
F value
FVH
    fulminant viral hepatitis
FVL
    flexible videolaparoscope
FVM
    familial visceral myopathy
FVN
    familial visceral neuropathy
Fx1A antibody
fyn protein

NOTES

G

G protein
G protein disease
G syndrome
gabapentin
gabexate mesylate
Gabriel proctoscope
gadolinium
    g. chelate
    g. EOB-DTPA (Gd-EOB-DTPA)
gadolinium-enhancement magnetic resonance
Gadolite oral suspension
GAG
    glycosaminoglycan
gag
    Millard mouth g.
    mouth g.
    g. reflex
    g. response
GAGUA
    glycosaminoglycans uronate
gain
    interdialytic weight g. (IDWG)
    symptomatic fluid g.
    weight g.
gait
    broad-based g.
    g. disturbance
    favored g.
    parkinsonian g.
    spastic g.
    steppage g.
    Trendelenburg g.
    unsteady g.
galactitol
galactodes
Galacto-Light assay
galactoma
galactopexy
galactose-1-phosphate uridyltransferase
galactose elimination capacity (GEC)
galactose-free diet
galactosemia
    Indiana variant g.
    Rennes variant g.
galactosidase
    beta g.
galactosyltransferase isoenzyme II
galacturia
galanin antiserum
Galant reflex
Galeati gland
galeni
    porus g.

galenic preparation
GALF
    glycyrrhetinic acidlike factor
gall
    g. duct
    g. duct spoon
gallamine
gallbladder (GB)
    adenomyoma of g.
    g. adenomyomatosis
    g. bag positioner
    g. bed
    bilobed g.
    g. calculus
    g. carcinoma
    cholesterolosis of g.
    chronically inflamed g.
    g. contraction
    Courvoisier g.
    dilated g.
    g. displacement
    g. dome
    double g.
    duplicated g.
    g. dysmotility
    edematous g.
    g. ejection fraction (GBEF)
    g. ejection rate (GBER)
    g. emptying-refilling curve
    empyema of g.
    endoscopic transpapillary catheterization of g. (ETCG)
    g. filling
    fish-scale g.
    floating g.
    g. function
    g. function test
    g. fundus
    gangrene of g.
    hourglass constriction of g.
    g. hydrops
    g. ileus
    inflamed g.
    infundibulum of g.
    g. lift
    mobile g.
    mucocele of g.
    multiseptate g.
    nonfunctioning g.
    nonvisualization of g.
    notch of g.
    palpable g.
    perforation of g.
    porcelain g.
    robin's egg-blue g.

gallbladder *(continued)*
   g. scan
   g. scoop
   g. series (GBS)
   g. sludge
   g. stasis
   stasis g.
   g. stone
   strawberry g.
   thick-walled g.
   thin-walled g.
   g. torsion
   torsion of g.
   trauma of g.
   g. trauma
   g. trocar
   g. varix
   g. volume
   g. wall
   g. wall abscess
   wandering g.
Gallie transplant
gallinaginis
   caput g.
gallium
   g. imaging
   g. nitrate
   g. scan
gallium-67
gallop rhythm
Galloway-Mowat syndrome (GMS)
gallows-type retractor
gallstone
   asymptomatic g.
   bilirubin pigment g.
   black pigment g.
   brown pigment g.
   calcified g.
   cholesterol-containing g.
   g. colic
   dissolution of g.
   faceted g.
   floating g.
   g. forceps
   g. formation
   g. ileus
   g. incidence
   innocent g.
   intragastric g.
   g. migration
   mixed-cholesterol g.
   mulberry g.
   g. pancreatitis
   g. pattern
   pigmented g.
   g. probe
   radiolucent g.
   retained g.
   silent g.
   symptomatic g.
   unextractable g.
gallstone-solubilizing agent
Gal 4 protein
GALT
   gastrointestinal-associated lymphoid tissue
   gut-associated lymphoepithelial tissue
   gut-associated lymphoid tissue
galvanic probe
Gambee
   G. anastomosis
   G. stitch
   G. suture
Gambian sleeping sickness
Gambro
   G. AK10 machine
   G. dialyzer
   G. FH88H filter
   G. Lundia Minor artificial kidney
gamete
   g. intrafallopian transfer (GIFT)
   g. micromanipulation
gametic
gametocidal
gametocide
gametocyst
gamma
   g. emission
   g. fetoprotein
   g. globulin
   g. globulin therapy
   g. heavy chain disease
   g. interferon
   g. light chain
   nucleocapsid antigen-stimulated interferon g.
   g. scintillation camera
   g. seminoprotein
   g. split-sling wrap
   g. transverse colon loop
gamma-aminobutyric
   g.-a. acid
   g.-a. acid accumulation
   g.-a. acidergic neuron
gammaglobulin
   antithymocyte g. (ATGAM)
gamma-glutamyltransferase (GGT)
   serum g.-g.
gamma-glutamyltransferase level
gamma-glutamyl transpeptidase (GGTP)
gamma-lyase
   cystathionine g.-l.
Gammatone II gamma camera
gammopathy
   monoclonal g.
Gamna
   G. disease
   G. nodule

Ganau criteria
ganciclovir
Gandy-Gamna nodule
ganglial
ganglion, pl. **ganglia**
    basal ganglia
    celiac-superior mesenteric ganglia
    g. cell loss
    dorsal root g.
    enteric g.
    intramural g.
    nodose g.
    subserous g.
    Troisier g.
ganglionated plexus
ganglioneuroblastoma
ganglioneuroma
    adrenal cortex g.
ganglioneuromatosis
ganglion-free muscle strip
ganglioside
    GM3 g.
gangraenosa
    balanitis g.
gangrene
    cecal g.
    Fournier g.
    g. of gallbladder
    gas g.
    ischemic penile g.
gangrenosum
    ecthyma g.
    pyoderma g. (PG)
gangrenous
    g. appendicitis
    g. appendix
    g. balanitis
    g. bowel
    g. cholecystitis
    g. colon
    g. cystitis
    g. ischemic colitis
    g. ischemic enterocolitis
    g. necrosis
GAN-19 needle
Gans
    incisura dextra of G.
Ganser diverticulum
Gantanol
    Azo G.
Gant clamp

Gantrisin
    Azo G.
gantry
GAP
    glans approximation procedure
    GAP test
gap
    anion g.
    glottic g.
    g. junction
    osmolarity g.
    stool osmotic g.
    underwater spark g.
    urinary anion g.
GAPD
    glyceraldehyde phosphate dehydrogenase
GAPDH
    glyceraldehyde phosphate dehydrogenase
    glyceraldehyde-3-phosphate dehydrogenase
Garamycin
garbled speech
GARD
    gastroesophageal antireflux device
Garden prognostic system
Gardner-Diamond syndrome
Gardnerella vaginalis
Gardner syndrome (GS)
gargle
    viscous Xylocaine g.
garnet
    holmium:yttrium aluminum g. (Ho:YAG)
Garren
    G. balloon
    G. gastric bubble
Garren-Edwards
    G.-E. balloon
    G.-E. gastric (GEG)
    G.-E. gastric bubble
Garrett dilator
Gartner
    G. duct
    G. duct cyst
gas
    g. abscess
    arterial blood g. (ABG)
    bowel g.
    g. chromatography
    g. chromatography/mass spectroscopy (GC/MS)
    colonic g.

NOTES

gas *(continued)*
    g. cupula
    g. cyst
    g. cystometry
    g. density line
    ethylene oxide g. (ETO)
    free subphrenic g.
    g. gangrene
    hydrogen g.
    g. isotope ratio mass spectrometry
    g. pattern
    g. sterilization
    g. thermometer
GaSampler collection system
GasBGon filter seat cushion
gas-bloat syndrome
gaseous
    g. cholecystitis
    g. distention
    g. pericholecystitis
gas-forming
    g.-f. liver abscess
    g.-f. organism in bowel wall
    g.-f. pyogenic liver infection
gasket
    United Surgical Seal-Tite g.
gasless
    g. laparoscopic approach
    g. laparoscopy
GASP
    gastric augment and single-pedicle tube
gas-producing food
gasserian syndrome
Gasser syndrome
gassiness
gassy
gaster
gastradenitis, gastroadenitis
gastralgia
gastrectasis, gastrectasia
gastrectomized patient
gastrectomy
    antecolic g.
    Billroth I, II g.
    completion g.
    distal g.
    esophagoproximal g.
    high subtotal g.
    Horsley g.
    partial g.
    physiologic g.
    Pólya g.
    proximal g.
    subtotal g.
    total g.
gastric
    g. accommodation test
    g. achlorhydria
    g. acid

g. acidity
g. acidity reduction
g. acid pump inhibitor
g. acid rebound
g. acid secretion
g. actinomycosis
g. adenocarcinoma
g. adenoma
g. adenopapillomatosis
g. air bubble
g. analysis
g. aneurysm
g. angiodysplasia
g. angioma
g. angiomyolipoma
g. anisakiasis
g. anoxia
g. antral erosion
g. antral sessile polyp
g. antral vascular ectasia (GAVE)
g. antrum
g. arteriography
g. arteriovenous malformation
g. artery
g. aspirate
g. aspiration
g. aspiration tube
g. atony
g. atresia
g. augment and single-pedicle tube (GASP)
g. bacterial overgrowth (GBO)
g. balloon
g. balloon implantation
g. bezoar
g. bladder
g. bladder replacement
g. bleeding time (GBT)
g. brush cytology
g. bypass (GBP)
g. bypass surgery
g. calculus
g. cancer
g. capacity
g. carcinoid
g. carcinoid tumor
g. carcinoma
g. carcinosarcoma
g. cardia
g. carditis
g. cell kinetics
g. channel
g. chloroma
g. chromoscopy
g. coin removal
g. colic
g. compression
g. content
g. crisis

g. cycle
g. cystic duplication
g. decompression
g. diet
g. dilation
g. distention
g. diverticulosis
g. duplication cyst
g. dysfunction
g. dyspepsia
g. effect
g. electrical dysrhythmia
g. electrical stimulation
g. emptying (GE)
g. emptying breath test (GEBT)
g. emptying delay
g. emptying half-time (GET1/2)
g. emptying scan
g. emptying scintigraphy
g. emptying time (GET)
g. epithelial cell infiltration
g. epithelial cell replication
g. feeding
g. first-pass metabolism of ethanol (GFPM)
g. fistula
g. fold
g. foreign body
g. fornix
g. foveola
g. foveolar epithelium
g. freezing
g. function test
g. fundus
g. fundus wrap
Garren-Edwards g. (GEG)
g. gland
g. hemorrhage
g. heterotopia
g. hyperacidity
g. hyperemia
g. hyperplastic polyp
g. hypersecretion
g. hypochlorhydria
g. hypomotility
g. hypothermia
g. hypothermia machine
g. ileus
g. impression
g. impression on liver
g. indigestion
g. inflammatory fibroid polyp

g. inhibitor factor
g. inhibitory peptide (GIP)
g. inhibitory polypeptide (GIP)
g. insufficiency
g. juice
g. Kaposi sarcoma
g. laryngeal mask airway (GLMA)
g. lavage
g. lavage tube
g. leiomyoma
g. leiomyosarcoma
g. lesion
g. lipoma
g. luminal pH
g. lymphoma
g. malaria
g. mass
g. mechanosensory threshold
g. metaplasia
g. metaplasia of duodenum
g. microenvironment
g. motility disorder
g. mucormycosis
g. mucosal atrophy
g. mucosal barrier
g. mucosal blood flow
g. mucosal damage
g. mucosal degradation
g. mucosal disease
g. mucosal ectopia
g. mucosal ectopia in rectum (GMER)
g. mucosal erosion
g. mucosal injury
g. mucosal laminin receptor
g. mucosal pattern classification
g. mucosal prolapse
g. mucus
g. muscularis mucosa
g. mycosis
g. myoelectrical activity
g. neobladder
g. neobladder procedure
g. neurasthenia
g. neurectomy
g. notch
g. omentum
g. outlet
g. outlet obstruction (GOO)
g. outline
g. oxyntic cell receptor
g. pacemaker cell

NOTES

gastric *(continued)*
- g. pacemaker region
- g. parietography
- g. partition
- g. peptide TFF1, TFF2
- g. perforation
- g. petechia
- g. pH monitor
- g. pigment
- g. pit
- g. pitting
- g. plasma
- g. plasmacytoma
- g. plexus
- g. pneumocystosis
- g. polypectomy
- g. polyposis
- g. pool
- g. pouch
- g. pseudolymphoma
- g. red spot
- g. remnant
- g. resection (GR)
- g. residuum
- g. retention (GR)
- g. rupture
- g. sclerosis
- g. secretory test
- g. sedative
- g. serosa
- g. stapling
- g. stasis
- g. stump
- g. syphilis
- g. tear
- g. teratoma
- g. tetany
- g. tone
- g. transit time
- g. transposition
- g. trauma
- g. tuberculosis
- g. ulcer
- g. ulceration
- g. urease activity
- g. variceal ligation
- g. varix
- g. varix bleeding
- g. vascular ectasia (GVE)
- g. vein
- g. venacaval shunt
- g. vertigo
- g. volume
- g. volvulus
- g. window
- g. xanthoma
- g. xanthomatosis

gastrica
- achylia g.
- adenasthenia g.
- area g.
- myasthenia g.
- myxorrhea g.
- zymosis g.

gastricae
- areae g.
- fibrae oblique g.
- foveolae g.
- rugae g.
- sordes g.

gastrici
- folliculi lymphatici g.

gastric-juice ammonia assay
gastric-type surface epithelium
gastricum
- corpus g.

gastricus
- fundus g.
- liquor g.
- status g.
- succus g.

Gastrimmune
gastrin
- antral g.
- basic g. (BG)
- g. cell
- g. cell function
- g. cell hyperfunction
- fasting serum g.
- g. gene
- g. mRNA
- g. mRNA:G-cell density
- g. mRNA level
- g. mRNA species
- g. receptor
- G. RIA kit II
- serum g.
- g. stain
- g. stimulation test

gastrin-17
gastrinoma
- duodenal g.
- g. triangle

gastrin-releasing
- g.-r. peptide (GRP)
- g.-r. peptide/bombesin

gastrin-secreting
- g.-s. cell
- g.-s. non beta islet cell tumor

gastritis
- active chronic g.
- acute erosive g. (AEG)
- acute hemorrhagic g.
- alcoholic hemorrhagic g.
- alkaline reflux g.
- antral atrophic g. (AAG)
- antral-predominant g.
- antrum g.

gastritis · gastrocolic

aspirin-induced g.
atrophic g.
autoimmune metaplastic atrophic g. (AMAG)
bile reflux g.
bleeding g.
Campylobacter pyloridis g.
catarrhal g.
chemical g.
chronic active g.
chronic atrophic g. (CAG)
chronic cystic g.
chronic erosive g.
chronic follicular g.
chronic interstitial g.
chronic nonimmune g.
chronic superficial g. (CSG)
cirrhotic g.
corpus g.
corrosive g.
g. cystica polyposa
g. cystic profunda
diffuse antral g. (DAG)
diffuse varioliform g.
drug-induced g.
emphysematous g.
endoscopic atrophic g.
endoscopic enterogastric reflux g.
endoscopic erythematous/exudative g.
endoscopic hemorrhagic g.
endoscopic raised erosive g.
endoscopic rugal hyperplastic g.
environmental metaplastic atrophic g. (EMAG)
eosinophilic g.
erosive g.
erosive-hemorrhagic g.
exfoliative g.
follicular g.
fundal g.
fundic atrophic g. (FAG)
fundic gland g.
giant hypertrophic g.
g. granulomatosa fibroplastica
granulomatous g.
Helicobacter pylori-induced g.
hemorrhagic g.
histological chronic active g.
hyperpeptic g.
hypertrophic lymphocytic g. (HLG)
idiopathic chronic erosive g.

interstitial g.
isolated granulomatous g.
lymphocytic g. (LG)
metaplastic atrophic g.
multifocal atrophic g. (MAG)
mycotic g.
nonautoimmune fundic atrophic g.
nonerosive nonspecific g.
nonspecific erosive g.
oxyntic mucosal g.
phlegmonous g.
polypous g.
postgastrectomy g.
postoperative g.
proliferative hypertrophic g.
pseudomembranous g.
purulent g.
radiation g.
reflux bile g.
severe g.
specific g.
stress g.
superficial g.
suppurative g.
Sydney classification of g.
syphilitic g.
toxic g.
tuberculous g.
type A, B g.
type A, B antral g.
ulcerative g.
uremic g.
varioliform g.
g. varioliformis
verrucous g.
viral g.
zonal g.
gastritis-associated peptic ulcer disease
gastroadenitis (*var. of* gastradenitis)
gastroadynamic
gastroalbumorrhea
gastroanastomosis
gastroatonia
gastroblennorrhea
gastrocamera
    Olympus GTF-A g.
gastrocardiac syndrome
Gastroccult test
gastrocele
gastrochronorrhea
gastrocolic
    g. fistula

NOTES

gastrocolic *(continued)*
    g. ligament
    g. omentum
    g. reflex
gastrocolitis
gastrocolostomy
gastrocutaneous
    g. fistula
    g. fistulous tract
gastrocystoplasty
gastrodiaphanoscopy
gastrodiaphany
gastroduodenal
    g. angiodysplasia
    g. artery (GDA)
    g. artery complex
    g. carcinoid
    g. Crohn disease
    g. double ulcer
    g. dyspepsia
    g. fistula
    g. hypertrophy
    g. lumen
    g. misperfusion
    g. mucosa
    g. mucosal injury
    g. mucosal protection
gastroduodenal-to-renal
    g.-t.-r. artery bypass
    g.-t.-r. artery bypass graft
gastroduodenectomy
gastroduodenitis
    neutrophilic g.
gastroduodenoenterostomy
gastroduodenopancreatectomy
gastroduodenoscopy
    Billroth g.
gastroduodenostomy
    Billroth I g.
    Jaboulay g.
gastrodynia
gastroenteralgia
gastroenteric fistula
gastroenteritis
    acute g. (AGE)
    acute infectious nonbacterial g.
    astrovirus g.
    Calicivirus g.
    Coronavirus g.
    endemic nonbacterial infantile g.
    eosinophilic g. (EG, EGE, EOG)
    epidemic nonbacterial g.
    infantile g.
    infectious g.
    nonbacterial g.
    Norwalk g.
    rotavirus g.
    viral g.
    winter g.

gastroenteroanastomosis
gastroenterocolitis
gastroenterocolostomy
gastroenterologic
gastroenterologist
gastroenterology
    American College of G. (ACG)
gastroenteropancreatic (GEP)
    g. tumor
gastroenteropathy
    g. detection
    eosinophilic g.
    protein-losing g.
gastroenteroplasty
gastroenteroptosis
gastroenterostomy (GE)
    Balfour g.
    Billroth g. type I, II
    Braun-Jaboulay g.
    Courvoisier g.
    Finney g.
    Heineke-Mikulicz g.
    Hill esophageal g.
    Hofmeister g.
    percutaneous g. (PGE)
    Pólya g.
    Roux-en-Y g.
    Schoemaker g.
    truncal vagotomy and g.
gastroenterotomy
gastroepiploic
    g. arcade
    g. artery (GEA, GEPA)
    g. blood vessel
gastroesophageal (GE)
    g. antireflux device (GARD)
    g. hernia
    g. incompetence
    g. junction
    g. reflux (GER)
    g. reflux disease (GERD)
    g. reflux scan
    g. scintigraphy
    g. scintiscan
    g. sphincter
    g. variceal plexus
    g. varix type 1, 2
gastroesophagitis
gastroesophagostomy
    cervical g.
gastrogastrostomy
gastrogavage
gastrogenic diarrhea
gastrogenous diarrhea
Gastrografin
    G. contrast medium
    G. enema
    G. GI series
    G. swallow

GastrograpH
    G. ambulatory pH monitoring system
    G. Mark III pH analyzer
gastrohepatic
    g. bare area
    g. ligament
    g. omentum
gastrohydrorrhea
gastroileac
    g. augmentation
    g. reflex
gastroileal reflex
gastroileitis
gastroileostomy
gastrointestinal (GI)
    g. absorption
    g. allergy
    g. assistant (GIA)
    g. autonomic nerve tumor
    g. biota
    g. bleed
    g. bleeding (GIB)
    g. blood loss test
    g. cancer
    g. cancer-associated antigen (GICA)
    g. complication
    g. cross
    g. endoscopic specialist
    g. endoscopy
    g. endothelium
    g. eosinophilic granuloma
    g. fiberscope
    g. fistula
    g. fungal ball
    g. hamartomatous polyp
    g. histoplasmosis
    g. immunodeficiency syndrome
    g. intubation
    g. Kaposi sarcoma
    g. lavage
    g. lesion
    g. lipoma
    g. motility
    g. myenteric plexus
    g. needle
    g. neuroendocrinology
    g. neurofibroma
    g. peptide hormone
    g. polyposis (GIP)
    g. reflux
    g. regularity peptide
    g. smooth muscle
    g. stoma
    g. stromal tumor (GIST)
    G. Symptom Rating Scale (GSRS)
    g. system (GIS)
    g. telangiectasia
    g. therapeutic system (GITS)
    g. tract (GIT)
    g. tract hemorrhage
    g. transit
    G. Tumor Study Group (GITSG, GTSG)
    upper g. (UGI)
gastrointestinal-associated lymphoid tissue (GALT)
gastrointestinalis
    mycetism g.
    pseudoleukemia g.
gastrojejunal
    g. constipation
    g. loop obstruction syndrome
gastrojejunocolic fistula
gastrojejunostomy
    antecolic long-loop isoperistaltic g.
    Billroth g. type I, II
    compression button g.
    Hofmeister-Shoemaker g.
    loop g.
    percutaneous endoscopic g. (PEG-J)
gastrokinesograph
gastrokinetic agent
gastrolavage
gastrolienal ligament
gastrolith
gastrolithiasis
gastrologist
gastrology
gastrolysis
Gastrolyte oral solution
gastromalacia
GastroMark
gastromegaly
gastromotor insufficiency
gastromycosis
gastromyotomy
gastromyxorrhea
gastronesteostomy
gastropancreatic
    g. fold
    g. ligament
    g. reflex
gastropancreatitis

NOTES

GastroPanel assay kit
gastroparalysis
gastroparesis
    diabetic g.
    g. diabeticorum
    idiopathic g.
    nondiabetic g.
    postvagotomy g.
    transient g.
gastroparietal
gastropathic
gastropathy
    aphthous g.
    benign hyperplastic g.
    cardiofundic g.
    chemical g.
    congestive hypertensive g.
    diabetic g.
    erosive g.
    erythematous g.
    hemorrhagic g.
    hypertensive g.
    hypertrophic hypersecretory g.
    idiopathic hypertrophic g.
    nonsteroidal antiinflammatory drug g.
    NSAID g.
    papulous g.
    portal hypertensive g. (PHG)
    prolapse g.
    protein-losing g.
    varioliform g.
gastroperiodynia
gastroperitonitis
gastropexy
    Boerema anterior g.
    Hill posterior g.
    Horsley g.
gastrophotography
gastrophrenic ligament
gastrophthisis
gastroplasty (GP)
    Collis g.
    Collis-Nissen g.
    Eckhout vertical g.
    fundus rotation g.
    Gomez horizontal g.
    greater curvature banded g.
    horizontal g.
    Laws g.
    Mason vertical banded g.
    Silastic ring vertical g.
    silicone elastomer ring vertical g. (SRVG)
    Stamm g.
    tubular vertical g.
    unbanded g.
    vertical banded g. (VBG)
    vertical ring g. (VRG)
    vertical Silastic ring g.
gastroplegia
gastroplication
    endoluminal g.
Gastro-Port II feeding device
gastroprokinetic
gastroprotection
    adaptive g.
gastroprotective
gastroptosis
gastropylorectomy
gastropyloric
Gastroreflex ambulatory pH monitor/recorder
gastrorenal shunt
gastrorrhagia
gastrorrhaphy
gastrorrhea continua chronica
gastrorrhexis
gastroschisis
    Silastic silo reduction of g.
gastroscope
    ACMI g.
    Benedict g.
    Bernstein g.
    Cameron omniangle g.
    Chevalier Jackson g.
    disposable-sheath flexible g.
    Eder g.
    Eder-Bernstein g.
    Eder-Chamberlin g.
    Eder-Hufford g.
    Eder-Palmer semiflexible g.
    Ellsner g.
    end-viewing g.
    Ewald g.
    FCS-ML II g.
    FGS-ML II g.
    fiberoptic g.
    flexible g.
    Fujinon EG-310D g.
    Fujinon EG-200FP g.
    Fujinon EG-410HR g.
    Fujinon GF-100PE g.
    GFC g.
    GFT Olympus g.
    Herman-Taylor g.
    Hirschowitz g.
    Housset-Debray g.
    Janeway g.
    Jenning-Streifeneder g.
    Kelling g.
    Krentz g.
    Mancke flex-rigid g.
    Mikulicz g.
    Olympus GIF-K-series g.
    Olympus GIFxP10 g.
    Olympus GIF-XQ30 flexible g.

gastroscope · gauge

Olympus 2T-2000 twin-channel therapeutic g.
Olympus XQ230 g.
pediatric g.
Pentax EUP-EC124 ultrasound g.
peroral g.
Q200 g.
Schindler semiflexible g.
Sielaff g.
Taylor g.
Tomenius g.
Universal g.
Wolf-Henning g.
Wolf-Knittlingen g.
Wolf-Schindler semiflexible g.
XQ230 Olympus g.

gastroscopic
gastroscopy
cap-fitted g.
high-magnification g.
infrared transillumination g.

Gastrosed
gastrosia fungosa
gastrosis
GastroSoft data reduction and prognostic software package
gastrospasm
Gastrospirillum hominis
gastrosplenic
g. ligament
g. omentum

gastrostaxis
gastrostenosis
gastrostogavage
gastrostolavage
gastrostomy
Beck g.
Beck-Jianu g.
g. bumper
button g.
g. button
CT-guided percutaneous endoscopic g.
DePage-Janeway g.
dual percutaneous endoscopic g. (DPEG)
endoscopic ultrasound-guided pancreatic g.
feeding g.
g. feeding
Glassman g.
Janeway g.

jejunal tube through percutaneous endoscopic g. (JETPEG)
Kader g.
Martin g.
Olympus g.
percutaneous g. (PG)
percutaneous endoscopic g. (PEG)
plug g.
Russell percutaneous endoscopic g.
g. scarring
Ssabanejew-Frank g.
Stamm g.
Surgitek One-Step percutaneous endoscopic g.
g. tube
g. tube migration
ultrasound-assisted percutaneous endoscopic g.
venting percutaneous g. (VPG)
Witzel g.

gastrosuccorrhea
digestive g.
g. mucosa

gastrotome
gastrotomy
gastrotonometer
gastrotonometry
gastrotoxic
gastrotoxin
gastrotropic
Gastrovist contrast medium
gastroxia
Gastrozepine
Gas-X
gate
method of g.'s
sampling g.

gatekeeper
g. gene
G. reflux repair system

Gatta prognostic system
Gaucher
G. cell
G. disease
G. splenomegaly

Gauderer-Ponsky PEG operation
Gauder Silicon PEG catheter
Gau gastric balloon
gauge
Chatillon Digital Force g.
Dacomed snap g.
g. of instrument

NOTES

gauge *(continued)*
    intraabdominal pressure g.
    LeVeen inflator with pressure g.
    snap g.
    Statham P23 strain g.

Gaur balloon distension technique

Gautier ureteroscope

gauze
    g. dressing
    Iodoform g.
    g. pack
    g. sponge
    Surgicel g.
    Vaseline g.
    Xeroform g.

gavage
    1090 G. bag
    g. feeding

Gavard muscle

GAVE
    gastric antral vascular ectasia
    GAVE syndrome

Gavin-Miller intestinal forceps

Gaviscon

Gaviscon-2

GAX
    glutaraldehyde cross-linked collagen

gay bowel syndrome

Gaymar water-circulating blanket

Gazayerli
    G. endoscopic retractor
    G. knot pusher

GB
    gallbladder
    GB virus C/hepatitis G virus (GBV-C/HGV)
    GB virus C/hepatitis G virus RNA (GBV-C/HGV-RNA)
    GB vol+ fluctuation

GBEF
    gallbladder ejection fraction

GBER
    gallbladder ejection rate

GBM
    glomerular basement membrane
    GBM collagen fiber
    perimesangial GBM
    GBM polyanion

GBO
    gastric bacterial overgrowth

GBP
    gastric bypass

GBS
    gallbladder series
    group B streptococcus

GBT
    gastric bleeding time

GBV-C/HGV
    GB virus C/hepatitis G virus

GBV-C/HGV-RNA
    GB virus C/hepatitis G virus RNA

GC
    gonococcus
    granular cast

GC-16
    Surgitek graduated cystocope GC-16

GCD
    giant colonic diverticulum

G-cell
    G-c. gastrin release
    G-c. hyperplasia

GC/MS
    gas chromatography/mass spectroscopy

G-CSF
    granulocyte colony-stimulating factor

GCS-HS
    glutamylcysteine synthetase heavy subunit

GCT
    giant cell transformation
    granular cell tumor

GCW
    glomerular capillary wall

GDA
    gastroduodenal artery
    GDA aneurysm

G:D-cell ratio

Gd-EOB-DTPA
    gadolinium EOB-DTPA

GDNF
    glial cell line-derived neurotrophic factor
    glial-derived neurotrophic factor

GDSS
    Glasgow Dyspepsia Severity Score

GE
    gastric emptying
    gastroenterostomy
    gastroesophageal
        GE junction
        GE reflux
        GE RT 3200 Advantage II

GEA
    gastroepiploic artery
    GEA graft

GEBT
    gastric emptying breath test

GEC
    galactose elimination capacity

Gee disease

Gee-Herter disease

Gee-Herter-Heubner
    G.-H.-H. disease
    G.-H.-H. syndrome

Geenan Endotorque guidewire

Gee-Thaysen disease

GEG
  Garren-Edwards gastric
  GEG bubble
gel
  agar g.
  agarose g.
  Betadine g.
  chondrocyte-alginate g.
  Contractubex g.
  Deflux injectable g.
  deletion and mutation detection enhancement g.
  dihydrotestosterone g.
  ferric hyaluronate g.
  g. filtration chromatography
  ILE-SORB absorbent g.
  IntraDose g.
  percutaneous testosterone g.
  polyacrylamide g.
  Sephacryl S-300 HR g.
  Simaal G. 2
  testosterone g. 1%
  viscoelastic g.
Gelamal
gelatin
  g. Hank buffered salt solution (GHBSS)
  g. resorcinol and formaldehyde (GRF)
  g. sponge
  g. sponge packing
gelatinous
  g. ascites
  g. nodule
gelatin-subbed slide
Gelcaps
  Anemagen OB G.
Gelclair
GELdose
  Zantac G.
Gelfoam
  G. cube
  G. embolization
  G. particle transarterial embolization treatment
Gellhorn pessary
Gelpi self-retaining retractor
gelsolin
  recombinant human g.
Gelusil
  open-label G.
Gelusil-II

Gelusil-M
Gély suture
gemcitabine HCl
Gemella
gemfibrozil
gemifloxacin
Gemini
  G. gall duct forceps
  G. paired wire helical basket
Gemzar
Genasense
gender
  g. effect
  g. reassignment
gender-matched control
gene
  g. A
  adenomatous polyposis coli g.
  ADPKD1 g.
  alpha g.
  angiotensin-converting enzyme g.
  APC tumor suppressor g.
  APOB g.
  apolipoprotein B g.
  ATP7A g.
  break cluster homology g.
  cagA g.
  cag PAI g.
  caretaker g.
  g. carrier
  C-beta g.
  c-Ha-ras g.
  G. Clean II kit
  COL4A3 g.
  COL4A4 g.
  COL4A5 g.
  DAZ g.
  DCC g.
  deleted in colon carcinoma g.
  DRB g.
  Fas g.
  FCC-COCA1 g.
  fucosyltransferase g.
  gastrin g.
  gatekeeper g.
  HDA-DR3 g.
  HFE g.
  HLA class II g.
  HLA-DQw2 g.
  HLA-DR3 g.
  hMLH1 g.
  human kidney chloride channel g.

NOTES

gene *(continued)*
  immunogenic g.
  integrase g.
  Jagged 1 g.
  KAL1 g.
  kallikreinlike g.
  Ki-ras g.
  KLF6 g.
  K-ras g.
  Kruppel-like factor 6 g.
  g. linkage
  LMP g.
  MCC g.
  MCH g.
  MDM2 g.
  MDR1 g.
  Menkes disease g.
  metastasis g.
  MLH1 g.
  MSH2 g.
  MTS1 g.
  MTS2 g.
  MUC-1 g.
  multidrug-resistance g. (MDR1)
  MutL g.
  MutS g.
  NM23 g.
  OB g.
  p15 g.
  P15/INK4B g.
  p16 g.
  p18 g.
  P21/WAF1 g.
  P27Kip1 g.
  p53 g.
  PAX2 g.
  PAX8 g.
  phospholipid export pump g. (MDR3)
  PKD1, *PKD2* g.
  polymorphic g.
  prodynorphin g.
  proenkephalin g.
  proopiomelanocortin g.
  Rb g.
  G. Screen nylon membrane filter
  serine threonine kinase g. 11
  SRY g.
  STK11 g.
  suppressor g.
  TAP g.
  TAP2 peptide transporter g.
  TGF-beta-1 g.
  g. therapy
  TNF-alpha g.
  TP40 g.
  TP53 g.
  tumor suppressor g.
  uromodulin g.
  vacuolating toxin g. A (VacA)
  V-alpha g.
  V-beta g.
  VHL g.
  von Hippel-Lindau g.
  WTI g.
gene-blotting study
gene-inductive effect
gene-linkage analysis (GLA)
general
  G. Electric Signa scanner
  g. endotracheal anesthesia (GETA)
  g. peptic ulcer
generalized
  g. abdominal tenderness
  g. distal renal tubular acidosis
  g. elastolysis
  g. glycogenosis
  g. peritonitis
general-practice urologist
generation
  anti-HCV antibody third g.
  Chiron RIBA HCV test system second g.
  interdialytic urea g.
  Ortho HCV ELISA test system second g.
generator
  banana plug dipolar g.
  electrohydraulic g.
  electrosurgical g.
  Endostat II bipolar/monopolar electrosurgical g.
  implantable pulse g. (IPG)
  isolated g.
  Itrel pulse g.
  Medstone STS shock wave g.
  microexplosive g.
  Northgate SD-100 EHL g.
  piezoelectric g.
  spark-gap shock wave g.
  Symmetry endobipolar g.
  Valleylab II g.
  Valleylab SSE2L g.
genetic
  g. aberration
  g. alteration
  g. code
  g. hemochromatosis (GH)
  g. heterogeneity
  g. marker
  g. predisposition
  g. susceptibility
  G.'s Systems microplate reader spectrophotometer
gene-transfer therapy
geniohyoid muscle
genistein

genital
- g. burn
- g. cord
- g. cryptococcosis
- g. differentiation
- g. dysplasia
- g. elephantiasis
- g. end bulb
- g. human papillomavirus
- g. mesonephros
- g. rash
- g. reconstruction
- g. scabies
- g. swelling
- g. tract
- g. tuberculosis
- g. ulcer
- g. wart

genitalia
- adolescent g.
- ambiguous external g.
- anomalous g.

genitocerebral evoked potential study
genitocrural
genitofemoral nerve
genitography
- retrograde g.

genitoinfectious
genitomesenteric band
genitoplasty
- feminizing g.
- masculinizing g.

genitourinary
- g. carcinoma
- g. fistula
- g. neoplasm
- g. prolapse
- g. region
- g. surgeon
- g. tract
- g. tuberculosis

genodermatosis
genome
- full-length viral g.
- retroviral g.

genome/ml
genomewide screen
genomic
- g. deoxyribonucleic acid
- g. DNA
- g. DNA probe
- g. imprinting
- g. instability
- g. sequence
- g. site

genotoxic
genotype
- ADPKD1 g.
- ADPKD2 g.
- hepatitis C virus g.
- g. III 2a
- g. II, III
- g. IV 2b
- g. V 3

Genta
- G. method
- G. stain

Gentafair
Gentamar
gentamicin sulfate
gentian violet
gentle
- G. Nature
- G. Touch colostomy appliance

genuine
- g. cystine stone
- g. stress incontinence (GSI)
- g. stress urinary incontinence (GSUI)

genu of pancreatic duct
Geocillin
geographic
- g. distribution
- g. tongue
- g. variance

Geopen
geophagia, geophagism, geophagy
geotrichosis
Geotrichum candidum
GEP
- gastroenteropancreatic

GEPA
- gastroepiploic artery

GER
- gastroesophageal reflux

Gerald forceps
GERD
- gastroesophageal reflux disease
- Enteryx technology for GERD
- Los Angeles classification of GERD
- RS associated with GERD

GERDcheck ambulatory esophageal pH monitoring system

NOTES

Gerhardt
    G. table
    G. test
geriatric
    g. constipation
    g. incontinence
    g. incontinence evaluation
    g. urinary tract infection
    g. urology
    g. voiding dysfunction
geriatrics
Geridium
Geriplex-FS
Gerlach valve
germ
    g. cell carcinoma
    g. cell hypoplasia
    g. cell neoplasm
    g. cell tumor
    g. layer
germander
germicide
    liquid chemical g. (LCG)
germinal
    g. center formation
    g. epithelium
germinomatous
germline mutation
Gerota
    G. capsule
    G. fascia
gestation
    ectopic g.
gestational
    g. diabetes
    g. thyrotoxicosis
    g. trophoblastic tumor (GTT)
GET
    gastric emptying time
GET1/2
    gastric emptying half-time
GETA
    general endotracheal anesthesia
GFC gastroscope
GFD
    gluten-free diet
GFP
    green fluorescent protein
GFPM
    gastric first-pass metabolism of ethanol
GFR
    glomerular filtration rate
        AmB-induced reduction GFR
        single-nephron GFR
GFS Mark II inflatable penile prosthesis
GFT Olympus gastroscope
GF-UM30P linear-oriented radial scanning echoendoscope
GF-UM2 radial-sector scan transducer
GF-UM3 radial-sector scan transducer
GF-UM20 radial-sector scan transducer
GFXTM Genomic blood DNA purification kit
GG
    Lactobacillus GG (LGG)
GGT
    gamma-glutamyltransferase
    GGT test
GGTP
    gamma-glutamyl transpeptidase
    GGTP liver function test
GGU
    giant gastric ulcer
GH
    genetic hemochromatosis
GHBSS
    gelatin Hank buffered salt solution
Ghedini-Weinberg serologic test
GHP
    growth hormone promoter
    ^{99m}Tc GHP
GI
    gastrointestinal
    Gingival Index
        GI bleeding of obscure origin
        GI bleeding scan
        GI cancer
        GI cocktail
        GI electrophysiology
        Imagent GI
        GI pacemaker cell
        GI tract
        GI tract flora
GIA
    gastrointestinal assistant
        GIA autosuture apparatus
        GIA autosuture device
        GIA instrument
        GIA stapler
Gianotti-Crosti syndrome
giant
    g. anorectal condyloma acuminatum
    g. cell
    g. cell adenocarcinoma
    g. cell hepatitis
    g. cell transformation (GCT)
    g. colon
    g. colonic diverticulum (GCD)
    g. diverticulosis
    g. fibrous mesothelioma
    g. gastric fold
    g. gastric polyp
    g. gastric ulcer (GGU)
    g. hypertrophic gastritis
    g. hypertrophy of gastric mucosa
    g. intestinal fluke
    g. migrating contraction (GMC)

g. mitochondria
g. molluscum contagiosum
g. nonpancreatic pseudocyst
g. peptic ulcer

Gianturco
G. coil
G. expandable self-expanding metallic biliary prosthesis
G. expandable self-expanding metallic biliary stent
G. metal urethral stent
G. Z stent

Gianturco-Rosch
G.-R. biliary Z stent
G.-R. self-expandable Z stent

Gianturco-Roubin flexible coil stent

Giardia
G. *duodenalis*
G. *intestinalis*
G. *lamblia*

giardiasis dysentery
giardin
GIB
gastrointestinal bleeding

Gibbon
G. hernia
G. hydrocele
G. indwelling ureteral stent

Gibbs-Donnan equilibrium
Gibson
G. excision
G. incision

Gibson-Balfour abdominal retractor
GICA
gastrointestinal cancer-associated antigen

Giemsa
G. method
G. stain

Giemsa-stained section
Gierke disease
GIF
glycosylation-inhibiting factor
GIF N30 fiberoptic pediatric endoscope
GIF XP20 endoscope
GIF XQ10 upper endoscope

GIF-HM fiberscope
GIF-Q240 upper digestive tract endoscope
GIFT
gamete intrafallopian transfer

GIF1T130
Olympus large-channel endoscope GIF1T130

gigantica
Fasciola g.

gigantism
acromegalic g.

Gigasept
Gilbert
G. cholemia
G. cystic duct forceps
G. disease
G. sign
G. syndrome

Gilbert-Behçet syndrome
Gilbert-Dreyfus syndrome
Gilchrist
G. ileocecal bladder
G. procedure

Gill renal tourniquet
Gilman-Abrams gastric tube
Gil-Vernet
G.-V. dorsal lumbotomy incision
G.-V. extended pyelolithotomy
G.-V. ileocecal cystoplasty
G.-V. ileocecal cystoplasty urinary diversion
G.-V. operation
G.-V. orthotopic urinary diversion
G.-V. position
G.-V. procedure
G.-V. retractor
G.-V. technique

ginger root
gingival
G. Index (GI)
g. papilloma

gingivostomatitis
herpetic g.

ginkgo
ginseng
Giordano-Giovannetti diet
Giordano sphincter
GIP
gastric inhibitory peptide
gastric inhibitory polypeptide
gastrointestinal polyposis

GIP/MEDI-Globe needle
Giraldes
organ of G.

NOTES

girdle
    Neptune g.
    shoulder g.
Gironcoli hernia
girth
    abdominal g.
GIS
    gastrointestinal system
GIST
    gastrointestinal stromal tumor
GIT
    gastrointestinal tract
Gitelman syndrome
GITS
    gastrointestinal therapeutic system
GITSG
    Gastrointestinal Tumor Study Group
Gittes
    G. bladder neck suspension
    G. needle
    G. technique
    G. urethral suspension procedure
    G. urethropexy
Gittes-Loughlin
    G.-L. bladder neck suspension
    G.-L. procedure
Given
    G. diagnostic imaging system
    G. imaging capsule/M2A capsule
    G. Imaging Ltd.
    G. M2A endoscopic videocapsule
    G. videocapsule system
GL
    glucagon
GLA
    gene-linkage analysis
glabella reflex
glabrata
    Candida g.
    Torulopsis g.
glabrous cirrhosis
Glahn test
gland
    accessory adrenal g.
    accessory parotid g.
    accessory sex g.
    accessory thyroid g.
    acid g.
    adrenal g.
    Albarran g.
    anal intramuscular g.
    Bartholin g.
    biliary g.
    Brunner g.
    bulbourethral g.
    cardiac-type g.
    Cowper g.
    esophageal ectopic sebaceous g.
    esophageal mucosal g.
    Galeati g.
    gastric g.
    hilum of suprarenal g.
    Home g.
    Lieberkühn g.
    Littré g.
    Luschka cystic g.
    medulla of suprarenal g.
    metaplastic gastric fundic g.
    middle g.
    misplaced g.
    mucous g.
    mucus-secreting g.
    oxyntic g.
    paraurethral g.
    periductal g.
    periurethral g.
    preputial g.
    pyloric g.
    Skene g.
    suprarenal g.
    trapped prostate g.
    urethral g.
    vestibular g.
    von Ebner g.
glandula, pl. **glandulae**
glandular
    g. cystitis
    g. metaplasia
    g. structure
glandularis
    cystitis g.
    pyelitis g.
    ureteritis g.
    urethritis g.
glandule
glandulectomy
glandulopexy
glandulous
glans
    g. approximation procedure (GAP)
    conical g.
    g. hyperemia
    g. penis
    g. penis papilla
glansplasty
    meatal advancement and g. (MAGPI)
glanular hypospadias
glanuloplasty
Glasgow
    G. classification of choledocholithiasis
    G. coma scale
    G. criteria for severity of pancreatitis
    G. Dyspepsia Severity Score (GDSS)

glass
    g. penile prosthesis
    g. pH electrode
Glasser gastrostomy tube
Glassman
    G. basket
    G. brush
    G. gastrostomy
    G. noncrushing gastrointestinal clamp
    G. stone extractor
Glassman-Allis intestinal forceps
Glaxo
    G. stain
    G. Wellcome protocol S3BA3003
Glazyme APF-EIA-TEST test
GLDH
    glutamate dehydrogenase
Gleason
    G. cancer grade
    G. grading system
    G. score
gleet
gleety
Gleevec
Glenn
    G. diverticulum forceps
    G. technique
Glenn-Anderson
    G.-A. advancement
    G.-A. technique
    G.-A. ureteroneocystostomy
gliadin
    g. ELISA
    g. IgA
    wheat g.
gliadin-specific T-cell clone
glial cell line-derived neurotrophic factor (GDNF)
glial-derived neurotrophic factor (GDNF)
glibornuride
gliclazide
glidewire
    angle-tip G.
    G. Gold surgical guidewire
    Terumo G.
Glidex coated Percuflex catheter
glimepiride
glioblastoma multiforme
glioma-polyposis syndrome
glipizide

glischruria
Glisson
    G. capsule
    G. cirrhosis
    G. sphincter
glissonitis
glitter cell
GLMA
    gastric laryngeal mask airway
global sclerosis
globi (*pl. of* globus)
globoside
globular
    g. albuminuria
    g. hyalin
    g. proteinuria
globulin
    alpha-1 g.
    alpha-1-antitrypsin g.
    antilymphocyte g.
    antithymocyte g. (ATG)
    Bence Jones g.
    cytomegalovirus immune g.
    g. fraction
    gamma g.
    hepatitis B hyperimmune g.
    human hepatitis B immune g.
    immune serum g.
    lymphocyte immune g. (LIG)
    Minnesota antilymphocyte g.
    prophylactic gamma g.
    sex hormone-binding g. (SHBG)
    testosterone-binding g.
    testosterone-estrogen-binding g.
    tetanus g.
    thyroxine-binding g.
globulinuria
globus, pl. **globi**
    esophageal g.
    g. hystericus
    g. major
    g. major epididymidis
    g. minor
    g. minor epididymidis
glomerular, glomerulose
    g. accumulation
    g. arteriole
    g. basement membrane (GBM)
    g. basement membrane disease
    g. capillary
    g. capillary healing
    g. capillary hypertension

NOTES

glomerular *(continued)*
- g. capillary pressure
- g. capillary wall (GCW)
- g. cell culture
- g. cell proliferation
- g. contractile cell
- g. crescent
- g. cyst
- g. endothelial myxovirus-like microtubular inclusion
- g. endotheliosis
- g. epithelial cell
- g. epithelial cell toxin puromycin aminonucleoside
- g. extracellular matrix
- g. fibronectin mRNA
- g. filtration
- g. filtration rate (GFR)
- g. hematuria
- g. hypercellularity
- g. hyperfiltration
- g. hypertrophy
- g. injury
- g. ischemia
- g. macrophage infiltration
- g. mesangium
- g. metabolism
- g. microvascular thrombosis
- g. morphology
- g. necrosis
- g. neutrophil infiltration
- g. podocyte
- proliferating g.
- g. proteinuria
- g. sclerosis
- g. tip lesion (GTL)
- g. tuft
- g. ultrafiltrate
- g. ultrafiltration
- g. ultrafiltration coefficient

glomerulation
glomeruli (*pl. of* glomerulus)
glomerulitis
glomerulocapillary
glomerulocapsular nephritis
glomerulocystic kidney disease
glomerulonephritis, pl. **glomerulonephritides (GN)**
- acute g. (AGN)
- acute mesangial proliferative g.
- acute poststreptococcal g. (APSGN)
- anti-GBM g.
- antiglomerular basement membrane g.
- antithymocyte antibody-induced g.
- biopsy-verified chronic g.
- chronic g. (CG, CGN)
- chronic membranous g. (CMGN)
- chronic renal failure g.
- complement-mediated experimental g.
- crescentic g.
- diffuse proliferative g.
- Ellis types 1, 2 g.
- experimental g.
- fibrillary g.
- focal necrotizing g.
- focal proliferative g.
- idiopathic crescentic g.
- idiopathic membranous g.
- idiopathic rapidly progressive g. (IRPGN)
- IgA g.
- immune complex g. (IC-GN)
- immunotactoid g.
- membranoproliferative g. type I, II (MPGN)
- membranous g. (MGN)
- mesangiocapillary g.
- mesangioproliferative g.
- necrotizing crescentic g. (NCGN)
- pauciimmune antineutrophil cytoplasmic antibody-associated g.
- pauciimmune crescentic g.
- postinfectious g.
- poststreptococcal g. (PSGN)
- poststreptococcal acute g.
- proliferative g.
- rapidly progressive g. (RPGN)
- recurrent focal sclerosing g.
- tropical mesangiocapillary g.
- type I mesangiocapillary g.

glomerulopathy
- Adriamycin g.
- amyloidlike g.
- collagenofibrotic g.
- collapsing g.
- immunotactoid g. (ITGP)
- inflammatory g.
- lipoprotein g.
- nonamyloid g.
- proteinuric g.
- toxic g.

glomerulosa
- zona g.

glomerulosclerosis
- diffuse diabetic g.
- focal segmental g. (FSGS)
- segmental g.

glomerulose (*var. of* glomerular)
glomerulotubular balance
glomerulus, pl. **glomeruli**
- afferent vessel of g.
- amyloidotic g.
- atubular g.
- capsula glomeruli
- human g.
- kidney glomeruli

glomerulus · glutamine

malpighian glomeruli
obsolescent g.
pooled glomeruli
renal glomeruli
Ruysch glomeruli
vas afferens glomeruli
vas efferens glomeruli

glomus tumor
glossitis
Rider-Moeller g.

glossodynia
Glo-tip biliary catheter
glottic
g. gap
g. spasm

glove
SensiCare synthetic powder-free surgical g.
Tactyl 1 g.

GLPT
glutamate pyruvate transaminase

glucagon (GL)
g. precipitation
g. stain

glucagon-evoked gastric dysrhythmia
glucagonoma syndrome
gluceptate
erythromycin g.

glucoamylase
maltase g.

glucocerebrosidase
glucocorticoid
g. kinase
g. response element (GRE)
g. treatment

glucocorticoid-induced
g.-i. hypercalcemia
g.-i. hypercalcemic nephrolithiasis

gluconate
calcium g.
iron g.
quinidine g.

gluconeogenesis
gluconeogenesis-associated enzyme
gluconeogenic-competent human proximal tubule cell
gluconeogenic pathway
glucoreceptor
glucose
G. Analyzer II test
control g.

CSF g.
g. excretion
filtered g.
g. intolerance
luminal g.
g. test
g. tolerance
g. transport
g. transporter
g. uptake
urinary g.

glucose-6-phosphatase deficiency
glucose-6-phosphate isomerase
glucose-dependent insulinotropic peptide
glucose-galactose malabsorption
glucosuria
renal g.

Glucotrol
glucuronate
trimetrexate g.

glucuronidase
glucuronidation
glucuronide
glucuronosyltransferase
uridine diphosphate g. (UDPGT)

glucuronyl
g. transferase
g. transferase deficiency

glue
cyanoacrylate g.
fibrin g.
hemostatic surgical g.
tissue g.

glutamate
g. dehydrogenase (GLDH)
g. pyruvate transaminase (GLPT)

glutamic
g. acid
g. acid hydrochloride

glutamic-oxaloacetic transaminase (GOT)
glutamic-pyruvic transaminase (GPT)
glutaminase
mitochondrial phosphate-dependent g.
phosphate-dependent g. (PDG)
phosphate-independent g. (PIG)

glutamine
g. aminotransferase pathway
CSF g.
g. nitrogen
g. test

NOTES

glutamylcysteine synthetase heavy subunit (GCS-HS)
glutamyl transpeptidase (GTP)
glutaral
glutaraldehyde
    activated alkaline g.
    g. alarm
    g. cross-linked collagen (GAX)
    g. cross-linked collagen injection
glutaraldehyde-induced proctitis
glutathione (GSH)
    g. metabolism
    g. peroxidase
    g. redox cycle
    g. S-transferase (GST)
    g. S-transferase M1
    g. S-transferase pi
    g. transferase
gluteal
    g. artery
    g. fold
    g. nerve
gluten
    g. challenge
    dietary g.
    g. enteropathy
    g. sensitivity
    g. solution
    wheat g.
gluten-dependent population
gluten-free diet (GFD)
gluten-rich diet
gluten-sensitive
    g.-s. diarrhea
    g.-s. enteropathy (GSE)
gluteus
    g. maximus
    g. maximus transposition
glyburide
glycated albumin
glyceraldehyde-3-phosphate dehydrogenase (GAPDH, G3PDH)
glyceraldehyde phosphate dehydrogenase (GAPD, GAPDH)
glycerin
    g. enema
    g. suppository
glycerol
Glycerol-T
glycerylphosphorylcholine
    alpha g.
glyceryl trinitrate (GTN)
glycine
glycocalyx
    podocyte g.
glycochenodeoxycholate
glycogen
    g. inclusion
    g. nephrosis
    g. phosphorylase
    g. storage disease
glycogenic acanthosis
glycogenosis
    brancher deficiency g.
    generalized g.
    hepatophosphorylase-deficiency g.
    hepatorenal g.
    type III g.
glycogen-rich cystadenoma
glycol
    ethylene g.
    polyethylene g. (PEG)
    polyethylene g. 600
glycolate
glycolipid
    mucin-type g.
glycolysis
    aerobic g.
    anaerobic g.
glycolytic
    g. enzyme
    g. inhibition
glycoprotein
    g. accumulation
    acidic epididymal g.
    alpha-1-acid g.
    B2 g. I
    dimeric acidic g. (DAG)
    heterodimeric g.
    microfil-associated g. (MAGP)
    N-linked g.
    TAG-72 g.
    viral g.
glycoprotein-2
    sulfated g.-2 (SGP-2)
glycoprotein-producing tumor
glycopyrrolate test
glycosaminoglycan (GAG)
    g. heparin
    g. layer
    g.'s uronate (GAGUA)
glycosaminoglycan-degrading enzyme
glycosidase
glycoside
    anthracene g.
    cardiac g.
glycosphingolipid
glycosuria
    alimentary g.
    digestive g.
glycosylated phosphoprotein
glycosylation
    g. of EPO
    nonenzymatic g.
    g. process
glycosylation-inhibiting factor (GIF)
glycosyltransferase
glycyl prolinuria

glycyltryptophan test
glycyrrhetinic acidlike factor (GALF)
glycyrrhiza
 syrup of g.
Glynazan
glyoxylate
Glypressin
GMC
 giant migrating contraction
GM-CSF
 granulocyte-macrophage colony-stimulating factor
  GM-CSF cytokine
Gmelin test
GMER
 gastric mucosal ectopia in rectum
GM3 ganglioside
G91-9215 monocrystant antimony pH catheter
GMP
 guanosine 5′-monophosphate
GMS
 Galloway-Mowat syndrome
GN
 glomerulonephritis
gnawing pain
GNG phase imaging
GNRF
 guanine nucleotide-releasing factor
GnRH
 gonadotropin-releasing hormone
goat
 g. antirabbit HRP conjugate
 g. model
goblet
 g. cell
 g. cell hyperplasia
 g. cell metaplasia
Goelet retractor
goiter
 nontoxic g.
gold
 cationic colloidal g. (CCG)
 7C Gold urine test
 g. compound
 G. deep surgery forceps
 g. nephropathy
 G. Probe
 G. Probe Direct bipolar hemostasis catheter
 G. Probe electrocoagulation
 G. Probe electrohemostasis catheter
 g. salt
 g. seed implant
 g. seed implantation technique
gold-198 (^{198}Au)
Goldberg Anorectic Attitude scale
Goldblatt
 G. clamp
 G. hypertension
 G. kidney
 G. phenomenon
Goldenhar syndrome
Goldman classification of operative risk
Goldschmiedt technique
Goldstein
 G. disease
 G. hematemesis
 G. Microspike approximator clamp
 G. Microspike approximator clamp for vasoepididymostomy
 G. Microspike approximator clamp for vasovasostomy
Goldston syndrome
Goldwasser suture carrier
golf-hole configuration
Golgi
 G. apparatus
 G. complex
 G. vesicle
Goligher
 G. extraperitoneal ileostomy
 G. modification
 G. retractor
GoLYTELY
 G. bowel preparation
 G. solution
Gomco
 G. suction
 G. suction tube
 G. umbilical clamp
Gomez
 G. fundoplasty
 G. horizontal gastroplasty
 G. horizontal gastroplasty with reinforced stoma
Gompertzian tumor kinetics
gonad
 dysgenetic g.
 intersex g.
 streak g.
 vanishing g.
gonadal
 g. artery

NOTES

gonadal *(continued)*
    g. differentiation
    g. dysgenesis
    g. ligament
    g. vein
    g. vein valve
    g. vessel
gonadectomize
gonadectomy
gonadial
gonadoblastoma
gonadoliberin
gonadopathy
gonadotherapy
gonadotoxic
gonadotoxicity
    chemotherapy g.
gonadotroph
gonadotropin, gonadotrophin
    human chorionic g. (HCG)
    human menopausal g.
gonadotropin-releasing
    g.-r. hormone (GnRH)
    g.-r. hormone deficiency
    g.-r. hormone pulsatile secretion
    g.-r. hormone test
gonaduct
Gonal-F
gonangiectomy
gondii
    Toxoplasma g.
gonecyst
gonecystic calculus
gonecystis
gonecystitis
gonecystolith
gonecystopyosis
gonococcal
    g. perihepatis pelvic inflammatory disease
    g. proctitis
    g. urethritis (GU)
gonococcus (GC)
gonocyte
    seminiferous tubule g.
gononephrotome
gonophore
gonorrhea
    rectal g.
gonorrheal
    g. bubo
    g. proctitis
    g. urethritis
gonorrhoeae
    Neisseria g.
GOO
    gastric outlet obstruction

good
    g. performance unit
    g. voiding
Goodpasture
    G. disease
    G. epitope
    G. reactivity
    G. syndrome
Goodsall rule
Goodwin
    G. cup-patch principle
    G. technique
    G. technique ureterocolonic anastomosis
Goodwin-Hohenfellner technique
Goodwin-Scott technique
Gopalan syndrome
GOR
    antibody to GOR (anti-GOR)
Gordon
    G. disease
    G. syndrome
gordonae
    Mycobacterium g.
Gore-Tex
    G.-T. ACUSEAL cardiovascular patch
    G.-T. catheter
    G.-T. graft
    G.-T. sling reinforcement
    G.-T. soft tissue patch
    G.-T. strip
gorge
gorget
    probe g.
    Teale g.
Gorlin basal cell nevus syndrome
Gorlin-Chaudhry-Moss syndrome
goserelin acetate
Gosset appendectomy retractor
GOT
    glutamic-oxaloacetic transaminase
Gothic arch formation
Gott
    G. shunt
    G. tube
Gottron sign
gouge
    Capener g.
Gould
    G. inverted mattress suture
    G. polygraph gastric motility measuring device
    G. pressure monitor
    G. pressure transducer
Goulding procedure
Gouley catheter
gout

gouty
    g. kidney
    g. proteinuria
    g. urethritis
    g. urine
Gowers
    G. attack
    G. sign
    G. syndrome
Goyrand hernia
GP
    gastroplasty
G3PDH
    glyceraldehyde-3-phosphate dehydrogenase
        G3PDH CDNA probe
        G3PDH mRNA species
GPL unit
gp330 receptor
GPT
    glutamic-pyruvic transaminase
GR
    gastric resection
    gastric retention
        GR drug class
Grabstald Memorial staging system
gracilis
    g. muscle
    g. muscle flap
    g. musculocutaneous unit
    g. myocutaneous neovagina
    g. neosphincter
graciloplasty
    direct nerve stimulation g.
    dynamic urinary g. (DUG)
    intramuscular perineural stimulation g.
    stimulated g.
grade
    g. 4 cystocele
    Gleason cancer g.
    hemorrhoid g.
    Hetzel-Dent esophagitis g.
    high g. (HG)
    Matts g. 1–4
    M.D. Anderson g.
    mucosal PMN g.
    Roenigk g.
    Savary-Miller II g.
    tumor g.
graded
    g. alcohol
    g. esophageal balloon distention test
gradient
    A-a g.
    acinar g.
    albumin g.
    biliary-duodenal pressure g.
    duodenobiliary pressure g.
    g. echo
    hepatic venous pressure g. (HVPG)
    serum-ascites albumin g. (SAAG)
    transcapillary hydrostatic pressure g.
    transmural hydrostatic pressure g.
    transtubular potassium g. (TTKG)
gradient recalled acquisition in steady state (GRASS)
grading
    Edmondson g. (EdGr)
    histologic g.
    tumor g.
graft
    aortic g.
    aortoenteric g.
    aortohepatic arterial g.
    aortorenal bypass g.
    g. atherosclerosis
    autogenous tunica vaginalis g.
    g. bed
    biologic collagen-based tissue-matrix g.
    bladder mucosal g.
    bovine g.
    branched vascular g.
    buccal mucosal patch g.
    bypass g.
    C g.
    cadaveric pericardial g.
    cadaveric segmental g.
    Dacron interposition g.
    Diastat vascular access g.
    dorsal vein patch g.
    free-GEPA g.
    free jejunal g.
    full-thickness g.
    g. function
    gastroduodenal-to-renal artery bypass g.
    GEA g.
    Gore-Tex g.
    hepatic-to-renal artery saphenous vein bypass g.
    HLA identical kidney g.

NOTES

graft *(continued)*
    Horton-Devine dermal g.
    iliac-to-renal artery bypass g.
    Impra g.
    INTERING vascular g.
    interposition Dacron g.
    live-donor segmental g.
    loop forearm g.
    g. loss
    Marlex g.
    Martius g.
    meshed g.
    mucosal g.
    omental pedicle flap g.
    g. parenchymal cell
    patch g.
    pedicle g.
    pedicled omental g.
    g. placement
    portacaval H g.
    postauricular Wolfe g.
    prosthetic arterial g.
    quality of kidney g.
    reduced-size g.
    renal artery g.
    segmental liver g.
    seromuscular intestinal patch g.
    skin g.
    g. spatulation
    splenorenal bypass g.
    split-thickness skin g.
    g. substitute
    superior mesenteric to renal artery saphenous vein bypass g.
    sural nerve g.
    Surgisis Gold hernia repair g.
    g. survival
    synthetic vascular g.
    Thiersch g.
    Thiersch-Duplay tube g.
    tube g.
    tubed free skin g.
    vascular access g. (VAG)
    Vectra hemodialysis access g.
    V-Y sliding skin g.
    Y-V sliding skin g.
graft-enteric fistula
grafting
    endovascular stent g.
graft-versus-host disease (GVHD)
Graham
    G. catheter
    G. closure
    G. closure with omental pouch
    G. deep surgery scissors
    G. plication
    G. scale for drug-induced gastric damage
    G. test

grain density
Gram
    G. stain
    G. stain of stool
    G. stain of stool test
gram-negative
    g.-n. bacterium
    g.-n. rod
    g.-n. sepsis
gram-positive
    g.-p. bacterium
    g.-p. organism
    g.-p. sepsis
gram-stain morphology
granddaughter cyst
granisetron
granny knot
Grant gallbladder retractor
granular
    g. cast (GC)
    g. cell myoblastoma
    g. cell tumor (GCT)
    g. induration
    g. kidney
granularity
granulation
    healing by g.
granule
    acidophilic PAS-positive g.
    acrosomal g.
    Birbeck g.
    carcinoid secretory g.
    DiPAS-positive g.
    Fordyce g.
    hemosiderin g.
    Kretz g.
    mucin g.
    perichromatin g.
    Weibel-Palade g.
    zymogen g.
granulocyte
    g. colony-stimulating factor (G-CSF)
    g. count
    g. exocytosis
granulocyte-macrophage colony-stimulating factor (GM-CSF)
granulocytic
    g. sarcoma
    g. sarcoma of stomach
granulocytopenia
granuloma
    amebic g.
    barium g.
    caseating g.
    eosinophilic g.
    epithelioid g.
    gastrointestinal eosinophilic g.
    hepatic g.

g. inguinale
noncaseating tuberclelike g.
nonnecrotizing g.
plasma cell g.
portal zone g.
pulmonary g.
pyogenic g.
sperm g.
stone g.
suture g.
umbilical g.

granulomatis
Calymmatobacterium g.

granulomatosa
Miescher cheilitis g.

granulomatosis
lipophagia g.
lipophagic intestinal g.
Wegener g.

granulomatous
g. bowel disease
g. cheilitis
g. cholangitis
g. enteritis
g. enterocolitis
g. gastritis
g. hepatitis
g. ileitis
g. peritonitis
g. prostatitis
g. transmural colitis

granulosa
appendicitis g.
g. cell tumor
urethritis g.

granulosa-theca cell tumor
granulosus
Echinococcus g.

granzyme B
grapefruit diet
grapelike cyst
Graser diverticulum
grasp
g. biopsy
palmar g.
plantar g.
g. tripod forceps

grasper
Allis tooth g.
atraumatic g.
bowel g.

four-pronged polyp g.
laparoscopic g.
Polaris g.
polyp g.
three-pronged g.
traumatic locking g.
tripod g.
umbilical port g.

grasping
g. forceps
g. instrument

GRASS
gradient recalled acquisition in steady state

Grass
G. force displacement fluid collector
G. Model SIU5A stimulation isolation unit
G. Model S9 stimulator

Grassi
nerve of G.

Graves
G. disease
G. technique

gravidarum
cholestatic hepatosis icterus g.
hyperemesis g.
icterus g.
nephritis g.

gravid uterus
gravimetric
g. technique
g. weighing

gravis
colitis g.
enteritis g.
icterus g.
myasthenia g.

gravity
g. cavernosometry
g. cystogram
urinalysis specific g.
g. urinary incontinence
urinary specific g.
urine specific g.

gravity-dependent drainage
gravity-induced erosion
Grawitz
G. cachexia
G. tumor

NOTES

gray
    G. cystic duct forceps
    g. scale

gray-scale
    g.-s. imaging
    g.-s. sonography
    g.-s. ultrasonography
    g.-s. ultrasound

GRE
    glucocorticoid response element

great
    g. epiploon
    g. lacuna
    g. pancreatic artery

greater
    g. celandine
    g. curvature banded gastroplasty
    g. curvature of stomach
    g. curvature ulcer
    g. curve position
    g. omentum
    g. peritoneal sac
    g. sciatic foramen

greedy bowel

green
    G. cystic duct forceps
    g. fluorescent protein (GFP)
    indocyanine g.
    g. Mersilene suture
    g. sputum
    g. stool

Greenen
    G. Endotorque
    G. pancreatic stent

Greene retractor

Greenfield
    G. caval catheter
    G. filter

Greenville gastric bypass

Greenwald
    G. Control Tip cystoscopic electrode
    G. needle
    G. Roth Grip-Tip suture guide
    G. sound

Greer EZ Access drainage pouch
Gregoir-Lich procedure
Greishaber self-retaining retractor
Grey
    G. Turner disease
    G. Turner sign
    G. Turner sign of retroperitoneal hemorrhage

GRF
    gelatin resorcinol and formaldehyde

GRFoma
Grice suture needle
gridiron incision
Griess test

Griffen Roux-en-Y bypass
Griffith point
Grimelius
    G. silver stain
    G. staining
    G. technique

Grimelius-positive cell

grip
    hand g. (HG)
    hook g.
    power g.
    precision g.
    three-finger g.
    two-finger g.

Grip-Tip suture guide
griseofulvin
grit-free solution
gritty tumor
G-RNA
Grocco sign
Grocott methenamine silver stain
groin incision
Grondahl-Finney esophagogastroplasty

groove
    anal intersphincteric g.
    esophageal g.
    innominate g.
    intersphincteric g.
    Liebermeister g.
    oval-form colonic g.
    g. pancreatitis
    paracolic g.
    radial g.
    spindle colonic g.

grooved director

grooving
    transurethral g. of prostate

gross
    g. deformity
    G. disease
    g. hematuria
    G. test

ground-glass
    g.-g. appearance
    g.-g. cell
    g.-g. hepatocytes

group
    ABH blood g.
    ABO blood g.
    antibiotic g.
    Astra/Merck G.
    Benelux Multicentre Trial Study G.
    g. B streptococcus (GBS)
    Canadian Urology Oncology G. (CUOG)
    crossreactive g. (CREG)
    g. C rotavirus
    Eastern Cooperative Oncology G. (ECOG)

Gastrointestinal Tumor Study G. (GITSG, GTSG)
hydroxyl g.
International Germ Cell Cancer Collaborative G. (IGCCCG)
Laparoscopic Colorectal Surgery G. (LCSSG)
Leuprolide Depot Neoadjuvant Prostate Cancer Study G.
Lewis blood g.
nadolol g.
National Prostatic Cancer Treatment G. (NPCTG)
National Wilms Tumor Study G. (NWTSG)
permixon g.
phytyl g.
population-based control g.
radical resection g.

growth
cancer cell g.
g. of coagulase-negative *Staphylococcus*
g. factor
g. factor beta
g. factor isoform
fungating g.
g. hormone deficiency
g. hormone promoter (GHP)
g. regulation
somatic g.

GRP
gastrin-releasing peptide

Gruber-Landzert fossa

Grüntzig, Gruentzig
G. balloon
G. balloon catheter
G. balloon dilation
G. dilator

Grynfeltt
G. hernia
G. triangle

GS
Gardner syndrome

GSA
guanidinosuccinic acid
technetium GSA

GSE
gluten-sensitive enteropathy

G&S Electroejaculator

GSH
glutathione
GSH prodrug

GSI
genuine stress incontinence

GSRS
Gastrointestinal Symptom Rating Scale

GST
glutathione S-transferase

GSUI
genuine stress urinary incontinence

GTL
glomerular tip lesion

GTL-16 gastric carcinoma cell

GTN
glyceryl trinitrate

GTP
glutamyl transpeptidase
guanosine triphosphate

GTPase-activating protein
GTP-dependent signaling protein
GTP-regulatory protein

GTSG
Gastrointestinal Tumor Study Group

GTT
gestational trophoblastic tumor

G tube

GU
gonococcal urethritis

guaiac
bicolor g. (BG)
g. gum
g. test

guaiac-impregnated slide
guaiac-negative stool
guaiac-positive stool
guanabenz
guanadrel
guanethidine
parenteral g.

guanfacine
guanidine thiocyanate
guanidinium thiocyanate buffer
guanidino compound
guanidinosuccinic acid (GSA)
guanine
dihydroxypropoxymethyl g. (DHPG)
g. nucleotide
g. nucleotide-regulatory protein
g. nucleotide-releasing factor (GNRF)

guanoclor

NOTES

guanosine
- g. monophosphate
- g. 5′-monophosphate (GMP)
- g. monophosphate pathway
- g. triphosphate (GTP)

guanoxan
guanylate cyclase
guanylyl cyclase
guarding
- abdominal g.
- involuntary g.
- muscle g.
- g. reflex
- g. sign
- voluntary g.

guard-ring tocodynamometer
guar gum
gubernacular
- g. cord
- g. vein

gubernaculum
- chorda g.

Guenzberg test
Guerin
- valve of G.

guidance
- choledochoscopic g.
- endoscopic g.
- fluoroscopic g.

guide
- catheter g.
- Coons g.
- Greenwald Roth Grip-Tip suture g.
- Grip-Tip suture g.
- image g. (IG)
- J-wire g.
- light g. (LG)
- Lunderquist-Ring torque g.
- master image g.
- Roth Grip-Tip suture g.
- soft-tipped wire g.
- suture g.
- TFE-coated wire g.
- tracer Hybrid wire g.

guided
- g. fine-needle pass
- g. percutaneous drainage
- g. transcutaneous biopsy

guided-needle aspiration cytology
guide-eye instrument
guideline
- Appropriate Use of Gastrointestinal Endoscopy g.'s
- string g.

guidewire (*See also* wire)
- Amplatz Super Stiff g.
- Bard Director g.
- Bentson floppy-tipped g.
- Bentson-type Glidewire g.
- cannula with preloaded g.
- Conceptus Robust g.
- Eder-Puestow g.
- ERCP g.
- g. exchange
- FasTrac hydrophilic coated g.
- flexible-tip g.
- floppy-tipped g.
- Geenan Endotorque g.
- Glidewire Gold surgical g.
- HPC g.
- hydrophilic-coated g.
- hydrophilic polymer-coated steerable g.
- Hydro Plus coated g.
- Jagwire g.
- Lumina g.
- Lunderquist g.
- Microvasive angled hydrophilic g.
- Microvasive Geenen Endotorque g.
- Microvasive Glidewire g.
- g. and minisnare technique
- nonconductive g.
- olive over g.
- g. passage
- Pathfinder exchange g.
- Placer g.
- slipper-tipped g.
- g. sphincterotomy
- Teflon-coated g.
- Terumo hydrophilic g.
- Terumo/Meditech g.
- Terumo-Radiofocus hydrophilic polymer-coated g.
- Wilson-Cook Protector g.
- Wilson-Cook THSF-series g.
- Wilson-Cook Tracer g.
- Zebra exchange g.

guidewire/basket lasso
guiding catheter
Guillain-Barré syndrome
guillotine
- g. incision
- g. needle biopsy

gullet
Gull renal epistaxis
gum
- guaiac g.
- guar g.
- Karaya g.

gumma
gummatous necrosis
gummosa
- periarteritis g.

gun
- Bard Biopty g.
- biopsy g.
- Biopty g.
- Cook biopsy g.

EEA stapler g.
introducer g.
Mentor g.
modified caulking g.
Moss T-anchor introducer g.
spring loaded biopsy g.
gun-barrel enterostomy
gunpowder lesion
gurgle
gurgling bowel sounds
Gussenbauer suture
gustatory
g. hyperesthesia
g. hypoesthesia
g. sweating
gustatory-salivary reflex
gut
artificial g.
caffeine g.
g. colonization
congenital malrotation of g.
g. flora
g. hormone
nervous g.
plain g.
g. rest
gut-associated
g.-a. lymphoepithelial tissue (GALT)
g.-a. lymphoid tissue (GALT)

gut-hormone profile
gutter
lateral g.
left g.
paracolic g.
right g.
guttered T tube
Guyon
G. sign
G. sound
GVAX pancreatic cancer vaccine
GVE
gastric vascular ectasia
GVHD
graft-versus-host disease
Gymnodinium breve
gynandroblastoma
Gynecare TVT support system
gynecologic laparoscopy
gynecomastia
gynecomastia-aspermatogenesis syndrome
Gyromitra
Gyrus
G. bipolar electrode
G. endourology system

NOTES

H2
  histamine-2
    H2 blocker
    H2 breath test
    H2 receptor
    H2 receptor antagonist (H2RA)
    H2 receptor-blocker
    H2 receptor-blocking drug
HA
  hyaluronan
HAA
  hepatitis-associated antigen
HAART
  highly active antiretroviral therapy
Haberer
  H. abdominal spatula
  H. intestinal clamp
  H. intestinal forceps
  vena marginalis epididymis of H.
habit
  bowel h.
  dietary h.
  drinking h.
habitus
  body h.
  marfanoid h.
Hadefield-Clarke syndrome
Hadera continent reservoir
Hadju-Cheney acroosteolysis syndrome
HAE
  hereditary angioedema
HAEC
  Hirschsprung-associated enterocolitis
haeckelii
  Psorospermium h.
haematobium
  Schistosoma h.
haemolyticus
  Haemophilus h.
Haemophilus
  H. ducreyi
  H. haemolyticus
  H. influenzae
haemorrhagica
  achylia gastrica h.
Hafnia alvei
hafniae
  Enterobacter h.
Hagner operation
HAI
  hepatic arterial infusion
  histological activity index
Hailey-Hailey disease
hair
  h. ball
  digital manipulation of pubic h.
  Frey h.
hairy
  h. leukoplakia
  h. tongue
HAL
  hand-assisted laparoscopy
Halban procedure
Halcion
Haldane effect
Haldane-Priestly tube
Hald-Bradley classification
Haldol
Hale
  H. colloidal iron stain
  H. colloidal iron technique
Haley's M-O
HALF
  hyperacute liver failure
half-body irradiation
half-Fourier acquisition single-shot turbo spin-echo (HASTE)
half-hitch knot
half-life
half-normal saline
half-strength feeding
half-time
  gastric emptying h.-t. (GET1/2)
haliphagia
halitosis
Hallberg biliointestinal bypass
Halle point
Haller
  crypt of H.
HALNU
  hand-assisted laparoscopic nephroureterectomy
halo effect
haloperidol
halothane hepatotoxicity
halothane-induced
  h.-i. disease
  h.-i. hepatitis
HALS
  hand-assisted laparoscopic surgery
Halsted
  H. anastomosis
  H. forceps
  H. hemostat
  H. hernioplasty
  H. inguinal herniorrhaphy
  H. interrupted mattress suture
  H. interrupted quilt suture
  H. method
  H. operation

Halsted-Bassini
    H.-B. hernia repair
    H.-B. herniorrhaphy
HALT-C
    hepatitis C antiviral long-term treatment to prevent cirrhosis
    HALT-C study
Haltran
Ham
    H. F12 medium
    H. test
hamartoma
    ampullary h.
    angiomatous lymphoid h.
    Brunner gland h.
    colonic h.
    cystic h.
    duodenal wall h.
    mesenchymal h.
    pancreatic h.
    Peutz-Jeghers h.
    renal h.
hamartomatous
    h. gastric polyp
    h. lesion
    h. polyposis
Hamilton deep surgery forceps
Hamilton-Thorn motility analyzer
Hammock
    H. technique
    H. technique urinary diversion
hammock
    omental h.
Hampton
    H. line
    H. sign
hand
    h. grip (HG)
    h. temperature
hand-assisted
    h.-a. laparoscopic nephroureterectomy (HALNU)
    h.-a. laparoscopic sigmoidectomy
    h.-a. laparoscopic surgery (HALS)
    h.-a. laparoscopy (HAL)
handheld retractor
Handi-Cath catheter kit
handling
    renal tubular sodium h.
    tubular sodium h.
HandPort system
handsewn anastomosis
Haney
    H. needle driver
    H. retractor
Hanger test
hanging-drop culture
hanging panniculus

Hank
    H. balanced salt solution (HBSS)
    H. buffer solution
Hanley
    H. method
    H. rectal bladder procedure
Hanot
    H. cirrhosis
    H. disease
    H. syndrome
Hanot-Chauffard syndrome
Hanot-Rössle syndrome
Hansel stain
Hansenula fabianii
H2-antagonist therapy
Hantavirus
HAP
    hepatic arterial-dominant phase
    high-amplitude peristalsis
    HAP image
hapatotoxic range
HAPC
    high-amplitude contraction
HA-PI
    hepatic arterial pulsatility index
haploid cell
haplotype
    DQ2 h.
    DR7 h.
    histocompatibility h.
    HLA DQ2 h.
    HLA DR17 h.
haptocorrin degradation
haptoglobin
    serum h.
Hara classification of gallbladder inflammation
hard
    h. adhesion
    h. sonolucent plastic cone
    h. stool
harderoporphyria
harderoporphyrinogen
Harley disease
harmonic
    h. scalpel
    h. scalpel coagulating shears
Harnal
harpoon extraction
Harrington
    H. Deaver retractor
    H. esophageal diverticulectomy
    H. forceps
    H. splanchnic retractor
Harrington-Mayo scissors
Harris
    H. band
    H. hematoxylin
    H. segregator

    H. tube
    H. tube suction
Harris-Benedict energy requirement equation
Harrison spot test
hartford
    Salmonella h.
Hartmann
    H. closure of rectum
    H. colostomy
    H. fossa
    H. operation
    H. point
    H. pouch
    H. procedure
    H. reconstruction technique
    H. solution
Hartnup
    H. disease
    H. disorder
    H. syndrome
Harvard pump
harvest
harvester
    Arandel cell h.
    Brandel cell h.
harvesting en bloc
Harvey
    H. and Bradshaw criteria
    H. Stone clamp
Harvey-Bradshaw index
Hashimoto
    H. struma
    H. thyroiditis
Hashizume endoscopic ligator kit
Hashmat shunt
Hashmat-Waterhouse shunt
Haslinger esophagoscope
Hasson
    H. bullet-tip forceps
    H. method
    H. needle-nose forceps
    H. open laparoscopy cannula
    H. ring forceps
    H. spike-tooth forceps
    H. trocar
HASTE
    half-Fourier acquisition single-shot turbo spin-echo
    HASTE sequence
HAstV
    human *Astrovirus*

HAT
    hepatic artery thrombosis
hatching
    blastocyst h.
    h. test
H+-ATPase
    vacuolar H+-ATPase
Haudek sign
Hauri technique
Hausted all-purpose chair
haustra (*pl. of* haustrum)
haustral
    h. blunting
    h. crest
    h. fold
    h. indentation
    h. marking
    h. pattern
    h. pouch
haustration
haustrum, pl. **haustra**
    cecal h.
    haustra coli
    haustra of colon
Hautmann ileal neobladder
HAV
    hepatitis A virus
Havrix
Hawaii
    H. agent
    H. virus
Hawes-Pallister-Landor syndrome
Hayem
    H. icterus
    H. jaundice
Hayes
    H. anterior resection clamp
    H. colon clamp
Hayflick phenomenon
Hay test
HB
    histamine blocker
    Tagamet HB
HBAg
    hepatitis B antigen
HBcAb
    hepatitis B core antibody
HBcAg
    hepatitis B core antigen
    HBcAg immunostaining
    recombinant HBcAg (rHBcAg)

NOTES

HBeAb, HbeAb
    hepatitis Be antibody
        HBeAb antibody
HBeAg, HbeAg
    hepatitis B early antigen
        HBeAg antigen
        HBeAg immunological study
        HBeAg positive
        purified HBeAg
HBe antibody
HB-EGF
    heparin-binding epidermal growth factor
HBIG
    hepatitis B immunoglobulin
HBOT
    hyperbaric oxygen therapy
HBsAb
    hepatitis B surface antibody
HBsAg
    hepatitis B surface antigen
        HBsAg immunological study
        HBsAg subtype
HBsAg-negative anti-HCV-negative chronic liver disease
HBSS
    Hank balanced salt solution
HBV
    hepatitis B virus
        HBV Engerix-B
        HBV genomic DNA
        HBV virion
HBV-associated DNA polymerase
HBV-specific T cell
HBVV
    hepatitis B virus vaccine
HC-1
    hydrocortisone
HCA
    hepatocellular adenoma
HCC
    hepatocellular carcinoma
HCG
    human chorionic gonadotropin
HCl
    hydrochloric acid
    hydrochloride
        alfuzosin HCl
        alosetron HCl
        alprostadil/prazosin HCl
        atrasentan HCl
        benazepril HCl
        gemcitabine HCl
        liposomal daunorubicin HCl
        lomefloxacin HCl
        1% pramoxine HCl
        sibutramine HCl
        sulamserod HCl
        tamsulosin HCl
        Tris HCl
        Vancocin HCl
        vardenafil HCl
HCN
    high calorie and nitrogen
        Isocal HCN
HCO^{3-}
    bicarbonate
        luminal HCO^{3-}
        peritubular HCO^{3-}
        HCO^{3-} reabsorption
HCP
    hereditary coproporphyria
HCS
    hematocystic spot
HCTZ
    hydrochlorothiazide
HCTZ-TA
    hydrochlorothiazide-triamterene
HCV
    hepatitis C virus
        HCV antibody
        HCV DupliType test
        HCV EIA II
        HCV ELISA test
        HCV genotype 1b
        HCV protein
        HCV QuantaSure Plus
        HCV QuantaSure Plus test
        HCV RNA
HD
    hemodialysis
HDA-DR3 gene
HDAg
    hepatitis D antigen
HDC
    high-dose chemotherapy
    histidine decarboxylase
H disease
HDL
    high-density lipoprotein
HDLC
    high-density lipoprotein cholesterol
H63D mutation
HDV
    hepatitis delta virus
    hepatitis D virus
HDVD
    high-definition video display
HE
    hepatic encephalopathy
H&E
    hematoxylin and eosin
        H&E stain
head
    Medusa h.
    h. of pancreas
    pancreatic h.
    h. symptom

headlamp
    Keeler Magnalite h.
head-mounted device
healed
    h. ulcer
    h. yellow atrophy
healing
    delayed primary intention h.
    durable h.
    h. by first intention
    glomerular capillary h.
    h. by granulation
    h. per primam intentionem
    h. per secundam intentionem
    h. by primary intention
    h. by secondary intention
    h. by second intention
    wound h.
health
    National Institutes of H. (NIH)
    h. outcome
health-related quality of life (HRQOL)
Healy intestinal forceps
Heaney
    H. clamp
    H. retractor
heaped-up edge
heart
    H. Outcomes Prevention Evaluation (HOPE)
    h. rate monitoring
    h. transplant
    h. transplantation
    Wistar-Kyoto h.
HeartBar Orange Drink
heartbeating simulator
heartburn
    nocturnal h.
    h. of pregnancy
    h. relief formula (HRF)
    spontaneous h.
    symptoms of chronic h.
heart-kidney transplant
heart-lung machine
heat
    h. exchanger
    h. probe
    h. probe thermocoagulation
    h. shock protein (HSP)
    h. therapy
heater
    h. probe (HP)
    h. probe coagulation
    h. probe therapy
    h. probe thermocoagulation
    telescope h.
heat-inactivated fetal calf serum
heating
    preferential h.
heat-labile
    h.-l. enterotoxin
    h.-l. factor (HLF)
    h.-l. toxin (LT)
heat-stable enterotoxin (ST)
heat-sterilized by autoclave
heaves
    dry h.
heavy
    h. chain deposition
    h. chain deposition disease
    h. silk suture
Hebra disease
Hectorol injection
hedrocele
heel tap test
HE9 fibroblast
Hegar
    H. intrarectal bougie
    H. rectal dilator
h-EGF
    human epidermal growth factor
Heibronn technique
heidelberg
    Salmonella h.
Heidenhain
    H. cell
    H. pouch
Heifitz clip
heilmannii
    Helicobacter h.
Heimlich maneuver
Heineke-Mikulicz
    H.-M. fashion
    H.-M. gastroenterostomy
    H.-M. incision
    H.-M. operation
    H.-M. principle
    H.-M. pyloroplasty
    H.-M. strictureplasty
Heiss
    H. flexible endoscopic scissors
    H. loop
Heister
    H. diverticulum

NOTES

Heister *(continued)*
    H. fold
    spiral valve of H.
    H. valve
Heitz-Boyer procedure
HeLa cell
helical
    H. basket
    h. coil
    h. computed tomography
    h. CT
    h. fashion
helical-ridged ureteral stent
Helicide
helicine artery
Helicobacter
    H. bilis
    H. cinaedi
    H. felis
    H. fennelliae
    H. heilmannii
    H. hepaticus
    H. pylori (HP)
    H. pylori breath excretion test
    H. pylori-induced gastritis
    H. pylori-like organism (HPLO)
    H. pylori stool antigen EIA
    H. pylori stool assay
***Helicobacter*-induced gastric injury**
Helicoblot 2.1 test
Helicosol
Helidac therapy
heliotrope sign
Heliotropium
Helisal
    H. Rapid Blood diagnostic kit
    H. rapid blood test
helium insufflation
helium-neon laser
Helivax vaccine
helix-loop-helix protein
helix-turn-helix protein
Heller
    H. cardiomyotomy
    H. esophagomyotomy
    H. myotomy
    H. operation
Heller-Belsey correction of achalasia of esophagus
Heller-Dor procedure
Heller-Nelson syndrome
Heller-Nissen correction of achalasia of esophagus
HELLP
    hemolysis, elevated liver enzymes, and low platelet count
        HELLP syndrome
Helmholtz double-surface coil
helminthemesis

helminthiasis
helminthic
    h. abscess
    h. appendicitis
    h. dysentery
    h. infection
    h. pseudotumor
helminthism
Helmstein balloon
helper T cell
Helvetius ligament
Hemaccel
hemagglutination
    indirect h. (IHA)
hemangioblastoma
    cerebral h.
    spinal h.
hemangioblastomatosis
    cerebelloretinal h.
    von Hippel-Lindau cerebellar h.
hemangioendothelial sarcoma
hemangioepithelioma
hemangioma
    capillary h.
    cavernous h.
    cutaneous h.
    hepatic h.
    h. laser treatment
    polypoid colorectal cavernous h.
    renal h.
    scrotal h.
    strawberry h.
    urethral h.
    vascular h.
hemangiomatosis
    duodenal h.
    splenic capillary h.
hemangiopericytoma
hemangiosarcoma
Hemaseel APR kit fibrin sealant
hematemesis
    Goldstein h.
Hematest test
hematin cast
hematobilia evacuation
hematocele
hematocelia (*var. of* hematocoelia)
hematochezia
    severe h.
hematochyluria
hematocoelia, hematocelia
hematocolpos
hematocrit
    hemoglobin and h. (H&H)
    multivariate analysis of h.
hematocystic spot (HCS)
hematocystis
hematocyturia
hematogenic metastasis

hematogenous
    h. micrometastasis
    h. proteinuria
    h. pyelitis
    h. pyelonephritis
    h. spread of infection
hematologic
    h. abnormality
    h. complication
    h. study
hematological stain
hematoma
    butterfly h.
    duodenal h.
    esophageal intramural h.
    expanding retroperitoneal h.
    intrahepatic h.
    intramural duodenal h. (IDH)
    kidney h.
    mesenteric h.
    parenchymal h.
    perianal h.
    perinephric h.
    perirenal h.
    pulsatile h.
    rectus abdominis h.
    rectus sheath h. (RSH)
    renal h.
    retroperitoneal h.
    septal h.
    subcapsular h.
    warfarin-associated subcapsular h.
    wound h.
hematometrocolpos
hematomphalocele
hematonephrosis
hematopathology
hematopoiesis
    extramedullary h.
    hepatic extramedullary h.
hematopoietic
    h. cell
    h. cell transplantation
    h. lineage
hematoporphyrin
    h. derivative (HpD)
    h. derivative therapy
hematoscheocele
hematospermatocele
hematospermia
hematoxylin
    h. and eosin (H&E)
    h. and eosin stain
    Harris h.
hematuresis
hematuria
    adolescent stress h.
    angioneurotic h.
    anticoagulant-induced h.
    benign familial h.
    endemic h.
    essential h.
    exercise-induced h.
    familial benign h.
    glomerular h.
    gross h.
    idiopathic h.
    initial h.
    macroscopic h.
    microscopic h.
    nonglomerular h.
    painful h.
    painless h.
    renal h.
    stress h.
    terminal h.
    total h.
    urethral h.
    vesical h.
    h. with clots
hematuria-dysuria syndrome
HemaWipe test
heme
    h. pigment-induced acute tubular necrosis
    h. test
heme-albumin
    intravenous h.-a.
heme-negative stool
heme-porphyrin assay
heme-positive
    h.-p. NG aspirate
    h.-p. stool
HemeSelect
hemiacidrin irrigation
hemianopsia
hemiballismus
hemiblock
    anterior h.
hemibody irradiation
hemicolectomy
    laparoscopic-assisted h.
hemicolon
hemicrypt column

NOTES

hemifundoplication
    Toupet h.
hemigastrectomy and vagotomy (H&V)
hemihepatectomy
hemihypertrophy
hemi-Kock
    h.-K. neobladder
    h.-K. pouch
    h.-K. procedure
    h.-K. system
    urethral h.-K.
    h.-K. urinary diversion
heminephrectomy
heminephroureterectomy
hemiorchiectomy
hemiparesis
hemiplegia
hemipylorectomy
hemipyonephrosis
hemiscrotectomy
hemiscrotum
hemispherium, pl. **hemispheria**
    h. bulbi urethra
hemi-T
    h.-T augmentation
    h.-T augmentation procedure
hemizona assay
hemobilia
Hemoccult
    H. II
    H. II card
    H. II test
    H. Sensa
    H. Sensa developer
    H. Sensa slide
    H. Sensa test
hemocholecyst
hemochromatosis
    African h.
    C282Y h.
    Desferal Mesylate challenge for h.
    genetic h. (GH)
    hereditary h. (HH)
    hereditary human leukocyte antigen-linked h.
    idiopathic h.
    non-HFE h.
    perinatal h.
    precirrhotic h.
hemochromatotic cirrhosis
hemoclip
    Hx-5LR-1 h.
hemoclipping
    h. application device
    endoscopic h.
hemoconcentration
hemocrit
    increased h.
hemoculture
hemocyanin
    keyhole limpet h. (KLH)
Hemocyte-F
    H.-F elixir
    H.-F tablet
Hemocyte Plus tablet
hemocytometer
hemodiafiltration
    continuous arteriovenous h. (CAVHDF)
    continuous venovenous h. (CVVHDF)
    double-chamber h.
    online h.
hemodialysis (HD)
    h. air embolism
    continuous arteriovenous h. (CAVHD)
    continuous venovenous h. (CVVHD)
    conventional h.
    cool-temperature h.
    daily h.
    dermatosis of h.
    frequent h.
    intermittent h. (IHD)
    nocturnal h.
    h. patient
    h. population
    sequential ultrafiltration h.
    simplified nocturnal home h. (SNHHD)
    single-pass h.
    sorbent h.
    standard h.
    h. vascular access
    venovenous continuous h.
hemodialysis-associated
    h.-a. anemia
    h.-a. ascites
hemodialyzer
    ALTRA-FLUX h.
    1550 Baxter h.
    2008E h.
    ultrafiltration h.
hemoductal pancreatitis
hemodynamics
    erection h.
    hepatic arterial h.
    intraglomerular h.
    intrarenal h.
    renal h.
hemofilter
hemofiltration
    arteriovenous h.
    continuous arteriovenous h. (CAVH)
    continuous venovenous h. (CVVH)
    simultaneous hemodialysis and h.

hemofiltration · hemorrhagic

h. therapy (HFT)
venovenous h.
hemoflagellate parasite
hemoglobin
    carbamylated h.
    h. content index (IHb)
    h. and hematocrit (H&H)
    mean corpuscular h. (MCH)
    mucosal blood h.
hemoglobinemia
    paroxysmal nocturnal h.
hemoglobinopathy
    sickle h.
hemoglobinuria
    intermittent h.
    paroxysmal nocturnal h. (PNH)
Hemoject
    H. injection catheter
    H. needle
hemolysin
hemolysis
    h., elevated liver enzymes, and low platelet count (HELLP)
    sulfasalazine-induced oxidative h.
hemolytic
    h. anemia
    h. jaundice
    h. splenomegaly
    h. streptococcus
hemolytic-uremic syndrome (HUS)
hemonephrosis
hemoperfusion
    albumin-coated resin h.
    charcoal h.
    hepatic venous isolation by direct h. (HVI-DHP)
    h. with charcoal
hemopericardium
hemoperitoneum
Hemophan membrane
hemophilia
    renal h.
hemophiliac
hemoptysis
hemopyelectasis, hemopyelectasia
HemoQuant
    H. assay
    H. fecal blood test
hemorrhage
    acute nonvariceal upper gastrointestinal h.
    adrenal h.
    bland pulmonary h.
    colonic h.
    concealed h.
    h. control
    diffuse alveolar h. (DAH)
    diverticular h.
    endoscopic stigmata of h.
    esophageal variceal h. (EVH)
    exsanguinating h.
    fetal adrenal gland h.
    gastric h.
    gastrointestinal tract h.
    Grey Turner sign of retroperitoneal h.
    hepatic h.
    h. in inflammatory bowel disease
    internal h.
    intestinal h.
    intraabdominal h.
    intracranial h.
    intramural intestinal h.
    intraperitoneal h.
    kidney h.
    lower gastrointestinal h.
    neonatal adrenal gland h.
    nonvariceal upper GI h.
    pancreatitis-related h.
    postgastrectomy h.
    postpolypectomy h.
    refractory variceal h.
    renal cyst h.
    retroperitoneal h.
    stigmata of recent h. (SRH)
    stress ulcer h.
    subcapsular h.
    subconjunctival h.
    subepithelial h.
    submucosal gastric h.
    torrential h.
    upper GI h. (UGIH)
    variceal h.
hemorrhagic
    h. ascites
    h. colitis
    h. cystitis
    h. dengue
    h. diarrhea
    h. enteritis
    h. enterocolitis
    h. fever
    h. fever with renal syndrome
    h. gastritis

NOTES

hemorrhagic *(continued)*
  h. gastropathy
  h. hypotension
  h. necrotizing pancreatitis
  h. nephritis
  h. nephrosonephritis
  h. radiation injury
  h. speck
  h. telangiectasia
hemorrhoid
  bleeding h.
  cloverleaf excision of h.
  combined h.'s
  dilation of h.
  external h.
  h. grade
  internal h.
  ligation of h.
  Lord dilation of h.
  mixed h.'s
  mucocutaneous h.'s
  necrotic h.
  prolapsed internal h.
  prolapsing fourth-degree h.
  h. reduction
  rubber band ligation of h.
  strangulated h.
  thrombosed internal and
    external h.'s
hemorrhoidal
  h. banding
  h. clamp
  h. cushion
  h. plexus
  h. prolapse
  h. sclerotherapy
  h. tag
  h. zone
hemorrhoidectomy
  ambulatory h.
  closed h.
  diathermy h.
  Ferguson h.
  laser h.
  Longo h.
  Lord method of h.
  Milligan-Morgan h.
  modified Whitehead h.
  open h.
  radical h.
  semiopen h.
  stapled h.
  sutured h.
HemoSelect test
hemosiderin
  h. deposit
  h. granule
hemosiderin-laden macrophage
hemosiderosis

hemospermia
  h. spuria
  h. vera
HemoSplit catheter
hemostasis
  endoscopic h.
hemostat
  Carmalt h.
  Crile h.
  curved h.
  Endo-Assist disposable h.
  Endo-Avitene microfibrillar
    collagen h.
  Halsted h.
  Kelly h.
  Kocher h.
  microfibrillar collagen h. (MCH)
  Mixter h.
  mosquito h.
  Ochsner h.
  Rochester-Péan h.
  Westphal h.
hemostatic
  h. agent
  h. bond strength
  h. clamp
  h. surgical glue
  h. suture
  h. therapy
hemosuccus pancreaticus
HemoTherapies liver dialysis unit
hemothorax
hemotympanum
Hemovac Suction Standard drain
hemp seed calculus
hemuresis
Henderson-Hasselbalch equation
Hendren
  H. clamp
  H. technique
Henke triangle
Henle
  H. ampulla
  H. band
  H. internal cremaster
  internal cremaster of H.
  loop of H. (LH)
  H. loop
  H. sphincter
  H. tubule
Henning sign
Henoch-Schönlein purpura
Henry approach
henselae
  Bartonella h.
Hensing fold
Hepa
  Amino Mel H.
Hepadnaviridae

hepadnavirus
Hepahydrin
Hepaplastin test
hepar
    h. adiposum
    h. lobatum
heparan sulfate proteoglycan (HSPG)
heparin
    h. bolus
    glycosaminoglycan h.
    intravesical h.
    low molecular weight h. (LMWH)
heparinase
heparin-binding
    h.-b. epidermal growth factor (HB-EGF)
    h.-b. growth factor-1
heparin-induced
    h.-i. lipolysis
    h.-i. thrombocytopenia (HIT)
heparinization
    regional h.
heparinized saline
hepatalgia
HepatAmine amino acid solution
HepatAssist Liver Support System
hepatectomy
    donor h.
    extended right h.
    partial h.
    recipient h.
    triple-lobe h.
hepatic
    h. abnormality
    h. abscess
    h. adenoma
    h. adhesion
    h. allograft
    h. amebiasis
    h. amyloidosis
    h. angiomatosis
    h. angiosarcoma
    h. architecture
    h. arterial-dominant phase (HAP)
    h. arterial hemodynamics
    h. arterial infusion (HAI)
    h. arterial infusion chemotherapy
    h. arterial pulsatility index (HA-PI)
    h. arterial vascular resistance
    h. arteriogram
    h. arteriography
    h. artery
    h. artery aneurysm
    h. artery infusion pump
    h. artery ligation
    h. artery thrombosis (HAT)
    h. bed
    h. bifurcation
    h. blood flow
    h. blood pool scan
    h. calculus
    h. candidal infection
    h. capsule
    h. capsulitis
    h. circulation
    h. cirrhosis
    h. clearance
    h. clonorchiasis
    h. colic
    h. coma
    h. congestion
    h. copper overload
    h. cord
    h. cystadenoma
    h. cystic disease
    h. deformability
    h. diverticulum
    h. duct
    h. duct stone
    h. dullness
    h. echinococcal cyst
    h. echinococcosis
    h. edge
    h. encephalopathy (HE)
    h. endothelialis
    h. extramedullary hematopoiesis
    h. fascioliasis
    h. fibrosis
    h. fistula
    h. flexure
    h. flexure of colon
    h. funiculus
    h. funiculus of Rauber
    h. glycogen store
    h. granuloma
    h. hemangioma
    h. hemorrhage
    h. hilar region
    h. hilum
    h. Hodgkin disease
    h. hydrothorax
    h. hypoxia
    h. insufficiency
    h. intermittent fever

NOTES

hepatic *(continued)*
    h. iron concentration (HIC)
    h. iron index (HII)
    h. lectin
    h. leiomyosarcoma
    h. ligament
    h. lipase (HL)
    h. lobectomy
    h. malignancy
    h. malondialdehyde content
    h. mass lesion
    h. metabolism
    h. metastatic disease
    h. 3-methylglutaryl coenzyme A reductase (HMG-CoA)
    h. osteodystrophy
    h. outflow tract
    h. parenchyma
    h. peliosis
    h. perfusion index (HPI)
    h. phosphorylase deficiency
    h. porphyria
    h. resection
    h. rudiment
    h. rupture
    h. sarcoidosis
    h. schistosomiasis
    h. sclerosis
    h. segmentectomy
    h. sinusoid
    h. span
    h. steatosis
    h. stellate cell (HSC)
    h. stimulatory substance (HSS)
    h. subcellular element
    h. subsegmentectomy
    h. telangiectasia
    h. toxemia
    h. trauma
    h. triad
    h. triglyceride lipase (HTGL)
    h. tumor
    h. tumor index (HTI)
    h. uptake
    h. urea
    h. uroporphyrinogen decarboxylase activity
    h. vein (HV)
    h. vein catheterization
    h. vein injury
    h. vein occlusion
    h. vein thrombosis
    h. vein wedge pressure
    h. venogram
    h. venography
    h. venoocclusive disease
    h. venous isolation by direct hemoperfusion (HVI-DHP)
    h. venous outflow
    h. venous outflow obstruction (HVOO)
    h. venous pressure
    h. venous pressure gradient (HVPG)
    h. venous pressure gradient reduction
    h. venous web disease
    h. venule
    h. web
    h. web dilation
    h. wedge pressure
hepatica
    facies h.
    Fasciola h.
Hepatic-Aid powdered feeding
hepatic-alveolar echinococcosis
hepaticocholedochostomy
hepaticocystic junction
hepaticodochotomy
hepaticoduodenostomy
hepaticoenterostomy
hepaticogastrostomy
hepaticojejunal anastomosis
hepaticojejunostomy
    Roux-en-Y h.
hepaticoliasis
hepaticolithotomy
hepaticolithotripsy
hepaticopulmonary fistula
hepaticostomy
hepaticotomy
hepatic-to-renal
    h.-t.-r. artery saphenous vein bypass
    h.-t.-r. artery saphenous vein bypass graft
hepaticus
    fetor h.
    Helicobacter h.
    peliosis h.
hepatis
    area nuda h.
    facies diaphragmatica h.
    facies inferior h.
    facies posterior h.
    facies superior h.
    facies visceralis h.
    impressio esophagealis h.
    incisura vesicae felleae h.
    ligamentum teres h.
    peliosis h.
    pons h.
    ponticulus h.
    porta h.
hepatitic
hepatitis, pl. **hepatitides**
    h. A
    active chronic h.

acute h. (AH)
acute alcoholic h.
acute mononucleosis-like h.
acute parenchymatous h.
acute self-limited h.
acute viral h. (AVH)
h. A inactivated & hepatitis B recombinant vaccine
alcoholic h. (AH)
amebic h.
anesthetic h.
anicteric viral h.
autoimmune h. (AIH)
h. A virus (HAV)
h. B
h. B antigen (HBAg)
h. B core antibody (HBcAb)
h. B core antigen (HBcAg)
h. B DNA detection
h. Be antibody (HBeAb, HbeAb)
h. Be antigen
h. B early antigen (HBeAg, HbeAg)
h. B hyperimmune globulin
h. B immunoglobulin (HBIG)
h. B-like DNA
h. B-like DNA virus
bloodborne non-A non-B h.
h. B surface antibody (HBsAb)
h. B surface antigen (HBsAg)
h. B surface antigen subdeterminant
h. B virus (HBV)
h. B virus-encoded antigen
h. B virus vaccine (HBVV)
h. C
h. C antiviral long-term treatment to prevent cirrhosis (HALT-C)
capsula fibrosa h.
h. carrier
cholangiolitic h.
cholestatic viral h.
chronic h. (CH)
chronic active h. (CAH)
chronic active viral h. (CAVH)
chronic active viral h. non-A non-B (CAVH-NAB)
chronic active viral h., type B (CAVH-B)
chronic aggressive h. (CAH)
chronic autoimmune h.
chronic benign h. (CBH)

chronic fibrosing h.
chronic interstitial h.
chronic lobular h. (CLH)
chronic persistent h. (CPH)
chronic progressive h.
chronic type B h.
chronic viral h.
cryptogenic chronic h.
h. C viremia
h. C virus (HCV)
h. C virus-associated venoocclusive disease
h. C virus DupliType test
h. C virus enzyme immunoassay
h. C virus genotype
h. C virus RNA
h. C virus RNA detection
cytomegalovirus h.
h. D
h. D antigen (HDAg)
delta agent h.
h. delta virus (HDV)
de novo autoimmune h.
drug-induced h.
h. D superinfection
h. D virus (HDV)
h. E
ENANB h.
enterically transmitted non-A non-B h. (ET-NANBH)
epidemic h.
h. E virus (HEV)
h. F
familial h.
fatty liver h.
fibrosing cholestatic h. B
flucloxacillin-induced delayed cholestatic h.
fulminant h. A–E
fulminant viral h. (FVH)
giant cell h.
granulomatous h.
h. G virus (HGV)
halothane-induced h.
herpetic h.
hyperglobulinemic h.
idiopathic autoimmune chronic h.
inapparent h.
h. infection A–E
infectious h.
interface h.
intrahepatic h.

NOTES

hepatitis *(continued)*
    ischemic h.
    isoniazid-induced h.
    lobular h.
    long incubation h.
    lupoid h.
    malarial h.
    MS-1, -2 h.
    murine h.
    NANB h.
    neonatal h.
    newborn h.
    non-A–E h.
    non-A–G fulminant h.
    non-A non-B h.
    non-A non-B, non-C h.
    non-A non-B posttransfusion h.
    nonspecific reactive h.
    normal carrier h.
    occult h.
    oxacillin-associated anicteric h.
    persistent chronic h.
    persistent viral h. (PVH)
    persistent viral h. non-A, non-B (PVH-NANB)
    persistent viral h. type B (PVH-B)
    plasma cell h.
    posttransfusion h.
    quiescent h.
    h. serologic marker
    serum h.
    short incubation h.
    spontaneous reactivation of h.
    subacute h.
    subclinical h.
    superimposed alcoholic h.
    syphilitic h.
    terbutaline h.
    toxic h.
    transfusion h.
    transfusion-associated h.
    h. type 1
    type 1, 2 autoimmune h.
    viral h.
    viral h. type A, B
    virus A, B h.
hepatitis-associated antigen (HAA)
Hepatix device
hepatization
hepatobiliary
    h. capsule
    h. cholescintigraphy
    h. fibropolycystic disease
    h. malignancy
    h. manifestation
    h. scan
    h. scintigraphy
    h. tract disease
    h. tree

hepatoblastoma
hepatocanalicular
    h. cholestasis
    h. jaundice
hepatocarcinogenesis
hepatocarcinogenic
hepatocarcinoma
    fibrolamellar h.
hepatocele
hepatocellular
    h. adenoma (HCA)
    h. adnexa
    h. atypia
    h. ballooning
    h. basolateral plasma membrane fluidity
    h. carcinoma (HCC)
    h. cholestasis
    h. death
    h. disease
    h. injury
    h. jaundice
    h. necrosis
    h. protein
hepatocerebral degeneration
hepatocholangeitis
hepatocholangiocarcinoma
hepatocholangiocystoduodenostomy
hepatocholangioduodenostomy
hepatocholangioenterostomy
hepatocholangiogastrostomy
hepatocholangiojejunostomy
hepatocholangiostomy
hepatocholangitis
hepatocirrhosis
hepatocolic ligament
hepatocystic
Hepatocystis
hepatocystocolic ligament
hepatocyte
    ballooned h.
    ballooning degeneration of h.
    cobblestone pattern of h.
    ground-glass h.
    h. growth factor (HGF)
    lipid-laden h.
    h. lysosome
    h. necrosis
    periportal h.
    polygonal h.
    porcine h.
    h. proliferation inhibitor (HPI)
    h. protein synthesis
    pseudoductular transformation of h.
    h. transplantation
hepatocytes
hepatocyte-type cytokeratin
hepatocytic cord

hepatoduodenal
    h. ligament
    h. reflection
hepatoduodenal-peritoneal reflection
hepatoduodenostomy
hepatodynia
hepatodysentery
hepatoenterostomy
hepatofugal
    h. arterioportal shunt
    h. flow
    h. portosystemic venous shunt
hepatogastric ligament
hepatogastroduodenal ligament
hepatogastroenterology
hepatogenic, hepatogenous
    h. jaundice
hepatography
hepatohemia
hepatoid adenocarcinoma
hepatoiminodiacetic acid (HIDA)
hepatojugular reflux
hepatolenticular
    h. degeneration
    h. disease
hepatolith
hepatolithectomy
hepatolithiasis
hepatologist
hepatology
hepatoma
    fibrolamellar h.
hepatomegaly
    congestive h.
hepatomphalocele
hepatomphalos
hepatonephoric syndrome
hepatonephromegaly
hepatopancreatica
    ampulla h.
hepatopancreatic fold
hepatopancreatoduodenectomy
hepatopathic
hepatopathy
    radiation h.
hepatopetal flow
hepatopexy
hepatophosphorylase-deficiency glycogenosis
hepatophrenic ligament
hepatopleural fistula
hepatoportal sclerosis

hepatoportoenterostomy
    Kasai-type h.
hepatoptosis
hepatopulmonary syndrome (HPS)
hepatorenal
    h. angle
    h. bypass
    h. glycogenosis
    h. ligament
    h. space of Morison
    h. syndrome (HRS)
hepatorrhagia
hepatorrhaphy
hepatorrhea
hepatorrhexis
hepatoscopy
hepatosplenic T-cell lymphoma
hepatosplenomegaly
hepatosplenopathy
hepatostomy
hepatotherapy
hepatotomy
hepatotoxemia
hepatotoxic
hepatotoxicity
    acetaminophen h.
    Amanita mushroom h.
    anesthetic h.
    anticonvulsant agent h.
    antidepressant drug h.
    antidiabetic agent h.
    antineoplastic drug h.
    antipsychotic drug h.
    antithyroid drug h.
    carbamazepine h.
    cardiovascular drug h.
    chemotherapeutic agent h.
    cocaine h.
    cyclosporine A-induced h.
    drug h.
    erythromycin estolate h.
    halothane h.
    hydrazide h.
    nitrofurantoin h.
    2-nitropropane h.
    phenylbutazone h.
    potentiation of drug h.
    valproic acid h.
    yellow phosphorus h.
hepatotoxin
hepatoumbilical ligament
Hep-B-Gammagee

NOTES

HepBzyme
HEPES
    H. buffer
    H. solution
hepG2 cell
Heprofile ELISA
Hepsera
heptacarboxyl
heptahelical receptor protein
Heptalac
Heptavax-B
Heptazyme
HEPTIMAX hepatitis C viral load test
HER-2/neu oncogene
heracleifolia
    Cimicifuga h.
herald
    h. bleed
    h. patch
Herbgels
    BioFIT H.
Herculink Plus biliary stent
hereditary
    h. angioedema (HAE)
    h. coproporphyria (HCP)
    h. flat adenoma syndrome (HFAS)
    h. fructose intolerance
    h. hemochromatosis (HH)
    h. hemorrhagic telangiectasia (HHT)
    h. human leukocyte antigen-linked hemochromatosis
    h. internal anal sphincter myopathy
    h. nephritis
    h. nonpolyposis colon cancer (HNPCC)
    h. nonpolyposis colorectal cancer
    h. nonpolyposis colorectal cancer syndrome
    h. nonpolyposis colorectal carcinoma
    h. osteoonychodysplasia
    h. pancreatitis (HP)
    h. papillary renal cancer (HPRC)
    h. prostate cancer 1 locus (HPC-1)
    h. spastic paraplegia voiding dysfunction
    h. tyrosinemia
Hering
    canal of H.
Herlitz junctional epidermolysis bullosa
Hermansky-Pudlak syndrome
Herman-Taylor gastroscope
hermaphroditism, hermaphroditismus
hermetically
hernia, pl. **herniae**
    abdominal wall h.
    acquired h.
    antevesical h.
    axial hiatal h.

Barth h.
Béclard h.
bladder h.
Bochdalek h.
cecal h.
Cheatle-Henry h.
Cloquet h.
combined hiatal h.
congenital diaphragmatic h.
Cooper h.
diaphragmatic h. (DH)
direct inguinal h.
duodenojejunal h.
easily reducible h.
enterocele-like central h.
epigastric h.
femoral h.
foramen of Bochdalek h.
funicular inguinal h.
gastroesophageal h.
Gibbon h.
Gironcoli h.
Goyrand h.
Grynfeltt h.
Hesselbach h.
Hey h.
hiatal h.
Holthouse h.
h. hydrocele
incarcerated intrathoracic h.
h. incarceration
incisional h.
incomplete h.
indirect inguinal h.
inguinal h. (IH)
inguinofemoral h.
inguinoscrotal h.
inguinosuperficial h.
interstitial h.
intraepiploic h.
intrailiac h.
irreducible h.
h. knife
Krönlein h.
Larrey h.
lateral ventral h.
Laugier h.
Lesgaft h.
levator ani h.
Littré h.
Madden repair of incisional h.
Maydl h.
mesenteric h.
mesentericoparietal h.
mesocolic h.
metachronous contralateral hernias
Morgagni h.
multiorgan h.
obturator h.

occult levator ani h.
pantaloon h.
paracolostomy h.
paraduodenal h.
paraesophageal diaphragmatic h.
paraesophageal hiatal h.
paraesophageal h. type I, II
parahiatal h.
paraileostomal h.
parapubic h.
parastomal h.
parietal h.
h. pouch
properitoneal h.
reducible h.
h. repair
retrograde h.
retroperitoneal h.
retrosternal h.
Richter h.
Rieux h.
right inguinal h. (RIH)
Rokitansky h.
rolling hiatal h.
h. sac
sciatic h.
scrotal h.
sliding esophageal hiatal h.
spigelian h.
h. stapler
strangulated h.
traumatic diaphragmatic h.
Treitz h.
umbilical h.
ureteral h.
h. uteri inguinale
Velpeau h.
ventral h.
vesicle h.
voluminous hiatus h.
w h.

hernial defect
herniated preperitoneal fat
herniation
    paracolostomy h.
    ureteroneocystostomy h.
hernioenterotomy
herniolaparotomy
hernioplasty
    Cooper ligament h.
    Halsted h.
    Lichtenstein open tension-free mesh h.
    mesh-plug h.
    open mesh-plug h.

herniorrhaphy
    Anson-McVay femoral h.
    Bassini inguinal h.
    Halsted-Bassini h.
    Halsted inguinal h.
    Hill hiatus h.
    Lichtenstein h.
    Macewen h.
    Madden incisional h.
    McVay h.
    pants-over-vest h.
    Ponka h.
    Shouldice inguinal h.
    ventral h.
    vest-over-pants h.

herniotome
    Cooper h.
herniotomy
herpangina
herpes
    anorectal h.
    h. labialis
    h. pharyngitis
    h. progenitalis
    h. simplex
    h. simplex esophagitis
    h. simplex infection
    h. simplex virus (HSV)
    h. simplex virus-thymidine kinase (HSK-tk)
    h. zoster
    h. zoster virus
herpesvirus
    Kaposi sarcoma-associated h.
    h. simplex (HVS)
herpetic
    h. esophagitis
    h. gingivostomatitis
    h. hepatitis
    h. stomatitis
    h. ulcer
herpetiform esophagitis
herpetiformis
    dermatitis h. (DH)
Herrick kidney clamp
herring worm
herring-worm disease
Hers disease

NOTES

Herter
    H. disease
    H. infantilism
Herter-Heubner disease
Herzberg test
hesitancy
    urinary h.
Hesselbach
    H. hernia
    H. ligament
    H. triangle
Hess operation
HETE
    hydroxyeicosatetraenoic acid
heterochromatin
heteroconjugate
    antilymphocyte h.
heterodimer
heterodimeric
    h. glycoprotein
    h. protein
heteroduplex analysis
heterogeneity
    cancer cell h.
    genetic h.
    intratumoral h.
heterogeneous
    h. pseudocyst
    h. texture
heterologous
    h. anti-GBM antibody
    h. liver perfusion
heterotopia, heterotopy
    fundic gland h.
    gastric h.
heterotopic
    h. cylindric ciliated epithelium
    h. diversion
    h. gastric mucosa
    h. pancreas
heterotopic-aberrant pancreas
heterotopy (*var. of* heterotopia)
heterotrimer
heterotrimeric G protein
heterozygosity
heterozygote
heterozygous
    h. DR5
    h. ornithine transcarbamylase (HOTC)
HE-TUMT
    high-energy transurethral microwave thermotherapy
Hetzel-Dent
    H.-D. classification
    H.-D. esophagitis grade
    H.-D. scale
Heubner-Herter disease

HEV
    hepatitis E virus
Hewlett-Packard IVUS imaging system
Hexabrix
Hexacrol Phosphate
hexagon snare
hexamethonium bromide
hexobarbital
hexocyclium
hexokinase (HK)
Hexvix
Hey
    H. hernia
    H. ligament
Heyde syndrome
Heyer-Schulte
    H.-S. Small-Carrion sizing set
    H.-S. stent
Heymann
    H. antibody
    H. nephritis
    H. nephritis antigenic complex (HNAC)
    H. nephrosis
HFAS
    hereditary flat adenoma syndrome
HFE **gene**
HFT
    hemofiltration therapy
HFU
    high-intensity focused ultrasound
HFUPS
    high-frequency ultrasound probe sonography
HG
    hand grip
    high grade
        Cobe Centrysystem dialyzer 400 HG
HgCl2
    mercury chloride
HGD
    high-grade dysplasia
HGF
    hepatocyte growth factor
    human growth factor
        recombinant HGF
HGF-stimulated renal epithelial cell
HGV
    hepatitis G virus
HH
    hereditary hemochromatosis
H&H
    hemoglobin and hematocrit
H3 histone
HHM
    humoral hypercalcemia of malignancy
HHT
    hereditary hemorrhagic telangiectasia

HIAA
  hydroxyindoleacetic acid
5-HIAA
  5-hydroxyindoleacetic acid
hiatal
  h. esophagism
  h. hernia
hiatus
  aortic h.
  diaphragmatic h.
  h. hernia
  patulous h.
  vaginal h.
  vena cava h.
Hibiclens
Hibidil solution
Hibistat
Hibond N+ nylon membrane
HIC
  hepatic iron concentration
hiccup, hiccough, pl. **hiccups**
HIDA
  hepatoiminodiacetic acid
  HIDA scan
  ^{99m}Tc HIDA
hidden antigen
hidradenitis suppurativa
hiemis
  hyperemesis h.
HIFU
  high-intensity focused ultrasound
Higgins India ink
high
  h. abdominal plain film
  h. anion gap metabolic acidosis
  h. calorie
  h. calorie and nitrogen (HCN)
  h. enema
  h. failure rate
  h. false-positive rate
  h. fundal lesion
  h. grade (HG)
  h. intermuscular abscess
  h. intraluminal pressure
  h. ligation
  h. ligation of hernia sac
  h. lithotomy
  h. neurological lesion
  h. nitrogen (HN)
  h. rectal washout
  h. resting anal pressure
  h. risk for endocarditis
  h. small bowel obstruction
  h. subtotal gastrectomy
  h. testis
  h. transection
  h. transection of inferior mesenteric artery
high-affinity
  h.-a. low-capacity system
  h.-a. receptor
  h.-a. sodium-dependent phosphate transport system
high-altitude endoscopy
high-amplitude
  h.-a. contraction (HAPC)
  h.-a. peristalsis (HAP)
high-bulk, low-fat diet
high-calcium dialysate
high-calorie diet
high-carbohydrate diet
high-ceiling diuretic
high-compliance latex balloon
high-definition video display (HDVD)
high-density
  h.-d. lipoprotein (HDL)
  h.-d. lipoprotein cholesterol (HDLC)
  V33W h.-d. endocavity probe
high-diameter dilator
high-dose
  h.-d. chemotherapy (HDC)
  h.-d. consensus interferon
  h.-d. intravenous urography
  h.-d. IVU
  h.-d. pulse steroid
high-echoic area
high-efficiency dialysis
high-ending vagina
high-energy
  h.-e. amplitude
  h.-e. modification
  h.-e. protocol
  h.-e. transurethral microwave thermotherapy (HE-TUMT)
  h.-e. TUMT
higher
  h. host susceptibility
  h. incidence of rejection
high-fat diet
high-fiber diet
high-flow priapism
high-flux
  h.-f. dialysis
  h.-f. dialysis membrane

NOTES

high-flux *(continued)*
    h.-f. dialyzer
    h.-f. polysulfone
    h.-f. polysulfone membrane
high-frequency
    h.-f. electrosurgical current
    h.-f. endosonography
    h.-f. hemostatic forceps
    h.-f. intraluminal ultrasound
    h.-f. miniprobe
    h.-f. ultrasound probe sonography (HFUPS)
high-grade
    h.-g. cholestasis
    h.-g. dysplasia (HGD)
    h.-g. hydronephrosis
    h.-g. obstruction
    h.-g. synchronous colon cancer
    h.-g. tumor
high-intensity
    h.-i. focused ultrasonography
    h.-i. focused ultrasound (HFU, HIFU)
high-level disinfection (HLD)
highlight
    human genome h.
high-loop cutaneous ureterostomy
highly
    h. active antiretroviral therapy (HAART)
    h. selective group of patients
    h. selective vagotomy
high-lying side
high-magnification
    h.-m. colonoscopy
    h.-m. endoscopy
    h.-m. gastroscopy
Highmore
    H. body
    H. corpus
Highmori
    corpus H.
high-pass filtering
high-performance liquid chromatography (HPLC)
high-pitched bowel sounds
high-power
    h.-p. field (hpf)
    h.-p. photomicrograph
high-pressure
    h.-p. antireflux barrier
    h.-p. arterial baroreceptor
    h.-p. inflatable prosthesis cylinder
    h.-p. liquid chromatography (HPLC)
    h.-p. zone (HPZ)
high-protein diet
high-resolution
    h.-r. endoluminal sonography (HRES)
    h.-r. endoscopy
    h.-r. real-time scanner
    h.-r. ultrasonography
high-riding bladder
high-roughage diet
high-sensitivity collimator
high-speed electrical tissue morcellator
high-starch diet
high-velocity flow
HII
    hepatic iron index
hila (*pl. of* hilum)
hilar
    h. bile duct stenting
    h. carcinoma
    h. cholangiocarcinoma
    h. clamp
    h. mass
    h. plate
    h. retractor
    h. structure scar tissue
hill
    H. antireflux operation
    h. diarrhea
    H. esophageal antireflux repair
    H. esophageal fundoplication
    H. esophageal gastroenterostomy
    H. hiatus hernia repair
    H. hiatus herniorrhaphy
    H. median arcuate repair
    H. posterior gastropexy
    H. rectal retractor
Hill-Ferguson rectal retractor
Hilton white line
hilum, pl. **hila**
    hepatic h.
    renal h.
    h. renale
    h. renalis
    splenic h.
    h. stimulation
    h. of suprarenal gland
hilus
    liver h.
    renal h.
hindgut
    h. carcinoid
    h. dysfunction
    h. pattern
hind kidney
Hind-SITE 20/20 system
Hinkle-James rectal speculum
Hinman
    H. procedure
    H. reflux
    H. syndrome
Hinman-Allen syndrome
Hippel-Lindau syndrome
hippocratic succussion

Hippuran clearance technique
hippurate
    methenamine h.
hippuric acid
Hiprex
hirschfeldii
    Salmonella h.
Hirschmann
    H. anoscope
    H. pile clamp
    H. speculum
Hirschowitz
    H. endoscope
    H. gastroduodenal fiberscope
    H. gastroscope
Hirschsprung-associated enterocolitis (HAEC)
Hirschsprung disease
hirsute papilloma of penis
hirsutism
    adrenal h.
hirsutoid papilloma
His
    angle of H.
    bundle of H.
Hismanal
Histalog stimulation test
histamine
    h. blocker (HB)
    h. dihydrochloride
    h. fish poisoning
    h. H2 antagonist
    h. test
histamine-2 (H2)
    h.-2 receptor antagonist (H2RA)
histamine-fast
histamine-producing mast cell
histamine-releasing factor (HRF)
histamine-resistant achlorhydria
histaminergic type 2 receptor
histatin
histidine
    h. decarboxylase (HDC)
    h. residue
histidine decarboxylase (HDC)
histiocyte
    pigmented h.
histiocytic lymphoma
histiocytoma
    fibrous h.
    kidney malignant fibrous h.

histiocytosis
    Langerhans cell h.
    malignant h.
Histoacryl injection
histochemical pattern
histochemical-ultrastructural analysis
histochemistry
histocompatibility
    h. antigen
    h. complex
    h. haplotype
    h. testing
histocytochemical technique
Histofine
    H. SAB kit
    H. SAB-PO kit
histogram flattening
histologic
    h. anal canal
    h. cirrhosis
    h. damage
    h. diagnosis
    h. grading
    h. patchiness
    h. sign
histological
    h. activity index (HAI)
    h. chronic active gastritis
    h. esophagitis
histology
    bladder h.
histolytica
    Entamoeba h.
histometry
histomorphometric
histone
    H3 h.
histopathologic
    h. criterion
    h. nature of tumor
histopathology
    renal h.
Histoplasma capsulatum
histoplasmosis
    disseminated h.
    duodenal h.
    gastrointestinal h.
    intestinal h.
    mediastinal h.
    recurrent colonic h.
history
    positive family h.

NOTES

history (continued)
    psychosexual h.
    significant clinical h.
histrelin implant
histrionic personality
HIT
    heparin-induced thrombocytopenia
Hitachi
    H. 717 analyzer
    H. 737 autoanalyzer
    H. F-2000 fluorescence spectrophotometer
hitch
    psoas h.
hit-skip distribution
HIV
    human immunodeficiency virus
    HIV infection
    HIV P24 antigen
HIV-1 enteropathy
HIVAN
    human immunodeficiency virus-associated nephropathy
hive
Hi-Vegi-Lip
HK
    hexokinase
    HK enzyme
hK3
H+/K+-ATPase
    H+/K+-ATPase acid pump inhibitor
    H+/K+-ATPase enzyme system
H-K-ATPase proton pump
HL
    hepatic lipase
HLA
    human leukocyte antigen
    HLA class II phenotype
    HLA class II restricted
    HLA class II-restricted interferon-gamma
    HLA class II-restricted T-cell epitope
    HLA DQ2 haplotype
    HLA DR
    HLA DR3
    HLA DR4
    HLA DR17 haplotype
    HLA identical kidney graft
    HLA mismatch
    solubilized HLA
    HLA typing
    HLA typing immunological study
HLA-A, B
HLA-B8
HLA **class II gene**
HLA-DP allele
HLA-DQ2
    HLA-DQ2 marker
    HLA-DQ2 molecule
HLA-DQ8 marker
HLA-DQ typing
HLA-DQw2 **gene**
HLA-DR
    HLA-DR antigen
    HLA-DR DNA typing
    HLA-DR matching
HLA-DR+
HLA-DR2 subtyping
HLA-DR3 **gene**
HLA-identical sibling
HLA-matched kidney
HLD
    high-level disinfection
HLF
    heat-labile factor
    HLF cell
HLG
    hypertrophic lymphocytic gastritis
HM4
    HM4 lithotriptor
^{1}**H magnetic resonance spectroscopy**
HMB-45
    HMB-45 monoclonal antibody
    HMB-45 monoclonal antibody marker
HM-CAP serological test
HMG-CoA
    hepatic 3-methylglutaryl coenzyme A reductase
hMLH1 **gene**
HN
    high nitrogen
    hypertensive nephrosclerosis
    HN feeding
HNAC
    Heymann nephritis antigenic complex
H-600 normothermic irrigation
HNPCC
    hereditary nonpolyposis colon cancer
hobnailed cell
hobnail liver
Hochenegg operation
hockey-stick incision
Hodge intestinal decompression tube
Hodgkin disease
Hodgson
    H. technique of modified Lich procedure
    H. XX procedure
hoe
    Joe h.
Hoefer GS 300 laser densitometer
Hoehn and Yahr stage
Hoesch test
Hoffmann-Steinberg gastric reservoir

Hofmeister
    H. anastomosis
    H. gastroenterostomy
    H. operation
    H. procedure
    H. technique
Hofmeister-Pólya anastomosis
Hofmeister-Shoemaker gastrojejunostomy
Hogan/Geenen criteria
Hoguet maneuver
H_2O_2-induced injury
holder
    Adson needle h.
    Bihrle dorsal clamp-T-C needle h.
    Bookler swivel-ball laparoscope h.
    Bovie h.
    Capillary System slide h.
    Cath-Secure catheter h.
    Crile-Wood needle h.
    Dale Foley catheter h.
    DeMartel-Wolfson clamp h.
    diamond-jaw needle h.
    Endo-Assist disposable needle h.
    Jacobson needle h.
    Kilner needle h.
    Lloyd-Davis knee and leg h.
    Mason needle h.
    Mayo-Hegar needle h.
    microneedle h.
    microvascular needle h.
    needle h.
    Sarot needle h.
    Stratte needle h.
    T-C needle h.
    Young needle h.
hold-up
    bolus h.-u.
Holinger esophagoscope
Hollander test
Hollande solution
Hollenhorst plaque
hollisae
    Vibrio h.
Hollister
    H. Convex insert
    H. First Choice pouch
    H. Guardian F skin barrier
    H. Holligard pouch
    H. irrigator drain
    H. Karaya 5 ostomy pouch
    H. Karaya Seal pouch
    H. Premium paste
    H. Premium pouch
    H. urostomy bag
hollow-fiber dialyzer
hollow viscus
holmium
    h. laser
    h. laser resection of prostate (HoLRP)
holmium-aluminum-garnet lithotripsy
holmium:YAG laser
holmium:yttrium aluminum garnet (Ho:YAG)
holodiastolic
Hologic densitometer
holosystolic
HoLRP
    holmium laser resection of prostate
Holter
    H. Pediatric Pump 903, 907
    H. valve
    vesicovaginal H.
Holthouse hernia
Holt-Oram syndrome
Holyoke
    H. brief
    H. pants
homatropine methylbromide
home
    H. Care Simplimatt Plus zoned foam mattress
    h. dialysis
    H. gland
    H. lobe
    h. parenteral nutrition (HPN)
    h. screening test
    h. uroflowmetry
homeostasis
    calcium h.
    calcium-phosphate h.
    sodium h.
homeostatic therapy
Homer Wright rosette
HomeSelect test
homing
    lymphoblast h.
hominis
    Blastocystis h.
    Gastrospirillum h.
    Mycoplasma h.
    Trichomonas h.
homocladic anastomosis

NOTES

homocysteine
    h. level
    plasma h.
    protein-bound h.
    total h. (tHcy)
homocystinuria
homodimer
homodimerization
    ligand-dependent receptor h.
homogenate
    cecal h.
    fecal h.
    mucosal h.
    sphincter of Oddi h.
homogeneity
    assumption of h.
homogenous, homogeneous
    h. ablation
    h. cooling
    h. nucleation
    h. radioimmunoassay
    h. texture
homologous
    h. protein overload disease
    h. serum jaundice
homosexual rectal trauma
homotransplant
homotransplantation
    renal h.
homovanillic acid (HVA)
homozygote
homozygous sickle cell anemia
honeycomb
    h. mucosa
    h. pattern
honeymoon cystitis
hood
    latex h.
hooded prepuce
hook
    Adson dissecting h.
    Barr fistula h.
    cold knife h.
    Crile nerve h.
    crypt h.
    Dandy nerve h.
    h. forceps
    h. grip
    Joseph h.
    h. knife
    Neivert polyp h.
    nerve h.
    Pratt crypt h.
    Pratt rectal h.
    Pucci-Seed h.
    Rosser crypt h.
    h. scissors
    Shambaugh fistula h.
    Stewart crypt h.
    Whitaker h.
hooked catheter
hooklet
    hydatid h.
hook-tip laparoscopic electrode
hookworm disease
Hooper deep surgery scissors
HOPE
    Heart Outcomes Prevention Evaluation
    HOPE study
Hopkins
    H. II rod lens
    H. rod-lens system for rigid choledochoscope
    H. symptom checklist
    H. telescope
hordein
hordeolum
Horizon prostatic stent
horizontal
    h. electrophoresis
    h. folds of rectum
    h. gastroplasty
    h. mattress suture
    h. transmission
hormonal
    h. downstaging
    h. therapy
hormone
    adrenocorticotropic h. (ACTH)
    h. antagonist
    antidiuretic h. (ADH)
    corticotropin-releasing h. (CRH)
    endothelium-derived relaxing h.
    enteric h.
    follicle-stimulating h. (FSH)
    gastrointestinal peptide h.
    gonadotropin-releasing h. (GnRH)
    gut h.
    human menopausal h.
    international unit of male h.
    luteinizing h. (LH)
    luteinizing hormone follicle-stimulating h. (LH-FSH)
    luteinizing hormone releasing h. (LHRH)
    parathyroid h. (PTH)
    peptide h.
    plasma parathyroid h. (PTH)
    h. receptor
    secosteroid h.
    syndrome of inappropriate secretion of antidiuretic h. (SIADH)
    thyroid h.
    thyrotropin-releasing h.
hormone-secreting tumor syndrome
hormone-stimulated cAMP synthesis

horn
    anterior h.
    H. sign
Horner syndrome
horseradish peroxidase-conjugated anti-rabbit IgG
horseshoe
    h. abscess
    h. anomaly of pancreatic duct
    h. communication
    h. configuration
    h. fistula
    h. kidney
    h. track
Horsley
    H. anastomosis
    H. gastrectomy
    H. gastropexy
    H. pyloroplasty
    H. suture
hortobezoar
Horton-Devine
    H.-D. dermal graft
    H.-D. flip-flap hypospadias repair
    H.-D. operation
    H.-D. procedure
hose-pipe appearance of terminal ileum
Hospal Biospal filter
Hospital Anxiety and Depression Inventory
hospital-based clinic
host
    h. factor
    immunocompetent h.
    immunocompromised h.
    h. side
    h. tyrosine phosphorylation
hostility score
HOT
    Hypertension Optimal Treatment
    HOT trial
hot
    h. appendix
    h. biopsy
    h. biopsy forceps
    h. biopsy monopolar coagulation
    h. biopsy technique
    h. defect
    h. flexible forceps
    h. spot
    h. squeeze
    h. wire balloon

HOTC
    heterozygous ornithine transcarbamylase
Hounsfield unit (HU)
hour
24-hour
    24-h. ambulatory esophageal pH monitoring
    24-h. ambulatory gastric pH monitor
    24-h. ambulatory manometry study
    24-h. ambulatory pH-metry
    24-h. ambulatory pH test
    24-h. creatinine clearance
    24-h. esophageal pH probe
    24-h. fecal fat excretion
    24-h. gastric acidity test
    24-h. home pH-metry
    24-h. intraesophageal pH study
    24-h. spectrophotometric bilirubin monitoring
    24-h. urine collection
72-hour fecal fat test
hourglass
    h. constriction of gallbladder
    h. contraction
    h. deformity
    h. narrowing
    h. stomach
    h. stricture
12-hour home pad test
hourly scratching activity (HSA)
House
    H. advancement anoplasty
    H. sliding advancement flap
Housset-Debray gastroscope
Houston
    H. muscle
    valve of H.
    H. valve
Howard test
Howel-Evans syndrome
Howell
    H. needle
    H. Rotatable BII papillotome
Howell-Jolly body
Howmedica slit catheter
Howship-Romberg sign
Ho:YAG
    holmium:yttrium aluminum garnet
HP
    heater probe
    Helicobacter pylori

NOTES

HP (*continued*)
    hereditary pancreatitis
    hyperplastic polyp
        HP Chek screening system
        Ku-Zyme HP
        HP thermocoagulation
HPA
    hypothalamic-pituitary-adrenal
    hypothalamic-pituitary axis
HPC
    hydrophilic-coated
        HPC guidewire
HPC-1
    hereditary prostate cancer 1 locus
HPC-2 standard needle knife
HpD
    hematoporphyrin derivative
        HpD dye
        low-dose HpD
hpf
    high-power field
Hpfast rapid urease test
HPI
    hepatic perfusion index
    hepatocyte proliferation inhibitor
HPLC
    high-performance liquid chromatography
    high-pressure liquid chromatography
        HPLC fluorescence assay
HPLO
    Helicobacter pylori-like organism
HPN
    home parenteral nutrition
HP-NAP
    neutrophil-activating protein of *Helicobacter pylori*
HP7754 pneumohydraulic capillary infusion system
HPRC
    hereditary papillary renal cancer
        HPRC syndrome
HPRT
HPS
    hepatopulmonary syndrome
    hypertrophic pyloric stenosis
HpSA
    Premier Platinum HpSA
    HpSA test
HPT
    human proximal tubule
    hyperparathyroidism
Hp-test
    Jatrox Hp-t.
HPUS
    hydrogen peroxide ultrasound
HPV
    human papillomavirus
HPV 16
    human papillomavirus 16
    H. pylori SA test
HPZ
    high-pressure zone
16HR
    Synectics PC Polygraf 16HR
H2RA
    histamine-2 receptor antagonist
    H2 receptor antagonist
HRARE
    hybrid rapid acquisition with relaxation enhancement
H2-receptor antagonist therapy
H-related protein
HRES
    high-resolution endoluminal sonography
HRF
    heartburn relief formula
    histamine-releasing factor
        Maalox HRF
HRQOL
    health-related quality of life
HRS
    hepatorenal syndrome
HSA
    hourly scratching activity
HSC
    hepatic stellate cell
HSE
    hypertonic saline-epinephrine
        HSE solution
H-shaped
    H-s. ileal pouch-anal anastomosis
    H-s. tilt tag
HSK-tk
    herpes simplex virus-thymidine kinase
HSP
    heat shock protein
HSP-70
    HSP-70 cDNA
    HSP-70 messenger ribonucleoprotein acid level
    HSP-70 mRNA
HSPG
    heparan sulfate proteoglycan
HSS
    hepatic stimulatory substance
HSV
    herpes simplex virus
5-HT
    5-hydroxytryptamine
    serotonin
        5-HT test
HT-29 cell
5-HT4 agonist
HTGL
    hepatic triglyceride lipase
5-HT$_3$, 5-HT$_4$ antagonist
H-thymidine
3H-thymidine

[³H]thymidine uptake
HTI
    hepatic tumor index
HTLV-I
    human T-cell leukemia virus type I
        antibody to HTLV-I (anti-HTLV-I)
HTLV-I-associated myelopathy
HTP
    hydroxytryptophan
    hypothromboplastinemia
        Bio-Gel HTP
H-type fistula
HU
    Hounsfield unit
Huan
    Jin Bu H.
HuCV
    human enteric calcivirus
Hueter maneuver
Huggins operation
Huibregtse biliary stent
Huibregtse-Katon papillotome
Hulka clip
hum
    venous h.
human
    h. adenovirus 12
    h. apo A-I DNA probe
    h. *Astrovirus* (HAstV)
    h. case report
    h. chorionic gonadotropin (HCG)
    h. chromosome 6
    h. cytochrome P-450 enzyme system
    h. cytotoxic T cell
    h. enteric calcivirus (HuCV)
    h. epidermal growth factor (h-EGF)
    h. fibronectin cDNA probe
    h. gastrin probe
    h. genome highlight
    h. glandular kallikrein 3
    h. glomerulus
    h. growth factor (HGF)
    h. gut bacterium
    h. hepatitis B immune globulin
    h. immunodeficiency virus (HIV)
    h. immunodeficiency virus-associated nephropathy (HIVAN)
    h. insulin
    h. intestinal epithelial Coco-2 cell
    h. kidney chloride channel gene
    h. leukocyte antigen (HLA)
    h. leukocyte antigen renal allograft
    h. lymphoblastoid interferon (L-IFN)
    h. lymphocyte chromosomal aberration test
    h. lyophilized dura cystoplasty
    h. menopausal gonadotropin
    h. menopausal hormone
    h. motilin receptor
    h. papillomavirus (HPV)
    h. papillomavirus 16 (HPV 16)
    h. PDGF receptor
    h. proximal tubule (HPT)
    h. recombinant erythropoietin
    h. recombinant TGF
    h. serum albumin
    h. serum I-FABP
    h. serum jaundice
    h. synovial fibroblast
    h. T-cell leukemia virus type I (HTLV-I)
    h. T-cell lymphotrophic virus type I, II
    h. thrombin concentrate
    h. umbilical vein endothelial cell (HUVEC)
humanized
    h. anti-CD3 monoclonal antibody
    h. monoclonal antibody
humeral neck
Humicade
humoral
    h. antibody response
    h. arm
    h. hypercalcemia of malignancy (HHM)
    h. immunity
    h. immunodeficiency disorder
hump
    diaphragmatic h.
    dromedary h.
hunger
    h. contractions
    h. pain
hungry bone syndrome
Hunner
    H. interstitial cystitis
    H. stricture
    H. ulcer
Hunt
    H. colostomy clamp
    H. test

NOTES

hunterian chancre
Hunter line
Hunt-Lawrence pouch
Hunt-Limo-Basto gastric reservoir
Hurst
    H. bougienage
    H. bullet-tip dilator
    H. mercury bougie
    H. mercury-filled dilator
Hurst-Tucker pneumatic dilator
Hurst-type bougie
Hurwitz
    H. dialysis catheter
    H. esophageal clamp
    H. intestinal clamp
HUS
    hemolytic-uremic syndrome
husband
    artificial insemination h. (AIH)
Huschke ligament
husk
    ispaghula h.
Hutch diverticulum
Hutinel disease
HUVEC
    human umbilical vein endothelial cell
HV
    hepatic vein
H&V
    hemigastrectomy and vagotomy
HVA
    homovanillic acid
HVI-DHP
    hepatic venous isolation by direct hemoperfusion
HVOO
    hepatic venous outflow obstruction
HVPG
    hepatic venous pressure gradient
HVR1
    hypervariable region 1
HVS
    herpesvirus simplex
HWA 486
    leflunomide
HX-5/6-1 endoscopic clipping device
Hx-5LR-1 hemoclip
Hyalgan
hyalin
    alcoholic h.
    globular h.
hyaline
    h. arteriolar nephrosclerosis
    h. cast
    Mallory h.
hyalinized stroma

hyalinosis
    arteriolar h.
hyaluronan (HA)
    polysaccharide h.
hyaluronate
    sodium h.
hyaluronic
    h. acid
    h. acid concentration
hyaluronidase activity
hybridization
    dot-blot h.
    fluorescence in situ h. (FISH)
    nucleic acid h.
    quantitative liquid h.
    reverse dot h.
    sequence-sequence oligonucleotide h.
    in situ h.
    Southern blot h.
hybridoma-derived monoclonal antibody
hybrid rapid acquisition with relaxation enhancement (HRARE)
Hybritech
    H. method
    H. PSA scan
    H. Tandem prostate-pecific antigen assay
    H. Tandem PSA ratio test
    H. Tandem-R assay kit
    H. Tandem-R PSA assay
Hy-Cal calorie supplement
Hycamtin
hycanthone mesylate
hydatid
    h. cyst
    h. cyst disease
    h. cyst intrahepatic rupture
    h. hooklet
    Morgagni h.
    h. resonance
    h. sand
hydatidiform mole
hydatidocele
hydatidosis
    renal h.
hydatidosus
    polypus h.
hydatiduria
Hydeltrasol
Hydeltra-T.B.A.
Hydergine
Hyde shunt
Hydra
    H. Vision Es urological imaging system
    H. Vision IV urology system
    H. Vision Plus DR urological imaging system
hydraeroperitoneum

hydragogue diuretic
hydralazine
hydramnios
    acute h.
hydrargyria, hydrargyrism
hydrate
    chloral h.
hydrated
    h. gelatinous coat
    h. pyelogram
hydration
    intravenous h.
hydraulic
    h. abdominal concussion
    h. capillary infusion system
    h. hinge penile prosthesis
hydrazide hepatotoxicity
hydrazine sulfate
Hydrea
hydremic
    h. ascites
    h. nephritis
hydrepigastrium
hydrindantin
hydro
    Cutinova H.
    H. Plus coated guidewire
    H. Plus stent
hydroappendix
hydrobilirubin
hydrobromide
hydrocalycosis
hydrocele
    abdominoscrotal h.
    communicating h.
    congenital h.
    cord h.
    Dupuytren h.
    encysted h.
    h. feminae
    filarial h.
    funicular h.
    Gibbon h.
    hernia h.
    Maunoir h.
    meconium h.
    h. muliebris
    noncommunicating h.
    Nuck h.
    postoperative h.
    h. repair
    simple h.
    h. wall
hydrocelectomy
    h. bottle procedure
    h. dartos pouch procedure
    h. plication technique
    h. scleral therapy
hydrocephalus
    normal-pressure h.
hydrochloric
    h. acid (HCl)
    h. acid secretion
    h. acid test
hydrochloride (HCl)
    alosetron h.
    amiloride h.
    amitriptyline h.
    bethanechol h.
    bupivacaine h.
    buspirone h.
    ciprofloxacin h.
    colestipol h.
    desipramine h.
    flavoxate h.
    fluoxetine h.
    glutamic acid h.
    hydroxyzine h.
    imipramine h.
    irinotecan h.
    lomefloxacin h.
    meperidine h.
    midazolam h.
    nefazodone h.
    oxyphencyclimine h.
    papaverine h.
    phenazopyridine h.
    phenoxybenzamine h.
    1% pramoxine h.
    prazosin h.
    procaine h.
    propoxyphene h.
    pseudoephedrine h.
    quinine urea h.
    ranitidine h.
    sevelamer h.
    tetracycline h.
    thioridazine h.
    tocainide h.
    tolazoline h.
    trospium h.

NOTES

hydrochloride *(continued)*
  vancomycin h.
  yohimbine h.
hydrochlorothiazide (HCTZ)
  h. and reserpine
  h. and spironolactone
  h. and triamterene
hydrochlorothiazide-triamterene (HCTZ-TA)
hydrocholecystis
hydrocholeretic drug
Hydrocil Instant
hydrocirsocele
hydrocodone
hydrocolpos
hydrocortisone (HC-1)
  1% h.
  h. acetate
  h. acetate rectal aerosol
  h. enema
  h. foam
Hydrocortone Acetate
hydrodilation
hydrodistention
  bladder h.
HydroDIURIL
Hydroflex
  H. penile implant
  H. penile prosthesis
  H. sphincter
hydroflumethiazide
hydrogen
  h. adenosine triphosphatase
  h. breath test
  h. gas
  h. gas clearance
  h. gas clearance technique
  h. ion
  h. ion concentration (pH)
  h. ion production
  h. peroxide
  h. peroxide enema
  h. peroxide ultrasound (HPUS)
hydrography
  MR h.
hydrohematonephrosis
hydrohepatosis
hydrolase
  carboxylic ester h. (CEH)
  lactase-phlorizin h. (LPH)
hydrolysis
  brush-border h.
  intragastric h.
  urea h.
hydrolyze
hydrolyzed
  h. in ethanol
  h. whey formula
Hydromer-coated polyurethane stent

Hydromer grafted catheter
hydrometrocolpos
hydromorphone
Hydromox
Hydromox-R
hydronephrosis
  bilateral h.
  evaluation of symptomatic h.
  high-grade h.
  prenatal fetal h.
  significant h.
  h. in utero
hydronephrotic
hydroosmotic action of vascopressin
hydropancreatosis
Hydro-Par
hydroperinephrosis
hydroperitoneum
hydroperitonia
hydroperoxide
  lipid h.
hydrophila
  Aeromonas h.
hydrophilic
  h. polymer-coated steerable guidewire
  h. wire
hydrophilic-coated (HPC)
  h.-c. guidewire
hydrophilicity
hydrophobic binding region
hydrophone
  needle h.
hydropic nephrosis
hydropigenous nephritis
hydropneumoperitoneum
hydropneumothorax
Hydropres
Hydropres-25, 50
hydrops
  h. abdominis
  gallbladder h.
  nonimmune h.
hydropyonephrosis
hydrorachis
hydrosarcocele
hydroscheocele
Hydro-Serp
Hydroserpine
hydrostatic
  h. balloon
  h. balloon catheter
  h. balloon dilation
  h. decompression
  h. dilator
  h. pressure
  h. pressure therapy
  h. ultrafiltration

hydrothorax
    cirrhotic h.
    hepatic h.
Hydro-T Tabs
hydroureter
hydroureteronephrosis
hydroureterosis
hydrouria (var. of hydruria)
Hydroxacen
hydroxide
    aluminum h.
    ammonium h.
    magnesium h.
hydroxyapatite
6-hydroxybenzoate
hydroxychloroquine
18-hydroxycorticosterone
18-hydroxycortisol
hydroxyeicosatetraenoic acid (HETE)
20-hydroxyeicosatetraenoic acid
5-hydroxyindoleacetic acid (5-HIAA)
hydroxyindoleacetic acid (HIAA)
hydroxyl
    h. group
    h. radical
    h. radical scavenger
hydroxylamine
hydroxylase
hydroxylated vitamin D
hydroxyl-free radical
3-hydroxy-3-methylglutaric aciduria
hydroxyquinoline
hydroxystilbamidine
5-hydroxytryptamine (5-HT)
hydroxytryptophan (HTP)
hydroxyurea
25-hydroxyvitamin
    25-h. D
    25-h. D3 (25(OH)D3)
    25-h. D level
hydroxyzine hydrochloride
hydruria, hydrouria
hydruric
hygiene
    h. hypothesis
    perianal h.
Hygroton
hymen
    imperforate h.
hymenal band
hymenolepiasis

Hymenolepis
    H. diminuta
    H. nana
hymenotomy
hyodeoxycholate
hyodysenteriae
    Serpulina h.
hyointestinalis
    Campylobacter h.
hyoscine butylbromide
hyoscyamine
    sublingual h.
    h. sulfate
    h. sulfate orally disintegrating tablet
Hyosophen
hypanakinesia, hypanakinesis
Hypaque
    H. contrast medium
    H. enema
    H. swallow
hypazoturic nephropathy
hyperabduction
hyperabsorption
hyperacid
hyperacidity
    gastric h.
hyperactive
    h. bowel sounds
    h. rectosigmoid junction
hyperactivity
    detrusor h.
hyperacute
    h. graft-versus-host disease
    h. liver failure (HALF)
    h. rejection
hyperadiposis
hyperaldosteronism
    familial h.
    primary h.
    secondary h.
hyperalgesia
    colonic h.
    selective jejunal h.
    visceral h.
hyperalimentation
    central h.
    intravenous h. (IVH)
    parenteral h.
    peripheral h.
hyperalimentosis
hyperalkalinity

NOTES

hyperaminoaciduria
hyperammonemia
hyperammonemic syndrome
hyperamylasemia
hyperanakinesia
hyperandrogenism
hyperbaric
    h. oxygen
    h. oxygen chamber
    h. oxygen therapy (HBOT)
    h. oxygen toxicity
hyperbetalipoproteinemia
hyperbilirubinemia
    congenital h.
    conjugated h.
    constitutional h.
    familial unconjugated h.
    idiopathic unconjugated h.
    neonatal conjugated h.
    unconjugated h.
hypercalcemia
    familial hypocalciuric h. (FHH)
    glucocorticoid-induced h.
    iatrogenic h.
    h. of malignancy
hypercalcemic
    h. nephrolithiasis
    h. nephropathy
hypercalciuria
    absorptive h.
    idiopathic h. (IH)
    renal h.
    resorptive h.
hypercaloric diet
hypercarbia
hypercatabolic
hypercatharsis
hypercathartic
hypercellularity
    glomerular h.
    interstitial h.
    mesangial h.
hyperchloremia
hyperchloremic metabolic acidosis
hyperchlorhydria
hypercholecystokininemia
hypercholesterolemia
    familial h.
hypercholesterolemic cadaveric renal transplant
hypercholesterolia
hypercholia
hyperchromatic nucleus
hyperchylia
hyperchylomicronemia
    familial h.
hypercoagulability
hypercoagulable state
hypercontinence

hypercontinent
hypercontractile external sphincter response
hyperdense
hyperdibasic aminoaciduria
hyperdiploidy
hyperdistention
hyperdiuresis
hyperdopaminemia
hyperdynamic
    h. circulation
    h. ileus
    h. precordium
    h. syndrome
hypereccrisia
hypereccritic
hyperechoic
    h. shadowing
    h. spot
    h. stranding
hyperemesis
    h. gravidarum
    h. hiemis
hyperemetic
hyperemia
    gastric h.
    glans h.
    postprandial portal h.
    reactive h.
    splanchnic h.
hyperemic
    h. border zone
    h. mucosa
hypereosinophilia syndrome
hyperesthesia
    cutaneous h.
    gustatory h.
hyperesthetic
hyperferremia
hyperferritinemia
hyperfibrinogenemia
hyperfiltration
    capillary h.
    glomerular h.
    h. injury
    renal h.
    h. theory
hyperfractionated radiation therapy
hyperfunction
    adrenal cortex h.
    antral gastrin cell h.
    gastrin cell h.
hyperganglionosis
hypergastrinemia
    clinical h.
    h. with acid hypersecretion
hypergenitalism
hyperglobulinemic hepatitis
hyperglycemia

hyperglycemic clamping
hyperglyceridemia
    exogenous h.
hyperglycogenolysis
hypergonadotropic hypogonadism
HyperHep
hyperhepatia
hyperhidrosis
hyperhomocystinemia
hyperhydrochloria, hyperhydrochloridia
hypericin
    intravascular instillation of h.
hyperinfection
hyperingestion
hyperinsulinemia
    euglycemic h.
hyperinsulinism
    alimentary h.
hyperkalemia
hyperkaluria
hyperkeratosis
    esophageal h.
    h. palmaris et plantaris
hyperkinesis, hyperkinesia
    esophageal h.
    paroxysmal anal h.
hyperleydigism
hyperlipidemia, hyperlipemia
    carbohydrate-induced h.
    combined fat- and carbohydrate-induced h.
    familial combined h.
    familial fat-induced h.
    familial hypercholesterolemia with h.
    idiopathic h.
    mixed h.
hyperlipoproteinemia
    acquired h.
    familial h. type II
hyperlithic
hyperlithuria
hypermagnesemia
hypermetabolic state
hypermobile kidney
hypermobility
    bladder neck h.
    urethral h.
hypermotility
hypernatremia
    hypervolemic h.
    hypovolemic h.

hypernephritis
hypernephroid
hypernephroma
hypernephronia
hypernutrition
hyperorchidism
hyperorexia
hyperosmolar
    h. liquid
    h. perfusate
hyperosmolarity
    extracellular h.
hyperosmotic
    h. feeding
    h. laxative
    h. nonketotic dehydration
    h. urine
hyperoxaluria
    absorptive h.
    acquired h.
    enteric h.
    idiopathic h.
    mild h.
    primary h. type I, II (PH-I)
hyperoxaluric stone
hyperpancreatism
hyperpancreorrhea
hyperparathyroidism (HPT)
    primary h. (PrHPT)
    secondary h.
    tertiary h.
hyperpepsia
hyperpepsinemia
hyperpepsinia
hyperpepsinogenemia
hyperpeptic gastritis
hyperperfusion
hyperperistalsis
hyperphagia
    weight loss with h.
hyperphagic
hyperphosphatemia
hyperpipecolatemia
hyperplasia
    adenomatous h. (AH)
    adrenal zona glomerulosa h.
    antral G-cell h.
    atypical adenomatous h. (AAH)
    benign prostatic h. (BPH)
    biliary epithelia h.
    bilobar h.
    Brunner gland h.

NOTES

hyperplasia *(continued)*
    colonic nodular lymphoid h.
    congenital adrenal h. (CAH)
    crypt h.
    diffuse nodular h. (DNH)
    ductal epithelial h.
    duodenal lymphonodular h.
    ECL cell h.
    ECL hypertrophy and h.
    fibromuscular h.
    flat h.
    focal lymphoid h. (FLH)
    focal nodular h. (FNH)
    follicular lymphoid h.
    foveolar h.
    G-cell h.
    goblet cell h.
    incomplete basal cell h.
    insulin h.
    intimal h.
    islet cell h.
    lymphonodular h.
    median lobe h.
    mesonephric h.
    mesothelial h. (MH)
    musculomucoid intimal h.
    myointimal h.
    neointimal h.
    nodular lymphoid h. (NLH)
    nodular regenerative h. (NRH)
    nonantral endocrine cell h.
    papillary h.
    parathyroid h.
    polypoid gastric rugal h.
    polypoid lymphoid h.
    polypoid lymphomatous h.
    postatrophic h.
    prostate gland benign h.
    prostatic h.
    Rokitansky-Aschoff sinus h.
    symptomatic benign prostatic h.
    trilobar h.
hyperplasiogenic polyp
hyperplastic
    h. adenomatous polyp
    h. arteriolar nephrosclerosis
    h. cholecystosis
    h. dystrophy
    h. epithelial gastric polyp
    h. foveolar epithelium
    h. gastric polyp
    h. nodule
    h. obesity
    h. polyp (HP)
    h. polyposis
hyperplasticity
hyperpolarization
    membrane h.

hyperprebetalipoproteinemia
    familial hyperbetalipoproteinemia and h.
    familial hyperchylomicronemia with h.
hyperprochoresis
hyperprolactinemia
hyperproliferation
hyperproteinemia
hyperproteosis
hyperprotidic diet
hyperpyrexia
hyperreflexia
    autonomic h.
    degree of h.
    detrusor h.
    neurogenic h.
    pathogenesis of h.
hyperreflexic
    h. bladder
    h. motor urge incontinence
hyperreninemia
hyperreninemic
hyperresonance
hyperresonant abdomen
hyperresponsiveness
hyperrugosity
hypersalivation
hypersecreting tumor
hypersecretion
    acid h.
    cortisol h.
    gastric h.
    hypergastrinemia with acid h.
    h. obstruction hypothesis
    salivary h.
hyperselective embolization
hypersensitive esophagus
hypersensitivity
    h. angiitis
    antiepileptic drug h.
    cholestatic h.
    delayed-type h. (DTH)
    paraaminosalicylate h.
    phenindione h.
    h. reaction
    visceral h.
hyperspectral imaging
hypersplenism
hypersthenuria
hyperstimulation
hypersuprarenalism
hypertension
    accelerated h.
    African-American Study of Kidney Disease and H. (AASK)
    allograft-mediated h.
    angiotensin-dependent h.
    concomitant h.

hypertension · hypoactive

dietary approach to stop h. (DASH)
ductal h.
extrahepatic portal venous h.
glomerular capillary h.
Goldblatt h.
idiopathic portal h. (IPH)
impact of donor h.
intraglomerular h.
intrahepatic portal h.
isolated systolic h. (ISH)
JNC VI classification of h.
Joint National Committee Sixth Report classification of h.
lithotripsy-induced h.
noncirrhotic portal h.
H. Optimal Treatment (HOT)
H. Optimal Treatment trial
pancreatic ductal h.
portal h. (PHT)
portopulmonary h.
presinusoidal intrahepatic portal h.
refractory h.
renal h.
renin-mediated renovascular h.
renovascular h.
h. resistance axis
salt-sensitive h.
secondary h.
splenoportal h.
systemic h.

hypertensive
h. autosomal-dominant polycystic kidney disease
h. end-organ damage
h. gastropathy
h. lower esophageal sphincter
h. lower esophageal sphincter syndrome
h. nephrosclerosis (HN)
h. renal injury

hypertestosteronism
hyperthermia
malignant h.
microwave h.
transrectal prostatic h. (TPH)

hyperthyroidism
hyperthyroxinemia
hypertonia
anal canal h.

hypertonic
h. bladder
h. crystalloid
h. infusion
h. saline
h. saline-epinephrine (HSE)
h. saline-epinephrine solution

hypertonicity
hypertransaminasemia
cryptogenic h.

hypertrichosis lanuginosa acquisita
hypertriglyceridemia
familial h.

hypertrophic
h. cirrhosis
h. hypersecretory gastropathy
h. lymphocytic gastritis (HLG)
h. obesity
h. osteoarthropathy
h. pyloric stenosis (HPS)
h. pylorus

hypertrophy
benign prostatic h. (BPH)
Billroth h.
bilobar h.
h. of column of Bertin
compensatory testicular h.
crypt h.
gastroduodenal h.
glomerular h.
muscle h.
prostatic h.
renal h.
renovascular h.
rugal h.
symptomatic benign prostatic h.
trilobar h.

hypertyrosinemia
hyperuricemia
hyperuricuria
hypervariable
h. deoxyribonucleic acid
h. region 1 (HVR1)

hypervolemia
hypervolemic hypernatremia
hyphema, hyphemia
intertropical h.
tropical h.

Hypnovel
%HYPO
percentage of hypochromic red cells

hypoacidity
luminal h.

hypoactive bowel sounds

NOTES

hypoactivity
hypoalbuminemia
hypoalbuminemic patient
hypoaldosteronism
    hyporeninemic h.
    isolated h.
hypoalimentation
hypoandrogenism
hypobetalipoproteinemia
hypobicarbonatemia
hypocalcemia
    asymptomatic h.
    familial hypocalciuric h.
hypocapnia
hypochloremia
hypochloremic hypokalemic metabolic alkalosis
hypochlorhydria
    epidemic h.
    gastric h.
hypochlorhydric cirrhosis
hypochloruric nephropathy
hypocholia
hypochondria (*pl. of* hypochondrium)
hypochondriac
    h. fossa
    h. region
hypochondriacal patient
hypochondriasis
hypochondrium, pl. **hypochondria**
hypochromic
    h. microcytic anemia
    h. red cell
hypochylia
hypocitraturia
hypocomplementemia
hypocontractile detrusor
hypocontractility
    detrusor h.
hypocupremia
hypocystotomy
hypodiaphragmatic
hypodiploidy
hypodipsia
hypoeccrisis
hypoeccritic
hypoechoic
    h. cancer
    h. lesion
    h. periphery
    h. ringed layer
    h. thickening
hypoesthesia
    gustatory h.
hypoestrogenic urethritis
hypoestrogenism
hypofibrinogenemia
hypofunction
hypogammaglobulinemia
hypogammaglobulinemic
hypoganglionosis of colon
hypogastric
    h. artery
    h. artery aneurysm
    h. fiber
    h. nerve
    h. node
    h. papillary zone
    h. plexus
    h. region
    h. vessel
hypogastrium
hypogastrocele
hypogastroschisis
hypogenetic nephritis
hypogenitalism
hypogeusia
hypoglycemia
    alcohol-induced h.
    postprandial h.
hypoglycin
    acetyl coenzyme h. A
hypogonadal state
hypogonadism
    hypergonadotropic h.
hypohepatia
hypohydrochloria
hypokalemia
    diuretic-induced h.
hypokalemic
    h. metabolic alkalosis
    h. nephropathy
    h. nephrosis
    h. renal tubular acidosis
hypokaluria
hypolactasia
    adult h.
hypoleydigism
hypomagnesemia
hypomagnesuria
hypometabolic
hypometabolism
hypomethylation
    DNA h.
hypomotility
    esophageal h.
    gastric h.
hypomyxia
hyponatremia
    dilutional h.
    early signs of dilutional h.
    euvolemic h.
    thiazide-induced h.
hypoorchidism
hypoosmotic urine
hypopancreatism
hypopancreorrhea
hypoparathyroidism

hypopepsia
hypopepsinia
hypoperfusion
    renal h.
hypoperistalsis syndrome
hypoperistaltic
hypopharyngeal
    h. cancer
    h. diverticulum
hypopharynx
hypophosphatasia
hypophosphatemia
    X-linked h. (XLH)
hypophosphatemic rickets
hypophosphaturia
hypophrenic
hypophysectomy
hypoplasia
    bile duct h.
    bladder h.
    congenital h.
    corpus spongiosum h.
    erythroid h.
    exocrine pancreatic h.
    germ cell h.
    intrahepatic biliary duct h.
    oligonephronic h.
    prostate gland h.
    thymic h.
    unilateral renal h.
hypoplastic
    h. blind-ending spermatic vessel
    h. glomerulocystic disease
    h. kidney
hypoposia
hypoproteinemia
hypoproteinosis
hypoprothrombinemia
hypopyon
hyporeninemic hypoaldosteronism
hyporesponsiveness
    cardiac beta-adrenoreceptor h.
    erythropoietin h.
hypospadiac
hypospadias
    anterior h.
    balanic h.
    complex h.
    concealed h.
    coronal h.
    female h.
    glanular h.
    middle h.
    penile h.
    penoscrotal h.
    perineal h.
    posterior h.
    pseudovaginal perineoscrotal h.
    scrotal h.
    subcoronal h.
hypospermatogenesis
hyposplenism
hypostasis
hypostatic
hyposthenuria
    renal h.
hyposuprarenalism
hypotension
    dialysis-associated h.
    hemorrhagic h.
    intradialytic h. (IDH)
    systemic h.
hypotestosteronism
hypothalamic-pituitary-adrenal (HPA)
hypothalamic-pituitary axis (HPA)
hypothalamic-pituitary-testicular-penile axis
hypothalamic suppression
hypothalamus
hypothenar eminence
hypothermia
    gastric h.
    intraoperative kidney h.
    renal h.
hypothermic
    h. effect
    h. pulsatile perfusion
    h. storage
hypothesis
    affinity-avidity h.
    cumulative damage h.
    hygiene h.
    hypersecretion obstruction h.
    iron shuttle h.
    Keller h.
hypothromboplastinemia (HTP)
hypothyroidism
hypotonia
    rectal h.
hypotonic
    h. bladder
    h. duodenography
hypouremia
hypouresis

NOTES

hypouricemia
hypouricuria
hypourocrinia
hypoventilation
    benzodiazepine-induced h.
    sedation-induced h.
hypovolemia
    nephrosis with h.
    nephrosis without h.
    watery diarrhea, hypokalemia, and h. (WDHH)
hypovolemic
    h. anemia
    h. hypernatremia
    h. shock
    h. variance
hypoxanthine-guanine phosphoribosyltransferase deficiency
hypoxemia
hypoxia
    hepatic h.
    pericentral h.

hypoxia-induced rhabdomyolysis
Hypoxis rooperi
Hyrtl sphincter
hysterectomy
hysteresis
hysterical vomiting
hystericus
    globus h.
hysterocele
hysterocystopexy
hysterosacropexy
    Ivalon sponge h.
    polyvinyl alcohol sponge h.
hysterosalpingectomy
    laparoscopic h.
hysteroscopy
Hy-Tape
Hytrin Dosepak
Hyzine-50

I-125
    iodine-125
        I-125 iothalamate clearance
I-131
    iodine-131
^{131}I
    ^{131}I paraaminohippuric acid
^{125}I
    ^{125}I albumin
IA
    intraarterial
I-alpha-hydroxyvitamin D3
IAS
    internal anal sphincter
    intraabdominal sepsis
iatrogenic
    i. chymobilia
    i. coagulopathy
    i. colitis
    i. enterocele
    i. hypercalcemia
    i. hypercalcemic nephrolithiasis
    i. immunodeficiency syndrome
    i. intraoperative ureteral injury
    i. malabsorption
    i. pancreatic trauma
    i. pneumothorax
    i. prostatourethral-rectal fistula
    i. rectourethral fistula
    i. tumor perforation
    i. urolithiasis
IBB
    intestinal brush border
IBC
    iron-binding capacity
IBD
    inflammatory bowel disease
IBDQ
    Inflammatory Bowel Disease Questionnaire
ibotenic acid
IBS
    inflammatory bowel syndrome
    irritable bowel syndrome
IBStat
ibuprofen
IBW
    ideal body weight
IC
    indeterminate colitis
    intracisternal
    irritable colon
IC351

ICA
    islet cell antibody
        ICA test
ICAM-1
    intercellular adhesion molecule-1
    intracellular adhesion molecule inhibitor
ICC
    interstitial cells of Cajal
ICDB
    Interstitial Cystitis Data Base
ice
    i. cooling
    i. slush
    i. water test
ice-cold sucrose buffer
iced
    i. intestine
    i. lactated Ringer solution
    i. saline
    i. saline lavage
IceSeeds
ice-water swallow
ICF
    intracellular fluid
ICG
    indocyanine green dye
        ICG clearance
        ICG test
IC-GN
    immune complex glomerulonephritis
ICGN
    ICR strain-derived glomerular nephritis
ichthyismus exanthematicus
ICIT
    intracavernosal injection therapy
ICL
    intracorporeal laser lithotripsy
icodextrin 7.5% peritoneal dialysis solution
ICP
    intrahepatic cholestasis of pregnancy
ICR strain-derived glomerular nephritis (ICGN)
ICS
    International Continence Society
ICSF
    idiopathic calcium (renal) stone formation
ICSI
    intracytoplasmic sperm injection
ICT
    isolated cortical tubule
ictal
icteric
    i. necrosis

icteric *(continued)*
    i. sclerae
    i. skin
icterogenic
icterohepatitis
icteroid
icterus
    benign familial i.
    conjunctival i.
    i. gravidarum
    i. gravis
    Hayem i.
    i. melas
    i. neonatorum
    i. praecox
    scleral i.
icterus
ictometer
ictus
ID
    inner diameter
    intraduodenal
I&D
    incision and drainage
IDA
    iminodiacetic acid
idarubicin
IDD
    intraluminal duodenal diverticulum
IDDM
    insulin-dependent diabetes mellitus
IDE
    insulin-degrading enzyme
ideal
    i. body weight (IBW)
    i. patient profile
identification
    colonic lesion i.
    lesion i.
identified
IDH
    intradialytic hypotension
    intramural duodenal hematoma
idiopathic
    i. achalasia
    i. adulthood ductopenia
    i. ascites
    i. autoimmune cholangitis
    i. autoimmune chronic hepatitis
    i. bile acid malabsorption
    i. calcium (renal) stone formation (ICSF)
    i. chronic erosion
    i. chronic erosive gastritis
    i. colitis
    i. constipation
    i. crescentic glomerulonephritis
    i. diffuse ulcerative nongranulomatous enteritis
    i. edema
    i. enteropathy
    i. esophageal ulcer (IEU)
    i. fibrosing pancreatitis
    i. fibrous retroperitonitis
    i. gastric acid secretion
    i. gastroparesis
    i. hematuria
    i. hemochromatosis
    i. hypercalciuria (IH)
    i. hypereosinophilic syndrome (IHES)
    i. hyperlipidemia
    i. hyperoxaluria
    i. hypertrophic gastropathy
    i. hypertrophic pyloric stenosis
    i. hypocomplementemic interstitial nephritis
    i. infertility
    i. inflammatory bowel disease (IIBD)
    i. intestinal pseudoobstruction
    i. megacolon
    i. megarectum
    i. membranous glomerulonephritis
    i. nephralgia
    i. nephrotic syndrome
    i. nonfamilial visceral neuropathy
    i. obstruction
    i. portal hypertension (IPH)
    i. proctitis
    i. proctocolitis
    i. rapidly progressive glomerulonephritis (IRPGN)
    i. recurrent pancreatitis (IRP)
    i. retroperitoneal fibrosis
    i. steatorrhea
    i. thrombocytopenic purpura
    i. unconjugated hyperbilirubinemia
    i. varix
    i. volvulus
idiotype-anti-idiotype interaction
idioventricular
IDL
    intermediate density lipoprotein
IDPN
    intradialytic parenteral nutrition
idremcinal
IDST
    intraductal secretin test
IDUS
    intraductal ultrasonography
    intraductal ultrasound
IDWG
    interdialytic weight gain
IEBD
    intraesophageal balloon distention
IEC-6 cell

IED
 immune-enhancing diet
IEHL
 intracorporeal electrohydraulic lithotripsy
IEL
 intraepithelial leukocyte
 intraepithelial lymphocyte
  IEL T cell
IEM
 ineffective esophageal motility
IEU
 idiopathic esophageal ulcer
IF
 intrinsic factor
I-FABP
 intestinal fatty acid-binding protein
  human serum I-FABP
IFE
 immunofixation electrophoresis
Ifex, Taxol, Platinol (ITP)
IFN
  IFN alfa
   interferon-alpha
  IFN alfa therapy
  IFN alpha-2b therapy
IFN-gamma
 interferon-gamma
IFOBT
 immunological fecal occult blood test
IFP
 inflammatory fibroid polyp
IG
 image guide
 intragastric
  IG bundle
Ig
 immunoglobulin
IgA
 immunoglobulin A
  IgA deficiency
  dimeric IgA
  IgA EMA
  endomysial IgA
  gliadin IgA
  IgA glomerulonephritis
  IgA immunological study
  jejunal IgA
  IgA kappa-chain myeloma
  IgA nephropathy
  IgA neuropathy
  IgA polymerization
  secretory IgA (sIgA)
  IgA tTG
  IgA tTG assay
IgA1
 immunoglobulin A1
IgA2
 immunoglobulin A2
IgA-antigliadin
IgA-producing cell
IGCCCG
 International Germ Cell Cancer Collaborative Group
  IGCCCG classification
IgD
 immunoglobulin D
IgE
 immunoglobulin E
IGF
 insulinlike growth factor
IGF-1
 insulinlike growth factor-1
  exogenous IGF-1
IGF-2
 insulinlike growth factor-2
IGF-binding protein-1 mRNA
IGFBP-1
 insulinlike growth factor-binding protein-1
IGF-BP3 complex
IGF-1R
  IGF-1R mRNA
  IGF-1R RNA
IgG
 immunoglobulin G
  IgG AGA
  IgG alpha-gliadin antibody
  IgG anti-HAV-positive
  horseradish peroxidase-conjugated anti-rabbit IgG
  IgG immunological study
  polyclonal IgG
  IgG reticulin antibody
  IgG serology
IgG1
 immunoglobulin G1
IgG2a
 immunoglobulin G2a
  IgG2a antibody
IgG-producing cell
Iglesias
  I. fiberoptic resectoscope
  I. method of aspiration

NOTES

IgM
    immunoglobulin M
        IgM anti-HAV
        IgM anti-HAV antibody
        IgM anti-HBc antibody
        anti-*Helicobacter pylori* IgM
        IgM immunological study
        monoclonal IgM
        IgM nephropathy

IgM-antigliadin
IgM-HA antibody
IgM-HEV antibody titer
IGP
    injection gold probe
IGV
    isolated gastric varices type 1, 2
IH
    idiopathic hypercalciuria
    inguinal hernia
IHA
    indirect hemagglutination
    intrahepatic atresia
        IHA determination
IHb
    hemoglobin content index
IHD
    intermittent hemodialysis
IHES
    idiopathic hypereosinophilic syndrome
IHPS
    infantile hypertrophic pyloric stenosis
IIBD
    idiopathic inflammatory bowel disease
IIEF
    International Index of Erectile Function
IIF
    indirect immunofluorescence
[^{123}I]IMP
    iodoamphetamine
[^{123}I]iodoamphetamine radionuclide
I-IV
    Bismuth classification, types I-IV
IJ
    intrajejunal
IK allele
IkBa protein
IL
    ileum
    interleukin
IL-1
    interleukin-1
IL-2
    interleukin-2
IL-6
    interleukin-6
IL-8
    interleukin-8

IL-10
    interleukin-10
        recombinant IL-10
ILA surgical stapler
ILC
    interstitial laser coagulation
ILDL
    intermediate low-density lipoprotein
ileac
ileal
    i. artery
    i. artery stent
    i. atresia
    i. biopsy
    i. bladder
    i. blood vessel
    i. brake
    i. conduit urinary diversion
    i. crypt
    i. duplication cyst
    i. effluent
    i. follicle
    i. ileoscopy
    i. inflow tract
    i. interposition
    i. intestinal antireflux valve
    i. J pouch
    i. loop
    i. loopography
    i. low-pressure bladder substitute pouch
    i. Malone cecostomy
    i. neobladder
    i. neobladder urinary diversion
    i. neobladder urinary pouch
    i. nipple valve
    i. orthotopic bladder substitute
    i. outflow tract
    i. papilla
    i. patch ureteroplasty
    i. pouch-anal anastomosis (IPAA)
    i. pouch-distal rectal anastomosis
    i. pullthrough
    i. reflux
    i. resection (IR)
    i. reservoir
    i. reservoir construction
    i. reservoir evacuation
    i. segment (IS)
    i. sleeve
    i. S pouch
    i. spout
    i. stasis
    i. ureter
    i. ureteral substitution
    i. urinary conduit
    i. varix
    i. W pouch

ilealis
    frenulum valvae i.
    ostium valvae i.
    papilla i.
    valva i.
ileectomy
ilei
    arteriae i.
ileitis
    backwash i.
    Crohn i.
    distal i.
    granulomatous i.
    Meckel i.
    obstructive dysfunctional i.
    pouch i.
    prestomal i.
    regional i. (RI)
    terminal i.
ileoanal
    i. anastomosis
    i. endorectal pullthrough
    i. pouch
    i. pullthrough procedure
    i. reservoir
ileoascending colostomy
ileocaecalis
    frenulum valvae i.
    papilla i.
    valva i.
ileocecal
    i. bladder
    i. continent urinary reservoir
    i. cutaneous diversion
    i. fat pad
    i. insufficiency
    i. intestinal antireflux valve
    i. intussusception
    i. junction
    i. papilla
    i. pouch
    i. region
    i. resection
    i. segment
    i. segment transposition
    i. sphincter
    i. syndrome
    i. tuberculosis
    i. ureterosigmoidostomy
ileocecale
    ostium i.
ileocecalis
    plica i.
ileocecocystoplasty bladder augmentation
ileocecostomy
ileocolectomy
ileocolic
    i. anastomosis
    i. artery
    i. disease
    i. fold
    i. intussusception
    i. plexus
    i. resection
    i. urinary diversion
    i. vessel
ileocolica
    arteria i.
ileocolitis
    Crohn i.
    transmural i.
    tuberculous i.
    i. ulcerosa chronica
ileocolonic
    i. bladder
    i. Crohn disease
    i. neobladder
    i. pouch
    i. pouch urinary diversion
    i. transit
ileocolonoscopy
ileocolostomy
    end-loop i.
    LeDuc-Camey i.
ileocolotomy
ileoconduit
ileocystoplasty
    Camey i.
    clam i.
    LeDuc-Camey i.
ileocystostomy
    cutaneous i.
ileoentectropy
ileogastric reflex
ileogastrostomy
ileogram
ileography
    endoscopic retrograde i.
ileoileal intussusception
ileoileostomy
ileojejunitis

NOTES

ileopexy
ileoproctostomy (IP)
ileorectal anastomosis (IRA)
ileorectostomy
ileorenal bypass
ileorrhaphy
ileoscopy
    ileal i.
ileosigmoid
    i. anastomosis
    i. colostomy
    i. fistula
    i. knot
ileosigmoidostomy
ileostogram
ileostomate
ileostomist
ileostomy
    i. bag
    Bishop-Koop i.
    blow-hole i.
    Brooke i.
    i. closure
    continent i.
    i. cup
    Dennis-Brooke i.
    i. diarrhea
    diversionary i.
    diverting loop i.
    double-barrel i.
    i. effluent
    end i.
    end-loop i.
    Goligher extraperitoneal i.
    incontinent i.
    J-loop i.
    Kock continent i.
    Kock reservoir i.
    loop i. (LI)
    loop end i.
    mucosal i.
    permanent loop i.
    pouched i.
    i. rod
    split i.
    i. stoma
    temporary loop i.
    terminal i.
    Turnbull end-loop i.
ileotomy
ileotransverse
    i. colon anastomosis
    i. colostomy
ileotransversostomy
ileovesical
    i. anastomosis
    i. fistula
ileovesicostomy
    continent i.
    incontinent i.
    laparoscopic-assisted ileocystoplasty and i.
    laparoscopy-assisted ileocystoplasty and i.
    transverse retubularized i.
    Yang-Monti i.
ILE-SORB absorbent gel
ileum (IL)
    antimesenteric border of distal i.
    collapsed i.
    duplex i.
    hose-pipe appearance of terminal i.
    neoterminal i.
    i. nipple
    terminal i.
ileus
    adhesive i.
    adynamic i.
    colonic i.
    dynamic i.
    focal i.
    gallbladder i.
    gallstone i.
    gastric i.
    hyperdynamic i.
    mechanical i.
    meconium i.
    occlusive i.
    paralytic i.
    i. paralyticus
    postoperative i.
    spastic i.
    i. subparta
    terminal i.
    verminous i.
iLEX skin protectant paste
ilia (*pl. of* ilium)
iliac
    i. artery
    i. artery aneurysm
    i. artery embolization
    i. bend
    i. colon
    i. crest
    i. fossa
    i. roll
    i. spine
    i. vein
iliac-to-renal artery bypass graft
iliacus muscle
iliococcygeus muscle
iliocolotomy
iliohypogastric nerve
ilioinguinal
    i. nerve
    i. ring
iliopectineal line

iliopsoas
    i. ring
    i. sign
    i. test
^{131}I-lipiodol isotope
ilium, pl. **ilia**
ILL
    intracorporeal laser lithotripsy
illness
    food-borne i. (FBI)
    severe morbid i.
illuminated St. Mark retractor
illumination system
ilodecakin
Ilopan
iloprost
Ilosone
Ilotysin
Ilozyme
IL-2,-3,-4,-6,-8 receptors
ILS
    intraluminal stapler
ILUS
    intraluminal ultrasound
        ILUS catheter
IM
    intramuscular
    Rocephin IM
IMA
    inferior mesenteric artery
image
    i. analysis
    axial i.
    B-mode ultrasound i.
    i. cytometry
    i. guide (IG)
    i. guide bundle
    HAP i.
    longitudinal i.
    point-counting i.
    probe i.
    i. processing
    sagittal i.
    thumbnail i.
    transverse i.
    T1-weighted i.
    T2-weighted i.
image-guided therapy
Imagent GI
image-processing unit
imager
    Tesla Signa MR i.

imaging
    i. algorithm
    anorectal i.
    bladder i.
    i. bladder support
    B-mode i.
    color flow Doppler i.
    complete urological i.
    Doppler color flow i.
    endoanal magnetic resonance i.
    endorectal coil magnetic resonance i.
    endoscopic ultrasonographic i.
    functional magnetic resonance i. (fMRI)
    gallium i.
    GNG phase i.
    gray-scale i.
    hyperspectral i.
    internet-based digital i.
    LaparoScan laparoscopic ultrasonic i.
    magnetic endoscopic i.
    magnetic resonance i. (MRI)
    i. method
    narrow-band i.
    nuclear hepatobiliary i.
    parathyroid i.
    photodynamic i.
    planar i.
    radiolabeled i.
    radionuclide renal i.
    renal helical CT i.
    RHCT i.
    sonoelasticity i.
    technetium i.
    i. technology
    thallium i.
    thermal i.
    transcutaneous ultrasound i.
    uniplanar i.
imaging-guided minimally invasive procedure
imatinib mesylate
imbalance
    acid-base i.
imbedded microtransducer
imbricate
IMC-C225
    Cetuximab
IMCD
    inner medullary collecting duct

NOTES

IMED 430 enteral feeding pump
Imerslund syndrome
imidazole aminoaciduria
imidazolecarboxamide
imidoacetic acid radioactive agent
imiglucerase
iminodiacetic acid (IDA)
iminoglycinuria
imipenem
imipenem-cilastatin
imipramine hydrochloride
imiquimod
immature teratoma
IMMC
    intestinal mucosal mast cell
    intravesical mitomycin C
immediate blush
immersion
    i. cooling
    water i.
immitis
    Candida i.
immotile cilia syndrome
ImmTher
Immu-4
Immudia-HemSp
IMMULITE
    I. 2000 anti-HBc IgM analyzer
    I. 2000 anti-HBs analyzer
    I. 2000 free PSA assay
    I. 2000 HBsAg immunoanalyzer
    I. HBsAg immunoassay analyzer
    I. 2000 third-generation PSA assay
immune
    i. complex glomerulonephritis (IC-GN)
    i. deficiency
    i. electron microscopy
    i. rabbit antibody
    i. response
    i. serum (IS)
    i. serum globulin
    i. suppression
    i. system
immune-enhancing diet (IED)
immune-mediated
    i.-m. infertility
    i.-m. interstitial nephritis
    i.-m. reaction
immunity
    acquired i.
    adaptive i.
    cell-mediated i.
    cellular i.
    humoral i.
    immunologic i.
    innate i.
    natural i.
    nonimmunologic i.

immunization
    DNA i.
    parenteral i.
immunoadsorption
immunoanalyzer
    Elecsys 1010 and 2010 i.
    IMMULITE 2000 HBsAg i.
immunoassay
    Abbott TDx monoclonal fluorescence polarization i.
    Cytoscreen Human Eotaxin i.
    Elecsys anti-HBs i.
    enzyme i. (EIA)
    hepatitis C virus enzyme i.
    Magic Lite chemiluminometric i.
    microparticle enzyme i. (MEIA)
    rapid enzyme i.
    second-generation enzyme i. (EIA-2)
    TDX fluorescent polarization i.
immunobead assay
immunobead-reacting antigen
immunobiology
immunoblot test
ImmunoCard
    I. serum antibody test
    I. STAT!
    I. STAT! Rotavirus test
immunocompetency
immunocompetent host
immunocompromised host
ImmunoCyt
    I. test
immunocyte
immunocytochemical stain
immunocytochemistry
    vacuolar-type proton pump i.
immunocytology
immunodeficiency
    acquired i.
    common variable i. (CVI)
    i. disease
    severe combined i. (SCID)
immunodepression
immunodiffusion
    radial i.
    i. test
immunodominant T-cell epitope
immunoelectrophoresis
immunoenhancing
immunofixation electrophoresis (IFE)
immunofluorescence
    indirect i. (IIF)
    i. microscopy
    negative i.
immunofluorescent antibody test
immunogen
    enteric i.

immunogenic gene
immunoglobulin (Ig)
    i. A (IgA)
    i. A1 (IgA1)
    i. A2 (IgA2)
    i. A endomysial antibody
    i. A nephropathy
    anti-gp330 i. G
    i. A transglutaminase antibody
    biliary i.
    i. D (IgD)
    i. E (IgE)
    i. G (IgG)
    i. G1 (IgG1)
    i. G2a (IgG2a)
    i. G2a antibody
    i. G antigliadin antibody
    i. G clearance
    hepatitis B i. (HBIG)
    intravenous i. (IVIg)
    i. M (IgM)
    i. neuropathy
    secretory i. A
    i. superfamily adhesion molecule
immunohistochemical
    i. detection
    i. method
    i. stain
    i. staining
immunohistochemistry
    p53 i.
immunohistology
Immuno I complex PSA test
immunologic
    i. abnormality
    i. immunity
immunological
    i. fecal occult blood test (IFOBT)
    i. rapid urease test
immunology
    intestinal i.
immunomodulatory
    i. action
    i. gene therapy
immunonephelometry
immunoneutralization
immunoperoxidase
    light and electron i.
    i. stain
    i. staining
    i. staining technique
immunophenotypical profiling of patient

immunopositivity
immunoprecipitation
immunoproliferative small intestinal disease (IPSID)
immunoradiometric assay (IRMA)
immunoreactive
    i. methionine-enkephalin (IRME)
    i. trypsin enzyme
    i. trypsinogen (IRT)
immunoreactive methionine-enkephalin (IRME)
immunoreactivity
    cholecystokinin-like i. (CCK-LI)
    PYY-like i.
    vasoactive intestinal polypeptide i. (VIP-IR)
immunoregulator
immunoregulatory drug
immunoscintigraphy
    ^{111}In-CYT-103 i.
immunosorbent
immunostain
immunostaining
    Fas i.
    HBcAg i.
    in situ i.
    i. technique
    i. of transversely sectioned tubule
immunosuppressant
    antiproliferative i.
    cornerstone i.
immunosuppressed patient
immunosuppression
    posttransplant i.
immunosuppressive
    i. agent
    i. drug
    i. regimen
    i. therapy
immunosurveillance
immunotactoid
    i. glomerulonephritis
    i. glomerulopathy (ITGP)
immunotherapy
    adoptive i.
    BCG i.
    intravesical i.
    Pacis BCG bladder cancer i.
    specific i.
immunotyping
Imodium A-D

NOTES

impact
    i. of donor hypertension
    I. lithotriptor system
    i. of microwave antennas on treatment outcome
    I. nutritional supplement

impacted
    i. ampullary stone
    i. calculus
    i. cystic duct
    i. feces
    i. stool
    i. ureteral stone

impaction
    acute esophageal food i. (AEFI)
    endoscope i.
    fecal i.
    food bolus i.
    meat i.
    rectal i.
    stone and basket i.

impactor
    electromechanical i. (EMI)
    stone i.

impaired
    i. cell differentiation
    i. colonic motor function
    i. gastric absorption
    i. lecithin synthesis
    i. regeneration syndrome (IRS)
    i. urinary concentrating ability

impairment
    anabolic steroid spermatogenesis i.
    ethanol-specific i.
    memory i.

impar
    i. hypogastric plexus
    plexus of i.
    plexus hypogastric i.

impassable ureter

impedance
    i. epigastrography
    intraluminal electrical i.
    i. planimetry
    i. plethysmography (IPG)
    rectal i.

impedancometry
    intraluminal electrical i.
    multiple intraluminal i.'s

imperforate
    i. anus
    i. hymen

implant
    Alpha I penile i.
    BrachySeed Pd-103 i.
    Contigen Bard collagen i.
    Deflux injectable i.
    Deflux system i.
    Dynaflex penile i.
    Enteryx i.
    i. erosion
    Flexi-Flate penile i.
    gold seed i.
    histrelin i.
    Hydroflex penile i.
    iridium 192 wire i.
    islet cell i.
    Jonas i.
    leuprolide acetate i.
    Lifecath peritoneal i.
    Macroplastique i.
    malleable i.
    palladium-103 seed i.
    penile i.
    Rapid Strand i.
    i. reabsorption
    retropubic i.
    Septopal i.
    Surgitek Flexi-Flate II penile i.
    testicular i.
    transperineal seed i.
    Zoladex i.

implantable
    i. neuromodulation system
    i. penile venous compression device
    i. pulse generator (IPG)

implantation
    artificial genitourinary sphincter i.
    artificial urinary sphincter i.
    bulbous urethral cuff i.
    Enteryx i.
    gastric balloon i.
    intracavitary i.
    i. metastasis
    metastatic i.
    percutaneous transperineal seed i.
    i. of prosthetic material
    radioactive seed i.
    real-time 3-D biplanar transperineal prostate i.
    second-cuff i.
    ureter i.
    ureterointestinal i.

implication
    clinical i.

importance
    preeminent diagnostic i.

important risk factor

impotence
    arteriogenic i.
    diabetic i.
    ejaculatory i.
    Esteem advanced vacuum therapy for i.
    functional i.
    organic i.
    orgastic i.

paretic i.
psychic i.
psychogenic i.
secondary i.
symptomatic i.
vasculogenic i.
venogenic i.
venous leak i.

impotentia
i. coeundi
i. erigendi

Impra graft

impressio, pl. **impressiones**
i. esophagealis hepatis

impression
colic i.
colon i.
digastric i.
duodenal i.
esophageal i.
gastric i.
liver i.
renal i.
suprarenal i.

Impress Softpatch

imprinting
genomic i.

improved
i. graft survival
i. visualization

improvement
clinical i.
i. in patient recovery
subjective i.

IMPT
intensity-modulated proton therapy

IMRT
intensity-modulated radiation therapy

Imuran

IMV
inferior mesenteric vein

IMx
I. Hg assay
I. PSA system

In
indium

in
in situ
in situ end labeling (ISEL)
in situ hybridization
in situ immunostaining
in utero programming
in vitro
in vitro clearance
in vitro compatibility
in vitro fertilization
in vitro incubation
in vitro model
in vitro synergism
in vivo
in vivo clearance
in vivo microscopy
in vivo veritas

inactivated pepsin (IP)

inactivation
oncogene i.

inactive
i. Crohn disease
i. schistosomiasis

inactivity
physical i.

inadequate
i. bowel preparation
i. dilation

inadvertent enterotomy

in-and-out catheterization

inanimate simulator

inanition fever

inapparent hepatitis

Inapsine

inborn error of metabolism

inbreeding coefficient

incarcerated
i. bowel
i. intrathoracic hernia
i. omentum
i. prolapse
i. snare

incarceration
colon i.
colonoscopy-related i.
hernia i.
penile i.
i. symptom

InCare PRES 9300 system

incentive spirometry

incidence
i. of acute rejection
angle of i.
i. of bacteremia
gallstone i.

incidental
i. adenoma

incidental *(continued)*
    i. appendectomy
    i. splenectomy
incidentaloma
    adrenal gland i.
incipient
    i. nephropathy
    i. proteinuria
Incise Pouch
incision
    Amussat i.
    anterolateral thoracotomy i.
    apron skin i.
    Battle i.
    Battle-Jalaguier-Kammerer i.
    Bevan abdominal i.
    bilateral subcostal i.
    bilateral transabdominal i.
    bucket-handle i.
    burrowing i.
    buttonhole i.
    celiotomy i.
    Cheatle-Henry i.
    Cherney i.
    chevron i.
    choledochotomy i.
    circumumbilical i.
    cold knife i.
    Connell i.
    cruciate i.
    Czerny-Kocher-Perthes i.
    darting i.
    Deaver i.
    dorsal lumbotomy i.
    i. and drainage (I&D)
    eleventh rib flank i.
    eleventh rib transperitoneal i.
    elliptical i.
    endopyelotomy i.
    endoscopic i.
    endourological cold-knife i.
    enterotomy i.
    epigastric i.
    extended left subcostal i.
    fishmouth i.
    flank i.
    four-quadrant i.
    Gibson i.
    Gil-Vernet dorsal lumbotomy i.
    gridiron i.
    groin i.
    guillotine i.
    Heineke-Mikulicz i.
    hockey-stick i.
    infraumbilical i.
    inguinal i.
    inverted-U abdominal i.
    Joel-Cohen i.
    Kammerer-Battle i.
    Kehr i.
    Kocher i.
    LaRoque herniorrhaphy i.
    less morbid lower abdominal transverse i.
    i. line
    lower abdominal transverse i.
    low transverse i.
    lumbodorsal i.
    lumbotomy i.
    Mallard i.
    McBurney i.
    median i.
    midabdominal transverse i.
    midline lower abdominal i.
    midline upper abdominal i.
    minilaparotomy i.
    mini-Pfannenstiel i.
    modified Gibson i.
    muscle-cutting i.
    muscle-splitting i.
    oblique i.
    omega-shaped i.
    paramedian i.
    pararectus i.
    perineal i.
    Pfannenstiel i.
    plaque i.
    posterior transthoracic i.
    precut i.
    pyelotomy i.
    radial i.
    relaxing i.
    Rockey-Davis i.
    Salmon backcut i.
    Sanders i.
    Schuchardt relaxing i.
    smiling i.
    stab i.
    stepladder i. technique
    steri-stripped i.
    subcostal flank i.
    subcostal transperitoneal i.
    supracostal i.
    surgical i.
    teardrop i.
    thoracoabdominal i.
    transperitoneal anterior subcostal i. (TASI)
    transpubic i.
    transurethral i. (TUI)
    transverse semilunar skin i.
    Turner-Warwick i.
    unilateral subcostal i.
    vertical midline i.
    Wangensteen i.
    xiphoid-to-pubis midline abdominal i.

incision · incontinentia

xiphoid-to-umbilicus i.
Y-shaped i.
incisional
   i. biopsy
   i. corporoplasty
   i. hernia
incisor
incisura
   i. angularis
   i. dextra of Gans
   i. vesicae felleae hepatis
inclusion
   i. body
   concentric hyaline i.
   i. cyst
   glomerular endothelial myxovirus-like microtubular i.
   glycogen i.
   intracytoplasmic tuboreticular i. (TRI)
   tubuloreticular i. (TRI)
incompatible
   ABO i.
incompetence
   gastroesophageal i.
   LES i.
   neurogenic sphincteric i.
incompetent
   i. ileocecal valve
   i. sphincter
incomplete
   i. basal cell hyperplasia
   i. cirrhosis
   i. duplication
   i. hernia
   i. pancreas divisum (IPD)
   i. passage
   i. polypectomy
   i. rectal prolapse
   i. relaxation
   i. voiding
inconspicuous penis
incontinence
   adolescent i.
   anal i.
   anatomic stress i.
   anterior fecal i.
   bladder i.
   Blaivas classification of urinary i.
   bowel i.
   continuous i.
   daytime i.

diurnal i.
double i.
extraurethral i.
fecal i.
flatus i.
functional i.
genuine stress i. (GSI)
genuine stress urinary i. (GSUI)
geriatric i.
gravity urinary i.
hyperreflexic motor urge i.
ischemic fecal i.
mixed i.
Miyazaki-Bonney test for stress i.
neurogenic refractory urge i.
nocturnal i.
overflow fecal i.
pad test for urinary i.
paradoxical i.
paralytic i.
passive i.
postprostatectomy i.
posttraumatic i.
postvoid i.
rectal i.
recurrent stress i.
reflex i.
refractory motor urge i.
i. related
Resident Assessment Protocol for i.
i. score
secondary i.
sphincteric i.
stool i.
stress i. type 0, I, II, III
stress urinary i. (SUI)
i. surgery
Teflon paste injection for i.
transdermal oxybutynin for urinary i.
unconscious i.
urge i.
urgency i.
urinary exertional i.
urinary stress i.
incontinent
   i. epispadias
   i. ileostomy
   i. ileovesicostomy
incontinentia
   i. alvi
   i. urinae

NOTES

incoordination
    pharyngeal-UES i.
Incorporated
    Enteron Pharmaceuticals, I.
increased
    i. bladder permeability
    i. clinical demand
    i. hemocrit
    i. peritoneal clearance
    i. in proportion
    i. risk of penile carcinoma
incretin
incrustation
    stent i.
incrusted cystitis
incubation
    in vitro i.
incurable cancer
Incystene
^{111}**In-CYT-103 immunoscintigraphy**
indapamide
indentation
    haustral i.
indentifiable intrascrotal lesion
independent
    i. positive predictive factor
    i. predictor
    i. risk factor
Inderal
Indermil adhesive
indeterminate colitis (IC)
index, pl. **indices**
    American Urological Association symptom i.
    apoptotic i.
    AUA Symptom I.
    biliary saturation i.
    body mass i. (BMI)
    Bouchard i.
    BPH impact i. (BII)
    brachial pressure i.
    Broder i.
    cardiac output/cardiac i. (CO/CI)
    CD activity i.
    i. of cell proliferation
    cholesterol saturation i. (CSI)
    Clinical Activity I. (CAI)
    clitoral i.
    creatinine height i. (CHI)
    Crohn Disease Activity I. (CDAI)
    detrusor activity i.
    Doppler perfusion i. (DPI)
    frequency-duration i. (FDI)
    Functional Bowel Disorder Severity I. (FBDSI)
    Gingival I. (GI)
    Harvey-Bradshaw i.
    hemoglobin content i. (IHb)
    hepatic arterial pulsatility i. (HAPI)
    hepatic iron i. (HII)
    hepatic perfusion i. (HPI)
    hepatic tumor i. (HTI)
    histological activity i. (HAI)
    insulin sensitivity i.
    intrarenal resistive i.
    Karnofsky i.
    Knodell i.
    Kruger i.
    Maine Medical Assessment Program i.
    i. of malnutrition
    mean shunt i.
    mitosis-karyorrhexis i. (MKI)
    mitotic i.
    MMAP i.
    modified Barthel degree of disability i.
    Multidimensional Fatigue I. (MFI)
    National Institutes of Health Chronic Prostatitis Symptom I. (NIH-CPSI)
    Nepean Dyspepsia I. (NDI)
    nutritional i.
    obesity i.
    obstruction i.
    oxygen saturation i. (ISO_2)
    parietal cell i.
    PCNA-labeling i.
    Pediatric Crohn Disease Activity I. (PCDAI)
    Penetrating Abdominal Trauma I. (PATI)
    penile-brachial i. (PBI)
    penile-brachial pressure i. (PBPI)
    Perianal Crohn Disease Activity I. (PDAI)
    portal shunt i. (PSI)
    portal vein congestive i. (PVCI)
    postthaw sperm motility i.
    Pouchitis Disease Activity I. (PDAI)
    p_2 penile-brachial i.
    prognostic nutritional i. (PNI)
    PSA free/total i.
    Psychological General Well-Being I. (PGWBI)
    pulsatility i.
    Quetelet BMI i.
    renal failure i.
    renal resistive i.
    renovascular resistance i. (RVRI)
    resistive i. (RI)
    role of the resistive i.
    saturation i. (SI)
    Sexual Function I. (SFI)
    solute removal i.

spleen i.
symptom problem i. (SPI)
symptom sensitivity i.
symptom severity i. (SSI)
systemic vascular resistance i. (SVRI)
thymidine-labeling i.
transition zone i.
Truelove-Witts i.
tumor proliferative i.
uroflow i.
van Hees i.
van Hees Activity I. (VHAI)

India
    I. ink
    I. ink tattoo

Indiana
    I. continent reservoir
    I. continent reservoir urinary diversion
    I. urinary pouch
    I. variant galactosemia

Indian sickness

indican
    urinary i.

indication
    clinical i.
    primary i.
    i.'s for stenting

indicator
    prognostic i.
    i. of reactive oxygen species formation

indices (*pl. of* index)

Indiclor

indifferent electrode

indigenous amebiasis

indigestion
    acid i.
    fat i.
    gastric i.
    intestinal i.
    nervous i.

indigitation

indigo
    i. calculus
    i. carmine
    i. carmine dye
    i. carmine stain
    i. carmine-stained normal saline
    I. diffuse fiber
    I. LaserOptic treatment system
    I. Optima laser
    I. Optima laser system

indinavir calculus

indinavir-induced nephrolithiasis

indirect
    i. bilirubin
    i. hemagglutination (IHA)
    i. hemagglutination determination
    i. hernia sac
    i. immunofluorescence (IIF)
    i. immunofluorescence assay
    i. immunolocalization technique
    i. inguinal hernia

indispensable diagnostic modality

indium (In)
    i. 64-labeled white blood cell scan
    i. leukocyte scan
    i. pentetreotide

indium-111
    i. DTPA
    i. murine anti-CEA monoclonal antibody
    i. pentetreotide

[111]indium-labeled autologous leukocyte test

indium-labeled leukocyte scan

individual
    intermediate cystinuric i.
    i. parameter

individualization

Indocin

indocyanine
    i. green
    i. green clearance
    i. green dye (ICG)

indolalkylamine alkaloid

indole

indolent
    i. bubo
    i. radiation-induced rectal ulcer

indomethacin

indomethacin-induced mucosal damage

indoramin

indoxyl

indoxyluria

induced nitric oxide synthase (iNOS)

inducer
    interferon i.

induction
    c-fos i.

indurated appendix

NOTES

induration
　bowel wall i.
　fibroid i.
　granular i.
indurative nephritis
industrial toxin
indwelling
　i. stomal device
　i. ureteral stent
　i. urinary catheter
ineffective
　i. colonic propulsion
　i. erythropoiesis
　i. esophageal motility (IEM)
inertia
　colonic i.
inevitable postoperative pain
infancy
　melanotic neuroectodermal tumor of i. (MNTI)
infant
　i. esophagoscope
　i. reflex
　very low birth weight i.
infantile
　i. celiac disease
　i. colic
　i. diarrhea
　i. food protein-induced enterocolitis syndrome
　i. gastroenteritis
　i. hypertrophic pyloric stenosis (IHPS)
　i. leishmaniasis
　i. nephrotic syndrome
　i. pellagra
　i. polycystic disease (IPCD)
infantilism
　Herter i.
　sexual i.
infantis
　Bifidobacterium i.
　Salmonella i.
infantum
　cholera i.
　Leishmania i.
　Leishmania donovani i.
infarct
　bile i.
　bilirubin i.
　Brewer i.
　small bowel i.
　uric acid i.
　Zahn i.
infarcted bowel
infarction
　acute nonocclusive bowel i.
　intestinal i.
　mesenteric i.
　myocardial i.
　nonocclusive intestinal i.
　occlusive i.
　omental i.
　segmental ileal i.
　segmental testicular i.
　small intestinal i.
　total i.
infected
　i. bile duct
　i. pseudocyst
　i. pancreatic necrosis (IPN)
　i. tract
infection
　active systemic bacterial i.
　adenovirus i.
　i. after renal transplantation
　antifungal esophageal i.
　antifungal-resistant opportunistic i.
　Aspergillus i.
　asymptomatic urinary tract i. (AUTI)
　bacterial i.
　biomaterial-associated i.
　bladder *Candida* i.
　bloodstream i. (BSI)
　i. calculus
　Candida i.
　candidal i.
　catheter-related bloodstream i. (CR-BSI)
　catheter tunnel i.
　Chlamydia trachomatis i.
　CMV i.
　coliform urinary i.
　coxsackievirus i. A, B
　cryptosporidial i.
　cytomegalovirus i.
　deep-seated fungal i.
　dengue hemorrhagic fever i.
　dermatophyte i.
　device-related urinary tract i.
　dialysis access i.
　disseminated CMV i.
　domiciliary urinary tract i.
　echovirus i.
　enteric i.
　epididymal i.
　Epstein-Barr viral i.
　esophageal fungal i.
　exit site i.
　extrapulmonary *Pneumocystis carinii* i.
　fungal i.
　gas-forming pyogenic liver i.
　geriatric urinary tract i.
　helminthic i.
　hematogenous spread of i.
　hepatic candidal i.

hepatitis i. A–E
herpes simplex i.
HIV i.
intestinal i.
intraabdominal i.
isolated urinary tract i.
liver cyst i.
metasynchronous bacterial urinary tract i.
monilial i.
multiple hepatitis virus i.'s
Mycobacterium i.
necrotizing i.
nematode i.
nosocomial fungal i.
nosocomial urinary tract i.
opportunistic i.
parasitic i.
pediatric urinary tract i.
perianal i.
perineal i.
peristomal i.
peritoneal fungal i.
pneumococcal i.
polymicrobial i.
Polyomavirus i.
postsplenectomy i.
preventing urinary tract i.
recurrent urinary tract i.
renal allograft i.
renal cyst i.
retroperitoneal i.
retrovirus i.
rotavirus i.
seminal vesicle i.
i. stone
strongyloid i.
synchronous urinary tract i.
torulopsis i.
tunnel i.
uncomplicated urinary tract i.
unresolved urinary tract i.
urinary tract i. (UTI)
varicella-zoster i.
Vibrio fetus i.
viral i.
whipworm i.
wound i.
infection-prevention device
infection-related interstitial nephritis
infectious
    i. avian nephrosis

i. colitis
i. complication
i. esophagitis
i. gastroenteritis
i. hepatitis
i. jaundice
i. mononucleosis heterophil antibody
i. nosocomial diarrhea
i. pancreatic necrosis
i. splenomegaly
i. viral diarrhea
infective
i. endocarditis
i. jaundice
i. splenomegaly
INFeD
Infergen
inferior
i. aberrant ductule
i. adrenal vein
i. anal nerve
i. anal plexus
arteria epigastrica i.
arteria mesenterica i.
arteria pancreatica i.
arteria rectalis i.
i. digital fossa
i. duodenal fold
i. extremity
i. fascia
fascia diaphragmatis pelvis i.
flexura duodeni i.
i. hemorrhoidal artery
i. hypogastric plexus
i. mesenteric artery (IMA)
i. mesenteric vein (IMV)
i. pancreatic artery
i. pancreaticoduodenal artery
i. phrenic artery
plica duodenalis i.
i. pole
i. rectal nerve
i. rectal vein
i. vena cava (IVC)
i. vena cava thrombosis
ventral posterior i. (VPI)
inferiores
arteriae pancreaticoduodenales i.
inferomedial
infertility
i. androgeny

NOTES

infertility *(continued)*
    idiopathic i.
    immune-mediated i.
    tubal i.
infestation
    Ascaris i.
    biliary i.
    Fasciola hepatica i.
    parasitic i.
infiltrate
    chronic inflammatory cell i.
    lobular inflammatory i.
    lobular mononuclear cell i.
    MN i.
    mononuclear histiocytic portal i.
    PMN i.
    polymorphonuclear inflammatory i.
    sparse inflammatory i.
infiltrating
    i. adenocarcinoma
    i. inflammatory cell
    i. T cell
infiltration
    bacterial mucosal i.
    cellular i.
    colonic i.
    fat i.
    focal fatty i.
    gastric epithelial cell i.
    glomerular macrophage i.
    glomerular neutrophil i.
    lymphohistiocytic i.
    massive malignant i.
    neutrophilic i.
    panmucosal inflammatory cell i.
    perirectal fat i.
    plasma cell portal i.
    portal plasma cell i.
    serosal i.
    tumor i.
infiltrative
    i. disease
    i. lymphoma
inflamed
    i. appendix
    i. diverticulum
    i. gallbladder
    i. mucosa
inflammation
    cervical i.
    evidence of i.
    Hara classification of gallbladder i.
    interstitial i.
    intralobular i.
    kidney i.
    i. marker
    microbiliary i.
    parenchymal i.
    periportal i.
    portal eosinophilic i.
    portal tract i.
    refractory pouch i.
    transmural i.
    traumatic i.
    tubulointerstitial i.
    vaginal i.
inflammatoria
    dysphagia i.
inflammatory
    i. bowel disease (IBD)
    I. Bowel Disease Questionnaire (IBDQ)
    i. bowel syndrome (IBS)
    i. colitis
    i. diarrhea
    i. fibroid polyp (IFP)
    i. glomerulopathy
    i. pancreatitis
    i. polyp-fold complex (IPFC)
    i. prostatic mass (IPM)
    i. pseudotumor
    i. reaction
    i. renal mass
    i. response
inflatable penile prosthesis (IPP)
inflated rubber cylinder
inflator
    LeVeen i.
InflatoRing
infliximab IV infusion
influenzae
    Haemophilus i.
influenza virus
influx
    Rb i.
infold
infolding
    complex papillary i.
infracolic compartment
infradiaphragmatic radiotherapy
infragastric pancreoscopy
infrahepatic vena cava
inframammary region
inframesocolic compartment
infraorbital
infrared
    i. coagulation
    i. coagulator
    i. endoscopy
    i. photocoagulation (IRC)
    i. spectroscopy
    i. transillumination gastroscopy
    i. videoendoscope
infrarenal template procedure
infraumbilical
    i. incision
    i. mound
infravesical prostatic obstruction

infrequent
    i. defecation
    i. voider-lazy bladder syndrome
Infumorph
infundibular
    i. neck
    i. stenosis
    i. width
infundibuliform
infundibulopelvic
    i. angle
    i. ligament
    i. stenosis
infundibuloplasty
infundibulum
    i. of bile duct
    caliceal i.
    i. of gallbladder
    lower i.
    single midline caliceal i.
Infusaid
    I. chemotherapy implantable pump
    I. hepatic pump
infuser
    UROS i.
infusion
    acid i.
    atropine i.
    Avastin IV i.
    BabyBIG powder for IV i.
    bladder i.
    circadian-shaped i.
    citrate i.
    continuous ambulatory i.
    hepatic arterial i. (HAI)
    hypertonic i.
    infliximab IV i.
    Infuvite Pediatric IV i.
    insulin/glucagon i.
    intraarterial vasopressin i.
    intraduodenal lipid i.
    intravariceal i.
    intravenous urea i.
    intravenous vasopressin i.
    lipid i.
    monooctanoin i.
    multiple vitamins for i.
    i. nephrotomography
    Normosol-M IV i.
    pentagastrin i.
    Protonix IV powder for i.
    i. pump (IP)
    i. pyelography
    Remicade IV i.
    saline i.
    solvent i.
    total dose i.
    transcatheter arterial i.
    vasopressin i.
Infuvite Pediatric IV infusion
ingested
    i. foreign body
    i. foreign object
ingestion
    acid i.
    alkali i.
    battery i.
    button battery i.
    caustic i.
    cocaine package i.
    fish bone i.
    foreign body i.
    lye i.
    mercuric oxide battery i.
    razor blade i.
    safety pin i.
Ingold M3, M4 glass electrode pH monitor
ingrowth
    mesodermal i.
    i. of tumor
inguinal
    i. adenopathy
    i. bulge
    i. canal
    i. cord
    i. crease
    i. crease compound nevus
    i. cryptorchidism
    i. floor
    i. fold
    i. hernia (IH)
    i. incision
    i. laparoscopy
    i. ligament
    i. ligament of Blumberg
    i. lymphadenopathy
    i. lymph node
    i. reservoir inserter
    i. ring
    i. sphincter
    i. triangle
    i. varicocelectomy

NOTES

inguinale
    granuloma i.
    hernia uteri i.
inguinoabdominal
inguinocrural
inguinofemoral hernia
inguinoperitoneal
inguinoscrotal hernia
inguinosuperficial hernia
inhalation aerosol
inhaler
    Allis i.
    Vanceril i.
inherent to linkage
inheritance
    kallikrein i.
inherited defect
inhibin
    beta i.
inhibition
    alcohol dehydrogenase i.
    5-alpha-reductase i.
    antisense DNA i.
    i. assay
    bladder i.
    COX-1, -2 i.
    cyclooxygenase i.
    deglutitive i.
    detrusor muscle i.
    effect of i.
    glycolytic i.
    laminin receptor i.
    lipoxygenase i.
    micturition reflex i.
    presynaptic i.
    renin i.
    secretory leukocyte proteinase i. (SLPI)
    spinobulbospinal micturition reflex i.
inhibitor
    ACE i.
    alkaline protease i. (API)
    alpha-glucosidase i.
    5-alpha-reductase i.
    angiotensin-converting enzyme i. (ACEI)
    aromatase i.
    ATPase i.
    azasteroid i.
    calcineurin i.
    carbonic anhydrase i. (CAI)
    C-1 esterase i.
    chain-terminating i.
    collagen synthesis i.
    COX-2 i.
    cyclin-dependent kinase i.
    cyclooxygenase i.
    cyclooxygenase-2 i.
    cytolysis i.
    familial lipoprotein lipase i.
    gastric acid pump i.
    hepatocyte proliferation i. (HPI)
    H+/K+-ATPase acid pump i.
    inter-alpha-trypsin i. (ITI)
    intracellular adhesion molecule i. (ICAM-1)
    lipoxygenase i.
    5-lipoxygenase i.
    metalloproteinase i.
    monoamine oxidase i.
    nitric oxide synthase i.
    nonnucleoside reverse transcription i. (NNRTI)
    pancreatic secretory trypsin i. (PSTI)
    phosphodiesterase i.
    plasminogen activator i. (PAI)
    plasminogen activator i. type 1, 2 (PAI-1, -2)
    protease i.
    proteinase i.
    proton pump i. (PPI)
    purine synthesis i.
    rapamycin i.
    rectoanal i.
    RNAse i.
    sertraline serotonin reuptake i.
    serum alpha$_1$-protease i.
    topoisomerase I i.
    trypsin i.
    tumor-derived angiogenic i.
    urinary trypsin i.
    wheat amylase i.
inhibitory
    i. effect
    i. intestinointestinal reflex
    i. postsynaptic potential (IPSP)
    i. syndrome
inhomogeneity of parenchyma
inhomogeneous hyperechoic mass
initial
    i. broad-spectrum therapy
    i. clinical experience
    i. hematuria
    i. in-plan record
    i. proximal diversion
    i. treatment
initiation
    micturition reflex manual i.
    voiding i.
initiative
    Dialysis Outcomes Quality I. (DOQI)
    Kidney Disease Outcomes Quality I. (K/DOQI)
    National Kidney Foundation-Data Outcomes Quality I. (NKF-DOQI)

InjecAid · injury

InjecAid system
injectable
i. ester
Macroplastique i.
injection
adrenalin i.
Albunex i.
Antizol for i.
BayGam IM i.
BCG live intravesical i.
Benzacot I.
botulinum toxin i.
BTX i.
Camptosar i.
i. catheter
collagen i.
corpus cavernosum papaverine i.
cyanoacrylate i.
cyanocobalamin i.
daptomycin for i.
depot i.
diazepam emulsified i.
Dibent I.
doxercalciferol i.
Eligard sustained-release subcu i.
endoscopic botulinum toxin i.
endoscopic epinephrine i.
endoscopic India ink i.
endoscopic ultrasound-guided fine-needle i.
endosonographically targeted i.
enoxaparin sodium i.
ERxin multicomponent penile i.
ethanol i.
etoposide i.
fibrin i.
follitropin alfa for i.
glutaraldehyde cross-linked collagen i.
i. gold probe (IGP)
Hectorol i.
Histoacryl i.
intracytoplasmic sperm i. (ICSI)
intralesional steroid i.
intraperitoneal i.
intrasphincteric botulinum toxin i.
intravariceal i.
iopamidol i.
iron sucrose i.
lipiodol i.
local depot i.
meropenem for i.
moxisylyte i.
mycophenolate mofetil intravenous for i.
2-octyl cyanoacrylate i.
papaverine i.
paravariceal i.
PEG-interferon alfa-2b powder for i.
PEG-Intron powder for i.
percutaneous ethanol i. (PEI)
periurethral collagen i.
PGE_1 i.
Plenaxis powder for IM i.
polidocanol i.
Polytef i.
polytetrafluoroethylene paste i.
polytetrafluoroethylene periurethral i.
Renovist I.
sclerosant i.
i. sclerosis
i. sclerotherapy
sham i.
i. site
sodium hyaluronate i.
sodium morrhuate i.
sodium tetradecyl i.
somatropin i.
submucosal saline i.
submucosal Teflon i.
subureteric Teflon i. (STING)
synthetic porcine secretin for i.
tangential colonic submucosal i.
^{99m}Tc DISIDA contrast i.
technetium 99m Exametazime i.
i. therapy
Tisseel fibrin sealant i.
transduodenal i.
trigger point i.
Twinrix IM i.
zoledronic acid for i.
Zometa for i.
Zorbtive powder for subcu i.
injector
Olympus i.
Teflon i.
Virag i.
InjecTx cystoscope
injured allograft
injury
acid i.
Ajmalin liver i.
alcohol-induced gastric i.

NOTES

injury *(continued)*
  alkaline i.
  antecedent pancreatic i.
  bile salt i.
  bladder i.
  blast i.
  bowel i.
  cavernous artery i.
  cell-mediated hepatic i.
  closed i.
  comparison of depth of tissue i.
  diaphragmatic i.
  drug-induced acute hepatic i.
  duodenal i.
  emetogenic i.
  gastric mucosal i.
  gastroduodenal mucosal i.
  glomerular i.
  Helicobacter-induced gastric i.
  hemorrhagic radiation i.
  hepatic vein i.
  hepatocellular i.
  H_2O_2-induced i.
  hyperfiltration i.
  hypertensive renal i.
  iatrogenic intraoperative ureteral i.
  intestinal radiation i.
  ischemia-reperfusion i.
  juxtahepatic venous i.
  liver transplantation preservation i.
  major deceleration i.
  medication-induced i.
  microangiopathic renal i.
  mitochondrial i.
  mucosal i.
  NSAID-induced gastric i.
  NSAID-induced intestinal i.
  obstetric i.
  open i.
  oxidant i.
  oxidative cell i.
  pancreatic i.
  paraquat-induced upper gastrointestinal i.
  pill-induced esophageal i.
  pinch i.
  PMN-mediated endothelial cell i.
  radiation i.
  rectal i.
  renovascular i.
  reperfusion i.
  spinal cord i. (SCI)
  splenic i.
  straddle i.
  stress-related mucosal i.
  treatment of nonspecific inflammatory i.
  tubular epithelial cell i.
  tubular morphologic i.
  tubulointerstitial i.
  ureteral i.
  urethra blowout i.
  vascular i.
ink
  autoclaved India i.
  China i.
  Higgins India i.
  India i.
  Koh-I-Noor Universal India i.
  osmolarity of i.
  Pelikan brand India i.
  solution-diluted India i.
inlay
  Turner-Warwick i.
Inlay-Tabs
  Ursinus I.-T.
inlet
  esophageal i.
  i. patch
  i. patch mucosa
  i. port
  i. pouch (IP)
  thoracic i.
[111]In-leukocyte technique
in-line blood gas monitor
innate immunity
inner
  i. crossbar
  i. diameter (ID)
  i. medulla
  i. medullary collecting duct (IMCD)
innervation
  adrenal gland i.
  afferent i.
  bladder i.
  cholinergic i.
  intrinsic excitatory i.
  kidney i.
  pelvis i.
  prostate gland i.
  rectal i.
  seminal vesicle i.
  serosal afferent i.
  striated muscle i.
innocens
  Serpulina i.
innocent gallstone
innocuous
Innoflex variable-stiffness colonoscope
Inno-LiPA assay
innominate
  i. bone
  i. groove
Innova home incontinence therapy system
inoculated medium
inoculum size

inorganic iodine
iNOS
 induced nitric oxide synthase
inositol
 i. lipid
 i. ring
 i. triphosphate
 i. 1,4,5-triphosphate (IP3)
 i. 1,4,5-triphosphate Ca2+
In-111 pentetreotide
input
 fast cholinergic i.
 nociceptive sensory i.
insemination
 intrauterine i. (IUI)
 subzonal i. (SUZI)
insensible loss of water
insert
 FemSoft i.
 Hollister Convex i.
 Nu-Hope Convex i.
 Reliance urinary control i.
 Sur-Fit Natura disposable convex i.
 United Surgical Convex i.
 urinary control urethral i.
inserter
 Furlow cylinder i.
 inguinal reservoir i.
insertion
 biliary endoprosthesis i.
 chromosome i.
 flatus tube i.
 jejunal tube i.
 J-tube i.
 i. mutation
 PEG i.
 Sengstaken-Blakemore tube i.
 subclavian catheter i.
 i. tube
InSIGHT
 I. manometry
 I. manometry system
insignificant
 clinically i.
insipidus
 congenital nephrogenic diabetes i. (CNDI)
 diabetes i.
 nephrogenic diabetes i. (NDI)
 neurogenic diabetes i.
insorption
inspiration

inspiratory
inspissated
 i. bile
 i. bile syndrome
 i. feces
 i. sump syndrome
instability
 bladder postcystourethropexy i.
 chromosome i.
 detrusor i. (DI)
 detrusor muscle i.
 genomic i.
 microsatellite i. (MSI)
instant
 i. camera
 Hydrocil I.
 i. photography
instantaneous clearance
InStent EsophaCoil stent
instillation
 intravesical i.
 i. therapy
instituted GI bleeding management program
institutional
 i. colon
 i. dysentery
institutionalized patient
instrument
 Accurate Surgical and Scientific I.'s (ASSI)
 Bard Biopty i.
 Bard BladderScan bladder volume i.
 biopsy i.
 BIP biopsy i.
 i. count
 CRIT-LINE i.
 Digestive Health Status I. (DHSI)
 Dilamezinsert urologic i.
 DMI urologic i.
 Duette double-lumen ERCP i.
 endosonography i.
 ERBE electrical coagulation i.
 ERBE electrical cutting i.
 gauge of i.
 GIA i.
 grasping i.
 guide-eye i.
 mechanical radial-scanning i.
 oblique forward-viewing i.
 PCEE automated anastomotic i.

NOTES

instrument *(continued)*
  quality of life i.
  Quinton suction biopsy i.
  Radiometer 85 i.
  Roboprep G i.
  Sharpoint cutting i.
  slotted i.
  small-diameter endosonographic i.
  spring-loaded-type biopsy i.
  standardized i.
instrumentation
  biliary i.
  Karl Storz i.
  Microvasive i.
  retrograde i.
instrument-track seeding
insufficiency
  acute renal i. (ARI)
  adrenal i.
  Angiotensin-Converting Enzyme Inhibition in Progressive Renal I. (AIPRI)
  chronic renal i. (CRI)
  exocrine pancreatic i. (EPI)
  gastric i.
  gastromotor i.
  hepatic i.
  ileocecal i.
  pancreatic exocrine i.
  primary adrenal i.
  progressive renal i.
  pyloric i.
  renal i.
  underlying chronic renal i.
  vascular i.
  velopharyngeal i. (VPI)
insufflation
  air i.
  colonic i.
  helium i.
  i. of stomach
insufflator
  carbon dioxide i.
  nitrous oxide i.
  PROTOCO$_2$L i.
Insuflon insulin delivery device
insular structure
insulated
  i. curved scissors
  i. straight scissors
insulated-tip electrosurgical knife
insulation-tipped electrosurgical knife
insulin
  human i.
  i. hyperplasia
  Lente i.
  NPH i.
  protamine zinc i.
  i. reaction
  i. receptor-related receptor
  i. resistance
  i. resistance syndrome
  Semilente i.
  i. sensitivity index
  i. stain
  Ultralente i.
insulin-degrading enzyme (IDE)
insulin-dependent
  i.-d. diabetes
  i.-d. diabetes mellitus (IDDM)
insulin/glucagon
  i./g. infusion
  putative hepatotrophic factors i./g.
insulinlike
  i. growth factor (IGF)
  i. growth factor-1 (IGF-1)
  i. growth factor-2 (IGF-2)
  i. growth factor-binding protein-1 (IGFBP-1)
insulinoma
insulinopenia
insulin-transferrin-sodium selenite
insulin-treated diabetic
insult
  ischemic i.
intact
  i. hormone assay
  i. proprioception
  i. PTH
intake
  caloric i.
  clandestine i.
  daily protein i. (DPI)
  dietary energy i.
  i. and output (I&O)
Intal
integrase gene
integrated
  i. assessment
  i. automatic stone-tissue detection system
  i. clearance
  i. genomic map
integrating spherical power meter
integrin
  alpha-3-beta-1 i.
  alpha-5-beta-1 i.
  B1, B2 i.
  beta-1 chain i.
  i. mediated
  membrane-spanning i.
integrity
  mucosal i.
integument
intensified radiographic imaging system (IRIS)
intensity
  fluorescence i.

fluorescent light i. (FLI)
light fluorescent i.
intensity-modulated
i.-m. proton therapy (IMPT)
i.-m. radiation therapy (IMRT)
intention
delayed primary i.
healing by first i.
healing by primary i.
healing by second i.
healing by secondary i.
i. to treat (ITT)
intentional injection of Enteryx
intentionem
healing per primam i.
healing per secundam i.
interaction
bacterial host i.
cell-cell i.
cervical mucus-sperm i.
crystal-cell i.
crystal-phospholipid i.
idiotype-anti-idiotype i.
shock wave-gas bubble i.
vasoactive peptide-cytokine i.
interactive video technology (IVT)
inter-alpha inhibitor family
inter-alpha-trypsin inhibitor (ITI)
intercalated cell
intercalatum
Schistosoma i.
intercapillary nephrosclerosis
INTERCEED absorbable adhesion barrier
intercellular
i. adhesion molecule-1 (ICAM-1)
i. space
Intercept
I. esophagus microcoil
I. prostate microcoil
I. urethra microcoil
interceptive conditioning
Interceptor M3 triple-channel solid-state monitor
intercolonoscopy
interconversion
intercostal
i. pedicle esophagogastropexy
i. scan
i. space

intercourse
receptive anal i.
interdialytic
i. urea generation
i. weight gain (IDWG)
interdigestive
i. antroduodenal motility
i. migrating motor complex
i. myoelectric complex
interdigitate
interdigitating teeth
interface
fluid-air i.
i. hepatitis
interference
bacterial i.
i. barrier filter
catheter bacterial i.
interferential electrical stimulation
interferon
i. alfa-2a
i. alfacon-1
i. alfa-n1
i. alfa-n3
i. alpha
alpha i.
i. alpha-2b therapy
i. alpha therapy
beta i.
consensus i. (CIFN)
gamma i.
i. gamma stimulation
high-dose consensus i.
human lymphoblastoid i. (L-IFN)
i. inducer
low-dose i.
pegylated i.
recombinant human alfa i.
i. treatment
type I i.
alpha-2-a-interferon
interferon-beta
interferon-alpha (IFN alfa)
i.-a. 2-beta
interferon-gamma (IFN-gamma)
basal i.-g.
HLA class II-restricted i.-g.
interferon-stimulated regulatory element (ISRE)
interfoveolar muscle

NOTES

Intergel
    I. adhesion prevention solution
    I. irrigating solution
Intergroup Rhabdomyosarcoma Study (IRS)
interhaustral
    i. fold
    i. septum
interiliacus
    plexus i.
INTERING vascular graft
interlabial
    i. rhabdomyosarcoma
    i. sarcoma botryoid
interleukin (IL)
interleukin-1 (IL-1)
    i. receptor antagonist
interleukin-2 (IL-2)
    i. receptor-blocking agent
    recombinant i.
    serum i.
interleukin-6 (IL-6)
    serum i.
interleukin-8 (IL-8)
    serum i.
interleukin-10 (IL-10)
interleukin-1b urinary marker
interlobar
    i. renal artery
    i. vein
interlobular
    i. bile duct
    i. fibrosis
interlobulares
    ductuli i.
interlocking
    i. detachable coils
    i. ligature
interloop abscess
intermedia
    Yersinia i.
intermediate
    i. biomarker
    i. cystinuric individual
    i. density lipoprotein (IDL)
    i. fasting
    i. filament bundle
    i. junction
    i. low-density lipoprotein (ILDL)
    malignant teratoma, i. (MTI)
    i. mesenteric lymph node
    i. polyposis
    i. space
    thiol i.
intermedius
    Citrobacter i.
intermesenteric abscess
intermicrovillar area

intermittens
    dyspragia i.
intermittent
    i. calcitriol therapy
    i. catheterization
    i. click
    i. diarrhea
    i. drip feeding
    i. hemodialysis (IHD)
    i. hemoglobinuria
    i. hepatic fever
    i. hormone therapy
    i. obstruction
    i. pain
    i. positive-pressure breathing (IPPB)
    i. proteinuria
    i. pulse
    i. self-catheterization (ISC)
    i. self-obturation
    i. suctioning
interna
    elastica i.
    fascia spermatica i.
    lamina rara i. (LRI)
internal
    i. abdominal fascia
    i. abdominal ring
    i. absorption
    i. anal sphincter (IAS)
    i. biliary drainage
    i. biliary lavage
    i. biliary stent
    i. cremaster of Henle
    i. fiberoptic cable
    i. hemorrhage
    i. hemorrhoid
    i. iliac artery
    i. iliac vein
    i. inguinal ring
    i. oblique
    i. oblique fascia
    i. oblique muscle
    I. Ostomy Association (IOA)
    i. procidentia
    i. proctotomy
    i. pudendal artery
    i. pudendal vein
    i. rectal sphincter
    i. ribosome entry site (IRES)
    i. rotation
    i. septation
    i. spermatic fascia
    i. spermatic vessel
    i. sphincterotomy
    i. urethrotomy
international
    i. androgen unit
    I. Association for Enterostomal Therapy

I. Autoimmune Hepatitis Group score
I. Biomedical Mode 745-100 microcapillary infusion system
I. Continence Society (ICS)
I. Continence Society classification of voiding dysfunction
I. Continence Society voiding function classification
I. Germ Cell Cancer Collaborative Group (IGCCCG)
I. Germ Cell Cancer Collaborative Group classification
I. Index of Erectile Function (IIEF)
I. Prognostic Index score
I. Prostate Symptom Score (IPSS)
i. unit of male hormone
i. units per liter (IU/L)

internet-based digital imaging
interneuron
    enteric i.
internist tumor
internodal strand
internuclear ophthalmoplegia
internum
    orificium urethrae externum i.
    ostium urethrae i.
interobserver reliability
interosseous
interpersonal sensitivity
interphase PBMC
interpolar region
interposition
    colonic i.
    i. Dacron graft
    i. flap of omentum
    ileal i.
    jejunal pouch i. (JPI)
    omental i.
    i. operation
interrogans
    Leptospira i.
interrupted
    i. manual mucomucosal absorbable suture
    i. seromuscular suture
intersex
    i. condition
    i. gonad
intersexual
    adult i.

intersexuality
intersphincteric
    i. anal fistula
    i. anorectal space
    i. groove
    i. perirectal abscess
    i. plane
    i. rectal dissection
    i. resection
    i. sulcus
InterStim device
interstitial
    i. brachytherapy
    i. cells of Cajal (ICC)
    i. cell tumor of testis
    i. collagenase
    i. cystitis
    I. Cystitis Data Base (ICDB)
    i. diffusion
    i. diode
    i. fibroblast
    i. fibrosis
    i. gastritis
    i. hernia
    i. hypercellularity
    i. immunocompetent cell
    i. inflammation
    i. irradiation
    i. laser coagulation (ILC)
    i. mononuclear cell
    i. pancreatitis
    i. photodynamic therapy
    i. rejection
    i. scarlatinal nephritis
    i. syphilitic nephritis
    i. volume
interstitium
    medullary i.
    renal i.
intersymphyseal
    i. bar
    i. stitch
intertriginous region
intertrigo
    candidal i.
intertropical hyphema
interureteral
interureteric ridge
interval
    i. appendectomy
    confidence i. (CI)

NOTES

intervention
    angiographic i.
    endoscopic i.
    urological i.
interventional
    i. technique
    i. uroradiology
interventricular defect
interview
intestinal
    i. absorption
    i. absorptive cell
    i. adaptation
    i. amebiasis
    i. anastomosis
    i. angina
    i. anthrax
    i. antireflux valve
    i. atony
    i. atresia
    i. atrophy
    i. bacterium
    i. bag
    i. biopsy
    i. brush border (IBB)
    i. bypass
    i. calculus
    i. capillariasis
    i. clamp
    i. colic
    i. colonization
    i. concretion
    i. content
    i. decompression
    i. distention
    i. distomiasis
    i. diverticulum
    i. emphysema
    i. endocrine cell
    i. endoscopy
    i. enterocyte
    i. epithelial cell
    i. fatty acid-binding protein (I-FABP)
    i. fistula
    i. fixation
    i. flora
    i. hemorrhage
    i. histoplasmosis
    i. immunology
    i. indigestion
    i. infarction
    i. infection
    i. intoxication
    i. intussusception
    i. ischemia
    i. juice
    i. lactase deficiency
    i. lamina propria
    i. lipodystrophy
    i. loop
    i. lumen
    i. lymphangiectasia
    i. malrotation
    i. metaplasia type I–III
    i. motility disorder
    i. mucosa
    i. mucosal mast cell (IMMC)
    i. myiasis
    i. myoneurosis
    i. myxoneurosis
    i. necrosis
    i. obstruction (IO)
    i. parasite
    i. peptide
    i. peptide TFF3
    i. perforation
    i. perfusion
    i. permeability
    i. permeability measurement
    i. phlebectasia
    i. pneumatosis
    i. polyposis
    i. polyposis-cutaneous pigmentation syndrome
    i. prolapse
    i. protozoa
    i. pseudoobstruction
    i. radiation injury
    i. schistosomiasis
    i. sedative
    i. sling
    i. sling placement
    i. spirochete
    i. stasis
    i. stasis syndrome
    i. steatorrhea
    i. stenosis
    i. stricture
    i. surgery
    i. tract
    i. transit study
    i. tuberculosis
    i. ureteral replacement
    i. viability
    i. villous architecture
    i. villus
    i. volvulus
    i. web
intestinalis, pl. **intestinales**
    arteriae intestinales
    dyspragia intermittens angiosclerotica i.
    Encephalitozoon i.
    Giardia i.
    lipodystrophia i.
    mycosis i.
    myxorrhea i.

pneumatosis cystoides i. (PCI)
sepsis i.
Septata i.
trunci intestinales
intestine
bacterial metabolism in i.
blind i.
Crohn small i.
distal i. (DI)
empty i.
iced i.
jejunoileal i.
kink in i.
malrotation of i.
mesenterial i.
milking of i.
papillary adenoma of large i.
segmental i.
small i.
straight i.
villous coat of small i.
intestinofugal neuron
intestinogastric reflex
intestinointestinal
intestinorum
pneumatosis cystoides i.
intimal
i. fibroplasia
i. hyperplasia
intimin
intolerance
dietary protein i.
disaccharide i.
fatty food i.
fructose i.
glucose i.
hereditary fructose i.
lactose i.
intoxication
acute methanol i.
alcohol i.
drug i.
intestinal i.
metal i.
methanol i.
quinidine i.
systemic mercury i.
intraabdominal
i. abscess
i. actinomycosis
i. adhesion
i. bile leakage

i. desmoid tumor
i. hemorrhage
i. ileal reservoir
i. infection
i. mass
i. pressure
i. pressure gauge
i. sepsis (IAS)
i. transverse testicular ectopia
i. viscus
intraanal
i. electromyography
i. pressure
i. wart
intraaortic endovascular sonography
intraappendicular
intraarterial (IA)
i. chemotherapy
i. chemotherapy catheter
i. digital subtraction angiography
i. vasopressin infusion
intraassay precision
intraballoon pressure
intrabulbar fossa
intracapillary thrombosis
intracapsular dissection
intracavernosal
i. injection therapy (ICIT)
i. injection treatment
i. pressure
intracavernous
i. injection and stimulation test
i. injection therapy
intracavitary
i. application brachytherapy
i. implantation
i. radiation boost therapy
i. topical therapy
i. transducer
intracellular
i. acidity
i. acification
i. adhesion molecule inhibitor (ICAM-1)
i. buffering
i. fluid (ICF)
i. flush effect
i. pH
i. pool
i. potassium
i. signaling system

NOTES

intracellulare
    Mycobacterium i.
intracholedochal
    i. manometric catheter
    i. pressure
    i. stent
intracisternal (IC)
IntraCoil nitinol stent
intracolonic Kaposi sarcoma
intracorporeal
    i. anastomosis
    i. electrohydraulic lithotripsy (IEHL)
    i. injection therapy
    i. laser lithotripsy (ICL, ILL)
    i. lithotripsy
    i. lithotriptor
    i. needle breakage
    i. shock wave lithotripsy (ISWL)
    i. therapy of erectile dysfunction
intracranial
    i. hemorrhage
    i. pressure monitoring
intracrine negative feedback modulator
intractable
    i. constipation
    i. diarrhea
    i. tumor
    i. ulcer
    i. ulcerative colitis
    i. vomiting
intracuticular suture
intracystic epithelial proliferation
intracytoplasmic
    i. calcium
    i. CMV inclusion body
    i. mucin
    i. sperm injection (ICSI)
    i. tuboreticular inclusion (TRI)
intradermal
    i. suture
    i. tattooing technique
intradialytic
    i. hypotension (IDH)
    i. parenteral nutrition (IDPN)
    i. period
    i. symptom
intradiverticular papilla
IntraDose gel
Intraducer peritoneal cannula
intraductal
    i. cholangioscopy
    i. endoscope
    i. imaging catheter
    i. lithiasis
    i. mucin-hypersecreting neoplasm
    i. mucin-producing tumor
    i. oncocytic papillary neoplasm (IOPN)
    i. papillary-mucinous neoplasm (IPMN)
    i. papillary-mucinous tumor (IPMT)
    i. papillary and mucinous tumors
    i. papillary and mucinous tumors of pancreas (IPMY)
    i. papillary tumor (IPT)
    i. pressure
    i. secretin test (IDST)
    i. ultrasonography (IDUS)
    i. ultrasound (IDUS)
    i. ultrasound probe
intraduodenal (ID)
    i. lipid infusion
intraepiploic hernia
intraepithelial
    i. body
    i. cancer
    i. leukocyte (IEL)
    i. lymphocyte (IEL)
    i. lymphocytosis
intraesophageal
    i. acid test
    i. balloon distention (IEBD)
    i. peristaltic pressure
    i. pH
    i. pH monitoring (EpHM)
    i. pH test
    i. stent
    i. variceal pressure
intrafamilial clustering of *Helicobacter pylori*
intragastric (IG)
    i. acidity
    i. balloon
    i. bubble
    i. continuous pH-meter
    i. drip
    i. EGF
    i. gallstone
    i. hydrolysis
    i. pH
    i. pH mapping
    i. pH monitor record
    i. pressure
    i. volume
intraglandular fluid
intraglomerular
    i. hemodynamics
    i. hypertension
    i. mesangial cell
    i. pressure
intragraft
intrahaustral contraction ring
intrahepatic
    i. abscess
    i. antigen-dependent lymphocyte-hepatocyte
    i. artery-systemic shunt

intrahepatic · intraoperative

i. ascariasis
i. atresia (IHA)
i. AV fistula
i. bile duct
i. biliary cystic dilation
i. biliary duct hypoplasia
i. biliary stricture
i. cholangioenterostomy
i. cholangiojejunostomy
i. cholelithiasis
i. cholestasis
i. cholestasis of pregnancy (ICP)
i. ductal dilation
i. hematoma
i. hepatitis
i. invasion
i. lymphocyte
i. portal hypertension
i. portal obstruction
i. radicle
i. sclerosing cholangitis
i. spontaneous arterioportal fistula
i. stone

intrailiac hernia
intrajejunal (IJ)
intralesional
i. steroid injection
i. treatment

intralipid fat emulsion
intralobar
intralobular
i. fibrosis
i. inflammation

intraluminal
i. clot
i. cyst
i. distention
i. duodenal diverticulum (IDD)
i. electrical impedance
i. electrical impedancometry
i. esophageal pressure
i. filling defect
i. gas bubble
i. lipolysis
i. manometry
i. pH-pressure relationship
i. pouch
i. pressure recording
i. probe
i. proliferation
i. radiotherapy

i. reference electrode
i. Silastic esophageal stent
i. stapler (ILS)
i. stone
i. ultrasound (ILUS)
i. urethral pressure

intramembranous particle strand
intramesenteric
i. abscess
i. desmoid tumor

intramucosal
i. cancer
i. carcinoma
i. metastasis

intramural
i. air dissection
i. aneurysm
i. atheromatous disease
i. colonic air
i. diverticulum
i. duodenal hematoma (IDH)
i. fistulous tract
i. ganglion
i. incision technique
i. intestinal hemorrhage
i. lesion
i. microvessel density
i. secretory reflex
i. ureter

intramuscular (IM)
i. perineural stimulation graciloplasty

intranuclear CMV inclusion body
intraoperative
i. angiography
i. autologous transfusion
i. biliary endoscopy
i. cavernous nerve stimulation
i. cholangiogram
i. cholangiography (IOC)
i. complication
i. electron beam radiotherapy
i. enteroscopy (IOE)
i. findings
i. kidney hypothermia
i. mortality
i. penile erection
i. phlebography
i. radiation therapy (IORT)
i. radiotherapy (IORT)
i. ultrasonography (IOUS)

NOTES

intrapancreatic
    i. bile duct
    i. nerve
intrapapillary terminus
intraparavariceal procedure
intraparenchymal tumor
intrapelvic
    i. filling defect
    i. somatic fiber
intraperitoneal (IP)
    i. abscess
    i. adhesion
    i. air
    i. cavity
    i. hemorrhage
    i. hyperthermic chemotherapy (IPHC)
    i. hyperthermic perfusion (IPHP)
    i. injection
    i. onlay mesh hernia repair (IPOM)
    i. perforation
    i. viscus
    i. volume
intraportal endovascular ultrasonography (IPEUS)
intraportally
intraprostatic
    i. characteristic variation
    i. spiral
    i. stent
    i. temperature
    i. temperature-guided treatment
    i. temperature measurement
    i. vascularization
    i. vasculature
intrapulmonary shunting
intrarectal
    i. intussusception
    i. retroflexion
    i. ultrasonography
intrarenal (IR)
    i. calculus
    i. chemolysis
    i. collecting system
    i. distribution
    i. hemodynamics
    i. matrix-degrading enzyme cascade
    i. reflux
    i. renal artery aneurysm
    i. resistive index
    i. vascular thrombosis
IntraSonix TULIP laser device
intrasphincteric botulinum toxin injection
intrasplenic pseudocyst
IntraStent DoubleStrut biliary endoprosthesis
intratesticular cyst

intrathecal
    i. catheter
    i. chemotherapy
intrathoracic
    i. esophagogastroscopy
    i. esophagogastrostomy
    i. Nissen fundoplication
    i. stomach
intratubular
    i. germ cell neoplasia (ITGCN)
    i. obstruction
intratumoral heterogeneity
intraurethral
    i. coil
    i. PGE_1
    i. pressure
    i. prostaglandin suppository (IPS)
    i. swab specimen
    i. therapy of erectile dysfunction
intrauterine
    i. growth restriction (IUGR)
    i. insemination (IUI)
intravaginal
    i. electrical stimulation
    i. torsion
intravariceal
    i. ethanolamine oleate
    i. infusion
    i. injection
    i. injection sclerotherapy
    i. pressure
intravasation
intravascular
    i. instillation of hypericin
    i. lipolysis
    i. thrombosis
    i. ultrasound (IVUS)
    i. ultrasound catheter
    i. volume
    i. volume expansion
intravenous (I.V.)
    i. albumin
    botulism immune globuln i.
    i. cholangiogram (IVC)
    i. cholangiography (IVC)
    i. cholecystography
    i. drip
    i. drug abuse
    i. feeding
    i. heme-albumin
    i. H2 receptor antagonist (IVH2RA)
    i. hydration
    i. hyperalimentation (IVH)
    i. immunoglobulin (IVIg)
    i. lipid emulsion
    i. nitroglycerin
    i. nutrition (IVN)
    i. pyelogram (IVP)

i. pyelography (IVP)
i. renal angiography
i. secretin test
i. urea infusion
i. urogram (IVU)
i. urography (IVU)
i. vasopressin infusion
intravesical
    i. alum
    i. alum irrigation
    i. anastomosis
    i. bacillus Calmette-Guérin
    i. BCG
    i. capsaicin
    i. chemotherapy
    i. electromotive drug administration (EMDA)
    i. formalin
    i. heparin
    i. hyaluronic acid
    i. immunotherapy
    i. instillation
    i. migration
    i. oxybutynin
    i. pressure
    i. silver nitrate
    i. ureterocele
    i. ureterolysis
intravesical mitomycin C (IMMC)
intrinsic
    i. enzymatic activity
    i. excitatory innervation
    i. factor (IF)
    i. factor secretion
    finger i.
    i. proteinuria
    i. reflex
    i. sphincter deficiency (ISD)
    i. sphincter dysfunction (ISD)
    i. striated muscle of urethra
    i. striated sphincter
    i. ureteral stricture
    i. ureteropelvic junction obstruction
    i. urethral sphincter
introducer
    Atkinson i.
    Dumon-Gilliard prosthesis i.
    entrapment sack i.
    Furlow i.
    i. gun
    KeyMed Nottingham i.
    LapSac i.
    Nottingham KeyMed i.
    Nottingham semirigid i.
    pull-apart i.
    semirigid Nottingham i.
    i. set
    split-sheath i.
    Wilson-Cook prosthesis i.
introitus esophagi
Introl bladder neck support prosthesis
intromission
Intromit
Intron
    I. A multidose pen
    Rebetol with I.
Intropin
intubate
intubated ureterotomy
intubation
    catheter-guided endoscopic i. (CAGEIN)
    endotracheal i.
    enterocutaneous i.
    esophageal i.
    esophagogastric i.
    i. failure
    gastrointestinal i.
    nasal i.
    nasogastric i.
    nasotracheal i.
    oral i.
    orotracheal i.
    pyloric i.
    terminal ileum i. (TII)
intumescence
intumescent
intussuscepted
    i. ileal triple nipple
    i. nipple valve
intussusception
    agonic i.
    appendiceal i.
    bowel i.
    cecocolic i.
    colocolic i.
    double i.
    ileocecal i.
    ileocolic i.
    ileoileal i.
    intestinal i.
    intrarectal i.
    jejunogastric i.
    postmortem i.

NOTES

intussusception *(continued)*
    rectal i.
    retrograde i.
    sigmoidoanal i.
    triple i.
intussusceptum
intussuscipiens
inulin
    i. clearance
    plasma i.
    i. solution
Inutest test
invaginated membrane
invaginating ampulla of Vater
invagination
    i. of the ampulla
    stomal i.
    stump i.
    i. technique
InVance male sling procedure
Invanz
invariant
    kinetically i.
invasion
    i. of adjacent organ
    capillary-lymphatic i.
    dermatolymphatic i.
    intrahepatic i.
    neural i.
    periportal i.
    stromal i.
    vascular i.
    venous i.
    Wilms tumor capsule i.
invasive
    i. adenocarcinoma
    i. carcinoma
    i. colorectal polyp
    i. diagnostic test
    i. enteric pathogen
    i. procedure
    i. surgery
    i. transvaginal approach
invasiveness
    minimal i.
    i. of surgery
inventory
    Beck Depression I.
    Hospital Anxiety and Depression I.
    Minnesota Multiphasic Personality I. (MMPI)
    Ostomy Assessment I. (OAI)
    Urogenital Distress I. (UDI)
    Weekly Stress I. (WSI)
invermination
inversely proportional
Inversine
inversion
    i. appendectomy
    i. of bladder
    chromosome i.
inversion-ligation appendectomy
inversus
    abdominal situs i.
    situs i.
inverted
    i. diverticulum of colon
    i. papilloma
    i. sigmoid diverticulum
    i. testis
    i. U-pouch ileal reservoir
inverted-U
    i.-U. abdominal incision
    i.-U. pouch
inverted-V sign
inverter
    Mayo-Kelly appendix i.
inverting suture
investigation
    clinical i.
    Lapides cystometric i.
    radiological i.
    urodynamic i.
investing fascia
Invicorp
involuntary
    i. guarding
    i. reflex rigidity
involution
    prostate gland i.
involvement
    mediastinal i.
    multifocal i.
    renal i.
    tubercular i.
IO
    intestinal obstruction
I&O
    intake and output
IOA
    Internal Ostomy Association
IOC
    intraoperative cholangiography
iocetamic
    i. acid
    i. acid contrast medium
Iodamoeba buetschlii
iodide
    isopropamide i.
    Lugol i.
    i. nephropathy
    propidium i.
iodinated
    i. contrast agent
    i. contrast material
iodine
    i. dye
    i. hippurate scanning

inorganic i.
Lugol i.
i. scan
i. staining
iodine-123 iodoamphetamine
iodine-125 (I-125)
i. brachytherapy seed
iodine-131 (I-131)
radioactive i.
iodine-131-labeled metaiodobenzylguanidine
iodipamide
i. meglumine
i. meglumine contrast medium
sodium i.
iodism
iodoamphetamine ([^{123}I]IMP)
iodine-123 i.
iodoantipyrine clearance
iodochlorhydroxyquin
iodocholesterol scan
Iodoform gauze
iodohippurate
iodophor
iodopyracet
iodoquinol
IOE
intraoperative enteroscopy
iohexol
ion
i. beam-assisted deposition
i. channel
i. chromatography
hydrogen i.
i. laser
phosphate i. (PI)
Ionamin
ionizing radiation
ionomycin
ionophore
calcium i.
ion-sensitive field-effect transistor
ion-specific electrode
iontophoresis
ion-urea
phosphate i.-u. (PI-urea)
iopamidol
i. contrast imaging agent
i. injection
iopanoic
i. acid
i. acid contrast medium

IOPN
intraductal oncocytic papillary neoplasm
iopromide
IORT
intraoperative radiation therapy
intraoperative radiotherapy
IOT29, clone K20 monoclonal antibody
iothalamate
i. clearance
i. level
sodium i.
iothalamate-125
iothalamic acid
iotroxate
meglumine i.
IOUS
intraoperative ultrasonography
ioversol
ioxaglate
IP
ileoproctostomy
inactivated pepsin
infusion pump
inlet pouch
intraperitoneal
IP chemotherapy
IP3
inositol 1,4,5-triphosphate
IPAA
ileal pouch-anal anastomosis
IPCD
infantile polycystic disease
IPD
incomplete pancreas divisum
ipecac
i. abuse
i. syrup
ipecac-induced
i.-i. cardiotoxicity
i.-i. myopathy
i.-i. vomiting
IPEC-J2 cell
IPEUS
intraportal endovascular ultrasonography
IPFC
inflammatory polyp-fold complex
IPG
impedance plethysmography
implantable pulse generator
IPH
idiopathic portal hypertension

NOTES

IPHC
intraperitoneal hyperthermic chemotherapy
IPHP
intraperitoneal hyperthermic perfusion
I-Plant brachytherapy seed
IPM
inflammatory prostatic mass
IPMN
intraductal papillary-mucinous neoplasm
IPMT
intraductal papillary-mucinous tumor
IPMY
intraductal papillary and mucinous tumors of pancreas
IPN
infected pancreatic necrosis
ipodate contrast medium
IPOM
intraperitoneal onlay mesh hernia repair
IPP
inflatable penile prosthesis
IPPB
intermittent positive-pressure breathing
ipratropium
iproniazid
iproniazid-induced jaundice
iproplatin
IPS
intraurethral prostaglandin suppository
IPSID
immunoproliferative small intestinal disease
ipsilateral adrenalectomy
IPSP
inhibitory postsynaptic potential
IPSS
International Prostate Symptom Score
IPT
intraductal papillary tumor
IR
ileal resection
intrarenal
^{192}Ir
iridium 192
^{192}Ir wire
IRA
ileorectal anastomosis
IRC
infrared photocoagulation
IRES
internal ribosome entry site
iridectomy scar
iridium
i. 192 (^{192}Ir)
i. 192 loaded stent
i. prosthesis
i. ribbon
i. seed
i. 192 wire implant
irinotecan hydrochloride
IRIS
intensified radiographic imaging system
iritis
IRMA
immunoradiometric assay
IRME
immunoreactive methionine-enkephalin
iron (Fe)
i. deficiency
i. dextran
i. gluconate
i. nephropathy
oral i.
i. overload disorder
i. poisoning
serum i. (SI)
i. shuttle hypothesis
i. storage disease
i. store
i. sucrose
i. sucrose injection
iron-binding capacity (IBC)
iron-deficiency anemia
iron-dependent oxidant
Irospan
Vitelle I.
IRP
idiopathic recurrent pancreatitis
IRPGN
idiopathic rapidly progressive glomerulonephritis
irradiate
irradiated tumor vaccine
irradiation
i. effect
external-beam i.
i. failure
half-body i.
hemibody i.
interstitial i.
Nd:YAG laser i.
total body i. (TBI)
total lymphoid i. (TLI)
ultraviolet i.
irreducible hernia
irregular
i. amputated mucosal pattern
i. duct
i. pupil
i. rhythm
irregularity
cervical i.
irretrievable object
irrigant
Neosporin G.U. I.

irrigating
    i. fluid
    i. patient
irrigation
    acetohydroxamic acid i.
    bladder i.
    bowel i.
    catheter i.
    i. of colostomy
    continuous bladder i. (CBI)
    copious i.
    i. fluid absorption syndrome
    hemiacidrin i.
    H-600 normothermic i.
    intravesical alum i.
    pulsed i.
    rectal pulsed i.
    rectum i.
    Renacidin i.
    whole-gut i.
irrigation-suction
    postoperative i.-s.
irrigator
    Sur-Fit Natura Visi-Flow i.
irrigator/aspirator
    Nezhat-Dorsey i./a.
irritable
    i. bladder
    i. bowel syndrome (IBS)
    i. colon (IC)
    i. colon syndrome
    i. gut syndrome
    i. pouch syndrome
    i. stricture
    i. testis
irritant dermatitis
irritative
    i. diarrhea
    i. symptom
IRS
    impaired regeneration syndrome
    Intergroup Rhabdomyosarcoma Study
IRS-IV trial
IRT
    immunoreactive trypsinogen
IS
    ileal segment
    immune serum
Isaacs-Ludwig arteriole
ISC
    intermittent self-catheterization

ischemia
    acute gastric i.
    acute occlusive mesenteric i.
    atherosclerosis-induced cavernosal i.
    AVF-induced renal i.
    colonic i.
    glomerular i.
    intestinal i.
    kidney i.
    mesenteric i.
    midgut i.
    mucosal i.
    myocardial i.
    i. necrosis
    nonocclusive mesenteric i.
    outer medullary i.
    renal i.
    i. or sloughing of the flap
    tubular i.
    visceral i.
    warm i.
ischemia-reperfusion injury
ischemic
    i. bowel
    i. bowel disease
    i. colitis
    i. fecal incontinence
    i. hepatitis
    i. insult
    i. penile gangrene
    i. tubular cell death
    i. tubular damage
ischial tuberosity
ischioanal
ischiocavernosus muscle
ischiorectal
    i. abscess
    i. anorectal space
    i. aponeurosis
    i. excavation
    i. fascia
    i. fat
    i. fistula
    i. fossa
    i. fossa plane
    i. region
ischochymia
ISD
    intrinsic sphincter deficiency
    intrinsic sphincter dysfunction
ISEL
    in situ end labeling

NOTES

isethionate
    pentamidine i.
ISH
    isolated systolic hypertension
ISIS 2302
island
    buried vaginal i.
    i. flap procedure
    i. groin flap
    lipid i.
    mucosal i.
    i. pedicle flap
islet
    i. amyloid polypeptide
    i. cell
    i. cell adenoma
    i. cell antibody (ICA)
    i. cell carcinoma
    i. cell hyperplasia
    i. cell implant
    i. cell of Langerhans
    i. cell tumor
    Langerhans i.
Isletest-ICA
Ismelin
Is-5-Mn
    isosorbide-5-mononitrate
ISO$_2$
    oxygen saturation index
isoamyl alcohol
isoamylase
    salivary-type i.
ISOBAR barostat distension device
isobaric gastric distention
isobutyl 2-cyanoacrylate
Isocal
    I. HCN
    I. HCN liquid feeding
isocarboxazid
isodose contour
isoechoic
isoenzyme
    alkaline phosphatase i.
    galactosyltransferase i. II
    Regan i.
    serum pepsinogen i. I, II
isoflavone
isoflurane
isoform
    growth factor i.
isoiodide
isolate
isolated
    i. adenomatous lesion
    i. cortical tubule (ICT)
    i. cyst
    i. gastric varices type 1, 2 (IGV)
    i. generator
    i. granulomatous gastritis
    i. hepatocyte perfusion
    i. hypoaldosteronism
    i. renal mucormycosis
    i. retained antrum syndrome
    i. systolic hypertension (ISH)
    i. urinary tract infection
isolation
    body substance i. (BSI)
    category-specific i.
    i. defect
    disease-specific i.
isoleucine
    peptide histidine i. (PHI)
isomannide
IsoMed constant-flow infusion system
isomerase
    glucose-6-phosphate i.
isometric
    i. force
    i. tubular vacuolization
Isomil
    I. SF
    I. SF formula
isomotic lavage
isoniazid
isoniazid-induced hepatitis
isoosmolar liquid
isopentane
isoperistaltic
    i. anastomosis
    i. direction
    i. ileal reservoir
    i. strictureplasty
isoprenaline
isoprenologue
isopropamide iodide
isopropanol
isoproterenol
Isoptin
Isordil
isosorbide dinitrate
isosorbide-5-mononitrate (Is-5-Mn)
Isospora belli
isosporan parasite
isosporiasis
Isotein HN feeding
isotherm
    Langmuir adsorption i.
isothiocyanate
    fluorescein i. (FITC)
isotonic
    i. contraction
    i. feeding
    i. saline
isotope
    ^{131}I-lipiodol i.
    i. meal
    i. nephrography
    i. renal scan

i. renogram
i. renography
i. study
^{99m}Tc MAG-3 i.
technetium-99m mercaptoacetythiglycine i.
i. voiding cystourethrography (IVCU)
isotropic
    i. probe
    i. scan
isovaleric
    i. acid
    i. acidemia
isovolemic variance
Isovue
Isovue-300
isoxazole derivative
isoxsuprine
I-Soyalac formula
isozyme
    CYP i.
ispaghula husk
isradipine
Israel
    I. operation
    I. retractor
ISRE
    interferon-stimulated regulatory element
isthmectomy
isthmic
isthmus, pl. **isthmi**
    i. prostatae
    i. urethra
Isuprel
ISWL
    intracorporeal shock wave lithotripsy
itch
    jock i.
    swimmer's i.
iterative bifid branching system
ITGCN
    intratubular germ cell neoplasia
ITGP
    immunotactoid glomerulopathy
ITI
    inter-alpha-trypsin inhibitor
Ito
    I. cell
    I. cell sarcoma
ITP
    Ifex, Taxol, Platinol

itraconazole
Itrel pulse generator
ITT
    intention to treat
Iturelix
IUGR
    intrauterine growth restriction
IUI
    intrauterine insemination
IU/L
    international units per liter
I.V.
    intravenous
        I.V. fluid
        I.V. fluid therapy
        Merrem I.V.
        piggybacking of I.V.
        I.V. sedation
IVa
    Edmondson-Steiner histologic grading of hepatocellular I. I, II, III, IVa
IVAC needleless IV System
Ivalon
    I. sponge
    I. sponge hysterosacropexy
    I. sponge rectopexy
    I. sponge-wrap operation
    I. suture
Ivanissevitch ligation
IVC
    inferior vena cava
    intravenous cholangiogram
    intravenous cholangiography
IVCU
    isotope voiding cystourethrography
Ivemark syndrome
ivermectin
IVH
    intravenous hyperalimentation
IVH2RA
    intravenous H2 receptor antagonist
IVIg
    intravenous immunoglobulin
IVN
    intravenous nutrition
Ivor
    I. Lewis esophagogastrectomy
    I. Lewis two-stage subtotal esophagectomy

NOTES

IVP
   intravenous pyelogram
   intravenous pyelography
IVT
   interactive video technology
IVU
   intravenous urogram
   intravenous urography
     high-dose IVU
     one-shot IVU
IVUS
   intravascular ultrasound
   IVUS catheter

J
- J chain
- J line
- J needle
- J pelvic ileal pouch
- J pouch
- J reservoir
- J turn of scope
- J wire

Jaboulay
- J. button
- J. gastroduodenostomy
- J. procedure
- J. pyloroplasty

Jaboulay-Doyen-Winkleman
- J.-D.-W. operation
- J.-D.-W. technique

jackknife position

Jackson
- J. esophageal bougie
- J. esophagoscope
- J. membrane
- J. staging system
- J. veil

Jackson-Pratt
- J.-P. catheter
- J.-P. drain

jackstone calculus
Jacobson needle holder
Jacobs-Palmer laparoscope
Jacoby test
Jadassohn syndrome
Jaffe
- J. picrate reaction
- J. test

Jagged 1 gene
Jagwire guidewire
Jaksch test
Jamaican
- J. vomiting sickness
- J. vomiting syndrome

Jamshidi liver biopsy needle
Janeway
- J. gastroscope
- J. gastrostomy
- J. lesion

Jansen retractor
Jansen-type metaphyseal chondrodysplasia
Janus System III
Japanese
- J. cancer classification
- J. classification of cancer
- J. dysentery
- J. schistosomiasis

japonica
- cutaneous schistosomiasis j.
- schistosomiasis j.

japonicum
- *Schistosoma j.*

Jarit rotator
Jarvis
- J. hemorrhoid clamp
- J. hemorrhoid forceps
- J. pile clamp

Jass staging for rectal carcinoma
Jatrox
- J. *Helicobacter pylori* test
- J. Hp-test

jaundice
- acholuric j.
- benign postoperative j.
- black j.
- Budd j.
- catarrhal j.
- cholestatic j.
- chronic idiopathic j.
- cloxacillin-induced cholestatic j.
- Crigler-Najjar j.
- deep j.
- Epping j.
- familial chronic idiopathic j.
- familial nonhemolytic j.
- Hayem j.
- hemolytic j.
- hepatocanalicular j.
- hepatocellular j.
- hepatogenic j.
- homologous serum j.
- human serum j.
- infectious j.
- infective j.
- iproniazid-induced j.
- latent j.
- leptospiral j.
- malignant obstructive j.
- mechanical j.
- neonatal j.
- newborn j.
- nonhemolytic j.
- nonobstructive j.
- obstructive j.
- painless j.
- parenchymal j.
- physiologic j.
- regurgitation j.
- retention j.
- shrapnel-induced obstructive j.
- ticrynafen-induced j.

jaundiced skin

Jaworski
- J. body
- J. corpuscles
- J. test

jaw wiring

J/cm
joules per centimeter

J-curve effect

Jeffrey introducer set

jejunal
- j. bypass
- j. colonization
- j. crest
- j. cutaneous urinary diversion
- j. diverticulosis
- j. drainage and biopsy
- j. feeding tube
- j. gas infusion test
- j. gluten challenge
- j. IgA
- j. interposition of Henle loop
- j. limb
- j. pouch
- j. pouch interposition (JPI)
- j. syndrome
- j. tube insertion
- j. tube through percutaneous endoscopic gastrostomy (JETPEG)
- j. ulcer
- j. urinary conduit
- j. varix
- j. villus

jejunales
arteriae j.

jejunectomy

jejuni
Campylobacter j.

jejunitis
- nongranulomatous j.
- ulcerative j.

jejunocecostomy
ulcerative jejunitis j.

jejunocolic fistula

jejunocolostomy

jejunogastric intussusception

jejunoileal (JI)
- j. atresia
- j. bypass (JIB)
- j. bypass surgery
- j. fold pattern reversal
- j. intestine
- j. shunt

jejunoileitis
nongranulomatous ulcerative j.

jejunoileostomy
Roux-en-Y distal j.

jejunoileum

jejunojejunostomy

jejunoplasty

jejunorrhaphy

jejunostomy
- direct percutaneous j. (DPJ)
- j. elemental diet feeding
- endoscopic j.
- laparoscopic-guided feeding j.
- long Roux-en-Y pouch j.
- loop j.
- needle-catheter j.
- percutaneous endoscopic j. (PEJ)
- Roux-en-Y j.
- j. tract choledochoscopy
- j. tube
- j. tube feeding
- Witzel j.

jejunotomy

jejunum
- j. antigen
- proximal j.
- Roux-en-Y loop of j.

Jelco catheter

jelly
- Anestacon 2% lidocaine hydrochloride j.
- carboxymethylcellulose j.
- electrode j.
- lidocaine hydrochloride j.
- Lubraseptic j.
- Snap-It lubricating j.
- spermicidal j.
- Xylocaine j.

JEM-100B, 100S electron microscope

Jenamicin

Jendrassik-Grof method

Jenning-Streifeneder gastroscope

JEOL
- J. 100 CX electron microscope
- J. JSM 35 CF scanning electron microscope

jerk
- absent ankle j.
- ankle j.

Jesberg esophagoscope

jet
- j. nebulizer
- j. stream phenomenon
- ureteral j.

Jetco-Spray Cannula

jetlike bleeding

JETPEG
jejunal tube through percutaneous endoscopic gastrostomy

Jeune
- J. asphyxiating thoracic dystrophy
- J. syndrome

Jevity
- J. isotonic liquid nutrition
- J. tube feeding formula

jeweler's forceps

Jewett
    J. bladder carcinoma classification
    J. classification of bladder carcinoma
    J. sound
    J. staging system
Jewett classification of bladder carcinoma, O, A, B, C, D
Jewett-Strong system
Jewett-Whitmore Cancer Staging System
JF-200
    J. duodenoscope
    J. side-viewing videoendoscope
JF-20 side-viewing fiberoptic endoscope
JFB III endoscope
JF-IT20 duodenoscope
JG
    juxtaglomerular
J-hook tip laparoscopic electrode
JI
    jejunoileal
JIB
    jejunoileal bypass
Jin Bu Huan
J-loop ileostomy
J-Maxx stent
JNC VI classification of hypertension
Jobert de Lamballe suture
Job syndrome
jock itch
Joe hoe
Joel-Cohen incision
Johanson-Blizzard syndrome
Johne disease
Johns
    J. Hopkins gallbladder forceps
    J. Hopkins gallbladder retractor
    J. Hopkins prostate cancer grading system
Johnson
    J. esophagogastroscopy
    J. esophagogastrostomy
Johnson and Demeester Score
Johnson-DeMeester symptom score
Johnston buttonhole procedure
joint
    j. erythema
    J. National Committee Sixth Report classification of hypertension
Jolles test

Jonas
    J. implant
    J. penile prosthesis
Jones-Politano technique
Jones silver stain
Jonnesco
    J. fold
    J. fossa
    J. operation
Joseph
    J. hook
    J. syndrome
Joubert syndrome
joules per centimeter (J/cm)
Joyce-Loebl Magiscan image analysis system
JP
    juvenile polyposis
JPD
J-pexy
    omental J-p.
JPI
    jejunal pouch interposition
JPS
    juvenile polyposis syndrome
JR-St cell
J-scope esophagoscope
J-shaped
    J.-s. endoscope
    J.-s. ileal pouch
    J.-s. ileal pouch-anal anastomosis
    J.-s. ileal reservoir
JT1001 prostate cancer vaccine
J tube
J-tube insertion
J-type maneuver
Jubileum 2.0 single-use gastroesophageal pH probe
Judd
    J. cystoscope
    J. pyloroplasty
    J. ventral hernia repair
Judd-Allis intestinal forceps
Judd-DeMartel gallbladder forceps
jugular
juice
    acid-peptic j.
    duodenal j.
    gastric j.
    intestinal j.
    pancreatic j.
    pure pancreatic j. (PPJ)

NOTES

Julian
    J. cystoresectoscope
    J. splenorenal forceps
jumbo
    j. biopsy
    j. biopsy forceps
jumentosa
junction
    anomalous pancreatobiliary duct j. (APBDJ)
    anorectal j.
    cardioesophageal j. (CEJ)
    cardioesophageal mucosal j.
    choledochoduodenal j.
    choledochopancreatic ductal j.
    corticomedullary j.
    costochondral j.
    cystic-choledochal j.
    cysticohepatic j.
    desmosomal j.
    detrusor muscle protrusion j.
    duodenojejunal j. (DJJ)
    esophagogastric j.
    fundic-antral j.
    gap j.
    gastroesophageal j.
    hepaticocystic j.
    hyperactive rectosigmoid j.
    ileocecal j.
    intermediate j.
    mucosal j.
    NS3/NS4 j.
    NS4/NS5 j.
    pancreaticobiliary ductal j.
    pancreaticocholedochoductal j.
    patulous gastroesophageal j.
    penopubic j.
    penoscrotal j.
    pharyngoesophageal j.
    prostatovesical j.
    pyloroduodenal j.
    rectosigmoid j.
    saphenofemoral j.
    squamocolumnar j. (SCJ)
    squamocolumnar mucosal j.
    tracheoesophageal j.
    ureteropelvic j. (UPJ)
    ureterovesical j. (UVJ)
    urethrovesical j.
junctional
    j. cyst
    j. intestinal metaplasia
juvenile
    j. cirrhosis
    j. nephronophthisis
    j. nephronophthisis-medullary cystic disease
    j. polyposis (JP)
    j. polyposis coli
    j. polyposis syndrome (JPS)
    j. retention polyp
    j. xanthogranuloma
juxtacapillary process
juxtaglomerular (JG)
    j. apparatus
    j. apparatus tumor
    j. body
juxtahepatic venous injury
juxtamedullary
    j. arteriole
    j. renal corpuscle
juxtapapillary
    j. duodenal diverticulum
juxtaposed mesenteric lymph nodes
juxtapyloric ulcer
juxtaregional node
juxtavesical ureter
J-Vac
    J-Vac closed wound drainage
    J-Vac drain
    J-Vac suction reservoir
J-wave phenomenon
J-wire guide

K
    K antigen
    K diet
    K tube
K2
    vitamin K2
K-141
    Dianeal K-141
K+
    Ca^{2+}-activated K+
K562 erythroid line
kabure
Kader
    K. gastrostomy
    K. operation
KAL1 **gene**
kala azar
Kaleorid
kaliopenic nephropathy
Kaliscinski
    K. plication
    K. ureteral folding technique
kaliuretic diuretic
kallidin
kallikrein
    human glandular k. 3
    k. inheritance
    plasma k.
    tissue k.
    urinary k.
kallikreinlike gene
Kallmann syndrome
Kammerer-Battle incision
Kanagawa phenomenon
kanamycin nephropathy
Kane umbilical clamp
Kangaroo
    K. Delivery System
    K. 200, 330 enteral feeding pump
    K. 324 feeding pump
    K. gastrostomy tube
kansasii
    Mycobacterium k.
Kantor-Berci video laryngoscope
Kantor string sign
Kantrex
kanyemba
Kaodene
kaolin
Kaopectate
Kapectolin
Kaplan-Meier
    K.-M. analysis
    K.-M. curve
    K.-M. estimation
    K.-M. method
Kaposi
    K. sarcoma (KS)
    K. sarcoma-associated herpesvirus
kappa
    k. light chain
    k. receptor opioid agonist
Kapp-Beck colon clamp
Kapsinow test
KAR
    killer-activating receptor
Karaya
    K. gum
    K. 5 paste
    K. powder
    K. ring ileostomy appliance
    K. 5 seal
Karl
    K. Storz Calcutript
    K. Storz endoscope
    K. Storz flexible ureteropyeloscope
    K. Storz instrumentation
    K. Storz-Lutzeyer lithotriptor
Karmen unit
Karnofsky
    K. index
    K. performance status scale
    K. score
Karroo syndrome
Kartagener syndrome
karyometry
karyotype
    chromosome k.
Kasai
    K. classification for extrahepatic bile duct atresia
    K. operation
    K. peritoneal venous shunt
    K. portoenterostomy
    K. procedure
kasai
Kasai-type hepatoportoenterostomy
Kashin-Beck disease
Kashiwado test
Kaslow intestinal tube
Kasugai
    chronic pancreatitis of K.
    K. classification
Katayama
    K. disease
    K. fever
    K. syndrome
KATO-III cell
Kato test

Kaufman syndrome
Kawasaki syndrome
Kaye
    K. nephrostomy tamponade balloon
    K. tamponade balloon catheter
Kayexalate enema
Kayser-Fleischer ring
KB
    ketone body
KBR
    ketone body ratio
KC
    Kupffer cell
KCl
    potassium chloride
K+2 diet
32/67-kD laminin receptor
K/DOQI
    Kidney Disease Outcomes Quality Initiative
Kearns-Sayre syndrome (KSS)
Keeler
    K. Magnalite headlamp
    K. panoramic loupe
Keen Edge disposable biopsy forceps
Keflex
Keftab
Kefzol
Kegelcisor
Kegel pelvic muscle exercise
Kehr
    K. incision
    K. sign
    K. T tube
Keith needle
Kelami classification
Keller
    K. hydrodynamic hypothesis of sieving
    K. hypothesis
Kelling
    K. gastroscope
    K. test
Kelling-Madlener procedure
Kellogg's Castor Oil
Kelly
    K. abdominal retractor
    K. clamp
    K. cystoscope
    K. fistula scissors
    K. forceps
    K. hemostat
    K. operation
    K. plication
    K. plication procedure
    K. proctoscope
    K. rectal speculum
    K. sigmoidoscope
    K. sign
    K. sphincteroscope
Kelly-Kennedy modification
Kelly-Murphy forceps
Kelly-Stoeckel operation
Kelman
    K. air cystotome
    K. double-bladed cystotome
    K. knife-cannula cystotome
    K. knife cystotome
keloid
kelotomy
Kelsey pile clamp
Kemadrin
Kendall Foley catheter
Kennedy disease
Kent deep surgery forceps
Keofeed
    K. enteral feeding bag
    K. 500 enteral feeding pump
    K. II enteral feeding pump
    K. II feeding tube
keratin
    antibody to k.
keratinization
    single-cell k.
keratinocyte growth factor (KGF)
Keratinocyte-Serum-Free-Medium culture medium
keratitis
    seborrheic k.
keratoacanthoma
keratoderma blennorrhagica
keratosis, pl. **keratoses**
    k. blennorrhagica
    k. follicularis
    lacelike k.
keratotic pseudoepitheliomatous balanitis
Kerckring
    circular folds of K.
    K. fold
    valve of K.
kerion formation
Kerlix wrap
kernicterus
Kernig sign
Kerr kink
Keshan disease
Kessler-Kleinert suture
ketamine
ketanserin
keto
    k. acid
    k. acid-amino acid supplement
ketoacidosis
    diabetic k.
7-ketocholesterol
ketoconazole

ketogenesis
ketoglutaramate (KGM)
  alpha k.
ketoglutarate (KG)
  k. dehydrogenase (KGDH)
ketone
  k. body (KB)
  k. body ratio (KBR)
  k. body test
  urinary k.
ketoprofen analgesic therapy
ketorolac tromethamine
ketosteroid
17-ketosteroid
ketotifen
keyhole
  k. deformity
  k. limpet hemocyanin (KLH)
KeyMed
  K. advanced dilator
  K. advanced esophageal dilator set
  K. Atkinson endoprosthesis
  K. automatic reprocessor
  K. disposable variceal injection needle
  K. heater probe thermocoagulation
  K. Nottingham introducer
  K. unit
Key-Pred 25, 50
Keystone technique
KG
  ketoglutarate
  alpha-KG
KGDH
  ketoglutarate dehydrogenase
  alpha-KGDH
KGF
  keratinocyte growth factor
KGM
  ketoglutaramate
  alpha-KGM
KHB
  Krebs-Henseleit bicarbonate buffer
Ki-67 stain
Kidd cystoscope
kidney
  abdominal k.
  k. abscess
  k. adenoma
  adipose arteries of k.
  adipose capsule of k.
  k. adysplasia
  k. agenesis
  allocating cadaveric k.
  k. allograft
  amyloid k.
  k. amyloidosis
  k. angiomyolipoma
  k. aplasia
  k. arteriovenous fistula
  artificial k.
  k. ascent
  Ask-Upmark k.
  k. ballottement
  cadaver k.
  cake k.
  k. calcification
  k. calix
  k. carbuncle
  k. carcinoma
  k. carcinosarcoma
  k. clearance
  clear cell carcinoma of k.
  k. clear cell sarcoma
  coarsely granular k.
  k. collecting system
  congenital double k.
  congested k.
  k. cortex
  crush k.
  cyanotic k.
  k. cyst
  decapsulation of k.
  K. Disease Outcomes Quality Initiative (K/DOQI)
  disk k.
  donor k.
  k. donor
  Dow Hollow Fiber k. (DHFK)
  dump k.
  dwarf k.
  k. dysplasia
  dysplastic k.
  dystopic k.
  ectopic k.
  k. electrolyte clearance rate
  k. electrolyte excretion rate
  embryoma of k.
  k. failure
  fatty k.
  k. fibroma
  k. fibrosarcoma
  finely granular k.
  flea-bitten k.

NOTES

kidney (*continued*)
- Formad k.
- k. function
- fused k.
- Gambro Lundia Minor artificial k.
- k. Gerota fascia
- k. glomeruli
- k. glomerulocystic disease
- Goldblatt k.
- gouty k.
- granular k.
- k. hematoma
- k. hemorrhage
- hind k.
- HLA-matched k.
- horseshoe k.
- hypermobile k.
- hypoplastic k.
- k. inflammation
- k. innervation
- k. internal splint/stent (KISS)
- k. internal splint/stent catheter
- k. ischemia
- lardaceous k.
- k. leiomyosarcoma
- k. liposarcoma
- k.'s, liver, spleen (KLS)
- living donor k.
- k. lobe
- lumbar k.
- lump k.
- k. lymphoblastoma
- k. magnesium filtration
- malacoplakia of k.
- k. malacoplakia
- k. malignant fibrous histiocytoma
- k. mass
- maximal tubular excretory capacity of k.
- k. medulla
- medullary sponge k.
- mortar k.
- multicystic k. (MCK)
- multicystic dysplastic k. (MCDK)
- multilobar k.
- multilobular k.
- mural k.
- murine k.
- myelin k.
- myeloma k.
- k. nephroma
- nephropathia epidermica k.
- non-heart-beating donor k.
- obstructed k. (OBK)
- k. oncocytoma
- k. ossifying tumor
- k. osteogenic sarcoma
- Page k.
- palpable k.
- pancake k.
- k. pedicle clamp
- pelvic k.
- pole of k.
- presacral ectopic k.
- primordial k.
- k. pseudotumor
- k. punch
- putty k.
- pyramid of k.
- k. rhabdomyosarcoma
- Rokitansky k.
- Rose-Bradford k.
- sacciform k.
- k. scarring
- sclerotic k.
- k. shock wave effect
- sigmoid k.
- k. size
- soapy k.
- solitary k.
- k. stone
- supernumerary k.
- thoracic k.
- k. transillumination
- k. transplant
- k. transplantation
- k. transplant recipient
- unilateral fused k.
- unipapillary k.
- k.'s, ureters, bladder (KUB)
- k.'s, ureters, bladder radiography
- k. variant
- k. vascular pedicle
- k. vasculature
- k. weight (KW)
- k. worm

KidneyScreen at Home test
kidney-sparing operation
Kids
- Resource Just for K.

Kiernan space
killer
- natural k. (NK)
- k. T cell

killer-activating receptor (KAR)
Killian
- K. dehiscence
- K. rectal speculum
- K. suction tube
- K. triangle

Killian-Jamieson area
Killian-Lynch laryngoscope
Kilner needle holder
KilRoid single-handed ligator
Kim Care contour brief
Kimmelstiel-Wilson (KW)
- K.-W. disease
- K.-W. syndrome

Kimura disease
kinase
    conserved helix-loop-helix ubiquitous k. (CHUK)
    cyclin-dependent k. (CDK)
    extracellular signal-regulated protein k. (ERK)
    foal adhesion k.
    glucocorticoid k.
    herpes simplex virus-thymidine k. (HSK-tk)
    ligand-triggered protein tyrosine k.
    mitogen-activated protein k. (MAPK)
    muscle-brain isoenzyme of creatine k. (CK-MB)
    myosin light-chain k.
    protein k. A
    protein k. C (PKC)
    protein serine k.
    protein threonine k.
    protein tyrosine k.
    pyruvate k.
    serum k.
    serum pyruvate k. (SPK)
    tyrosine protein k.
3-kinase
    phosphoinositide 3-k.
    PI 3-k.
Kinesed
kinetic
    bromodeoxyuridine cell k.'s
    capacity-limited k.'s
    first-order k.'s
    k. gallbladder study
    gastric cell k.'s
    Gompertzian tumor k.'s
    Michaelis-Menten k.'s
    k. parameter
    urea k.'s
kinetically invariant
Kinevac
king
    K.'s College ALF criteria
    King technique
King-Armstrong unit
kinin
kink
    k. in bowel
    k. in intestine
    Kerr k.
Kinkiang fever

kinking
Kinnier Wilson disease
Ki-ras
    K.-r. gene
    K.-r. gene mutation
Kirchner diverticulum
Kirschner abdominal retractor
Kirsten-ras
    K.-r. oncogene
    K.-r. oncogen mutation
Kish urethral illuminate catheter
KISS
    kidney internal splint/stent
    KISS catheter
kissing
    k. prostatic lobes
    k. ulcers
kit
    Abbott HCV EIA 2nd generation k.
    Abbott HCV 2.0 test k.
    Bard-Stiegmann-Goff variceal ligation k.
    Bayer Versant HCV RNA 2.0 assay test k.
    BCA-1 protein assay k.
    BIO 101 MERmaid DNAk.
    Boehringer k.
    Carey-Coons biliary endoprosthesis k.
    Cavilon diabetes foot care k.
    Coloplast irrigation k.
    Cytoscreen human interferon-gamma ELISA k.
    DNA labeling k.
    EIA k.
    Enteryx GERD procedure k.
    EZ Detect colorectal screening test k.
    FertilMARQ home diagnostic screening test k.
    Fix and Perm permeabilizing k.
    Flexiflo Inverta-PEG gastrostomy k.
    Flexiflo Lap J laparoscopic jejunostomy k.
    Flexiflo over-the-guidewire gastrostomy k.
    FlexSure in-office rapid serology test k.
    Gastrin RIA k. II
    GastroPanel assay k.
    Gene Clean II k.

NOTES

kit *(continued)*
    GFXTM Genomic blood DNA purification k.
    Hashizume endoscopic ligator k.
    Helisal Rapid Blood diagnostic k.
    Histofine SAB k.
    Histofine SAB-PO k.
    Hybritech Tandem-R assay k.
    MERmaid DNA k.
    Moss G-tube PEG k.
    Nichols IRMA k.
    OctreoScan k.
    Ott/Mayo Channel Sampling k.
    Percufix catheter cuff k.
    Predicta TGF-β1 k.
    propHiler urinary pH testing k.
    Pros-Check k.
    Pulse-Pak infusion k.
    Puregene DNA isolation k.
    PyloriTek *Helicobacter pylori* test k.
    QuickVue *H.* pylori gII test k.
    Random Primed DNA Labeling k.
    rapid urease testing k.
    RIA k.
    Russell gastrostomy k.
    RUT k.
    Sacks-Vine gastrostomy k.
    Serodia commercial k.
    Steigmann-Goff endoscopic ligator k.
    StoneRisk diagnostic monitoring k.
    Tandem-R assay k.
    UltraTag RBC k.
    Uri-Kit culture k.
    UriSite urine collection k.
    Uri-Three culture k.
    Vectastain ABC k.
    Versa-PEG gastrostomy k.
    Vesica percutaneous bladder neck suspension k.
    Vitros Immunodiagnostic Products HBsAg Confirmatory K.
    Wilson-Cook feeding tube k.
    XTRAX DNA commercial extraction k.

Kitano knot
Kiton red dye
Kittner dissector
Klatskin
    K. liver biopsy needle
    K. stenosis
    K. tumor
Klebanoff
    K. common duct bougie
    K. common duct sound
    K. gallstone scoop
Klebs disease

Klebsiella
    K. oxytoca
    K. pneumoniae
Kleinert
    K. pants
    K. Safe and Dry panty and pad system
Kleinschmidt appendectomy clamp
Klemm sign
Klemperer disease
Kleppinger forceps
KLF6
    Kruppel-like factor 6
    KLF6 gene
KLH
    keyhole limpet hemocyanin
KLH-ImmuneActivator
Klinefelter syndrome
Kling dressing
Klippel-Trenaunay-Weber syndrome
Klonopin
Klor-Con
    K.-C. 8, 10
    K.-C. M10, 20
KLS
    kidneys, liver, spleen
Km
    Michaelis constant
KMI 60 enteral feeding pump
Knack
knee-chest position
knee-elbow position
knife, pl. **knives**
    Bard-Parker k.
    k. blade
    cautery k.
    cold k.
    Collin k.
    Collings electrosurgery k.
    Desmarres paracentesis k.
    electrocautery k.
    k. electrode
    electrosurgical cutting k.
    endarterectomy k.
    hernia k.
    hook k.
    HPC-2 standard needle k.
    insulated-tip electrosurgical k.
    insulation-tipped electrosurgical k.
    Lempert paracentesis k.
    Mori k.
    needle k.
    optical laser k.
    optical urethrotome k.
    Orandi k.
    skin k.
    triangle-tipped k.
    urethrotome k.
knife-like pain

knob
  lateral deflection control k.
knobby process
knock
  pericardial k.
Knodell
  K. component
  K. criteria for histology activity
  K. index
  K. score
knot
  Aberdeen k.
  crochet k.
  curved-needle surgeon's k.
  externally releasable k.
  friction k.
  granny k.
  half-hitch k.
  ileosigmoid k.
  Kitano k.
  laparoscopic k.
  one-handed k.
  prelooped intracorporeal k.
  Roeder loop k.
  self-tightening slip k.
  square k.
  surgeon's k.
  Tim k.
knotting
  stochastic k.
knowledge
  Crohn and Colitis K. (CCKNOW)
  ever-increasing k.
  facile working k.
knuckle of colon
Ko-Airan maneuver
Kocher
  K. anastomosis
  K. clamp
  K. dilatation ulcer
  K. forceps
  K. gallbladder retractor
  K. hemostat
  K. incision
  K. maneuver
  K. operation
  K. pylorectomy
  K. ureterosigmoidostomy procedure
kocherization
Koch postulate
Kock
  K. continent ileostomy
  K. neobladder
  K. nipple
  K. nipple valve
  K. pouch cutaneous urinary diversion
  K. pouch modified procedure
  K. reservoir
  K. reservoir ileostomy
  K. technique
  K. urinary pouch
Kockogram
Kodak Ektachem 700 machine
Koenig, König
  K. syndrome
Koerte gallstone forceps
Koh-I-Noor Universal India ink
Kohlmeier-Degos disease
Kohlrausch valve
KOH smear
koilocytosis
Kollmann dilator
Kolmogorov-Smirnov test
kolypeptic
Kondremul
König (*var. of* Koenig)
Konigsberg
  K. catheter
  K. five-channel solid-state catheter assembly
  K. microtransducer
Konsyl
Konsyl-D
Koplik spot
Korean
  K. hemorrhagic fever
  K. hemorrhagic nephrosonephritis
Koro syndrome
Korsakoff syndrome
Kossa stain
Koyanagi technique for hypospadias repair
K-Pek
K-Phos Neutral
K-ras
  K.-r. gene
  K.-r. oncogene
Kraske
  K. operation
  K. parasacral approach
  K. position
  K. roll

NOTES

kraurosis
   penile k.
Krause
   K. arm rest
   K. ligament
Krazy Glue sclerosant
Krebs
   K. cycle
   K. solution
Krebs-Henseleit bicarbonate buffer (KHB)
Krebs-Ringer
   K.-R. bicarbonate buffer
   K.-R. solution
Kreha
   polysaccharide K. (PSK)
Krentz gastroscope
Kretz
   K. Combison 330 ultrasound scanner
   K. granule
   K. 311 ultrasound scanner
   K. ultrasound system
Kringle domain
Kristalose for oral solution
kristensenii
   Yersinia k.
Krokiewicz test
Kron
   K. bile duct dilator
   K. gall duct dilator
Krönlein hernia
Kropp
   K. bladder neck reconstruction
   K. cystourethroplasty
   K. operation
   K. procedure
   K. technique
Kruger index
Krukenberg
   K. tumor
   K. vein
Kruppel-like
   K.-l. factor 6 (KLF6)
   K.-l. factor 6 gene
krusei
   Candida k.
Kruskal-Wallis
   K.-W. analysis of variance
   K.-W. test

krypton laser
KS
   Kaposi sarcoma
KSG-504 CCK antagonist
KSS
   Kearns-Sayre syndrome
KTP
   potassium-titanyl phosphate
     KTP 532 laser
     KTP laser probe
     KTP laser prostatectomy
     Laserscope KTP 532
KTP/532 laser system
KTP/Nd:YAG laser treatment
K tube
Kt/V urea
KUB
   kidneys, ureters, bladder
     KUB radiography
Kudrox
Kugel hernia patch
Kulchitsky cell
Kumpe catheter
Kunkel syndrome
Kupffer
   K. cell (KC)
   K. cell sarcoma
Kussmaul
   K. breathing
   K. endoscope
Kutrase
Ku-Zyme
   K.-Z. HP
   K.-Z. HP pancreatic enzyme
Kveim test
KW
   kidney weight
   Kimmelstiel-Wilson
kwashiorkor
Kwell
Kyasanur Forest disease
kymography
   balloon k.
kyphoscoliosis
kyphosis
Kyrle disease
Kytril

LA
    long acting
    Los Angeles
    lupus anticoagulant
        LA classification
        Detrol LA
        Trelstar LA
L.A.
    long acting
        Dalalone L.A.
LAAL
    lower anterior axillary line
Labbe
    L. syndrome
    L. triangle
labeled red blood cell scan
labeling
    in situ end l. (ISEL)
    terminal uridine deoxynucleotide nick-end l. (TUNEL)
labetalol
labia (*pl. of* labium)
labialis
    herpes l.
labial ulceration
labile
    acid l.
labium, pl. **labia**
    l. inferius valvulae coli
    l. majus muscle
    l. minus muscle
    l. superius valvulae coli
    l. urethra
labor
    prolonged obstructed l.
laboratory
    l. abnormality
    surgical simulation virtual reality l.
    Venereal Disease Research L. (VDRL)
labyrinth
    cortical l.
    Ludwig l.
    renal l.
    Santorini l.
lab zymogen
lacelike keratosis
laceration
    concurrent hepatic l.
    longitudinal l.
    lower pole l.
    Mallory-Weiss l.
    rectal l.
    splenic l.
    vascular l.

Lachnospira
lacrimal duct probe
lactaciduria
Lactaid
lactaris
    Ruminococcus l.
lactase
    l. deficiency
    l. enzyme
lactase-ceramidase complex
lactase-phlorizin hydrolase (LPH)
lactate
    l. dehydrogenase (LDH)
    Ringer l.
lactated Ringer solution
lacteal
    central l.
    l. vessel
lactic
    l. acid
    l. acid dehydrogenase (LDH)
    l. acidosis
Lactinex
lactobacilli preparation
Lactobacillus
    L. acidophilus
    L. agilis
    L. bifidus
    L. bulgaricus
    L. casei
    L. GG (LGG)
    L. plantarum
    L. plantarum-fermented food
    L. plantarum-fermented oat
    L. plantarum 299v
    L. reuteri
    L. rhamnosus
lactobezoar
lactobionate
    erythromycin l.
lactoferrin
lacto-*N*-fucopentaose
    sialylated l.-N-f.
lactose
    disaccharide l.
    l. hydrogen breath testing (LHBT)
    l. intolerance
    l. malabsorption (LMA)
    l. maldigestor
    l. tolerance test
lactose-associated diarrhea
lactose-free
    l.-f. diet (LFD)
    l.-f. feeding
lactovegetarian

lactovegetarianism
Lactrase
lactulose
    l. breath test (LBT)
    l. enema
    l. solution
lactulose-mannitol
    l.-m. permeability test
    l.-m. ratio
lacuna, pl. **lacunae**
    great l.
    l. magna
    Morgagni lacunae
    l. of muscle
    l. of urethra
    urethral l.
lacunar abscess
lacunule
Ladd
    L. band
    L. correction of malrotation of bowel
    L. operation
    L. procedure
    L. syndrome
laddering
    DNA l.
Laënnec cirrhosis
Lafora body
LAGB
    Lap-Band adjustable gastric banding
    LAGB system
lag phase
Lahey
    L. aneurysm needle
    L. gall duct forceps
    L. liver transplant bag
Lahey-Babcock forceps
Laidley double-catheterizing cystoscope
Laird-McMahon anorectoplasty
LAK cell
lake
    bile l.
Lalonde hook forceps
LAMA
    laser-assisted microanastomosis
L-AmB
    liposomal-amphotericin B
Lambda Plus PDL 1, 2 laser system
Lambert-Eaton myasthenic syndrome
lamblia
    Giardia l.
lambliasis
lamina, pl. **laminae**
    basal l.
    l. densa
    l. muscularis mucosae
    proper l.
    l. propria
    l. propria of buccal mucosa
    l. propria lymphoid cell
    l. rara externa (LRE)
    l. rara interna (LRI)
    vascular l.
laminar cortical necrosis
laminated calcification
laminectomy
laminin
    destruction of l.
    l. receptor
    l. receptor inhibition
lamivudine
lamotrigine
lamp
    slit l.
    Wood l.
    xenon l.
Lancereaux nephritis
lancet-shaped biopsy forceps
lancinating pain
Landau
    L. reflex
    L. trocar
landmark
    bony l.
Landzert fossa
Lane
    L. band
    L. disease
    L. gastroenterostomy catheter
    L. gastroenterostomy clamp
    L. intestinal clamp
    L. intestinal forceps
    L. operation
Lange
    L. skinfold calipers
    L. test
Langerhans
    L. cell
    L. cell histiocytosis
    L. islet
    islet cell of L.
    L. lineage
Langer line
Langhans
    L. cell
    L. line
Langmuir adsorption isotherm
Lanoxin
lanreotide
lansoprazole
lansoprazole, amoxicillin, clarithromycin
lanthanum carbonate
Lanza scale
Lanz point
LAP
    leucine aminopeptidase

leukocyte alkaline phosphatase LAP test

lap
    laparotomy
        l. Nissen
        l. pad
        L. sac
        l. sponge
        l. tape

laparectomy
laparocele
laparocholecystotomy
laparocolectomy
laparocolostomy
laparocystectomy
laparoendoscopy
laparoenterostomy
Laparofan
laparoflator
    Weck High-Flow l.
laparogastroscopy
Laparolift system
LaparoLith
laparonephrectomy
laparorrhaphy
LaparoSAC single-use obturator and cannula
LaparoScan laparoscopic ultrasonic imaging
laparoscope
    50-degree Foroblique optic l.
    0-degree forward optic l.
    10-degree operating l.
    diagnostic l.
    EL2-LS2 flexible video l.
    flexible l. (FVL)
    Jacobs-Palmer l.
    Olympus A5256 l.
    operative l.

laparoscopic
    l. abdominoperineal excision
    l. abdominoperineal resection
    l. adjustable gastric banding
    l. adrenalectomy
    l. adrenal gland surgery
    l. Allis clamp
    l. antireflux surgery (LARS)
    l. appendectomy
    l. biopsy
    l. biopsy of liver
    l. bladder neck suspension
    l. bladder neck suture suspension procedure
    l. Burch urethropexy
    l. cannula
    l. cholecystectomy (LC)
    l. clip application
    l. colectomy
    l. colorectal cancer surgery
    L. Colorectal Surgery Group (LCSSG)
    l. colposuspension technique
    l. contact ultrasonography (LCU)
    l. cystoplasty
    l. cystourethropexy
    l. dismembered pyeloplasty
    l. gastric bypass
    l. grasper
    l. Heller myotomy
    l. hysterosalpingectomy
    l. intracorporeal ultrasound (LICU)
    l. knot
    l. laser-assisted autoaugmentation
    l. laser cholecystectomy (LLC)
    l. living donor nephrectomy
    l. lymphocelectomy
    l. lysis
    l. management
    l. marsupialization
    l. needle colposuspension
    l. needle driver
    l. Nissen and Toupet fundoplication
    l. orchiopexy
    l. partial nephrectomy (LPN)
    l. pelvic lymphadenectomy
    l. pelvic lymph node dissection (LPLND)
    l. photography
    l. promontofixation
    l. pyelolithotomy
    l. radical nephrectomy (LRN)
    l. radical nephroureterectomy
    l. radical prostatectomy
    l. renal artery aneurysm repair
    l. retraction system
    l. retropubic colposuspension
    l. scissors
    l. seromyotomy
    l. stapler
    l. stapling
    l. surgery in pediatric urology
    l. suture rectopexy
    l. tie clip

NOTES

laparoscopic *(continued)*
    l. transcystic duct exploration
    l. transcystic duct stenting of papilla
    l. transcystic papillotomy
    l. treatment of ureteropelvic junction obstruction
    l. trocar sleeve
    l. ultralow anterior resection
    l. ultrasound (LUS)
    l. ureteral reanastomosis
    l. ureterolithotomy
    l. ureterolysis
    l. urinary diversion procedure
    l. uterolysis
    l. vagotomy
    l. varicocelectomy
    l. varicocele repair
    l. varix ligation

laparoscopically
    l. assisted colorectal resection
    l. assisted panenteroscopy
    l. guided transcystic exploration

laparoscopic-assisted
    l.-a. approach
    l.-a. hemicolectomy
    l.-a. ileocystoplasty and ileovesicostomy

laparoscopic-guided feeding jejunostomy
laparoscopist
laparoscopy
    l. complication
    l. contraindication
    diagnostic l.
    double-puncture l.
    extraperitoneal l.
    flexible l.
    gasless l.
    gynecologic l.
    hand-assisted l. (HAL)
    inguinal l.
    l. in pediatric urology
    pulmonary gas embolism during l.
    robot-assisted l. (RAP)
    single-puncture l.
    standard l. (SL)
    subsequent diagnostic l.
    therapeutic l.
    l. trocar configuration
    l. trocar placement

laparoscopy-assisted ileocystoplasty and ileovesicostomy
laparoscopy-guided subhepatic cholecystostomy
Laparoshield laparoscopic smoke filtration system
LaparoSonic coagulating shears
laparosplenectomy
laparotomy (lap, LAP)
    emergency l.
    exploratory l.
    negative l.
    l. pack
    l. pad
    l. pad cover
    second-look l.
    l. sponge
    l. tape

laparotyphlotomy
Lap-Band
    L.-B. adjustable gastric banding (LAGB)
    L.-B. adjustable gastric banding system

Lapides
    L. classification
    L. classification of voiding dysfunction
    L. cystometric investigation
    L. test
    L. vesicostomy

Lapides-Ball urethropexy
Laplace
    L. forceps
    law of L.
    L. law

Lapra-Ty clip
Lapro-Clip
LapSac introducer
LapTie
LAR
    low anterior resection

LAR/CAA
    low anterior resection in combination with coloanal anastomosis

lardaceous kidney
large
    l. bowel
    l. bowel cancer
    l. bowel carcinoma
    l. bowel obstruction
    l. cell change (LCC)
    l. common duct stone
    l. forceps biopsy
    l. impacted ureteral stone
    l. needle size

large-bore
    l.-b. biliary endoprosthesis
    l.-b. cannula
    l.-b. catheter
    l.-b. double-pigtail stent
    l.-b. gastric lavage tube
    l.-b. heat probe
    l.-b. rigid esophagoscope
    l.-b. Tygon tubing

large-channel
    l.-c. endoscope
    l.-c. therapeutic duodenoscope

l.-c. video curvilinear echoendoscope
large-diameter bougie
large-droplet fatty liver
large-particle biopsy
large-volume paracentesis (LVP)
L-arginine
lari
  Campylobacter l.
Larodopa
LaRoque
  L. herniorrhaphy incision
  L. repair
  L. technique
Larrey hernia
Larrey-Weil disease
Larry
  L. rectal director
  L. rectal probe
LARS
  laparoscopic antireflux surgery
larval nephrosis
larva migrans
larvata
laryngeal
  l. carcinoma
  l. edema
  l. jack-assisted retrograde esophageal membranotomy
  l. jack technique
  l. vestibule
larynges (*pl. of* larynx)
laryngitis
  reflux l.
laryngopharyngectomy
laryngoscope
  Bullard intubating l.
  Kantor-Berci video l.
  Killian-Lynch l.
  Olympus ENF-P-series l.
  Ossoff-Karlan l.
laryngoscopy
  direct l.
laryngospasm
larynx, pl. **larynges**
LAS
  lymphadenopathy syndrome
laser
  l. ablation
  ADD'Stat l.
  l. adjustable silicone gastric banding (LASGB)

alexandrite l.
argon ion l.
argon pumped dye l.
balloon l.
Candela Model MDL 2000 l.
Candela 405-nm pulsed-dye l.
carbon dioxide l.
L. CHRP rigid fiberscope system
l. clipping
CO_2 l.
l. coagulation
Coherent model 90-K l.
coumarin dye l.
coumarin flashlamp-pumped pulsed-dye l.
l. desorption/ionization mass spectrometry
diode l.
Diomed l.
l. disk
l. Doppler flowmeter
l. Doppler velocimetry
dye l.
endoscopic pulsed-dye l.
erbium:YAG l.
flashlamp pumped-dye l.
FREDDY Nd:YAG l.
frequency-doubled-double pulse ND:YAG l.
helium-neon l.
l. hemorrhoidectomy
l. hemorrhoid excision
holmium l.
holmium:YAG l.
Indigo Optima l.
ion l.
krypton l.
KTP 532 l.
l. laparoscopic vagotomy
Lateralase l.
lateral-firing l.
Lithognost flash-lamp pulsed-dye l.
l. lithotripsy (LL)
l. lithotriptor
l. lithotriptor basket
LX-20 l.
medical l.
Medilas fiberTome l.
l. microscope
Molectron Nd:YAG l.
Myriadlase Side-Fire l.
Nd:YAG l.

NOTES

laser *(continued)*
    neodymium:yttrium garnet l.
    Olympus Nd:YAG l.
    OmniPulse MAX holmium l.
    l. partial nephrectomy
    l. photoablation
    l. photocoagulation
    l. photodestruction
    l. plume
    Prolase II lateral-firing Nd:YAG l.
    l. prostatectomy
    pulsed-dye l.
    pulsed-dye neodymium:YAG l.
    pulse dye l.
    Pulsolith l.
    pumped-dye l.
    Q-switched alexandrite l.
    Q-switched Nd:YAG l.
    rhodamine 6G dye l.
    l. sclerosis
    Side-Fire l.
    SLT contact MTRL l.
    l. surgery
    l. technology
    l. temperature
    l. therapy
    l. thermocoagulation
    l. tissue weld
    l. tissue welding
    l. tissue-welding solder
    Trimedyne holmium l.
    tunable pulsed-dye l.
    Ultraline l.
    ultrasound-guided l.
    Urolase l.
    l. vaporization
    VersaPulse PowerSuite dual-wavelength l.
    VersaPulse PowerSuite holmium l.
    VersaPulse Select l.
    visual endoscopically controlled l.
    l. welding technique
    l. writer
    YAG l.
    yttrium-aluminum-garnet l.
laser-assisted
    l.-a. endoscopic myotomy
    l.-a. microanastomosis (LAMA)
    l.-a. tissue-welding technique
laser-Doppler Periflux PF-3 probe
laser-guided biopsy
laser-induced
    l.-i. fluorescence spectroscopy (LIFS)
    l.-i. fragmentation
    l.-i. intracorporeal shock wave lithotripsy (LISL)
LaserMed laser pointer
laser-scanning confocal microscopy

Laserscope
    L. KTP 532
    L. YAG 1064
Lasersonic ACMI Ultraline
LaserSonics
    L. EndoBlade
    L. Nd:YAG Laserblade scalpel
laserthermia
lasertripsy
LaserTripter
    Candela MDA-200 L.
    L. MDL 3000
LASGB
    laser adjustable silicone gastric banding
Lashmet-Newburgh method
Lasix
L-asparaginase
Lassa hemorrhagic fever
lasso
    guidewire/basket l.
    l. snare
    l. technique
last-generation serologic ELISA test
lata *(pl. of* latum*)*
    fascia l.
latamoxef sodium
Latarjet
    nerve of L.
late
    l. dumping
    l. dumping syndrome
    l. graft dysfunction
latency
    pudendal nerve terminal motor l. (PNTML)
latent
    l. jaundice
    l. nephritis
late-onset
    l.-o. ataxia
    l.-o. hepatic failure
late-period filariasis
lateral
    l. abdominal region
    l. bending technique
    l. branch
    l. chordee
    l. cutaneous paresthesia
    l. cystocele
    l. decubitus
    l. decubitus position
    l. deflection control knob
    l. fossa
    l. fossa of preputial space
    l. gutter
    l. internal pelvic reservoir
    l. lithotomy
    l. lobe
    l. margin

l. node dissection
l. oblique fascia
l. pancreaticojejunostomy
l. prostatotomy
l. pyelography
l. rectal ligament
l. reflection of colon
l. sphincterotomy
l. ventral hernia
l. window technique

Lateralase laser
lateral-firing laser
lateralizing sensory deficit
lateral-lateral pouch
lateral-viewing endoscope
latex
l. agglutination assay
l. allergy
l. balloon
l. fixation test
l. hood
l. sclerosant

latex-base skin cement
latissimus
l. dorsi detrusor myoplasty
l. dorsi free flap
l. dorsi muscle

latum, pl. **lata**
condyloma l.
Diphyllobothrium l.
solvent-dehydrated cadaveric fascia lata

Latzko
L. partial colpocleisis
L. technique

Laubry-Soulle syndrome
laudanum
Laugier hernia
Launois-Cléret syndrome
Laurence-Moon-Bardet-Biedl syndrome
Laurence-Moon-Biedl syndrome
Lauren gastric carcinoma classification
lavage
abdominal l.
l. bowel preparation
cisapride-assisted l.
closed continuous l.
colonic l.
l. cytology
Easi-Lav l.
endoscopically guided segmental gut l.
external biliary l.
gastric l.
gastrointestinal l.
iced saline l.
internal biliary l.
isomotic l.
Lazarus-Nelson peritoneal l.
nasocystic catheter l.
nasogastric l.
norepinephrine l.
oral l.
oral colonic l. (OCL)
PEG l.
peritoneal l.
polyethylene glycol-based l.
rapid colonic l.
l. solution
stomach l.
l. and suction
Waterpik l.

lavage-induced
l.-i. cardiac asystole
l.-i. pill malabsorption

law
Bell l.
Courvoisier l.
Fitz l.
Laplace l.
l. of Laplace
Meyer-Weigert l.
Poiseuille l.
Poiseuille-Hagen l.
Salmon l.
Tait l.
Weigert-Meyer l.

lawn mower technique
Lawrence
L. Add-A-Cath
L. deep surgery forceps
L. gastric reservoir

Laws
L. gastroplasty
L. gastroplasty with Silastic collar-reinforced stoma

laxa
cutis l.

laxation
laxative
l. abuse
anthracene-type l.
anthraquinone l.
bulk l.

NOTES

laxative *(continued)*
    bulk-producing l.
    Ceo-Two l.
    contact l.
    emollient l.
    Fleet Phospho-soda buffered saline l.
    hyperosmotic l.
    lubricant l.
    osmotic l.
    saline l.
    sodium phosphate-based l.
    stimulant l.
    l. and stool softener softgel
    stool-softening l.
    surfactant l.
    Women's Gentle L.

LaxCaps
    Phillips L.

Laxinate 100

laxity
    ligamentous l.

Lax-Senna
    Black-Draught L.-S.

layer
    Bernard glandular l.
    echo-poor l.
    fascial l.
    germ l.
    glycosaminoglycan l.
    hypoechoic ringed l.
    seromuscular l.
    sonographic l.
    subcutaneous l.
    submucosal vaginal smooth musculofascial l.
    submucous l.
    subserosal l.

laying-open fistulotomy
lay-open method
Lazaro da Silva technique
Lazarus-Nelson
    L.-N. peritoneal lavage
    L.-N. technique

lazy bladder syndrome
LB 9501 luminometer
LBM
    lean body mass
LBT
    lactulose breath test
LC
    laparoscopic cholecystectomy
    liver cirrhosis
LCA
    lithocholic acid
    liver cell adenoma
LCA-DCA
    lithocholic acid-deoxycholic acid ratio
        LCA-DCA ratio

L-carnitine
    L.-c. capsule
    L.-c. tablet
LCAT
    lecithin-cholesterol acyltransferase
LCC
    large cell change
L-365,260 CCK antagonist
L-364,781 CCK antagonist
LCDD
    light-chain deposition disease
L cell
LC-EMR
    lift-and-cut endoscopic mucosal resection
LCFA
    long-chain fatty acid
LCG
    liquid chemical germicide
LCHAD
    long-chain 3-hydroxyacyl coenzyme A dehydrogenase
L-citrulline
lck protein
LCSSG
    Laparoscopic Colorectal Surgery Group
LCT
    long-chain triglyceride
LCU
    laparoscopic contact ultrasonography
LD
    living donor
LDH
    lactate dehydrogenase
    lactic acid dehydrogenase
        LDH enzyme
        LDH isoenzyme 5
        LDH level of ascitic fluid
        LDH test
LDL
    low-density lipoprotein
        LDL Direct test
        oxidized LDL
        LDL susceptibility
LDLC
    low-density lipoprotein cholesterol
LDLT
    living donor liver transplantation
LDP-02 antibody
LDS
    ligating and dividing stapler
        LDS stapler
LE cell
Le
    Le Bag
    Le Bag ileocolonic pouch
    Le Bag neobladder
    Le Bag pouch reservoir
    Le Bag urinary diversion
    Le Bag urinary pouch

Lea
    disialosyl L.
    monosialosyl L.
Leach technique
lead
    l. citrate
    l. citrate stain
    l. colic
    l. nephropathy
    l. poisoning
    l. wire
Leadbetter
    L. and Clarke technique
    L. and Clarke ureteral anastomosis
    L. cystourethroplasty
    L. ileal loop diversion
    L. maneuver
    L. modification technique
    L. procedure
    L. tunneling technique
Leadbetter-Politano
    L.-P. reimplantation
    L.-P. ureteroneocystostomy
    L.-P. ureterovesicoplasty
leading bar
lead-pipe
    l.-p. appearance
    l.-p. colon
leaf, pl. **leaves**
    chaparral l.
    l. of mesentery
leafless tree appearance
leaflike villus
leak
    anastomotic l.
    distal pouch l.
    lymphatic l.
    l. pressure
    proximal pouch l.
    renal calcium l.
leakage
    anastomotic l.
    biliary l.
    bilious l.
    l. bypass cable
    cavernovenous l.
    crural venous l.
    cystic duct l.
    intraabdominal bile l.
    postmicturition continuous l.
    postoperative biliary l.
    precipitant l.
    l. severity
    tube l.
    venous l.
leaking
leak-point pressure (LPP)
lean body mass (LBM)
learned enuresis
learning curve
leather-bottle stomach
leaves (*pl. of* leaf)
leaves of diaphragm
Leber amaurosis
Lebsche shears
lecimibide
lecithin
    polyunsaturated l.
lecithin-cholesterol acyltransferase (LCAT)
lectin
    hepatic l.
    l. reactivity
    l. staining
lecturescope
LeDuc
    L. fashion
    L. technique
    L. technique urinary diversion
    L. ureteral anastomosis
LeDuc-Camey
    L.-C. ileocolostomy
    L.-C. ileocystoplasty
leech
    mechanical l.
leflunomide (HWA 486, LFM)
LeFort
    L. procedure
    L. sound
left
    l. colon
    l. colonic flexure
    l. decubitus position
    l. gastroomental artery
    l. gutter
    l. hepatic duct (LHD)
    l. hepatic duct stricture
    l. hepatic lobe (LHL)
    l. hepatic vein (LHV)
    l. lateral decubitus position
    l. lower quadrant (LLQ)
    Monti-Malone, l.
    l. pancreaticogastric fold

NOTES

left (continued)
    l. upper quadrant (LUQ)
    l. ureter
left-sided
    l.-s. appendicitis
    l.-s. clonus
    l.-s. colitis
left-to-right subtotal pancreatectomy
Legionella pneumophila
Leigh disease
Leiner disease
leiomyoblastoma
leiomyoma, pl. **leiomyomata, leiomyomas**
    bizarre l.
    colonic l.
    duodenal l.
    epithelioid l.
    esophageal l.
    gastric l.
    parasitic l.
    l. of seminal vesicle
    testicular l.
    Zenker l.
leiomyosarcoma
    bladder l.
    gastric l.
    hepatic l.
    kidney l.
    low-grade l.
    paratesticular l.
    prostate gland l.
    rectal l.
    small intestine l.
    spermatic cord l.
Leishmania
    L. donovani chagasi
    L. donovani donovani
    L. donovani infantum
    L. esophagitis
    L. infantum
leishmanial enteritis
leishmaniasis, leishmaniosis
    infantile l.
    visceral l.
Lembert inverting seromuscular suture
lemostenosis
Lempert paracentesis knife
Lendrum stain
length
    anal canal l. (ACL)
    functional profile l.
    functional urethral l. (FUL)
    lower infundibular l.
    peripheral capillary filtration slit l.
    telomere l.
    total slit pore l.
l-ENK
    leucine-enkephalin
Lennhoff sign

lens
    120-degree l.
    Foroblique l.
    Hopkins II rod l.
    narrow l.
    objective l.
    right-angle l.
lenta
    cholangitis l.
Lente insulin
lentigines, electrocardiographic conduction abnormalities, ocular hypertelorism, pulmonary stenosis, abnormal genitalia, retardation of growth, and deafness (LEOPARD)
lentigo
Lentivirus
lentum
    Eubacterium l.
Leonard
    L. Arm
    L. deep surgery forceps
LEOPARD
    lentigines, electrocardiographic conduction abnormalities, ocular hypertelorism, pulmonary stenosis, abnormal genitalia, retardation of growth, and deafness
    LEOPARD syndrome
Leo test
leprae
    Mycobacterium l.
leprosy
leptin
    l. level
    recombinant methionyl human l. (r-metHuLeptin)
Leptospira interrogans
leptospiral
    l. jaundice
    l. nephritis
leptospirosis
leptum
    Clostridium l.
Leriche syndrome
LES
    lesser esophageal sphincter
    lower esophageal sphincter
        LES incompetence
        LES locator
        LES relaxation
        transient relaxation of LES
Lesch-Nyhan syndrome
Lescol
Leser-Trélat sign
Lesgaft
    L. hernia
    L. space
    L. triangle

lesion
- acetowhite l.
- acute gastric mucosal l.
- ampullary l.
- anal squamous intraepithelial l.
- angiodysplastic l.
- Antopol-Goldman l.
- aortoostial l.
- aphthous-type l.
- apple-core l.
- Armanni-Ebstein l.
- Baehr-Lohlein l.
- bilobed polypoid l.
- blanching of l.
- bleeding l.
- Bosniak l. category I–IV
- bull's eye l.
- Cameron l.
- cauda equina l.
- colonic vascular l.
- Councilman l.
- cutaneous l.
- Dieulafoy gastric l.
- doughnut l.
- duodenal l.
- dye sham intrarenal l.
- Ebstein l.
- echo-poor l.
- ectatic vascular l.
- exophytic l.
- extramural l.
- fingertip l.
- flat depressed l.
- flat elevated l.
- florid bile duct l.
- Forest I, II l.
- gastric l.
- gastrointestinal l.
- glomerular tip l. (GTL)
- gunpowder l.
- hamartomatous l.
- hepatic mass l.
- high fundal l.
- high neurological l.
- hypoechoic l.
- l. identification
- indentifiable intrascrotal l.
- intramural l.
- isolated adenomatous l.
- Janeway l.
- local glomerular l.
- localized l.
- Lohlein-Baehr l.
- lower motor neuron l.
- lumbar spinal cord l.
- lymphoepithelial l.
- macroorchidism l.
- macroscopic l.
- Mallory-Weiss l.
- mesenteric vascular l.
- metachronous l.
- metastatic l.
- minute polypoid l.
- mucosal l.
- mulberry l.
- multicentric l.
- napkin-ring annular l.
- neoplastic l.
- nodular l.
- nonerosive gastric mucosal l.
- nonneoplastic l.
- ocular l.
- pancreas l.
- pancreatic l.
- papillary l.
- penile l.
- perianal l.
- photon-deficient l.
- plaquelike l.
- pliable l.
- polypoid l.
- precancerous l.
- preoperative l.
- primary glomerular l.
- right-sided l.
- ringlike l.
- ruptured peliotic l.
- satellite l.
- scirrhous l.
- semipedunculated l.
- sessile l.
- short-segment l.
- significant liver l.
- skip l.
- space-occupying l.
- stenotic l.
- stress l.
- subglottic l.
- submucosal upper gastrointestinal tract l.
- synchronous l.
- target l.
- thrombic l.
- traumatic l.

NOTES

lesion *(continued)*
    trophic l.
    tubulovillar l.
    uremic gastrointestinal l.
    vascular l.
    vasculitic l.
    vegetative l.
    wire-loop l.

LESP
    lower esophageal sphincter pressure

LESR
    lower esophageal sphincter relaxation

lesser
    l. curvature of stomach
    l. curvature ulcer
    l. epiploon
    l. esophageal sphincter (LES)
    l. omentum
    l. pancreas
    l. peritoneal sac

less morbid lower abdominal transverse incision

Lester Martin modification of Duhamel operation

lethargic

LE-TUMT
    low-energy transurethral microwave thermotherapy

Leube test meal

leucine
    l. aminopeptidase (LAP)
    l. aminopeptidase test
    l. metabolism
    radiolabeled l.
    l. zipper
    l. zipper sequence

leucine-enkephalin (l-ENK)

Leucomax

leucovorin
    oxaliplatin, 5-fluorouracil, l.
    l. rescue

leu-enkephalin

leukemia
    acute lymphoblastic l.
    acute lymphocytic l.
    acute myelomonocytic l.
    chylous l.
    testicular l.

Leukeran

leukobilin

leukocyte
    l. adherence inhibition test
    l. alkaline phosphatase (LAP)
    l. alkaline phosphatase test
    chemotaxis of polymorphonuclear l.
    l. common antigen
    l. esterase
    l. esterase test
    fecal l.
    intraepithelial l. (IEL)
    peritoneal l.
    polymorphonuclear l. (PMNL)
    l. scintigraphy
    tether circulating l.
    l. trafficking
    WBC l.

leukocytoclastic vasculitis

leukocytosis

leukopenia
    acute l.

leukoplakia
    bladder l.
    hairy l.
    oral l.
    l. of penis

LEUKO-TEST

leukotriene
    l. A_4
    l. C_4
    cysteinyl l.
    l. D_4

leukourobilin

leu-peptide

leupeptin

Leuprogel

leuprolide
    l. acetate
    l. acetate implant
    l. acetate for injectable suspension
    L. Depot Neoadjuvant Prostate Cancer Study Group

Leutrol

Leuvectin

levamfetamine

levamisole

Levaquin

Levarterenol

Levatol

levator
    l. ani
    l. ani hernia
    l. ani muscle
    l. ani syndrome
    l. fascia
    l. plate
    l. span
    l. veli palatini muscle

Levbid

levcromakalim

LeVeen
    L. ascites shunt
    L. catheter
    L. inflation syringe
    L. inflator
    L. inflator with pressure gauge
    L. peritoneal shunt
    L. peritoneovenous shunt
    L. valve

level
- air-fluid l.
- Albarran deflecting l.
- alpha-1-antitrypsin l.
- alpha fetoprotein l.
- ammonia l.
- AMP l.
- anti-M2 antimitochondrial antibody l.
- blood alcohol l. (BAL)
- blood lead l. (BLL)
- blood urea l.
- breath ethane l.
- complement l.
- control l.
- des-gamma-carboxy prothrombin l.
- fasting C-peptide l.
- fasting serum gastrin l.
- fluid-debris l.
- gamma-glutamyltransferase l.
- gastrin mRNA l.
- homocysteine l.
- HSP-70 messenger ribonucleoprotein acid l.
- 25-hydroxyvitamin D l.
- iothalamate l.
- leptin l.
- lipoprotein X l.
- motilin plasma l.
- pathological resistive index l.
- pentane excretion l.
- pepsinogen l. A, B, C
- pericardial air-fluid l.
- polyamine l.
- protein C, S l.
- red blood cell folate l.
- serum eotaxin l.
- serum gastrin l.
- serum leptin l.
- serum urate l.
- somatostatin MRNA l.
- stairstep air-fluid l.
- theophylline l.
- thyroid-stimulating hormone l.
- transferrin saturation l.
- uric acid l.
- urinary cGMP l.
- whole-blood trough l.

Levin
- L. tube
- L. tube aspiration

Levitra

levocarnitine
levodopa/carbidopa
levodopa dopaminergic medication
levofloxacin
levorphanol
levothyroxine
levovirin
Levovist contrast agent
Levsinex Timecaps
Levsin/SL
levulose test
Lewis
- L. A blood group antigen
- L. acid
- L. blood group
- L. B, X, Y antigen
- L. classification for vascular anomalies of the gastrointestinal tract
- L. cystometer
- L. Y carbohydrate epitope

Lewis-Tanner esophagectomy procedure
Lewy syringe
lexipafant
Lexirin
Leyden disease
Leydig
- L. cell
- L. cell adenoma
- L. cell secretion
- L. cell secretory function
- L. cell tumor
- L. duct

leydigarche
LFD
- lactose-free diet
- low-fat diet

LFM
- leflunomide

LFS
- liver function series

LFT
- liver function tests

LG
- light guide
- lymphocytic gastritis
- LG bundle

LGD
- low-grade dysplasia

LGG
- *Lactobacillus* GG

NOTES

LGIB
 lower gastrointestinal bleeding
L-glutamine
L-glyceric aciduria
LGV
 lymphogranuloma venereum
LH
 loop of Henle
 luteinizing hormone
LHBT
 lactose hydrogen breath testing
LHD
 left hepatic duct
Lhermitte-Duclos disease
LH-FSH
 luteinizing hormone follicle-stimulating hormone
LHL
 left hepatic lobe
LHRH
 luteinizing hormone releasing hormone
LHV
 left hepatic vein
LI
 loop ileostomy
libera
 taenia l.
libidinal
libido
Librax
Libritabs
Lich
 L. extravesical technique
 L. procedure
 L. ureteral implantation for neobladder construction
lichen
 l. nitidus
 l. planus
 l. sclerosus
 l. sclerosus et atrophicus
 l. simplex chronicus
lichenoid reaction
Lich-Gregoire
 L.-G. anastomosis
 L.-G. repair
 L.-G. technique
 L.-G. ureterolysis
Lichtenstein
 L. hernia repair
 L. herniorrhaphy
 L. open tension-free mesh hernioplasty
LICU
 laparoscopic intracorporeal ultrasound
lidamidine
Liddle
 L. disease

 L. mutation
 L. syndrome
Lidex
lidocaine
 l. hydrochloride jelly
 l. topical anesthetic
 viscous l.
lidocaine-prilocaine cream
lidofenin
 ^{99m}Tc l.
Lidox
Lidoxide
Lieberkühn
 L. ampulla
 L. crypt
 L. follicle
 L. gland
Lieberman
 L. proctoscope
 L. sigmoidoscope
Liebermeister
 L. furrow
 L. groove
lieenulus (*var. of* lienculus)
lien
 l. accessorius
 l. mobilis
lienal artery
lienalis
 arteria l.
 penicilli arteriae l.
lienculus, lieenulus
lienectomy
lienis
 pulpa l.
 trabeculae l.
lienitis
lienocele
lienomalacia
lienomedullary
lienomyelogenous
lienomyelomalacia
lienopancreatic
lienopathy
lienophrenic ligament
lienorenal ligament
lienteric
 l. diarrhea
 l. stool
lientery
lienunculus
lieutaudi
 trigonum vesicae l.
Lieutaud uvula
LIFE
 light-induced fluorescence endoscopy
life
 l. cycle of *Echinococcus*

health-related quality of l. (HRQOL)
quality of l. (QOL)
Lifecath peritoneal implant
LifeJet catheter
lifelong obesity
Lifemed catheter
LifeSite hemodialysis access system
lifestyle
l. modification (LSM)
l. therapy
Life-Tech flowmeter
L-IFN
human lymphoblastoid interferon
Li-Fraumeni syndrome
LIFS
laser-induced fluorescence spectroscopy
lift
gallbladder l.
lift-and-cut
l.-a.-c. biopsy
l.-a.-c. endoscopic mucosal resection (LC-EMR)
l.-a.-c. method
l.-a.-c. technique
lifting sign
LIG
lymphocyte immune globulin
ligament
Arantius l.
Bellini l.
Camper l.
Carcassonne perineal l.
cardinal l.
cholecystoduodenal l.
Clado l.
Cooper l.
coronary l.
costovertebral l.
external l.
falciform l.
femoral l.
fissure of round l.
fundiform l.
gastrocolic l.
gastrohepatic l.
gastrolienal l.
gastropancreatic l.
gastrophrenic l.
gastrosplenic l.
gonadal l.
Helvetius l.

hepatic l.
hepatocolic l.
hepatocystocolic l.
hepatoduodenal l.
hepatogastric l.
hepatogastroduodenal l.
hepatophrenic l.
hepatorenal l.
hepatoumbilical l.
Hesselbach l.
Hey l.
Huschke l.
infundibulopelvic l.
inguinal l.
Krause l.
lateral rectal l.
lienophrenic l.
lienorenal l.
lumbodorsal l.
l. of Mackenrodt
medial umbilical l.
median arcuate l.
mucosal suspensory l.
periurethral l.
phrencolic l.
phrenicoesophageal l.
Poupart l.
pubocervical l.
puboprostatic l.
pubourethral l.
pubovesical l.
rectosacral l.
l. reflecting edge
reflecting edge of l.
round l.
sacrospinous l.
sacrotuberous l.
sacrouterine l.
shelving edge of Poupart l.
splenocolic l.
splenopancreatic l.
splenorenal l.
suspensory l.
l. of Treitz
triangular l.
umbilical l.
ureteropelvic l.
urethropelvic l.
uterosacral l.
vesical l.
ligamentous laxity
ligamentum, pl. **ligamenta**

NOTES

ligamentum *(continued)*
    l. teres
    l. teres cardiopexy
    l. teres hepatis
    l. venosum

ligand
    l. for ELAM-1
    reciprocal l.
    l. recognition

ligand-dependent receptor homodimerization

ligand-gated channel

ligandin

ligand-triggered
    l.-t. membrane guanylate cyclase
    l.-t. protein tyrosine kinase

ligase
    Thermus aquaticus DNA l.

ligated
    doubly l.
    suture l.

ligating and dividing stapler (LDS)

ligation
    band l.
    Barron l.
    bidirectional l.
    bile duct l. (BDL)
    detachable miniloop l.
    l. device
    Doppler-guided hemorrhoidal artery l. (DGHAL)
    elastic band l.
    endoscopic band l. (EBL)
    endoscopic detachable miniloop l.
    endoscopic esophagogastric variceal l.
    endoscopic hemorrhoid l. (EHL)
    endoscopic mucosal resection with l. (EMRL)
    endoscopic ultrasound-assisted band l.
    endoscopic variceal l. (EVL)
    endoscopic variceal band l.
    esophageal band l.
    gastric variceal l.
    l. of hemorrhoid
    hepatic artery l.
    high l.
    Ivanissevitch l.
    laparoscopic varix l.
    loop l.
    miniloop l.
    open retroperitoneal high l.
    penile vein l.
    postureteral l.
    retroflexed endoscopic multiple band l. (REMBL)
    rubber band l. (RBL)
    spermatic vein l.
    stump l.
    transesophageal l.
    transgastric l.
    triple rubber band l.
    tubal l.
    variceal band l.
    varix l.

ligator
    Bandito single-band l.
    Barron rubber band l.
    DDV l.
    endoscopic band l.
    KilRoid single-handed l.
    McGivney hemorrhoidal l.
    multiple band l.'s
    multiple-band l.
    NAMI DDV l.
    O'Regan hemorrhoid l.
    RapidFire multiple-band l.
    rubber band l. (RBL)
    Rudd Clinic hemorrhoidal l.
    Saeed multiband l.
    Saeed multiple l.
    Saeed six-shooter l.
    Speedband Superview l.
    Stiegmann-Goff Clearvue endoscopic l.
    Stiegmann-Goff variceal l.
    variceal l.
    Wilson-Cook l. 4, 6, 10 band

Ligat test

ligature
    elastic l.
    interlocking l.
    pursestring l.
    retroperitoneoscopic vein l.
    l. sign
    silk l.
    Surgiwip suture l.
    suture l.

light
    bili l.
    l. cable
    Cholestyramine L.
    l. electrocautery
    l. and electron immunoperoxidase
    l. and electron immunoperoxidase observation
    l. emitter
    l. flow
    fluorescence correlation spectroscopy magnifying l. (FCS-ML)
    l. fluorescent intensity
    l. guide (LG)
    l. guide bundle
    light-chain deposition disease (LCDD)
    l. micrographic study
    l. microscopy

l. monitoring probe
l. reflex
light-induced
    l.-i. autofluorescence spectroscopy
    l.-i. fluorescence endoscopy (LIFE)
Lightwood syndrome
Lignac
    L. disease
    L. syndrome
Lignac-Fanconi
    L.-F. disease
    L.-F. syndrome
lignan
likelihood ratio
Likert scale
Lillie intestinal forceps
limb
    afferent ileal l.
    afferent jejunal l.
    ascending l.
    blind l.
    l. deformity
    efferent l.
    jejunal l.
    Roux l.
    Roux-en-Y jejunal l.
    thick ascending l. (TAL)
    thin descending l.
    vertebral, anal, cardiac, tracheoesophageal fistula, renal, l. (VACTERL)
Limberg flap repair
limbus, pl. **limbi**
LIM 2537 cell
limerence
limit dextrinosis
limited
    l. economic lithotripsy
    l. intravenous pyleography
    l. obturator node dissection
    l. range of motion
limiting
    l. dilution assay
    l. plate
    l. plate erosion
limosum
    Eubacterium l.
limy bile
Lincoln deep surgery scissors
lincomycin
lindane

line
Aldrich-Mees l.
anocutaneous l.
anorectal l.
anterior axillary l. (AAL)
apoptosis in cell l.
arcuate l.
arterial l.
B-cell l.
Beacon surgical l.
Brödel l.
Cantlie l.
CaSki cell l.
cell l.
central venous pressure l.
colonic mucosal l.
Conradi l.
dentate l.
l. of Douglas
Dul45 cell l.
Freedom Clear long-seal male external catheter l.
Freedom Clear LS male external catheter l.
Freedom Clear sport-sheath male external catheter l.
Freedom Clear SS male external catheter l.
gas density l.
Hampton l.
Hilton white l.
Hunter l.
iliopectineal l.
incision l.
J l.
K562 erythroid l.
Langer l.
Langhans l.
lower anterior axillary l. (LAAL)
lower midclavicular l. (LMCL)
lymphoblastoid cell l.
midaxillary l.
midclavicular l. (MCL)
milkman's l.
mucosal l.
murine mesangial cell l.
myelomonocytic cell l.
neuronal cell l.
pararectal l.
pectinate l.
Poupart l.
pubic hair l.

NOTES

line *(continued)*
    pubococcygeal l.
    pubosacral l.
    Rex-Cantli-Serege l.
    Richter-Monroe l.
    Sergent white adrenal l.
    skin l.
    suture l.
    T-cell l.
    l. of Toldt
    total parenteral nutrition l.
    TPN l.
    transverse umbilical l.
    upper midclavicular l. (UMCL)
    white anococcygeal l.
    Z l.

linea
    l. alba
    l. nigra

lineage
    hematopoietic l.
    Langerhans l.

linear

linear-array
    l.-a. analog pain score
    l.-a. convex array scanner
    curved l.-a.
    l.-a. echoendoscope
    l.-a. erosion
    l.-a. fluorescein
    l.-a. gastric ulcer
    l.-a. mode
    l.-a. probe
    l.-a. proctotomy
    l.-a. regression
    l.-a. staple cutter
    l.-a. stapler
    l.-a. stapling device
    l.-a. streaks en face
    l.-a. transducer
    l.-a. ulceration

Lingeman
    L. 3-in-1 procedure drape
    L. TUR drape

lingua, pl. **linguae**
    pityriasis l.

lingual lipase

linguatuliasis

lingula

linitis
    l. plastica
    l. plastica carcinoma

link
    cytoskeletal l.

linkage
    gene l.
    inherent to l.

linked
    UV l.

Linnartz intestinal clamp
linoleic acid
linsidomine chlorohydrate
Linton
    L. shunt
    L. tourniquet clamp

Linton-Nachlas tube
Lioresal
Lipancreatin
LIP angle
liparocele
lipase
    bile salt-stimulated l. (BSSL)
    Cherry-Crandall method for testing serum l.
    colipase-dependent l.
    l. enzyme
    hepatic l. (HL)
    hepatic triglyceride l. (HTGL)
    lingual l.
    lipoprotein l. (LPL)
    pancreatic l.
    serum l.
    l. test

lipid
    l. bilayer
    biliary l.
    l. emulsion
    extracellular l.
    l. hydroperoxide
    l. infusion
    inositol l.
    l. island
    l. maldigestion
    membrane-based l.
    l. metabolism
    l. nephrosis
    l. oxidation rate
    l. peroxidation

lipid-laden
    l.-l. clear cell
    l.-l. hepatocyte

lipid-lowering drug
lipidosis
    ceramide lactoside l.
    Schwann cell l.

lipidosterol extract
lipid-to-protein ratio
lipiduria
lipiodol
    l. injection
    l. transarterial embolization treatment

lipoblastic sarcoma
lipoblastoma
lipocele
lipodystrophia intestinalis

lipodystrophy
    intestinal l.
    mesenteric l.
lipofection reagent
lipofuscin
lipogranuloma
    mesenteric l.
lipogranulomatosis
lipoidal
lipoid nephrosis (LN)
lipolysis
    heparin-induced l.
    intraluminal l.
    intravascular l.
    LPL-mediated l.
lipolytic enzyme
lipoma
    colonic l.
    l. of cord
    gastric l.
    gastrointestinal l.
    submucosal ileal l.
lipomalike tissue
lipomatosis
    pelvic l.
lipomatous
    l. ileocecal valve
    l. nephritis
    l. paranephritis
    l. tissue
lipomeningocele
lipomyelocystocele
lipomyelomeningocele
lipophagia granulomatosis
lipophagic intestinal granulomatosis
lipophagy
lipopolysaccharide (LPS)
lipoprotein
    apolipoprotein B-containing l.
    l. glomerulopathy
    high-density l. (HDL)
    intermediate density l. (IDL)
    intermediate low-density l. (ILDL)
    l. lipase (LPL)
    liver-specific membrane l. (LSP)
    low-density l. (LDL)
    l. metabolism
    oxidized l.
    oxidized low-density l. (Ox-LDL)
    very low density l. (VLDL)
    l. X
    l. X level

liposarcoma
    bladder l.
    kidney l.
    spermatic cord l.
liposclerotic mesenteritis
liposomal-amphotericin B (L-AmB)
liposomal daunorubicin HCl
Liposorber LA-15 System lithotriptor
Liposyn II fat emulsion solution
lipothymia
Lipoxide
lipoxin
lipoxygenase
    l. blockade
    l. inhibition
    l. inhibitor
    5-l. inhibitor
    l. pathway
Lipram-PN10
Lipshultz urology microsurgical set
liquefaciens
    Aeromonas l.
    Enterobacter l.
    Serratia l.
liquefaction
    semen l.
liquefactive necrosis
Liqui-Char
liquid
    l. antacid
    AntaGel L.
    l. chemical germicide (LCG)
    l. chromatographic assay
    l. diarrhea
    l. diet
    EMF oral l.
    l. emptying
    Enfamil Low Iron l.
    l. food dysphagia
    full l.'s (FL)
    hyperosmolar l.
    isoosmolar l.
    Nutrament oral l.
    Peptamen L.
    Peptic Relief l.
    Phenyl-Free oral l.
    L. Pred
    Resource Diabetic ready-to-use l.
    Resource Fruit Beverage ready-to-use l.
    Resource Just for Kids ready-to-use l.

NOTES

liquid *(continued)*
    Resource oral l.
    l. scintillation spectrometer
    l. stool
Liqui-Doss
Liqui-E
liquor
    l. entericus
    l. gastricus
    l. pancreaticus
    l. seminis
lisinopril
LISL
    laser-induced intracorporeal shock wave lithotripsy
list
    Mood Adjective Check L.
Listeria
    L. monocytogenes
    L. monocytogenes peritonitis
liter
    international units per l. (IU/L)
    millimoles per l. (mmol/L)
lithagogue
lithangiuria
lithectasy
lithectomy
lithiasis
    Crixivan l.
    intraductal l.
    renal l.
    urinary l.
lithium
    l. clearance (CLi)
    fractional excretion of l. (FELI)
lithocenosis
lithocholate
lithocholic
    l. acid (LCA)
    l. acid-deoxycholic acid ratio (LCA-DCA)
lithoclast
    Swiss L.
Lithoclast endoscopic lithotriptor
lithoclysmia
lithocystotomy
lithodialysis
lithogenesis
    urinary l.
lithogenic bile
Lithognost flash-lamp pulsed-dye laser
lithokonion
litholabe
litholapaxy
    Bigelow l.
litholysis
    chemical l.
litholyte
litholytic
lithometer
lithomyl
lithonephritis
lithonephrotomy
lithophone
lithoscope
Lithostar
    L. nonimmersion lithotriptor
    L. Plus
    L. Plus electromagnetic lithotriptor bidimensional x-ray focusing system
    Siemens L.
Lithostat
lithostathine molecule
lithotome
lithotomist
lithotomy
    bilateral l.
    dorsal l.
    high l.
    lateral l.
    Marian l.
    median l.
    mediolateral l.
    perineal l.
    l. position
    prerectal l.
    rectovesical l.
    suprapubic l.
    vaginal l.
    vesical l.
    vesicovaginal l.
lithotresis
    ultrasonic l.
lithotripsy
    alexandrite laser l.
    biliary l.
    blind l.
    contact l.
    coumarin green tunable dye laser l.
    cystoscopic electrohydraulic l.
    Dornier extracorporeal shock wave l.
    Dornier MPL 9000 gallstone l.
    electrohydraulic l. (EHL)
    electrohydraulic shock wave l. (ESWL)
    endoscopic-controlled l.
    endoscopic electrohydraulic l.
    endoscopic Ho:YAG l.
    endoscopic metallic stent l.
    endoscopic pulsed-dye laser l.
    external shock wave l.
    extracorporeal piezoelectric l. (EPL)
    extracorporeal piezoelectric shock wave l.
    holmium-aluminum-garnet l.

lithotripsy · lithotrity

    intracorporeal l.
    intracorporeal electrohydraulic l. (IEHL)
    intracorporeal laser l. (ICL, ILL)
    intracorporeal shock wave l. (ISWL)
    laser l. (LL)
    laser-induced intracorporeal shock wave l. (LISL)
    limited economic l.
    mechanical l.
    Medstone extracorporeal shock wave l.
    nonstented ureteroscopic l.
    pancreatoscopic laser l. (PSLL)
    peroral shock wave l. (PSWL)
    piezoelectric l.
    pneumatic l.
    pressure-regulated electrohydraulic l.
    l. retreatment
    shock wave l. (SWL)
    stented ureteroscopic l.
    l. table
    l. technology
    tunable dye laser l.
    ultrasonic l.
    ureteroscopic intracorporeal electrohydraulic l.
    visible-light l.

lithotripsy-induced hypertension
lithotripter
    dual-pulse l.
    Twinheads shock wave l.

lithotriptic
lithotriptor, lithotripter
    American endoscopy mechanical l.
    Breakstone l.
    Calcutript electrohydraulic l.
    Circon-ACMI l.
    Diasonics Therasonic l.
    Direx Tripter X-1 l.
    DoLi S extracorporeal shock wave l.
    Dornier compact l.
    Dornier gallstone l.
    Dornier HM3, HM4 electrohydraulic l.
    Dornier MPL 5000 l.
    DP-1 l.
    EDAP LT.01 l.
    effective l.
    electrohydraulic l.
    electromagnetic l.
    electropneumatic endoscopic l.
    extracorporeal piezoelectric l.
    extracorporeal shock wave l.
    HM4 l.
    intracorporeal l.
    Karl Storz-Lutzeyer l.
    laser l.
    Liposorber LA-15 System l.
    Lithoclast endoscopic l.
    Lithostar nonimmersion l.
    manual l.
    Medispec Econolith spark plug l.
    Medstone STS l.
    MFL 5000 l.
    Modulith SL 20 l.
    Northgate SD-3 dual-purpose l.
    Olympus BML-3Q, -4Q l.
    out-of-scope l.
    percutaneous ultrasonic l.
    piezoelectric shock wave l.
    Piezolith EPL l.
    Piezolith 2300, 2500 model l.
    pneumatic endoscopic l.
    Richard Wolf Piezolith l.
    second-generation l.
    shock wave l.
    Siemens Lithostar Plus System C l.
    Sonolith Praktis portable l.
    Sonotrode l.
    Swiss Lithoclast l.
    Technomed Sonolith 3000 l.
    Therasonics l.
    third-generation l.
    tubeless l.
    ultrasonic l.
    Waltz endoscopic l.
    water cushion l.
    Wilson-Cook mechanical l.
    Wolf Piezolith 2300 l.
    Wolf Sonolith l.

lithotriptoscope
lithotriptoscopy
lithotrite
    Lowsley l.
    Marmite l.
    Reliquet l.
    Rotolith l.
    Thompson l.
    Wolf l.

lithotrity

NOTES

lithous
Lithovac stone removal
lithoxiduria
lithuresis
lithureteria
litmus milk test
littoral
    l. cell
    l. cell angioma
Littré
    crypt of L.
    L. gland
    L. hernia
Livaditis circular myotomy
live
    l. attenuated virus
    BCG l.
    l. renal donation
live-donor
    l.-d. nephrectomy
    l.-d. segmental graft
liver
    l. abscess
    l. acinus
    acute fatty l.
    acute yellow atrophy of the l.
    l. Ah receptor
    albuminoid l.
    alcoholic fatty l.
    ballottable l.
    bare area of l.
    l. bed
    biliary cirrhotic l.
    l. biopsy
    l. breath
    l. cancer
    capsular cirrhosis of l.
    l. capsule
    cardiac impression on l.
    caudate eminence of l.
    caudate lobe of l.
    l. cell adenoma (LCA)
    l. cell carcinoma
    l. cell dysplasia
    l. cell plate
    centrilobular region of l.
    l. cirrhosis (LC)
    cirrhotic l.
    colic impression on l.
    cutdown l.
    cut surface of l.
    l. cyst infection
    l. death
    l. deposit
    l. dialysis system
    l. dialysis unit
    diaphragmatic surface of l.
    l. diet
    l. distribution
    dome of l.
    l. dullness
    duodenal impression on l.
    l. eater
    echogenic l.
    l. edge
    l. engorgement
    l. enzyme
    l. failure
    fatty l. (FL)
    fatty infiltration of l.
    l. fibrosis
    fibrous appendage of l.
    fibrous capsule of l.
    fibrous tunic of l.
    finely fatty foamy l.
    l. flap
    l. flap sign
    l. fluke
    foamy l.
    focal fatty infiltration of l.
    focal nonfatty infiltration of l.
    l. function profile
    l. function series (LFS)
    l. function tests (LFT)
    gastric impression on l.
    l. hilus
    hobnail l.
    l. hydatid disease
    l. impression
    l. iron store
    l., kidneys, spleen (LKS)
    laparoscopic biopsy of l.
    large-droplet fatty l.
    lobe of l.
    lobular architecture of l.
    l. lymphoma
    macrovesicular fatty l.
    l. meal
    l. membrane antigen
    l. metastasis
    nodular l.
    l. nodule
    noncirrhotic l.
    nonparasitic cyst of l.
    nutmeg l.
    L. Panel Plus 9
    l. parenchyma
    phlegmonous alcoholic fatty l.
    polycystic l.
    polycystic disease of l. (PDL)
    polylobar l.
    potato l.
    l. protein store
    pyogenic l.
    quadrate lobe of l.
    renal impression on l.
    l. resection
    sagittal fissure of l.

l. scan
segmentectomy of l.
shock l.
shrunken l.
l. sinusoid
small-droplet fatty l.
l. span
stasis l.
subacute atrophy of l.
subchronic atrophy of l.
suprarenal area of l.
tender l.
l. transplant
l. transplantation
l. transplantation preservation injury
l. trauma
undersurface of l.
undifferentiated embryonal sarcoma of l.
venoocclusive disease of l.
l. volume
wandering l.
yellow atrophy of l.

liver-adipose tissue cycle
liver-deprived epithelial clonic cell
liver-directed autoreactivity
liver-kidney
l.-k. microsomal antibody
l.-k. microsome (LKM)
liver-specific
l.-s. antigen
l.-s. membrane lipoprotein (LSP)
l.-s. protein
liver-spleen scan
living
l. adult-to-adult donor
l. donor (LD)
l. donor kidney
l. donor liver transplantation (LDLT)
l. donor transplant
l. related donor
l. unrelated donor (LURD)
Livingston triangle
livor mortis
LKB Optiphase 2 scintillation fluid
LKB-Wallac scintillation counter
LKM
liver-kidney microsome
LKM specificity
LKS
liver, kidneys, spleen

LL
laser lithotripsy
LLC
laparoscopic laser cholecystectomy
MedSlant LLC
LLC-PK1-FBPase+ cell
LLC-PK renal tubular cell
Lloyd-Davies
L.-D. stirrups
L.-D. Trendelenburg position
Lloyd-Davis
L.-D. knee and leg holder
L.-D. sigmoidoscope
Lloyd sign
LLQ
left lower quadrant
LMA
lactose malabsorption
LMCL
lower midclavicular line
LMP **gene**
LMW
low molecular weight
LMWH
low molecular weight heparin
LN
lipoid nephrosis
lupus nephritis
LNa
low sodium
LNaCl
low salt
L-NAME
N^G-nitro-L-arginine methyl ester
L-NMMA
N^G-monomethyl-L-arginine
L-N-monomethyl-arginine
load
osmotic l.
virus l.
loading
differential l.
methionine l.
peripheral l.
uniform l.
water l.
lobar
l. atrophy
l. nephronia
lobatum
hepar l.

NOTES

lobe
   caudate l.
   Home l.
   kidney l.
   kissing prostatic l.'s
   lateral l.
   left hepatic l. (LHL)
   l. of liver
   median l.
   predominant median l.
   quadrate l.
   renal l.
   Riedel l.
   right l.
lobectomy
   hepatic l.
lobi (*pl. of* **lobus**)
lobucavir
lobular
   l. architecture
   l. architecture of liver
   l. hepatitis
   l. inflammatory infiltrate
   l. mononuclear cell infiltrate
   l. necroinflammation
lobulated
   l. border
   l. filling defect
   l. mass
lobulation
   portal l.
lobule
   l. of pancreas
   portal l.
lobuli (*pl. of* **lobulus**)
lobulization
lobulose
lobulus, pl. **lobuli**
   lobuli testis
lobus, pl. **lobi**
local
   l. alcohol instillation effect
   l. anesthesia
   l. depot injection
   l. glomerular lesion
   l. recurrence
   l. scarring
localization
   bleeding site l.
   manometric l.
   pancreatic tumor l.
   target l.
localized
   l. amyloidosis
   l. lesion
   l. pain
localizing tenderness

locally
   l. acting paracrine effector
   l. made rapid urease test (LRUT)
location
   distant pH probe l.
   tumor l.
locator
   LES l.
   lower esophageal sphincter l.
LoCholest
loci (*pl. of* **locus**)
locker room syndrome
locking suture
lock stitch
lock-stitch suture
Lockwood-Allis intestinal forceps
LOCM
   low osmolar contrast medium
locomotor
locus, pl. **loci**
   hereditary prostate cancer 1 l. (HPC-1)
   tellurite resistance loci
Loeffler syndrome
Loewe (*var. of* **Löwe**)
Lofenalac formula
logarithmic rate
Logen
logger
   Digitrapper Gold MK III solid-state data l.
logistic regression analysis
log-rank test
Lohlein-Baehr lesion
Lohlein nephritis
loin
   l. pain
   l. pain hematuria syndrome (LPHS)
lollipop tree sign
Lomanate
lomefloxacin
   l. HCl
   l. hydrochloride
   l. TMP-SMX
Lomotil
lomustine
Lonalac
   L. feeding
   L. formula
Lone
   L. Star retractor
   L. Star self-retractor
long
   l. acting (LA, L.A.)
   l. anal sphincter
   l. incubation hepatitis
   l. intestinal tube
   l. intestinal tube decompression
   l. Roux-en-Y pouch jejunostomy

l. seal (LS)
l. terminal repeat (LTR)
l. vascular needle driver
Long45 endocutter
long-chain
  l.-c. acyl-CoA dehydrogenase deficiency
  l.-c. fatty acid (LCFA)
  l.-c. 3-hydroxyacyl coenzyme A dehydrogenase (LCHAD)
  l.-c. triglyceride (LCT)
longitudinal
  l. band of colon
  l. choledochotomy
  l. colostomy
  l. enterotomy
  l. esophageal stricture
  l. fasciculi of colon
  l. fissure
  l. image
  l. laceration
  l. myotomy
  l. nephrotomy of Boyce
  l. pancreaticojejunostomy
  l. subepithelial venous plexus
  l. ulcer
  l. view
longitudinalis
  plica l.
long-jaw disposable forceps
long-limb surgical bypass
Longmire operation
long-neck diverticulum
long-nosed
  l.-n. retriever snare
  l.-n. sphincterotome
Longo hemorrhoidectomy
long-segment
  l.-s. Barrett esophagus (LSBE)
  l.-s. CLE
long-term
  l.-t. antibiotic
  l.-t. catheter use
  l.-t. durability
  l.-t. effects of metabolic acidosis
  l.-t. followup data
  l.-t. graft destruction
  l.-t. indwelling catheter
  l.-t. low-dose maintenance chemoprophylaxis
  l.-t. outcome
  l.-t. outcome of urethroplasty

l.-t. renal functional effect
l.-t. result
l.-t. survival of renal allograft
longum
  Bifidobacterium l.
Lonox
loop
  afferent l.
  air-filled l.
  alpha-sigmoid l.
  autocrine reinforcing l.
  Biebl l.
  bipolar urological l.
  blind l.
  bowel l.
  Bradley l.
  brain stem-sacral l.
  l. caliber
  cerebral-sacral l.
  l. choledochojejunostomy
  closed afferent l.
  closed efferent l.
  colonic l.
  contiguous l.
  Cordonnier ureteroileal l.
  Davis l.
  diathermic l.
  l. diuretic
  double reverse alpha-sigmoid l.
  duodenal l.
  duodenal C l.
  efferent l.
  l. end ileostomy
  l. esophagojejunostomy
  l. forearm graft
  gamma transverse colon l.
  l. gastrojejunostomy
  Heiss l.
  Henle l.
  l. of Henle (LH)
  ileal l.
  l. ileostomy (LI)
  intestinal l.
  jejunal interposition of Henle l.
  l. jejunostomy
  l. ligation
  Maxon l.
  N l.
  N-shaped sigmoid l.
  ostomy l.
  l. ostomy bridge
  polyglactin monofilament l.

NOTES

loop *(continued)*
    polyglyconate monofilament l.
    puborectalis l.
    l. of redundant colon
    resectoscope l.
    reverse alpha-sigmoid l.
    Roeder l.
    Roux-en-Y l.
    sentinel l.
    sigmoid l.
    l. stoma
    Surgitite ligating l.
    l. suture
    transverse l.
    l. transverse colostomy
    Vapor Cut l.
    vesical-sacral-sphincter l.
    Wedge l.
looped cautery
looping of endoscope
loopogram
loopography
    ileal l.
    retrograde l.
loop-tipped electrode
loop-type
    l.-t. snare forceps
    l.-t. stone-crushing forceps
Looser-Milkman stria
loose stool
loperamide
Lopez enteral valve
Lopid
Lopressor
LoPresti fiberoptic esophagoscope
Lopurin
Lorabid
loracarbef
Lorad
    L. StereoGuide
    L. StereoGuide prone breast biopsy system
lorazepam
Lord
    L. dilation
    L. dilation of hemorrhoid
    L. method of hemorrhoidectomy
lordosis
    lumbar l.
Lorenzo oil
Lortat-Jacob hepatic resection
Los Angeles (LA)
    LA classification
    LA classification of GERD
    LA Classification grade A, B, C, D esophagitis
losartan
Losec

LoSo
    L. Prep
    L. Prep bowel cleansing solution
Losotron Plus
losoxantrone
loss
    autoimmune sensorineural hearing l.
    chronic gastrointestinal blood l.
    chronic GI blood l.
    cortical l.
    electrolyte l.
    estimated blood l. (EBL)
    fluid l.
    ganglion cell l.
    graft l.
    negligible blood l.
    nephron l.
    obligatory dialysate protein l.
    psoas l.
    sensory l.
    l. of sigmoid curve
    weight l.
Lotheissen-McVay technique
Lotrel
Lotrimin
Lotrisone
Lotronex tablet
loupe
    Keeler panoramic l.
    surgical l.
    wide-angled l.
lovastatin
Lovelace forceps
Lovenox
low
    l. anterior resection (LAR)
    l. anterior resection in combination with coloanal anastomosis (LAR/CAA)
    l. available carbohydrate diet
    l. coloanal anastomosis
    l. intermittent suction
    l. intersphincteric anal fistula
    l. molecular weight (LMW)
    l. molecular weight heparin (LMWH)
    l. molecular weight heparin (LMWH)
    l. molecular weight protein
    l. molecular weight protein ribonuclease
    l. osmolar contrast medium (LOCM)
    l. recurrence rate
    l. salt (LNaCl)
    l. small bowel obstruction
    l. sodium (LNa)
    l. tonicity

l. transverse incision
l. urethral pressure (LUP)
low-affinity high-capacity system
low-affinity transporter
low-calcium dialysate
low-calorie diet
low-compliance
    l.-c. balloon
    l.-c. bladder
    l.-c. perfusion pump
    l.-c. perfusion system
    l.-c. pneumohydraulic pump
low-density
    l.-d. lipoprotein (LDL)
    l.-d. lipoprotein cholesterol (LDLC)
    l.-d. lipoprotein susceptibility
low-dose
    l.-d. HpD
    l.-d. interferon
Löwe, Loewe
    L. disease
low-energy
    l.-e. program
    l.-e. protocol
    l.-e. transurethral microwave thermotherapy (LE-TUMT)
    l.-e. TUMT
lower
    l. abdominal reoperation
    l. abdominal transverse incision
    l. anterior axillary line (LAAL)
    l. energy treatment
    l. esophageal B ring
    l. esophageal contraction ring
    l. esophageal mucosal ring
    l. esophageal sphincter (LES)
    l. esophageal sphincter circular muscle
    l. esophageal sphincter locator
    l. esophageal sphincter pressure (LESP)
    l. esophageal sphincter relaxation (LESR)
    l. esophageal sphincter tone
    L. gall duct forceps
    l. gastrointestinal bleeding (LGIB)
    l. gastrointestinal hemorrhage
    l. GI bleeding
    l. GI tract foreign body
    l. infundibula diameter
    l. infundibular length
    l. infundibulopelvic angle
    l. infundibulum
    l. midclavicular line (LMCL)
    l. motor neuron bladder disorder
    l. motor neuron lesion
    l. nephron nephrosis
    l. panendoscopy
    l. pole laceration
    l. pole stone
    l. ureter
    l. ureteric calculus
    l. urinary tract dysfunction (LUTD)
    l. urinary tract symptom (LUTS)
    l. urinary tract symptomatology
Lowery method
lowest clearance
Lowe syndrome
low-fat diet (LFD)
low-fiber diet
low-flow priapism
low-flux
    l.-f. cuprophane membrane
    l.-f. dialysis membrane
    l.-f. polysulfone membrane
low-grade
    l.-g. dysplasia (LGD)
    l.-g. fever
    l.-g. leiomyosarcoma
    l.-g. positive smear
low-lactose diet
low-loop cutaneous ureterostomy
low-lying rectal cancer
low-magnification electron micrograph
Lown criteria
low-oxalate diet
low-pitched bowel sounds
low-power photomicrograph
low-pressure
    l.-p. bladder substitute
    l.-p. cardiopulmonary baroreceptor
    l.-p., low-flow voiding dysfunction
    l.-p. pouch
    l.-p. venous system
low-pulsatility arterial waveform
low-residue
    l.-r. diet
    l.-r. feeding
low-roughage diet
Lowsium
Lowsley
    L. lithotrite
    L. operation

NOTES

Lowsley *(continued)*
   L. retractor
   L. tractor
Lowsley-Peterson cystoscope
low-sodium diet
low-turnover osteomalacia (LTOM)
low-tyrosine, low-phenylalanine diet
low-volume sclerotherapy
loxiglumide
lozenge
   tetracaine l.
Lozol
LP
   lymphomatous polyposis
   AstraZeneca Pharmaceuticals LP
L-PAM
   L-phenylalanine mustard
LPH
   lactase-phlorizin hydrolase
LPHS
   loin pain hematuria syndrome
LPL
   lipoprotein lipase
LPL-mediated lipolysis
LPLND
   laparoscopic pelvic lymph node dissection
LPN
   laparoscopic partial nephrectomy
LPP
   leak-point pressure
LPS
   lipopolysaccharide
LRE
   lamina rara externa
L-rhamnose
LRI
   lamina rara interna
LRN
   laparoscopic radical nephrectomy
LRUT
   locally made rapid urease test
LS
   long seal
LSBE
   long-segment Barrett esophagus
LSBM
   lumbar spine bone mineral density
LSC 7000 curved-array transducer
LSD
   lysosomal storage disease
L-selectin
LSM
   lifestyle modification
LSP
   liver-specific membrane lipoprotein
LT
   heat-labile toxin

Ltd.
   Given Imaging L.
LTOM
   low-turnover osteomalacia
LTR
   long terminal repeat
Lubb syndrome
Lubraseptic jelly
lubricant
   l. laxative
   Surgilube l.
Lubri-Flex ureteral stent
lucent cyst
Lucey-Driscoll syndrome
Luder-Sheldon syndrome
Ludwig labyrinth
Luer
   L. hemorrhoid forceps
   L. syringe
Luer-Lok
   L.-L. connector
   L.-L. syringe
Lugol
   L. chromoendoscopy
   L. iodide
   L. iodine
   L. iodine solution
   L. solution stain
Lugol-combined upper gastrointestinal videoendoscopy
Lukes-Collins classification
lumbar
   l. appendicitis
   l. artery
   l. kidney
   l. lordosis
   l. nephrectomy
   l. nephrotomy
   l. plexus
   l. spinal cord lesion
   l. spine bone mineral density (LSBM)
   l. vein
lumbocolostomy
lumbocolotomy
lumbocostoabdominal triangle
lumbodorsal
   l. fascia
   l. incision
   l. ligament
lumbosacral
   l. fascia
   l. plexus
   l. trunk
lumbotomy
   dorsal l.
   l. incision

lumbricoides
    Ascaris l.
lumen, pl. **lumina**
    bile duct l.
    bowel l.
    cystic duct l.
    duct l.
    duodenal l.
    esophageal l.
    gastroduodenal l.
    intestinal l.
    rectal l.
    scalloped bowel l.
    l. of seminiferous tubule
    single l.
lumen-seeking catheter
lumen-to-bath sodium flux
lumina guidewire
luminal
    l. acid
    l. acid clearance
    l. amoxicillin
    l. antigliadin
    l. bulge
    l. candesartan
    l. CCK-releasing factor
    l. content
    l. contrast study
    l. Crohn disease
    l. diameter
    l. EGF
    l. glucose
    l. HCO^{3-}
    l. hypoacidity
    l. narrowing
    l. nutrition
    l. secretagogue
    l. sodium
    l. stenosis
luminol-enhanced chemiluminescence
luminometer
    LB 9501 l.
Lumi-Phos 530
lumpectomy
    endoscopic aspiration l. (EAL)
lump kidney
Lunar DPX total-body scanner
lunata
    Curvularia l.
lunatus
    penis l.
Lunderquist guidewire

Lunderquist-Ring torque guide
Lundh
    L. meal
    L. test
lung
    l. cancer
    l. disease
    l. dysplasia
    farmer's l.
    l. purpura
LUP
    low urethral pressure
lupoid hepatitis
Lupron Depot
lupus
    l. anticoagulant (LA)
    l. erythematosus
    l. nephritis (LN)
LUQ
    left upper quadrant
LURD
    living unrelated donor
LUS
    laparoscopic ultrasound
Luschka
    accessory duct of L.
    L. crypt
    L. cystic gland
    L. duct
lusoria
    arteria l.
    dysphagia l.
lusorian artery
LUTD
    lower urinary tract dysfunction
luteinized granulosa-theca cell tumor
luteinizing
    l. hormone (LH)
    l. hormone follicle-stimulating hormone (LH-FSH)
    l. hormone-follicle-stimulating hormone-releasing factor
    l. hormone releasing hormone (LHRH)
    l. hormone-releasing hormone antagonist
Lütkens sphincter
LUTS
    lower urinary tract symptom
Lutz automatic reprocessor
luxation
Luy segregator

NOTES

LVP
  large-volume paracentesis
lwoffi
  Acinetobacter l.
LX-20 laser
Lycopodium serratum
lye ingestion
Lyell
  L. disease
  L. syndrome
Lyme disease
lymph
  l. channel
  l. node
  l. node adenopathy
  l. node dissection
  l. node metastasis
  l. scrotum
  subcarinal l.
lymphadenectomy
  endocavitary pelvic l. (ECPL)
  extended pelvic l.
  laparoscopic pelvic l.
  mediastinal l.
  mesorectal l.
  minilaparotomy staging pelvic l.
  paraaortic l.
  pelvic l.
  prophylactic l.
  retroperitoneal l.
  thoracoabdominal retroperitoneal l.
  three-field l.
  two-field l.
lymphadenitis
lymphadenopathy
  cervical l.
  inguinal l.
  malignant peribiliary l.
  mediastinal l.
  perihepatic l.
  l. syndrome (LAS)
lymphangiectasia, lymphangiectasis
  congenital renal l.
  intestinal l.
  pancreatic l.
  peritoneal l.
  primary intestinal l. (PIL)
lymphangiogram
lymphangiography
lymphangioma
  scrotal l.
lymphangitic streak
lymphangitis
  penile sclerosing l.
  sclerosing l.
lymphapheresis
lymphatic
  l. channel
  l. leak
  l. metastasis
  l. microcyst
  l. obstruction
  l. package
  l. transport
  l. vessel
lymphatica
  folliculus l.
lymphedema
  filarial l.
lymphoblast homing
lymphoblastoid
  l. cell line
  l. interferon alpha
lymphoblastoma
  kidney l.
  renal l.
lymphocele
  l. aspiration
  l. internal drainage
  l. percutaneous drainage
  l. spontaneous regression
lymphocelectomy
  laparoscopic l.
  pelvic l.
lymphocyst
lymphocyte
  B l.
  CD8 l.
  CD45RO l.
  CD8+ T l.
  l. costimulatory molecule
  l. count
  crypt intraepithelial l. (cIEL)
  cytolytic T l. (CTL)
  l. cytotoxicity
  cytotoxic T l. (CTL)
  l. immune globulin (LIG)
  intraepithelial l. (IEL)
  intrahepatic l.
  l. migration
  naive B and T l.
  peripheral blood l. (PBL)
  sinusoidal l.
  T l.
  thymus-derived l.
  total l. (TTL)
  tumor-infiltrating l. (TIL)
  virgin l.
  WBC l.
lymphocyte-hepatocyte
  intrahepatic antigen-dependent l.-h.
lymphocyte-target cell
lymphocytic
  l. colitis
  l. gastritis (LG)
  l. vasculitis
lymphocytosis
  intraepithelial l.

lymphocytotoxic antibody
lymphocyturia
lymphoepithelial lesion
lymphogenic metastasis
lymphogranuloma venereum (LGV)
lymphography
lymphohemangioma
    bladder l.
lymphohistiocytic infiltration
lymphoid
    l. aggregate
    l. cholangitis
    l. component
    l. follicle
    l. interstitial pneumonia
    l. nodule
    l. polyp
    l. tumor
lymphokine-activated killer cell
lymphokine production
lymphoma
    benign l.
    bladder l.
    Burkitt l.
    colorectal l.
    cutaneous T-cell l.
    duodenal l.
    enteropathy-associated T-cell l. (EATCL)
    gastric l.
    hepatosplenic T-cell l.
    histiocytic l.
    infiltrative l.
    liver l.
    MALT l.
    marginal zone l.
    Mediterranean l.
    mucosa-associated lymphoid tissue l. (MALToma)
    nodular l.
    non-Hodgkin l. (NHL)
    penis l.
    polypoid l.
    primary B-cell l.
    primary gastric l. (PGL)
    primary hepatosplenic l. (PHSL)
    prostate gland l.
    retroperitoneal l.
    seminal vesicle l.
    small intestinal malignant l.
    small non-cleaved-cell l.
    T-cell l.
    testicular l.
    ulcerative l.
lymphomatosis
lymphomatous
    l. nodule
    l. polyposis (LP)
lymphomononuclear cell
lymphonodular hyperplasia
lymphonoduli (*pl. of* lymphonodulus)
lymphonodulus, pl. **lymphonoduli**
    L. splenici
lymphoplasmacytosis
lymphoproliferative
    l. disorder
    l. syndrome
lymphosarcoma
lymphoscintigraphy
lymphovascular permeation
Lynch syndrome II
LYOfoam dressing
Lyon
    L. ring
    L. ring-constrictive band
lyophilized dura mater for pubovaginal sling
Lyphocin
lysate
    depleted l.
lyse
lysine
lysinuria
lysis
    l. of adhesion
    colon tumor cell l.
    CTL-mediated l.
    laparoscopic l.
    mesangial l.
    tumor cell l.
lysolecithin
lysosomal
    l. accumulation
    l. enzyme
    l. membrane
    l. storage disease (LSD)
    l. swelling
lysosome
    hepatocyte l.
lysozyme
lysyl-bradykinin
lytic cocktail
Lytren electrolyte solution

NOTES

μV
microvolt
M
microfold
M antibody
M cell
M phase
M1
antibody to Leu M1
glutathione S-transferase M1
M10, 20
Klor-Con M10, 20
M20
M30
Zeiss morphomate M30
M344
antigen M344
M344 antigen
M2A
M. capsule/Given imaging capsule
M. Swallowable Imaging Capsule
MAA
macroaggregated albumin
malondialdehyde-acetaldehyde adducts
^{99m}Tc MAA
Maalox
M. Antacid/Calcium supplement
M. Anti-Gas Extra-Strength oral suspension
M. HRF
M. Plus
M. Quick Dissolve chewable tablet
M. spray
M. Therapeutic Concentrate
MAB
maximal androgen blockade
MAb, mAb
monoclonal antibody
anti-class II MAb
MAb IOT2-recognizing monomorphic DR determinant
MABP
mean arterial blood pressure
Macalister
valve of M.
Macaluso stent remover
MacConkey agar
Macdonald test
MACE
Malone antegrade continent enema
Macewen
M. hernia operation
M. herniorrhaphy

MACH1
metronidazole, amoxicillin, clarithromycin, *H. pylori*, one-week therapy
MACH1 study
Machado-Guerreiro test
Machida
M. choledochoscope
M. FCS-ML II magnifying colonoscope
machine
A2008 ABGII hemodialysis m.
Accuson-128 color flow Doppler m.
Belzer m.
endoscopic sewing m.
Endotek m.
Fresenius 2008H hemodialysis m.
Gambro AK10 m.
gastric hypothermia m.
heart-lung m.
Kodak Ektachem 700 m.
MOX TM-100 portable renal preservation m.
Narco esophageal motility m.
Nova II m.
perfusion m.
Phillips ultrasound m.
portable renal preservation m.
Primus Prostate M.
Mackenrodt
ligament of M.
Mackenzie
M. disease
M. point
MacLean test
Maclet magnetic ring
macroaggregated albumin (MAA)
macroalbuminuria
macroamylase
macroamylasemia
macroangiodynamic
macroangiopathic hemolytic anemia
Macrobid
macrocephaly
macrocrystal
macrocyclic triene
macrocyst
adrenocortical m.
Macrodantin
macrogenitosomia
macroglobulinemia
Waldenström m.

477

macrolide
   m. antibiotic
   m. antimicrobial
macromolecular
   m. secretion
   m. uronate (MMUA)
macromolecule
   radiolabeled m.
macronidia
macronodular cirrhosis
macroorchidism lesion
macropenis
macrophage
   bile-laden m.
   ceroid-laden m.
   m. colony-stimulating factor (M-CSF)
   hemosiderin-laden m.
   parasitizing m.
   peritoneal m.
macrophage-rich inflammatory response
macrophage-TGF-beta axis
macrophallus
Macroplastique
   M. implant
   M. implantation device
   M. injectable
   M. soft tissue synthetic bulking agent
macroprolactinoma
macroproteinuria
macroregenerative nodule
macroscopic
   m. hematuria
   m. lesion
   m. liver cyst
macrosomia
   fetal m.
macrosteatosis
macrothrombocyte
macrovascular disease
macrovesicular
   m. fat
   m. fatty liver
   m. steatosis
macula, pl. maculae
   m. densa
   m. densa cell
macular degeneration
macule
maculopapular
Madayag biopsy needle
Madden
   M. incisional herniorrhaphy
   M. intestinal clamp
   M. repair
   M. repair of incisional hernia
   M. technique
Maddrey discriminant function

Mad Hatter syndrome
Madigan prostatectomy
Madsen-Iversen
   M.-I. scale
   M.-I. scoring system
Madsen symptom score
mafenide acetate
Maffucci syndrome
MAG
   multifocal atrophic gastritis
MAG-3
   mercaptoacetyltriglycine
   MAG-3 renal scan
   TechneScan MAG-3
magaldrate
Magic Lite chemiluminometric immunoassay
magna
   arteria pancreatica m.
   Fascioloides m.
   lacuna m.
Magnacal liquid feeding
Magnascanner
   Picker Vista M.
MagneBind 200
MagneBind 300
MagneBind 400 RX
magnesia
   citrate of m.
   milk of m. (MOM)
   Phillips Milk of M.
magnesium
   m. ammonium phosphate
   m. ammonium phosphate urolithiasis
   m. carbonate
   m. citrate
   m. deficiency
   esomeprazole m.
   m. hydroxide
   m. metabolism
   m. oxide
   m. salt
   m. trisilicate
magnesium-induced diarrhea
magnet
   endoscopic gastroenteric anastomosis with m.'s
magnetic
   m. bore
   m. compression anastomosis
   m. endoscopic imaging
   m. internal ureteral stent
   m. resonance
   m. resonance angiography (MRA)
   m. resonance cholangiography (MRC)
   m. resonance cholangiopancreatography (MRCP)

m. resonance colography
m. resonance colonography (MRC)
m. resonance imaging (MRI)
m. resonance imaging thermometry
m. resonance pancreatography (MRP)
m. resonance spectroscopy (MRS)
m. resonance urography (MRU)
m. stimulation
m. susceptibility test

magnetization prepared-rapid gradient echo (MP-RAGE)
magnetoencephalography (MEG)
magnetometry
magnification
    m. chromoendoscopy
    m. endoscopy with acetic acid spraying

magnifying
    m. colonoscope
    m. colonoscopy
    m. endoscope
    m. endoscopy with narrow-band image system
    m. enteroscope

Mag-OX 400
MAGP
    microfil-associated glycoprotein
    MAGP microfibrillar protein

MAGPI
    meatal advancement and glansplasty
    meatal advancement, glanuloplasty, penoscrotal junction meatotomy
    MAGPI operation

Magsal tablet
mahogany-colored stool
Mahurkar catheter
MAI
    Mycobacterium avium-intracellulare

main
    m. pancreatic duct (MPD)
    m. pancreatic duct stent

Maine
    M. Medical Assessment Program (MMAP)
    M. Medical Assessment Program index

Mainstay urologic soft tissue anchor
maintenance treatment
Mainz
    M. pouch augmentation
    M. pouch cutaneous urinary diversion
    M. pouch II
    M. pouch operation
    M. pouch urinary reservoir
    M. urinary pouch

Mainz-type ureterosigmoidostomy
maitre
    tour de m.

Maixner cirrhosis
major
    curvatura gastrica m.
    curvatura ventriculi m.
    m. deceleration injury
    m. GI surgery
    globus m.
    m. histocompatibility complex (MHC)
    m. papilla
    papilla duodeni m.

majus
    Chelidonium m.
    omentum m.

Makkas operation
Makler
    M. cannula
    M. counting chamber
    M. insemination device
    M. sperm-counting device

malabsorption
    bile acid m. (BAM)
    m. disease
    D-xylose m.
    folate m.
    folic acid m.
    glucose-galactose m.
    iatrogenic m.
    idiopathic bile acid m.
    lactose m. (LMA)
    lavage-induced pill m.
    m. syndrome
    vitamin B_{12} m.

malabsorptive diarrhea
malacia
    tracheobronchial m.

malacoplakia, malakoplakia
    bladder m.
    kidney m.
    m. of kidney
    m. vesicae

malacotomy
maladaptive response

NOTES

maladjustment
    Structured and Scaled Interview to Assess M. (SSIAM)
Malakit *Helicobacter pylori* **Biolab**
malakoplakia (*var. of* malacoplakia)
malaria
    algid m.
    bilious remittent m.
    dysenteric algid m.
    falciparum m.
    gastric m.
    malignant tertian m.
    pernicious m.
    Plasmodium falciparum m.
    quartan m.
malariae
    Plasmodium m.
malarial
    m. dysentery
    m. hepatitis
    m. nephropathy
malate
malayi
    Brugia m.
maldescended testicle
maldescent
maldigestion
    lipid m.
maldigestion-absorption syndrome
maldigestive diarrhea
maldigestor
    lactose m.
male
    m. catheter
    m. epispadias
    m. escutcheon
    m. genitalia melanoma
    m. pelvis
    m. perineum
    m. predominance of urinary tract calculus
    m. sterility
    m. Turner syndrome
maleate
    methysergide m.
    perhexiline m.
    tegaserod m.
Malecot
    M. gastrostomy tube
    M. nephrostomy tube
    M. reentry catheter
    M. suprapubic catheter
malemission
malformation
    anorectal m.
    anus m.
    arteriovenous m. (AVM)
    bronchopulmonary foregut m.
    Chiari m.
    cloacal m.
    Dieulafoy vascular m.
    dysraphic m.
    gastric arteriovenous m.
    mermaid m.
    polypoid vascular m.
    pulmonary arteriovenous m.
    scrotal arteriovenous m.
    sink-trap m.
    submucosal arterial m.
    submucosal vascular m.
    vascular m.
malignancy
    bulky m.
    de novo m.
    detection of m.
    esophageal m.
    esophagocardial m.
    extracolonic m. (ECM)
    hepatic m.
    hepatobiliary m.
    humoral hypercalcemia of m. (HHM)
    hypercalcemia of m.
    nonskin m.
    pancreaticobiliary m.
    paratesticular m.
    periampullary m.
    peritoneal m.
malignancy-associated cellular marker
malignant
    m. acanthosis nigricans
    m. ascites
    m. atrophic papulosis
    m. B-cell syndrome
    m. biliary obstruction
    m. biliary obstructive disease
    m. cachexia
    m. carcinoid syndrome
    m. dysentery
    m. dysphagia
    m. dysplasia
    m. esophagopericardial fistula
    m. histiocytosis
    m. hyperthermia
    m. malnutrition
    m. melanoma
    m. meniscus sign
    m. mesenchymal tumor
    m. mesenchymoma
    m. nephrosclerosis
    m. nuclear structure
    m. obstructive jaundice
    m. pancreatic neoplasms
    m. peribiliary lymphadenopathy
    m. pheochromocytoma
    m. polyp
    m. potential
    m. pseudoachalasia

m. rectal stricture
m. renal mass
m. seeding
m. stenosis
m. teratoma (MT)
m. teratoma, intermediate (MTI)
m. teratoma, trophoblastic (MTT)
m. tertian malaria
m. ulcer

maljunction
pancreaticobiliary m.

mall
space of M.

Mallard incision
malleability
pelvic m.

malleable
m. blade
m. implant
m. prosthesis
m. retractor
m. scoop

Mallinckrodt catheter
Mallory
M. hyaline
M. hyaline body

Mallory-Azan stain
Mallory-Weiss
M.-W. laceration
M.-W. lesion
M.-W. mucosal rupture
M.-W. syndrome
M.-W. tear

malnourished
malnutrition
index of m.
malignant m.
protein-calorie m. (PCM)
protein-energy m.

malnutrition-related diabetes mellitus (MRDM)
malodorous
m. fluid
m. stool

malondialdehyde (MDA)
malondialdehyde-acetaldehyde adducts (MAA)
Malone
M. antegrade colonic enema
M. antegrade colonic enema stoma procedure
M. antegrade continence enema
M. antegrade continent enema (MACE)
M. antegrade continent enema channel
M. cecostomy
M. conduit
M. continent appendicostomy
M. principle

Maloney
M. bougie
M. dilation
M. mercury-filled esophageal dilator
M. tapered-tip dilator

Maloney-Hurst dilator
malpighian
m. body
m. corpuscles
m. glomeruli

malpighii
acinus renalis m.
acinus renis m.
stratum m.

Malpighi pyramid
malrotation
intestinal m.
m. of intestine
midgut volvulus with m.

MALT
mucosa-associated lymphoid tissue
MALT lymphoma

maltase glucoamylase
Maltese cross
MALToma
mucosa-associated lymphoid tissue lymphoma

maltophilia
Stenotrophomonas m.
Xanthomonas m.

maltose tetrapalmitate
Maltsupex
mammalgia
mammalian
m. cell membrane
m. transgenesis

mammillated
mammillation
mammilliform
mammose
managed conservatively
management
m. of adult urinary tract trauma

NOTES

management (continued)
    m. algorithm
    American Academy of Wound M. (AAWM)
    antibiotic m.
    conservative m.
    endoscopic m.
    endourologic m.
    foreign body m.
    laparoscopic m.
    mechanical endoscopic m.
    open m.
    seton m.
    stone m.
Manchester-Fothergill operation
Manchester virus
Manchurian hemorrhagic fever
Mancke flex-rigid gastroscope
Mandelamine
mandelate
    methenamine m.
mandelic acid
mandible
mandril set
maneuver
    alpha-loop m.
    avoidance m.
    bunching m.
    Credé m.
    experimental m.
    Fowler-Stephens m.
    Heimlich m.
    Hoguet m.
    Hueter m.
    J-type m.
    Ko-Airan m.
    Kocher m.
    Leadbetter m.
    Mattox m.
    Mendelsohn m.
    Müller m.
    peroral m.
    Prentiss m.
    Pringle m.
    straightening m.
    suppressive m.
    U-turn m.
    Valsalva m.
mangafodipir trisodium
manifestation
    extrahepatic m.
    frequent joint m.
    hepatobiliary m.
    otolaryngologic m.
    tissue m.
Manifold II slot-blot apparatus
manipulation
    antegrade ureteroscopic m.
    direct m.
    endoscopic stone m.
    pancreatic duct m.
    postureteroscopic m.
    transureteral endoscopic m.
mannan
    yeast strain m.
Mann-Bollman fistula
Manning criteria
mannitol
mannose-specific adhesion
Mann-Whitney rank sum test
Mann-Williamson
    M.-W. operation
    M.-W. ulcer
manofluorography (MFG)
manometer
manometric
    m. criteria
    m. evaluation
    m. feature
    m. findings
    m. localization
    m. pattern
    m. sensor
    m. study
manometry
    ambulatory m.
    anal vector m.
    aneroid m.
    anorectal m.
    antral m.
    antroduodenal m.
    antroduodenojejunal m.
    balloon reflex m.
    biliary m.
    m. catheter
    colonic m.
    computer-aided ambulatory gastrojejunal m.
    dry swallow on esophageal m.
    endoscopic m.
    endoscopic sphincter of Oddi m.
    ERCP m.
    esophageal m. (EM)
    InSIGHT m.
    intraluminal m.
    papillary m.
    perendoscopic m.
    PIP on esophageal m.
    point of respiratory reversal on esophageal m.
    pullthrough m.
    rectosigmoid m.
    sphincter of Oddi m. (SOM)
    transileostomy m.
Manson
    M. disease
    M. schistosomiasis
mansonelliasis

mansoni
    Schistosoma m.
    schistosomiasis m.
Mansson
    M. operation
    M. urinary pouch
Mantel-Haenszel test
manual lithotriptor
MAO
    maximal acid output
MAP
    mean arterial pressure
    MAP kinase signaling cascade
    systemic MAP
map
    acid-base m.
    integrated genomic m.
MAPK
    mitogen-activated protein kinase
maple-syrup urine disease (MSUD)
mapping
    anal m.
    bladder m.
    cavernous nerve m.
    intragastric pH m.
maprotiline
Maquet endoscopy table
Maranon syndrome
marantic endocarditis
marasmus
Marblen
Marburg virus
Marcaine block
marcescens
    Serratia m.
Marchand adrenals
Marchiafava-Micheli
    M.-M. disease
    M.-M. syndrome
Marcillin
Mardis soft stent
Mardi test
Marechal-Rosen test
Marezine
Marfan
    M. epigastric puncture
    M. syndrome
marfanoid habitus
margin
    anal m.
    cell-positive m.
    circumferential m.
    convex m.
    costal m.
    crenate m.
    cristate m.
    dentate m.
    disk m.
    dissection m.
    echogenic duct m.
    lateral m.
    medial m.
    obtuse m.
    positive m.
    subcostal m.
    superior m.
marginal
    m. artery of Drummond
    m. kidney donor
    m. ulcer
    m. zone lymphoma
margo, pl. margines
Marian
    M. lithotomy
    M. operation
marianum
    Silybum m.
Marie-Strumpell disease
marina
    Anisakis m.
Marinesco-Sjögren syndrome
Marinol
marinus
    vomitus m.
Marion disease
mark
    crosshatch m.
marked
    m. deterioration
    m. tube
marker
    anthropometric m.
    antigen m.
    biochemical m.
    biologic m.
    bone turnover m.
    B5 tumor m.
    CA 1-18 tumor m.
    CA 72-4 tumor m.
    cell cycle m.
    C100-3 hepatitis C m.
    chromosomal m.
    m. chromosome
    chromosome m.

NOTES

marker *(continued)*
    D4S231 m.
    D4S414 m.
    D16S84 m.
    D16S283 m.
    D16S291 m.
    DUPAN 2 tumor m.
    fecal m.
    fluid phase m.
    genetic m.
    hepatitis serologic m.
    HLA-DQ2 m.
    HLA-DQ8 m.
    HMB-45 monoclonal antibody m.
    inflammation m.
    interleukin-1b urinary m.
    malignancy-associated cellular m.
    molecular m.
    novel molecular m.'s
    OA-519 prognostic prostate carcinoma m.
    p-ANC genetic m.
    pancreatic cancer m.
    plasma membrane m.
    polycationic m.
    radiopaque m.
    serologic m.
    serum m.
    Spot endoscopic m.
    m. stitch
    surrogate m.
    tape m.
    m. transit study
    tumor m.
    viral hepatitis m.
markers for cancer
marking
    haustral m.
    red wale m.
Mark IV Moss decompression-feeding catheter
Markov model
Marlen
    M. double-faced adhesive disk
    M. Gas Relief drainage pouch
    M. Neoprene All-Flexible faceplate
    M. Odor-Ban ileostomy pouch
    M. Solo ileostomy pouch
    M. Zip Klosed pouch
Marlex
    M. band
    M. graft
    M. hernial repair
    M. mesh
    M. mesh abdominal rectopexy
    M. plug technique
Marmite lithotrite
marneffei
    Penicillium m.

Marogen
maroon blood
maroon-colored stool
marrow transplant recipient
MARS
    molecular adsorbents recirculating system
Marseille pancreatitis classification
Marshall
    M. and Tanner pubertal staging
    M. test
    M. U-stitch suture
Marshall-Bonney test
Marshall-Marchetti-Birch operation
Marshall-Marchetti-Krantz (MMK)
    M.-M.-K. cystourethropexy
    M.-M.-K. operation
    M.-M.-K. procedure
    M.-M.-K. urethropexy
Marshall-Marchetti test
Marsh classification
marshmallow
    barium-coated m.
    barium-impregnated m.
    m. bolus
marsupialization
    epididymis m.
    laparoscopic m.
    renal cyst m.
marsupium
Martel clamp
Martin
    M. anoplasty
    M. gastrostomy
    M. operation
Martin-Davis rectal speculum
Martius
    M. fascial sling
    M. fat pad
    M. graft
    M. labial fat pad flap
    M. operation
    M. scarlet blue stain
Martius-Harris operation
Martorell hypertensive ulcer
MAS
    mean allograft survival
    multiple anal sphincterotomies
masculinae
    crista urethralis m.
    ostium urethrae externum m.
masculinizing genitoplasty
masculinum
    ovarium m.
masculinus
    uterus m.
    utriculus m.
MASE
    microsurgical extraction of sperm from epididymis

mask · mastoiditis

mask
    Bili m.
    m. phenomenon
    Prohibit antifog face m.

Mason
    M. abdominotranssphincteric resection
    M. needle holder
    M. operation
    M. vertical banded gastroplasty

mass
    abdominal wall m.
    adjusted body m. (ABM)
    adnexal m.
    adrenal gland m.
    appendiceal m.
    asymptomatic m.
    body cell m. (BCM)
    colonic m.
    colorectal m.
    congenital renal m.
    cul-de-sac m.
    cystic m.
    discrete m.
    duodenal m.
    dysplasia-associated lesion or m. (DALM)
    esophageal m.
    exophytic m.
    expansile abdominal m.
    extramucosal m.
    extrarenal m.
    extrinsic m.
    flank m.
    fluctuant m.
    gastric m.
    hilar m.
    inflammatory prostatic m. (IPM)
    inflammatory renal m.
    inhomogeneous hyperechoic m.
    intraabdominal m.
    kidney m.
    lean body m. (LBM)
    lobulated m.
    malignant renal m.
    mediastinal m.
    mushroom-shaped m.
    neoplastic renal m.
    palpable m.
    parapancreatic m.
    parovarian m.
    periampullary m.
    perirectal m.
    m. peristalsis
    phlegmonous m.
    pleural m.
    polypoid m.
    pulsatile m.
    rectal m.
    renal m.
    salivary m.
    scrotal m.
    soft tissue m.
    submucosal m.
    testicular m.
    m. transfer area coefficient (MTAC)
    transformary m.
    traumatic renal m.
    tubular excretory m.
    vaginal m.
    vascular renal m.

massage
    prostatic m.

masse
    reduction en m.

masseter strength

Masset test

massive
    m. bowel resection syndrome
    m. colonic diverticular bleeding
    m. epithelial cell necrosis
    m. hepatic necrosis
    m. malignant infiltration

Masson
    M. trichrome
    M. trichrome stain
    M. trichrome staining technique

Masson-Fontana stain

mast
    m. cell
    m. cell degranulation

master
    m. duodenoscope
    m. IG bundle
    m. image guide
    M.'s intestinal clamp

MasterFlex pump

Masters-Schwartz liver clamp

masticatory-salivary reflex

Mastisol liquid surgical adhesive

mastocytosis
    systemic m.

mastoiditis

NOTES

masturbation
   traumatic m.
Masugi nephritis
matairesinol
matching
   donor/recipient race m.
   HLA-DR m.
   optimizing HLA m.
   optimizing human leukocyte antigen m.
material
   anastomotic m.
   biocompatible m.
   coarse m.
   coffee-grounds m. (CGM)
   congophilic m.
   Conray 60, 70, 280 contrast m.
   extravasated iodinated contrast m.
   fecal m.
   implantation of prosthetic m.
   iodinated contrast m.
   methods & m.'s
   microcrystalline m.
   polyglactin suture m.
   proteinaceous cast m.
   purulent m.
   suture m.
   Triangle gelatin-sealed sling m.
maternal
   m. age as risk factor
   m. morbidity
Mathews rectal speculum
Mathieu
   M. island onlay flap
   M. procedure
   M. technique
Mathieu-Horton-Devine flip-flap
matrices (*pl. of* matrix)
Matrigel
Matritech NMP22 test for bladder cancer
matrix, pl. **matrices**
   m. calculus
   m. deposition
   extracellular m. (ECM)
   glomerular extracellular m.
   m. metalloproteinase (MMP)
   m. metalloproteinase-7
   nuclear m.
   pericellular m. (PCM)
   prostate gland tissue m.
   TissueMend soft tissue repair m.
   m. urolithiasis
Matson operation
matted node
Mattox maneuver
mattress
   Bedge antireflux m.
   Home Care Simplimatt Plus zoned foam m.
   m. suture
Matts grade 1–4
maturation
   collagen m.
   mucosal barrier m.
   normal m.
   osteoclast m.
   stone m.
mature teratoma
maturing the stoma
maturity-onset diabetes of the youth (MODY)
matutinus
   vomitus m.
Mauch double-sheathed plastic wash pipe
Maunoir hydrocele
Maunsell-Weir operation
Maxamine
Maxaquin
Max-EPA capsule
Maxeran
MaxForce
   M. TTS biliary balloon dilatation catheter
   M. TTS high-performance balloon dilatation catheter
maximal
   m. acid output (MAO)
   m. androgen blockade (MAB)
   m. toleration (MT)
   tubular m. (Tm)
   m. tubular excretory capacity of kidney
maximum
   m. (anal) resting pressure (MRP)
   m. bladder capacity
   m. coagulative necrosis
   m. cystometric capacity
   m. detrusor pressure
   m. diameter
   m. free-flow rate
   m. squeeze pressure (MSP)
   m. tolerable volume (MTV)
   m. urethral closure pressure (MUCP)
   m. urinary flow rate
   m. vasal pressure (MVP)
maximus
   gluteus m.
Maxipeme
Maxisal with vitamin C
Maxisorb test plate
Maxolon
Maxon
   M. loop
   M. suture

Maxum reusable forceps
Maxzide
Maydl
    M. hernia
    M. operation
    M. procedure
    M. ureterosigmoidostomy
Mayer
    M. acid alum hematoxylin stain
    M. hematoxylin solution
Mayer-Rokitansky-Kuster-Hauser syndrome
Mayer-Rokitansky syndrome
May-Grünwald-Giemsa stain
Mayo
    M. abdominal clamp
    M. abdominal retractor
    M. bladder
    M. Clinic system for primary biliary cirrhosis
    M. common duct probe
    M. common duct scoop
    M. common duct spoon
    M. gallstone scoop
    M. grading system
    M. operation
    M. scissors
    M. stand
    M. trocar-point needle
Mayo-Adams appendectomy retractor
Mayo-Blake gallstone forceps
Mayo-Hegar needle holder
Mayo-Kelly appendix inverter
Mayo-Noble dissecting scissors
Mayo-Ochsner suction trocar cannula
Mayo-Péan forceps
Mayo-Robson
    M.-R. gallstone scoop
    M.-R. intestinal clamp
    M.-R. intestinal forceps
    M.-R. position
Mays operation
Mazicon
mazindol
Mazzariello-Caprini forceps
MBS
    modified barium swallow
MC
    mesangial cell
    methotrexate, cisplatin
MCA
    middle colic artery

MCAD
    medium-chain acyl-CoA dehydrogenase
McArdle syndrome
McBurney
    M. incision
    M. point
    M. retractor
    M. sign
MCC
    mutated colorectal carcinoma
    MCC gene
McCall culdoplasty
McCarthy
    M. electrode
    M. evacuator
    M. Foroblique panendoscope cystoscope
McCarthy-Campbell miniature cystoscope
McCleery-Miller intestinal clamp
McCormack gastric mucosal sign
McCort sign
McCrea
    M. cystoscope
    M. sound
McCune-Albright syndrome
MCD
    metastatic Crohn disease
MCDK
    multicystic dysplastic kidney
McDonald
    M. cerclage
    M. stone dissector
McDougal prostatectomy clamp
MCF-7 tumor
MCFA
    medium-chain fatty acid
McGaw
    M. plastic bottle
    M. volumetric pump
McGill
    M. forceps
    M. pain questionnaire
McGivney
    M. hemorrhoidal ligator
    M. hemorrhoid forceps
M-CH
    mitomycin adsorbed onto activated charcoal
MCH
    mean corpuscular hemoglobin
    microfibrillar collagen hemostat

NOTES

MCH (continued)
    Endo-Avitene MCH
    MCH gene
MCHA
    microsome antibody
MCHC
    mean corpuscular hemoglobin concentration
***m*-chlorophenyl-piperazine**
McIndoe procedure
McIntyre reverse cystotome
MCK
    multicystic kidney
MCL
    midclavicular line
    MCL port
McLean pile clamp
McNealey-Glassman-Mixter forceps
McNeer classification
McNemar ascites test
MCP
    membrane cofactor protein
    monocyte chemotactic protein
MCP-1
    monocyte chemoattractant protein-1
M-CSF
    macrophage colony-stimulating factor
MCT
    mean colonic transit
    medium-chain triglyceride
    medullary carcinoma of thyroid
    MCT oil
MCTD
    mixed connective tissue disease
MCU
    micturating cystourethrography
MCV
    mean corpuscular volume
    methotrexate, cisplatin, vinblastine
    molluscum contagiosum virus
McVay
    M. herniorrhaphy
    M. inguinal hernial repair
    M. operation
MD-60 contrast medium
MDA
    malondialdehyde
M.D. Anderson grade
MDCA
    mean distal contraction amplitude
MDCK epithelial cell
MDE
    mucinous ductal ectasia
MDLO
    metoclopramide, dexamethasone, lorazepam, ondansetron
***MDM2* gene**
MDP
    ^{99m}Tc MDP

MDR
    minimum daily requirement
MDR1
    multidrug-resistance gene
    MDR1 gene
MDR3
    phospholipid export pump gene
MDRD
    modification of diet in renal disease
MDS
    membrane-spanning domain
MDT
    mean dissolution time
    median detection threshold
    MDT renogram
Meadox Surgimed Doppler probe
MeAIB
    methylaminoisobutyric acid
MEA-I, II
    multiple endocrine adenomatosis type I, II
meal
    barium m.
    Boas test m.
    Boyden test m.
    butter m.
    Dock test m.
    double-contrast barium m.
    Ehrmann alcohol test m.
    Ewald test m.
    fatty m.
    Fischer test m.
    isotope m.
    Leube test m.
    liver m.
    Lundh m.
    motor test m.
    normal saline m.
    opaque m.
    pH standardized m.
    retention m.
    Riegel test m.
    Salzer test m.
    small bowel m.
    solid egg-white m.
    standard fatty m.
    ^{99m}Tc-sulfur colloid egg m.
    test m.
meal-related secretion pattern
meal-stimulated
    m.-s. acid output (MSAO)
    m.-s. pancreatic secretion
mean
    m. allograft survival (MAS)
    m. arterial blood pressure (MABP)
    m. arterial pressure (MAP)
    m. colonic transit (MCT)
    m. corpuscular hemoglobin (MCH)

m. corpuscular hemoglobin concentration (MCHC)
m. corpuscular volume (MCV)
m. dissolution time (MDT)
m. distal contraction amplitude (MDCA)
m. electrosurgical resistance
m. energy
m. input time (MIT)
m. prostatic volume
m. renal volume
m. resistance time (MRT)
m. shunt index
m. TIMP-1/GAPDH rate
m. TIMP-3-GAPDH ratio
m. transit time (MTT)
m. treatment duration
m. venous outflow (MVO)

Meares-Stamey technique
measure
antiendotoxin m.
cGy radiation m.
temporizing m.

measurement
anorectal m.
anthropometric m.
bulbocavernous reflex latency m.
Doppler ultrasound intestinal blood flow m.
intestinal permeability m.
intraprostatic temperature m.
microfluorometric m.
physiologic m.
planimetric m.
plasma bile acid m.
pressure m.
quantitative m.
rectal compliance m.
RigiScan m.
serum bile acid m.
standard m.
m. test
urethral pressure m.
Vector volume m.
velocity m.
voiding urethral pressure m. (VUPM)

measuring-mounting (MM)
m.-m. catheter

meatal
m. advancement

m. advancement and glansplasty (MAGPI)
m. advancement, glanuloplasty, penoscrotal junction meatotomy (MAGPI)
m. atresia
m. spreader
m. stenosis
m. stenosis after circumcision

meat impaction
meatoplasty
Stacke m.
V-flap m.

meatorrhaphy
meatoscope
meatoscopy
ureteral m.

meatotome
meatotomy
meatal advancement, glanuloplasty, penoscrotal junction m. (MAGPI)
m. scissors
ureteral m.
ventral m.
Y-V m.

meatus, pl. **meatus**
retrusive m.
urethral m.
m. urinarius

mebendazole
mebeverine
mebrofenin
mecamylamine
mecasermin
MeCCNU, Oncovin, fluorouracil (MOF)
mechanical
m. anastomosis
m. assist system
m. biliary obstruction
m. cystitis
m. diarrhea
m. duct obstruction
m. endoscopic management
m. extrahepatic obstruction
m. ileus
m. intestinal obstruction
m. jaundice
m. leech
m. lithotripsy
m. product
m. radial-scanning instrument
m. rotating probe

NOTES

mechanical *(continued)*
    m. small bowel obstruction
    m. stress wave
    m. ureteral dilation
    m. variceal compression
    m. ventilation

mechanism
    Albarran m.
    antireflux flap-valve m.
    cell-mediated m.
    countercurrent m.
    cyclooxygenase-dependent m.
    deglutition m.
    deranged hemostatic m.
    flap-valve m.
    Mitrofanoff m.
    neuroparacrine m.
    nonimmune m.
    peptidergic m.
    pinchcock m.
    renal autoregulatory m.
    sphincteric m.
    swallowing m.
    T-cell-dependent m.
    tubuloglomerular feedback m.
    urethral closure m.

mechanoreceptor dysfunction
mechanosensitive afferent
Mecholyl
mecillinam
Meckel
    M. diverticulitis
    M. diverticulum
    M. ileitis
    M. rod
    M. scan
    M. syndrome

Meckel-Gruber syndrome
meclizine
meclofenamate
    sodium m.

meconium
    m. hydrocele
    m. ileus
    m. ileus equivalent (MIE)
    m. peritonitis
    m. plug
    m. plug syndrome

Mectra tissue sample retainer
Medena tube
media (*pl. of* medium)
    serum-free conditional m.

medial
    m. fibroplasia
    m. margin
    m. preoptic area
    m. umbilical ligament

median
    m. arcuate ligament
    m. bar formation
    m. bar of Mercier
    m. detection threshold (MDT)
    m. follow-up
    m. furrow of the prostate
    m. incision
    m. lithotomy
    m. lobe
    m. lobe hyperplasia
    m. operative time
    m. raphe cyst

mediastinal
    m. crunch
    m. histoplasmosis
    m. involvement
    m. lymphadenectomy
    m. lymphadenopathy
    m. lymph node sampling
    m. mass
    m. pleura
    m. shift
    m. thickening
    m. tube
    m. tumor
    m. widening

mediastinitis
mediastinum
    m. germ cell tumor
    m. testis

mediated
    integrin m.
    plasmid m.

mediation
    autoimmune immunoglobulin m.

mediator
    mesenchymal inductive m.
    secreted m.

medical
    m. castration
    m. dilation
    m. evaluation
    m. food
    m. laser
    m. prevention
    m. prophylaxis
    m. resource
    m. therapy
    M. Therapy of Prostatic Symptoms (MTOPS)
    M. Therapy of Prostatic Symptoms trial
    m. vagotomy

medically induced achlorhydria
medicamentosus
    pseudopolyposis m.

Medicare patient
Medicated Urethral System for Erection (MUSE)

medication
    m. allergy
    anticholinergic m.
    m. bezoar
    bromocriptine dopaminergic m.
    carbidopa dopaminergic m.
    dopaminergic m.
    levodopa dopaminergic m.
    pergolide dopaminergic m.
    psychopharmacologic m.
    psychotropic m.
    m. teratogenesis
medication-associated
    m.-a. erection
    m.-a. suppression of gastric secretion
medication-induced injury
medicine
    American College of Physicians-American Society of Internal M. (ACP-ASIM)
    complementary and alternative m. (CAM)
    nuclear m. (NM)
    renal m.
    teratogenic m.
MediClenze hygiene and water therapy system
Medicone
Medicon-Jackson rectal forceps
medicus
    furor m.
Medicut
    M. cannula
    M. catheter
Mediflex-Gazayerli retractor
Mediflex MD-7 endoscopic video system
Medi-Ject
Medi-Jector Choice
Medilas fiberTome laser
Medina
    M. ileostomy catheter
    M. tube
mediolateral lithotomy
Mediplex Ultra tabule
medisect
Medisense Pen 2 glucose meter
Medispec Econolith spark plug lithotriptor
Medi-Tech
    M.-T. bipolar catheter
    M.-T. bipolar probe
    M.-T. steerable catheter
Mediterranean
    M. fever
    M. lymphoma
Meditron EL-100 Endolav
medium, pl. **media**
    Aeromonas media
    arteria colica media
    arteria rectalis media
    Balch 1 broth m.
    Baricon contrast m.
    Baroflave contrast m.
    Barosperse contrast m.
    Biligrafin contrast m.
    Biliscopin contrast m.
    Bilivist contrast m.
    Bilopaque contrast m.
    Biloptin contrast m.
    Campy-BAP culture m.
    Cary-Blair m.
    Cheetah radiopaque contrast m.
    chocolate agar m.
    Cholebrine contrast m.
    Cholografin contrast m.
    contrast m.
    culture m.
    dissociated m.
    Dulbecco modified Eagle m. (DMEM)
    Eagle minimal essential m. (EMEM)
    Earle m.
    extravasation of contrast m.
    Gastrografin contrast m.
    Gastrovist contrast m.
    Ham F12 m.
    Hypaque contrast m.
    inoculated m.
    iocetamic acid contrast m.
    iodipamide meglumine contrast m.
    iopanoic acid contrast m.
    ipodate contrast m.
    Keratinocyte-Serum-Free-Medium culture m.
    low osmolar contrast m. (LOCM)
    MD-60 contrast m.
    meglumine diatrizoate contrast m.
    meglumine iotroxate contrast m.
    Niopam contrast m.
    OCT m.
    Oragrafin contrast m.

NOTES

medium *(continued)*
    Reno-M contrast m.
    RPMI-1640 m.
    Selenite-F enrichment m.
    Skirrow m.
    sodium iodipamide contrast m.
    Solu-Biloptin contrast m.
    sorbitol-MacConkey m.
    Telepaque contrast m.
    Thorotrast contrast m.
    tyropanoate contrast m.
    Urografin 290 contrast m.
    Varibar oral contrast media
    water-soluble contrast m.
medium-chain
    m.-c. acyl-CoA dehydrogenase (MCAD)
    m.-c. acyl-CoA dehydrogenase deficiency
    m.-c. fatty acid (MCFA)
    m.-c. triglyceride (MCT)
medium-power photomicrograph
medium-term result
Medivator automatic reprocessor
Medoc-Celestin
    M.-C. endoprosthesis
    M.-C. pulsion tube
medorrhea
Medrad MRInnervu endorectal colon probe
Medralone
Medrol
medronate
    ^{99m}Tc m.
medroxyprogesterone acetate
MEDS
    microsurgical extraction of ductal sperm
MedSlant
    M. LLC
    M. therapeutic pillow
Medstone
    M. extracorporeal shock wave lithotripsy
    M. IRIS system
    M. STS lithotripsy system
    M. STS lithotriptor
    M. STS shock wave generator
Medtrax
    M. urology database
    M. urology software
Medtronic thin flexible antimony electrode
medulla, pl. **medullae**
    adrenal m.
    m. glandulae suprarenalis
    inner m.
    kidney m.
    outer m.
    renal m.
    suprarenal m.
    m. of suprarenal gland
medullaris
    conus m.
medullary
    m. carcinoma of thyroid (MCT)
    m. collecting duct
    m. cystic disease
    m. interstitial osmolality
    m. interstitium
    m. oxygenation
    m. pyramid
    m. sponge kidney
    m. thyroid carcinoma
medullation
medullectomy
medulloadrenal
medulloblastoma
medulloid
medullosuprarenoma
medusa, pl. **medusae**
    caput medusae
    M. head
Meeker gallbladder clamp
mefenamic acid
mefloquine
Mefoxin
Mefoxin-saline solution
MEG
    magnetoencephalography
megabladder
megacalycosis
Megace
megacolon
    acquired functional m.
    acute m.
    aganglionic m.
    congenital m.
    m. congenitum
    idiopathic m.
    toxic m.
megacystic
    m. mucinous neoplasm
    m. syndrome
megacystis
    bladder congenital m.
megacystis-megaureter
    m.-m. association
    m.-m. syndrome
megacystis-microcolon-intestinal hypoperistalsis syndrome
megaduodenum
megaesophagus
    Chagasic m.
megakaryocyte
megalin
Megalink biliary stent
megaloblastic anemia
megalocystis

megaloesophagus
megalogastria
megalopenis
megalophallus
megaloureter
megalourethra
megameatus
megameatus-intact prepuce (MIP)
megamitochondria
megarectum
    idiopathic m.
megasigmoid syndrome
megaureter
    m. classification
    obstructive m.
    primary obstructive m.
    primary refluxing m.
    secondary refluxing m.
    unilateral m.
megaurethra
megavitamin
megestrol acetate
meglumine
    m. diatrizoate
    m. diatrizoate contrast medium
    m. diatrizoate enema
    iodipamide m.
    m. iotroxate
    m. iotroxate contrast medium
    Urovist M.
MEGX
    monoethylglycinexylidide
MEIA
    microparticle enzyme immunoassay
Meigs syndrome
Meissner plexus
mekongi
    Schistosoma m.
    schistosomiasis m.
melaninogenicus
    Bacteroides m.
melanogaster
    Drosophila m.
melanoma
    adrenal gland m.
    bladder malignant m.
    familial atypical multiple-mole m. (FAMM)
    m. intratumor pressure
    male genitalia m.
    malignant m.
    metastatic m.

melanorrhagia
melanorrhea
melanosis
    m. coli
    penile m.
melanotic neuroectodermal tumor of infancy (MNTI)
melas
    icterus m.
melasma
    m. addisonii
    m. suprarenale
MELAS syndrome
melatonin
Melchior ileal neobladder
MELD
    Model for End-Stage Liver Disease
    MELD model
    MELD score
melena
    m. neonatorum
    m. spuria
    m. vera
melenemesis
melenic stool
melitensis
    Brucella m.
melituria
Melkersson-Rosenthal syndrome
mellitus
    diabetes m.
    insulin-dependent diabetes m. (IDDM)
    malnutrition-related diabetes m. (MRDM)
    noninsulin-dependent diabetes m. (NIDDM)
    posttransplant diabetes m. (PTDM)
    prevalence of diabetes m.
    risk factors of posttransplant diabetes m.
    streptozotocin-induced diabetes m.
    type 2 diabetes m.
meloxicam
melphalan
Meltzer-Lyon test
Meltzer sign
membranate
membrane
    abdominal m.
    antiglomerular basement m.
    antitubular basement m.

NOTES

membrane *(continued)*
- antral m.
- apical m.
- basement m.
- basolateral m. (BLM)
- biocompatible m.
- bioincompatible m.
- brush-border m. (BBM)
- m. catheter technique
- cell m.
- cellulose-based m.
- cellulose diacetate m.
- Chwalla m.
- cloacal m.
- m. cofactor protein (MCP)
- congenital pyloric m.
- croupous m.
- cuprophane m.
- m. current
- Debove m.
- dialyzer m.
- dry mucous m.
- m. effect
- elastic silicone m.
- false m.
- filtration slit m.
- glomerular basement m. (GBM)
- Hemophan m.
- Hibond N+ nylon m.
- high-flux dialysis m.
- high-flux polysulfone m.
- m. hyperpolarization.
- invaginated m.
- Jackson m.
- low-flux cuprophane m.
- low-flux dialysis m.
- low-flux polysulfone m.
- lysosomal m.
- mammalian cell m.
- microvillous m.
- moist mucous m.
- MSI nylon m.
- mucous m.
- NaK-ATPase m.
- nuclear m.
- m. oxygenator
- m. permeability
- m. peroxidation
- phrenoesophageal m.
- polymethylmethacrylate m.
- polysulfone m.
- porous filter m.
- posttransplant antiglomerular basement m.
- Preclude peritoneal m.
- prostate-specific m. (PSM)
- Seprafilm bioresorbable m.
- serous m.
- small intestinal m.
- thin basement m. (TBM)
- Toldt m.
- m. trafficking
- m. transport protein
- tubular basement m. (TBM)
- urea-impermeable m.
- urothelial basement m. (UBM)

membrane-attack complex
membrane-based lipid
membrane-bound multicomponent enzyme complex
membrane-coated SEMS
membrane-covered stent
membraneous urethral stricture
membrane-spanning
- m.-s. domain (MDS)
- m.-s. integrin

membranolysis
membranoproliferative glomerulonephritis type I, II (MPGN)
membranotomy
- laryngeal jack-assisted retrograde esophageal m.

membranous
- m. glomerulonephritis (MGN)
- m. nephropathy
- m. neuropathy
- m. urethra

membrum virile
Memokath catheter
memory
- m. impairment
- m. T cell
- m. wire

Memotherm
- M. colorectal stent
- M. endoscopic biliary stent
- M. Flexx biliary stent
- M. nitinol stent

MEN
- multiple endocrine neoplasia
  - MEN 2A
  - MEN 2B
  - MEN I syndrome

menaquinone (MK)
mendelian pattern
Mendelsohn maneuver
Mendez ultrasonic cystotome
Ménétrier disease
Menghini
- M. liver biopsy needle
- M. technique
- M. technique for percutaneous liver biopsy

Menghini-type coring bevel
Meni-D
Ménière disease
meningismus

meningitis
    pyogenic m.
meningomyelocele
meningosepticum
    Flavobacterium m.
meniscus sign
Menkes
    M. disease
    M. disease gene
    M. syndrome
menouria
MENS
    multiple endocrine neoplasia syndrome
mentagrophytes
    Trichophyton m.
Mentor
    M. Alpha 1 inflatable penile prosthesis
    M. Bioflex cylinder
    M. GFS penile prosthesis
    M. gun
    M. IPP penile prosthesis
    M. malleable penile prosthesis
    M. Mark II penile prosthesis
    M. nonhydrophilic PVC catheter
    M. Response VCD
    M. straight catheter
Mentor-Piston VCD
Mentor-Touch VCD
Menuet Compact urodynamic testing device
MEOS
    microsomal ethanol oxidizing system
mepenzolate bromide
meperidine
    m. conscious sedation
    m. hydrochloride
mephentermine
mepiperphenidol
meprobamate
mercaptan
mercaptoacetyltriglycine (MAG-3)
mercaptoethane sulfonate
2-mercaptoethanesulfonic acid (mesna)
6-mercaptopurine (6-MP)
Mercedes Benz sign
Mercier
    M. bar
    median bar of M.
    M. operation
mercurialism
mercurial nephrosis

mercuric
    m. chloride-induced ARF
    m. chloride-induced nephritis
    m. chloride nephrotoxicity
    m. oxide
    m. oxide battery ingestion
mercury
    m. bougienage treatment
    m. chloride (HgCl2)
    millimeters of m. (mmHg)
    m. poisoning
mercury-containing balloon
mercury-filled dilator
mercury-weighted
    m.-w. dilator
    m.-w. rubber bougie
    m.-w. tube
Meridia
merimepodib
Merindino operation
Meritene liquid feeding
MERmaid DNA kit
mermaid malformation
meropenem for injection
Merrem I.V.
Mersilene
    M. mesh
    M. for pubovaginal sling
    M. strut
    M. suture
    M. tape
merthiolate fresh stool examination
merycism
MES
    mucosal electrosensitivity
MESA
    microepididymal sperm aspiration
    microsurgical epididymal sperm aspiration
mesalamine
    m. enema
    m. rectal suppository
    m. sodium
mesalazine
mesangial
    m. angle
    m. cell (MC)
    cultured rat m.
    m. deposit
    m. hypercellularity
    m. lysis
    m. matrix expansion

NOTES

mesangial *(continued)*
- m. nephropathy
- m. pattern
- m. proliferation
- m. volume fraction

mesangiocapillary glomerulonephritis
mesangiolysis
mesangiolytic change
mesangioproliferative glomerulonephritis
mesangium
- extraglomerular m. (EGM)
- glomerular m.

mesaraica
- tabes m.

mesenchyma cell
mesenchymal
- m. change
- m. hamartoma
- m. inductive mediator
- m. protein

mesenchyme
- metanephrogenic m.

mesenchymoma
- benign m.
- malignant m.

mesenterectomy
mesenterial intestine
mesenteric
- m. adenitis
- m. angiogram
- m. apoplexy
- m. arterial embolism
- m. arterial thrombosis
- m. arteriography
- m. arteriovenous fistula
- m. artery
- m. artery constriction
- m. attachment
- m. attachments of colon
- m. circulation
- m. cyst
- m. defect
- m. fat stranding
- m. fibromatosis
- m. hematoma
- m. hernia
- m. infarction
- m. inflammatory venoocclusive disease (MIVOD)
- m. ischemia
- m. lipodystrophy
- m. lipogranuloma
- m. lymph node (MLN)
- m. panniculitis (MP)
- m. rupture
- m. sensory receptor
- m. steal syndrome
- m. tear
- m. triangle
- m. tumefaction
- m. varix
- m. vascular disease
- m. vascular lesion
- m. vascular occlusion
- m. vasculitis
- m. vein
- m. vein thrombosis (MVT)
- m. window

mesenterica
- tabes m.

mesentericoparietal hernia
mesenteriolum
mesenteriopexy
mesenteriorrhaphy
mesenteriplication
mesenteritis
- liposclerotic m.
- retractile m.
- sclerosing m.

mesenterium
mesenteroaxial gastric volvulus
mesenterorenal bypass
mesentery
- leaf of m.
- small intestine m. (SIM)

mesentorrhaphy
mesh
- Bard Visilex m.
- Dacron m.
- Dexon polyglycolic acid m.
- Marlex m.
- Mersilene m.
- PelviSoft m.
- polypropylene m.
- polytetrafluoroethylene m.
- Sperma-Tex preshaped m.
- m. stent
- m. stent prosthesis
- Surgipro m.
- synthetic m.
- Trelex m.
- Vicryl m.
- Visilex m.

meshed graft
mesher
- Collin m.

mesh-plug hernioplasty
mesna
- 2-mercaptoethanesulfonic acid

Mesnex
mesnili
- *Chilomastix* m.

mesoappendicitis
mesoappendix
mesoblastic nephroma
mesocaval
- m. anastomosis

m. H-graft shunt
m. interposition shunt
mesocecum
mesocolic
    m. band
    m. hernia
    m. shelf
mesocolica
    taenia m.
mesocolon
mesocolonic vessel
mesocolopexy
mesocoloplication
mesodermal ingrowth
mesogastric
mesogastrium
    dorsal m.
    ventral m.
mesoileum
mesometrium
mesonephric
    m. adenoma
    m. duct
    m. hyperplasia
    m. nephron
    m. remnant
    m. tubule
mesonephricus
    ductus m.
mesonephros, pl. **mesonephroi**
    caudal m.
    cranial m.
    genital m.
mesopexy
mesophilic bacterium
MESOR
    midline estimating statistic of rhythm
mesorectal
    m. excision
    m. lymphadenectomy
    m. tissue
mesorectum
mesoridazine
mesorrhaphy
mesosigmoid colon
mesosigmoidopexy
mesothelial
    m. hyperplasia (MH)
    m. metaplasia
mesothelioma
    benign cystic m.
    diffuse malignant m. (DMM)
    giant fibrous m.
    peritoneal m.
    well-differentiated papillary m. (WDPM)
mesotrypsin
message-2
    testosterone-repressed prostate m.-2 (TRPM-2)
messenger
    m. ribonucleic acid (mRNA)
    m. RNA (mRNA)
    m. RNA molecule
    T-cell second m.
    ureteral peristalsis second m.
Messerklinger endoscope
Mestinon
mesylate
    doxazosin m.
    gabexate m.
    hycanthone m.
    imatinib m.
    nafamostat m.
metaanalysis
metaanalytic review
metabolic
    m. abnormality
    m. acidosis
    m. alkalosis
    m. balance
    m. bone survey
    m. calculus
    m. complication
    m. consequences
    m. derangement
    m. disorder
    m. effect
    m. evaluation
    m. liver disease
    m. predictor
    m. range
    m. rate
    m. stone
    m. stone disease
    m. therapy
metabolism
    albumin m.
    basal m. (BM)
    bile salt m. (BSM)
    calcium m.
    citrate m.
    cortisol m.
    cystine m.

NOTES

metabolism *(continued)*
    drug m.
    first-pass m. (FPM)
    glomerular m.
    glutathione m.
    hepatic m.
    inborn error of m.
    leucine m.
    lipid m.
    lipoprotein m.
    magnesium m.
    oxalate m.
    phosphorus m.
    protein m.
    sulfur amino acid m.
    tryptophan m.
metabolite
    arachidonic acid m.
    cyclooxygenase m.
    cytochrome P450 m.
    reactive oxygen m.
    toxic m.
metachromatic dye
metachronous
    m. adenoma
    m. colon cancer
    m. contralateral hernias
    m. lesion
    m. neoplasia
    m. small bowel adenocarcinoma
    m. tumor
metadysentery
MetaFluor system
Metagonimus yokogawai
Metahydrin
metaicteric
metaiodobenzylguanidine (MIBG)
    iodine-131-labeled m.
metal
    m. ball-tip catheter
    m. bar retractor
    m. clip
    m. intoxication
    m. olive
    m. olive dilator
    m. sound
    m. stent
    m. wing clamp
metallic
    m. biliary stent
    m. biliary stent migration
    m. embolus
    self-expanding m. (SEM)
    m. staple
    m. stent placement
metallic-tip catheter
metalloenzyme
metalloproteinase
    m. inhibitor
    matrix m. (MMP)
    tissue m. (TIMP)
    tissue inhibitor of m.
    tissue inhibitor of m.-2 (TIMP-2)
metalloproteinase-7
    matrix m.
metallothionein
metal-tipped stent pusher
metal-weighted Silastic feeding tube
metal Z stent
metamorphosis
    fatty m.
Metamucil
metanephric
    m. tubule
    m. vesicle
metanephrine
metanephrogenic mesenchyme
metanephros, pl. **metanephroi**
metaplasia
    Barrett m.
    bladder squamous m.
    cardia intestinal m. (CIM)
    colonic m.
    columnar m.
    gastric m.
    glandular m.
    goblet cell m.
    intestinal m. type I–III
    junctional intestinal m.
    mesothelial m.
    myeloid m.
    osseous m.
    pancreatic acinar m. (PAM)
    pyloric m. (PYME)
    specialized intestinal m. (SIM)
metaplasia-dysplasia-carcinoma sequence
metaplastic
    m. atrophic gastritis
    m. epithelium
    m. gastric fundic gland
    m. ossification
    m. polyp
metaproterenol
metaraminol
metastasis, pl. **metastases**
    bleeding jejunal m.
    brain m.
    colonic m.
    cutaneous m.
    diffuse m.
    disseminated m.
    distant m.
    duodenal m.
    extrahepatic m. (EHM)
    extralymphatic m.
    m. gene
    hematogenic m.
    implantation m.

    intramucosal m.
    liver m.
    lymphatic m.
    lymph node m.
    lymphogenic m.
    neoplasm m.
    paraesophagogastric lymph node m.
    percutaneous image-guided thermal ablation of hepatic m.
    port site m.
    m. suppression
    tumor, nodes, metastases (TNM)

metastasis
    bone m.

metastatic
    m. adenocarcinoma
    m. cancer
    m. carcinoid syndrome
    m. cascade
    m. cholangiocarcinoma
    m. complication
    m. Crohn disease (MCD)
    m. dissemination
    m. fat necrosis
    m. implantation
    m. lesion
    m. melanoma
    m. neuroblastoma
    m. orchitis
    m. prostatic carcinoma
    m. renal cell carcinoma (MRCC)

Metastron
metasulfobenzoate
    prednisolone m.

metasynchronous bacterial urinary tract infection
Metatensin
metaxalone
met-enkephalin
    methionine-enkephalin met-enkephalin peptide
    plasma met-enkephalin

meteorism
meter
    Aleo m.
    Fisher Accumet pH m.
    integrating spherical power m.
    Medisense Pen 2 glucose m.
    One Touch blood glucose m.
    Synectics 6000 digital pH-meter m.

metformin
methacholine

methacrylate
    methyl m.

methadone
methamphetamine
methane (CH4) excretor
methanethiol
Methanobrevibacter smithii
methanogen
methanogenesis
methanogenic archaea
methanol intoxication
methantheline bromide
methapyrilene
methdilazine
Methedrine
methemalbumin
methemoglobinemia
methenamine
    m. hippurate
    m. mandelate

methicillin
methicillin-resistant *Staphylococcus aureus* **(MRSA)**
methimazole
Methiodal
methionine-enkephalin (met-enkephalin)
    immunoreactive m.-e. (IRME)

methionine loading
methionine-rich food
methixene
method
    ablate-and-chip m.
    acid guanidine thiocyanate-phenol-chloroform m.
    acid hematin m.
    Addis m.
    Albert-Lembert m.
    anthrone m.
    avidin-biotin-peroxidase complex m.
    barostat m.
    Beck m.
    Bence Jones protein m.
    Benedict and Franke m.
    Benedict-Talbot body surface area m.
    Bertrand m.
    Biogenex antigen retrieval m.
    Brown and Wickham pressure profile m.
    cap m.
    cholesterol-cholesteroloxidase-phenol 4-aminophenazone m.

NOTES

method (continued)
- cinefluoroscopic m.
- Cockroft m.
- dye scattering m.
- efficacious noninvasive anesthesia-independent first-line m.
- ellipsoid m.
- endoscopic mucosal resection, cap m. (EMRC)
- endoscopic mucosal resection, tube m. (EMRT)
- Esbach m.
- Essed plication m.
- Fishberg m.
- Folin-Benedict-Myers m.
- Folin-Denis m.
- Folin gravimetric m.
- m. of Gates
- Genta m.
- Giemsa m.
- Halsted m.
- Hanley m.
- Hasson m.
- Hybritech m.
- imaging m.
- immunohistochemical m.
- Jendrassik-Grof m.
- Kaplan-Meier m.
- Lashmet-Newburgh m.
- lay-open m.
- lift-and-cut m.
- Lowery m.
- Metzer-Boyce m.
- microwave-assisted streptavidin-biotin peroxidase m.
- Morison m.
- noninvasive m.
- Okamoto m.
- Papanicolaou m.
- Parker-Kerr closed m.
- partial hood assisted lift-and-cut m.
- Patterson-Parker m.
- pause-squeeze m.
- Payr m.
- percutaneous sampling m.
- Permutit m.
- phosphotungstic acid-magnesium chloride precipitation m.
- pull m.
- Quimby m.
- radiochromium-labeled erythrocyte m.
- Reddick-Saye m.
- Rehfuss m.
- Schwartz m.
- Sengstaken-Blakemore m.
- Shohl-Pedley m.
- Sjöqvist m.
- Stachrom AT III routine chromogenic m.
- standard radioenzymatic m.
- suck-and-cut m.
- Sumner m.
- technically elaborate m.
- thermally active m.
- thiourea-resorcinol m.
- trapezoid m.
- triangulation stapling m.
- turn-and-suction m.
- two-devices-in-one-channel m.
- Volhard-Fahr m.
- Warthin-Starry m.
- Waterston m.
- Wheeless m.
- Woolf m.

methods & materials
methotrexate (MTX)
- m., cisplatin (MC)
- m., cisplatin, vinblastine (MCV)
- m., vinblastine, Adriamycin, cisplatin (MVAC, M-VAC)
- m., vinblastine, epirubicin, cisplatin (M-VEC)

methotrimeprazine
methoxamine
methoxsalen
methoxyflurane anesthesia
methoxyphenamine
methscopolamine bromide
methyclothiazide
methyl
- m. CCNU
- m. methacrylate
- 5-methyl cytosine
- m. red test
- m. salicylate

methylaminoisobutyric acid (MeAIB)
methylate
- phentolamine m.

methylatropine nitrate
methylbromide
- anisotropine m.
- homatropine m.

methylcellulose
methylcitric
- 2-m. acid

methyldopa
- parenteral m.

methyldopate
methylene
- m. blue
- m. blue chromoendoscopy
- m. blue dye
- m. blue enema
- m. blue stain
- 5,10-m.-tetrahydrofolate reductase (MTHFR)

methylhistamine
3-methylhistidine
    urinary 3-m.
methylmalonic acid
methylnaltrexone (MNTX)
methylnitrate
    atropine m.
methylphenidate
1-methyl-4-phenyl-1,2,3,6-
    tetrahydropyridine (MTPT)
6-methylprednisolone
methylprednisolone acetate
methylsulfate
    diphemanil m.
    neostigmine m.
methyl-*tert*-butyl
    m.-t.-b. ether (MTBE)
    m.-t.-b. ether therapy
methyltestosterone
methyltestosterone-induced cholestasis
methysergide maleate
Meticorten
meticulous dissection
Metizol
metoclopramide
    m., dexamethasone, lorazepam, ondansetron (MDLO)
    m. premedication
metoclopramide, dexamethasone, lorazepam, ondansetron (MDLO)
metocurine
metolazone
metoprolol tartrate
metreleptin
Metricide disinfectant
metrifonate
metrizamide
metrizoate
MetroGel
metronidazole
    m., amoxicillin, clarithromycin, *H. pylori*, one-week therapy (MACH1)
    omeprazole, amoxicillin, m. (OAM)
metronidazole-resistant strain
Metryl 500
metschnikovii
    Vibrio m.
metyrapone stimulation test
metyrosine
Metzenbaum scissors

Metzer-Boyce method
Meulengracht diet
Mevacor
Mewissen infusion catheter
Mexican hat sign
mexiletine
Meyenburg complex
Meyer-Weigert law
mezlocillin
MFG
    manofluorography
MFI
    Multidimensional Fatigue Index
MFL 5000 lithotriptor
mg
    milligram
MGN
    membranous glomerulonephritis
MGUS
    monoclonal gammopathy of undetermined significance
MH
    mesothelial hyperplasia
MHC
    major histocompatibility complex
        MHC class I, II antigen
MHC-bound
MHV
    middle hepatic vein
3.5–10 MHz curved-array transducer
Mi-Acid
MIAD
    mild idiopathic adulthood biliary ductopenia
Miami pouch
MIB-1
    monoclonal antibody MIB-1
    MIB-1 staining
MIBG
    metaiodobenzylguanidine
MIC
    minimal inhibitory concentration
    MIC gastroenteric tube
    MIC gastrostomy tube
micaceous growth of penis
mica operation
micellar solubilization
micelle formation
Michaelis constant (Km)
Michaelis-Gutmann body
Michaelis-Menten kinetics

NOTES

Michal
    M. II technique
    M. procedure I, II
Michel clip
Michigan
    M. intestinal forceps
    M. Kidney Registry
Mick
    M. prostate template
    M. TP-200 applicator
MIC-Key
    M.-K. G gastrostomy tube
    M.-K. J gastrostomy tube
miconazole
Micral urine dipstick test
Micro-6 ureteroscope
microabscess
microacini
microadenoma
microaerophilic organism
microalbuminuria
microanastomosis
    laser-assisted m. (LAMA)
microaneurysm
microangiopathic renal injury
microangiopathy
    diabetic m.
    tacrolimus-associated m.
    thrombotic m.
microballoon probe
microbial
    m. approach
    m. ecology
microbial biofilm
microbiliary inflammation
microbiology
microbiota
microcalcification
microcalculus, pl. **microcalculi**
microcalix
microcatheter
    FasTracker 325 coaxial m.
Microcell chamber
microcephaly
microchimerism
    donor hematopoietic cell m.
    donor-type m.
microchromoendoscopy
microclimate
    acid m.
Micrococcus
microcoil
    Intercept esophagus m.
    Intercept prostate m.
    Intercept urethra m.
Microcoleus
microcolitis
microcolon
microcrystal

microcrystalline material
microcyst
    lymphatic m.
microcystic disease of renal medulla
microdensitometer
    Vickers M85a m.
microdroplet fat deposition
Microelectrode
    M. MI-506 small-caliber pH electrode
    M. MI-506 small-caliber probe
microemulsion
    cyclosporine for m.
microenvironment
    gastric m.
microepididymal sperm aspiration (MESA)
microerosion
microexplosive generator
microfibril
microfibrillar
    m. collagen hemostat (MCH)
    m. protein (MP)
microfilament bundle
microfilariasis
microfil-associated glycoprotein (MAGP)
microfilter
    Minnpure m.
microflora
    colonic m.
microfluorometric measurement
microfold (M)
    m. cell
microgastria
microgenitalism
Microglass pH electrode
microgram
micrograph
    low-magnification electron m.
Microgyn II urinary incontinence device
microhamartoma, pl. **microhamartomata, microhamartomas**
    biliary m.
microhematuria
microimplant
    silicone m.
microlens cystourethroscope
microlith
microlithiasis
    common bile duct m. (CBDM)
    pulmonary alveolar m.
    testicular m.
microlithiasis-induced pancreatitis
MicroLyzer
    M. Gas analyzer
    M. model 12i
    M. model SC
    QuinTron M.

micromanipulation
    gamete m.
    oocyte m.
micrometastasis
    hematogenous m.
Micronase
microneedle holder
micronidia
micronized
    m. flavonidic fraction
    m. purified flavonoid fracture (MPFF)
micronodular cirrhosis
microparticle enzyme immunoassay (MEIA)
micropenis
microperforation
microperfusion study
microphallus
micropipette
micropuncture
    epididymis m.
    m. technique
microrchidia
micros
    Peptostreptococcus m.
microsatellite
    m. instability (MSI)
    m. stable (MSS)
microsatellite instability (MSI)
microscope
    dual-axis confocal m.
    ELMISKOP 101 electron m.
    JEM-100B, 100S electron m.
    JEOL 100 CX electron m.
    JEOL JSM 35 CF scanning electron m.
    laser m.
    Olympus BH2-epifluorescence m.
    Olympus BH2-RFCA reflecting m.
    Olympus BHT-2 m.
    Olympus CBK fluorescence m.
    Phillips CM 12 electron m.
    real-time confocal scanning laser m.
    scanning electron m.
    Zeiss Axiophot m.
    Zeiss IDO3 phase-contrast m.
    Zeiss S9 electron m.
microscopic
    m. colitis
    m. colitis syndrome
    m. epididymal sperm aspiration
    m. hematuria
    m. polyangiitis (MPA)
    m. urine examination
microscopy
    confocal laser scanning m.
    electron m.
    epifluorescence m.
    immune electron m.
    immunofluorescence m.
    laser-scanning confocal m.
    light m.
    paraffin-section light m.
    polarization m.
    rotary shadowing electron m.
    scanning electron m.
    scanning force m. (SFM)
    transmission electron m. (TEM)
    urinalysis sediment m.
    in vivo m.
microseminoprotein
    beta m.
MicroSkin ostomy pouch
microsomal
    m. damage
    m. ethanol oxidizing system (MEOS)
microsome
    m. antibody (MCHA)
    liver-kidney m. (LKM)
microsphere
    biodegradable m.
    Super-Bright m.
    ^{99m}Tc albumin m.
Microspike approximator clamp
Microsporidia
microsporidian
microsporidiosis
microsurgery
    rectal expander-assisted transanal endoscopic m. (RE-TEM)
    transanal endoscopic m. (TEM)
microsurgical
    m. denervation of spermatic cord
    m. epididymal sperm aspiration (MESA)
    m. epididymal sperm aspiration procedure
    m. epididymovasostomy (MSEV)
    m. extraction of ductal sperm (MEDS)

NOTES

microsurgical (continued)
  m. extraction of sperm from epididymis (MASE)
  m. inguinal varicocelectomy
microsuture
  Sharpoint m.
microtelangiectasia
microtendon
microtip
  m. sensor catheter
  m. transducer catheter
microtitration plate reader
microtrabecular hepatocellular carcinoma
microtransducer
  imbedded m.
  Konigsberg m.
  m. technique
microtubule (MT)
microvascular
  m. clamp
  m. flap
  m. needle holder
Microvasive
  M. Altertome
  M. angled hydrophilic guidewire
  M. ASAP 18
  M. balloon catheter
  M. biliary stent system
  M. CRE esophageal dilator
  M. disposable alligator-shaped forceps
  M. 5F mini-snare
  M. Geenen Endotorque guidewire
  M. Glidewire guidewire
  M. Gold probe bipolar electrocautery device
  M. instrumentation
  M. papillotome
  M. radial-jaw 3 biopsy forceps
  M. radial-jaw 1597-20 large-capacity biopsy forceps
  M. radial-jaw 31263-20 large-capacity biopsy forceps
  M. retrieval balloon
  M. Rigiflex balloon dilator
  M. Rigiflex through-the-scope balloon
  M. sclerotherapy needle
  M. Ultraflex esophageal stent system
  M. ultratome
microvesicular
  m. fat
  m. steatosis
microvillous membrane
microvillus, pl. **microvilli**
  m. inclusion disease
microvolt (μV)

microwave
  m. antenna design
  m. applicator
  m. coagulation
  endoscopic m.
  m. hyperthermia
  m. nonsurgical treatment
  m. therapy
  m. thermotherapy
  m. tissue coagulator
microwave-assisted streptavidin-biotin peroxidase method
microwell plate
miction
MIC-TJ transgastric jejunal tube
micturating
  m. cystogram
  m. cystourethrogram
  m. cystourethrography (MCU)
micturition
  m. cystourethrogram
  m. phase
  m. problem
  m. reflex
  m. reflex inhibition
  m. reflex manual initiation
midabdominal
  m. abscess
  m. transverse incision
  m. wall
Midamor
midaxillary line
midazolam
  m. conscious sedation
  m. hydrochloride
midclavicular line (MCL)
midcolon
middle
  m. adrenal artery
  m. colic artery (MCA)
  m. extrahepatic bile duct
  m. gland
  m. hemorrhoidal artery
  m. hepatic vein (MHV)
  m. hypospadias
  m. rectal fold
  m. rectal vein
  m. rectal venous plexus
  m. stomach
  m. ureter
midepigastric area
midepigastrium
midesophageal diverticulum
midesophagus
midgastric electrode
midgut
  m. ischemia
  m. volvulus
  m. volvulus with malrotation

midline
    m. abdominal crease
    m. estimating statistic of rhythm (MESOR)
    m. lower abdominal incision
    m. upper abdominal incision
midodrine
midrectal area
midregion PTH
midsigmoid colon
midstomach
midstream
    m. specimen of urine (MSU)
    m. urinalysis
midtransverse segment
midureteral calculus
midurethral support
MIE
    meconium ileus equivalent
Miescher cheilitis granulomatosa
MIF
    migration inhibition factor
mifepristone
miglitol
migraine
    abdominal m.
migrans
    larva m.
    visceral larva m.
migrating
    m. motor complex (MMC)
    m. myoelectric complex
migration
    aboral m.
    calculus m.
    electrode m.
    gallstone m.
    gastrostomy tube m.
    m. inhibition factor (MIF)
    intravesical m.
    lymphocyte m.
    metallic biliary stent m.
    retrograde m.
    stent m.
    tube m.
Mikulicz
    M. bag
    M. clamp
    M. colostomy
    M. drain
    M. drain technique
    M. gastroscope
    M. gastrostomy tube
    M. operation
    M. packing
    M. pad
    M. peritoneal forceps
    M. procedure
    M. pyloroplasty
    M. retractor
mil
    deltas per m.
mild
    m. distress
    m. hyperoxaluria
    m. idiopathic adulthood biliary ductopenia (MIAD)
    m. tubulitis
Miles
    M. abdominoperineal resection
    M. operation
    M. V.I.P. 300 vacuum infiltration processor
milia (*pl. of* milium)
miliaria rubra
miliary tuberculosis
milium, pl. **milia**
milk
    acidophilus m.
    m. diet
    m. of magnesia (MOM)
    m. protein antibody
    m. sickness
    m. thistle
milk-alkali syndrome
milking of intestine
Milkinol
milkman's line
milk-of-calcium bile
milk-sensitive colitis
milky
    m. ascites
    m. fluid
    m. urine
Millard mouth gag
Millar urodynamic catheter
Millen technique retropubic prostatectomy
Miller
    M. cystoscope
    M. Fisher syndrome
    M. rectal forceps
    M. rectal scissors
Miller-Abbott intestinal tube

NOTES

milleri
    Streptococcus m.
Miller-Senn retractor
Millex-GS pore-size filter
Millex-GV filter
Millie female urinal
Milligan-Morgan
    M.-M. hemorrhoidectomy
    M.-M. operation
    M.-M. technique for hemorrhoid treatment
milligram (mg)
millijoule (mJ)
milliliter (mL, ml)
millimeters of mercury (mmHg)
millimolar concentration
millimoles per liter (mmol/L)
Millin
    M. bladder retractor
    M. forceps
    M. T clamp
milliosmole/kilogram (mosm/kg)
Millipore filter
milliwatt (mW)
Mill-Rose
    M.-R. flexible endoscopic overtube
    M.-R. RiteBite biopsy forceps
milrinone
Milroy disease
MILTS
    Multicentre International Liver Tumor Study
mimic
    endocrine m.
mind-bladder syndrome
mineral
    divalent m.
    m. oil (M-O)
mineralocorticoid
mineralocorticoid-independent factor
Ming gastric carcinoma classification
miniature
    m. probe
    m. ultrasound suction device
miniaturized
    m. sheath
    m. ultrasound catheter probe
MiniBard catheter
minicap
    Coloplast flange m.
Miniguard adhesive patch
minihelical basket
minilaparatomy approach
minilaparoscope
    m. cholecystectomy
    Storz m.
minilaparotomy
    m. incision
    m. pelvic lymph node dissection
    m. restorative proctocolectomy
    m. staging pelvic lymphadenectomy
miniloop
    m. ligation
    Olympus HX-21L detachable m.
minimal
    m. access surgery
    m. change disease
    m. distending pressure
    m. inhibitory concentration (MIC)
    m. invasiveness
    m. transurethral resection of prostate (M-TURP)
minimal-access surgical skill
minimal-change
    m.-c. nephritic syndrome
    m.-c. nephrotic syndrome
minimal-lesion nephrotic syndrome
minimally
    m. invasive approach
    m. invasive surgery
    m. invasive therapy
    m. invasive treatment
minimicrosphere
minimize patient morbidity
minimum daily requirement (MDR)
minipapillotome
miniperc
    minipercutaneous
    m. technique
minipercutaneous (miniperc)
    m. nephrolithotomy
mini-Pfannenstiel incision
minipouch
    Assura closed m.
    Coloplast m.
    Sur-Fit M.
Minipress
miniprobe
    high-frequency m.
minipump
    Alzer Model 2001 osmotic m.
miniscope
    Candela M.
    Circon-ACMI m.
    Wolfe m.
minisnare
    Microvasive 5F m.
mini-VAB
    vinblastine, actinomycin D, bleomycin
mink cell bioassay
Minnesota
    M. antilymphocyte globulin
    M. Multiphasic Personality Inventory (MMPI)
    M. tube
Minnpure microfilter
Minocin
minocycline

minor
    m. calix
    curvatura gastrica m.
    curvatura ventriculi m.
    globus m.
    m. papilla
    papilla duodeni m.
    m. papilla sphincterotomy
minoxidil
Mintezol
minus
    omentum m.
minute
    m. bleeding
    counts per m. (cpm, CPM)
    m. polypoid lesion
    30-m. transurethral microwave thermotherapy
    30-m. TUMT
30-minute
    30-m. transurethral microwave thermotherapy
    30-m. TUMT
minutissimum
    Corynebacterium m.
MIP
    megameatus-intact prepuce
mirabilis
    Proteus m.
MiraLax
Mirizzi syndrome
mirror-image artifact
misakiensis
    Streptomyces m.
miscellaneous urolithiasis
mismatch
    HLA m.
    V/Q m.
misonidazole
misoprostol protection
misperfusion
    gastroduodenal m.
misplaced gland
missed diagnosis
missense mutation
Mission
    M. vacuum constriction device
    M. vacuum erection device
    M. VCD, VED
Missouri catheter
Misstique female external urinary collector

Mistifier spray catheter
mistletoe
MIT
    mean input time
Mitchell
    M. technique
    M. technique for epispadias repair
Mitek bone anchor
Mithracin
mithramycin
mitis
    nephritis m.
mitochondrial
    m. antibody
    m. complex
    m. encephalomyopathy, lactic acidosis and strokelike episodes
    m. ethanol oxidase system
    m. fatty acid beta-oxidation
    m. glutamate dehydrogenase pathway
    m. immunological study
    m. injury
    m. neurogastrointestinal encephalomyopathy (MNGIE)
    m. neurogastrointestinal encephalomyopathy syndrome
    m. phosphate-dependent glutaminase
mitochondrian, pl. **mitochondria**
    giant mitochondria
mitogen
mitogen-activated protein kinase (MAPK)
mitogenic
    m. effect
    m. stimulation
    m. stimulus
mitomycin
    m. adsorbed onto activated charcoal (M-CH)
    m. C
    fluorouracil, Adriamycin, m. C (FAMe)
    5-fluorouracil, Adriamycin, m. C (FAM)
    m. transarterial embolization treatment
mitosis count
mitosis-karyorrhexis index (MKI)
mitotane

NOTES

mitotic
- m. activity
- m. index

mitoxantrone

Mitrofanoff
- M. appendicovesicostomy
- M. catheterizable channel
- M. catheterizable stoma
- M. conduit
- M. continent urinary diversion technique
- M. continent urinary stoma
- M. mechanism
- M. neourethra
- M. principle
- M. procedure
- M. solution
- M. tube
- M. valve

Mitrolan

Mitscherlich test

mittelschmerz

mivacurium chloride

MIVOD
- mesenteric inflammatory venoocclusive disease

mixed
- m. cirrhosis
- m. connective tissue disease (MCTD)
- m. connective tissue disorder
- m. essential cryoglobulinemia
- m. germ cell-sex cord stromal tumor
- m. germ cell tumor
- m. gonadal dysgenesis
- m. growth on culture
- m. hemorrhoids
- m. hyperlipidemia
- m. hyperplastic-adenomatous gastric polyp
- m. incontinence
- m. intralobular fibrosis
- m. leukocyte culture (MLC)
- m. rhabdomyosarcoma
- m. structure

mixed-cholesterol gallstone

Mixter
- M. clamp
- M. dilating probe
- M. dissector
- M. gallstone forceps
- M. hemostat

mixture
- amino acid-glucose m.
- citric acid bladder m.
- eutectic m.
- eutectic m. of local anesthetics (EMLA)
- sodium citrate and potassium citrate m.

Miyazaki-Bonney test for stress incontinence

mizoribine

mJ
- millijoule

MK
- menaquinone

MKI
- mitosis-karyorrhexis index

MKII automated scanner

MKIII
- Digitrapper MK III

mL, ml
- milliliter

MLC
- mixed leukocyte culture
- allogeneic MLC

MLH1 **gene**

MLN
- mesenteric lymph node

MLP
- multiple lymphomatous polyposis

MM
- measuring-mounting
- MM catheter

MMAP
- Maine Medical Assessment Program
- MMAP index

MMC
- migrating motor complex
- murine mesangial cell

MMF
- mycophenolate mofetil

mmHg
- millimeters of mercury

MMK
- Marshall-Marchetti-Krantz

mmol/L
- millimoles per liter

MMP
- matrix metalloproteinase

MMPI
- Minnesota Multiphasic Personality Inventory

MMR
- mutation mismatch repair

MMUA
- macromolecular uronate

MN
- mononuclear
- MN cell
- MN infiltrate

MNB
- monomicrobial nonneutrocytic bacterascites

MNE
- monosymptomatic nocturnal enuresis

MNGIE
  mitochondrial neurogastrointestinal encephalomyopathy
MNTI
  melanotic neuroectodermal tumor of infancy
MNTX
  methylnaltrexone
M-O
  mineral oil
    Haley's M-O
MoAb
  monoclonal antibody
Moban
Mobigesic
mobile gallbladder
mobilis
  lien m.
mobility
  electrophoretic m.
mobilization
  anorectal m.
  urogenital sinus m.
Mobin-Uddin umbrella
Moctanin
modality
  current treatment m.
  dialysis m.
  ever-expanding armamentarium of therapeutic m.'s
  indispensable diagnostic m.
  therapeutic m.
Modane
  M. Soft
  M. Versabran
mode
  autosomal-recessive m.
  linear m.
  radial m.
model
  ablation m.
  m. 500A gamma camera discriminator
  Cox regression m.
  dominant inheritance m.
  M. for End-Stage Liver Disease (MELD)
  m. 500F electromagnetic flowmeter
  goat m.
  m. IL 750 AA spectrophotometer
  Markov m.
  m. 3-60 mass spectroscopy
  m. 440 M1.5, M4 electrode
  pig colon m.
  m. 5500 vapor pressure osmometer
  in vitro m.
modeling
  penile m.
  urea kinetic m. (UKM)
moderate
  m. distress
  m. proteinuria
moderately differentiated adenoma
modification
  Al-Ghorab m.
  m. of diet in renal disease (MDRD)
  M. of Diet in Renal Disease trial
  evidence-based dietary/fluid m.
  Goligher m.
  high-energy m.
  Kelly-Kennedy m.
  lifestyle m. (LSM)
  Muzsnai m.
  posttranslational m.
  Pugh m.
  pylorus-preserving Whipple m. (PPW)
  Raz m.
  recent technical m.
  Walsh surgical m.
modified
  m. aspirating catheter
  m. barium swallow (MBS)
  m. Barthel degree of disability index
  m. Bismuth-Corlete classification
  m. Cantwell technique
  m. caulking gun
  m. Essed-Schroeder corporoplasty
  m. Gibson incision
  m. Hassan open technique
  m. Hetzel-Dent scale
  m. ileocecal valve
  m. Ingelman-Sundberg procedure
  m. Lich-Gregoir ureteroneocystostomy
  m. liver diet
  m. Lloyd-Davies position
  m. method of Pugh
  m. Minnesota tube
  m. Nesbit procedure
  m. Norfolk procedure
  m. penectomy

NOTES

modified *(continued)*
- m. Pereyra bladder neck suspension
- m. polyethylene dilator
- m. Sacks-Vine push-pull technique
- m. sham feeding
- m. thermal nitinol electrode
- m. Thiersch-Duplay technique
- m. transduodenal rendezvous procedure
- m. Vest technique
- m. Whitehead hemorrhoidectomy
- m. Young urethroplasty
- m. Z stent

modifier
- biologic response m. (BRM)

modulation
- antigenic m.
- obstruction-induced m.
- pressure amplitude m.

modulator
- intracrine negative feedback m.

Modulith
- M. SL 20 device for ESWL
- M. SL 20 lithotriptor

Moduretic

MODY
- maturity-onset diabetes of youth
- maturity-onset diabetes of the youth

Moersch esophagoscope

MOF
- MeCCNU, Oncovin, fluorouracil
- multiple organ failure

mofetil
- mycophenolate m. (MMF)

Mogen clamp

Mohr test

Mohs microsurgery technique

moiety
- steroid m.

moist
- m. laparotomy pack
- m. mucous membrane
- m. necrosis
- m. papule

Moi-Stir

molar pregnancy

mole
- hydatidiform m.
- repeated complete m.

Molectron Nd:YAG laser

molecular
- m. adsorbents recirculating system (MARS)
- m. basis of proteinuria
- m. cloning
- m. cloning and sequencing
- m. genetic alteration
- m. marker
- m. study
- m. typing
- m. weight (mol wt)

molecule
- adhesion m.
- CD4 m.
- CD8 m.
- cell-adhesion m.
- class I, II MHC m.
- extracellular matrix m.
- HLA-DQ2 m.
- immunoglobulin superfamily adhesion m.
- lithostathine m.
- lymphocyte costimulatory m.
- messenger RNA m.
- monocyte adhesion m.
- neural cell-adhesive m. (NCAM, N-CAM)

molecule-1
- endothelial leukocyte adhesion m.-1 (ELAM-1)
- intercellular adhesion m.-1 (ICAM-1)
- vascular cell adhesion m.-1 (VCAM-1)

molgramostim

molimen, pl. **molimina**

molindone

mollusc
- bivalve m.

molluscum
- m. contagiosum
- m. contagiosum virus (MCV)

Molnar disk

mol wt
- molecular weight

MOM
- milk of magnesia

Mondor phlebitis

Monfort
- M. abdominoplasty
- M. operation

mongolian spot

Monilia **esophagitis**

monilial
- m. esophagitis
- m. infection

moniliasis

Monistat

monitor
- Bravo pH M.
- Contimed II pelvic floor muscle m.
- Deltatrac Metabolic M.
- Dinamap Plus m.
- Dobbhoff biofeedback m.
- gastric pH m.
- Gould pressure m.
- 24-hour ambulatory gastric pH m.

monitor · monooxygenase

Ingold M3, M4 glass electrode pH m.
in-line blood gas m.
Interceptor M3 triple-channel solid-state m.
m. peptide
return electrode m. (REM)
RigiScan penile tumescence and rigidity m.
television m.
video m.

monitoring
ambulatory intraesophageal bilirubin m.
ambulatory intraesophageal pH m.
ambulatory urodynamic m.
clinical m.
cystometrographic m.
endoscopic m.
esophageal pH m.
fluoroscopic m.
heart rate m.
24-hour ambulatory esophageal pH m.
24-hour spectrophotometric bilirubin m.
intracranial pressure m.
intraesophageal pH m. (EpHM)
nocturnal penile tumescence m.
NPT m.
pH m.
self blood glucose m. (SBGM)
tumescence m.

monitor/recorder
Gastroreflex ambulatory pH m./r.

monoamine oxidase inhibitor
Monocal tablet
monocapsule
bismuth triple m.

Monocid
monoclonal
m. antibody (MAb, mAb, MoAb)
m. antibody BR96
m. antibody ED1
m. antibody MIB-1
m. antibody scintigraphic scan
m. antibody therapy
m. anti-DNA antibody
m. antigen
m. anti-HBc
4B4 m. antibody
19B7 m. antibody

m. gammopathy
m. gammopathy of undetermined significance (MGUS)
m. IgM
4KB5 m. antibody
m. light chain
m. proliferation
90Y-CYT-356 m. antibody

monoclonality by genetic analysis
Monocryl suture
monocyte
m. adhesion molecule
m. chemoattractant protein
m. chemoattractant protein-1 (MCP-1)
m. chemotactic protein (MCP)
WBC m.

monocytes/macrophages
monocytogenes
Listeria m.

Monodox
Monodral
monoethanolamine oleate
monoethylglycinexylidide (MEGX)
m. liver function tests

monofilament
m. absorbable suture
m. nylon suture
m. snare wire

monofocal papillary carcinoma
Mono-Gesic
monohydrate
cefadroxil m.
doxycycline m.
sodium phosphate monobasic m.

monohydroxy bile salt
monokine
monolayer
cobblestonelike m.

monomer
tissue m.

monomicrobial nonneutrocytic bacterascites (MNB)
mononephrous
mononuclear (MN)
m. cell recruitment
m. dyspepsia
m. histiocytic portal infiltrate

mononucleotide
flavin m.

monooctanoin infusion
monooxygenase pathway

NOTES

511

monophosphate
    5′-m.
    adenosine m. (AMP)
    cyclic adenosine m. (cAMP)
    5′-cyclic adenosine m. (cAMP)
    cyclic guanosine m. (cGMP)
    5′-cyclic guanosine m. (cGMP)
    guanosine m.
    guanosine 5′-m. (GMP)
monopodial
monopolar
    BICAP m.
    m. coagulation
    m. electrocautery
    m. electrocoagulation
    m. probe
    m. triple-hook active needle
monopole
monopolypoid adenoma
monosaccharide
Monoscopy locking trocar with Woodford spike
monosialoganglioside
monosialosyl Lea
monosodium urate
Monospot
monosymptomatic nocturnal enuresis (MNE)
monoterpene
monotherapy
    androgen ablative m.
    bicalutamide m.
    nonsteroidal antiandrogen m.
    sirolimus m.
mons
    m. plasty
    m. veneris
Montague
    M. proctoscope
    M. sigmoidoscope
Montezuma revenge
Montgomery
    M. abdominal strap
    M. salivary bypass tube
    M. strap dressing
    M. tape
Monti-Malone, left
Monti procedure
Monurol
Mood Adjective Check List
moon
    m. facies
    M. rectal retractor
Moore
    M. classification for vascular anomalies of gastrointestinal tract
    M. gallstone scoop
MOP-Videoplan morphometric system

Moraxella
    M. bovis
    M. nonliquefaciens
morbidity
    febrile m.
    maternal m.
    minimize patient m.
    operative m.
    m. of percutaneous nephrolithotomy
    perioperative m.
    postoperative m.
    reflux m.
    m. risk
    treatment m.
    uncorrected maternal m.
    uncorrected reflux m.
morbid obesity
morbus
    cholera m.
morcellated nephrectomy
morcellation
    m. technique
    vaginal m.
morcellator
    Cook tissue m.
    electric tissue m.
    high-speed electrical tissue m.
    tissue m.
morcellement operation
Moreno gastroenterostomy clamp
Morgagni
    M. appendix
    M. caruncle
    column of M.
    M. crypt
    foramen of M.
    fossa of M.
    M. fovea
    frenum of M.
    M. hernia
    M. hydatid
    M. lacunae
    M. retinaculum
    M. valve
morganii
    Proteus m.
Morganstern
    M. aspiration/injection system
    M. continuous-flow operating cystoscope
moribund
moricizine
Mori knife
Morison
    hepatorenal space of M.
    M. method
    M. pouch
morning diarrhea
Moro-Heisler diet

Moro reflex
morphea
morphine
    m. cholescintigraphy
    m. narcotic analgesic therapy
morphine-neostigmine test
morphogenesis
morphogenetic process
morphologic
    m. change
    m. stage
morphological
    m. change
    m. study of renal biopsy
morphology
    chromosome m.
    closed m.
    crystal m.
    Dogiel type I, II m.
    filamentous m.
    glomerular m.
    gram-stain m.
    open m.
morphometric criteria
morphometry
    nuclear m.
morrhuate
    m. sclerosant
    sodium m.
mortality
    cardiovascular m.
    intraoperative m.
    overall m.
    risk-adjusted m.
mortar kidney
mortis
    livor m.
    rigor m.
mosaic duodenal mucosal pattern
mosaicism
    XX male m.
Moschcowitz
    M. operation
    M. procedure
    M. vaginal prolapse repair
Moscontin
MOSD
    multiple organ system dysfunction
MOSF
    multiple organ system failure
Mosher
    M. bag
    M. dilator
    M. esophagoscope
mosm/kg
    milliosmole/kilogram
mosquito
    m. forceps
    m. hemostat
    m. hemostatic clamp
Moss
    M. gastrostomy tube
    M. G tube
    M. G-tube PEG kit
    M. Mark IV tube
    M. T-anchor introducer gun
Mosse syndrome
Mostofi-grade prostate cancer
mother
    m. cyst
    m. endoscopic retrograde cholangiopancreatoscopy system
mother-baby endoscope system
mother-baby-scope system
mother-daughter endoscope
mother-infant dyad
mother-to-infant transmission of hepatitis C virus
motif
    coiled-coil m.
    Patterson-Parker m.
motilide
motilin
    basal release of m.
    m. plasma level
motility
    m. agent
    altered sperm m.
    antropyloroduodenal m.
    colonic m.
    colorectal m.
    m. disorder
    disordered m.
    esophageal m.
    gastrointestinal m.
    ineffective esophageal m. (IEM)
    interdigestive antroduodenal m.
    neurohumoral control of m.
    prefreeze m.
    reduced m.
    sequential m.
    spermatozoon m.
    m. test
Motilium

NOTES

motion
- brownian m.
- full range of m.
- limited range of m.
- paradoxic m.
- passive range of m.
- m. picture camera
- range of m.
- m. sickness

motogenesis
motogenic
motoneuron
- enteric excitatory m.
- enteric inhibitory m.

motor
- m. activity
- m. endplate
- m. examination
- m. meal barium GI series
- m. neuron
- m. oil peritoneal fluid
- m. quiescence
- m. syringe
- m. test meal
- m. unit action potential
- m. urgency

Moto-Tool
- Dremel M.-T.

Motrin
mottled testis
moulage sign
mound
- infraumbilical m.

Moure esophagoscope
mouse
- peritoneal m.

Mousseau-Barbin prosthetic tube
mouth
- m. breathing
- Ceylon sore m.
- m. gag

mouthguard
- oxygenating m.
- Oxyguard oxygenating m.

movable testis
movement
- bowel m. (BM)
- dyscoordinate hyoid m.
- pelvic floor m.
- periodic leg m. (PLM)
- segmentation m.
- symmetric face m.
- tongue m.
- urethral catheter m.
- vermicular m.

moxalactam
moxisylyte injection
MOX TM-100 portable renal preservation machine

Moynihan
- M. artery forceps
- M. bile duct probe
- M. clamp
- M. gall duct forceps
- M. gallstone probe
- M. gallstone scoop
- M. technique
- M. test

MP
- mesenteric panniculitis
- microfibrillar protein

6-MP
- 6-mercaptopurine

MPA
- microscopic polyangiitis

MPD
- main pancreatic duct
  - MPD stent

MPEC
- multipolar electrocoagulation

MPFF
- micronized purified flavonoid fracture

MPGN
- membranoproliferative glomerulonephritis type I, II

M phase
MP-RAGE
- magnetization prepared-rapid gradient echo

MRA
- magnetic resonance angiography

MRC
- magnetic resonance cholangiography
- magnetic resonance colonography

MRCC
- metastatic renal cell carcinoma

MRCP
- magnetic resonance cholangiopancreatography
  - MRCP using HASTE with phased-array coil

MRDM
- malnutrition-related diabetes mellitus

MR hydrography
MRI
- magnetic resonance imaging
  - endorectal surface coil MRI
  - fast spin-echo acquisition MRI
  - rectal coil MRI
  - MRI scan
  - ultrafast MRI

mRNA
- messenger ribonucleic acid
- messenger RNA
  - AR mRNA
  - beta-actin mRNA
  - clusterin mRNA
  - cotransporter mRNA

COX mRNA
cyclooxygenase mRNA
gastrin mRNA
glomerular fibronectin mRNA
HSP-70 mRNA
IGF-binding protein-1 mRNA
IGF-1R mRNA
preproEt-1 mRNA
taurine cotransporter mRNA
TCT mRNA

MRP
magnetic resonance pancreatography
maximum (anal) resting pressure

MRP2
multidrug-resistance-associated protein-2

MRS
magnetic resonance spectroscopy

MRSA
methicillin-resistant *Staphylococcus aureus*

MRT
mean resistance time

MRU
magnetic resonance urography

MS-8
Pancrecarb MS-8

MS-1, -2 hepatitis

MSAO
meal-stimulated acid output

MS Classique balloon dilatation catheter

M-scope multibending scope

MSEV
microsurgical epididymovasostomy

MSH2 **gene**

MSI
microsatellite instability
MSI nylon membrane

MSOF
multiple-system organ failure
multisystem organ failure

MSP
maximum squeeze pressure

MSS
microsatellite stable

MSU
midstream specimen of urine

MSUD
maple-syrup urine disease

MT
malignant teratoma

maximal toleration
microtubule

MTAC
mass transfer area coefficient

MTBE
methyl-*tert*-butyl ether
MTBE gallstone dissolution
MTBE therapy

MTHFR
5,10-methylene-tetrahydrofolate reductase

m-THP-Chlorin

MTI
malignant teratoma, intermediate

MT20, MT24

MTOPS
Medical Therapy of Prostatic Symptoms
MTOPS trial

MTPT
1-methyl-4-phenyl-1,2,3,6-tetrahydropyridine

MTS1 **gene**

MTS2 **gene**

Mt. Sinai classification

MTT
malignant teratoma, trophoblastic
mean transit time

M-TURP
minimal transurethral resection of prostate

MTV
maximum tolerable volume

MTX
methotrexate

MU-3 monoclonal antibody

MUC
mucosal ulcerative colitis

MUC-1 **gene**

mucilaginous

mucin
m. granule
intracytoplasmic m.
m. polymer

mucin-hypersecreting
m.-h. carcinoma
m.-h. tumor

mucinous
m. adenocarcinoma
m. adenoma
m. carcinoma
m. cystadenoma
m. cystic neoplasm
m. cystic tumor

NOTES

mucinous *(continued)*
    m. ductal ectasia (MDE)
    m. pancreatic tumor
    m. tumor nodule
mucin-producing
    m.-p. adenocarcinoma
    m.-p. cancer
    m.-p. tumor
mucin-type glycolipid
Muckle-Wells syndrome
mucocele
    appendiceal m.
    m. of gallbladder
mucociliary clearance
mucocolitis
mucocutaneous
    m. hemorrhoid
    m. pigmentation of Peutz-Jeghers syndrome
mucoenteritis
mucoepidermoid carcinoma
mucoid
    m. secretion
    m. stool
mucolipidosis
mucolytic agent
mucolytic-antifoam solution
mucomembranous enteritis
Mucomyst
mucopolysaccharide
mucoprotein
    Tamm-Horsfall m. (THM)
mucopurulent
    m. cervicitis
    m. exudate
Mucorales
Mucor corymbifera
Mucoreae
mucormycosis
    m. esophagitis
    gastric m.
    isolated renal m.
    pulmonary m.
mucorrhea
mucosa, pl. **mucosae**
    antral m.
    antral-type m.
    antrofundal m.
    biopsy of gastric m.
    blanching of m.
    buccal m.
    burned-out m.
    cardiac stomach m.
    cardiac-type m.
    cobblestone m.
    cobblestoning of m.
    colitic m.
    colorectal m.
    columnar m.
    congested m.
    denuded m.
    duodenal m. (DM)
    dysplastic m.
    ectopic gastric m.
    edematous hyperemic m.
    esophageal m.
    foveolar gastric m.
    friable m.
    frog-spawnlike m.
    fundic m.
    gastric muscularis m.
    gastroduodenal m.
    gastrosuccorrhea m.
    giant hypertrophy of gastric m.
    heterotopic gastric m.
    honeycomb m.
    hyperemic m.
    inflamed m.
    inlet patch m.
    intestinal m.
    lamina muscularis mucosae
    lamina propria of buccal m.
    multifocal ectopic gastric m.
    muscularis m.
    neoanal m.
    normal-appearing m.
    oxyntic m.
    pyloric m.
    rectal m.
    rose thorn ulcer of m.
    sloughing of m.
    tethering of m.
    thumbprinting of m.
    tunica m.
    urothelial m.
    vaginal m.
mucosa-associated
    m.-a. lymphoid tissue (MALT)
    m.-a. lymphoid tissue lymphoma (MALToma)
mucosal
    m. abnormality
    m. abrasion
    m. adenocarcinoma
    m. aneuploidy
    m. angiography
    m. atrophy
    m. background
    m. banding
    m. barrier maturation
    m. biopsy
    m. bleeding
    m. blood flow
    m. blood hemoglobin
    m. border
    m. break
    m. bridge
    m. bridging

m. cell proliferation
m. cobblestoning
m. detachment
m. diverticulum
m. dysplasia
m. electrosensitivity (MES)
m. elevation
m. erosion
m. esophageal ring
m. fatty acid
m. fold
m. gastric ulcer
m. graft
m. guideline pattern
m. hexosamine content
m. homogenate
m. ileal diaphragm
m. ileostomy
m. injury
m. integrity
m. ischemia
m. island
m. junction
m. lesion
m. lesion of acid peptic disease
m. line
m. lymphoid follicle
m. nodularity
m. pallor
m. pit
m. plexus
m. PMN grade
m. polyp
m. proctectomy
m. prolapse
m. prolapse syndrome
m. prostaglandin synthesis
m. sleeve resection
m. stripping
m. suspensory ligament
m. tear
m. tongue
m. ulcerative colitis (MUC)
m. urease
m. vaccine
m. vascular dilation
m. vascular permeability
m. washout
m. web

mucosanguineous
mucosa-to-mucosa anastomosis

mucosectomy
　aspiration m.
　endoanal m.
　endoscopic aspiration m. (EAM)
　endoscopic oblique aspiration m.
　negative pressure-method ambulatory endoscopic esophageal m.
　rectal m.
　suck-and-cut m.
mucosector
　oblique aspiration m.
mucoserous
mucositis
mucous
　m. colic
　m. colitis
　m. crypt
　m. crypt of duodenum
　m. depletion
　m. diarrhea
　m. enteritis
　m. fistula
　m. gel thickness
　m. gland
　m. lake of stomach
　m. membrane
　m. membrane pemphigoid
　m. neck cell
　m. papule
　m. patch
　m. stool
　m. tunic
mucoviscidosis
MUCP
　maximum urethral closure pressure
mucronata
　Bertiella m.
mucus
　excess m.
　extruding m.
　gastric m.
　m. secretagogue
mucus-secreting
　m.-s. cell
　m.-s. gland
mud
　biliary m.
Mueller-Hinton-supplemented agar plate
muelleri
　ductus m.
Muir hemorrhoid forceps
Muir-Torre syndrome

NOTES

Mui Scientific pressurized capillary infusion system
mulberry
    m. calculus
    m. gallstone
    m. lesion
    m. stone
Mulholland sphincterotomy
muliebris
    hydrocele m.
    orificium urethrae externum m.
    testis m.
    urethra m.
mulleri
    Streptococcus m.
müllerian
    m. capsule
    m. duct
    m. duct cyst
    m. duct derivation syndrome
    m. duct, unilateral renal agenesis, and anomalies of cervicothoracic somites (MURCS)
    m. inhibiting factor
    m. remnant
Müller maneuver
multiacinar regenerative nodule
multiband ligating device
Multibite biopsy forceps
multicenter
    m. outcome
    m. prospective trial
    m. study
Multicentre International Liver Tumor Study (MILTS)
multicentricity
multicentric lesion
multichannel
    m. cystometry
    m. recorder
Multiclip
multicystic
    m. dysplastic kidney (MCDK)
    m. kidney (MCK)
    m. kidney disease
    m. renal dysplasia
Multidimensional Fatigue Index (MFI)
multidrug regimen
multidrug resistance associated protein
multidrug-resistance-associated protein-2 (MRP2)
multidrug-resistance gene (MDR1)
multifiber catheter
Multifire
    M. clip applicator
    M. Endo GIA stapling device
Multi-Flex stent
multifocal
    m. atrophic gastritis (MAG)
    m. bladder tumor
    m. ectopic gastric mucosa
    m. involvement
multiforme
    erythema m. (EM)
    glioblastoma m.
Multifunctional Opus surgical table
multigenic origin
Multikine
multiligand receptor
multiloaded clip applier
multiload occlusive clip applicator
multilobar kidney
multilobular
    m. cirrhosis
    m. kidney
multilocular
    m. crypt
    m. cyst
    m. cystic nephroma
multilocularis
    Echinococcus m.
multiloculated cyst
multilumen
    m. manometric catheter
    m. probe
multimodal protocol
multinucleated giant cell
multiorgan
    m. hernia
    m. system failure
multiple
    m. acute rejection episodes
    m. anal sphincterotomies (MAS)
    m. band ligators
    m. biopsies
    m. calices
    m. concentric rings sign
    m. data testing
    m. endocrine adenomatosis type I, II (MEA-I, II)
    m. endocrine neoplasia (MEN)
    m. endocrine neoplasia 1, 2A, 2B
    m. endocrine neoplasia syndrome (MENS)
    m. endoscopic biopsy specimens
    m. familial polyposis
    m. hamartoma syndrome
    m. hepatitis virus infections
    m. intraluminal impedancometries
    m. lymphomatous polyposis (MLP)
    m. myeloma
    m. nodules
    m. organ failure (MOF)
    m. organ failure syndrome
    m. organ system dysfunction (MOSD)
    m. organ system failure (MOSF)
    m. polyps

m. recurrent renal colic
m. sclerosis
m. sidehole manometric assembly
m. stones
m. surgical procedures
m. testing of data
m. vasovasotomies
m. vitamins for infusion
multiple-band ligator
multiple-system
　　m.-s. atrophy
　　m.-s. organ failure (MSOF)
multiplication
　　countercurrent m.
multiplier
　　countercurrent m.
multipolar
　　m. coagulation
　　m. electrocautery
　　m. electrocoagulation (MPEC)
　　m. neuron
Multipulse laser system
multiseptate gallbladder
multiseries
　　Pseudo-nitzschia m.
multispecific organic anion transporter
multisynaptic pathway
multisystem organ failure (MSOF)
multitargeted antifolate
multivariable logistic regression analysis
multivariate
　　m. analysis
　　m. analysis of hematocrit
multocida
　　Pasteurella m.
mumps
　　m. epididymitis
　　m. pancreatitis
Munchausen syndrome
Munich inclusion criteria
Munk disease
Munro point
mural
　　m. kidney
　　m. thrombus
MURCS
　　müllerian duct, unilateral renal agenesis, and anomalies of cervicothoracic somites
　　　　MURCS association
murine
　　m. B16 cell

B72.3 m. monoclonal antibody
m. hepatitis
m. kidney
m. lymphoid cell
m. mesangial cell (MMC)
m. mesangial cell line
m. Peyer patch
m. proximal tubule cell
3T3 m. fibroblast
muris
　　Cryptosporidium m.
　　Trichuris m.
murmur
　　continuous m.
　　Cruveilhier-Baumgarten m.
　　systolic m.
muromonab-CD3
Murphy
　　M. button
　　M. common duct dilator
　　M. drip
　　M. gallbladder retractor
　　M. kidney punch
　　M. sign
　　M. treatment
muscarine
muscarinic
　　m. activity
　　m. blockade
　　m. cholinergic agonist
　　m. receptor
muscimol
muscle
　　adductor brevis m.
　　adductor longus m.
　　aryepiglottic m.
　　m. atrophy
　　Bell m.
　　bladder neck detrusor m.
　　bladder smooth m.
　　Braune m.
　　bulbospongiosus m.
　　circular m.
　　coccygeus m.
　　colonic circular m.
　　cremaster m.
　　cremasteric m.
　　cricopharyngeus m.
　　dartos m.
　　diaphragmatic m.
　　digastric anterior m.
　　digastric posterior m.

NOTES

muscle *(continued)*
    electromyography of penile corpus cavernosum m.
    external anal sphincter m.
    external oblique m.
    external sphincter ani profundus m.
    m. filling
    gastrointestinal smooth m.
    Gavard m.
    geniohyoid m.
    gracilis m.
    m. guarding
    Houston m.
    m. hypertrophy
    iliacus m.
    iliococcygeus m.
    interfoveolar m.
    internal oblique m.
    ischiocavernosus m.
    labium majus m.
    labium minus m.
    lacuna of m.
    latissimus dorsi m.
    m. layer disease
    levator ani m.
    levator veli palatini m.
    lower esophageal sphincter circular m.
    mylohyoid m.
    oblique arytenoid m.
    obturator internus m.
    Ochsner m.
    organic m.
    palatoglossus m.
    palatopharyngeus m.
    paraspinous m.
    pectoralis m.
    pelvis m.
    perineal m.
    periurethral striated m.
    piriformis m.
    pleuroesophageal m.
    psoas m.
    puboanalis m.
    pubococcygeus m.
    puborectal m.
    puborectalis m.
    pubovisceral m.
    pyramidal m.
    rectococcygeus m.
    rectourethral m.
    rectourethralis m.
    rectus abdominis m.
    rhabdosphincter m.
    sacrospinalis m.
    m. sensory receptor
    serratus posterior m.
    smooth m.
    m. spasm
    styloglossus m.
    stylohyoid m.
    stylopharyngeus m.
    submucosal vaginal m.
    superficial trigonal m.
    suspensory m.
    tendinous arch of levator ani m.
    tensor veli palatini m.
    thyroarytenoid m.
    thyrohyoid m.
    transverse abdominis m.
    transversus abdominis m.
    transversus perinei m.
    urogenital sphincter m.
    vascular smooth m.
    visceral m.
    m. wasting
    Wilson m.

muscle-alginate complex
muscle-brain isoenzyme of creatine kinase (CK-MB)
muscle-cutting incision
muscle-filling procedure
muscle-splitting
    m.-s. incision
    m.-s. technique
muscular
    m. coat
    m. dystrophy
    m. esophageal ring
    m. tunic
muscularis
    m. externa
    m. mucosa
    m. propria
    tunica m.
    m. tunnel closure
muscularization of vein
musculature
    electrophysiology of gastric m.
    paraspinal m.
musculocutaneous flap
musculomucoid intimal hyperplasia
musculotropic relaxant
MUSE
    Medicated Urethral System for Erection
    MUSE urethral suppository
mushroom
    Amanita m.
    m. catheter
    Coprinus m.
    m. poisoning
mushroom-and-stem appearance
mushroom-shaped mass
mushy stool
musical bowel sounds
Musshoff modification of Ann Arbor classification

Mustarde
    M. hypospadias repair
    M. procedure
mustard seed
mutagenic effect
Mutamycin
mutated colorectal carcinoma (MCC)
mutation
    C282Y m.
    deletion m.
    endogenous m.
    germline m.
    H63D m.
    insertion m.
    Ki-ras gene m.
    Kirsten-ras oncogen m.
    Liddle m.
    m. mismatch repair (MMR)
    missense m.
    nontruncating m.
    p53 m.
    splice-cite m.
    transition m.
    transversion m.
mutichannel
MutL **gene**
MutS **gene**
Muzsnai modification
muzzled sperm
MVAC, M-VAC
    methotrexate, vinblastine, Adriamycin, cisplatin
M-VEC
    methotrexate, vinblastine, epirubicin, cisplatin
MVO
    mean venous outflow
MVP
    maximum vasal pressure
MVT
    mesenteric vein thrombosis
    acute MVT
mW
    milliwatt
myalgia
    tension m.
myasthenia
    m. gastrica
    m. gravis
mycelial
    m. antibody
    m. phase

mycetism, mycetismus
    m. gastrointestinalis
Mycin
mycobacteria (*pl. of* Mycobacterium)
mycobacterial
    m. antibody
    m. disease
    m. spheroplast
mycobacteriology
Mycobacterium, pl. **mycobacteria**
    M. avium
    M. avium complex
    M. avium-intracellulare (MAI)
    M. bovis
    M. bovis BCG
    M. fortuitum
    M. gordonae
    M. infection
    M. intracellulare
    M. kansasii
    M. leprae
    M. paratuberculosis
    M. phlei cellular extract
    Runyon group III mycobacteria
    M. smegmatis
    M. tuberculosis
    M. xenopi
mycogastritis
Mycolog-II
mycology
mycophenolate
    m. area
    m. mofetil (MMF)
    m. mofetil capsule
    m. mofetil intravenous for injection
    m. mofetil oral suspension
    m. mofetil tablet
mycoplasma
    M. hominis
    m. urethritis
mycoplasmal
mycosis, pl. **mycoses**
    endemic deep m.
    m. fungoides
    gastric m.
    m. intestinalis
Mycostatin
mycotic
    m. aneurysm
    m. gastritis
    m. prostatitis
Mycotrim triphasic culture system

NOTES

MycroMesh biomaterial
myectomy
    anorectal m.
    detrusor m.
myelin kidney
myelocele
myelocystocele
myelodysplasia
myelofibrosis
    primary m.
myelography
myeloid
    m. dentritic cell
    m. metaplasia
myelolipoma
    adrenal gland m.
myeloma
    IgA kappa-chain m.
    m. kidney
    multiple m.
    plasmablastic m.
    m. protein
myelomeningocele
myelomonocytic cell line
myelopathy
    HTLV-I-associated m.
myeloperoxidase
myeloperoxidase-H2O2-halide system
myelophthisic splenomegaly
myeloproliferative
    m. disease
    m. disorder
myelosuppression
myenteric
    m. ganglion cell
    m. plexus
    m. potential oscillation
    m. reflex
myentericus
    plexus m.
Myers bunching technique
Myers-Fine test
Mygel II
myiasis
    intestinal m.
Mylanta-II
Myles hemorrhoidal clamp
Mylicon
Mylius test
mylohyoid muscle
myoblastic myoma
myoblastoma
    bladder granular cell m.
    granular cell m.
myocardial
    m. infarction
    m. ischemia
    m. revascularization
myocelialgia

myoclonic encephalopathy
myoclonus
myoclonus-opsoclonus syndrome
myocutaneous flap
myoelectric activity
myoelectrical
myofibroblast
myofibroma
myogenic tumor
myoglobinuria
myointimal
    m. cell
    m. hyperplasia
Myojector
myolysis
myoma
    ball m.
    myoblastic m.
    red degeneration of uterine m.
myoneurosis
    colic m.
    intestinal m.
myopathy
    childhood visceral m. (CVM)
    familial visceral m. (FVM)
    hereditary internal anal
      sphincter m.
    ipecac-induced m.
    nemaline m.
    nonfamilial visceral m.
    schistosomal pelvic floor m.
    sporadic hollow visceral m.
myoplasty
    latissimus dorsi detrusor m.
myorrhaphy
myosin
    m. crossbridge
    detrusor muscle m.
    m. light-chain kinase
myotomy
    circular m.
    cricoid m.
    cricopharyngeal m.
    esophageal m.
    Heller m.
    laparoscopic Heller m.
    laser-assisted endoscopic m.
    Livaditis circular m.
    longitudinal m.
Myotonachol
myotonic muscular dystrophy
MyoTrac EMG
Myotrophin
Myphentol
Myriadlase Side-Fire laser
myringotomy tube
Mytelase
myxedema ascites
myxocystitis

myxofibroma
myxoglobulosis appendicitis
myxomembranous
    m. colitis
    m. enteritis

myxoneurosis
    intestinal m.
myxorrhea
    m. gastrica
    m. intestinalis

NOTES

¹³N
  ammonia-13
NA
  nalidixic acid
NAB
  nocturnal acid breakthrough
Nabi-HB
NABS
  normoactive bowel sounds
nabumetone
NABX
  needle aspiration biopsy
***N*-Ac-5-ASA**
  N-acetyl-5-ASA
***N*-acetyl-5-ASA (*N*-Ac-5-ASA)**
***N*-acetylated alpha-linked dipeptidase**
***N*-acetyl-beta-D-glucosaminidase**
***N*-acetyl-beta-glucosaminidase (NAG)**
N-acetylcysteine
***N*-acetyl-p-benzoquinoneimine (NAPQI)**
Nachlas gastrointestinal tube
Nachlas-Linton esophagogastric balloon tamponade device
Naclerio
  N. sign
  V sign of N.
NADH
  nicotinamide adenine dinucleotide
nadolol group
NADPH
  nicotinamide adenine dinucleotide phosphate
    NADPH diaphorase stain
    NADPH oxidase
NAE
  net acid excretion
naeslundii
  Actinomyces n.
NaF
  sodium fluorescein
nafamostat mesylate
nafcillin
NAFLD
  nonalcoholic fatty liver disease
nafoxidine
NAG
  N-acetyl-beta-glucosaminidase
  nonagglutinable
    NAG lysosomal marker enzyme
nagging pain
NA+-glucose cotransporter
Na+/H+
  amiloride-sensitive, electroneutral Na+/H+ antiporter

Na+/H+ antiporter
NA+/H+ antiporter activity
nail
  n. bed
  thickened n.
nail-patella syndrome
naive B and T lymphocyte
Nakao snare I, II
Na/K-ATPase
  N.-A. activity
  NaK-ATPase membrane
Nakayama test
naked fat sign
nalbuphine
Naldecon
nalidixic acid (NA)
NA+-linked cotransport system
Nallpen
nalmefene
naloxone hydrochloride
NAMI DDV ligator
nana
  Hymenolepis n.
NANB
  NANB hepatitis
NANC
  nonadrenergic noncholinergic
  NANC inhibitory transmitter
nandrolone decanoate
NaP
  sodium phosphate
naphazoline
naphthylamine
naphthylurea
  polysulfonated n.
napkin-ring annular lesion
nappe
NAPQI
  N-acetyl-p-benzoquinoneimine
NapraPAC
Naprosyn
naproxen sodium
NAPS
  nurse-administered propofol sedation
Naqua
Narcan
Narco
  N. Bio-Systems MMS 200 physiograph tracing
  N. Bio-Systems rectilinear recorder
  N. esophageal motility machine
narcotic
  n. analgesic
  n. bowel syndrome
Nardil

525

Nardi test
naris, pl. **nares**
narrow
    n. albumin gradient ascites
    n. lens
    n. substrate
narrow-band imaging
narrow-caliber duct
narrowing
    bird-beak n.
    discrete n.
    hourglass n.
    luminal n.
nasal
    Concentraid N.
    n. deformity
    n. discharge
    n. feeding
    n. intubation
    n. polyp
    n. trumpet
Nasalcrom
Nasalide
nascent macula densa
NASH
    nonalcoholic steatohepatitis
nasobiliary
    n. drain (NBD)
    n. drainage
    n. drainage catheter
    n. drain cholangiography
    n. tube
nasocystic
    n. catheter
    n. catheter lavage
    n. drain
    n. drainage tube
nasoduodenal feeding tube
nasoenteric
    n. feeding
    n. feeding tube
nasogastric (NG)
    n. aspirate
    n. decompression
    n. drainage
    n. feeding tube
    n. intubation
    n. lavage
    n. suction
    n. tube (NGT)
nasoileal tube
nasojejunal (NJ)
    n. feeding
    n. feeding tube
nasopancreatic
    n. catheter
    n. drainage

nasopharyngeal
    n. angiofibroma
    n. reflux
nasotracheal intubation
nasovesicular
    n. catheter
    n. catheter technique
NAT
    nucleic acid testing
natalizumab
nateglinide
Nathanson liver retractor
national
    N. Association of Anorexia Nervosa and Associated Disorders
    N. Cooperative Dialysis Study
    N. general purpose cystoscope
    N. Health and Nutrition Examination Survey (NHANES)
    N. Institute of Diabetes, Digestive and Kidney Disease (NIDDK)
    N. Institutes of Health (NIH)
    N. Institutes of Health Chronic Prostatitis Symptom Index (NIH-CPSI)
    N. Kidney Foundation-Data Outcomes Quality Initiative (NKF-DOQI)
    n. Prostatic Cancer Project
    N. Prostatic Cancer Treatment Group (NPCTG)
    N. Wilms Tumor Study Group (NWTSG)
native
    n. kidney function
    n. pancreatic secretin receptor
    n. renal biopsy
    n. urethra
    n. valve bacterial endocarditis
NA+ transport system
natriuresis
    pressure n.
natriuretic peptide receptor (NPR)
natural
    n. immunity
    n. killer (NK)
    n. killer cell
    N. stool formula
nature
    Gentle N.
Naturetin
Naturlose
nausea
    chemotherapy-induced n.
    epidemic n.
    postprandial n.
    n. and vomiting (N&V)
    n., vomiting, diarrhea (NVD)
nauseant

nauseate
nauseated
nausea, vomiting, diarrhea (NVD)
nauseous
Navane
navel
> blue n.

navicular abdomen
navicularis
> fossa n.
> valvula fossae n.

Navigator flexible endoscope
Navy single-layer everting anastomosis
NBC
> nephroblastomatosis complex
> nonbacterial cystitis

NBD
> nasobiliary drain
> nucleotide-binding domain

N-benzoyl-L-tyrosyl-P-aminobenzoic
> N-b.-L.-t.-P.-a. acid
> N-b.-L.-t.-P.-a. acid excretion test

NBNC CLD
> non-B non-C chronic liver disease

NBP
> nonbacterial prostatitis

NBT
> nitroblue tetrazolium

NBT-PABA
> nitroblue tetrazolium-paraaminobenzoic acid
> NBT-PABA test

N-butl-2-cyanoacrylate
N-butyl cyanoacrylate
NBVV
> nonbleeding visible vessel

NC
> nephrocalcin

N-cadherin
NCAM, N-CAM
> neural cell-adhesive molecule

NCB
> needle core biopsy

NCCP
> noncardiac chest pain

NCCT
> noncontrast helical computed tomography

NCGN
> necrotizing crescentic glomerulonephritis

NCPF
> noncirrhotic portal fibrosis

NCT
> number connection test

N-demethylation
NDF
> new differentiation factor

NDI
> Nepean Dyspepsia Index
> nephrogenic diabetes insipidus
> X-linked recessive NDI

Nd:YAG
> Nd:YAG laser
> Nd:YAG laser irradiation
> Nd:YAG laser photoablation
> Nd:YAG laser therapy

near-infrared
> n.-i. electronic endoscope
> n.-i. Raman spectroscopy

nebulizer
> jet n.

nebulous urine
NEC
> necrotizing enterocolitis

Necator americanus
necatoriasis
neck
> bladder n.
> humeral n.
> infundibular n.
> n. of pancreas
> tonic n.
> transurethral incision of bladder n. (TUIBN)
> vesical n.

necroinflammation
> lobular n.

necroinflammatory activity
necrolysis
> toxic epidermal n. (TEN)

necrolytic
> n. migratory erythema
> n. migratory erythema syndrome

necropsy
necropurulent appendicitis
necrosectomy
necrosis, pl. **necroses**
> acute sclerosing hyaline n. (ASHN)
> acute tubular n. (ATN)
> arterial wall n.
> avascular n.
> Balser fatty n.
> biliary piecemeal n.
> bowel n.

NOTES

necrosis *(continued)*
  bridging hepatic n.
  calpain in acute tubular n.
  caseating n.
  cecal n.
  cell n.
  central n.
  centrilobular acidophilic n.
  centrizonal n.
  cheesy n.
  coagulation n.
  coagulative n.
  colliquative n.
  colonic n.
  confluent hepatic n.
  distal renal tubular n.
  drug-induced acute tubular n.
  electrocoagulation n.
  enzymatic fat n.
  ethanol-induced tumor n. (ETN)
  fatty n.
  fibrinoid n.
  fibrosing piecemeal n.
  focal hepatocellular n.
  gangrenous n.
  glomerular n.
  gummatous n.
  heme pigment-induced acute tubular n.
  hepatocellular n.
  hepatocyte n.
  icteric n.
  infected pancreatic n.
  infectious pancreatic n.
  intestinal n.
  ischemia n.
  laminar cortical n.
  liquefactive n.
  massive epithelial cell n.
  massive hepatic n.
  maximum coagulative n.
  metastatic fat n.
  moist n.
  nephrotoxic tubular n.
  pancreatic glandular n.
  papillary n.
  patchy n.
  penile n.
  pericentral n.
  peripancreatic n.
  peripheral n.
  perivenular confluent n.
  piecemeal n.
  postischemic tubular n.
  pressure n.
  progressive emphysematous n.
  puromycin aminonucleoside n.
  renal coagulation n.
  n. of renal papilla
  renal papillary n. (RPN)
  renal tubular n.
  renocortical n.
  scrotal fat n.
  septic n.
  spinal cord n.
  spontaneous penile ischemic n.
  sterile pancreatic n.
  strangulation n.
  subacute hepatic n.
  submassive hepatic n.
  tissue n.
  tubular n.
  tumor n.
necrospermia
necrotic
  n. cirrhosis
  n. hemorrhagic colitis
  n. hemorrhoid
  n. tissue
  n. ulceration
necroticans
  enteritis n.
necrotizing
  n. bowel vasculitis
  n. crescentic glomerulonephritis (NCGN)
  n. enterocolitis (NEC)
  n. fasciitis
  n. fasciitis of scrotum
  n. infection
  n. pancreatitis
  n. vasculitis of bowel
necrozoospermia
needle
  n. ablation
  Articulator injection n.
  ASAP channel-cut automated biopsy n.
  ASAP prostate biopsy n.
  aspirating n.
  n. aspiration biopsy (NABX)
  n. aspiration cytology
  Baldwin perineum n.
  Bassini n.
  B-D Safety-Gard n.
  bicurved n.
  n. biopsy diagnosis
  Biopty cut n.
  BIP high-speed multibiopsy n.
  n. bladder neck suspension
  blunt n.
  butterfly n.
  Carr-Locke injection n.
  CE-24 n.
  Chiba n.
  Childs-Phillips intestinal plication n.
  circle n.
  Colapinto n.

needle · needle-knife

concentric n.
n. core biopsy (NCB)
Corson n.
n. count
curved transjugular n.
cutting LR n.
diathermic precut n.
n. driver
Durrani dorsal vein complex ligation n.
EchoTip Ultra endoscopic n.
n. electrode
n. electrode electromyography
electrosurgical n.
EUSN-1 EchoTip n.
Ferguson n.
fine n.
flexible aspiration n.
Franseen n.
French eye n.
GAN-19 n.
gastrointestinal n.
Gittes n.
Greenwald n.
Grice suture n.
Hemoject n.
n. holder
Howell n.
n. hydrophone
J n.
Jamshidi liver biopsy n.
Keith n.
KeyMed disposable variceal injection n.
Klatskin liver biopsy n.
n. knife
Lahey aneurysm n.
Madayag biopsy n.
Mayo trocar-point n.
Menghini liver biopsy n.
Microvasive sclerotherapy n.
monopolar triple-hook active n.
noncutting n.
Nottingham colposuspension n.
Olympus NM-K-series sclerotherapy n.
Olympus NM-L-series n.
Olympus reusable oval-cup forceps with n.
optical n.
n. papillotome
Pentax prototype n.
Pereyra n.
pneumoperitoneum n.
Promex biopsy n.
PS-2 n.
Quick-Core n.
reusable forceps with n.
n. root
Safety AV fistula n.
sclerotherapy n.
Securcut aspiration biopsy n.
Seldinger gastrostomy n.
Silverman n.
Silverman-Boeker n.
single-use maximum-capacity radial jaw with n.
skinny Chiba n.
smaller gauge n.
Spinelli biopsy n.
Stamey n.
Stifcore transbronchial aspiration n.
Sure-Cut biopsy n.
n. suspension procedure
suture-release n.
swaged n.
swaged-on n.
tapered n.
through-the-scope injection n.
n. tracheoesophageal puncture
n. tract
Tru-Cut biopsy n.
Tru Taper Ethalloy n.
TT-3 n.
Turner-Warwick n.
Variject n.
Veress n.
Vim-Silverman biopsy n.
Williams n.
winged steel n.
Yang n.

needle-catheter jejunostomy
needle-knife
n.-k. electrocautery (NKE)
n.-k. endoscopic pancreatic sphincterotomy
n.-k. fistulotome
n.-k. fistulotomy (NKF)
n.-k. papillotome
n.-k. papillotomy (NKP)
n.-k. precut papillotomy (NKPP)
n.-k. sphincterotome
n.-k. technique
n.-k. wire

NOTES

needleless system
needlescope device
needlescopic adrenalectomy
needle-tip
    n.-t. catheter
    n.-t. laparoscopic electrode
needle-tipped sphincterotome
needle-track seeding
nefazodone hydrochloride
negative
    n. anatomical factor
    n. core biopsy specimen
    n. immunofluorescence
    n. laparotomy
    n. nitrogen balance
    n. predictive value (NPV)
    n. pressure-controlled tube
    n. pressure-method ambulatory endoscopic esophageal mucosectomy
    n. pressure overtube
negative-pressure tube
NegGram
negligible blood loss
negro
    vomito n.
Negus rigid esophagoscope
Neil-Moore electrode
Neisseria gonorrhoeae
Neisser syringe
Neivert polyp hook
Nélaton
    N. catheter
    N. fold
    N. rubber tube drain
    N. sphincter
nelfinavir
Nellcor Durasensor adult oxygen transducer
Nelson
    N. forceps
    N. scissors
    N. syndrome
nemaline myopathy
nematode infection
nematodiasis
Nembutal
NEMD
    nonspecific esophageal motility disorder
neoadjuvant
    n. androgen derivation therapy
    n. antiandrogenic treatment
    n. chemoradiation
    n. chemotherapy
    n. hormonal ablation therapy
    n. hormonal deprivation
    n. total androgen ablation
neoanal
    n. function
    n. mucosa
    n. sphincter
neobladder
    Camey n.
    decompensated n.
    gastric n.
    Hautmann ileal n.
    hemi-Kock n.
    ileal n.
    ileocolonic n.
    Kock n.
    Le Bag n.
    Melchior ileal n.
    orthotopic ileal n.
    sigmoid n.
    Studer n.
    W-stapled ileal n.
neobladder-urethra anastomosis
neocholangiole
Neocholex
neocystostomy
    ureteral n.
    ureteroileal n.
neodymium:YAG laser therapy
neodymium:yttrium-aluminum-garnet
neodymium:yttrium garnet laser
neoformans
    Candida n.
    Cryptococcus n.
neointimal hyperplasia
Neo-Lax
Neoloid
neomeatus
Neomed electrocautery
neomembrane
neomycin
neonatal
    n. adrenal gland hemorrhage
    n. arginine vasopressin
    n. cholestasis
    n. conjugated hyperbilirubinemia
    n. exstrophic bladder repair
    n. hepatitis
    n. jaundice
    n. oliguria
neonate
    amino acid excretion in n.
    aminoaciduria in n.
neonatorum
    icterus n.
    melena n.
    volvulus n.
neopenis
neophallus
neoplasia
    anal intraepithelial n. (AIN)
    cervical intraepithelial n. (CIN)
    colonic n.
    distal n.

intratubular germ cell n. (ITGCN)
metachronous n.
multiple endocrine n. (MEN)
multiple endocrine n. 1, 2A, 2B
penile intraepithelial n.
predictors of proximal n.
preinvasive urothelial n.
prostatic intraepithelial n. (PIN)
n. risk

neoplasm
anal n.
bladder n.
colorectal n.
extragonadal germ cell n.
genitourinary n.
germ cell n.
intraductal mucin-hypersecreting n.
intraductal oncocytic papillary n. (IOPN)
intraductal papillary-mucinous n. (IPMN)
malignant pancreatic n.
megacystic mucinous n.
n. metastasis
mucinous cystic n.
nonseminomatous germ cell n.
paratesticular n.
periampullary n.
prostatic n.
retroperitoneal n.
n. staging
stomach n.
urothelial n.
vascular n.

neoplastic
n. cell proliferation
n. cyst
n. disease
n. lesion
n. origin
n. polyp
n. potential
n. renal mass
n. tissue
n. transformation

Neopterin
Neoral
neorectal emptying
neorectum
neoscrotum
neosphincter
Acticon n.

gracilis n.
stimulated gracilis n.
Neosporin G.U. Irrigant
neostigmine methylsulfate
neostomy
neoterminal ileum
neotransformation
papillomatous n.
neoumbilicus
neourethra
Mitrofanoff n.
Neo-Vadrin
neovagina
n. construction
gracilis myocutaneous n.
skin graft n.
neovascular bundle
neovascularization
Nepean Dyspepsia Index (NDI)
nephelometry
nephradenoma
nephralgia
idiopathic n.
nephralgic
NephrAmine
nephrectomize
nephrectomized
nephrectomy
abdominal n.
adjunctive n.
adjuvant n.
n. allograft
anterior n.
apical polar n.
Balkan n.
bilateral n.
cytoreductive n.
difficult n.
donor n.
extracorporeal partial n.
extraperitoneal laparoscopic n.
extraperitoneal supracostal live-donor n.
flank n.
laparoscopic living donor n.
laparoscopic partial n. (LPN)
laparoscopic radical n. (LRN)
laser partial n.
live-donor n.
lumbar n.
morcellated n.
palliative n.

NOTES

nephrectomy *(continued)*
    paraperitoneal n.
    partial polar n.
    perifascial n.
    polar segmental n.
    posterior n.
    radical n.
    retroperitoneoscopic n.
    simple n.
    transperitoneal laparoscopic n. (TLN)
    transplant n.
    unilateral n.

nephredema
nephrelcosis
nephremia
nephremphraxis
nephric
nephridium
nephritic
    n. calculus
    n. edema
    n. sediment
    n. syndrome

nephritis, pl. **nephritides**
    acute focal bacterial n. (AFBN)
    acute interstitial n. (AIN)
    acute serum sickness n.
    acute suppurative n.
    albuminous n.
    allergic interstitial n.
    anaphylactoid purpura n.
    antiglomerular basement membrane antibody n.
    antiglomerular basement membrane-negative crescentric glomerular n.
    anti-Thy-1 n.
    autoimmune interstitial n.
    bacterial n.
    Balkan n.
    capsular n.
    n. caseosa
    caseous n.
    catarrhal n.
    cheesy n.
    chloroazotemic n.
    clostridial n.
    crescentic n.
    croupous n.
    degenerative n.
    diffuse suppurative n.
    n. dolorosa
    dropsical n.
    embolic n.
    epidemic n.
    exudative n.
    fibrolipomatous n.
    fibrous n.
    focal bacterial n.
    glomerulocapsular n.
    n. gravidarum
    hemorrhagic n.
    hereditary n.
    Heymann n.
    hydremic n.
    hydropigenous n.
    hypogenetic n.
    ICR strain-derived glomerular n. (ICGN)
    idiopathic hypocomplementemic interstitial n.
    immune-mediated interstitial n.
    indurative n.
    infection-related interstitial n.
    interstitial scarlatinal n.
    interstitial syphilitic n.
    Lancereaux n.
    latent n.
    leptospiral n.
    lipomatous n.
    Lohlein n.
    lupus n. (LN)
    Masugi n.
    mercuric chloride-induced n.
    n. mitis
    nephrotoxic n. (NTN)
    nephrotoxic antiglomerular basement membrane antibody n.
    nephrotoxic serum n.
    parenchymatous n.
    passive Heymann n. (PHN)
    pauciimmune glomerular n.
    phenacetin n.
    pneumococcus n.
    potassium-losing n.
    n. of pregnancy
    productive n.
    salt-losing n.
    saturnine n.
    scarlatinal n.
    serum n.
    shunt n.
    silent lupus n.
    Steblay n.
    subacute n.
    suppurative cortical n.
    syphilitic n.
    tartrate n.
    transfusion n.
    trench n.
    tuberculous n.
    tubulointerstitial n. (TIN)
    vascular n.
    Volhard n.
    war n.
    water-losing n.

nephritogenic
    n. antigen
    n. epitope
nephroabdominal
nephroangiosclerosis
nephroblastoma
nephroblastomatosis complex (NBC)
nephrocalcin (NC)
nephrocalcinosis
    calcium phosphate n.
nephrocapsectomy
nephrocardiac
nephrocele
nephrocelom
nephrocolic
nephrocolopexy
nephrocoloptosis
nephrocystanastomosis
nephroerysipelas
nephrogastric
nephrogenic, nephrogenetic
    n. adenoma
    n. ascites
    n. cord
    n. diabetes insipidus (NDI)
    n. rest
    n. ridge
    n. zone
nephrogenous
    n. albuminuria
    n. dialysis ascites
    n. proteinuria
nephrogram
    delayed n.
    diffuse patchy n.
    rim n.
    soap-bubble n.
nephrography
    isotope n.
nephrohemia
nephrohydrosis
nephrohypertrophy
nephroid
nephrolith
nephrolithiasis
    autosomally inherited form of n.
    calcium oxalate n.
    N. Clinical Guidelines Panel
    glucocorticoid-induced hypercalcemic n.
    hypercalcemic n.
    iatrogenic hypercalcemic n.
    indinavir-induced n.
    percutaneous n.
    X-linked recessive n. (XRN)
nephrolitholapaxy
    percutaneous n.
nephrolithotomy
    anatrophic n.
    minipercutaneous n.
    morbidity of percutaneous n.
    percutaneous n. (PCN, PCNL, PNL)
    simultaneous bilateral percutaneous n. (SBPN)
nephrolithotripsy
    percutaneous n. (PCNL)
nephrologist
nephrology
nephrolysin
nephrolysis
nephrolytic
nephroma
    congenital mesoblastic n.
    cystic n.
    embryonal n.
    kidney n.
    mesoblastic n.
    multilocular cystic n.
nephromalacia
nephromegaly
nephron
    aldosterone-sensitive distal n.
    n. loss
    mesonephric n.
    n. plasma flow
    proximal n.
    n. segment
    n. transport
    N. underdosing
nephroncus
nephronia
    lobar n.
nephronophthisis, nephrophthisis
    familial juvenile n.
    juvenile n.
nephron-sparing surgery
nephroparalysis
nephropathia
    n. epidemica
    n. epidermica kidney
nephropathic
nephropathy
    acute hypokalemic n.

NOTES

nephropathy *(continued)*
    acute urate n.
    acute uric acid n.
    Adriamycin n.
    amphotericin B n.
    amyloid n.
    analgesic n.
    Balkan n.
    Berger n.
    bismuth n.
    cadmium n.
    carbon tetrachloride n.
    cast n.
    chronic allograft n.
    chronic hypokalemic n.
    chronic urate n.
    cisplatin n. (CPN)
    copper n.
    C1q n.
    Danubian endemic familial n.
    diabetic n.
    dropsical n.
    epidemic n.
    gold n.
    human immunodeficiency virus-associated n. (HIVAN)
    hypazoturic n.
    hypercalcemic n.
    hypochloruric n.
    hypokalemic n.
    IgA n.
    IgM n.
    immunoglobulin A n.
    incipient n.
    iodide n.
    iron n.
    kaliopenic n.
    kanamycin n.
    lead n.
    malarial n.
    membranous n.
    mesangial n.
    nonnephrotic immunoglobulin A n.
    obstructive n.
    overt n.
    oxalate n.
    phenacetin n.
    polymyxin n.
    n. of potassium depletion
    proteinuric n.
    puromycin aminonucleoside n. (PAN)
    Ramipril Efficacy in N. (REIN)
    reflux n.
    salt-losing n.
    sickle cell n.
    silver n.
    sodium-wasting n.
    streptomycin n.
    sulfonamide n.
    tetracycline n.
    toxic n.
    tropical n.
    tubular n.
    tubulointerstitial n.
    urate n.
    uric acid n.
    vascular n.
nephropexy
nephrophagiasis
nephrophthisis *(var. of* nephronophthisis)
nephropoietic
nephropoietin
nephroptosis, nephroptosia
nephropyelitis
nephropyelography
nephropyelolithotomy
nephropyeloplasty
nephropyosis
nephrorrhagia
nephrorrhaphy
nephrosclerosis
    arteriolar n.
    benign n.
    hyaline arteriolar n.
    hyperplastic arteriolar n.
    hypertensive n. (HN)
    intercapillary n.
    malignant n.
    senile n.
nephroscope
    flexible n.
    rigid n.
    n. sheath
    steerable n.
    Storz n.
    Wolf percutaneous universal n.
nephroscopy
    anatrophic n.
    antegrade n.
    flexible n.
    second-look flexible n.
nephrosis
    acute n.
    Adriamycin-induced n.
    amyloid n.
    cholemic n.
    congenital n.
    Epstein n.
    familial n.
    glycogen n.
    Heymann n.
    hydropic n.
    hypokalemic n.
    infectious avian n.
    larval n.
    lipid n.
    lipoid n. (LN)

lower nephron n.
mercurial n.
osmotic n.
pure n.
puromycin aminonucleoside n. (PAN)
steroid-dependent idiopathic n.
steroid-resistant idiopathic n.
steroid-sensitive idiopathic n.
vacuolar n.
n. with hypovolemia
n. without hypovolemia

nephrosonephritis
hemorrhagic n.
Korean hemorrhagic n.

nephrosplenopexy
nephrostogram
nephrostolithotomy
percutaneous n. (PCNL)

nephrostomy
n. catheter
percutaneous n.
retrograde n.
n. tract
n. tube

nephrotic
n. edema
n. syndrome

nephrotomic cavity
nephrotomogram
nephrotomography
infusion n.

nephrotomy
abdominal n.
anatrophic n.
lumbar n.
n. tube

nephrotoxic
n. acute renal failure
n. antiglomerular basement membrane antibody nephritis
n. antiserum
n. nephritis (NTN)
n. serum nephritis
n. tubular necrosis

nephrotoxicity
cadmium-induced n.
cyclosporine n.
mercuric chloride n.

nephrotoxin
nephrotropic
nephrotuberculosis

nephrotyphoid
nephroureteral stent
nephroureterectasis
nephroureterectomy
Beer n.
bilateral n.
hand-assisted laparoscopic n. (HALNU)
laparoscopic radical n.
radical n.
transperitoneal laparoscopic n.
n. with en bloc removal of cuff of bladder

nephroureterocystectomy
nephroureteroscopy
virtual n.

nephrourography
nephrovesical stent
Nephrox Suspension
Nepro diet supplement
Neptune girdle
NERD
nonerosive reflux disease

Nernst equation
nerve
afferent renal n.
anterior scrotal n.
n. block
cavernosal n.
cavernous n.
n. conduction study
n. cooling
criminal n.
dorsal n. of penis
n. entrapment syndrome
extrapudendal pelvic n.
femoral n.
genitofemoral n.
gluteal n.
n. of Grassi
n. growth factor (NGF)
n. growth factor receptor (NGFR)
n. hook
hypogastric n.
iliohypogastric n.
ilioinguinal n.
inferior anal n.
inferior rectal n.
intrapancreatic n.
n. of Latarjet
noncholinergic n.
obturator n.

NOTES

nerve *(continued)*
    pelvic autonomic n.
    perineal n.
    posterior scrotal n.
    postganglionic cholinergic n.
    postganglionic sympathetic n.
    pudendal pelvic n.
    rectal n.
    renal afferent n.
    renal sympathetic n.
    saphenous n.
    sciatic n.
    somatic peripheral n.
    splanchnic n.
    subcostal n.
    transcutaneous n.
    n. transsection
    vagus n.
nerve-sparing
    n.-s. lymph node dissection
    n.-s. radical retropubic prostatectomy
nervi (*pl. of* nervus)
nervosa
    anorexia n. (AN)
    bulimia n.
    dysphagia n.
nervosus
    singultus gastricus n.
nervous
    n. bladder
    n. dyspepsia
    n. eructation
    n. gut
    n. indigestion
    n. urine
    n. vomiting
nervus, pl. **nervi**
    nervi erigentes
Nesbit
    N. corporeal
    N. cystoscope
    N. operation
    N. plication
    N. technique
    N. technique ureterocolonic anastomosis
    N. tuck procedure
nesidiectomy
nesidioblastoma
NESP
    Novel erythropoiesis-stimulating protein
nest
    Brunn epithelial n.
NET
    neuroendocrine tumor
net
    n. acid excretion (NAE)
    rotatable Roth retrieval n.
    Roth polyp retrieval n.
    ureteric retrieval n.
netilmicin
Netromycin
network
    capillary n.
    Pentax EndoNet digital endoscopy n.
    trans-Golgi n.
    vascular collateral n.
Neubauer and Fischer test
Neukomm test
Neu-Laxova syndrome
Neu oncoprotein
neural
    n. cell-adhesive molecule (NCAM, N-CAM)
    n. control
    n. growth factor receptor (NGFR)
    n. invasion
    n. nodule
    n. pathway
    n. plexus
neuraminidase
neuraminidase-treated sheep erythrocyte
neurapraxia
neurasthenia
    gastric n.
neurectomy
    gastric n.
neurinoma
neuroaminidase
neuroanatomy
neuroblastoma
    cervical n.
    metastatic n.
    olfactory bulb n.
    paravertebral n.
    presacral n.
    n. staging
    n. subcutaneous nodule
neuroblockage
neurocutaneous syndrome
neurodegenerative disorder
neuroectodermal dysplasia
neuroendocrine
    n. cell
    n. tumor (NET)
neuroendocrinology
    gastrointestinal n.
neurofibroma
    bladder n.
    duodenal n.
    gastrointestinal n.
    plexiform n.
    von Recklinghausen gastric n.
neurofibromatosis (NF)
    familial intestinal n.
    von Recklinghausen n.

neurofilament protein triplet
neurogastroenterology
neurogenic
    n. bladder
    n. bladder disease
    n. diabetes insipidus
    n. disorder
    n. dysphagia
    n. erectile dysfunction
    n. hyperreflexia
    n. intestinal obstruction
    n. refractory urge incontinence
    n. secretory diarrhea
    n. sphincteric incompetence
    n. tumor
neurogram
    pudendal n.
neurohumoral
    n. control of motility
    n. disease
    n. excitation state
    n. factor
neurohumoral-immune axis
neurohypophysis
neuroimmune dysfunction
neurokinin A, B
neurologic
    n. complication
    n. deficit
    n. disorder
neurolysis
    celiac plexus n. (CPN)
    CT-guided celiac plexus n.
    endoscopic ultrasound-guided celiac plexus n.
    endosonography-guided celiac plexus n.
    EUS-guided celiac plexus n.
neurolytic
    n. celiac plexus block
    n. drug
neuroma
neuromedin U
neuromodulation
    chronic sacral n.
    efficacy of n.
    percutaneous sacral nerve root n.
    sacral nerve n.
    sacral root n.
    subchronic sacral n.
    n. work

neuron
    adrenergic n.
    afferent n.
    alpha motor n.
    argyrophilic and argyrophobic n.'s
    bipolar n.
    cholinergic n.
    enteric vasodilator n.
    final motor n.
    gamma-aminobutyric acidergic n.
    intestinofugal n.
    motor n.
    multipolar n.
    nonadrenergic n.
    noncholinergic n.
    parasympathetic postganglionic n.
    parasympathetic preganglionic n.
    peptidergic n.
    S n.
    sensory n.
    serotoninergic n.
    unipolar n.
    upper motor n.
    vagal input n.
    vagal preganglionic n.
neuronal cell line
neuronoma
    VIP-secreting n.
neuron-specific enolase (NSE)
neuroparacrine mechanism
neuropathic
    n. bladder
    n. cystinosis
    n. voiding dysfunction
neuropathy
    autonomic n.
    cyclosporine-induced optic n.
    diabetic autonomic n.
    familial visceral n. (FVN)
    idiopathic nonfamilial visceral n.
    IgA n.
    immunoglobulin n.
    membranous n.
    optic n.
    pigment n.
    polyradicular n.
    pudendal n.
    reflux n.
    topical n.
    vasculitic n.
    visceral n.
neuropeptide Y (NPY)

NOTES

neuropharmacology
neurophysiologic recording
neurophysiology
    pelvic floor n.
neuroplasticity
neuropsychotropic drug
neurosis, pl. **neuroses**
    bladder n.
neurospinal dysraphism
neurosteroid
neurostimulation
    root n.
    sacral n.
    transcutaneous sacral n.
neurotensin
neurotensinoma
neurotransmitter
    noncholinergic n.
neurotrophin
neurotropic
neuroureterectomy
neurourological
neurturin
neutral
    n. endopeptidase
    K-Phos N.
neutralophile
Neutra-Phos
Neutra-Phos-K
Neutrexin
neutrocytic ascites
neutron
neutropenia
neutropenic
    n. colitis
    n. typhlitis
neutrophil
    n. chemotactic peptide
    n. dysfunction
    n. elastase
    polymorphonuclear n. (PMNN)
    WBC n.
neutrophil-activating protein of *Helicobacter pylori* (HP-NAP)
neutrophilia
neutrophilic
    n. cryptitis
    n. dermatosis
    n. gastroduodenitis
    n. infiltration
neutropic virus
nevi (*pl. of* nevus)
Neville tracheal reconstruction prosthesis
nevirapine
nevus, pl. **nevi**
    n. flammeus
    inguinal crease compound n.
    pigmented n.
    spider n.

new
    n. chemotherapy combinations for advanced bladder cancer
    n. differentiation factor (NDF)
newborn
    n. hepatitis
    n. jaundice
newcastle
    Shigella n.
Newman proctoscope
newport
    Salmonella n.
NexACT
Nexium triple therapy
nexus
Nezhat-Dorsey irrigator/aspirator
NF
    neurofibromatosis
    nitrofurazone Foley
NF-KB
    nuclear factor kappa B
***N*-formyl-methionyl-leucyl-phenylalanine (fMLP, FMLP)**
NG
    nasogastric
    NG suction
NGD-95-1 antiobesity compound
NGF
    nerve growth factor
NGFR
    nerve growth factor receptor
    neural growth factor receptor
^{15}N-glutamine
NGT
    nasogastric tube
NH2-terminal SH2 domain
NHANES
    National Health and Nutrition Examination Survey
NHL
    non-Hodgkin lymphoma
NHS
    Nurses' Health study
niacin deficiency
nialamide
Nibblit
nicardipine
niche sign
Nichols-Condon bowel preparation
Nichols IRMA kit
nick end-labeling
niclosamide
Nicolet SM-300 stimulator
Nicorette
nicotinamide
    n. adenine dinucleotide (NADH)
    n. adenine dinucleotide phosphate (NADPH)
nicotine

nicotinic
- n. agonist
- n. receptor
- n. receptor blocker

NIDDK
National Institute of Diabetes, Digestive and Kidney Disease

NIDDM
noninsulin-dependent diabetes mellitus

nidogen
Niemann-Pick disease
Niemeier gallbladder perforation
nifedipine
- n. extended release
- n. ointment
- topical n.

Niferex-150
Niflex PEG-based lavage fluid
nifurtimox
niger
- vomitus n.

nigericin
nightly intermittent peritoneal dialysis (NIPD)
nighttime polyuria
nigra
- linea n.

nigricans
- acanthosis n.
- malignant acanthosis n.

NIH
National Institutes of Health
- NIH Classification Category I acute bacterial prostatitis
- NIH Classification Category II chronic bacterial prostatitis
- NIH Classification Category III inflammatory and noninflammatory chronic pelvic pain
- NIH Classification Category I–IV
- NIH Classification Category IV asymptomatic inflammatory prostatitis
- NIH Classification System for Prostatitis

NIH-CPSI
National Institutes of Health Chronic Prostatitis Symptom Index
- NIH-CPSI prostatitis classification
- NIH-CPSI type I–IV

NIHF
nonimmune hydrops fetalis

Nihon
- N. Kohden polygraph
- N. tocodynamometer

nihonkaiense
- *Diphyllobothrium n.*

Nilandron
nil disease
Nilstat
nilutamide
nimesulide
nimodipine
Ninhydrin
Niopam contrast medium
NIPD
nightly intermittent peritoneal dialysis

nipple
- antireflux n.
- antirefluxing n.
- continence n.
- n. discharge
- ileum n.
- intussuscepted ileal triple n.
- Kock n.
- pigmented n.
- n. slippage
- split-cuff n.
- ureteral split-cuff n.
- n. valve

nippled stoma
Nippostrongylus brasiliensis
Nipride
niridazole
Nisbet
- N. chancre
- N. disease

nisoldipine
N-isopropyl-p-iodoamphetamine
- biodistribution of N.-i.-p.-i.

Nissen
- N. antireflux operation
- N. 360-degree wrap fundoplication
- N. fundoplication wrap
- N. gall duct forceps
- lap N.
- N. laparoscopic fundoplication
- N. repair

Nissenkorn stent
nitazoxanide
nitidus
- lichen n.

nitinol
- n. basket

NOTES

nitinol *(continued)*
    n. mesh-covered frame
    n. mesh stent
    n. wire
nitisinone
Niti-S stent
nitrate
    gallium n.
    intravesical silver n.
    methylatropine n.
    organic n.
    silver n.
nitrate-induced venodilation
nitrazepam
nitrendipine
nitric
    n. oxide (NO)
    n. oxide-blocked sphincter relaxation
    n. oxide donor
    n. oxide-releasing nonsteroidal antiinflammatory drugs (NO-NSAIDs)
    n. oxide-releasing NSAIDS
    n. oxide synthase inhibitor
    n. oxide synthetase
nitrite
    amyl n.
    dietary n.
    n. test
4-nitrobiphenyl
nitroblue
    n. tetrazolium (NBT)
    n. tetrazolium-paraaminobenzoic acid (NBT-PABA)
9-nitrocamptothecin
nitrocellulose filter
nitrofigilis
    Acrobacter n.
nitrofuran
nitrofurantoin hepatotoxicity
nitrofurazone Foley (NF)
nitrogen
    n. balance
    blood urea n. (BUN)
    glutamine n.
    high n. (HN)
    high calorie and n. (HCN)
    n. overload
    n. partition test
    n. retention test
    serum urea n. (SUN)
    total body n. (TBN)
    urea n. (UN)
    urine urea n. (UUN)
nitrogenous waste
nitroglycerin
    intravenous n.
    n. ointment
    vasopressin with n.
nitroimidazole
2-nitropropane hepatotoxicity
nitroprusside
    sodium n. (SNP)
4-nitroquinolin-1-oxide-induced tumor (4NOQ)
nitrosamine
    carcinogenic n.
nitroso compound
nitrosourea
Nitrostat
nitrous
    n. oxide
    n. oxide insufflator
nizatidine
Nizoral
NJ
    nasojejunal
    NJ feeding tube
NK
    natural killer
    NK cell
NK1, NK2 tachykinin receptor
NKE
    needle-knife electrocautery
NKF
    needle-knife fistulotomy
NKF-DOQI
    National Kidney Foundation-Data Outcomes Quality Initiative
NKP
    needle-knife papillotomy
NKPP
    needle-knife precut papillotomy
NLH
    nodular lymphoid hyperplasia
N-linked glycoprotein
N loop
NLV
    Norwalk-like virus
NM
    nuclear medicine
NM23 **gene**
N^G**-monomethyl-L-arginine (L-NMMA)**
NMP
    nuclear matrix protein-22
NMP22
    NMP22 BladderChek
    NMP22 BladderChek test
NMP-22
    nuclear matrix protein-22
NMR
    nuclear magnetic resonance
N-myc oncogene
N^G**-nitro-L-arginine methyl ester (L-NAME)**
N-nitrosamine

NNRTI
nonnucleoside reverse transcription inhibitor
NO
nitric oxide
Noble
N. bowel plication
N. surgical plication of bowel
Nocardia otitidis-caviarum
nociceptin/orphanin FQ (N/OFQ)
nociceptive
n. sensory input
n. stimulation
n. structure
nociceptor
nocte
ranitidine n.
nocturia
age-related n.
nocturnal
n. acid breakthrough (NAB)
n. acid reflux
n. diarrhea
n. emission
n. enuresis
n. erection
n. gastric reflux
n. heartburn
n. hemodialysis
n. incontinence
n. pain
n. penile tumescence (NPT)
n. penile tumescence monitoring
n. polyuria
n. regurgitation
n. tumescence self-monitoring
node
celiac lymph n.
n. of Cloquet
n. dissection
n. distribution
Ewald n.
hypogastric n.
inguinal lymph n.
intermediate mesenteric lymph n.
juxtaposed mesenteric lymph n.'s
juxtaregional n.
lymph n.
matted n.
mesenteric lymph n. (MLN)
obturator lymph n.
Osler n.
pelvic lymph n.
perigastric n.
retrorectal lymph n.
sentinel n.
shotty lymph n.'s
Sister Mary Joseph lymph n.
subcarinal n.
succulent mesenteric lymph n.
Troisier n.
Virchow sentinel n.
Virchow-Troisier n.
nodosa
periarteritis n.
polyarteritis n.
vasitis n.
nodose ganglion
nodosum
erythema n.
nodular
n. hyperplasia of prostate
n. lesion
n. liver
n. lymphoid hyperplasia (NLH)
n. lymphoma
n. pancreatitis
n. regenerative hyperplasia (NRH)
n. transformation
n. transitional cell carcinoma
nodularity
antral n.
coarse n.
mucosal n.
surface n.
nodulated
nodulation
nodule
cecal mucosal n.
colonic lymphoid n.
daughter n.
discrete n.
Gamna n.
Gandy-Gamna n.
gelatinous n.
hyperplastic n.
liver n.
lymphoid n.
lymphomatous n.
macroregenerative n.
mucinous tumor n.
multiacinar regenerative n.
multiple n.'s
neural n.

nodule *(continued)*
    neuroblastoma subcutaneous n.
    pentastomum denticulatum n.
    peritoneal n.
    prostatic n.
    regenerative cirrhotic n.
    siderotic n.
    Sister Mary Joseph n.
    spindle cell n.
    surface n.
    thyroid n.
    yellow n.
nodule-in-nodule pattern
N/OFQ
    nociceptin/orphanin FQ
nolatrexed dihydrochloride
Nolvadex
nomenclature
    anorectal n.
nomogram
    A Bayesian n.
    Abrams-Griffith n.
    Schäfer n.
    Siroky n.
non-A
    n.-A non-B
    n.-A non-B hepatitis
    n.-A non-B, non-C hepatitis
    n.-A non-B posttransfusion hepatitis
nonabsorbable
    n. disaccharide
    n. suture
nonadherent clot
nonadhesive dressing
nonadrenergic
    n. neuron
    n. noncholinergic (NANC)
    n. noncholinergic inhibitory transmitter
non-A–E hepatitis
non-A–G
    n.-A-G chronic liver disease
    n.-A-G fulminant hepatitis
nonagglutinable (NAG)
nonalcoholic
    n. fatty liver disease (NAFLD)
    n. steatohepatitis (NASH)
nonalpha nonbeta pancreatic islet cell
nonamyloid glomerulopathy
nonaneuploid tumor
nonanion-gap metabolic acidosis
nonantibiotic colitis
nonantigen-expressing target cell
nonantral endocrine cell hyperplasia
nonapoptotic pathway
NO-naproxen
nonatrophic pangastritis
nonautoimmune fundic atrophic gastritis

nonazotemic
    n. cirrhosis
    n. patient
non-B
    enterically transmitted non-A n.-B (ENANB)
    n.-B islet cell tumor
    n.-B non-C chronic liver disease (NBNC CLD)
    n.-B, non-C CLD
nonbacterial
    n. cystitis (NBC)
    n. gastroenteritis
    n. prostatitis (NBP)
nonbench surgery
nonbilious vomitus
nonbiodegradable
nonbleeding visible vessel (NBVV)
nonbloody stool
non-breath-hold MR cholangiography
nonbuckling erection
noncalcareous renal calculus
noncalcified stone
noncalculous disease
noncardiac chest pain (NCCP)
noncaseating tuberclelike granuloma
noncerebral vasculopathy
non-CH4 excretor
noncholecystokinin substance
noncholinergic
    n. nerve
    n. neuron
    n. neurotransmitter
    nonadrenergic n. (NANC)
nonchylous ascites
noncirrhotic
    n. liver
    n. portal fibrosis (NCPF)
    n. portal hypertension
noncleaved B cell
noncollagen protein
noncommunicating
    n. biliary cyst
    n. diverticulum
    n. hydrocele
    n. polycystic disease
noncompliance
nonconductive guidewire
nonconfluent
noncontrast
    n. computerized tomography
    n. helical computed tomography (NCCT)
noncontributory
noncrushing bowel clamp
noncutting needle
nondiabetic
    n. gastroparesis

n. neurogenic erectile dysfunction
n. proteinuric renal disease
nondilating reflux
nondismembered anastomosis
nondisseminated intestinal threadworm
nondistended abdomen
nondistensible
nonenzymatic glycosylation
nonenzymic reaction
nonepithelial cyst
nonerosive
n. esophagitis
n. gastric mucosal lesion
n. gastroesophageal reflux disease
n. nonspecific gastritis
n. reflux disease (NERD)
nonestrogen supplemented
nonfamilial
n. gastrointestinal polyposis
n. intestinal pseudoobstruction
n. visceral myopathy
nonferromagnetic MR endoscope XGIF-MR30
nonfixed cancer
nonfluctuant
nonfunction
primary graft n.
nonfunctional pituitary tumor
nonfunctioning gallbladder
nonfusion
nonganglionated plexus
nongangrenous sigmoid volvulus
non-gas-forming liver abscess
nongene carrier
nongenomic
nongerm cell carcinoma
nonglomerular hematuria
nonglycated albumin
nongonococcal urethritis
nongranulomatous
n. jejunitis
n. ulcerative jejunoileitis
nonhealing ulcer
non-heart-beating
n.-h.-b. donor kidney
n.-h.-b. donor protocol
nonhemolytic
n. jaundice
n. *Streptococcus*
nonhemolyzed blood
non-HFE hemochromatosis
non-Hodgkin lymphoma (NHL)

nonhyperfunctioning adrenocortical adenoma
nonicteric
n. sclerae
n. skin
nonimmune
n. factor
n. hydrops
n. hydrops fetalis (NIHF)
nonimmune mechanism
nonimmunocompromised
nonimmunologic immunity
nonimmunosuppressed
noninflamed peripheral tissue
noninsulin-dependent diabetes mellitus (NIDDM)
nonintussuscepted valve
noninvasive
n. assessment of urinary flow
n. diagnosis
n. diagnostic test
n. intraanal electromyography
n. method
n. tumor
n. urodynamic test
nonionizing radiation
nonirrigating
n. descending colostomy
n. patient
nonischemic tubule
nonkeratinizing squamous epithelium
nonliquefaciens
Moraxella n.
nonmalleable pelvis
nonmalodorous fluid
nonmetallic
nonmyeloablative allogeneic peripheral blood stem cell transplantation
nonnecrotizing granuloma
nonnegligible number
Nonnenbruch syndrome
nonneoplastic
n. lesion
n. polyp
nonnephrotic immunoglobulin A nephropathy
nonnephrotoxic drug
nonneurogenic
n. neurogenic bladder
n. voiding dysfunction
nonnuclear fraction

NOTES

nonnucleoside reverse transcription inhibitor (NNRTI)
NONOate
    spermine N.
nonobstructive
    n. hepatic parenchymal disease
    n. jaundice
nonocclusive
    n. intestinal infarction
    n. mesenteric ischemia
    n. mesenteric thrombosis
nonoliguric acute renal failure
nonorgan confined disease
nonorganic dyspepsia
nonoxynol-9
nonpalpable cryptorchidism
nonparametric Wilcoxon statistic
nonparasitic
    n. cyst of liver
    n. splenic cyst
nonparticulate radiation
nonpathogenic *Escherichia coli*
nonpeptidyl agonist
nonperforated
    n. appendicitis
    n. appendix
nonpitting
nonpliable
nonplicated appendicocystostomy
nonpolar region
nonpolypoid adenoma
nonpolyposis colorectal cancer
nonpruritic
nonradioactive ^{13}C test
nonreactive pupil
nonreflux esophagitis
nonrefluxing colon conduit
nonrehydrated
    n. guaiac examination
    n. guaiac examination of rectum
nonrosetted cell
NO-NSAIDs
    nitric oxide-releasing nonsteroidal antiinflammatory drugs
nonsecreting pituitary tumor
nonsecretory sigmoid cystoplasty
nonseminomatous
    n. germ cell neoplasm
    n. germ cell tumor (NSGCT)
    n. testicular carcinoma
nonskin malignancy
nonsmall cell lung carcinoma
nonspecific
    n. colitis
    n. erosive gastritis
    n. esophageal motility disorder (NEMD)
    n. esophagitis
    n. gas pattern

    n. reactive hepatitis
    n. ulcerative proctitis
    n. urethritis (NSU)
nonstented ureteroscopic lithotripsy
nonsteroidal
    n. antiandrogen monotherapy
    n. antiinflammatory agent (NSAIA)
    n. antiinflammatory drug (NSAID)
    n. antiinflammatory drug gastropathy
    n. antiinflammatory drug-induced intestinal stricture
nonstrenuous activity
nonstructural protein 4 (NSP4)
nonstruvite
    n. calculus
    n. stone
nonsulfated bile acid
nonsuppurative destructive cholangitis
non–swallow-associated relaxation
nontarget tissue
non-T-cell fraction
nontoxic goiter
nontransected pancreatic duct
nontropical sprue
nontruncating mutation
nontuberculous mycobacteria-associated enterocolitis
nontumorous epithelium
nontyphoidal
    n. *Salmonella*
    n. salmonellosis
nonulcer
    n. dyspepsia (NUD)
    n. dysplasia
nonulcerative interstitial cystitis
nonvariceal upper GI hemorrhage
nonvenereal bubo
nonviable tissue
nonvisualization of gallbladder
nonvoiding patient
Noonan syndrome
noose
    Dormia n.
4NOQ
    4-nitroquinolin-1-oxide-induced tumor
noradrenaline
    serum n.
no rejection (NR)
norepinephrine lavage
norethandrolone
Norflex
norfloxacin
Norfolk technique
normal
    n. anatomy
    n. appendix
    n. asymptomatic volunteer
    bowel sounds n. (BSN)

n. carrier hepatitis
n. detrusor contractility
eversion n.
n. flora
n. maturation
palpably n.
n. penile size
n. saline meal
n. saline solution
normal-appearing mucosa
normal-caliber duct
normalized
    n. protein catabolic rate (NPCR)
    n. protein nitrogen appearance (nPNA)
normal-pressure hydrocephalus
normeperidine
Nor-Mil
normoacidity
normoactive bowel sounds (NABS)
normoamylasemia
normocephalic
normochlorhydria
normochromic
normocytic
Normodyne
normoglycemia
normokalemia
normoproliferative
Normosol-M IV infusion
normospermatogenic sterility
normotensive
Normotest test
normothermia
normothermic effect
Noroxin
Norplant
Norpramin
Nor-tet Oral
Northern blot analysis
Northgate
    N. SD-3 dual-purpose lithotriptor
    N. SD-100 EHL generator
nortriptyline
Norvasc
Norwalk
    N. agent
    N. gastroenteritis
    N. virus
Norwalk-like virus (NLV)
Norwegian cholestasis
Norwich

Norwood rectal snare
no-scalpel
    n.-s. vasectomy
    n.-s. vasectomy fixator ring clamp forceps
    n.-s. vasectomy instrument set
nosocomial
    n. fungal infection
    n. urinary tract infection
nostras
    cholera n.
nostril blood
notch
    n. of gallbladder
    gastric n.
    splenic n.
note
    percussion n.
notification of tumor
Nottingham
    N. colposuspension needle
    N. KeyMed introducer
    N. KeyMed introducing device
    N. One-Step tapered dilator
    N. semirigid introducer
    N. ureteral dilator
Nova II machine
Novamine amino acid
Novantrone
Novarel
novel
    N. erythropoiesis-stimulating protein (NESP)
    n. molecular markers
    n. tableted purgative
novo
    de n.
Novocain
NovolinPen device
NPCR
    normalized protein catabolic rate
NPCTG
    National Prostatic Cancer Treatment Group
NPH insulin
nPNA
    normalized protein nitrogen appearance
NPR
    natriuretic peptide receptor
NPT
    nocturnal penile tumescence
    NPT monitoring

NOTES

NPV
  negative predictive value
NPY
  neuropeptide Y
NR
  no rejection
NRH
  nodular regenerative hyperplasia
NS2, NS3, NS4, NS5 protein
NS3/NS4 junction
NS4/NS5 junction
NSAIA
  nonsteroidal antiinflammatory agent
NSAID
  nonsteroidal antiinflammatory drug
    NSAID gastropathy
    nitric oxide-releasing NSAIDS
NSAID-induced
  N.-i. gastric injury
  N.-i. intestinal injury
NSE
  neuron-specific enolase
NSGCT
  nonseminomatous germ cell tumor
N-shaped sigmoid loop
NSP4
  nonstructural protein 4
NSU
  nonspecific urethritis
NT
  nucleation time
N-terminal
  N-t. fragment
  N-t. propeptide of type III procollagen
NTN
  nephrotoxic nephritis
N-trimethylsilylimidazole
NTZ Long-Acting Nasal Solution
nuchal rigidity
Nuck
  canal of N.
  diverticulum of N.
  N. hydrocele
nuclear
  n. bleeding scan
  n. enema
  n. factor kappa B (NF-KB)
  n. factor kappa B transcription factor protein
  n. fraction
  n. fragment
  n. hepatobiliary imaging
  n. hyperchromasia and pleomorphism
  n. isotope scan
  n. magnetic resonance (NMR)
  n. matrix
  n. matrix alteration
  n. matrix protein-22 (NMP, NMP-22)
  n. medicine (NM)
  n. medicine scan
  n. membrane
  n. morphometry
  n. protein cyclin proliferating cell nuclear antigen
  n. roundness factor
  n. sclerosis
  n. transcriptional activation
nuclear-tagged
  n.-t. cell
  n.-t. red blood cell bleeding study
nuclear-to-cytoplasmic size ratio
nucleation
  epitaxial n.
  homogenous n.
  n. time (NT)
nucleic
  n. acid
  n. acid hybridization
  n. acid testing (NAT)
nucleocapsid
  n. antigen-specific
  n. antigen-stimulated interferon gamma
nucleoside
nucleosome
nucleotidase
  5' n.
5' nucleotidase
nucleotide
  adenosine n.
  guanine n.
nucleotide-binding domain (NBD)
nucleus
  n. ambiguus
  cigar-shaped hyperchromatic n.
  elongated pseudostratified n.
  hyperchromatic n.
  Onuf n.
  paraventricular n. (PVN)
  pyknotic n.
  n. raphe obscurus
  n. solitarius
  n. of solitary tract
  n. tractus solitarii
  n. tractus solitarius
NUD
  nonulcer dyspepsia
Nu-Hope
  N.-H. Adhesive waterproof skin barrier
  N.-H. cleaning solvent
  N.-H. Convex insert
  N.-H. hole cutter
  N.-H. ileostomy pouch
  N.-H. Karaya powder

N.-H. neonatal and preemie pouch
N.-H. Nu-Self drainable pouch
N.-H. pouch cover
N.-H. Protective Skin Barrier
N.-H. tubing
N.-H. urinary pouch
N.-H. urine collection bottle
N.-H. urostomy pouch
NuLev orally disintegrating tablet
null cell tumor
Nullo deodorant tablet
NuLYTELY enema
number
    n. connection test (NCT)
    nonnegligible n.
    shock n.
    wave n.
numbness
numerous plant extracts
Nupercainal ointment
Nuport PEG tube
nurse-administered propofol sedation (NAPS)
nurse cell formation
Nurses' Health study (NHS)
Nursoy formula
Nussbaum
    N. experiment
    N. intestinal clamp
    N. intestinal forceps
nutcracker esophagus
Nu-Tetra
Nu-Tip laparoscopic scissors
nutmeg liver
nutraceutical
Nutrament oral liquid
Nutramigen formula
NutraPrep
    N. bowel cleansing solution
    N. colonoscopy preparation
    N. food
Nutricia
nutrient enema
nutrition
    enteral n. (EN)
    European Society of Pediatric Gastroenterology, Hepatology, and N. (ESPGHAN)
    home parenteral n. (HPN)
    intradialytic parenteral n. (IDPN)
    intravenous n. (IVN)
    Jevity isotonic liquid n.
    luminal n.
    Nutri-Vent liquid n.
    parenteral n.
    Peptamen liquid n.
    perioperative n.
    Replete liquid n.
    support parenteral n. (SPN)
    total enteral n. (TEN)
    total parenteral n. (TPN)
    total peripheral parenteral n. (TPPN)
nutritional
    n. assessment
    n. cirrhosis
    n. deficiency
    n. dropsy
    n. index
    n. pancreatitis
    n. status
    n. support
    n. therapy
nutritive
nutriture
Nutri-Vent liquid nutrition
Nutromat Pad S feeding pump
Nutropin
Nuttall liver retractor
Nuvion
Nuviva
nux vomica
N&V
    nausea and vomiting
NVD
    nausea, vomiting, diarrhea
NWTSG
    National Wilms Tumor Study Group
nycturia
Nyhus-Nelson gastric decompression and jejunal feeding tube
Nyhus procedure
nylidrin
nylon tissue biopsy bag
Nymox urinary test
nystagmus
nystatin suspension
Nystex
Nytilax

NOTES

O1
: *Vibrio cholera O1*

O139
: *Vibrio cholera O139*

O_2
: oxygen
  fMLP-stimulated O_2
  PMA-stimulated O_2

OA-519 prognostic prostate carcinoma marker

OAC
: omeprazole, amoxicillin, clarithromycin

OAE
: open-access endoscopy

OAI
: Ostomy Assessment Inventory

OAM
: omeprazole, amoxicillin, metronidazole

O antigen

OASIS
: One Action Stent Introduction System

Oasis
: O. pusher tube system
  O. stent

oasthouse urine disease

oat
: o. cell
  o. cell carcinoma
  Lactobacillus plantarum-
      fermented o.

oatmeal
: colloidal o.

OB-10 Comfort bite block

OBA
: oral bile acid

O'Beirne sphincter

obesity
: adult-onset o.
  alimentary o.
  endogenous o.
  exogenous o.
  hyperplastic o.
  hypertrophic o.
  o. hypoventilation syndrome (OHS)
  o. index
  lifelong o.
  morbid o.

obeum
: *Ruminococcus o.*

OB gene

object
: foreign o.
  ingested foreign o.
  irretrievable o.
  radiolucent o.

objective
: o. lens
  o. vertigo

objectivity
: degree of o.

OBK
: obstructed kidney

obligate anaerobe

obligatory dialysate protein loss

oblique
: aponeurosis of external o.
  aponeurosis of internal o.
  o. arytenoid muscle
  o. aspiration mucosector
  external o.
  o. fibers of stomach
  o. fluoroscopy
  o. forward-viewing instrument
  o. gastric fiber
  o. incision
  internal o.
  o. mucosectomy device tip
  o. obturator
  o. viewing echoendoscope
  o. viewing endoscope

obliterans
: appendicitis o.
  arteriosclerosis o.
  balanitis xerotica o. (BXO)
  endophlebitis hepatica o.

obliterated varix

obliteration
: balloon-occluded retrograde
      transvenous o. (B-RTO)
  endoscopic extirpation cicatricial o.
  percutaneous transhepatic o.
  o. of psoas shadow

obscured ureteral orifice

obscure gastrointestinal bleeding

obscurus
: nucleus raphe o.

observation
: electron immunoperoxidase o.
  light and electron
      immunoperoxidase o.

observational followup study

obsolescent glomerulus

obstetric injury

obstipation

obstipum
: abdomen o.

obstructed
: o. collecting system
  o. kidney (OBK)

obstructed *(continued)*
- o. pelvis
- o. testis

obstructing
- o. cancer
- o. rectosigmoidal carcinoma

obstruction
- acquired ureteropelvic junction o.
- acute extrarenal o.
- adynamic intestinal o.
- airflow o.
- airway o.
- benign prostatic o. (BPO)
- bilateral ureteral o. (BUO)
- o. of bile flow
- biliary tract o.
- bladder neck o.
- bladder outflow o.
- bladder outlet o. (BOO)
- bowel o.
- bronchial o.
- *Brugia* lymphatic o.
- calix o.
- cerumen o.
- closed-loop intestinal o.
- clot-induced urinary tract o.
- colonic o.
- common bile duct o.
- complete bowel o.
- congenital ureteropelvic junction o.
- ductal o.
- duodenal o.
- o. duodenum
- ejaculatory duct o.
- epididymis o.
- esophageal o.
- extrahepatic bile duct o.
- extrahepatic biliary o.
- extrahepatic portal vein o. (EHPVO)
- extrinsic ureteral o.
- extrinsic ureteropelvic junction o.
- false colonic o.
- fecal o.
- food bolus o.
- functional cystic duct o.
- gastric outlet o. (GOO)
- hepatic venous outflow o. (HVOO)
- high-grade o.
- high small bowel o.
- idiopathic o.
- o. index
- infravesical prostatic o.
- intermittent o.
- intestinal o. (IO)
- intrahepatic portal o.
- intratubular o.
- intrinsic ureteropelvic junction o.
- laparoscopic treatment of ureteropelvic junction o.
- large bowel o.
- low small bowel o.
- lymphatic o.
- malignant biliary o.
- mechanical biliary o.
- mechanical duct o.
- mechanical extrahepatic o.
- mechanical intestinal o.
- mechanical small bowel o.
- neurogenic intestinal o.
- oliguric o.
- outflow o.
- outlet o.
- palliation of malignant large bowel o.
- paralytic colonic o.
- paralytic intestinal o.
- partial bile outflow o.
- partial bowel o.
- partial ureteral o.
- portal vein o.
- postoperative ureteral o.
- posturethral suspension o.
- primary ureteropelvic junction o.
- prolonged partial ureteral o.
- prostatic outlet o. (POO)
- pyloric outlet o.
- pyloroduodenal o.
- renal o.
- renovascular o.
- secondary ureteropelvic junction o.
- seminal vesicle o.
- shrapnel-induced biliary o.
- simple mechanical o.
- small bowel o. (SBO)
- splenic vein o. (SVO)
- strangulated bowel o.
- tubular o.
- unilateral ureteral o. (UUO)
- ureteral o.
- ureteric o.
- ureteropelvic junction o.
- ureterovesical o.
- urethral o.
- urinary o.
- urodynamic o.
- vas deferens o.

obstruction-induced modulation

obstructive
- o. anuria
- o. appendicitis
- o. biliary cirrhosis
- o. change
- o. cholangitis
- o. defecation
- o. dysfunctional ileitis
- o. gastroduodenal Crohn disease

o. jaundice
o. megaureter
o. nephropathy
o. pancreatitis
o. sleep apnea
o. uropathy
obtunded
obturation
obturator
    Alcock-Timberlake o.
    o. artery
    blunt-tipped o.
    Endopath Optiview laparoscopic o.
    o. hernia
    o. internus muscle
    o. lymphatic chain
    o. lymph node
    o. nerve
    oblique o.
    Optiview o.
    o. shelf cystourethropexy
    o. sign
    o. test
    Timberlake o.
    o. vein
obtuse margin
OCBF
    outer cortical blood flow
occipital
occiput
occluded shunt
occludens
    zonula o.
occlusion
    o. balloon
    balloon ureteral o.
    o. cholangiogram
    enteromesenteric o.
    hepatic vein o.
    mesenteric vascular o.
    portal triad o.
    retinal artery o.
    retinal vein o.
    o. of TIPS
    tourniquet o.
    urethral o.
occlusive
    o. azoospermia
    o. clamp
    o. collodion dressing
    o. ileus
    o. infarction

occult
    o. blood
    o. filariasis
    o. gastrointestinal bleeding
    o. hepatitis
    o. levator ani hernia
    o. spinal dysraphism
occupational
    o. toxin
    o. toxin exposure
OCG
    oral cholecystogram
Ochoa syndrome
Ochsner
    O. clamp
    O. flexible spiral gallstone probe
    O. forceps
    O. gallbladder probe
    O. gallbladder trocar
    O. hemostat
    O. muscle
    O. retractor
    O. ring
    O. treatment
Ockerblad-Boari flap
OCL
    oral colonic lavage
    OCL bowel preparation
OCLG
    osteoclast-like giant cell
10 o'clock selector catheter
O'Connor drape
OCP
    ova, cysts, and parasites
OCT
    optical coherence tomography
    OCT medium
octahedral-shaped dihydrate
Octamide
octanoic acid breath test
octapeptide
    cholecystokinin o. (CCK-8, CCK-OP)
OctreoScan
    O. kit
    O. scintigraphy
octreotide
    o. acetate
    o. acetate for injectable suspension
    o. effect
    somatostatin analog o.
octreotide-induced hepatic toxicity

NOTES

OCTT
    orocecal transit time
2-octyl cyanoacrylate injection
Ocuflox
ocular
    o. abnormality
    o. lesion
oculocerebrorenal
    o. dystrophy
    o. syndrome
oculopharyngeal muscular dystrophy
OD
    outer diameter
    overdose
        Xatral OD
ODC
    ornithine decarboxylase
Oddi
    denervated sphincter of O.
    sphincter of O. (SO)
O'Donoghue cystourethroscope
odor
    breath o.
    foul-smelling o.
    fruity o.
odorant
O'Duffy criteria
odynophagia
OEC-Diasonics 9400 fluoroscopy C-arm system
OEIS
    omphalocele, exstrophy of bladder, imperforate anus, and spinal abnormalities
        OEIS complex
Oerskovia
OES
    Olympus endoscopy system
        OES 4000 resectoscope
Oettingen abdominal retractor
office-based esophageal screening
offset-lens ureteroscope
ofloxacin
Ogen
Ogilvie syndrome
O'Hanlon intestinal clamp
Ohara disease
O'Hara forceps
25(OH)D3
    25-hydroxyvitamin D3
OHS
    obesity hypoventilation syndrome
oil
    arachis o.
    castor o.
    cottonseed o.
    fish o.
    Fleet Enema Mineral O.
    Fleet Flavored Castor O.
    Kellogg's Castor O.
    Lorenzo o.
    mineral o. (M-O)
    olive o.
    pennyroyal o.
    peppermint o.
    radioopaque iodized o.
    o. red O stain
    o. retention enema
    seabuckthorn seed o.
    silicone-based o.
oily stool
ointment
    Calmoseptine o.
    Ethezyme debriding o.
    nifedipine o.
    nitroglycerin o.
    Nupercainal o.
    Panafil o.
    Pazo Hemorrhoidal O.
    Tucks o.
OK432 streptococcal suspension
okadaic acid
Okamoto method
OK cell
OKT3
    Ortho-Kung T
    OKT3 anti-T-cell antibody
    OKT3 monoclonal antibody
    Orthoclone OKT3
OKT4 cell
OKT8 cell
Okuda transhepatic obliteration of varix
Olbert balloon dilator
Oldfield syndrome
Olean
oleandomycin
oleate
    intravariceal ethanolamine o.
    monoethanolamine o.
oleic acid
Olestra fat substitute
olfactory bulb neuroblastoma
oligoasthenospermia
oligoasthenoteratospermia
oligoasthenoteratozoospermia
oligoazoospermia
oligocholia
oligochylia
oligochymia
oligocilia
oligohydramnios complex
oligohydruria
oligomeganephronia
oligomerize
oligometric complex
oligonecrospermia
oligonephronic hypoplasia

oligonucleotide · Olympus

oligonucleotide
    antisense o.
    o. probe
    specific o.
oligopepsia
oligopeptide
oligophosphaturia
oligosaccharidase
oligosaccharide
oligosaccharide-binding membrane protein
oligospermatic
oligospermia, oligospermatism
oligosymptomatic ADPKD
oligosynaptic pathway
oligoteratoasthenozoospermia (OTA)
    o. syndrome
oligozoospermia, oligozoospermatism
oliguria, oliguresia, oliguresis
    neonatal o.
oliguric
    o. obstruction
    o. renal failure
olive
    Eder-Puestow o.
    expandable o.
    metal o.
    o. oil
    o. over guidewire
    palpable pyloric o.
    Savary-Gilliard metal o.
    o. shaped
olive-tipped
    o.-t. catheter
    o.-t. plastic dilator
OLS
    ouabainlike substance
olsalazine-S
olsalazine sodium
Olsen cholangiogram clamp
OLT
    orthotopic liver transplant
oltipraz
Olympus
    O. adapter
    O. A5256 laparoscope
    O. alligator-jaw endoscopic forceps
    O. Aloka EU-MI ultrasound gastrointestinal fiberscope
    O. Aloka GF-EU-series endoscope
    O. automatic reprocessor
    O. basket-type endoscopic forceps

    O. BH2-epifluorescence microscope
    O. BH2-RFCA reflecting microscope
    O. BHT-2 microscope
    O. BML-3Q, -4Q lithotriptor
    O. CBK fluorescence microscope
    O. CD-20Z heater probe
    O. CD-Z-series heat probe thermocoagulator
    O. CF 2301 endoscope
    O. CF-20 fibercolonoscope
    O. CF-HM-series magnifying colonoscope
    O. CF-L-series flexible sigmoidoscope
    O. CF-MB/LB colonoscope
    O. CF-MB-M colonoscope
    O. CF-MB-series colonoscope
    O. CF-OSF-series flexible sigmoidoscope
    O. CF24OZI colonoscope
    O. CF-PL-series colonoscope
    O. CF-P20S fiberoptic colonoscope
    O. CF100S sigmoidoscope
    O. CF100TL
    O. CF-1T100L colonoscope
    O. CF-TL-series forward-viewing videocolonoscope
    O. CF-1T100L videocolonoscope
    O. CF-100TL videocolonoscope
    O. CF-T-series colonoscope
    O. CF-TVL-series colonoscope
    O. CF-UHM-series colonoscope
    O. CF-UM3 colonoscope
    O. CF-UM3 flexible echocolonoscope
    O. CF-UM-series echoendoscope
    O. CF-UM20 ultrasonic endoscope
    O. CF-UM20 ultrasound endoscope
    O. CF-VL-series colonoscope
    O. CF-200Z colonoscope
    O. CF-200Z endoscope
    O. CG-P-series colonofiberscope
    O. CHF-P20 choledochoscope
    O. CHF-Q10 cholangioscope
    O. clip-fixing device
    O. CLV10 fiberscope light source
    O. CLV-series fiberoptic system
    O. CLV-U 20 endoscopic halogen light source
    O. 215-cm enteroscope
    O. continuous flow resectoscope

NOTES

Olympus *(continued)*
- O. CV-series colonoscope
- O. CV-series endoscope
- O. CYF-3 OES cystofiberscope
- O. cytology brush
- O. DES-series endoscope
- O. EF-series esophagoscope
- O. endoscopy system (OES)
- O. Endo-Therapy disposable biopsy forceps
- O. ENF-P2 scope
- O. ENF-P-series laryngoscope
- O. EUM-20 echoendoscope
- O. EUM-20 endoscope
- O. EU-M30S endoscopic ultrasonography receiver
- O. EU-M-series endosonography image processor
- O. Europe ETD automated endoscope washer
- O. EUS-series endoscope
- O. EVIS 140
- O. EVIS color computer chip system
- O. EVIS Q-series endoscope
- O. EVIS Q-200V
- O. EVIS 140 Q videoendoscope
- O. EVIS videocolonoscope
- O. EW-series fiberoptic duodenoscope
- O. FB-20C endoscopic forceps
- O. FB-25K endoscopic forceps
- O. FBK-13 forceps
- O. FB-24U biopsy forceps
- O. FG-12U wide-mouth forceps
- O. fiberoptic cystoscope
- O. FK-13-1 biopsy forceps
- O. FS-K-series endoscopic suture-cutting forceps
- O. gastrostomy
- O. GF-EU1 gastrointestinal fiberscope
- O. GF-series videoendoscope
- O. GF-UC30P echoendoscope
- O. GF-UCT30P linear-array echoendoscope
- O. GF-UM30P echoendoscope
- O. GF-UM30P endoscope
- O. GF-UM30P linear scanning probe
- O. GF-UM29 radial scanner echoendoscope
- O. GF-UM20 radial scanning endoscope
- O. GF-UM3 ultrasonic endoscope
- O. GF-UM20 ultrasound endoscope
- O. GF-UM3, -UM20 system
- O. GIF-D2 endoscope
- O. GIF-D-series panendoscope
- O. GIF20 echoendoscope
- O. GIF-EUM2 echoendoscope
- O. GIF-HM-series endoscope
- O. GIF-J-series endoscope
- O. GIF-K-series gastroscope
- O. GIF-P endoscope
- O. GIF-Q200 endoscope
- O. GIF-Q30 fiberscope
- O. GIF-series double-channel therapeutic videoendoscope
- O. GIF-series echoendoscope
- O. GIF-SQ-series videoendoscope
- O. GIF-1T10 echoendoscope
- O. GIF-2T10 endoscope
- O. GIF-2T200 endoscope
- O. GIF-T-series endoscope
- O. GIF-T-series videoendoscope
- O. GIFxP10 gastroscope
- O. GIF-XP-series endoscope
- O. GIF-XQ240 endoscope
- O. GIF-XQ30 flexible gastroscope
- O. GIF-XQ-series panendoscope
- O. GIF-XQ200 videogastroscope
- O. GIF-XQ230 videogastroscope
- O. GIF-XQ240 videogastroscope
- O. GIF-XV-series endoscope
- O. GIF-200Z videoendoscope
- O. grasping rat-tooth forceps
- O. GTF-A gastrocamera
- O. heater probe unit
- O. heat probe
- O. hot biopsy forceps
- O. HX-21L detachable miniloop
- O. injector
- O. intracavity transducer
- O. JF-series videoduodenoscope
- O. JF-series videoendoscope
- O. JF1T endoscope
- O. JF1T10 fiberoptic duodenoscope
- O. JF-T-series endoscope
- O. JF-TV-series endoscope
- O. JF-UM20 echoendoscope
- O. JF-V-series endoscope
- O. JF-V-series videoduodenoscope
- O. JT-series videoduodenoscope
- O. large-channel endoscope GIF1T130
- O. linear-array echoendoscope
- O. LUS-1 rigid device
- O. LUS-2 ultrasonic energy rigid device
- O. magnetic extractor forceps
- O. MAJ363 FNA needle system
- O. minisnare forceps
- O. monopolar cannula
- O. Nd:YAG laser
- O. needle-knife papillotome
- O. NM-K-series sclerotherapy needle

Olympus · OME

O. NM-L-series needle
O. OES fiberscope
O. OM-2 camera with SM-45 enlarging adapter
O. OM-1 reflex camera
O. OM-series endoscopic camera
O. One-Step Button
O. one-step button gastrostomy tube
O. OSF flexible sigmoidoscope
O. OSF scope
O. OSP fluorescence measuring system
O. OTV-S-series miniature camera
O. P20
O. PCF-130L videocolonoscope
O. PCF-100 pediatric colonoscope
O. PCF-130 pediatric colonoscope
O. PCF-series pediatric colonoscope
O. pelican-type endoscopic forceps
O. PJF endoscope
O. PJF-series pediatric duodenoscope
O. PJF-series pediatric endoscope
O. PSD-10 electrosurgical blend current
O. P-series endoscope
O. PW-1L wash catheter
O. PW-5V spray catheter
O. Q200 videoendoscope
O. rat-tooth endoscopic forceps
O. reusable oval-cup forceps
O. reusable oval-cup forceps with needle
O. rubber-tip endoscopic forceps
O. SCA-series endoscopic camera
O. SD-5L semicircular snare
O. shark-tooth endoscopic forceps
O. SIF-10 enteroscope
O. SIF-M magnifying colonoscope
O. SIF-M-series video enteroscope
O. SIF-Q240 enteroscope
O. SIF-SW fiberoptic endoscope
O. SIF-SW-series video enteroscope
O. SIF-100 video push endoscope
O. SIF-100 video push enteroscope
O. SIG-100L videoenteroscope
O. sphincterotome
O. spray catheter PW-5V
O. SP-series image analyzer
O. S-20-20R probe
O. SSIF-series videoenteroscope

O. stone retrieval basket
O. 2T100 endoscope
O. TJF-10, -100, -200 duodenoscope
O. TJF-100 endoscope
O. tripod-type endoscopic forceps
O. 2T-2000 twin-channel therapeutic gastroscope
O. UES-series snare cautery device
O. ultrasonic esophagoprobe
O. ultrathin balloon-fitted ultrasound probe
O. UM-F30-20R probe
O. UM-20 radial echoendoscope
O. UM-2R, -3R probe
O. UM-R-series miniature ultrasonic probe
O. UM-series endoscope
O. UM-S30-25R probe
O. UM-1W endoscopic probe
O. UM-W-series endoscopic probe
O. URF-P2 translaparoscopic choledochofiberscope
O. URF type P2 flexible ureteroscope
O. videoendoscopy system
O. videourology procedure system
O. V-series endoscope
O. VU-M2 echoendoscope
O. W-shaped endoscopic forceps
O. XCF-XK-series endoscope
O. XCHF-37 choledochoscope
O. XGF-UCT30 endoscope
O. XIF-UM3 echoendoscope
O. XK-series oblique-viewing flexible fiberscope
O. XMP-U2 catheter echoprobe
O. XP-series endoscope
O. XQ230 gastroscope
O. XQ-200, XQ-230 video endoscope
O. XSIF-series videoenteroscope
O. Zoom endoscope

omapatrilat

Ombrédanne
O. forceps
O. operation

OMC
omeprazole, metronidazole, clarithromycin

OME
omeprazole

NOTES

OmegaPort access port
omega-shaped
    o.-s. epiglottis
    o.-s. incision
omenta (*pl. of* omentum)
omental
    o. adhesion
    o. band
    o. bursitis
    o. cyst
    o. enterocleisis
    o. foramen
    o. hammock
    o. infarction
    o. interposition
    o. J-pexy
    o. patch
    o. pedicle
    o. pedicle flap
    o. pedicle flap graft
    o. plug
    o. studding
    o. tuberosity
    o. vein
    o. wrapping
omentale
    foramen o.
omentalis
    taenia o.
omentectomy
omentitis
omentofixation
omentopexy
omentoplasty
    pedicled o.
    pelvic o.
omentorrhaphy
omentovolvulus
omentum, pl. **omenta**
    bowel adherent to o.
    colic o.
    gastric o.
    gastrocolic o.
    gastrohepatic o.
    gastrosplenic o.
    greater o.
    incarcerated o.
    interposition flap of o.
    lesser o.
    o. majus
    o. majus flap procedure
    o. minus
    pancreaticosplenic o.
    pedicled o.
    splenogastric o.
omentumectomy
omeprazole (OME)
    o., amoxicillin, clarithromycin (OAC)
    o., amoxicillin, metronidazole (OAM)
    o., metronidazole, clarithromycin (OMC)
    o. test
    o. therapy
omeprazole/amoxicillin
omeprazole-clarithromycin-amoxicillin therapy
Omnicef
Omnicide disinfectant
Omni-LapoTract support system
OMNILINK 0.018, 0.035 biliary stent
Omnipaque
Omnipen
Omnipen-N
OmniPhase penile prosthesis
OMNI Prep
OmniPulse MAX holmium laser
Omnitract retractor
omphalectomy
omphalocele
omphalocele, exstrophy of bladder, imperforate anus, and spinal abnormalities (OEIS)
omphalocele repair
Onchocerca volvulus
onchocerciasis
oncoantigen 519
oncocytoma
    kidney o.
    renal o.
oncocytomatosis
oncofetal protein
oncogene
    c-jun o.
    c-met o.
    c-myc o.
    HER-2/neu o.
    o. inactivation
    Kirsten-ras o.
    K-ras o.
    N-myc o.
    polyoma middle T o.
    ras p21 o.
    sarcoma virus o.
oncogene-induced carcinogenesis
oncological
    o. outcome
    o. radicality
oncologic principle
On-Command catheter
oncoprotein
    c-ErbB-2/Neu o.
    Neu o.
    viral o.
OncoScint
    O. CR103
    O. CR/OV

O. CR/OV carcinoma localization scintigraphy (OncoScint CR/OV)
OncoSeed
OncoSpect
ondansetron
metoclopramide, dexamethasone, lorazepam, o. (MDLO)
one
O. Action Stent Introduction System (OASIS)
O. Touch blood glucose meter
one-handed knot
one-hour office pad test
oneirogmus
one-minute endoscopy room test
one-piece
o.-p. disposable plug
o.-p. ostomy pouch
one-session crossover study
one-shot
o.-s. intravenous urography
o.-s. IVU
one-stage
o.-s. hypospadias repair
o.-s. procedure
o.-s. reaction
o.-s. urethroplasty
One-Step
O.-S. gastric button
Surgitek O.-S. (SOS)
onion-skinning
onlay
o. island flap
o. island flap urethroplasty
o. technique
onlay-tube-onlay urethroplasty technique
online hemodiafiltration
onset
o. of dysphagia
o. of pain
ontogeny
Onuf nucleus
Oochoristica
oocyst
Cryptosporidium o.
oocyte micromanipulation
oolemma
oophorectomy
ooplasm
ooze
oozing blood

O&P
ova and parasites
O&P test
opacification
opacified
organs o.
opacify
opaque
o. meal
Sur-Fit Natura closed-end pouch, o.
open
o. adrenalectomy
o. biopsy
bowels not o. (BNO)
o. cystotomy
o. drainage
o. electrocautery snare
o. hemorrhoidectomy
o. injury
o. management
o. mesh-plug hernioplasty
o. morphology
o. pyelolithotomy
o. pyelotomy
o. radical prostatectomy
o. renal descent
o. retroperitoneal high ligation
o. sphincterotome
o. stone surgery
o. transurethral resection
o. ulcer
o. wound
open-access endoscopy (OAE)
open-ended
o.-e. ostomy pouch
o.-e. ureteral catheter
o.-e. vasectomy
open-end flow-through radiopaque tip
opener
potassium channel o.
opening
appendiceal o.
epispadiac o.
open-label Gelusil
operating
operating frequency
operation (*See also* procedure, repair)
Abbe small bowel o.
Aldridge o.
Alexander-Adams o.
Allingham o.
Amussat o.

NOTES

operation · operation

operation *(continued)*
    Andrews o.
    antireflux o.
    Aylett o.
    Bacon-Babcock rectovaginal fistula o.
    Baldy-Webster o.
    Ball o.
    bariatric o.
    Bassini o.
    Bates o.
    Battle o.
    Belfield o.
    Belsey Mark IV antireflux o.
    Belsey Mark V o.
    Bennett o.
    Bergenhem o.
    Best o.
    Bevan o.
    Bigelow o.
    Billroth I, II o.
    Bloch-Paul-Mikulicz o.
    Bloodgood o.
    Boari o.
    Bottini o.
    bottle o.
    Bozeman o.
    Bricker o.
    Browne o.
    Brunschwig o.
    Calot o.
    Camey I, II o.
    Cecil o.
    Child o.
    Civiale o.
    Clark o.
    Cock o.
    Collis antireflux o.
    Crespo o.
    Delorme rectal prolapse o.
    Deming o.
    Denis Browne o.
    Dittel o.
    Doppler o.
    Doyen o.
    Duhamel o.
    Duplay o.
    Edebohls o.
    Everett-TeLinde o.
    eversion o.
    Finney o.
    Foley o.
    Franco o.
    Frank o.
    Fredet-Ramstedt o.
    Freyer o.
    Fuller o.
    Furlow-Fisher modification of Virag 1 o.
    Gauderer-Ponsky PEG o.
    Gil-Vernet o.
    Hagner o.
    Halsted o.
    Hartmann o.
    Heineke-Mikulicz o.
    Heller o.
    Hess o.
    Hill antireflux o.
    Hochenegg o.
    Hofmeister o.
    Horton-Devine o.
    Huggins o.
    interposition o.
    Israel o.
    Ivalon sponge-wrap o.
    Jaboulay-Doyen-Winkleman o.
    Jonnesco o.
    Kader o.
    Kasai o.
    Kelly o.
    Kelly-Stoeckel o.
    kidney-sparing o.
    Kocher o.
    Kraske o.
    Kropp o.
    Ladd o.
    Lane o.
    Lester Martin modification of Duhamel o.
    Longmire o.
    Lowsley o.
    Macewen hernia o.
    MAGPI o.
    Mainz pouch o.
    Makkas o.
    Manchester-Fothergill o.
    Mann-Williamson o.
    Mansson o.
    Marian o.
    Marshall-Marchetti-Birch o.
    Marshall-Marchetti-Krantz o.
    Martin o.
    Martius o.
    Martius-Harris o.
    Mason o.
    Matson o.
    Maunsell-Weir o.
    Maydl o.
    Mayo o.
    Mays o.
    McVay o.
    Mercier o.
    Merindino o.
    mica o.
    Mikulicz o.
    Miles o.
    Milligan-Morgan o.
    Monfort o.

morcellement o.
Moschcowitz o.
Nesbit o.
Nissen antireflux o.
Ombrédanne o.
orthotopic hemi-Kock o.
Palomo o.
Payne o.
Petersen o.
Pickrell o.
Pólya o.
pubovaginal o.
Puestow-Gillesby o.
Ramstedt o.
Raz sling o.
repeat o.
restorative proctocolectomy o.
Rigaud o.
Ripstein rectal prolapse o.
Roux-en-Y o.
Rovsing o.
sacrofixation o.
Scott o.
scrotal pouch o.
second-look o.
sling o.
Smith-Boyce o.
Soave o.
sphincter-preserving o. (SPO)
Spivack o.
Ssabanejew-Frank o.
staging o.
Steinach o.
Stoppa o.
string o.
Swenson o.
Tanner o.
Thal fundic patch o.
Thiersch anal incontinence o.
Torek o.
transection and devascularization o.
Tuffier o.
Turnbull multiple ostomy o.
Turner-Warwick o.
van Hook o.
Vidal o.
Virag o.
Vogel o.
Volkmann o.
Voronoff o.
Wangensteen o.
Waugh-Clagett o.
Wheelhouse o.
Whipple o.
White o.
Whitehead o.
Wood o.
Young o.
Young-Dees o.
Young-Dees-Leadbetter o.
operative
    o. cholangiogram
    o. cholangiography
    o. choledochoscopy
    o. decompression
    o. laparoscope
    o. morbidity
    o. mortality rate
    o. staging
    o. time
ophthalmoplegia
    internuclear o.
opiate
    o. antagonist
    o. receptor
opioid
    o. antagonist
    o. antidiarrheal
    antisecretory o.
    endogenous o.
    o. peptide
    o. receptor agonist (ORA)
opioid-mediated pruritus
opisthorchiasis
Opisthorchis
    O. felineus
    O. sinensis
    O. viverrini
Opitz-Frias syndrome
opium
    deodorized tincture of o. (DTO)
Opmilas 144 Plus laser system
opportunistic
    o. complication
    o. infection
opposure
Op-Site dressing
opsonic activity
opsonization
opsonized zymosan
optic
    o. neuropathy
    Wappler cystoscope with microlens o.'s

NOTES

optical
- o. coherence tomography (OCT)
- o. crystallography
- o. esophagoscope
- o. fiber
- o. laser knife
- o. multichannel analyzer system
- o. needle
- o. switch
- o. ureterotome
- o. urethrotome knife

Optilume prostate balloon dilator

optimal
- o. diagnostic accuracy
- O. Regimen Cures *Helicobacter*-Induced Dyspepsia (ORCHID)
- o. shock wave rate

Optimental
optimization
optimizing
- o. HLA matching
- o. human leukocyte antigen matching

optimum cooling range
option
- therapeutic o.

Optiray
Optiview obturator
Opti-Vue plastic barrel
OPUS-1
- Ausonics OPUS-1

ORA
- opioid receptor agonist

Oracit
orad
- o. propagation
- o. side

Oragrafin contrast medium
oral
- o. alkalinization
- Ansaid O.
- o. barium suspension
- o. bile acid (OBA)
- Cartrol O.
- Ceftin O.
- o. cholecystogram (OCG)
- o. cholecystography
- o. colonic lavage (OCL)
- o. disease
- o. intubation
- o. iron
- o. iron preparation
- o. lavage
- o. leukoplakia
- Nor-tet O.
- Permitil O.
- Protostat O.
- o. purge
- o. rehydration
- o. rehydration solution (ORS)
- o. rehydration therapy (ORT)
- o. suction catheter
- Sumycin O.
- o. therapy of erectile dysfunction
- o. thermometer
- o. thrush
- o. tolerance
- o. transmission
- o. ulcer

Oralgen
Oramide
Orandi
- O. knife
- O. technique

orange bezoar
orange-colored tonsil
Orasone
OraSure salivary collection device
Orathecin
OraVax vaccine
orbiculare
- *Pityrosporon* o.

orbital
- o. depression
- o. exenteration gastroscopic access technique

Orcein stain
orchalis
orchectomy (*var. of* orchiectomy)
orchialgia, orchidalgia, orchioneuralgia
orchiatrophy
orchichorea
ORCHID
- Optimal Regimen Cures *Helicobacter*-Induced Dyspepsia
- ORCHID study

orchid
- calix o.

orchidalgia (*var. of* orchialgia)
orchidectomy (*var. of* orchiectomy)
orchidic
orchiditis (*var. of* orchitis)
orchidoepididymectomy
orchidometer
- Prader o.
- punched-out o.
- Test-Size o.

orchidopexy (*var. of* orchiopexy)
orchidoptosis
orchidorrhaphy
orchidotherapy
orchidotomy (*var. of* orchiotomy)
orchiectomy, orchectomy, orchidectomy
- partial o.
- prophylactic o.
- radical inguinal o.

orchiencephaloma
orchiepididymitis

orchilytic, orchitolytic
orchiocatabasis
orchiocele
orchiococcus
orchiodynia
orchiomyeloma
orchioncus
orchioneuralgia (*var. of* orchialgia)
orchiopathy
orchiopexy, orchidopexy
    Bevan o.
    Cabot-Nesbit o.
    eversion o.
    Fowler-Stephens o.
    laparoscopic o.
    Prentiss o.
    prophylactic o.
    scrotal pouch o.
    staged o.
    standard o.
    Torek o.
    transseptal o.
    two-step o.
    vasal pedicle o.
orchioplasty
orchiorrhaphy
orchiotherapy
orchiotomy, orchidotomy, orchotomy
orchis
orchitic
orchitis, orchiditis
    filarial o.
    metastatic o.
    o. parotidea
    Salmonella enteritidis o.
    spermatogenic granulomatous o.
    traumatic o.
    o. variolosa
orchitolytic (*var. of* orchilytic)
orchotomy (*var. of* orchiotomy)
orciprenaline
O'Regan
    O. hemorrhoid ligator
    O. procedure
Oresus Potentest test
Oretic
Oreticyl
Orfadin capsule
organ
    o. allocation policy
    artificial o.
    o. donation

    o. function
    o. of Giraldes
    invasion of adjacent o.
    O. Procurement Program
    radiosensitive o.
    o. transplantation
    well-matched o.
    o. of Zuckerkandl
organelle
organic
    o. conditioning film
    o. impotence
    o. muscle
    o. neurologic disease
    o. nitrate
organism
    Campylobacter-like o. (CLO)
    enteropathic o.
    gram-positive o.
    Helicobacter pylori-like o. (HPLO)
    microaerophilic o.
    pyogenic o.
    resistant o.
    terrestrial o.
    urea splitting o.
organization
    World Health O. (WHO)
organized germinal center
organoaxial gastric volvulus
organogenesis
organomegaly
organoscopy
organs opacified
orgastic impotence
Oriental
    O. cholangiohepatitis
    O. schistosomiasis
orienting reflex
orifice
    appendiceal o.
    bell-shaped o.
    biliary o.
    duodenal o.
    epispadiac o.
    fistulous o.
    obscured ureteral o.
    pancreatic o.
    papillary o.
    sharp-edged o.
    ureteral o.
orificial
orificium, pl. **orificia**

NOTES

orificium *(continued)*
    o. urethrae externum internum
    o. urethrae externum muliebris
    o. urethrae externum virilis
origin
    GI bleeding of obscure o.
    multigenic o.
    neoplastic o.
    O. trocar
O ring
Orion model EA 940 ion analyzer
orlistat
Ormond
    O. disease
    O. syndrome
ornidazole
ornithine
    o. carbamoyl transferase deficiency
    o. decarboxylase (ODC)
ornithine-aspartate
orocecal transit time (OCTT)
oroesophageal overtube
orogastric Ewald tube
oropharyngeal
    o. carcinoma
    o. damage
    o. dysphagia
    o. tube
ororespiratory tract
orosomucoid
orotracheal intubation
orphenadrine
Orr
    O. automatic reprocessor
    O. gall duct forceps
    O. rectal prolapse repair
Orr-Loygue transabdominal proctopexy
ORS
    oral rehydration solution
ORT
    oral rehydration therapy
Ortho
    O. Diagnostic System
    O. HCV 2.0 ELISA test system for hepatitis C
    O. HCV ELISA test system second generation
orthochromatic dye
Orthoclone OKT3
Orthohepadnavirus
Ortho-Kung T (OKT3)
Orthopara-DDD
orthophosphate
orthoplasty
    penile o.
orthostatic
    o. change
    o. proteinuria
orthostatism

orthotopic
    o. appendicocystostomy
    o. bladder
    o. bladder augmentation
    o. bladder substitution
    o. colonic reservoir
    o. continent reservoir
    o. hemi-Kock operation
    o. ileal neobladder
    o. liver transplant (OLT)
    o. reconstruction
    o. remodeled ileocolonic reservoir
    o. ureterocele
    o. urinary diversion
    o. voiding
    o. voiding pouch
Orthotripter
    OssaTron O.
orthovoltage teletherapy
Orthoxine
Orudis
Orzel
OS
    overall survival
OSB gastrostomy device
Osbon
    O. ErecAid VCD
    O. pressure-point tension ring
Os-Cal
oscheal
oscheitis
oschelephantiasis
oscheocele
oscheohydrocele
oscheolith
oscheoma
oscheoncus
oscheoplasty
oscillation
    myenteric potential o.
oscillatory potential
oscilloscope
    Tektronix digital o.
OSI-774
    erlotinib
Osler
    O. II syndrome
    O. node
Osler-Weber-Rendu
    O.-W.-R. disease
    O.-W.-R. syndrome
    O.-W.-R. telangiectasia
Osmette osmometer
osmium tetroxide
Osmoglyn
osmolality
    body fluid o.
    diurnal urine o.
    medullary interstitial o.

osmolality · 12-O-tetradecanoylphorbol-13-acetate

plasma o.
urine o.
osmolar clearance
osmolarity
  different o.
  o. gap
  o. of ink
  serum o.
  urine o. (Uosm)
Osmolite HN enteral feeding
osmolyte
osmometer
  model 5500 vapor pressure o.
  Osmette o.
osmoreceptor
OSMO reverse osmosis unit
osmotherapy
osmotic
  o. cathartic
  o. demyelination syndrome
  o. diarrhea
  o. diuresis
  o. diuretic
  o. laxative
  o. load
  o. nephrosis
  o. stimulus
  o. threshold for thirst
OssaTron
  O. Orthotripter
  O. shock wave therapy
osseous metaplasia
ossification
  metaplastic o.
Ossoff-Karlan laryngoscope
osteitis pubis
osteoarthropathy
  hypertrophic o.
osteoblast-derived
osteoblast-like proliferation
osteocalcin
osteoclast
  acid phosphate o.
  o. maturation
osteoclast-activating factor
osteoclast-like giant cell (OCLG)
osteodystrophy
  Albright hereditary o. (AHO)
  azotemic o.
  hepatic o.
  renal o.

osteogenic
  o. differentiation
  o. sarcoma
osteomalacia
  dialysis o.
  low-turnover o. (LTOM)
osteomyelitis
osteoonychodysplasia
  hereditary o.
osteopenia
osteophyte
  esophageal o.
osteopontin
osteoporosis
osteosarcoma
  bladder o.
osteotomy
  anterior innominate o.
  Dickson o.
  pelvic o.
ostia (*pl. of* ostium)
ostial
  o. artery atherosclerosis
  o. atherosclerotic plaque
ostiomeatal
ostium, pl. **ostia**
  o. appendicis vermiformis
  o. ileocecale
  o. pyloricum
  o. urethrae externum feminae
  o. urethrae externum masculinae
  o. urethrae internum
  o. valvae ilealis
ostomate
ostomy
  o. appliance
  O. Assessment Inventory (OAI)
  o. bag
  ConvaTec Durahesive Wafer o.
  o. loop
  o. skin
  o. takedown
ostreotoxism
O'Sullivan-O'Connor abdominal retractor
O'Sullivan scoring system
OTA
  oligoteratoasthenozoospermia
12-O-tetradecanoylphorbol-13-acetate (TPA, tPA)
  phorbol ester 12-O.-t.-13-a.

NOTES

Otis
    O. anoscope
    O. sound
    O. urethrotome
    O. urethrotomy
otitidis-caviarum
    Nocardia o.-c.
otolaryngologic manifestation
Otrivin
Ott/Mayo Channel Sampling kit
ouabain
ouabainlike substance (OLS)
out
    coring o.
outcome
    o. of cadaveric renal allograft
    o. equivalent to open surgery
    favorable o.
    health o.
    impact of microwave antennas on treatment o.
    long-term o.
    multicenter o.
    oncological o.
    poor long-term o.
    o. predictor
    primary o.
    o. and process assessment
    short-term survival o.
outer
    o. cortical blood flow (OCBF)
    o. crossbar
    o. diameter (OD)
    o. inflammatory protein
    o. medulla
    o. medullary collecting duct
    o. medullary ischemia
outflow
    hepatic venous o.
    mean venous o. (MVO)
    o. obstruction
    pulmonary o.
    o. tract
    vagal efferent o.
outlet
    bladder o.
    o. delay
    o. dysfunction
    gastric o.
    o. obstruction
    o. obstruction constipation
    pyloric o.
outlier syndrome
outline
    gastric o.
out-of-scope lithotriptor
outpatient endoscopy
output
    basal acid o. (BAO)
    bile phospholipid o. (BPO)
    bile salt o. (BSO)
    biliary cholesterol o. (BCO)
    cardiac o.
    intake and o. (I&O)
    maximal acid o. (MAO)
    meal-stimulated acid o. (MSAO)
    peak acid o. (PAO)
    urinary o.
outstanding anatomical detail
ova (*pl. of* ovum)
oval
    o. esophagoscope
    o. fat body
    o. snare
ovalbumin
oval-form colonic groove
ovalis
    fossa o.
oval-open esophagoscope
ovaria (*pl. of* ovarium)
ovarian
    o. artery
    o. cancer
    o. carcinoma
    o. dermoid cyst
    o. disease
    o. endometrioma
    o. enlargement
    o. fibroma
    o. hyperstimulation syndrome
    o. overstimulation syndrome
    o. remnant syndrome
    o. teratoma
    o. vein syndrome
ovarii
    stroma o.
    struma o.
    tunica albuginea o.
ovarium, pl. **ovaria**
    o. masculinum
ovary
    streak o.
ovatus
    Bacteroides o.
overactive bladder
overactivity
    detrusor muscle o.
overall
    o. mortality
    o. survival (OS)
over-and-over suture
overdistention, overdistension
    bladder o.
overdose (OD)
    acetaminophen o.
overdosing
overexpression
    p53 o.

overflow
    o. aminoaciduria
    o. fecal incontinence
    o. proteinuria
    o. theory
overgrowth
    bacterial o.
    candidal o.
    gastric bacterial o. (GBO)
    small intestine bacterial o. (SIBO)
    tube o.
    tumor o.
    yeast o.
overlapping sphincteroplasty
overlap syndrome
overload
    African iron o.
    hepatic copper o.
    nitrogen o.
    transfusional iron o.
    volume o.
overlying clot
overproduction
    oxalate o.
overreactive puborectalis
oversedation
over-the-endoscope Witzel dilator
over-the-wire
    o.-t.-w. balloon catheter
    o.-t.-w. set
    o.-t.-w. technique
overt nephropathy
overtube
    Christopher-Williams o.
    flexible endoscopic o.
    Mill-Rose flexible endoscopic o.
    negative pressure o.
    oroesophageal o.
    rotational colonoscope o.
    o. sheath
    split o.
    Steigmann-Goff endoscopic ligature o.
    Williams varix injection o.
oviductal fluid
oviduct epithelium
ovoid fungus
ovotestis, ovotestes
ovum, pl. **ova**
    ova, cysts, and parasites (OCP)
    ova and parasites (O&P)
oxacillin

oxacillin-associated anicteric hepatitis
oxalate
    calcium o.
    o. calculus
    o. crystal
    dietary o.
    o. intestinal absorption
    o. metabolism
    o. nephropathy
    o. overproduction
    urinary o.
oxalic acid
oxaliplatin, 5-fluorouracil, leucovorin
oxaloacetate
Oxalobacter formigenes
oxalosis
    primary o.
oxaluria
    calcium o.
    enteric o.
oxamniquine
oxandrolone treatment
oxaprozin
oxatomide
oxazepam
oxcarbazepine
oxidant
    o. injury
    iron-dependent o.
oxidant-trapping potential
oxidase
    o. cytosolic factor
    diamine o.
    NADPH o.
    xanthine o.
oxidation
    arachidonic acid o.
    substrate o.
    xanthine o.
oxidative
    o. burst
    o. cell injury
    o. phosphorylation
    slow-twitch o.
    o. stress
oxidative-glycolytic fiber
oxide
    deuterium o.
    donor of nitric o.
    endothelium-derived nitric o. (EDNO)
    ethylene o.

NOTES

oxide *(continued)*
    magnesium o.
    mercuric o.
    nitric o. (NO)
    nitrous o.
    propylene o.
    ultrasmall superparamagnetic iron o. (USPIO)
oxidized
    o. LDL
    o. lipoprotein
    o. low-density lipoprotein (Ox-LDL)
oxidoreductase activity
oxime
    sugar o.
oximetry
    pulse o.
oxine
Ox-LDL
    oxidized low-density lipoprotein
oxpentifylline
oxybutynin
    o. chloride
    intravesical o.
    o. transdermal patch
    o. transdermal system
Oxycel cotton
oxychlorosene sodium
oxycodone
oxygen (O_2)
    blood gas on o.
    o. desaturation
    fractional percentage of inspired o. (FIO_2)
    hyperbaric o.
    o. radical
    o. saturation
    o. saturation index (ISO_2)
oxygen-15
oxygenating mouthguard
oxygenation
    medullary o.
oxygenator
    membrane o.
oxygen-derived free radical
oxygen-free radical
Oxyguard oxygenating mouthguard
oxymorphone
oxyntic
    o. cell
    o. gland
    o. mucosa
    o. mucosal gastritis
oxyphenbutazone
oxyphencyclimine hydrochloride
oxyphenonium
oxytoca
    Klebsiella o.
oxytocin
Oxytrol transdermal system
Oxyuris

P
    P blood group system
    P cell
P-32, ³²P
    phosphorus-32
p53
    p53 allelotyping
    p53 antibody
    p53 assay
    p53 expression
    p53 immunohistochemical stain
    p53 immunohistochemistry
    p53 mutation
    p53 nuclear protein
    p53 nuclear staining
    p53 overexpression
    p53 protein
    p53 protooncogene
    p53 reactivity
    p53 tumor-suppressor gene analysis
P27Kip1 **gene**
p15 **gene**
P15/INK4B **gene**
p16 **gene**
p18 **gene**
P21/WAF1 **gene**
P23b Statham pressure transducer
P24 antigen
P450 function
p47, p67 cytosolic protein
p53 **gene**
PA
    plasminogen activator
PAA
    periampullary adenoma
10Pa Amicon chamber
PAb
    protein antibody
        PAb 1801 monoclonal antibody
PABA
    paraaminobenzoic acid
        PABA test
PACAP
    pituitary adenylate cyclase-activating polypeptide
paced rhythm
pacemaker
    p. cell
        Enterra gastrointestinal p.
pachycholia
pachychymia
pacificum
    Diphyllobothrium p.
pacinian corpuscle

Pacis BCG bladder cancer immunotherapy
pack
    gauze p.
    laparotomy p.
    moist laparotomy p.
    petrolatum gauze p.
    Rheumatrex dose p.
package
    GastroSoft data reduction and prognostic software p.
    lymphatic p.
Packard Auto-Gamma 5650 analyzer
packed red blood cells
packet
    single-dose p.
packing
    Adaptic p.
    p. forceps
    p. fraction
    gelatin sponge p.
    Mikulicz p.
paclitaxel
    polyglutamate p.
Pacquin ureterolysis
pad
    abdominal fat p.
    abdominal laparotomy p.
    Active Living incontinence p.
    antimesenteric fat p.
    bed p.
    bulbocavernosus fat p.
    p. cover
    dinner p.
    esophagogastric fat p.
    fat p.
    ileocecal fat p.
    lap p.
    laparotomy p.
    Martius fat p.
    Mikulicz p.
    perineal p.
    Sani-Pads medicated cleansing p.
    p. testing
    p. test for urinary incontinence
    p. urinary incontinence test
padding
    absorbent p.
    Spenco p.
PADS
    pain-associated disability syndrome
Padua bladder urinary pouch
Paecilomyces
PAF
    platelet-activating factor

Pagano
- P. technique ureterocolonic anastomosis
- P. ureteral anastomosis

PAGE
- polyacrylamide gel electrophoresis

Page kidney

Pagenstecher circle

Paget
- P. disease of perianal area
- P. extramammary disease
- P. perianal disease

pagetoid

Pagitane

PAH
- paraaminohippurate
- paraaminohippuric
  - PAH acid
  - PAH clearance

PAI
- plasminogen activator inhibitor

PAI-1, -2
- plasminogen activator inhibitor type 1, 2

pain
- abdominal p.
- acute flank p.
- ameliorate p.
- biliary tract p. (BTP)
- bladder p.
- boring p.
- burning p.
- chest p.
- colicky abdominal p.
- constricting p.
- p. control
- crampy abdominal p.
- deep p.
- diffuse p.
- drug-induced p.
- dull p.
- epicritic p.
- epigastric p.
- exacerbation of p.
- exertion-induced p.
- exquisite p.
- p. fiber
- flank p.
- functional p.
- gnawing p.
- hunger p.
- inevitable postoperative p.
- intermittent p.
- knife-like p.
- lancinating p.
- localized p.
- loin p.
- nagging p.
- NIH Classification Category III inflammatory and noninflammatory chronic pelvic p.
- nocturnal p.
- noncardiac chest p. (NCCP)
- onset of p.
- palliation of p.
- parietal p.
- perianal p.
- perirectal p.
- poorly localized p.
- postligation p.
- postprandial p.
- posture-dependent p.
- protopathic p.
- radiating p.
- rebound p.
- recurrent abdominal p. (RAP)
- referred p.
- remission of p.
- retrosternal chest p.
- sciatica-like p.
- scrotal p.
- severe p.
- somatic p.
- steady p.
- sudden onset of p.
- tearing p.
- testicular p.
- triangle of p.
- unrelenting p.
- unrelieved p.
- unremitting p.
- visceral p.

pain-associated disability syndrome (PADS)

painful
- p. defecation
- p. hematuria

painless
- p. hematuria
- p. jaundice
- p. rectal bleeding

pain-predominant irritable bowel syndrome

paint
- Castellani p.

painter's colic

Pak
- Trovan/Zithromax Compliance P.

palate
- cleft p.
- smoker's p.

palatine pillar

palatinus
- torus p.

palatoglossus muscle

palatopharyngeal fold

palatopharyngeus muscle

Palco enuretic alarm system
pale
    p. cell
    p. stool
Paleolithic diet
palindrome
palindromic rheumatism
palisade-type vein
palladium-103
    p.-103 seed implant
    transperineal p.-103
palliation
    p. of malignant large bowel obstruction
    p. of pain
palliative
    p. cystectomy
    p. decompression
    p. exeresis
    p. nephrectomy
    p. surgery
    p. therapy
pallidum
    Treponema p.
pallidus
    raphe p.
pallor
    cachectic p.
    mucosal p.
palmar
    p. erythema
    p. grasp
palmaris
    tylosis p.
palmatus
    penis p.
Palmaz
    P. balloon-expandable stent
    P. Corinthian biliary stent and delivery system
    P. Corinthian stent
Palmaz-Schatz biliary stent
Palmer acid test for peptic ulcer
palmin test
palmitin test
Palomo
    P. operation
    P. procedure
    P. technique
palonosetron
palpable
    p. adenopathy
    p. cord
    p. gallbladder
    p. kidney
    p. mass
    p. pyloric olive
    p. rib diastasis
    p. stool
palpably normal
palpating probe
palpation
    bladder p.
    p. in epigastrium
    p. tenderness
palpatory proteinuria
palpebrae
    paraphimosis p.
palsy
    cerebral p.
PAM
    pancreatic acinar metaplasia
Pamelor
Pamine Forte
p-aminohippuric acid
Pamisyl
pamoate
    pyrantel p.
pampiniformis
    plexus p.
pampiniform plexus
pampinocele
PAN
    puromycin aminonucleoside nephropathy
    puromycin aminonucleoside nephrosis
panacinar
    p. disease
    p. emphysema
Panafil ointment
pan-bud anomaly
p-ANC
    perinuclear antineutrophil cytoplasmic
    p-ANC genetic marker
p-ANCA
    perinuclear antineutrophil cytoplasmic antibody
pancake kidney
pancolectomy
pancolitis
    steroid-responsive p.
pancolonoscopy
pancreas
    aberrant p.
    p. accessorium

NOTES

pancreas *(continued)*
    accessory p.
    acinarization of p.
    anlage of p.
    annular p.
    Aselli p.
    capsule of p.
    Christmas tree appearance of p.
    divided p.
    p. divisum (PD)
    ectopic p.
    endoscopic retrograde parenchymography of p. (ERPP)
    exocrine p.
    fibrocystic disease of p.
    fibrofatty infiltration of p.
    head of p.
    heterotopic p.
    heterotopic-aberrant p.
    intraductal papillary and mucinous tumors of p. (IPMY)
    p. lesion
    lesser p.
    lobule of p.
    neck of p.
    solid and cystic tumors of p. (SCTP)
    tail of p.
    p. transplantation
    unciform p.
    uncinate process of p.
    Willis p.
    Winslow p.
Pancrease MT 4, 10, 16, 20
pancreas-kidney transplant
pancreatalgia
pancreatectomy, pancreectomy
    distal p.
    en bloc distal p.
    left-to-right subtotal p.
    partial p.
    subtotal p.
    total p.
    Whipple p.
pancreatic
    p. acinar cell
    p. acinar cell carcinoma
    p. acinar metaplasia (PAM)
    p. acinus
    p. agenesis
    p. alpha-amylase
    p. amylase
    p. ascariasis
    p. ascites
    p. bladder
    p. blood flow
    p. calcification
    p. calculus
    p. cancer (PC)
    p. cancer marker
    p. carcinoma (PCA)
    p. cholera
    p. cholera syndrome
    p. colic
    p. cutaneous fistula
    p. cyst
    p. diabetes
    p. diastase
    p. disease
    p. diverticulum
    p. duct
    p. ductal hypertension
    p. ductal morphological change
    p. duct-choledochus channel
    p. duct disruption
    p. duct encasement
    p. duct manipulation
    p. ductogram
    p. duct pressure (PDP)
    p. duct to pseudocyst
    p. duct sphincter (PDS)
    p. duct sphincterotomy
    p. duct stent
    p. duct stone
    p. duct stricture
    p. endopeptidase
    p. endoprosthesis
    p. enema
    p. enzyme replacement therapy
    p. exocrine dysfunction
    p. exocrine insufficiency
    p. exopeptidase
    p. fibrosis
    p. flare
    p. fluid collection (PFC)
    p. glandular necrosis
    p. hamartoma
    p. head
    p. injury
    p. intraluminal radiation therapy
    p. islet cell
    p. islet cell carcinoma
    p. islet cell transplantation
    p. islet cell tumor
    p. isoamylase enzyme
    p. juice
    p. lesion
    p. lipase
    p. lipase deficiency
    p. lymphangiectasia
    p. mucinous cystadenocarcinoma
    p. oncofetal antigen (POA)
    p. orifice
    p. papillary stenosis
    p. parenchyma
    p. phlegmon
    p. polypeptide (PP)

p. polypeptide-secreting tumor (PPoma)
p. polypeptide stain
p. pseudocyst
p. pseudocyst abscess
p. pseudocystogastrostomy
p. rendezvous
p. rest
p. sarcoidosis
p. secretory flow rate (PSFR)
p. secretory test
p. secretory trypsin inhibitor (PSTI)
p. sepsis
p. sepsis in acute pancreatitis
p. sphincteroplasty
p. steatorrhea
p. stone protein (PSP)
p. tail resection
p. transpapillary stenting
p. trauma
p. tree
p. tumor diagnosis
p. tumor localization

pancreatica
achylia p.
diarrhea p.
p. magna artery
sialorrhea p.

pancreaticobiliary
p. common channel
p. disease
p. ductal junction
p. ductal system
p. endoscopy
p. malignancy
p. maljunction
p. reflux
p. septum
p. sphincter
p. stricture
p. tract
p. tree

pancreaticocholedochoductal junction
pancreaticocystostomy
pancreaticoduodenal
anterosuperior p. (ASPD)
p. arteriography
p. transplantation
p. vein
p. venous drainage

pancreaticoduodenectomy
pylorus-sparing p.
Whipple p.
pancreaticoduodenostomy
Child p.
Dennis-Varco p.
Waugh-Clagett p.
Whipple p.
pancreaticogastric anastomosis
pancreaticogastrostomy
pancreaticohepatic syndrome
pancreaticojejunostomy
caudal p.
Duval distal p.
lateral p.
longitudinal p.
Puestow p.
Roux-en-Y p.
p. stenosis
pancreaticopleural fistula
pancreaticosplenic omentum
pancreatic-portal vein fistula
pancreaticus
ansa p.
ductus p.
hemosuccus p.
liquor p.
succus p.
pancreatin
pancreatis
arteria caudae p.
caput p.
corpus p.
facies anterior p.
facies inferior p.
facies posterior p.
pancreatitis
acquired p.
acute edematous p. (AEP)
acute gallstone p. (AGP)
acute hemorrhagic p.
acute recurrent p. (ARP)
acute relapsing p.
alcoholic p.
alcohol-induced p.
biliary p.
calcareous p.
calcific p.
calcifying p.
capsula p.
centrilobular p.
chronic p. (CP)

NOTES

pancreatitis *(continued)*
   chronic alcoholic p. (CAP)
   chronic alcohol-induced p.
   chronic calcifying p. (CCP)
   chronic fibrosing p.
   chronic relapsing p.
   coagulopathy p.
   diffuse p.
   drug-induced acute p.
   edematous p.
   endoscopic sphincterotomy-induced p.
   familial p.
   focal p.
   fulminating p.
   gallstone p.
   Glasgow criteria for severity of p.
   groove p.
   hemoductal p.
   hemorrhagic necrotizing p.
   hereditary p. (HP)
   idiopathic fibrosing p.
   idiopathic recurrent p. (IRP)
   inflammatory p.
   interstitial p.
   microlithiasis-induced p.
   mumps p.
   necrotizing p.
   nodular p.
   nutritional p.
   obstructive p.
   pancreatic sepsis in acute p.
   pentamidine-induced p.
   perilobar p.
   phlegmonous p.
   post-ERCP-induced p.
   postprocedure p.
   purulent p.
   Ranson criteria for severity of p.
   recurrent p.
   relapsing acute p.
   segmentary p.
   tropical calcific p.
   ventral chronic calcific p.
pancreatitis-related
   p.-r. bleeding
   p.-r. hemorrhage
pancreatobiliary
   p. canal
   p. region
pancreatocholangiography
   retrograde p.
pancreatocholecystostomy
pancreatoduodenal cancer
pancreatoduodenectomy
   pylorus-preserving p. (PPPD)
pancreatoduodenostomy
pancreatogastrostomy

pancreatogenous, pancreatogenic
   p. diarrhea
pancreatogram
   rat-tail appearance on p.
   retrograde p.
pancreatography
   dye-injection endoscopic retrograde p.
   endoscopic digital p. (EDP)
   endoscopic retrograde p. (ERP)
   magnetic resonance p. (MRP)
   retrograde p.
   three-dimensional CT p. (3-DCTP)
pancreatojejunostomy
   cystolateral p.
   retrocolic end-to-end p.
pancreatolith, pancreolith
pancreatolithectomy
pancreatolithiasis
pancreatolithotomy
pancreatolysis, pancreolysis
pancreatolytic, pancreolytic
pancreatomegaly
pancreatomy *(var. of* pancreatotomy*)*
pancreatopathy
pancreatoscope
   peroral electronic p. (PEPS)
   ultrathin p.
pancreatoscopic laser lithotripsy (PSLL)
pancreatoscopy
   peroral p. (POPS)
pancreatotomy, pancreatomy
Pancrecarb MS-8
pancreectomy *(var. of* pancreatectomy*)*
pancrelipase
pancreolith *(var. of* pancreatolith*)*
pancreolysis *(var. of* pancreatolysis*)*
pancreolytic *(var. of* pancreatolytic*)*
pancreopathy
pancreoprivic
pancreoscopy
   infragastric p.
pancreozymin
Pancrex
pancuronium
Panda gastrostomy feeding tube
pandysautonomia
panel
   Nephrolithiasis Clinical Guidelines P.
panel-reactive antibody (PRA)
panendoscope
   cap-fitted p.
   flexible forward-viewing p.
   Olympus GIF-D-series p.
   Olympus GIF-XQ-series p.
   Storz p.
   Wolf rigid p.

panendoscopy
  fiberoptic p.
  lower p.
  primary p.
  upper gastrointestinal p.
panenteroscopy
  laparoscopically assisted p.
Paneth cell
pangastritis
  atrophic p.
  nonatrophic p.
panlobular emphysema
panmalabsorption
panmucosal inflammatory cell infiltration
panmural cystitis
Panmycin
panniculalgia
panniculectomy
panniculitis
  mesenteric p. (MP)
  scrotal p.
panniculus, pl. panniculi
  hanging p.
pannus
panostotic fibrous dysplasia
Panoview rod-lens ureteroscope
panproctocolectomy
pantaloon hernia
Pantoloc+
Pantoloc tablet
Pantopaque
pantoprazole
  p. sodium
  p. sodium delayed-release tablet
pantothenic
  p. acid
  p. acid deficiency-induced colitis
pants
  Ashton p.
  Dignity incontinence p.
  Endo p.
  Holyoke p.
  Kleinert p.
  Suretys p.
  Ultrafem p.
pants-over-vest
  p.-o.-v. hernia repair
  p.-o.-v. herniorrhaphy
Panzer gallbladder scissors
PAO
  peak acid output

PAOGRP
  peak acid output after gastrin-releasing peptide
PAOPg
  peak acid output after pentagastrin stimulation
PAP
  prostatic acid phosphatase
  pulmonary artery pressure
papain
Papanicolaou
  P. method
  P. smear
  P. stain
  P. test
papaverine
  p. hydrochloride
  p. injection
PAP-HT25 cell
papilla, pl. papillae
  balloon dilation of p.
  ballooning of p.
  bile p.
  bulging p.
  duodenal p.
  p. duodeni major
  p. duodeni minor
  foliate papillae
  frenulum of duodenal p.
  fungiform p.
  glans penis p.
  ileal p.
  p. ilealis
  p. ileocaecalis
  ileocecal p.
  intradiverticular p.
  laparoscopic transcystic duct stenting of p.
  major p.
  minor p.
  necrosis of renal p.
  patulous p.
  renal p.
  p. of Santorini
  sloughed p.
  Suda classification type I, II, III of p.
  vallate p.
  p. of Vater
papillary
  p. adenocarcinoma
  p. adenoma

papillary *(continued)*
    p. adenoma of large intestine
    p. cystitis
    p. gastric carcinoma
    p. hyperplasia
    p. lesion
    p. manometry
    p. necrosis
    p. orifice
    p. renal cancer
    p. renal cell carcinoma
    p. stenosis
    p. tip
    p. transitional cell carcinoma
papillate
papillation
papillectomy
    balloon catheter-assisted endoscopic snare p.
papilledema
papilliferous
papilliform
papillitis
papilloma
    bladder inverted p.
    esophageal squamous p.
    gingival p.
    hirsutoid p.
    inverted p.
    p. of renal pelvis
    sporadic gingival p.
    squamous cell p. (SCP)
    p. venereum
    villous p.
papilloma-carcinoma sequence
papillomatosis
    biliary p.
    p. of intrahepatic bile duct
papillomatous neotransformation
papillomavirus
    genital human p.
    human p. (HPV)
    human p. 16 (HPV 16)
papillotome
    30-30 p.
    Accuratome precurved p.
    Bard Companion p.
    Classen-Demling p.
    Cremer-Ikeda p.
    double-lumen tapered-tip p.
    dual-lumen p.
    Erlangen p.
    Frimberger-Karpiel 12 o'clock p.
    Howell Rotatable BII p.
    Huibregtse-Katon p.
    Microvasive p.
    needle p.
    needle-knife p.
    Olympus needle-knife p.
    Piggyback needle-knife p.
    precut p.
    shark fin p.
    Swenson p.
    Wilson-Cook p.
    Wiltek p.
papillotome/sphincterotome
    Zimmon p./s.
papillotomy
    access p.
    endoscopic p. (EPT)
    Erlangen pull-type precut p.
    laparoscopic transcystic p.
    needle-knife p. (NKP)
    needle-knife precut p. (NKPP)
    precut p.
Pap-Kaps
papular acrodermatitis of childhood
papule
    Bowen p.
    moist p.
    mucous p.
    pearly penile p.
papulosis
    bowenoid p.
    malignant atrophic p.
papulosquamous disorder
papulous gastropathy
Paque
    E-Z P.
Paquin
    P. repair
    P. technique
    P. ureteral reimplantation
PAR
    postanesthesia recovery
paraaminobenzoic acid (PABA)
paraaminohippurate (PAH)
    p. clearance
paraaminohippuric (PAH)
    p. acid
    p. acid synthetase
paraaminosalicylate hypersensitivity
para-ANC antibody
paraaortic
    p. lymphadenectomy
    p. region
parabola
paracancerous tissue
paracecal appendix
paracellular
    p. flux
    p. pathway
    p. route
paracentesis
    abdominal p.
    diagnostic p.
    large-volume p. (LVP)
paracervical tenderness

paracetamol
    p. absorption
    p. absorption test
    p. acute liver failure
parachute reflex
Paracoccidioides brasiliensis
paracoccidioidomycosis
paracolic
    p. abscess
    p. groove
    p. gutter
paracollicular biopsy
paracolostomy
    p. hernia
    p. herniation
paraconal fascia
paracrine
    p. cell
    p. factor
    p. peptide
paradigm
    Sternberg p.
paradoxical
    p. diarrhea
    p. incontinence
    p. puborectalis contraction
    p. renal response
    p. sphincter reaction
paradoxic motion
paradoxus
    pulsus p.
paraductal adenopathy
paraduodenal
    p. fold
    p. hernia
    p. pseudocyst
paradysenteriae
    Shigella p.
paraesophageal
    p. collateral vein
    p. diaphragmatic hernia
    p. hernia type I, II
    p. hiatal hernia
    p. varix
paraesophagogastric
    p. devascularization
    p. lymph node metastasis
paraexstrophy skin flap
paraffin-embedded
    p.-e. specimen
    p.-e. tissue
paraffinoma

paraffin-section light microscopy
paraformaldehyde
parafrenal abscess
paraganglioma
paragastric pseudocyst
paragenitalis
paraglobulinuria
parahaemolyticus
    Vibrio p.
parahiatal hernia
paraileostomal hernia
paraisopropyliminodiacetic acid (PIPIDA)
parakeratosis
parallel plate dialyzer
paralysis, pl. **paralyses**
    esophageal p.
paralytic
    p. colonic obstruction
    p. ileus
    p. incontinence
    p. intestinal obstruction
    p. secretion
    p. shellfish poisoning
paralytica
    dysphagia p.
paralyticus
    ileus p.
parameatal-based flap
paramedian incision
parameter
    anthropomorphic p.
    chronobiological p.
    clinical p.
    clotting p.
    DIC p.
    individual p.
    kinetic p.
    prostate-specific antigen-based p.
    PSA-based p.
    quality-of-life p.
    specific clinical p.
    urodynamic p.
    valuable additional p.
    vascular p.
    voiding p.
paraneoplastic
    p. dermatomyositis
    p. syndrome
paranephric abscess
paranephritis
    lipomatous p.
paranephroma

NOTES

paranitroaniline release
paranitrophenol phosphate
parapancreatic mass
paraparesis
    spastic p.
    tropical spastic p.
parapelvic cyst
paraperitoneal nephrectomy
paraphimosis palpebrae
paraplegia
paraproctitis
paraprostatitis
paraproteinemia
parapubic hernia
paraquat
paraquat-induced upper gastrointestinal injury
pararectal
    p. abscess
    p. fistula
    p. line
    p. pouch
pararectus incision
pararotovirus
parasagittal plane
parasite
    p. examination
    hemoflagellate p.
    intestinal p.
    isosporan p.
    ova and p.'s (O&P)
    ova, cysts, and p.'s (OCP)
    protozoan p.
    stool for ova and p.'s
    urinalysis sediment microscopy p.
parasitemia
parasitic
    p. chylocele
    p. cyst
    p. infection
    p. infestation
    p. leiomyoma
    p. liver disease
    p. peritonitis
    p. prostatitis
parasitizing macrophage
parasitology
paraspinal musculature
paraspinous
    p. aspect
    p. muscle
parastomal hernia
parasympathetic
    p. postganglionic neuron
    p. preganglionic neuron
    p. projection
parasympatholytic drug
parasympathomimetic
    p. agent

    p. anticholinesterase
    p. drug
paratesticular
    p. fat
    p. leiomyosarcoma
    p. malignancy
    p. neoplasm
    p. rhabdomyosarcoma
    p. tumor
parathyroid
    p. disease
    p. hormone (PTH)
    p. hormone-related polypeptide
    p. hyperplasia
    p. imaging
paratuberculosis
    Mycobacterium p.
paratyphi
    Salmonella p. A, B, C
paraumbilical
    p. vein
    p. vein tumor (PUVT)
paraureteric
paraurethra
paraurethral
    p. cyst
    p. gland
paraurethrales
paraurethritis
paravaginal
    p. fascial repair
    p. pedicle
paravariceal
    p. fibrosis
    p. injection
    p. sclerotherapy
paraventricular nucleus (PVN)
paravertebral neuroblastoma
paravesical
    p. fossa
    p. pouch
paregoric
parenchyma
    allograft p.
    hepatic p.
    inhomogeneity of p.
    liver p.
    pancreatic p.
    renal p.
parenchymal
    p. atrophy
    p. collapse
    p. damage
    p. hematoma
    p. inflammation
    p. jaundice
    p. liver disease
    p. tissue
    p. tumor

parenchymal-sparing surgery
parenchymatous
    p. acute renal failure
    p. nephritis
parenchymography
    endoscopic retrograde p. (ERP)
parenteral
    p. alimentation
    p. diarrhea
    p. feeding
    p. guanethidine
    p. hyperalimentation
    p. immunization
    p. methyldopa
    p. nutrition
paresthesia
    lateral cutaneous p.
paretic impotence
pargyline
paries, pl. **parietes**
parietal
    p. cell
    p. cell index
    p. cell vagotomy (PCV)
    p. epithelium
    p. fistula
    p. hernia
    p. pain
    p. peritoneum
Parietex composite mesh for hernia surgery
parietitis
parietocolic fold
parietography
    gastric p.
parietosplanchnic
PARIET therapy
Paris renal adenocarcinoma
Parker-Kerr
    P.-K. closed method
    P.-K. closed method of end-to-end enteroenterostomy
    P.-K. intestinal clamp
    P.-K. suture
Parker retractor
Parkinson disease
parkinsonian gait
Parks
    P. ileal reservoir
    P. ileoanal anastomosis
    P. ileoanal reservoir
    P. ileostomy pouch

    P. method of anal fistulotomy
    P. partial sphincterotomy
    P. retractor
    P. staged fistulotomy
Parnate
paromomycin
paromphalocele
paronychia
parorchidium
parotidea
    orchitis p.
parotid gland enlargement
parovarian
    p. cyst
    p. mass
paroxetine
paroxysmal
    p. anal hyperkinesis
    p. motor disease
    p. nocturnal hemoglobinemia
    p. nocturnal hemoglobinuria (PNH)
Parsidol
partial
    p. adrenalectomy
    p. bile outflow obstruction
    p. bladder denervation
    p. bowel obstruction
    p. cystectomy
    p. enterocele
    p. external biliary diversion
    p. fasting
    p. fundoplication
    p. gastrectomy
    p. hepatectomy
    p. hood assisted lift-and-cut method
    p. ileal bypass
    p. nephrogenic diabetes insipidus phenotype
    p. orchidectomy
    p. pancreatectomy
    p. penectomy
    p. polar nephrectomy
    p. thromboplastin time (PTT)
    p. ureteral obstruction
    p. villous atrophy (PVA)
    p. water bath and water cushion
    p. zonal dissection (PZD)
partialocclusion clamp
particle
    Dane p.
    food p.
    viruslike p. (VLP)

NOTES

particulate
- p. radiation
- p. silicone
- p. stool

Partington-Rochelle procedure
Partin table
partition
- gastric p.

partitioning
- abdominal p.

paruresis
parvum
- *Corynebacterium* p.
- *Cryptosporidium* p.
- *Diphyllobothrium* p.

PAS
- periodic acid-Schiff
- PAS stain
- PAS test

PAS-AB
- periodic acid-Schiff-Alcian blue

pass
- guided fine-needle p.

passage
- biliary p.
- P. biliary dilatation catheter
- p. of flatus per vagina
- guidewire p.
- incomplete p.
- p. pressure
- spontaneous fragment p.
- spontaneous stone p.
- p. of stool

passer
- Carter-Thomason suture p.
- Protect-a-Pass suture p.

passion flower
passive
- p. chest drainage
- p. congestion
- p. Heymann nephritis (PHN)
- p. incontinence
- p. range of motion

Passport Balloon-on-a-Wire dilatation catheter
paste
- Anatrast barium sulfate p.
- barium p.
- Coloplast skin barrier p.
- Hollister Premium p.
- iLEX skin protectant p.
- Karaya 5 p.
- sandy skin-prepping p.
- Stomahesive p.

Pasteurella multocida
past pointing
PAT
- prophylactic antibiotic treatment

PAT1
- putative anion transporter

patch
- Androderm testosterone transdermal p.
- aortic p.
- bladder p.
- Bowen p.
- Carrel aortic p.
- p. clamp technique
- colic p.
- colonic p.
- estradiol transdermal p.
- Gore-Tex ACUSEAL cardiovascular p.
- Gore-Tex soft tissue p.
- p. graft
- p. graft urethroplasty
- herald p.
- inlet p.
- Kugel hernia p.
- Miniguard adhesive p.
- mucous p.
- murine Peyer p.
- omental p.
- oxybutynin transdermal p.
- Peyer p.
- Rutkow sutureless plug and p.
- schistosomiasis sandy p.
- shagreen p.
- Testoderm p.
- testosterone p.
- vein p.
- white p.

patchiness
- endoscopic p.
- histologic p.

patchy
- p. colitis
- p. colonic ulceration
- p. necrosis

patella disease
patency
- biliary stent p.
- p. rate
- stent p.

patent
- p. airway
- p. processus vaginalis
- p. urachus
- p. urethra

Paterson-Brown-Kelly syndrome
Paterson-Kelly syndrome
pathergy phenomenon
Pathfinder
- P. exchange guidewire
- P. wire

Pathilon

pathogen
    bloodborne p.
    enteric p.
    invasive enteric p.
    prokaryotic p.
    protozoan p.
    zoonotic food-borne p.

pathogenesis
    bacterial p.
    p. of hyperreflexia

pathogenetic factor
pathogenic bacterium
pathogenicity
pathognomonic feature
pathologic
    p. reflux
    p. substaging

pathological
    p. diagnosis
    p. hypersecretory condition
    p. resistive index level

pathology
    extravesical p.
    renal p.
    thoracic aortic p.

pathomechanism
pathophysiology of condition
pathway
    activation of programmed cell death p.
    antigen-dependent p.
    antigen-independent p.
    beta-oxidation p.
    care p.
    cholehepatic shunt p.
    cyclooxygenase p.
    gluconeogenic p.
    glutamine aminotransferase p.
    guanosine monophosphate p.
    lipoxygenase p.
    mitochondrial glutamate dehydrogenase p.
    monooxygenase p.
    multisynaptic p.
    neural p.
    nonapoptotic p.
    oligosynaptic p.
    paracellular p.
    polyol p.
    receptor-mediated endocytosis p.
    renal transduction p.
    signal transduction p.
    transcellular p.
    transduction p.
    WNT/wingless signaling p.

PATI
    Penetrating Abdominal Trauma Index

patient
    p. analgesia
    asymptomatic hemodialysis p.
    benefit for the p.
    Child class A–C p.
    cholestasis p.
    comparison of rates of appropriate EGD long-term management of p.'s
    consecutive asymptomatic p.'s
    cystinuric p.
    diabetic p.
    endoscopically normal p.
    European primary sclerosing cholangitis p.
    p. factor
    factors influencing colonic involvement in p.'s
    false negative rate in high-risk p.
    gastrectomized p.
    hemodialysis p.
    highly selective group of p.'s
    hypoalbuminemic p.
    hypochondriacal p.
    immunophenotypical profiling of p.
    immunosuppressed p.
    institutionalized p.
    irrigating p.
    Medicare p.
    nonazotemic p.
    nonirrigating p.
    nonvoiding p.
    p. positioning
    posttransplant p.
    renal transplant p.
    p. satisfaction
    seminal oxidative stress in p.
    shock p.
    stone-forming p.
    tube-fed p.
    unobstructed p.

patient-controlled
    p.-c. analgesia
    p.-c. sedation (PCS)

pattern
    abdominal wall venous p.
    anhaustral colonic gas p.

NOTES

pattern *(continued)*
    circadian testosterone p.
    cobblestone p.
    colonic mucosal p.
    complex calyceal p.
    crow's foot p.
    cytometric p.
    DNA ploidy p.
    echo p.
    fasted-to-fed p.
    fasting motor p.
    fed motor p.
    fine gastric mucosal p.
    fine reticular p.
    fold p.
    gallstone p.
    gas p.
    haustral p.
    hindgut p.
    histochemical p.
    honeycomb p.
    irregular amputated mucosal p.
    manometric p.
    meal-related secretion p.
    mendelian p.
    mesangial p.
    mosaic duodenal mucosal p.
    mucosal guideline p.
    nodule-in-nodule p.
    nonspecific gas p.
    propulsive motor p.
    punctate fluorescence p.
    Quimby p.
    reticulonodular p.
    rugal p.
    sausage-string p.
    segment-specific expression p.
    snake-skin mucosal p.
    sonographic gallstone p.
    spongy p.
    trabecular sinusoidal p.
    vascular p.
    venous p.
    Wilms tumor tubuloglomerular p.

Patterson-Parker
    P.-P. method
    P.-P. motif

patulous
    p. anus
    p. cardia
    p. gastroesophageal junction
    p. hiatus
    p. papilla
    p. pylorus

Pauchet procedure

pauciimmune
    p. antineutrophil cytoplasmic antibody-associated glomerulonephritis
    p. crescentic glomerulonephritis
    p. glomerular nephritis

paucity
    bile duct p.
    p. of clinical data

Paul-Mikulicz resection

Paul-Mixter tube

paupae
    Trichinella p.

pause-squeeze method

Pavabid

Pavacap

Pavacen

Pavatine

PAX2 **gene**

PAX8 **gene**

Payne-DeWind jejunoileal bypass

Payne operation

Payr
    P. disease
    P. method
    P. pyloric clamp
    P. pyloric forceps
    P. syndrome

Pazo Hemorrhoidal Ointment

PBC
    primary biliary cirrhosis

PBC-associated antibody

PBD
    percutaneous biliary drainage

PBG
    porphobilinogen

PBG-D
    porphobilinogen deaminase

PBI
    penile-brachial index

PBL
    peripheral blood lymphocyte

PBMC
    peripheral blood mononuclear cell
        interphase PBMC

PBNS
    percutaneous bladder neck stabilization
    percutaneous bladder neck suspension

PBPI
    penile-brachial pressure index

PBS
    phosphate-buffered saline

PBS-Tween buffer

PBTE
    percutaneous transhepatic liver biopsy with tract embolization

PC
    pancreatic cancer
    principal cell
        PC Polygraf HR device

PC10 monoclonal antibody

PCA
    pancreatic carcinoma

PCa
    prostate cancer
P-Cadherin
PCAR
    presumed circle area ratio
PCC
    peripheral cholangiocarcinoma
    pneumatosis cystoides coli
PCCL
    percutaneous cholecystolithotomy
PCD
    pneumatic compression device
    postparacentesis circulatory dysfunction
PCDAI
    Pediatric Crohn Disease Activity Index
PCEE automated anastomotic instrument
PCF-140L pediatric colonoscope
PCI
    pneumatosis cystoides intestinalis
PCIVOT
    Prostate Cancer Intervention Versus Observation Trial
PCLD
    polycystic liver disease
PCM
    pericellular matrix
    protein-calorie malnutrition
PCN
    percutaneous nephrolithotomy
PCNA
    proliferating cell nuclear antigen
PCNA-labeling index
PCNL
    percutaneous nephrolithotomy
    percutaneous nephrolithotripsy
    percutaneous nephrostolithotomy
PCP
    Pneumocystis carinii pneumonia
PCPS
    peroral cholangiopancreatoscopy
PCR
    polymerase chain reaction
    protein catabolic rate
PCRC
    primary colorectal cancer
PCR-SSCP
    polymerase chain reaction-based single-stranded conformation polymorphism
PCS
    patient-controlled sedation
    peroral cholangioscopy
    portacaval shunt
    postcholecystectomy syndrome
PCT
    porphyria cutanea tarda
    portacaval transposition
    proximal convoluted tubule
PCTCL
    percutaneous transhepatic cholecystolithotomy
PCV
    parietal cell vagotomy
PCWP
    pulmonary capillary wedge pressure
PD
    pancreas divisum
    peritoneal dialysis
    potential difference
    prostatodynia
PDAI
    Perianal Crohn Disease Activity Index
    Pouchitis Disease Activity Index
PDB
    preperitoneal distention balloon
PDC
    peritoneal dialysis catheter
PDE
    peritoneal dialysis effluent
    phosphodiesterase
PDE5
    PDE5 inhibitor
PDG
    phosphate-dependent glutaminase
PDGF
    platelet-derived growth factor
PDH
    pyruvate dehydrogenase
PDL
    polycystic disease of liver
PDP
    pancreatic duct pressure
PDS
    pancreatic duct sphincter
    PDS Vicryl suture
PDT
    photodynamic therapy
    Photofrin PDT
PE
    pharyngoesophageal
    platinum, etoposide
    portal embolization
peak
    p. acid output (PAO)

NOTES

peak (*continued*)
   p. acid output after gastrin-releasing peptide (PAOGRP)
   p. acid output after pentagastrin stimulation (PAOPg)
   p. flow
   p. flow rate (PFR)
   p. pressure
   pressure p.
   p. response
   p. secretory flow rate (PSFR)
   p. secretory flow rate test
   p. urinary flow study
   p. uroflow

Péan
   P. clamp
   P. forceps

peanut
   p. agglutinin (PNA)
   p. dissector
   p. sponge

pearly
   p. papule of penis
   p. penile papule

Pearson
   P. product correlation
   P. syndrome

pea soup stool
peau d'orange
PEB
   platinum, etoposide, bleomycin

Pecqueti
   receptaculum P.

pecten
   anal p.
   p. of anal canal
   p. analis
   p. band

pectenitis
pectenotomy
pectin
pectinate line
pectin-base skin barrier
pectiniforme
   septum p.

pectoralis muscle
pectoriloquy
   whispered p.

pectus excavatum
pedal
   p. control venography
   p. edema
   suction foot p.

Pedialyte RS electrolyte solution
Pediapred
PediaSure with Fiber
pediatric
   p. carcinoma
   p. colonoscope
   p. colonoscopy
   P. Crohn Disease Activity Index (PCDAI)
   p. cryptococcal epididymoorchitis
   p. endoscope
   p. endoscopy
   p. end-stage liver disease (PELD)
   p. esophagogastroduodenoscopy
   p. feeding tube
   p. fiberscope
   p. gastroscope
   p. nasogastric tube
   P. Peritoneal Dialysis Study consortium
   p. stirrups
   p. stone disease
   p. urinary tract infection
   p. urolithiasis
   p. urology
   p. voiding dysfunction

Pediazole
pedicle
   p. clamp
   p. flap urethroplasty
   p. graft
   p. island flap
   kidney vascular p.
   p. muscle flap
   omental p.
   paravaginal p.
   renal p.
   vascular p.

pedicled
   p. omental graft
   p. omentoplasty
   p. omentum
   p. penile skin urethroplasty

pediculicide
pediculosis pubis
Pedi PEG tube
pedunculated
   p. angiodysplasia
   p. polyp

pedunculation
peel-away introducer sheath
peeping testis
Pee Wee low-profile gastrostomy tube
pefloxacin
PEG
   percutaneous endoscopic gastrostomy
   polyethylene glycol
   Bard PEG
   PEG bumper
   complete replacement PEG
   CT-guided PEG
   20F PEG tube
   PEG insertion
   PEG lavage
   Ponsky-Gauderer type PEG

PEG pull
PEG push
replacement PEG
Sacks-Vine-type PEG
Sandoz Caluso 22F, 28F super PEG
PEG tube

peg
  rete p.

PEG-3500 solution
PEG-400 tube
PEG-assisted decompression
Pegasys
PEG-ELS
  polyethylene glycol electrolyte lavage solution

PEG-interferon
  PEG-i. alfa-2a
  PEG-i. alfa-2b powder for injection

PEG-Intron powder for injection
PEG-J
  percutaneous endoscopic gastrojejunostomy

PEG-JET
  percutaneous endoscopic gastrostomy and jejunal extension tube
  PEG-JET placement

pegylated interferon
pegylation
PEI
  percutaneous ethanol injection
  polyethylenimine
  PEI therapy

PEJ
  percutaneous endoscopic jejunostomy
  PEJ tube

PELD
  pediatric end-stage liver disease
  PELD score

pelican biopsy forceps
Pelikan brand India ink
peliosis
  bacillary p.
  hepatic p.
  p. hepaticus
  p. hepatis

pellagra
  infantile p.

pellagroid
pellagrous
pellet
  p. artifact
  radiopaque p.
  ^{99m}Tc-labeled Amberlite p.

pelleted stool
pellicular enteritis
pellucida
  zona p. (ZP)

pelves (*pl. of* pelvis)
pelvic
  p. abscess
  p. adhesion
  p. anatomy
  p. appendicitis
  p. autonomic nerve
  p. brim
  p. colon
  p. colonic surgery
  p. colon of Waldeyer
  p. diaphragm
  p. discontinuity
  p. dissection
  p. evisceration
  p. exenteration
  p. fascia
  p. floor
  p. floor descent
  p. floor disorder
  p. floor dysfunction
  p. floor dyssynergia
  p. floor electrical stimulation
  p. floor electromyography
  p. floor exercise (PFE)
  p. floor movement
  p. floor muscle exercise
  p. floor neurophysiology
  p. floor rehabilitation
  p. floor relaxation
  p. floor syndrome
  p. girdle relaxation (PGR)
  p. ileal reservoir construction
  p. ileal reservoir volume
  p. inflammatory disease (PID)
  p. kidney
  p. lipomatosis
  p. lymphadenectomy
  p. lymph node
  p. lymphocelectomy
  p. malleability
  p. muscle strength
  p. muscle training
  p. nerve plexus
  p. omentoplasty
  p. osteotomy

NOTES

pelvic *(continued)*
- p. peritoneum
- p. phased-array coil (PPA)
- p. pole
- p. pouch
- p. pouchoscopy
- p. pouch procedure
- p. prolapse
- p. sepsis
- p. sidewall
- p. stone
- p. ultrasonography
- p. ureter

pelvicaliceal
- p. stasis
- p. system

pelvicus
- plexus p.

pelviectasis
pelvilithotomy
pelvioileoneocystostomy
pelviolithotomy
pelvioneocystostomy
pelvioneostomy
pelvioperitonitis
pelvioplasty
pelvioradiography, pelviradiography
pelviostomy
pelviotomy
pelviperitonitis
pelviradiography *(var. of pelvioradiography)*
pelvirectal
- p. abscess
- p. achalasia
- p. fistula

pelviroentgenography
pelvis, pl. **pelves**
- arcus tendineus fasciae p.
- bifid renal p.
- bony p.
- cavum p.
- coccygeal p.
- extrarenal renal p.
- fascia p.
- female p.
- p. fracture
- p. innervation
- male p.
- p. muscle
- nonmalleable p.
- obstructed p.
- papilloma of renal p.
- pseudospider p.
- renal p.
- spider p.
- split p.
- subepithelial hematoma of renal p.

pelviscope

pelviscopic clip ligation technique
PelviSoft mesh
pelviureteroradiography
pelvocaliectasis
Pemberton sigmoid clamp
pemoline
pemphigoid
- benign mucous membrane p. (BMMP)
- bullous p.
- mucous membrane p.

pemphigus
- benign familial p.
- p. foliaceus
- p. vulgaris

PE-MV balloon dilatation catheter
pen
- Intron A multidose p.

penbutolol
pencil
- cautery p.
- electrocautery p.

pencillike stool
pencil-tipped electrode
pendetide
- satumomab p.

pendulous
- p. abdomen
- p. urethra

penectomy
- modified p.
- partial p.

penes *(pl. of penis)*
Penetrak
penetrans
- ulcus p.

penetrating
- p. abdominal trauma
- P. Abdominal Trauma Index (PATI)
- p. pancreatic trauma
- p. ulcer
- p. wound

penetration
- capsular p.
- splenic p.

Penetrex
Pen-F half-frame camera
penial
penicillamine
D-penicillamine
penicilli *(pl. of penicillus)*
penicilliary
penicillin
- benzathine p.
- beta-lactamase-resistant p.
- procaine p.

penicillin-streptomycin

Penicillium
   P. citrinum
   P. marneffei
penicillus, pl. **penicilli**
   penicilli arteriae lienalis
   penicilli arteriae splenicae
penile
   p. amputation
   p. anomaly
   p. arteriography
   p. artery
   p. biothesiometry
   p. blood pressure
   p. body
   p. carcinoma
   p. clamp
   p. crus
   p. curvature
   p. cyst
   p. deformity
   p. Doppler
   p. duplex ultrasonography
   p. edema
   p. enlargement
   p. epispadias
   p. erection
   p. extensibility
   p. fibromatosis
   p. fibrosis
   p. hypospadias
   p. implant
   p. incarceration
   p. injection testing
   p. injection therapy
   p. intraepithelial neoplasia
   p. island flap
   p. kraurosis
   p. lesion
   p. melanosis
   p. modeling
   p. necrosis
   p. orthoplasty
   p. plethysmography
   p. prosthesis
   p. prosthesis mechanical problem
   p. prothesis reliability
   p. pulse volume recording
   p. raphe
   p. reconstruction
   p. reconstructive surgery
   p. reflex
   p. revascularization
   p. root
   p. rupture
   p. schwannoma
   p. sclerosing lymphangitis
   p. sensitivity
   p. shaft degloving
   p. synechia
   p. torsion
   p. tuberculosis
   p. turgescence
   p. urethra
   p. vascular function assessment
   p. vein ligation
   p. vein occlusion therapy
   p. venous ligation surgery
   p. vibratory stimulation
penile-brachial
   p.-b. index (PBI)
   p.-b. pressure index (PBPI)
penis, pl. **penes**
   adolescent p.
   albuginea p.
   angiofibroma of p.
   bifid p.
   bulbus p.
   buried p.
   p. captivus
   carcinoma in situ of glans p.
   chordeic p.
   clubbed p.
   collum glandis p.
   concealed p.
   corona glandis p.
   corpus spongiosum p.
   crus p.
   cutaneous horn of p.
   dorsum of p.
   double p.
   dystrophic p.
   emissary vein of p.
   flaccid p.
   p. fracture
   frenulum of prepuce p.
   frenulum preputii p.
   glans p.
   hirsute papilloma of p.
   inconspicuous p.
   leukoplakia of p.
   p. lunatus
   p. lymphoma
   micaceous growth of p.
   p. palmatus

NOTES

penis *(continued)*
    pearly papule of p.
    p. plastica
    preputium p.
    prosthetic p.
    pseudoepitheliomatous micaceous growths of p.
    psoriasis of p.
    radix p.
    raphe p.
    p. reconstruction
    p. reflex
    retractile concealed p.
    p. sarcoma
    scapus p.
    septum glandis p.
    septum of glans p.
    p. syringoma
    trabeculae of corpora cavernosa of p.
    trabeculae corporis spongiosi p.
    trabeculae corporum cavernosorum p.
    trabeculae of corpus spongiosum of p.
    trapped p.
    venae cavernosae p.
    ventrum of p.
    webbed p.
penischisis
penitis
Penn
    P. pouch
    P. umbilical scissors
Pennington
    P. clamp
    P. forceps
    P. rectal speculum
pennyroyal oil
penoplasty
penopubic
    p. epispadias
    p. junction
penoscrotal
    p. hypospadias
    p. junction
    p. transposition
    p. transposition complex
    p. trapping
    p. webbing
penotomy
Penrose
    P. seton
    P. sump drain
pentagastrin (PG)
    p. gastric secretory test
    p. infusion
    p. infusion test
    p. provocative test
    p. stimulated analysis test
pentamidine-induced pancreatitis
pentamidine isethionate
pentane excretion level
pentapiperium
Pentasa
pentastomiasis
pentastomum
    p. denticulatum
    p. denticulatum nodule
Pentax
    P. duodenoscope
    P. EC-series videoendoscope
    P. EG-2901, -2940, -3800 endoscope
    P. EG-2900 videogastroscope
    P. EndoNet
    P. EndoNet digital endoscopy network
    P. endoscopic camera
    P. ESI-2000 fiberoptic endoscope
    P. EUP-EC124 ultrasound gastroscope
    P. FC-series colonoscope
    P. FD-series videoendoscope
    P. FG-32UA
    P. FG-36-UX linear-array echoendoscope
    P. FG-38X endoscope
    P. fiberscope
    P. FS-series flexible fiberoptic video sigmoidoscope
    P. linear-array echoendoscope
    P. prototype needle
    P. VSB-2000 fiberoptic endoscope
    P. VSB-P2900 pediatric colonoscope
    P. VSB-P-series enteroscope
Pentax/Hitachi FG-32UA
pentazocine
pentetreotide
    In-111 p.
    indium p.
    indium-111 p.
penthienate
pentolinium
pentopril
pentosan
    p. polysulfate sodium
    p. sodium polysulfate
    p. sulfate
pentose phosphate shunt
pentosuria
pentoxifylline
Pento-X syndrome
Pen-Vee K
peotomy

Pepcid
    P. AC
    P. Complete
    P. RPD
PEPCK
    phosphoenolpyruvate carboxykinase
peplomycin
pepo
    Cucurbita p.
peppermint oil
PEPS
    peroral electronic pancreatoscope
pepsic (*var. of* peptic)
pepsin
    inactivated p. (IP)
    p. secretion
pepsinogen
    p. A-C ratio
    p. level A, B, C
pepstatin
Peptamen liquid nutrition
Peptavlon stimulation test
Peptic
    P. Relief
    P. Relief chewable tablet
    P. Relief liquid
peptic, pepsic
    p. cell
    p. cell receptor
    p. disease
    p. esophageal stricture
    p. esophagitis
    p. reflux
    p. reflux disease
    p. ulcer
    p. ulcer bleeding
    p. ulcer disease (PUD)
peptidase
peptide
    adrenomedullin 52-amino acid p.
    28-amino acid p.
    antibody to core p. 9 (anti-CP9)
    antibody to core p. 10 (anti-CP10)
    antral p.
    atrial natriuretic p. (ANP)
    brain-gut p.
    brain natriuretic p. (BNP)
    calcitonin gene-related p. (CGRP)
    cellular p.
    chemotactic p.
    C-type atrial natriuretic p. (C-ANP)
    C-type natriuretic p. (CNP)
    gastrin-releasing p. (GRP)
    gastrointestinal regularity p.
    glucose-dependent insulinotropic p.
    p. HI
    p. histidine isoleucine (PHI)
    p. hormone
    intestinal p.
    p. mass fingerprinting
    met-enkephalin p.
    monitor p.
    neutrophil chemotactic p.
    opioid p.
    paracrine p.
    peak acid output after gastrin-releasing p. (PAOGRP)
    plasma atrial natriuretic p.
    posttranslational processing of p.
    regulatory p.
    somatostatin p.
    trefoil p.
    trypsinogen activation p.
    p. tyrosine
    urinary trypsinogen activation p.
    vasoactive intestinal p. (VIP)
    vasoconstrictor p.
    p. YY (PYY)
peptide/bombesin
    gastrin-releasing p./b.
peptidergic
    p. mechanism
    p. neuron
Pepto-Bismol
peptone
Peptostreptococcus micros
per
    p. anum
    p. anum bleeding
    p. anum intersphincteric rectal dissection
    p. rectal portal scintigraphy
    p. rectum
Perceived Stress Scale (PSS)
percent
    p. reduction in urea (PRU)
    p. transferrin saturation
percentage
    p. frequency of bacteremia
    p. of hypochromic red cells (%HYPO)
Percival gastric balloon
Percodan

NOTES

Percoll
- P. bead
- P. filter

Percufix catheter cuff kit

Percuflex
- P. Amsterdam stent
- P. biliary stent
- P. catheter
- P. endopyelotomy stent
- P. Plus ureteral stent

percussion
- dullness to p.
- p. note
- p. tenderness

percutaneous
- p. abscess drainage
- p. antegrade biliary drainage
- p. antegrade pyelography
- p. antegrade urography
- p. bacille Calmette-Guérin administration
- p. balloon aspiration
- p. balloon dilation
- p. biliary bypass
- p. biliary drainage (PBD)
- p. bladder neck stabilization (PBNS)
- p. bladder neck suspension (PBNS)
- p. catheter cecostomy
- p. cholecystolithotomy (PCCL)
- p. choledochoscopy
- p. CT-guided aspiration
- p. debulking
- p. drainage of epididymal abscess
- p. embolization therapy
- p. endopyeloplasty
- p. endopyeloureterotomy
- p. endoscopic cecostomy
- p. endoscopic gastrojejunostomy (PEG-J)
- p. endoscopic gastrostomy (PEG)
- p. endoscopic gastrostomy and jejunal extension tube (PEG-JET)
- p. endoscopic gastrostomy and jejunal extension tube placement
- p. endoscopic jejunostomy (PEJ)
- p. endoscopic placement of jejunal tube
- p. endoscopic removal
- p. epididymal sperm aspiration
- p. ethanol injection (PEI)
- p. ethanol injection therapy
- p. femoral vein catheter
- p. fetal cystoscopy
- p. fine-needle pancreatic biopsy
- p. gastroenterostomy (PGE)
- p. gastrostomy (PG)
- p. hepatobiliary cholangiography
- p. image-guided thermal ablation of hepatic metastasis
- p. liver biopsy (PLB)
- p. native renal biopsy
- p. needle aspiration
- p. needle bladder neck suspension
- p. nephrolithiasis
- p. nephrolitholapaxy
- p. nephrolithotomy (PCN, PCNL, PNL)
- p. nephrolithotripsy (PCNL)
- p. nephrostolithotomy (PCNL)
- p. nephrostomy
- p. nephrostomy Malecot catheter
- p. nephrostomy tube placement
- p. nerve evaluation (PNE)
- p. pancreas biopsy
- p. pressure ureteral perfusion test
- p. procedure
- p. radical cryosurgical ablation of prostate
- p. radiofrequency ablation
- p. removal of bezoar
- p. resection
- p. sacral nerve root neuromodulation
- p. sampling method
- p. stent
- P. Stoller Afferent Nerve Stimulation System
- p. stone removal
- p. testosterone gel
- p. transcatheter perfusion
- p. transhepatic approach
- p. transhepatic biliary drainage (PTBD)
- p. transhepatic biliary drainage catheter
- p. transhepatic cholangiodrainage (PTCD)
- p. transhepatic cholangiogram (PTC, PTHC)
- p. transhepatic cholangiography (PTC, PTHC)
- p. transhepatic cholangioscopy (PTCS)
- p. transhepatic cholecystolithotomy (PCTCL)
- p. transhepatic cholecystoscopy (PTCC)
- p. transhepatic cholecystostomy
- p. transhepatic choledochoscopic electrohydraulic
- p. transhepatic decompression
- p. transhepatic drainage (PTD)
- p. transhepatic liver biopsy with tract embolization (PBTE)
- p. transhepatic obliteration

p. transhepatic obliteration of esophageal varix
p. transhepatic pigtail catheter
p. transhepatic portography (PTP)
p. transluminal angioplasty (PTA)
p. transluminal balloon angioplasty
p. transluminal renal angioplasty (PTRA)
p. transperineal seed implantation
p. ultrasonic lithotriptor
p. vasectomy
p. vasography

Percy intestinal forceps
Percy-Wolfson gallbladder retractor
Perdiem Plain
perendoscopic manometry
Pereyra
P. bladder neck suspension
P. ligature carrier
P. needle
P. procedure

Pereyra-Raz cystourethropexy
PerFix Marlex mesh plug
perflubron
perforate
perforated
p. acid peptic ulcer
p. appendicitis
p. appendix
p. carcinoma
p. cholecystitis
p. diverticulum
p. nasal septum
p. ulcer disease
p. viscus

perforating
p. aneurysm
p. diverticulitis
p. forceps
p. ulcer

perforation
appendiceal p.
barogenic p.
bladder p.
bowel p.
cecal p.
p. of colon
colonic p.
ductal system p.
duodenal ulcer p. (DUP)
endoscopic sphincterotomy-induced duodenal p.

eosinophilic ileal p.
esophageal p.
p. of gallbladder
gastric p.
iatrogenic tumor p.
intestinal p.
intraperitoneal p.
Niemeier gallbladder p.
peritoneal p.
polyethylene p.
prepyloric p.
pyloroduodenal p.
resistant to electrosurgical p.
retroduodenal p.
retroperitoneal p.
stercoraceous p.

perforin
performance characteristic
Performa ultrasound system
perfringens
Clostridium p.
perfusate
p. bag
esophageal p.
hyperosmolar p.
p. solution

perfusion
allogenic liver p.
p. cannula
CCD p.
con A/anti-con A p.
continuous hypothermic pulsatile p.
p. cooling
extracorporeal liver p. (ECLP)
extracorporeal whole-organ p.
ex vivo p.
heterologous liver p.
p. hypothermia technique
hypothermic pulsatile p.
intestinal p.
intraperitoneal hyperthermic p. (IPHP)
isolated hepatocyte p.
p. machine
percutaneous transcatheter p.
plasma p.
skin p.
p. study
transcatheter p.
transvenous p.
trickle p.

pergolide dopaminergic medication

NOTES

perhexiline maleate
Periactin
periadvential tissue
periampullary
    p. adenoma (PAA)
    p. carcinoma
    p. duodenal diverticulum
    p. duodenal tumor
    p. malignancy
    p. mass
    p. neoplasm
    p. pseudotumor
perianal
    p. anorectal space
    p. area
    p. condyloma
    p. Crohn disease
    P. Crohn Disease Activity Index (PDAI)
    p. edema
    p. and enterourethral fistulae
    p. fistula
    p. fistula abscess
    p. hematoma
    p. hygiene
    p. infection
    p. lesion
    p. pain
    p. region
    p. sepsis
    p. skin tag
    p. soak
    p. wart
periappendicitis decidualis
periarteritis
    p. gummosa
    p. nodosa
pericapillary diffusion
pericardial
    p. air-fluid level
    p. decompression
    p. knock
pericarditis
    constrictive p.
pericecal abscess
pericellular matrix (PCM)
pericentral
    p. cholestasis
    p. fibrosis
    p. hypoxia
    p. necrosis
    p. pyridine nucleotide fluorescence
pericholangiolar
pericholangitis
pericholecystic
    p. abscess
    p. edema
    p. stranding

pericholecystitis
    gaseous p.
perichromatin granule
Peri-Colace
pericolic, pericolonic
    p. abscess
    p. fat
    p. membrane syndrome
    p. phlegmon
    p. stercoraceous
pericolitis
pericolonic (*var. of* pericolic)
pericolostomy area
pericostal suture
pericrypt eosinophilic enterocolitis
pericystitis
perididymis
perididymitis
peridiverticular
peridiverticulitis
    phlegmonous p.
periductal
    p. fibrosis
    p. gland
periesophageal collateral vein
periesophagitis
    chronic p.
perifascial nephrectomy
perigastric node
periglandular nonspecific inflammatory reaction
periglomerular space
perihepatic
    p. adhesion
    p. lymphadenopathy
perihepatitis syndrome
perihilar cholangiocarcinoma
periileal
perikaryon
perilobar pancreatitis
perilobular
    p. duct
    p. fibrosis
perimedial fibroplasia
perimesangial GBM
perimolysis, perimylolysis
perinatal
    p. hemochromatosis
    p. torsion
    p. urology
perindopril
perinea (*pl. of* perineum)
perineal
    p. abscess
    p. approach
    p. body
    p. Crohn disease
    p. descent
    p. drain

p. fascia
p. flexure
p. hypospadias
p. impact trauma
p. incision
p. infection
p. lithotomy
p. muscle
p. nerve
p. nerve terminal motor latency test
p. pad
p. polyp
p. pouch
p. prostatectomy
p. raphe
p. rectosigmoidectomy
p. region
p. section
p. sensation
p. sinus
p. sinus tract
p. skin tag
p. tendon
p. ulcer
p. urethrostomy
p. urethrotomy
p. urinary fistula

perinealis
raphe p.

perinei
raphe p.

perineobulbar
p. detrusor facilitative reflex
p. detrusor inhibitory reflex

perineodetrusor inhibitory reflex

perineometer
Peritron Precision P.

perineometry

perineorrhaphy

perineostomy

perineotomy

perinephretic fibrosis

perinephric
p. abscess
p. fat
p. fluid collection
p. hematoma
p. stranding
p. tissue

perinephrium

perineum, pl. **perinea**
anterior p.
bulging of p.
female p.
male p.
posterior p.
raphe of p.
watering-can p.
water pot p.

perinuclear
p. antineutrophil cytoplasmic (p-ANC)
p. antineutrophil cytoplasmic antibody (p-ANCA)
p. intracellular staining

period
dwell p.
intradialytic p.
pH-monitoring p.

periodic
p. abdominalgia
p. acid-Schiff (PAS)
p. acid-Schiff-Alcian blue (PAS-AB)
p. acid-Schiff-Alcian blue combination stain
p. acid-Schiff stain
p. acid-Schiff test
p. leg movement (PLM)
p. peritonitis
p. polyserositis
p. vomiting

periodicity
circadian p.

perioperative
p. antibiotic
p. data
p. morbidity
p. nutrition
p. risk
p. vomiting

peripancreatic
p. area
p. fibrosis
p. fluid
p. fluid collection
p. necrosis

peripapillary diverticulum

peripartum
p. endoscopy
p. symphysis separation

peripelvic
p. cyst

NOTES

peripelvic *(continued)*
    p. extravasation
    p. fat
peripenial
peripheral
    p. acinar vein
    p. adrenergic agent
    p. arterial vasodilation theory
    p. arthritis
    p. bile duct
    p. bladder denervation
    p. blood lymphocyte (PBL)
    p. blood mononuclear cell (PBMC)
    p. capillary filtration slit length
    p. cholangiocarcinoma (PCC)
    p. extremity edema
    p. hyperalimentation
    p. intrahepatic cholangiocarcinoma
    p. intravenous alimentation
    p. leukocyte count
    p. loading
    p. necrosis
    p. nerve evaluation (PNE)
    p. nerve evaluation test
    p. T cell
    p. vascular
    p. vascular resistance
    p. vasodilatation
    p. venous thrombosis
    p. zone
periphery
    hypoechoic p.
Periplast sealant
peripolesis
periportal
    p. area
    p. cirrhosis
    p. fibrosis
    p. hepatocyte
    p. inflammation
    p. invasion
    p. pyridine nucleotide fluorescence
    p. sinusoidal dilation
periportal-perisinusoidal fibrosis
periprandial
periprostatic
    p. block
    p. tissue
perirectal
    p. abscess
    p. fat
    p. fat infiltration
    p. fistula
    p. mass
    p. pain
perirenal
    p. abscess
    p. fascia
    p. fat
    p. hematoma
perisigmoid colon
perisinusoidal
    p. cell
    p. fibrin deposition
    p. fibrosis
    p. space
perispermatitis serosa
perisplenitis
    fibropurulent p.
peristalsis
    absent p.
    antegrade p.
    antral p.
    decreased p.
    disrupted p.
    esophageal p.
    high-amplitude p. (HAP)
    mass p.
    retrograde p.
    reversed p.
    secondary p.
    visible p.
peristaltic
    p. anastomosis
    p. contraction
    p. pump
    p. reflex
    p. rush
    p. unrest
    p. wave
peristomal
    p. area
    p. infection
    p. skin
    p. varix
peritomy
peritoneal
    p. access
    p. adenocarcinoma
    p. adhesion
    p. anatomy
    p. aspiration
    p. attachment
    p. autoplasty
    p. band
    p. biopsy
    p. blastomycosis
    p. button
    p. carcinoma
    p. carcinomatosis
    p. cavity
    p. cavity abscess
    p. deposit
    p. dialysate
    p. dialysis (PD)
    p. dialysis catheter (PDC)

p. dialysis creatinine clearance target
p. dialysis effluent (PDE)
p. dialysis urea removal
p. dropsy
p. encapsulation
p. equilibration test (PET)
p. fluid
p. friction rub
p. fungal infection
p. lavage
p. leukocyte
p. lymphangiectasia
p. macrophage
p. malignancy
p. membrane permeability
p. membrane solute transport capacity
p. membrane transport
p. mesothelial cell
p. mesothelioma
p. mouse
p. nodule
p. perforation
p. reflection
p. sac
p. seeding
p. sign
p. soilage
p. solute transport
p. space
p. studding
p. tap
p. toilet
p. transfusion
p. tuberculosis
p. vein
p. window

peritoneal-anal distance
peritoneal-atrial shunt
peritonealgia
peritonealis
    cavitas p.
peritonealize
peritonectomize
peritonei
    carcinomatosis p.
    pseudomyxoma p.
peritoneocaval shunt
peritoneocentesis
peritoneoclysis
peritoneogram

peritoneography
peritoneojugular shunt
peritoneopathy
peritoneopexy
peritoneoplasty
peritoneoscope
peritoneoscopy
peritoneotomy
peritoneovenous
    p. shunt (PVS)
    p. shunt patency scan
peritoneum
    abdominal p.
    p. lateral umbilical fold
    p. medial fold
    p. median fold
    parietal p.
    pelvic p.
    visceral p.
peritonism
peritonitis
    adhesive p.
    bacterial p.
    barium p.
    benign paroxysmal p.
    bile p.
    Candida p.
    chemical p.
    chylous p.
    coccidioidal p.
    Coccidioides immitis p.
    p. deformans
    exudative p.
    fecal p.
    fungal p.
    generalized p.
    granulomatous p.
    Listeria monocytogenes p.
    meconium p.
    parasitic p.
    periodic p.
    postsclerotherapy bacterial p.
    primary p.
    sclerosing encapsulating p.
    secondary bacterial p.
    Sgambati test for p.
    spontaneous bacterial p. (SBP)
    starch granulomatous p.
    sterile p.
    subacute nonspecific p.
    tuberculous p.
peritonize

NOTES

Peritron Precision Perineometer
peritubular
    p. capillary
    p. fluid
    p. HCO^{3-}
    p. myoid cell
    p. sodium
perityphlitis actinomycotica
periumbilical
    p. port
    p. region
periureteral
    p. abscess
    p. fibrosis
    p. stone
    p. stranding
periureteric
periureteritis plastica
periurethral
    p. abscess
    p. bulking agent
    p. collagen injection
    p. gland
    p. injection therapy
    p. ligament
    p. spongiofibrosis
    p. striated muscle
    p. transurethral microwave thermotherapy (P-TUMT)
    p. vein
periurethritis
perivascular
    p. fibroblast
    p. plexus
    p. sheath
perivascularis
    capsula fibrosa p.
peri-Vaterian therapeutic endoscopic procedure
perivenular
    p. confluent necrosis
    p. fibrosis
perivesical fat
perivesicular
perivesiculitis
Perkin-Elmer
    P.-E. model 5000 atomic absorption spectrophotometer
    P.-E. 9600 thermal cycler
Perls
    P. reaction
    P. stain
Perma-Hand silk suture
Permalume covering
permanent
    p. end colostomy
    p. loop ileostomy
    p. section
    p. stoma
    p. urinary
permanganate
    potassium p.
PermCath
    P. dual-lumen catheter
    Quinton P.
permeability
    capillary p.
    colonic p.
    increased bladder p.
    intestinal p.
    membrane p.
    mucosal vascular p.
    peritoneal membrane p.
    tight junction p.
    urea p.
    water p.
permeable
permeation
    lymphovascular p.
permethrin
Permitil Oral
permixon group
permselectivity
Permutit method
pernasal cholangiogram
pernicious
    p. anemia
    p. malaria
    p. vomiting
    p. vomiting of pregnancy
peroral
    p. approach
    p. bougienage
    p. cholangiopancreatoscopy (PCPS)
    p. cholangioscopy (PCS)
    p. electronic pancreatoscope (PEPS)
    p. endoprosthesis
    p. endoscopy
    p. esophageal dilation
    p. gastroscope
    p. jejunal biopsy
    p. maneuver
    p. pancreatoscopy (POPS)
    p. pneumocolon examination
    p. retrograde pancreaticobiliary ductography
    p. shock wave lithotripsy (PSWL)
peroxidase
    endogenous p.
    glutathione p.
    p. stain
peroxidase-conjugated streptavidin
peroxidation
    lipid p.
    membrane p.
peroxide
    hydrogen p.

peroxisome proliferator-activated receptor (PPAR)
peroxynitrite-induced colitis
perphenazine
PerQ SANS
Perry bag
PerryMeter anal electromyographic sensor EPS-21
Persantine
persimmon bezoar
persistent
    p. chronic hepatitis
    p. cloaca
    p. müllerian duct syndrome
    p. postmolar gestational trophoblastic tumor
    p. proteinuria
    p. pylorospasm
    p. symptom
    p. viral hepatitis (PVH)
    p. viral hepatitis non-A, non-B (PVH-NANB)
    p. viral hepatitis type B (PVH-B)
    p. vomiting
personal
    P. EMG trainer
    p. experience
    p. preference
    P. Scanner TM 18 bedside real-time ultrasonography system
personality
    histrionic p.
    ulcer-prone p.
personalized program
pertechnetate
    ^{99m}Tc sodium p.
    technetium-99m p.
Pertik diverticulum
Pertofrane
pertussin
    p. toxin
    p. toxin-sensitive G protein
pertussis
PERV
    porcine endogenous retrovirus
perversion
    taste p.
perversus
    situs p.
perverted appetite
pessary
    bladder neck support p.
    Gellhorn p.
    Smith-Hodge p.
pestis
    Yersinia p.
PET
    peritoneal equilibration test
    positron emission tomography
    PET dialysate volume
    PET scan
petechia, pl. **petechiae**
    gastric p.
petechial
    p. angioma
    p. rash
Petersen
    P. bag
    P. operation
pethidine premedication
Petit triangle
petrificans
    urethritis p.
petrolatum gauze pack
Pettenkofer test
Petz clamp
Peumus boldus
Peutz-Jeghers
    P.-J. gastrointestinal polyposis
    P.-J. hamartoma
    P.-J. polyp
    P.-J. syndrome (PJS)
Peyer
    aggregated lymphatic follicles of P.
    P. patch
Peyronie
    P. disease
    P. plaque
Pezzer
    P. catheter
    P. drain
Pfannenstiel incision
PFC
    pancreatic fluid collection
PFE
    pelvic floor exercise
PFGE
    pulsed-field gel electrophoresis
PFIC
    progressive familial intrahepatic cholestasis
PFR
    peak flow rate

NOTES

PFS
    pressure-flow study
        Adriamycin PFS
Pfuhl sign
PFV
    portal vein blood flow velocity
PG
    pentagastrin
    percutaneous gastrostomy
    prostaglandin
    pyoderma gangrenosum
        Amogel PG
        serum PG
PGE
    percutaneous gastroenterostomy
PGE2
    prostaglandin E2
        exogenous PGE2
        ratio of PGF2-alpha PGE2
PGE$_1$
    prostaglandin E
        PGE$_1$ injection
        intraurethral PGE$_1$
PGF2-alpha
    prostaglandin F2-alpha
PGG
    prostaglandin G
PGG2 endoperoxide
PGH
    prostaglandin H
PGH2 endoperoxide
PGI2
    prostaglandin I2
PGL
    primary gastric lymphoma
PGR
    pelvic girdle relaxation
        symptom-giving PGR
PGV
    proximal gastric vagotomy
PGWBI
    Psychological General Well-Being Index
pH
    hydrogen ion concentration
        blood pH
        pH electrode placement
        gastric luminal pH
        pH holding time
        intracellular pH
        intraesophageal pH
        intragastric pH
        pH monitoring
        pH probe
        pH recording
        pH standardized meal
        pH test
        pH threshold
        urinalysis pH
        urinary pH

pH4
PH30 protein
Phadebas angiotensin-I test
phage type
phagocyte
    bactericidal function of p.
    p. respiratory burst
phagocytic
    p. respiratory burst oxidase complex
    p. stellate cell
phagocytosis
phagosome
phallalgia
phallanastrophe
phallaneurysm
phallectomy
phalli (*pl. of* phallus)
phallic construction
phallitis
phalloarteriography
phallocampsis
phallocrypsis
phallodynia
phalloncus
phalloplasty
    reconstructive p.
phalloplethysmography (PPG)
phallorrhagia
phallorrhea
phallotomy
phallus, pl. **phalli**
phantom
    phantom ulcer
    P. 5 Plus ST balloon dilatation catheter
pharmacoangiography
pharmacoarteriography
pharmacocavernosogram
pharmacocavernosography
pharmacocavernosometry
pharmacoduplex ultrasonography
pharmacodynamic
pharmacokinetic
    everolimus p.'s
    famotidine p.'s
pharmacological
    p. agent
    p. treatment
pharmacologically induced erection
pharmacomechanical coupling
PharmaSeed
    P. I-125 brachytherapy
    P. iodine-125 seed
    P. palladium-103 seed
pharyngeal
    p. anesthesia
    p. diverticulum
    p. exudate

p. pouch
p. pouch syndrome
p. tear
p. tunic
p. wall
pharyngeal-UES incoordination
pharynges (*pl. of* pharynx)
pharyngitis
herpes p.
pharyngobasilar tunic
pharyngoesophageal (PE)
p. diverticulectomy
p. diverticulum
p. function
p. junction
p. sphincter
p. tear
pharyngoesophagogastroduodenoscopy
pharyngolaryngoesophagectomy
pharynx, pl. **pharynges**
phase
complement-independent autologous p.
hepatic arterial-dominant p. (HAP)
p. II contraction
p. II, III marrow transplant recipient
lag p.
M p.
micturition p.
mycelial p.
predialysis p.
pre-S p.
prolonged expiratory p.
reservoir p.
skin graft imbibition p.
skin graft inoculation p.
phasic
p. contractile activity
p. contraction
p. fluctuation on squeeze
p. wave duration
p. wave sequence
phasic-free tone variation
Phazyme
Phazyme-95, -125
Phazyme-PB
PHBD
predominant hyperparathyroid bone disease
pHCV31 antigen
pHCV34 antigen

phenacetin
p. nephritis
p. nephropathy
phenazopyridine
p. hydrochloric acid
p. hydrochloride
sulfamethoxazole and p.
sulfisoxazole and p.
phencyclidine abuse
phendimetrazine
phenelzine
Phenergan
phen-fen diet
phenindamine
phenindione hypersensitivity
phenmetrazine
phenobarbital
phenol
aqueous p.
p. II
p. red chromoendoscopy
Phenolax
phenolphthalein
phenolsulfonphthalein
phenoltetrachlorophthalein test
phenomenon, pl. **phenomena**
bicalutamide withdrawal p.
capillary-leak p.
cloud p.
common cavity p.
disappearing p.
dystonic p.
first-set p.
Goldblatt p.
Hayflick p.
jet stream p.
J-wave p.
Kanagawa p.
mask p.
pathergy p.
Schramm p.
second-set p.
walking stick p.
yo-yo weight-fluctuation p.
phenothiazine
phenotype
antigenic p.
B cellular p.
CD4 p.
CD8 p.
codominant p.
HLA class II p.

NOTES

phenotype *(continued)*
    p.'s of mast cells
    partial nephrogenic diabetes insipidus p.
    Potter p.
    replication error p.
    slow bilirubin glucuronidation p.
    ZZ p.
phenotypic
    p. sex
    p. study
Phenoxine
Phenoxodial
phenoxodiol
phenoxybenzamine hydrochloride
phenoxymethylpenicillin
phenprocoumon
phentermine
phentolamine
    p. methylate
    p. test
phentosanpolysulfate
phenylacetate
phenylalanine
L-phenylalanine mustard (L-PAM)
phenylbutazone hepatotoxicity
phenylephrine
phenylethyl alcohol agar
phenylethylamine N-methyl transferase (PNMT)
Phenyl-Free oral liquid
phenylhydrazine
phenyl-methane-sulfonyl fluoride
phenylpropanolamine
phenylpropylmethylamine
phenytoin
pheochromocytoma
    bilateral p.
    bladder p.
    ectopic p.
    familial p.
    malignant p.
    retroperitoneal laparoscopic adrenalectomy for p.
PHG
    portal hypertensive gastropathy
PHI
    peptide histidine isoleucine
PH-I
    primary hyperoxaluria type I, II
Philadelphia chromosome
philippinensis
    Capillaria p.
Phillips
    P. catheter
    P. CM 12 electron microscope
    P. LaxCaps
    P. Milk of Magnesia
    P. rectal clamp
    P. ultrasound machine
phimosiectomy
phimosis
    adult p.
phimotic
pH-Informer Deltron probe
pHisoHex scrub
PHIV
    portal hypertensive intestinal vasculopathy
PHLA
    postheparin lipolytic activity
phlebectasia
    intestinal p.
phlebitis
    enterocolic lymphocytic p. (ELP)
    Mondor p.
phlebography
    intraoperative p.
phlebolith
phleborheography
phleborrheograph
    Cranley p.
phlebosclerosis
    chronic ischemic colonic lesion caused by p. (CICLP)
phlegmon
    diverticular p.
    pancreatic p.
    pericolic p.
phlegmonous
    p. abscess
    p. adenitis
    p. alcoholic fatty liver
    p. change
    p. enteritis
    p. gastritis
    p. mass
    p. pancreatitis
    p. peridiverticulitis
phlorizin
pH-manometry probe
pH-meter
    intragastric continuous pH-m.
pH-metric testing
pH-metry
    esophagogastric pH-m.
    24-hour ambulatory pH-m.
    24-hour home pH-m.
pH-monitoring period
PHN
    passive Heymann nephritis
pholedrine
phonoenterography
    computerized p.
phonorenogram

phorbol
    p. ester 12-O-tetradecanoylphorbol-13-acetate
    p. ester TPA
    p. myristate acetate (PMA)
PhosLo
Phosphaljel
phosphatase
    alkaline p. (ALP, AP)
    alkaline phosphatase-antialkaline p. (APAAP)
    Bessey-Lowry unit for alkaline p.
    bone alkaline p. (BAP)
    bone-specific alkaline p. (BALP)
    leukocyte alkaline p. (LAP)
    phosphorylase p.
    placental alkaline p. (PIAP)
    prostate-specific acid p.
    prostatic acid p. (PAP)
    protein tyrosine p.
    total serum prostatic acid p. (TSPAP)
phosphate
    aluminum p.
    p. binder therapy
    calcium hydrogen p.
    cellulose p.
    chloroquine p.
    p. crystal
    dexamethasone sodium p.
    dietary p.
    disopyramide p. (DP)
    elemental p.
    p. enema
    estramustine p.
    fludarabine p.
    Hexacrol P.
    p. ion (PI)
    p. ion-urea (PI-urea)
    magnesium ammonium p.
    nicotinamide adenine dinucleotide p. (NADPH)
    paranitrophenol p.
    phosphatidylinositol p. (PI4P)
    potassium p.
    potassium-titanyl p. (KTP)
    pyridoxal p.
    renal p.
    serum p.
    sodium p. (NaP)
    sodium cellulose p.

phosphate-buffered
    p.-b. saline (PBS)
    p.-b. saline solution
phosphate-dependent glutaminase (PDG)
phosphate-independent glutaminase (PIG)
phosphatidylethanolamine
phosphatidylinositol (PI)
    p. phosphate (PI4P)
phosphatidylinositol 4,5-bisphosphate (PI4,5P2)
phosphatidylserine
phosphaturia
phosphodiester
phosphodiesterase (PDE)
    p. inhibitor
phosphoenolpyruvate carboxykinase (PEPCK)
phosphofructokinase
phosphoglucomutase
phosphoinositide 3-kinase
phosphokinase
    creatine p. (CPK)
phospholipase
    p. A2 (PLA2)
    p. A2 catalytic activity
    p. C (PLC)
    p. D
phospholipid
    p. bilayer
    p. export pump gene (MDR3)
    p. ratio
    serum p.
phospholipidase A
phospholipid-bound choline concentration
phospholipidosis
phosphonoformate
phosphopeptidomannan (PPM)
phosphoprotein
    glycosylated p.
phosphoramidite chemistry
phosphoribosyltransferase
    adenine p. (APRT)
phosphorous-31 magnetic resonance spectroscopy
phosphorus
    dietary p.
    p. metabolism
    p. poisoning
    serum p.
    tubular reabsorption of p.
phosphorus-32 (P-32, ^{32}P)

NOTES

phosphorylase
- brain-type glycogen p. (BGP)
- glycogen p.
- p. phosphatase
- uridine p.

phosphorylated growth factor receptor

phosphorylation
- host tyrosine p.
- oxidative p.
- p. protein
- protein p.
- *src* p.
- tyrosine p.

phosphorylcholine

Phospho-soda
- P.-s. enema
- Fleet P.-s.

phosphotungstic acid-magnesium chloride precipitation method

phosphotyrosine antibody

phosphotyrosine-SH2 binding

phosphotyrosyl protein profile

photoablation
- laser p.
- Nd:YAG laser p.

photoaffinity

photochemical ablation

photochemotherapy

photocoagulation
- infrared p. (IRC)
- laser p.
- transendoscopic laser p.
- p. treatment

photodestruction
- laser p.

photodiode

photodocumentation

photodynamic
- p. diagnosis (PPD)
- p. imaging
- p. therapy (PDT)

Photofrin
- P. derivative
- P. PDT

photogastroscope

photography
- endoscopic p.
- instant p.
- laparoscopic p.
- television p.

photoirradiation

photometer
- Anthos ht II automatic p.
- TUR-Cue p.

photometry
- flame p.

photomicrograph
- p. of colonoscopic biopsy specimen
- high-power p.
- low-power p.
- medium-power p.
- p. of specimen staining

photomicrography

photomultiplier
- EMI 9813B p.
- p. tube

photon-deficient lesion

photophobia

photoradiation therapy

Photoscan-3 hematoporphyrin derivative

photoselective vaporization of prostate

photosensitivity

photosensitizer
- porphyrin p.

photosensitizing hemoporphyrin derivative

photothermal laser ablation

PHP
- pseudohypoparathyroidism

phrenalgia

phrenectomy

phrenemphraxis

phrenic artery

phrenicectomize

phrenicectomy

phreniclasia, phreniclasis

phrenicocolic (*var. of* phrenocolic)

phrenicoesophageal ligament

phrenicoexeresis

phreniconeurectomy

phrenicotomy

phrenicotripsy

phrenocolic, phrenicocolic
- p. ligament

phrenocolopexy

phrenodynia

phrenoesophageal membrane

phrenogastric

phrenoglottic

phrenohepatic

phrenoplegia

phrenoptosis

phrenospasm

phrenosplenic

phrygian
- p. cap
- p. cap deformity

pH-sensitive radiotelemetry capsule

PHS I, II
- Physicians' Health Study I, II

PHSL
- primary hepatosplenic lymphoma
- B-cell PHSL

PHT
- portal hypertension

phthiriasis

Phthirus pubis

Phycomycetes

phycomycosis
phyllodes
   cystosarcoma p.
phylloquinone
phylogenetic tree
physalopteriasis
physic
physical
   p. examination
   p. examination findings
   p. inactivity
physician
   P.'s Health Study I, II (PHS I, II)
   treating p.
Physick pouch
physicochemical basis of gallstone formation
physiograph
physiologic
   p. gastrectomy
   p. jaundice
   p. measurement
   p. pH solution
   p. reflux test (PRT)
   p. role in acid secretion
   p. salt solution (PSS)
   p. scaling
   p. testosterone-replacement therapy
physiological
   p. condition
   p. trophic effect
physiology
   anorectal p.
   renal p.
   p. testing
physiotherapy
   chest p.
physostigmine
phytobezoar
phytochemical
phytoestrogen
phytoestrogen-induced menstrual cycle disturbance
phytohemagglutinin
phytonadione
phytopharmaceutical
phytosterolemia
phytotherapy
phytyl group
PI
   phosphate ion
   phosphatidylinositol
   PI 3-kinase
   PI surgical stapler
pi
   glutathione S-transferase p.
PI-30 stapler
PI-90 double-headed stapler
PIAP
   placental alkaline phosphatase
pica
Picchini syndrome
pick
   P. cell
   P. testicular adenoma
   tubular adenoma of P.
   P. tubular adenoma
Picker Vista Magnascanner
picket fence appearance
Pickrell operation
pickwickian syndrome
picobirnavirus
Picoprep-3
Picornaviridae
picornavirus
picosulfate
   sodium p.
picture-frame vertebra
PID
   pelvic inflammatory disease
piecemeal
   p. necrosis
   p. polypectomy
   p. resection
Pierre Robin syndrome
Piersol point
piezoelectric
   p. crystal
   p. generator
   p. lithotripsy
   p. shock wave
   p. shock wave lithotriptor
   p. transducer
piezoelectrically generated ultrasound
Piezolith
   P. EPL
   P. EPL lithotriptor
   P. 2300, 2500 model lithotriptor
PIG
   phosphate-independent glutaminase
pig colon model
piggyback
   p. liver transplantation
   P. needle-knife papillotome

NOTES

piggybacking · piriform

piggybacking of I.V.
pigment
    gastric p.
    p. neuropathy
    p. stone
pigmentary cirrhosis
pigmentation
pigmented
    p. gallstone
    p. histiocyte
    p. nevus
    p. nipple
    p. protuberance
pigment-laden Kupffer cell
pigmentosa
    urticaria p.
pigmenturia
pIgR
    polyimmunoglobulin receptor
pigtail
    p. biliary stent
    p. catheter
    p. endoprosthesis
    p. nephrostomy tube
    3/4-p. plastic endoprosthesis
PIL
    primary intestinal lymphangiectasia
pile, pl. piles
    bleeding p.
    prostatic p.
    sentinel p.
    thrombosed p.
pileuse
    tumeur p.
pilimiction
pili torti et canaliculus
pillar
    palatine p.
pill esophagitis
pill-induced
    p.-i. esophageal injury
    p.-i. esophagitis
pillow
    Bedge p.
    MedSlant therapeutic p.
    Sand-Eze EGD p.
    p. sign
pilonidal
    p. cyst
    p. cystectomy
    p. perirectal abscess
    p. sinus
    p. sinus disease
pilosicoli
    Serpulina p.
pilot study
pimagedine
pimelorrhea

PIN
    prostatic intraepithelial neoplasia
pinacidil
pinch
    p. biopsy
    diaphragmatic p.
    p. forceps
    p. injury
pinchcock
    diaphragmatic p.
    p. effect
    p. mechanism
pindolol
pineapple test
pine cone appearance of bladder
pineoblastoma
pinguecula
pinocytosis
    fluid-phase p.
    p. vacuole
pinpoint pupil
Pin-Rid
pinwheel appearance
pinworm
Pin-X
PIP
    pressure inversion point
    PIP on esophageal manometry
PI4P
    phosphatidylinositol phosphate
PI4,5P2
    phosphatidylinositol 4,5-bisphosphate
pipe
    endoscopic washing p.
    Mauch double-sheathed plastic wash p.
pipecuronium
pipenzolate
piperacillin sodium
piperazine citrate
piperidolate
piperoxan
pipestem
    p. cirrhosis
    p. stool
PIPIDA
    paraisopropyliminodiacetic acid
    PIPIDA hepatobiliary scan
    ^{99m}Tc PIPIDA
Pippi-Salle technique
Pipracil
PIR
    pressure increment rate
pirenzepine
piretanide
piriform
    p. fossa
    p. pooling
    p. sinus

piriformis
  p. artery
  p. muscle
piritramide
piritrexim
piroxicam
piston-type syringe
pit
  anal p.
  p. cell
  clathrin-coated p.
  colonic p.
  Frey gastric p.
  gastric p.
  mucosal p.
  postanal p.
pitfall
  potential p.
Pitres sign
Pitressin
pitting
  anal p.
  colonic p.
  p. edema
  gastric p.
pituitary
  p. adenoma
  p. adenylate cyclase-activating polypeptide (PACAP)
  p. tumor
pituitary-gonadal axis
pityriasis
  p. lingua
  p. rotunda
Pityrosporon orbiculare
PI-urea
  phosphate ion-urea
pivalate derivative
PIVKA
  protein in vitamin K absence
PIVKA-II
  prothrombin induced by vitamin K absence or antagonist-II
    PIVKA-II antagonist
    PIVKA-II EIA kit for hepatocellular carcinoma
PIVOT
  Prostate Cancer Intervention Versus Observation Trial
pivoxil
  cefditoren p.
PiZZ alpha-1-antitrypsin deficiency

PJS
  Peutz-Jeghers syndrome
PKC
  protein kinase C
***PKD1*, *PKD2* gene**
PLA2
  phospholipase A2
placebo
  p. effect
  p. therapy
placebo-controlled trial
placement
  band p.
  dilator p.
  electrode p.
  endoscopic biliary stent p.
  endotracheal tube p.
  feeding tube p.
  five-port fan p.
  four-port diamond p.
  graft p.
  intestinal sling p.
  laparoscopy trocar p.
  metallic stent p.
  PEG-JET p.
  percutaneous endoscopic gastrostomy and jejunal extension tube p.
  percutaneous nephrostomy tube p.
  pH electrode p.
  posttreatment p.
  radiologic biliary stent p.
  tube p.
  ultrasound-assisted PEG p.
  ureteral stent p.
  wire-guided p.
placental alkaline phosphatase (PIAP)
Placer guidewire
plain
  p. abdominal radiography
  p. catgut suture
  p. film
  p. film of abdomen
  p. gut
  p. gut suture
  Perdiem P.
  p. radiograph
planar
  p. imaging
  p. xanthoma
plane
  Addison clinical p.'s
  Camper p.

NOTES

plane *(continued)*
    cleavage p.
    p. of dissection
    intersphincteric p.
    ischiorectal fossa p.
    parasagittal p.
    p. of Treves
planimeter
planimetric measurement
planimetry
    impedance p.
    rectal impedance p.
planktonic bacterium
planning
    preintervention p.
Plantago ovata **seed**
plantar grasp
plantaris
    hyperkeratosis palmaris et p.
    tylosis palmaris et p.
plantarum
    Lactobacillus p.
planuria
planus
    lichen p.
plaque
    atherosclerotic p.
    augmentation p.
    Hollenhorst p.
    p. incision
    ostial atherosclerotic p.
    Peyronie p.
    Randall p.
    stone p.
plaquelike
    p. lesion
    p. linear defect
    p. thickening
plasma
    p. albumin
    p. ammonia
    p. androgen
    p. apo B-48
    p. atrial natriuretic peptide
    p. bile acid measurement
    p. bubble
    p. caffeine concentration
    p. catecholamine
    p. cell
    p. cell balanitis
    p. cell granuloma
    p. cell hepatitis
    p. cell portal infiltration
    p. clearance
    p. cloud
    p. cortisol
    p. creatinine
    cryoprecipitated p.
    dialysis to p.
    p. enzyme
    p. exchange
    p. fibronectin
    p. flow
    fresh frozen p. (FFP)
    gastric p.
    p. gastrin concentration
    p. homocysteine
    p. inulin
    p. ionized calcium
    p. kallikrein
    p. membrane marker
    p. met-enkephalin
    p. norepinephrine concentration
    p. oncotic pressure
    p. osmolality
    p. parathyroid hormone (PTH)
    p. perfusion
    p. protein
    p. protein fraction
    p. renin
    p. renin activity (PRA)
    p. renin activity captopril test
    p. renin concentration
    seminal p. C3
    p. tonicity
    p. ultrafiltrate
    p. urea
    p. urea concentration
    p. viscosity
    p. volume
    p. volume depletion
    p. volume expansion
plasma-activated
    p.-a. complement 3 (C3a)
    p.-a. complement 4 (C4a)
    p.-a. complement 5 (C5a)
plasmablastic myeloma
plasmacellularis
    balanitis circumscripta p.
plasmacytoma
    bladder p.
    extramedullary p.
    gastric p.
    radioresistant gastric p.
plasmacytosis
plasma-free choline concentration
PlasmaKinetic
    P. radiofrequency energy delivery
    P. surgery
plasmalogen
Plasma-Lyte
Plasmanate
plasmapheresis
    therapeutic p.
plasmid
    p. mediated
    p. profile
    p. profile role

plasminogen
  p. activator (PA)
  p. activator inhibitor (PAI)
  p. activator inhibitor type 1, 2 (PAI-1, -2)
  functional p.
plasmodium
  encapsulated p.
  P. falciparum
  P. falciparum malaria
  P. malariae
Plastibell circumcision
plastica
  linitis p.
  penis p.
  periureteritis p.
  rectal linitis p. (RLP)
plastic endoprosthesis
plasty
  bladder neck Y-V p.
  Foley Y-V p.
  mons p.
  posterior bladder flap p.
  V-Y p.
  Y-V p.
plate
  anal p.
  bladder p.
  blood agar p.
  bowel p.
  brain-heart infusion p.
  cloacal p.
  exstrophic bladder p.
  hilar p.
  levator p.
  limiting p.
  liver cell p.
  Maxisorb test p.
  microwell p.
  Mueller-Hinton-supplemented agar p.
  Skirrow agar p.
  Sur-Fit Natura irrigation adapter face p.
  trigonal p.
  urethral p.
plateau
  dieting p.
  p. response
platelet
  p. abnormality
  p. activation
  p. count
  p. dysfunction
  p. factor 4
  p. glycoprotein 2b3a receptor antagonist
  p. transfusion
platelet-activating factor (PAF)
platelet-derived growth factor (PDGF)
Platinol
  etoposide, Adriamycin, P. (EAP)
  5-fluorouracil, Adriamycin, P. (FAP)
  fluorouracil, leucovorin rescue, Adriamycin, P. (FLAP)
  Ifex, Taxol, P. (ITP)
  VePesid, ifosfamide (with mesna rescue), P. (VIP)
platinum
  cyclophosphamide, Velban, actinomycin D, bleomycin, p. (VAB-VI)
  p., etoposide (PE)
  p., etoposide, bleomycin (PEB)
  Velban, actinomycin D, bleomycin, p. (VAB-II)
  p., Velban, bleomycin (PVB)
platinum-based consolidation chemotherapy
platysma
PLB
  percutaneous liver biopsy
PLC
  phospholipase C
PLC-50 linear stapler
PLC-PRF 5 cell
PLD
  polycystic liver disease
pleating of small bowel
Pleatman sac
Plegine
pleiotropic
Plenaxis powder for IM injection
pleomorphic
  p. destructive cholangitis
  p. rhabdomyosarcoma
pleomorphism
  nuclear hyperchromasia and p.
Plesiomonas shigelloides
plethora
plethoric
plethysmography
  impedance p. (IPG)
  penile p.

NOTES

pleura
    mediastinal p.
pleural
    p. mass
    p. rub
    p. tube
pleuritis
    bile p.
pleurobiliary fistula
pleurocholecystitis
pleuroesophageal muscle
pleuroperitoneal
    p. canal
    p. foramen
    p. sinus
pleurovisceral
plexiform neurofibroma
plexus, pl. **plexuses**
    Auerbach and Meissner p.
    Auerbach mesenteric p.
    biliary p.
    celiac p.
    colonic myenteric p.
    cystic p.
    deep muscular p.
    distal venous p.
    esophageal p.
    extrapancreatic nerve p.
    fundic p.
    ganglionated p.
    gastric p.
    gastroesophageal variceal p.
    gastrointestinal myenteric p.
    hemorrhoidal p.
    hypogastric p.
    p. hypogastric impar
    ileocolic p.
    p. of impar
    impar hypogastric p.
    inferior anal p.
    inferior hypogastric p.
    p. interiliacus
    longitudinal subepithelial venous p.
    lumbar p.
    lumbosacral p.
    Meissner p.
    middle rectal venous p.
    mucosal p.
    myenteric p.
    p. myentericus
    neural p.
    nonganglionated p.
    pampiniform p.
    p. pampiniformis
    pelvic nerve p.
    p. pelvicus
    perivascular p.
    preprostatic p.
    prostaticovesical p.
    p. prostaticus
    proximal venous p.
    rectal p.
    p. renalis
    sacral p.
    Santorini venous p.
    spermatic p.
    p. spermaticus
    submucosal venous p.
    submucous p.
    submuscular p.
    suburothelial nerve p.
    superior hypogastric nerve p.
    superior rectal venous p.
    suprarenal p.
    testicular p.
    p. testicularis
    thyreoideus impar p.
    ureteric p.
    p. uretericus
    vascular p.
    p. venosus
    vesical p.
    p. vesicale
    p. vesicalis
    vesicoprostatic p.
pliable lesion
plica, pl. **plicae**
    plicae circulares
    p. duodenalis inferior
    p. duodenalis superior
    p. epigastrica
    p. ileocecalis
    p. longitudinalis
    p. pubovesicalis
    Rathke p.
    p. umbilicalis
    p. vesicalis transversa
plicae (*pl. of* plica)
plicamycin
plicated appendicocystostomy
plication
    Bard endoscope transesophageal endoscopic p.
    Child-Phillips bowel p.
    dorsal curve p.
    fundal p.
    Graham p.
    Kaliscinski p.
    Kelly p.
    Nesbit p.
    Noble bowel p.
    Rehne-Delorme p.
    Starr p.
    suture p.
    p. suture
    transgastric p.
    transmesenteric p.
    tunica albuginea p.

PLM
  periodic leg movement
ploidy
  p. analysis
  chromosome p.
plot
  Eadie-Hofstee p.
pluck technique
plug
  bile p.
  canalicular bile p.
  Coloplast conseal p.
  p. gastrostomy
  meconium p.
  omental p.
  one-piece disposable p.
  PerFix Marlex mesh p.
  protein p.
  urethral p.
plugged liver biopsy
plumbism
plume
  laser p.
Plummer
  P. bag
  P. dilator
  P. treatment
Plummer-Vinson syndrome
plus
  Bayer P.
  Charcoal P.
  Ensure P.
  HCV QuantaSure P.
  Lithostar P.
  Losotron P.
  Maalox P.
  Pyridium P.
  Resource P.
  Riopan P.
  RX Herculink P.
  Therevac P.
  Titralac P.
PMA
  phorbol myristate acetate
PMA-stimulated O_2
PMC
  pontine micturition center
  pseudomembranous colitis
PMMA
  polymethylmethacrylate
  PMMA bead

PMME
  primary malignant melanoma of esophagus
PMN
  polymorphonuclear
  PMN cell
  PMN chemotaxis assay
  PMN infiltrate
  PMN leukocyte
  PMN oxidative burst capacity
  uremic PMN
PMN-elastase
  fecal PMN-e.
PMNL
  polymorphonuclear leukocyte
PMN-mediated endothelial cell injury
PMNN
  polymorphonuclear neutrophil
P-Mod-S factor
PN
  pyelonephritis
PNA
  peanut agglutinin
PNCA
  proliferating nuclear cell antigen
PNE
  percutaneous nerve evaluation
  peripheral nerve evaluation
  PNE test
PNET
  primitive neuroectodermal tumor
pneumatic
  p. bag
  p. bag dilation of esophagus
  p. bag esophageal dilation
  p. balloon catheter dilation
  p. balloon dilator
  p. compression device (PCD)
  p. endoscopic lithotriptor
  p. leg pump
  p. lithotripsy
pneumatinuria (*var. of* pneumaturia)
pneumatocele
  scrotal p.
pneumatosis
  p. cystoides coli (PCC)
  p. cystoides intestinalis (PCI)
  p. cystoides intestinorum
  intestinal p.
pneumaturia, pneumatinuria
pneumobilia absent
pneumocholecystitis

NOTES

pneumococcal infection
pneumococcus nephritis
pneumocolon
    spiral computed tomography p.
Pneumocystis
    P. carinii
    P. carinii pneumonia (PCP)
pneumocystosis
    gastric p.
pneumodissection
pneumoenteritis
pneumogastrography
pneumography
    retroperitoneal p.
pneumohydraulic capillary infusion system
pneumohydroperitoneum
pneumokidney
pneumomediastinum
pneumonectomy
pneumonia
    aspiration p.
    lymphoid interstitial p.
    Pneumocystis carinii p. (PCP)
    Proteus p.
    Pseudomonas aeruginosa p.
    Pseudomonas pseudomallei p.
pneumoniae
    Klebsiella p.
pneumonitis
    radiation p.
pneumopenis
pneumopericardium
pneumoperitoneum
    benign p.
    p. needle
    stent-induced p.
    tension p.
pneumoperitonitis
pneumophila
    Legionella p.
pneumopyelography
pneumoradiography
    retroperitoneal p.
pneumoretroperitoneum
pneumoscrotum
Pneumo Sleeve
pneumostatic dilation
pneumothorax
    iatrogenic p.
    tension p.
PNH
    paroxysmal nocturnal hemoglobinuria
PNI
    prognostic nutritional index
PNL
    percutaneous nephrolithotomy
PNMT
    phenylethylamine N-methyl transferase
PNTML
    pudendal nerve terminal motor latency
POA
    pancreatic oncofetal antigen
        POA test
Pockel cell
pocketed calculus
podagra
podocalyxin
podocin
podocyte
    glomerular p.
    p. glycocalyx
podocyte-specific protein
podofilox solution
podophyllin
podophyllotoxin
POEMS
    polyneuropathy, organomegaly, endocrinopathy, monoclonal protein, and skin changes
        POEMS syndrome
poikilocyte
    teardrop p.
point
    Addison p.
    APACHE-II p.
    bleeding p.
    Boas p.
    Brewer p.
    Cannon p.
    Chauffard p.
    Desjardins p.
    dorsal p.
    F2 focal p.
    Griffith p.
    Halle p.
    Hartmann p.
    Lanz p.
    Mackenzie p.
    McBurney p.
    Munro p.
    Piersol p.
    pressure inversion p. (PIP)
    Ramond p.
    respiratory inversion p. (RIP)
    p. of respiratory reversal on esophageal manometry
    Robson p.
    Sudeck critical p.
    p. tenderness
    Voillemier p.
point-counting image
pointed condyloma
pointer
    LaserMed laser p.
POINTER computer program
pointing
    past p.

Poiseuille-Hagen law
Poiseuille law
poison
poisoning
    ackee fruit p.
    acute lead p.
    acute mercury p.
    Amanita phalloides mushroom p.
    bacterial food p.
    chronic lead p.
    chronic mercury p.
    ciguatera fish p.
    excitotoxic food p.
    ferrous salt p.
    food p.
    histamine fish p.
    iron p.
    lead p.
    mercury p.
    mushroom p.
    paralytic shellfish p.
    phosphorus p.
    Salmonella food p.
    scombroid fish p.
    Staphylococcus food p.
    thallium p.
Poisson regression
Polachrome 35-mm slide system
Poland syndrome
polar
    p. artery
    p. body
    P. enteral feeding bag
    p. region
    p. segmental nephrectomy
    p. sheathed flagella
Polaris grasper
polarization microscopy
polarized
    p. glucose transporter
    p. standing reflex
polarographic study
Polaroid
    P. camera
    P. endocamera EC-3
    P. SX-70 with ACMI adapter
pole
    caudal p.
    cranial p.
    inferior p.
    p. of kidney
    pelvic p.

Polhemus-Schafer-Ivemark syndrome
policy
    organ allocation p.
polidocanol
    p. injection
    p. injection therapy
    p. sclerosant
poliomyelitis
POLIP
    polyneuropathy, ophthalmoplegia, leukoencephalopathy, and intestinal pseudoobstruction
    POLIP syndrome
Politano-Leadbetter
    P.-L. anastomosis
    P.-L. technique
    P.-L. tunnel creation
    P.-L. ureterolysis
    P.-L. ureteroneocystostomy
polka fever
Pollack ureteral catheter
pollakiuria
pollen extract
Pólya
    P. anastomosis
    P. gastrectomy
    P. gastroenterostomy
    P. operation
    P. technique
polyacrylamide
    p. gel
    p. gel electrophoresis (PAGE)
polyamine
    p. level
    p. spermine
polyangiitis
    microscopic p. (MPA)
polyanion
    GBM p.
polyantibiotic chemotherapy
polyarteritis nodosa
polyarthritis
    seronegative p.
polycationic
    p. histochemical probe
    p. marker
polychemotherapy
polychloruria
Polycillin-N
Polycitra
Polycitra-K, -LC

NOTES

polyclonal
    p. epidermal growth factor antibody
    p. IgG
Polycose glucose supplement
polycystic
    p. chronic esophagitis
    p. disease of liver (PDL)
    p. kidney disease
    p. liver
    p. liver disease (PCLD, PLD)
polycystin-1, -2
polycythemia vera
Polydek suture
polydimethylsiloxane
polydioxan
polydioxanone suture
polydipsia
    psychogenic p.
polyester-reinforced Dacron tape
polyestradiol phosphate therapy
polyethylene
    p. balloon dilator
    p. cannula
    p. catheter
    p. endoprosthesis
    p. glycol (PEG)
    p. glycol 600
    p. glycol-based lavage
    p. glycol electrolyte lavage solution (PEG-ELS)
    p. perforation
    p. stent
    p. tube
polyethylenimine (PEI)
Polyflex stent
Poly GIA stapler
polyglactin
    p. monofilament loop
    p. suture
    p. suture material
polyglecaprone 25 suture
polyglutamate
    p. folate
    p. paclitaxel
polyglycolic
    p. acid
    p. acid collar
    p. acid suture
polyglyconate
    p. monofilament loop
    p. staple
    p. suture
polygonal hepatocyte
polygraph
    Nihon Kohden p.
polyhydramnios
polyimmunoglobulin receptor (pIgR)
poly-L-lysine-coated glass slide
polylobar liver
polymer
    mucin p.
    silicone p.
polymerase
    p. chain reaction (PCR)
    p. chain reaction-based single-stranded conformation polymorphism (PCR-SSCP)
    p. chain reaction technology
    DNA p.
    HBV-associated DNA p.
    Taq p.
polymerization
    IgA p.
polymethylmethacrylate (PMMA)
    p. membrane
polymicrobial
    p. bacterascites
    p. biofilm
    p. infection
polymorphic
    p. gene
    p. reticulosis
polymorphism
    ACE gene p.
    aldosterone synthase p.
    angiotensin-converting enzyme gene p.
    angiotensin I-converting enzyme insertion/deletion p.
    CARD15 p.
    deletion p.
    DNA p.
    polymerase chain reaction-based single-stranded conformation p. (PCR-SSCP)
    restriction fragment length p. (RFLP, RLP)
polymorphonuclear (PMN)
    p. cell
    p. inflammatory infiltrate
    p. leukocyte (PMNL)
    p. neutrophil (PMNN)
Polymox
polymyositis
polymyositis-dermatomyositis
polymyxin
    p. B
    p. nephropathy
polyneuropathy
    arsenical p.
    familial amyloid p. (FAP)
    p., ophthalmoplegia, leukoencephalopathy, and intestinal pseudoobstruction (POLIP)
    p., organomegaly, endocrinopathy, monoclonal protein, and skin changes (POEMS)

polyol pathway
polyoma middle T oncogene
polyomavirus
Polyomavirus **infection**
polyorchidism, polyorchism
polyostotic fibrous dysphasia
polyp
    adenomatous p. (AP)
    adenomatous colorectal p.
    adenomatous gastric p.
    antral p.
    benign adenomatous p.
    bleeding p.
    broad-based p.
    cervical p.
    cholesterol p.
    cloacogenic p.
    colonic p.
    colorectal p.
    diminutive adenomatous p.
    diminutive colonic p.
    diminutive hyperplastic p.
    duodenal p.
    elusive p.
    eroded p.
    esophageal p.
    fibroid p.
    fibrovascular p.
    filiform p.
    fundic gland p.
    gastric antral sessile p.
    gastric hyperplastic p.
    gastric inflammatory fibroid p.
    gastrointestinal hamartomatous p.
    giant gastric p.
    p. grasper
    hamartomatous gastric p.
    hyperplasiogenic p.
    hyperplastic p. (HP)
    hyperplastic adenomatous p.
    hyperplastic epithelial gastric p.
    hyperplastic gastric p.
    inflammatory fibroid p. (IFP)
    invasive colorectal p.
    juvenile retention p.
    lymphoid p.
    malignant p.
    metaplastic p.
    mixed hyperplastic-adenomatous gastric p.
    mucosal p.
    multiple p.'s
    nasal p.
    neoplastic p.
    nonneoplastic p.
    pedunculated p.
    perineal p.
    Peutz-Jeghers p.
    polypoid p.
    postinflammatory p.
    prepyloric p.
    prostatic urethral p.
    rectal p.
    p. relocation
    retention p.
    sentinel hyperplastic p.
    sessile p.
    small inflammatory p.
    p. stalk
    synchronous p.
    tuberculosis p.
    tubular p.
    tubulovillous p.
    villoglandular p.
    villous p.
polypectomized
polypectomy
    colonoscopic p.
    duodenal endoscopic p.
    electrosurgical snare p.
    endoscopic sessile p.
    gastric p.
    incomplete p.
    piecemeal p.
    saline-assisted p. (SAP)
    snare p.
    p. snare
    p. stump
polypeptide
    gastric inhibitory p. (GIP)
    p. growth factor
    islet amyloid p.
    pancreatic p. (PP)
    parathyroid hormone-related p.
    pituitary adenylate cyclase-activating p. (PACAP)
    vasoactive intestinal p. (VIP)
polyphagia
polyphosphate
    ^{99m}Tc p.
polyphosphoinositide
polypiform
polypoid
    p. cancer

NOTES

polypoid *(continued)*
- p. carcinoma
- p. colorectal cavernous hemangioma
- p. dysplasia
- p. excrescence
- p. exophytic nonulcerating carcinosarcoma
- p. filling defect
- p. gastric rugal hyperplasia
- p. lesion
- p. lymphoid hyperplasia
- p. lymphoma
- p. lymphomatous hyperplasia
- p. mass
- p. polyp
- p. tumor
- p. urethritis
- p. vascular malformation

polyposa
- colitis p.
- enteritis p.
- gastritis cystica p.

polyposis
- adenomatous p.
- cap p.
- p. coli
- colonic p.
- dense p.
- diffuse hyperplastic p.
- diffuse mucosal p.
- duodenal p.
- familial adenomatous p. (FAP)
- familial colorectal p.
- familial gastrointestinal p.
- familial hamartomatous p.
- familial intestinal p.
- familial juvenile p. (FJP)
- filiform p.
- florid p.
- gastric p.
- gastrointestinal p. (GIP)
- hamartomatous p.
- hyperplastic p.
- intermediate p.
- intestinal p.
- juvenile p. (JP)
- lymphomatous p. (LP)
- multiple familial p.
- multiple lymphomatous p. (MLP)
- nonfamilial gastrointestinal p.
- Peutz-Jeghers gastrointestinal p.
- sparse p.
- p. syndrome
- p. ventriculi

polypous gastritis
polyprenoic acid
Polyprep centrifugation

polypropylene
- p. mesh
- p. suture

polypus
- p. cysticus
- p. hydatidosus

polyradicular neuropathy
polyribosome
polysaccharide
- p. antigen
- p. capsule
- p. hyaluronan
- p. Kreha (PSK)

polysaccharide-iron complex
polyserositis
- familial paroxysmal p. (FPP)
- familial recurrent p.
- periodic p.

polysome
- endoplasmic reticulum-bound p.

polysomnography
polyspermy, polyspermia
polysplenia syndrome
polystyrene sodium sulfonate
polysulfate
- pentosan sodium p.
- sodium pentosan p.

polysulfonated naphthylurea
polysulfone
- 760 p. dialyzer
- F60S p.
- high-flux p.
- p. membrane

polysynaptic reflex
Polytef injection
polytetrafluoroethylene (PTFE)
- p. mesh
- p. paste injection
- p. periurethral injection
- p. sock

Polytrac Gomez retractor
polytropous enteronitis
polyunsaturated lecithin
polyurethane
- p. nasoenteric catheter
- p. stent

polyurethane-covered metallic stent
polyuria
- nighttime p.
- nocturnal p.

polyvinyl
- p. alcohol
- p. alcohol sponge
- p. alcohol sponge hysterosacropexy
- p. bougie
- p. chloride (PVC)
- p. chloride catheter
- p. dilator
- p. tubing

POMC
    proopiomelanocortin
Pompe disease
Pondimin
Ponka
    P. herniorrhaphy
    P. technique herniorrhaphy anesthesia
    P. technique for local anesthesia
pons hepatis
Ponsky
    P. pull
    P. technique
Ponsky-Gauderer type PEG
ponticulus, pl. **ponticuli**
    p. hepatis
pontine micturition center (PMC)
pontine-sacral reflex
POO
    prostatic outlet obstruction
pool
    abdominal p.
    bile acid p.
    gastric p.
    intracellular p.
pooled
    p. glomeruli
    p. saliva
Poole suction tube
pooling
    piriform p.
    vallecular p.
    venous p.
poor
    p. long-term efficacy
    p. long-term outcome
    p. long-term result
    p. risk
    p. surgical risk case
poorly
    p. compliant bladder
    p. differentiated adenoma
    p. localized pain
popliteal
    p. swelling
    p. tenderness
pop-off suture
Poppel sign
POPS
    peroral pancreatoscopy
population
    challenging patient p.
    gluten-dependent p.
    hemodialysis p.
    susceptible p.
population-based control group
porcelain gallbladder
porcine
    p. carboxypeptidase B
    p. dermis for pubovaginal sling
    p. endogenous retrovirus (PERV)
    p. hepatocyte
pore
    filtration slit p.'s
    shuntlike p.
porfimer sodium
Porges catheter
pori (*pl. of* porus)
porin channel protein
pork tapeworm
porotomy
porous filter membrane
porphobilinogen (PBG)
    p. deaminase (PBG-D)
porphyria
    acute intermittent p. (AIP)
    p. cutanea tarda (PCT)
    hepatic p.
    variegate p. (VP)
porphyrin photosensitizer
porphyrinuria, porphyruria
port
    BardPort implanted p.
    inlet p.
    MCL p.
    OmegaPort access p.
    periumbilical p.
    p. site metastasis
    subcostal p.
    suprapubic p.
    umbilical p.
porta
    p. hepatis
    p. renis
portable
    p. digital data recorder
    p. perfused manometric system
    p. renal preservation machine
Port-A-Cath catheter
portacaval
    p. anastomosis
    p. H graft
    p. H-graft shunt

NOTES

portacaval *(continued)*
    p. shunt (PCS)
    p. transposition (PCT)
Portagen
    P. diet
    P. feeding
    P. formula
Port-A-Germ anaerobic transport vial
portal
    p. azygous collateral
    p. block
    p. blood velocity
    p. canal
    p. cannula
    p. catheter
    p. circulation
    p. cirrhosis
    p. decompression
    p. embolization (PE)
    p. eosinophilic inflammation
    p. fissure
    p. hypertension (PHT)
    p. hypertensive gastropathy (PHG)
    p. hypertensive intestinal vasculopathy (PHIV)
    p. hypotensive drug
    p. lobulation
    p. lobule
    p. perfusion defect
    p. plasma cell infiltration
    p. portography
    p. pyemia
    p. shunt index (PSI)
    p. tract
    p. tract fibrosis
    p. tract inflammation
    p. triad
    p. triaditis
    p. triad occlusion
    p. trunk
    p. vascular bed
    p. vein (PV)
    p. vein blood flow velocity (PFV)
    p. vein congestive index (PVCI)
    p. vein obstruction
    p. vein thrombi
    p. vein thrombosis (PVT)
    p. venous pressure (PVP)
    p. venous system
    p. venous velocity (PVV)
    p. venule
    p. zone
    p. zone granuloma
portal-collateral circulation
portal-systemic *(var. of* portosystemic*)*
portal-to-portal
    p.-t.-p. bridging
    p.-t.-p. fibrosis
Porter duodenal forceps

portoenterostomy
    Kasai p.
portography
    arterial p.
    computed tomography arterial p.
    computed tomography during arterial p. (CTAP, CT-AP)
    CT during arterial p. (CTAP, CT-AP)
    percutaneous transhepatic p. (PTP)
    portal p.
    splenic p.
    transhepatic p.
    umbilical p.
portopulmonary
    p. hypertension
    p. shunt
portosystemic, portal-systemic
    p. encephalopathy (PSE)
    p. shunt
    p. shunting (PSS)
    p. shunt surgery
PortSaver PercLoop device
Portsmouth predictor equation
porus, pl. **pori**
    p. galeni
position
    anterior oblique p.
    body p.
    Buie p.
    cervical p.
    curved flank p.
    decubitus p.
    dorsal lithotomy p.
    dorsosacral p.
    Edebohls p.
    Elliot p.
    final p.
    flank p.
    forward-viewing p.
    Fowler p.
    frogleg p.
    Gil-Vernet p.
    greater curve p.
    jackknife p.
    knee-chest p.
    knee-elbow p.
    Kraske p.
    lateral decubitus p.
    left decubitus p.
    left lateral decubitus p.
    lithotomy p.
    Lloyd-Davies Trendelenburg p.
    Mayo-Robson p.
    modified Lloyd-Davies p.
    prone split-leg p.
    reverse Trendelenburg p.
    right anterior oblique p.
    Robson p.

Scultetus p.
semioblique p.
Sims p.
ski p.
subclavian p.
supine p.
Trendelenburg p.
positional obstructive uropathy
positioner
gallbladder bag p.
positioning
automated endoscopic system for optimal p. (AESOP)
flank roll p.
patient p.
positive
antigen p.
p. bowel sounds
p. culture result
extradomain A p. (EDA+)
p. family history
p. margin
p. nitrogen balance
p. predictive value (PPV)
p. secretin stimulation study
positive-pressure urethrography (PPUG)
Positrap
P. miniretrieval basket
P. retriever
P. three-prong nonretracting grasping forceps
positron
p. camera
p. emission tomography (PET)
p. emission tomography scan
P. Plus cushion
Posner attention test
post
p. hoc test
p. jejunoileal bypass hepatic disease
p. rubber band sepsis
status p. (SP, S/P)
postage stamp penile tumescence test
postanal
p. dimpling
p. pit
p. repair
postanesthesia recovery (PAR)
postatrophic hyperplasia
postauricular Wolfe graft
postautoclave contamination

postbiopsy
p. fistula
p. vascular complication
postbulbar duodenal ulcer
postcaval ureter
postcecal abscess
postchemotherapy surgery
postcholangitic stricture
postcholecystectomy
p. flatulent dyspepsia
p. syndrome (PCS)
postcholecystitis adhesion
postcibal symptom
postcoagulation syndrome
postcoital test
postcolonoscopy distention syndrome
postcricoid
p. area
p. web
postdialysis urea rebound
postdilation meglumine diatrizoate
postdystrophic scarring
postendoscopic cholangitis
postendoscopy
postenteritis syndrome
post-ERCP-induced pancreatitis
posterior
p. abdominal wall
anterior and p. (A&P)
arteria caecalis p.
arteria gastrica p.
arteria pancreaticoduodenalis superior p.
p. bladder flap plasty
p. duodenal ulcer
p. extremity
p. fissure
p. flap vaginoplasty
p. hypospadias
p. lumbar approach
p. mediastinal adenopathy
p. nephrectomy
p. pararenal compartment
p. pelvic exenteration
p. perineum
p. rectopexy
p. rectus sheath
p. renal fascia
p. sagittal anorectoplasty
p. sagittal and three-flap anoplasty
p. scrotal nerve
p. transthoracic incision

NOTES

posterior *(continued)*
- p. urethra
- p. urethral valve type I–IV (PUV)

posterolateral
posterorsuperior pancreaticoduodenal artery
postevacuation
- p. film
- p. view

post-fatty meal cholecystography
postfundoplication syndrome
postganglionic
- p. cholinergic nerve
- p. sympathetic nerve

postgastrectomy
- p. bleed
- p. cancer
- p. dysfunction
- p. gastritis
- p. hemorrhage
- p. stasis
- p. syndrome

postglomerular arteriole
postheparin lipolytic activity (PHLA)
posthepatic, posthepatitic
- p. cirrhosis

posthepatitis aplastic anemia
posthetomy
posthioplasty
posthitis
postholith
posthysterectomy vaginal prolapse
postictal
postinfectious glomerulonephritis
postinfective glomerulonephritis
postinflammatory
- p. contracture
- p. polyp
- p. traction

postischemic
- p. acute renal failure
- p. tubular necrosis

postligation
- p. discomfort
- p. pain
- p. ulcer

postmenopausal
postmicturition
- p. continuous leakage
- p. dribble

postmortem intussusception
postmyotomy reflux
postnasal drip
postnecrotic
- p. cirrhosis
- p. scarring

postnephrectomized
postobstructive diuresis

postoperative
- p. abscess
- p. adhesion
- p. advance
- p. alloantigen-dependent
- p. analgesia requirement
- p. anticoagulation therapy
- p. autologous transfusion
- p. biliary leakage
- p. cholangiography
- p. choledochoscopy
- p. cholesterol embolism
- p. complication
- p. evaluation
- p. gastritis
- p. hydrocele
- p. ileus
- p. irrigation-suction
- p. irrigation-suction drainage
- p. morbidity
- p. pleurobiliary fistula
- p. recurrent bleeding rate
- p. reflux
- p. regimen for oral early feeding (PROEF)
- p. retroperitoneal fibrosis
- p. stricture
- p. ureteral obstruction
- p. urinary retention
- p. vomiting

postoperatively
fluid intake p.

postparacentesis circulatory dysfunction (PCD)
postpartum constipation
postperfusion
postpolypectomy
- p. bleed
- p. coagulation syndrome
- p. hemorrhage

postprandial
- p. distention
- p. fullness
- p. hypoglycemia
- p. nausea
- p. pain
- p. portal hyperemia
- p. vomiting

postprocedure pancreatitis
postprostatectomy
- p. hemostatic catheter
- p. incontinence

postpyloric feeding tube
postreceptor signaling of parietal cell
postrema
area p.

postrenal
- p. albuminuria

p. anuria
p. proteinuria
postsclerotherapy bacterial peritonitis
postsecretory processing
postshunt encephalopathy
postsphincterotomy
p. ductography
p. ERCP cannulation
postsplenectomy infection
poststreptococcal
p. acute glomerulonephritis
p. glomerulonephritis (PSGN)
postsurgical
p. change
p. endoscopy
p. gastric stasis
p. recurrent ulcer
posttest score
postthaw sperm motility index
postthrombotic syndrome
post-TNM stage I, II, III, IV
posttransfusion hepatitis
posttranslational
p. modification
p. processing of peptide
posttransplant
p. antiglomerular basement membrane
p. diabetes mellitus (PTDM)
p. immunosuppression
p. immunosuppression therapy
p. lymphoproliferative disorder (PTLD)
p. patient
p. renal dysfunction
posttransplantation
p. cholangitis
p. survival rate
posttransurethral microwave thermotherapy prostatitis-like syndrome
posttraumatic
p. autotransplantation
p. incontinence
p. pancreatic-cutaneous fistula
p. posterior urethral stricture
posttreatment
p. discomfort
p. placement
post-TUMT prostatitis-like syndrome
posttussive vomiting

postulate
Koch p.
postural
p. quantitative analysis of acid exposure
p. regurgitation
p. stimulation test (PST)
posture-dependent pain
postureteral ligation
postureteroscopic manipulation
posture test
posturethral suspension obstruction
posturing
decerebrate p.
decorticate p.
posturography
computerized dynamic p. (CDP)
post-UUO time
Pos-T-Vac
P.-T-V. vacuum erection device
P.-T-V. VCD
postvagotomy
p. diarrhea
p. dysphagia
p. gastroparesis
p. syndrome
postvoid
p. dribble
p. dribbling of urine
p. incontinence
p. radiography
p. residual (PVR)
p. residual urine
postvoiding cystogram (PVC)
Potaba
potassium
aminobenzoate p.
p. balance
p. bicarbonate
p. channel
p. channel opener
p. chloride (KCl)
p. citrate
p. conductance
p. cyanide
p. deficiency
p. depletion
dietary p.
p. electrolyte
extracellular p.
fractional excretion of p. (FEFEK)
p. hydroxide smear

NOTES

potassium *(continued)*
    intracellular p.
    p. permanganate
    p. phosphate
    p. sensitivity test (PST)
potassium-binding resin
potassium-canrenoate antagonist
potassium-losing nephritis
potassium-sparing diuretic
potassium-titanyl phosphate (KTP)
potato liver
potency
    erectile p.
    failed recovery of p.
    recovery of sexual p.
    sexual p.
potential
    p. complication
    p. difference (PD)
    evoked p.
    excitatory junction p. (EJP)
    excitatory postsynaptic p. (EPSP)
    p. fusion protein
    inhibitory postsynaptic p. (IPSP)
    malignant p.
    motor unit action p.
    neoplastic p.
    oscillatory p.
    oxidant-trapping p.
    p. pitfall
    pudendal-evoked p.
    redox p.
    resting membrane p.
    p. role for simethicone in bowel preparation
    short-lasting afterhyperpolarizing p.
    spike p.
    stromal tumor of unknown malignant p. (STUMP)
    threshold p.
    p. toxicity
    visual evoked p.
potentiation
    alcohol p.
    p. of drug hepatotoxicity
Potter
    P. disease
    P. facies
    P. phenotype
    P. syndrome
Potts
    P. forceps
    P. scissors
Potts-Smith
    P.-S. forceps
    P.-S. scissors
pouch
    abdominovesical p.
    anal p.
    Assura convex drainable p.
    Assura convex urostomy p.
    Assura pediatric p.
    Assura standard drainable p.
    banded gastroplasty with divided p.
    Bard closed-end adhesive p.
    Bard drainage adhesive p.
    Bard Extra Ileo B p.
    Bard security p.
    Barnett p.
    Benchekroun p.
    p. biopsy
    bladder replacement urinary p.
    blind upper esophageal p.
    Bricker p.
    bulky colonic p.
    Camey urinary p.
    catheterization p.
    closed-end ostomy p.
    colonic J p.
    Coloplast closed p.
    Coloplast drainable p.
    Coloplast flange p.
    coloplasty p.
    p. configuration
    continent ileal reservoir catheterization p.
    ConvaTec colostomy p.
    ConvaTec Little One Sur-Fit p.
    ConvaTec Sur-Fit two-piece p.
    Cymed Micro Skin one-piece drainage p.
    Dansac Karaya Seal one-piece drainage p.
    Dansac Standard Ileo p.
    Denis Browne p.
    double-loop p.
    Douglas p.
    drainable ostomy p.
    Duke p.
    endorectal ileal p.
    p. excision
    p. failure
    First-Choice drainable p.
    p. fistula
    Florida urinary p.
    Fobi p.
    p. former
    fundal p.
    gastric p.
    Graham closure with omental p.
    Greer EZ Access drainage p.
    Hartmann p.
    haustral p.
    Heidenhain p.
    hemi-Kock p.
    hernia p.
    Hollister First Choice p.
    Hollister Holligard p.

Hollister Karaya 5 ostomy p.
Hollister Karaya Seal p.
Hollister Premium p.
Hunt-Lawrence p.
ileal J p.
ileal low-pressure bladder substitute p.
ileal neobladder urinary p.
ileal S p.
ileal W p.
p. ileitis
ileoanal p.
ileocecal p.
ileocolonic p.
Incise P.
Indiana urinary p.
inlet p. (IP)
intraluminal p.
inverted-U p.
J p.
jejunal p.
J pelvic ileal p.
J-shaped ileal p.
Kock urinary p.
lateral-lateral p.
Le Bag ileocolonic p.
Le Bag urinary p.
low-pressure p.
Mainz p. II
Mainz urinary p.
Mansson urinary p.
Marlen Gas Relief drainage p.
Marlen Odor-Ban ileostomy p.
Marlen Solo ileostomy p.
Marlen Zip Klosed p.
Miami p.
MicroSkin ostomy p.
Morison p.
Nu-Hope ileostomy p.
Nu-Hope neonatal and preemie p.
Nu-Hope Nu-Self drainable p.
Nu-Hope urinary p.
Nu-Hope urostomy p.
one-piece ostomy p.
open-ended ostomy p.
orthotopic voiding p.
Padua bladder urinary p.
pararectal p.
paravesical p.
Parks ileostomy p.
pelvic p.
Penn p.
perineal p.
pharyngeal p.
Physick p.
protease p.
RapiSeal p.
rectal p.
rectouterine p.
rectovaginal p.
rectovesical p.
renal p.
right colon p.
Rowland p.
S p.
sigma rectum p.
sigmoid p.
sigmoid-rectum p.
S pelvic ileal p.
S-shaped p.
Studer p.
superficial inguinal p.
Sur-Fit Natura flexible wafer and drainable p.
Sur-Fit Natura urostomy p.
Tena p.
terminal ileal p.
three-limb S p.
three-loop ileal p.
triple-loop p.
two-loop J-shaped ileal p.
two-piece ostomy p.
U p.
UCLA catheterization p.
p. ulceration
United Bongort Lifestyle p.
United Max-E drainable p.
United Surgical Bongort Lifestyle p.
United Surgical Featherlite ileostomy p.
United Surgical Shear Plus drainable p.
United Surgical Soft & Secure p.
vesica ileale p.
vesicouterine p.
VPI nonadhesive open-end p.
W p.
Willis p.
W pelvic ileal p.
W-shaped p.
Zenker p.
pouch-anal anastomosis
pouched ileostomy

NOTES

pouchitis
    chronic active p.
    P. Disease Activity Index (PDAI)
    episode of p.
    refractory p.
    wastebasket p.
pouchocele
pouchogram
pouchography
    evacuation p.
pouchoscopy
    pelvic p.
pouch-specific complication
Poupart
    P. ligament
    P. ligament shelving edge
    P. line
Pourchez XpressO hemodialysis catheter
povidone-iodine
    p.-i. enema
    p.-i. wash
powder
    BCAD 2 p.
    BC Cold P.
    Karaya p.
    Nu-Hope Karaya p.
    p. pyelogram
    Resource Arginaid p.
    Secretin-Ferring P.
    Seidlitz p.
    Sween Micro Guard p.
power
    p. Doppler ultrasound
    p. grip
PP
    pancreatic polypeptide
PP65
    PP65 antigenemia
    PP65 antigenemia assay
PPA
    pelvic phased-array coil
PPAF
    progressive perivenular alcoholic fibrosis
PPAR
    peroxisome proliferator-activated receptor
PPC
    prostatic pressure coefficient
PPD
    photodynamic diagnosis
    purified protein derivative test
        PPD immunological study
        PPD test
p_2 penile-brachial index
PPG
    phalloplethysmography
PPI
    proton pump inhibitor
        PPI triple therapy

PP-immunoreactive cell
PPJ
    pure pancreatic juice
PPM
    phosphopeptidomannan
PPoma
    pancreatic polypeptide-secreting tumor
    pure PPoma
PPPD
    pylorus-preserving pancreatoduodenectomy
PPTT
    prepubertal testicular tumor
PPUG
    positive-pressure urethrography
PPV
    positive predictive value
PPW
    pylorus-preserving Whipple modification
PRA
    panel-reactive antibody
    plasma renin activity
Prader orchidometer
Prader-Willi syndrome
praeacutus
    Bacteroides p.
praecox
    ejaculatio p.
    icterus p.
praeputii
    smegma p.
Praktis
    Sonolith P.
pralidoxime
pramlintide
1% pramoxine hydrochloride
Prandase
Prandin
Pratt
    P. anoscope
    P. bivalve retractor
    P. crypt hook
    P. rectal hook
    P. rectal probe
    P. rectal scissors
    P. rectal speculum
pravastatin
praziquantel
prazosin hydrochloride
PRCA
    pure red cell aplasia
preampullary portion of bile duct
preauricular
prebiotic
precaliceal canalicular ectasia
precancerous lesion
prechylomicron transport vesicle
precipitancy

precipitant
    p. leakage
    p. urination
precipitation
    glucagon p.
precirrhosis
precirrhotic hemochromatosis
precision
    p. grip
    intraassay p.
    P. Isotein HN powdered feeding
    P. Isotonic powdered feeding
    P. LR powdered feeding
    P. office TUNA system
    P. QID glucose monitoring system
    P. SpeedTac transvaginal anchor system
    P. Tack transvaginal anchor system
    P. Twist transvaginal anchor system
Precision-HN, -LR
Precisor
    P. Direct Bite biopsy forceps
    P. disposable biopsy forceps
Preclude peritoneal membrane
precordium
    hyperdynamic p.
precore mutant strain
Precose
precursor
    androgen p.
    benign neoplastic p.
    T-helper p.
precut
    p. incision
    p. papillotome
    p. papillotomy
    p. sphincterotome
    p. sphincterotomy
pred
    Liquid P.
predialysis
    p. phase
    p. plasma phosphate concentration
Predicta TGF-β1 kit
predictive value
predictor
    independent p.
    metabolic p.
    outcome p.
    p.'s of proximal neoplasia
predigested protein formula

predigestion
    diastase p.
predisposition
    familial p.
    genetic p.
prednisolone
    p. enema
    p. metasulfobenzoate
prednisone
prednisone-colchicine combination
predominant
    p. hyperparathyroid bone disease (PHBD)
    p. median lobe
preeclamptic liver disease
preeminent diagnostic importance
preendoscopy
preesophageal dysphagia
preexisting
    p. discomfort
    p. disease
preferential heating
prefreeze
    p. motility
    p. semen analysis
Pregestimil formula
preglomerular
    p. arteriole
    p. vasculature
pregnancy
    abdominal ectopic p.
    acute fatty liver of p. (AFLP)
    cholestasis of p.
    ectopic sigmoid p.
    fatty liver of p.
    heartburn of p.
    intrahepatic cholestasis of p. (ICP)
    molar p.
    nephritis of p.
    pernicious vomiting of p.
    pyelonephritis of p.
    recurrent molar p.
    subacute fatty liver of p.
    toxemia of p.
    tubal ectopic p.
    ureteral calculi in p.
    voluntary interruption of p. (VIP)
    p. wastage
pregnant uterus
pregnenolone
Prehn sign
preintervention planning

NOTES

preinvasive urothelial neoplasia
prekallikrein
Prelief
preliminary
    p. baseline descriptive statistic
    p. findings
Prelone
prelooped intracorporeal knot
Preludin
Premarin
Premasol
premature
    p. ejaculation
    p. stop codon
prematurity
    retinopathy of p.
premedication
    metoclopramide p.
    pethidine p.
    viscous lidocaine p.
premenarchal
premicturition pressure
Premier
    P. Platinum HpSA
    P. Platinum HpSA test
Premium
    P. Barrier
    P. CEEA circular stapler
    P. Plus CEEA disposable stapler
Premix-Slip
Prempree modification staging system
prenatal
    p. diagnosis
    p. fetal hydronephrosis
    p. ultrasonography
Prentice-Wilcoxon test
Prentiss
    P. maneuver
    P. orchiopexy
preoperative
    p. advance
    p. antibiotic
    p. function
    p. lesion
    p. tumor treatment
prep
  preparation
    LoSo Prep
    OMNI Prep
    Sween Prep
    United Skin Prep
prepancreatic anlagen
prepapillary bile duct
preparation (prep)
    bowel p.
    Brown dietary method for colon p.
    colonic purge p.
    Colonlite bowel p.
    CoLyte bowel p.
    cytocentrifuge p.
    Dulcolax bowel p.
    electrolyte p.
    Emulsoil bowel p.
    Evac-Q-Kwik bowel p.
    Fleet bowel p.
    galenic p.
    GoLYTELY bowel p.
    P. H
    inadequate bowel p.
    lactobacillus p.
    lavage bowel p.
    Nichols-Condon bowel p.
    NutraPrep colonoscopy p.
    OCL bowel p.
    oral iron p.
    potential role for simethicone in bowel p.
    renal proximal tubule p.
    Touch p.
    Tridrate bowel p.
    X-Prep bowel p.
prepatent-period filariasis
prepenile dislocation of scrotum
preperfusion
preperitoneal
    p. abscess
    p. anesthesia
    p. approach
    p. distention balloon (PDB)
    p. fat
    p. space
    transabdominal p. (TAPP)
preproenkephalin
preproEt-1 mRNA
preprostatic
    p. plexus
    p. sphincter
    p. urethra
prepubertal testicular tumor (PPTT)
prepuce
    hooded p.
    megameatus-intact p. (MIP)
    ventral apron p.
preputial
    p. adhesion
    p. calculus
    p. collar
    p. continent vesicostomy
    p. gland
    p. stenosis
    p. transverse island flap and glans channel
preputiotomy
preputium
    p. clitoridis
    p. penis
prepyloric
    p. antral diaphragm

p. antrum
p. atresia
p. gastric ulcer
p. perforation
p. polyp
p. sphincter
prerectal lithotomy
prerenal
p. anuria
p. azotemia
presacral
p. cyst
p. ectopic kidney
p. neuroblastoma
p. rectopexy
p. space
p. teratoma
p. tumor
presbyesophagus
prescribed clearance
presentation
rectocele p.
specific stone p.
trismus p.
preservation
bladder p.
cadaver renal p.
extracorporeal renal p.
renal p.
simple cold storage p.
p. time
p. times effect
p. of uterus
presinusoidal intrahepatic portal hypertension
pre-S phase
pressure
abdominal leak-point p. (ALPP)
ambulatory blood p.
p. amplitude modulation
anal sphincter squeeze p.
basal anal canal p.
basal anal sphincter p.
bile duct p.
biliary tract p.
bladder p. (BP)
bladder intravesical p.
blood p. (BP)
cavernosal systolic p.
cavernous artery occlusion p.
central venous p. (CVP)
cerebral perfusion p. (CPP)

choledochal basal p.
closing p.
colloid osmotic p.
cybernetic regulation of blood p.
detrusor muscle leak-point p.
p. diverticulum
p. dressing
dynamic closure p.
end-expiratory intragastric p.
end-filling p.
esophageal peristaltic p.
p. flow analysis
free hepatic venous p. (FHVP)
glomerular capillary p.
hepatic vein wedge p.
hepatic venous p.
hepatic wedge p.
high intraluminal p.
high resting anal p.
hydrostatic p.
p. increment rate (PIR)
intraabdominal p.
intraanal p.
intraballoon p.
intracavernosal p.
intracholedochal p.
intraductal p.
intraesophageal peristaltic p.
intraesophageal variceal p.
intragastric p.
intraglomerular p.
intraluminal esophageal p.
intraluminal urethral p.
intraurethral p.
intravariceal p.
intravesical p.
p. inversion point (PIP)
leak p.
leak-point p. (LPP)
lower esophageal sphincter p. (LESP)
low urethral p. (LUP)
maximum (anal) resting p. (MRP)
maximum detrusor p.
maximum squeeze p. (MSP)
maximum urethral closure p. (MUCP)
maximum vasal p. (MVP)
mean arterial p. (MAP)
mean arterial blood p. (MABP)
p. measurement
melanoma intratumor p.

NOTES

pressure *(continued)*
- minimal distending p.
- p. natriuresis
- p. necrosis
- pancreatic duct p. (PDP)
- passage p.
- peak p.
- p. peak
- penile blood p.
- plasma oncotic p.
- portal venous p. (PVP)
- premicturition p.
- proximal p.
- pulmonary artery p. (PAP)
- pulmonary capillary wedge p. (PCWP)
- renal perfusion p.
- resting anal sphincter p.
- sinusoidal capillary p.
- p. sore
- sphincter of Oddi p. (SOP)
- splanchnic capillary p.
- squeeze p.
- static closure p.
- p. study
- systemic arterial p.
- p. transducer
- transglomerular hydrostatic filtration p.
- transmembrane hydraulic p.
- p. transmission ratio (PTR)
- ureteral p.
- urethral closure p.
- Valsalva leak-point p. (VLPP)
- variceal p.
- voiding p.
- wedge p.
- wedged hepatic venous p. (WHVP)
- Whitaker perfusion p.

pressure-flow
- p.-f. electromyography study
- p.-f. micturition study
- p.-f. study (PFS)

pressure-injected bovine collagen
pressure-point tension ring
pressure-regulated electrohydraulic lithotripsy
pressure-specific bladder capacity
prestomal ileitis
presumed circle area ratio (PCAR)
presumptive sphincter
presurgical medical evaluation
presynaptic inhibition
preternatural anus
pretest global rating score
pretransplant evaluation
pretreatment serum creatinine
preureteral iliac artery
preurethritis

Prevacare total solution skin care spray
Prevacid Packet powder for oral suspension
Prevail protective underwear
prevalence
- cholelithiasis p.
- p. of diabetes mellitus
- p. of low glomerular filtration rate

Prevalite
preventing urinary tract infection
prevention
- acute pancreatitis p.
- Centers for Disease Control and P. (CDC)
- p. of first bleeding
- medical p.
- somatostatin p.

preventive intravesical therapy
prevertebral fascia
previous in vitro result
Prevpac triple therapy
PRF
- pulse repetition frequency

PrHPT
- primary hyperparathyroidism

priapism
- arterial p.
- drug-induced p.
- high-flow p.
- low-flow p.
- secondary p.
- stuttering p.
- Winter shunt for p.

priapitis
priapus
prilocaine
Prilosec
primaquine
primary
- p. adrenal insufficiency
- p. advantage of self-management
- p. anastomosis
- p. antiphospholipid syndrome
- p. arteriovenous fistula
- p. B-cell lymphoma
- p. biliary cirrhosis (PBC)
- p. case
- p. ciliary dyskinesia
- p. closure
- p. colorectal cancer (PCRC)
- p. contraction
- p. diagnostic endoscopy
- p. fistulotomy
- p. gastric lymphoma (PGL)
- p. gastric lymphoma staging
- p. glomerular disease
- p. glomerular lesion
- p. graft nonfunction
- p. hepatosplenic lymphoma (PHSL)

primary · probe

p. hyperaldosteronism
p. hyperoxaluria type I, II (PH-I)
p. hyperparathyroidism (PrHPT)
p. indication
p. infection of ascetic fluid
p. intestinal lymphangiectasia (PIL)
p. lung carcinoma
p. malignant melanoma of esophagus (PMME)
p. myelofibrosis
p. obstructive megaureter
p. outcome
p. oxalosis
p. panendoscopy
p. perineal hypospadias surgery
p. peristaltic wave
p. peritonitis
p. procedure
p. prophylaxis
p. pseudoobstruction syndrome
p. refluxing megaureter
p. renal calculus
p. sclerosing cholangitis (PSC)
p. spermatocyte
p. staging of testicular tumor
p. sterility
p. suture
p. syphilis
p. transitional cell carcinoma
p. tuberculosis
p. ureteropelvic junction obstruction
p. urinary diversion
p. vesicoureteral reflex

primed cell
primidone
priming
    androgen p.
primitive neuroectodermal tumor (PNET)
primordial kidney
Primus
    P. Prostate Machine
    P. transrectal thermography
principal cell (PC)
Principen
principle
    Boari-Ockerblad p.
    continent catheterizable appendicovesicostomy using Mitrofanoff p.
    countercurrent multiplier p.
    detubularization p.

flap valve p.
Goodwin cup-patch p.
Heineke-Mikulicz p.
Malone p.
Mitrofanoff p.
oncologic p.
Sarfeh p.
Seldinger p.
Yang-Monti p.

Pringle maneuver
prior negative inguinal exploration
Priscoline
privilege
    bathroom p.
proapoptotic effect
probable long-term kidney damage
PROBACTRIX
proband
Pro-Banthine
probe
    AcuNav steerable phased vector-array ultrasound catheter p.
    Aloka MP-PN ultrasound p.
    ambulatory p.
    antisense RNA p.
    Bakes p.
    Barr fistula p.
    Beckman 39042 pH p.
    beta-actin cDNA p.
    BICAP bipolar hemostasis p.
    BICAP electrocoagulation p.
    BICAP electrode p.
    BICAP endoscopic p.
    biliary balloon p.
    Bilitec 2000 intraluminal fiberoptic p.
    biotinylated DNA p.
    biplane sector p.
    Bipolar Circumactive P. (BICAP)
    Bipolar EndoStasis p. (BESP)
    bipolar hemostasis p.
    blunt p.
    Buie fistula p.
    bullet p.
    caliber p.
    Cameron-Miller monopolar p.
    catheter p.
    catheter-based ultrasound p.
    cDNA p.
    coagulation p.
    CO_2 laser p.
    contact p.

NOTES

probe *(continued)*
- continuously perfused p.
- Corson needle electrosurgical p.
- C-Trak p.
- cystic fibrosis gene p.
- Desjardins gallbladder p.
- Desjardins gall duct p.
- Desjardins gallstone p.
- p. dilator
- Dobbhoff bipolar coagulation p.
- Doppler p.
- dot-plotted p.
- Earle rectal p.
- EHL p.
- eight-channel cross-sectional anal sphincter p.
- electrode p.
- electrohydraulic lithotripsy p.
- electrosurgical monopolar spatula p.
- end-fire transrectal p.
- endoanal p.
- endorectal p.
- endoscopic BICAP p.
- endoscopic Doppler p.
- endoscopic heat p.
- endoscopic ultrasound p.
- EndoSound ultrasound p.
- Fenger gallbladder p.
- fistula p.
- Fluhrer rectal p.
- Fogarty biliary p.
- front-loading ultrasound p. (FLUP)
- gallstone p.
- galvanic p.
- genomic DNA p.
- Gold P.
- p. gorget
- G3PDH CDNA p.
- p. and groove director
- heat p.
- heater p. (HP)
- 24-hour esophageal pH p.
- human apo A-I DNA p.
- human fibronectin cDNA p.
- human gastrin p.
- p. image
- injection gold p. (IGP)
- intraductal ultrasound p.
- intraluminal p.
- isotropic p.
- Jubileum 2.0 single-use gastroesophageal pH p.
- KTP laser p.
- lacrimal duct p.
- large-bore heat p.
- Larry rectal p.
- laser-Doppler Periflux PF-3 p.
- light monitoring p.
- linear p.
- Mayo common duct p.
- Meadox Surgimed Doppler p.
- mechanical rotating p.
- Medi-Tech bipolar p.
- Medrad MRInnervu endorectal colon p.
- microballoon p.
- Microelectrode MI-506 small-caliber p.
- miniature p.
- miniaturized ultrasound catheter p.
- Mixter dilating p.
- monopolar p.
- Moynihan bile duct p.
- Moynihan gallstone p.
- multilumen p.
- Ochsner flexible spiral gallstone p.
- Ochsner gallbladder p.
- oligonucleotide p.
- Olympus CD-20Z heater p.
- Olympus GF-UM30P linear scanning p.
- Olympus heat p.
- Olympus S-20-20R p.
- Olympus ultrathin balloon-fitted ultrasound p.
- Olympus UM-F30-20R p.
- Olympus UM-2R, -3R p.
- Olympus UM-R-series miniature ultrasonic p.
- Olympus UM-S30-25R p.
- Olympus UM-1W endoscopic p.
- Olympus UM-W-series endoscopic p.
- palpating p.
- pH p.
- pH-Informer Deltron p.
- pH-manometry p.
- polycationic histochemical p.
- Pratt rectal p.
- Radiometer GK2803C pH p.
- rectal p.
- reflectance spectrophotometric p.
- RNA p.
- rotating Bruel and Kjaer p.
- Sandhill P32 pH antimony p.
- silver p.
- Sonocath ultrasound p.
- stimulation p.
- tactile p.
- through-the-scope catheter p.
- Transonics Systems flow p.
- transrectal p.
- triple-balloon p.
- tumor p.
- ultrasonic lithotriptor p.
- ultrasound catheter p. (UCP)
- virtual colonoscopy Side Fire APC p.

V33W high-density endocavity p.
water p.
probenecid
probenecid-containing solution
probenecid-inhibited organic anion transport system
Probiotica
probiotic therapy
problem
    bone marrow transplantation-related p.
    clinical p.
    micturition p.
    penile prosthesis mechanical p.
probucol
procainamide
procainamide-induced systemic lupus erythematosus
procaine
    p. hydrochloride
    p. penicillin
Pro-Cal-Sof
Procaltrol
procarbazine
Procardia XL
procedural amnesia
procedure (*See also* operation, repair)
    abdominal p.
    ACE p.
    Acucise retrograde p.
    Acucise RP outpatient p.
    Al-Ghorab p.
    Altemeier p.
    alternative endourological p.
    antegrade continence enema p.
    antiincontinence p.
    antireflux p.
    Asopa p.
    auxiliary p.
    Ball p.
    Barcat p.
    basket p.
    Belsey Mark IV p.
    Bengt-Johanson p.
    bladder chimney p.
    Bloodgood p.
    Boari bladder flap p.
    bowel refashioning p.
    Boyce-Vest p.
    Burch p.
    butterfly endoluminal gastroplasty p.
    bypass p.
    Camey p.
    Campbell p.
    CaverMap p.
    cecal imbrication p.
    Cecil p.
    Chester-Winter p.
    Cleveland Clinic weighted scale of endoscopic p.'s
    Cohen antireflux p.
    colon p.
    complex renal p.
    coring-out p.
    corporal plication p.
    corporal rotation p.
    dartos pouch p.
    DAWG p.
    Delorme p.
    Devine-Devine p.
    Duckett p.
    Duhamel pullthrough p.
    Duval p.
    Ebbehoj p.
    endorectal pullthrough p.
    endoscopy p.
    endourological p.
    Enteryx p.
    esophageal sling p.
    Essed surgical p.
    flap valve antireflux p.
    flip-flap p.
    Fowler-Stephens p.
    Frykman-Goldberg p.
    full Monti p.
    Fungi-Fluor p.
    gastric neobladder p.
    Gilchrist p.
    Gil-Vernet p.
    Gittes-Loughlin p.
    Gittes urethral suspension p.
    glans approximation p. (GAP)
    Goulding p.
    Gregoir-Lich p.
    Halban p.
    Hanley rectal bladder p.
    Hartmann p.
    Heitz-Boyer p.
    Heller-Dor p.
    hemi-Kock p.
    hemi-T augmentation p.
    Hinman p.
    Hodgson technique of modified Lich p.

NOTES

procedure *(continued)*
  Hodgson XX p.
  Hofmeister p.
  Horton-Devine p.
  hydrocelectomy bottle p.
  hydrocelectomy dartos pouch p.
  ileoanal pull-through p.
  imaging-guided minimally invasive p.
  infrarenal template p.
  intraparavariceal p.
  InVance male sling p.
  invasive p.
  island flap p.
  Jaboulay p.
  Johnston buttonhole p.
  Kasai p.
  Kelling-Madlener p.
  Kelly plication p.
  Kocher ureterosigmoidostomy p.
  Kock pouch modified p.
  Kropp p.
  Ladd p.
  laparoscopic bladder neck suture suspension p.
  laparoscopic urinary diversion p.
  Leadbetter p.
  LeFort p.
  Lewis-Tanner esophagectomy p.
  Lich p.
  Malone antegrade colonic enema stoma p.
  Marshall-Marchetti-Krantz p.
  Mathieu p.
  Maydl p.
  McIndoe p.
  Michal p. I, II
  microsurgical epididymal sperm aspiration p.
  Mikulicz p.
  Mitrofanoff p.
  modified Ingelman-Sundberg p.
  modified Nesbit p.
  modified Norfolk p.
  modified transduodenal rendezvous p.
  Monti p.
  Moschcowitz p.
  multiple surgical p.'s
  muscle-filling p.
  Mustarde p.
  needle suspension p.
  Nesbit tuck p.
  Nyhus p.
  omentum majus flap p.
  one-stage p.
  O'Regan p.
  Palomo p.
  Partington-Rochelle p.
  Pauchet p.
  pelvic pouch p.
  percutaneous p.
  Pereyra p.
  peri-Vaterian therapeutic endoscopic p.
  primary p.
  promontofixation p.
  ProstRcision p.
  pubovaginal sling p.
  Puestow p.
  Puestow-Gillesby p.
  pullthrough p.
  Ransley p.
  Raz p.
  Reichel-Pólya stomach p.
  repeat p.
  retropubic needle suspension p.
  Richardson p.
  Righini p.
  Ripstein p.
  Rives-Stoppa p.
  routine outpatient p.
  Roux-en-Y p.
  Salle p.
  Schoemaker p.
  Schwartz-Pregenzer urethropexy p.
  Secca p.
  selective tubal occlusion p. (STOP)
  simultaneous Malone antegrade continent enema and Mitrofanoff p.
  sling p.
  Snow p.
  Soave abdominal pullthrough p.
  SPARC p.
  Spence p.
  sphincter-saving p.
  Stamey p.
  Stamey-Martius p.
  Sting p.
  Stretta p.
  Studer pouch p.
  suburethral rectus fascial sling p.
  Sugiura esophageal varices p.
  surgical p.
  takedown of pelvic sling p.
  tension-free vaginal tape p.
  Thiersch p.
  Thiersch-Duplay proximal tube p.
  Thompson p.
  TIPS p.
  Toupet p.
  transhepatic antegrade biliary drainage p.
  transjugular intrahepatic portacaval shunt p.
  transvaginal Burch p.
  TVT p.

untethering p.
upper gastrointestinal p.
ureteral patch p.
vaginal flap reconstruction and pubovaginal sling p.
vaginal needle suspension p.
vaginal wall sling p.
Van de Kamer fecal fat p.
Vesica sling p.
Walsh p.
Whipple p.
Winter p.
Womack p.
York-Mason p.
Young-Dees p.

process
epithelial regenerative p.
fingerlike epithelial p.
foot p. (FP)
glycosylation p.
juxtacapillary p.
knobby p.
morphogenetic p.
signal transduction p.
sodium-linked p.
spinous p.
transverse p.
uncinate p.

processing
image p.
postsecretory p.
swim-up p.

processor
Miles V.I.P. 300 vacuum infiltration p.
Olympus EU-M-series endosonography image p.
ThinPrep P.

processus vaginalis
prochlorperazine suppository
ProCide disinfectant
procidentia
anal p.
internal p.
rectal p.
p. recti

procoagulant
procollagen
C-terminal propeptide of type I p.
N-terminal propeptide of type III p.

ProCon incontinence device

Procrit
proctalgia fugax
proctectasia
proctectomy
mucosal p.

proctitis
acute p.
allergic p.
bleeding p.
chronic radiation p.
chronic ulcerative p.
Dean stage I, II radiation p.
diversion p.
epidemic gangrenous p.
factitial p.
glutaraldehyde-induced p.
gonococcal p.
gonorrheal p.
idiopathic p.
nonspecific ulcerative p.
radiation p.
traumatic p.
ulcerative p.

proctoclysis
proctocolectomy
minilaparotomy restorative p.
restorative p. (RP, RPC)
single-stage total p.
totally stapled restorative p. (TSRPC)

proctocolitis
aphthoid p.
idiopathic p.
radiation p.
venereal p.

proctocolonoscopy
ProctoCream-HC
proctocystocele
proctocystoplasty
proctocystotomy
Proctofoam
Proctofoam-HC
proctogram
balloon p.
defecating p.

proctography
dynamic p.
evacuation p.
quantitative scintigraphic evacuation p.

proctoperineoplasty

proctopexy
    Orr-Loygue transabdominal p.
proctoplasty
proctoptosis
Proctor-Livingston
    P.-L. endoprosthesis
    P.-L. tube
proctorrhaphy
proctoscope
    Boehm p.
    Gabriel p.
    Kelly p.
    Lieberman p.
    Montague p.
    Newman p.
    Salvati p.
    Vernon-David p.
proctoscopy
    rigid p.
proctosigmoidectomy
proctosigmoiditis
    refractory p.
proctosigmoidoscope
    ACMI fiberoptic p.
proctosigmoidoscopy
    rigid p.
proctospasm
proctostenosis
proctotomy
    external p.
    internal p.
    linear p.
proctovalvotomy
procyclidine
Prodium
prodromal symptom
prodrome
prodrug
    GSH p.
product
    Amadori p.
    Biomedical Instruments and P.'s (BIP)
    fibrin/fibrinogen degradation p. (FDP)
    fibrinogen degradation p.
    fibrin split p. (FSP)
    mechanical p.
    secretory p.
    thermodynamic solubility p.
production
    ammonia p.
    autoantibody p.
    chylomicron p.
    creatinine p.
    hydrogen ion p.
    lymphokine p.
    spermatozoon p.
    superoxide p.
    unilateral renin p.
productive nephritis
productus
    Ruminococcus p.
prodynorphin gene
PROEF
    postoperative regimen for oral early feeding
proenkephalin gene
profile
    ASTRA p.
    cytokine p.
    emerging p.
    gut-hormone p.
    ideal patient p.
    liver function p.
    P. pediatric polypectomy snare
    phosphotyrosyl protein p.
    plasmid p.
    resting urethral pressure p.
    sickness impact p.
    side-effect p.
    spicule in p.
    StoneRisk diagnostic p.
    stress urethral pressure p.
    urethral closure pressure p.
    urethral pressure p. (UPP)
profiled dialysis
profilometry
    urethral pressure p.
profound acid reduction
profunda
    colitis cystica p. (CCP)
    fascia penis p.
    gastritis cystic p.
profuse vomiting
progenitalis
    herpes p.
progestational agent
progesteronal agent
progesterone
progesterone-associated colitis
prognostic
    p. factor
    p. indicator
    p. nutritional index (PNI)
    p. significance
    p. tool
prograde technique
Prograf
program
    CLIM computer p.
    instituted GI bleeding management p.
    low-energy p.
    Maine Medical Assessment P. (MMAP)
    Organ Procurement P.

program · proliferation

personalized p.
POINTER computer p.
Stat-View computer p.
stone-prevention p.
surveillance p.
Synectics computer p.
VariSeed 7.0 software computer p.

programming
    in utero p.

progression
    p. factor
    renal p.

progression-free survival

progressive
    p. diet
    p. dysphagia
    p. emphysematous necrosis
    p. familial cirrhosis
    p. familial intrahepatic cholestasis (PFIC)
    p. perivenular alcoholic fibrosis (PPAF)
    p. renal dysfunction
    p. renal insufficiency
    p. suppurative cholangitis
    p. systemic sclerosis (PSS)
    p. toxicity

Prohibit antifog face mask
proinflammatory cytokine
project
    Captopril Prevention P. (CAPPP)
    National Prostatic Cancer P.

projectile vomiting
projection
    afferent p.
    Chassard-Lapiné p.
    parasympathetic p.
    single-shot voxel p.
    sympathetic p.

prokaryotic pathogen
prokinetic
    p. agent
    p. drug
    p. effect
    p. therapy

prolactin
Prolamine
prolapse
    anal p.
    bladder p.
    concomitant p.
    Delorme operation for rectal p.
    external anorectal mucosal p.
    Frykman-Goldberg operation for rectal p.
    gastric mucosal p.
    p. gastropathy
    genitourinary p.
    hemorrhoidal p.
    incarcerated p.
    incomplete rectal p.
    intestinal p.
    mucosal p.
    pelvic p.
    posthysterectomy vaginal p.
    rectal p.
    stomal p.
    sudden valve p.
    ureterocele p.
    urethral p.
    urogenital p.
    vaginal p.
    valve p.
    Well operation for rectal p.

prolapsed
    p. bowel
    p. internal hemorrhoid
    p. rectum
    p. stoma

prolapsing fourth-degree hemorrhoid
Prolase
    Cytocare P. II
    P. II lateral-firing Nd:YAG laser

Pro-Lax
Prolene suture
Proleukin
Prolieve microwave therapy system
proliferans
    angiocholitis p.
    cholecystitis glandularis p.

proliferating
    p. cell nuclear antigen (PCNA)
    p. glomerular
    p. nuclear cell antigen (PNCA)
    p. state
    p. tubular cell

proliferation
    bile duct p.
    cell p.
    cellular p.
    colonic epithelial p.
    cystic epithelial p.
    diffuse mesangial p.
    DNA p.

NOTES

proliferation *(continued)*
    extraglandular endocrine cell p.
    p. of gastric epithelium
    glomerular cell p.
    index of cell p.
    intracystic epithelial p.
    intraluminal p.
    mesangial p.
    monoclonal p.
    mucosal cell p.
    neoplastic cell p.
    osteoblast-like p.
    p. of prostatic tissue
    rectal cell p.

proliferative
    p. glomerulonephritis
    p. hypertrophic gastritis
    p. inflammatory atrophy

prolinuria
    glycyl p.

Prolixin

prolonged
    p. expiratory phase
    p. obstructed labor
    p. partial ureteral obstruction

Proloprim

promazine

promethazine

Prometheus First Step inflammatory bowel disease screening assay

Promex biopsy needle

promontofixation
    laparoscopic p.
    p. procedure

promontory
    sacral p.

promoter
    growth hormone p. (GHP)

prompt GI consult

promulgated

Pronase

pronation

pronator drift

pronephros

prone split-leg position

Pronestyl

pronucleus, pl. **pronuclei**

proopiomelanocortin (POMC)
    p. gene

propafenone

propagated antroduodenal contraction

propagation
    p. of contraction
    orad p.

propantheline bromide

propendens
    venter p.

proper
    p. hepatic artery
    p. lamina
    p. transurethral resection of intramural ureter
    p. tunic

properitoneal
    p. fat
    p. flank stripe
    p. hernia

property
    similar psychometric p.'s
    structural p.

prophecy
    self-fulfilling p.

propHiler urinary pH testing kit

prophylactic
    p. antibiotic
    p. antibiotic treatment (PAT)
    p. cephalosporin
    p. cholecystectomy
    p. device
    p. gamma globulin
    p. lymphadenectomy
    p. orchiectomy
    p. orchiopexy
    p. sclerotherapy
    p. urethritis

prophylaxis, pl. **prophylaxes**
    antibiotic p.
    antimicrobial p.
    continuous p.
    medical p.
    primary p.
    secondary p.
    stress ulcer p.
    stricture p.

propidium iodide

propionate
    testosterone p.

Propionibacterium acnes

propiverine

propofol

proporphyria
    erythropoietic p. (EPP)

proportional
    inversely p.

proportionate reduction

propoxyphene hydrochloride

propranolol

propria
    arteria hepatica p.
    intestinal lamina p.
    lamina p.
    muscularis p.
    ratio of mucosa to submucosa to muscularis p.
    tunica p.
    underlying muscularis p.

proprioception
    intact p.

Propulsid
propulsion
    colonic p.
    ineffective colonic p.
propulsive
    p. motor pattern
    p. wave
propylene oxide
propylhexedrine
propylthiouracil (PTU)
prorenin
    serine protease-activated p.
Proscan
    P. ultrasound imaging system
    P. ultrasound unit
Proscar
Pros-Check
    P.-C. kit
    P.-C. PSA assay
Prosed/DS
Proshield Plus skin protectant
ProSobee liquid formula
prospective
    p. blinded study of diagnostic esophagoscopy
    p. clinical trial
    p. comparison
    p. evaluation
    p. multicenter randomized trial
    p. multicenter study
    p. randomized controlled trial
prospermia
Prostacoil stent
prostacyclin
prostaglandin (PG)
    p. 1
    p. analog
    colonic p.
    cytoprotective p.
    p. E (PGE_1)
    p. E2 (PGE2)
    p. F
    p. F2-alpha (PGF2-alpha)
    p. G (PGG)
    p. H (PGH)
    p. I2 (PGI2)
    renal p.
    renal vasodilator p.
    p. supplementation
    p. synthesis
Prostakath urethral stent
Prostalase laser system

ProstaLund
    P. CoreTherm system
    P. feedback treatment
prostanoid
    p. formation
    p. synthesis
ProstaScint scan
ProstaSeed I-125 seed
prostata
prostatae
    isthmus p.
prostatalgia
prostate
    atypical small acinar proliferation of p. (ASAP)
    p. balloon dilator
    boggy p.
    p. cancer (PCa)
    P. Cancer Intervention Versus Observation Trial (PCIVOT, PIVOT)
    carcinoma of p. (CAP)
    coagulation and hemostatic resection of p. (CHRP)
    contact laser vaporization of p. (CLVP)
    Costello laser ablation of p.
    cryosurgical ablation of p. (CSAP)
    ductal adenocarcinoma of p.
    enlarged p.
    funnel-neck p.
    p. gland benign hyperplasia
    p. gland biopsy
    p. gland C3 complement
    p. gland color flow Doppler examination
    p. gland cross-section
    p. gland cytoskeleton
    p. gland electrovaporization
    p. gland hypoplasia
    p. gland innervation
    p. gland involution
    p. gland leiomyosarcoma
    p. gland lymphoma
    p. gland needle ablation
    p. gland peripheral zone
    p. gland periurethral zone
    p. gland prostate-specific membrane antigen
    p. gland sarcoma
    p. gland secretion
    p. gland small cell carcinoma

NOTES

prostate *(continued)*
    p. gland stroma
    p. gland stromal cell
    p. gland tissue matrix
    p. gland transition zone
    p. gland transurethral balloon dilation
    p. gland transurethral resection
    holmium laser resection of p. (HoLRP)
    median furrow of the p.
    minimal transurethral resection of p. (M-TURP)
    nodular hyperplasia of p.
    percutaneous radical cryosurgical ablation of p.
    photoselective vaporization of p.
    prostatisme sans p.
    p. rhabdomyosarcoma
    salvage cryoablation of p.
    thick-loop transurethral resection of p.
    total transurethral resection of p. (T-TURP)
    transurethral electrovaporization of p. (TUVP, TVP)
    transurethral evaporation of p. (TUEP)
    transurethral grooving of p.
    transurethral incision of p. (TUIP)
    transurethral laser incision of p.
    transurethral needle ablation of p.
    transurethral resection of p. (TURP)
    transurethral vaporization of p. (TUVP)
    transurethral vaporization-resection of p. (TUVRP)
    visual laser ablation of p. (VLAP)
    p. volume
prostatectomy
    anatomical radical retropubic p.
    cavernosal nerve-sparing radical p.
    KTP laser p.
    laparoscopic radical p.
    laser p.
    Madigan p.
    Millen technique retropubic p.
    nerve-sparing radical retropubic p.
    open radical p.
    perineal p.
    pubic p.
    radical perineal p.
    radical retropubic p. (RRP)
    radical transcoccygeal p.
    retropubic ascending radical p.
    salvage p.
    Stanford radical retropubic p.
    suprapubic p.
    total perineal p.
    transurethral ablative p.
    transurethral balloon laserthermia p.
    transurethral ultrasound-guided laser-induced p. (TULIP)
    visual laser-assisted p. (VLAP)
    Walsh radical retropubic p.
prostate-specific
    p.-s. acid phosphatase
    p.-s. antigen (PSA)
    p.-s. antigen-based parameter
    p.-s. antigen bound to alpha-1 antichymotrypsin (PSA-ACT)
    p.-s. antigen density (PSAD)
    p.-s. antigen density of transition zone (PSA-TZ)
    p.-s. antigen velocity (PSAV)
    p.-s. membrane (PSM)
    p.-s. membrane antigen (PSMA)
Prostathermer
    Biodan P.
    P. 99D
    P. device
    P. prostatic hyperthermia system
prostatic
    p. abscess
    p. acid phosphatase (PAP)
    p. adenocarcinoma
    p. adenoma
    p. antibacterial factor
    p. artery
    p. block
    p. calculus
    p. capsule
    p. catheter
    p. chip
    p. cryptococcosis
    p. fascia
    p. fossa
    p. hyperplasia
    p. hypertrophy
    p. intraepithelial neoplasia (PIN)
    p. massage
    p. mesonephric remnant
    p. neoplasm
    p. nodule
    p. outlet obstruction (POO)
    p. pile
    p. pressure coefficient (PPC)
    p. sinus
    p. stent
    p. thermal treatment
    p. tuberculosis
    p. urethra
    p. urethral polyp
    p. urethral transitional cell carcinoma
    p. utricle
    p. volume

prostatica
    ductuli p.
    vesica p.
prostatici
    ductus p.
prostaticovesical plexus
prostaticovesiculectomy
prostaticus
    plexus p.
    utriculus p.
prostatism
    silent p.
    vesical p.
prostatisme sans prostate
prostatitic
prostatitis
    bacterial p.
    chemical p.
    chronic abacterial p.
    chronic bacterial p. (CBP)
    chronic nonbacterial p. (CNP)
    diagnosis of bacterial p.
    granulomatous p.
    mycotic p.
    NIH Classification Category I acute bacterial p.
    NIH Classification Category II chronic bacterial p.
    NIH Classification Category IV asymptomatic inflammatory p.
    NIH Classification System for P.
    nonbacterial p. (NBP)
    parasitic p.
    tuberculous p.
prostatocystitis
prostatocystotomy
prostatodynia (PD)
prostatography
prostatolith
prostatolithotomy
prostatomegaly
prostatometer
prostatomy (*var. of* prostatotomy)
prostatomyomectomy
prostatorrhea
prostatoseminal vesiculectomy
prostatotomy, prostatomy
    lateral p.
prostatotoxin
prostatourethral fistula
prostatourethral-rectal fistula
prostatovesical junction

prostatovesiculectomy
prostatovesiculitis
Prostatron
    P. microwave system
    P. transurethral thermotherapy device
prostatropin
prosthesis, pl. **prostheses**
    Alpha I inflatable penile p.
    Ambicor penile p.
    AMS controlled-expansion penile p.
    AMS Hydroflex penile p.
    AMS inflatable 700 penile p.
    AMS malleable 600 penile p.
    AMS Sphincter 800 Urinary P.
    Amsterdam-type p.
    AMS three-piece inflatable penile p.
    AMS Ultrex penile p.
    Angelchik antireflux p.
    Angelchik ring p.
    antireflux p.
    Atkinson p.
    balloon tamponade p.
    biliary p.
    bilioduodenal p.
    bladder neck support p.
    Celestin p.
    composite p.
    covered self-expanding p.
    CXM p.
    CX Plus p.
    Dacron p.
    Dilamezinsert penile p.
    double-pigtail p.
    Dura-II positionable penile p.
    Duraphase inflatable penile p.
    Dynaflex penile p.
    ERCP conventional p.
    EsophaCoil p.
    esophageal p.
    Finney Flexirod penile p.
    Flexi-Flate I, II penile p.
    Flexirod penile p.
    GFS Mark II inflatable penile p.
    Gianturco expandable self-expanding metallic biliary p.
    glass penile p.
    hydraulic hinge penile p.
    Hydroflex penile p.
    inflatable penile p. (IPP)
    Introl bladder neck support p.

NOTES

prosthesis *(continued)*
    iridium p.
    Jonas penile p.
    malleable p.
    Mentor Alpha 1 inflatable penile p.
    Mentor GFS penile p.
    Mentor IPP penile p.
    Mentor malleable penile p.
    Mentor Mark II penile p.
    mesh stent p.
    Neville tracheal reconstruction p.
    OmniPhase penile p.
    penile p.
    Scott AMS inflatable penile p.
    silicone donut p.
    silicone self-expanding p.
    Small-Carrion penile p.
    Subrini penile p.
    testicular p.
    Ultraflex esophageal p.
    Ultrex Plus penile p.
    Uni-Flate 1000 penile p.
    Unitary inflatable penile p.
    urethral stent p.
    UroLume Endourethral Wallstent p.
    UroLume urethral p.
    valved voice p.
    Wallstent esophageal p.
    Wilson-Cook plastic p.

prosthesis-related seroma formation

prosthetic
    p. arterial graft
    p. bladder
    p. penis
    p. testis
    p. utricle cyst

prosthetist

Prosthex sponge

Prostigmin

ProstRcision
    P. procedure
    P. treatment

ProTack
    P. stapler
    P. tacking device

Protalba-R

protamine
    p. sulfate
    p. zinc insulin

protease
    p. inhibitor
    p. pouch
    serine p.
    V8 p.

proteasome

protectant
    Proshield Plus skin p.

Protect-a-Pass suture passer

protection
    antibody-mediated p.
    gastroduodenal mucosal p.
    misoprostol p.

protective probiotic flora

protector plus wire

protein
    A-4 p.
    acute phase p.
    adenovirus-12 viral p.
    aldosterone-induced p. (AIP)
    androgen-binding p.
    p. antibody (PAb)
    antibody to c100 p.
    anti-Tamm-Horsfall p.
    ascitic fluid total p. (AFTP)
    band 3 p.
    basement membrane p.
    Bence Jones p.
    bladder cancer-specific nuclear matrix p. (BCLA-4)
    bone morphogenic p.
    p. C
    cagA p.
    calcium-binding p.
    calcium-regulated p.
    calcium-specific binding p.
    p. catabolic rate (PCR)
    CD3 p.
    CD4 p.
    CD8 p.
    CD2-associated p.
    CDC42 p.
    cholesterol ester transfer p. (CETP)
    c-met p.
    complement regulatory p.
    copper-binding p. (CBP)
    C-reactive p. (CRP)
    p. C, S deficiency
    CSF p.
    p. C, S level
    cytoplasmic adaptor p.
    cytotoxin-associated gene A p.
    p. depletion
    dietary p.
    dipstick p.
    downstream signaling p.
    E1b p.
    E1, E2, E6 p.
    E2F p.
    enzymatic p.
    eosinophil cationic p. (ECP)
    eosinophilic major basic p.
    eosinophil p. X (EPX)
    EP2-EP3 p.
    estramustine-binding p. (EMBP)
    EZH2 p.
    fatty acid-binding p. (FABP)
    fibronectin-binding p.

fyn p.
G p.
Gal 4 p.
green fluorescent p. (GFP)
GTPase-activating p.
GTP-dependent signaling p.
GTP-regulatory p.
guanine nucleotide-regulatory p.
HCV p.
heat shock p. (HSP)
helix-loop-helix p.
helix-turn-helix p.
hepatocellular p.
heptahelical receptor p.
heterodimeric p.
heterotrimeric G p.
H-related p.
IkBa p.
intestinal fatty acid-binding p. (I-FABP)
87kDa p.
p. kinase A
p. kinase C (PKC)
lck p.
liver-specific p.
low molecular weight p.
MAGP microfibrillar p.
membrane cofactor p. (MCP)
membrane transport p.
mesenchymal p.
p. metabolism
microfibrillar p. (MP)
monocyte chemoattractant p.
monocyte chemotactic p. (MCP)
multidrug resistance associated p.
myeloma p.
noncollagen p.
Novel erythropoiesis-stimulating p. (NESP)
NS2, NS3, NS4, NS5 p.
nuclear factor kappa B transcription factor p.
nuclear matrix p.-22 (NMP, NMP-22)
oligosaccharide-binding membrane p.
oncofetal p.
outer inflammatory p.
p53 p.
pancreatic stone p. (PSP)
pertussin toxin-sensitive G p.
PH30 p.
phosphorylation p.

p. phosphorylation
plasma p.
p. plug
p53 nuclear p.
podocyte-specific p.
porin channel p.
potential fusion p.
p47, p67 cytosolic p.
PTH-related p. (PTH-rP)
p21/Waf1 p.
rac p.
ras-related p.
Rb p.
receptor-associated p. (RAP)
replacement enzyme p.
p. restriction
retinoid-binding p.
retinol-binding p. (RBP)
rho p.
p. S
S-100 p.
salt transporting p.
scrapie p.
p. serine kinase
p. serine/threonine kinase activity
serum core p.
p. solder
STAR p.
steroidogenic acute regulatory p.
stress p.
p. supplement
surface p.
p. synthesis
Tamm-Horsfall p. (THP)
TATA-binding p.
T cell-specific p.
testicular androgen-binding p.
p. threonine kinase
tight junction membrane p.
toll-interleukin 1 receptor domain-containing adapter p. (TIRAP)
total p.
transmembrane p.
triglyceride-rich p.
p. tubular reabsorption
p. tyrosine kinase
p. tyrosine phosphatase
urinary marker p.
uronic acid-rich p.
vitamin D-binding p. (DBP)
p. in vitamin K absence (PIVKA)

NOTES

protein-1
    insulinlike growth factor-binding p.-1 (IGFBP-1)
    monocyte chemoattractant p.-1 (MCP-1)

protein-2
    multidrug-resistance-associated p.-2 (MRP2)

proteinaceous
    p. cast
    p. cast material

proteinase
    p. enzyme
    p. inhibitor

protein-bound homocysteine
protein-calorie malnutrition (PCM)
protein-energy malnutrition
protein-glutathione-S-transferase
    receptor-associated p.-g.-S-t.

protein-losing
    p.-l. enteropathy
    p.-l. gastroenteropathy
    p.-l. gastropathy

protein-mediated tubular toxicity
protein-overload proteinuria
protein-protein assay
proteinuria
    asymptomatic p.
    Bence Jones p.
    BSA-induced overload p.
    cardiac p.
    colliquative p.
    cyclic p.
    emulsion p.
    enterogenic p.
    febrile p.
    globular p.
    glomerular p.
    gouty p.
    hematogenous p.
    incipient p.
    intermittent p.
    intrinsic p.
    moderate p.
    molecular basis of p.
    nephrogenous p.
    orthostatic p.
    overflow p.
    palpatory p.
    persistent p.
    postrenal p.
    protein-overload p.
    residual p.
    p. test
    transient p.
    tubular p.

proteinuric
    p. glomerulopathy
    p. nephropathy
    p. state

proteoglycan
    p. biglycan
    p. decorin
    heparan sulfate p. (HSPG)

proteolysis
proteolytic
    p. degradation
    p. digestion
    p. enzyme

Proteus
    P. mirabilis
    P. morganii
    P. rettgeri
    Vibrio cholerae biotype *P.*
    P. vulgaris

Proteus **pneumonia**
prothrombin
    des-gamma-carboxy p. (DCP)
    p. induced by vitamin K absence or antagonist-II (PIVKA-II)
    p. time (PT)
    p. time/partial thromboplastin time (PT/PTT)

Protilase
pro time
protocol
    p. biopsy
    CISCA p.
    clinical p.
    Costello p.
    ELF chemotherapy p.
    Eulexin plus LHRH-A chemotherapy/radiation therapy p.
    high-energy p.
    low-energy p.
    multimodal p.
    non-heart-beating donor p.
    salvage p.
    software characteristics of treating p.
    Stanford p.
    surveillance p.
    treatment p.
    VAB-6 chemotherapy p.

PROTOCO$_2$L insufflator
Protocult test
proton
    p. flux
    p. magnetic resonance spectroscopy
    p. pump
    p. pump blocker
    p. pump inhibition therapy
    p. pump inhibitor (PPI)

protonated
proton-induced release of secretin

Protonix
    P. delayed-release tablet
    P. IV powder for infusion
protooncogene
    c-fos p.
    c-jun p.
    c-kit p. (CD117)
    c-myc p.
    p53 p.
    RET p.
protopathic pain
protoporphyria
    erythropoietic p.
protoporphyrin-9
Protostat Oral
prototype cholangioscope
protozoa
    intestinal p.
protozoan, protozoal
    p. abscess
    p. disease
    p. dysentery
    p. enteritis
    p. parasite
    p. pathogen
Protractor
protriptyline
protruding fat
protrusion
    anal p.
protuberance
    pigmented p.
protuberant
    p. abdomen
    p. carcinoma
Provera
Providencia
    P. alcalifaciens
    P. rettgeri
    P. stuartii
Provir
provocation
    edrophonium p.
provocative
    P. sensitivity balloon
    p. test
    p. testing
provoked cystometry
ProXeed dietary supplement
proxetil
    cefpodoxime p.

proximal
    p. bile duct
    p. convoluted tubule (PCT)
    p. gastrectomy
    p. gastric vagotomy (PGV)
    p. human colonic flora
    p. jejunum
    p. muscle weakness
    p. nephron
    p. pouch leak
    p. pressure
    p. renal tubular acidosis
    p. splenorenal shunt
    p. straight tubule (PST)
    p. superior mesenteric artery
    p. tubular cell
    p. tubular secretion of angiotensin
    p. tubule function
    p. ureteral calculus
    p. venous plexus
Proximate
    P. flexible linear stapler
    P. ILS SDH circular stapler
    P. intraluminal stapler
    P. linear cutter
Prozac
PRT
    physiologic reflux test
PRU
    percent reduction in urea
prucalopride
Prudoxin cream
Pruitt anoscope
Prulet
prune-belly syndrome category I-III
prune juice peritoneal fluid
prunetin
pruning
    p. abnormality
    p. sign
pruritic
pruritus
    p. ani
    opioid-mediated p.
    p. scroti
    uremic p.
PS-2 needle
PSA
    prostate-specific antigen
    PSA doubling time
    free PSA (fPSA)
    PSA free/total index

NOTES

PSA *(continued)*
    free-to-total PSA
    F:T PSA
    PSA RT-PCR
    total PSA (tPSA)
PSA4 prostate cancer test
PSA-ACT
    prostate-specific antigen bound to alpha-1 antichymotrypsin
PSA-based parameter
PSAD
    prostate-specific antigen density
PSA-TZ
    prostate-specific antigen density of transition zone
PSAV
    prostate-specific antigen velocity
PSC
    primary sclerosing cholangitis
PSE
    portosystemic encephalopathy
Pseudallescheria boydii
pseudoachalasia
    malignant p.
pseudoalcoholic liver disease
pseudoallergy
pseudoaneurysm
    p. formation
    ruptured p.
pseudoaneurysmal roof
pseudobile canaliculus
pseudo-Billroth I appearance
pseudocapsule
pseudocholangiocarcinoma sign
pseudochylous ascites
pseudocirrhosis
    cholangiodysplastic p.
pseudocolitis
pseudocolor fluorescence of Fura ed
pseudocryptorchism
pseudo-Cushing syndrome
pseudocyst
    p. communication
    drainage-resistant p.
    endosonography-guided drainage of pancreatic p.
    extramural p.
    extrapancreatic p.
    giant nonpancreatic p.
    heterogeneous p.
    infected p.
    intrasplenic p.
    pancreatic p.
    pancreatic duct to p.
    paraduodenal p.
    paragastric p.
    p. puncture
    retrogastric p.
    small p.
    uriniferous p.
pseudocystobiliary fistula
pseudocystogastrostomy
    pancreatic p.
pseudodefecation
pseudodeficiency rickets
pseudodelicatissima
    Pseudo-nitzschia p.
pseudodiverticulosis
    esophageal intramural p.
pseudodiverticulum
    urethral p.
pseudoductular transformation of hepatocyte
pseudodysentery
pseudodyssynergia
pseudoephedrine hydrochloride
pseudoepitheliomatous micaceous growths of penis
pseudoesophageal colic
pseudoexstrophy
pseudogout
pseudohermaphroditism
pseudohydronephrosis
pseudohyperkalemia
    familial p.
pseudohypha, pl. **pseudohyphae**
pseudohypoaldosteronism
    type I, II p.
pseudohyponatremia
pseudohypoparathyroidism (PHP)
pseudoileus
pseudoleukemia gastrointestinalis
pseudolipomatosis
pseudolithiasis
    ceftriaxone p.
pseudolymphoma
    gastric p.
pseudomelanosis
pseudomembrane
pseudomembranous
    p. colic
    p. colitis (PMC)
    p. enteritis
    p. enterocolitis
    p. gastritis
pseudomicrolithiasis
pseudomigration
Pseudomonas
    P. aeruginosa
    P. aeruginosa pneumonia
    P. pseudomallei pneumonia
Pseudomonas **exotoxin A**
pseudomononucleosis
pseudomyxoma peritonei
pseudoneurogenic bladder
Pseudo-nitzschia
    P.-n. australis

P.-n. multiseries
P.-n. pseudodelicatissima
P.-n. pungens
pseudoobstruction
    acute colonic p.
    bowel p.
    chronic idiopathic intestinal p. (CIIP)
    chronic intestinal p. (CIP, CIPO)
    colonic p.
    dolichocolon with p.
    familial intestinal p.
    idiopathic intestinal p.
    intestinal p.
    nonfamilial intestinal p.
    polyneuropathy, ophthalmoplegia, leukoencephalopathy, and intestinal p. (POLIP)
    p. syndrome
pseudopancreatic cholera syndrome
pseudoparallel channel sign
pseudopelade
pseudoperoxidase
pseudophimosis
pseudophytobezoar
pseudopodia
    tumorous p.
pseudopolyp
    chili-bean p.
pseudopolyposis medicamentosus
pseudo-prune-belly syndrome
pseudo-pseudohypoparathyroidism
pseudoresistance
pseudosac
pseudosacculation
pseudosarcoid
pseudosarcoma
    bladder p.
    p. of esophagus
pseudospider pelvis
pseudospiralis
    Trichinella p.
pseudostone
pseudostricture
pseudotubercle
pseudotuberculosis
    Yersinia p.
pseudotumor
    p. appearance
    helminthic p.
    inflammatory p.
    kidney p.
    periampullary p.
    urethral p.
pseudovaginal perineoscrotal hypospadias
pseudowatermelon esophagus
pseudo-Whipple disease
pseudoxanthoma elasticum
PSFR
    pancreatic secretory flow rate
    peak secretory flow rate
    PSFR test
PSGN
    poststreptococcal glomerulonephritis
PSI
    portal shunt index
psittaci
    Chlamydia p.
PSK
    polysaccharide Kreha
PSLL
    pancreatoscopic laser lithotripsy
PSM
    prostate-specific membrane
PSMA
    prostate-specific membrane antigen
psoas
    p. abscess
    p. fascia
    p. hitch
    p. loss
    p. muscle
    p. shadow
    p. sign
psorenteritis
psoriasis of penis
psoriatic arthropathy
Psorospermium haeckelii
PSP
    pancreatic stone protein
PSS
    Perceived Stress Scale
    physiologic salt solution
    portosystemic shunting
    progressive systemic sclerosis
PST
    postural stimulation test
    potassium sensitivity test
    proximal straight tubule
PSTI
    pancreatic secretory trypsin inhibitor
psuedocystolonic fistula
PSWL
    peroral shock wave lithotripsy

NOTES

psychic
- p. dysuria
- p. impotence

psychogenic
- p. constipation
- p. erectile dysfunction
- p. erection
- p. impotence
- p. polydipsia
- p. vomiting
- p. water drinking

psychologic
- p. dysfunction
- p. enuresis
- p. nonneuropathic bladder

psychological
- p. disorder
- p. factor
- P. General Well-Being Index (PGWBI)
- p. support

psychometric test
psychometry
psychopharmacologic medication
psychophysiologic testing
psychosexual
- p. history
- p. support
- p. therapy

psychosis
psychosomatic disorder
psychotropic
- p. drug
- p. medication

psychrophore
psyllium husk fiber
PT
- prothrombin time

PTA
- percutaneous transluminal angioplasty

PTBD
- percutaneous transhepatic biliary drainage
- PTBD catheter

PTC
- percutaneous transhepatic cholangiogram
- percutaneous transhepatic cholangiography

PTCC
- percutaneous transhepatic cholecystoscopy

PTCD
- percutaneous transhepatic cholangiodrainage

PTC-guided biopsy
PTCS
- percutaneous transhepatic cholangioscopy

PTD
- percutaneous transhepatic drainage

PTDM
- posttransplant diabetes mellitus

PTEN suppressor gene function
pteroylglutamic acid
pterygium
pterygoid depression
PTFE
- polytetrafluoroethylene

PTH
- parathyroid hormone
- plasma parathyroid hormone
  - carboxyterminal PTH
  - intact PTH
  - midregion PTH

PTHC
- percutaneous transhepatic cholangiogram
- percutaneous transhepatic cholangiography
- PTHC catheter

PTH-related protein (PTH-rP)
PTH-rP
- PTH-related protein
  - PTH-rP by immunoradiometric assay

PTLD
- posttransplant lymphoproliferative disorder

ptosis
- renal p.

PTP
- percutaneous transhepatic portography

PT/PTT
- prothrombin time/partial thromboplastin time

PTR
- pressure transmission ratio

PTRA
- percutaneous transluminal renal angioplasty

PTT
- partial thromboplastin time

PTU
- propylthiouracil

P-TUMT
- periurethral transurethral microwave thermotherapy

ptyocrinous cell
P-type amylase
puberty
pubic
- p. arch
- p. diastasis
- p. fixation
- p. hair line
- p. prostatectomy
- p. ramus
- p. symphysis
- p. tubercle

pubis
   body of p.
   osteitis p.
   pediculosis p.
   Phthirus p.
   symphysis p.
   symphysis ossium p.
published comparative trial
puboanalis muscle
pubocervical
   p. fascia
   p. ligament
pubococcygeal
   p. line
   p. muscle training
pubococcygeus muscle
puboprostatic
   p. ligament
   p. sling
puborectalis
   p. dysfunction
   dyskinetic p.
   p. loop
   p. muscle
   p. muscle function
   overreactive p.
   p. sling
   p. syndrome
puborectal muscle
pubosacral line
pubourethral
   p. ligament
   p. sling
pubovaginal
   p. operation
   p. sling
   p. sling procedure
pubovesicalis
   plica p.
pubovesical ligament
pubovesicocervical fascia
pubovisceral muscle
Pucci-Seed
   P.-S. hook
   P.-S. spatula
PUD
   peptic ulcer disease
pudding
   Ensure p.
   Sustacal p.
puddle sign
puddling on barium enema

pudenda (*pl. of* pudendum)
pudendal
   p. artery
   p. canal
   p. nerve function
   p. nerve terminal motor latency (PNTML)
   p. neurogram
   p. neuropathy
   p. pelvic nerve
   p. vein
   p. vessel
pudendal-anal reflex
pudendal-evoked potential
pudendum, pl. **pudenda**
   rima pudenda
puerperal septic pelvic vein thrombophlebitis
puerperium
Puestow
   P. pancreaticojejunostomy
   P. procedure
Puestow-Gillesby
   P.-G. operation
   P.-G. procedure
Pugh
   P. classification
   P. modification
   P. modification of Child criteria
   modified method of P.
Pugh-Child scoring system
pull
   complete PEG p.
   p. enteroscopy
   p. method
   PEG p.
   Ponsky p.
pull-apart introducer
pullthrough
   endorectal ileal p.
   ileal p.
   ileoanal endorectal p.
   p. manometry
   p. procedure
   rapid p. (RPT)
   sacroabdominoperineal p.
   Soave endorectal p.
   station p. (SPT)
   Swenson abdominal p.
   p. technique
pull-type sphincterotomy

NOTES

pulmonary
- p. alveolar microlithiasis
- p. arteriovenous malformation
- p. artery pressure (PAP)
- p. aspiration
- p. capillaritis
- p. capillary wedge pressure (PCWP)
- p. cavitation
- p. complication
- p. disorder
- p. edema
- p. embolism
- p. embolus
- p. gas embolism during laparoscopy
- p. granuloma
- p. methane excretion
- p. mucormycosis
- p. outflow

pulp
- splenic p.

pulpa
- p. lienis
- p. splenica

pulpar cell
pulpy testis
pulsatile
- p. hematoma
- p. mass

pulsatility index
pulse
- abdominal p.
- abrupt p.
- Altmann p.
- atrial liver p.
- Corrigan p.
- p. dye laser
- intermittent p.
- p. oximetry
- Quincke p.
- p. repetition frequency (PRF)
- p. spray catheter
- thready p.
- p. volume recording

pulsed
- p. Doppler
- p. Doppler ultrasound
- p. irrigation
- p. Solu-Medrol

pulsed-dye
- p.-d. laser
- p.-d. laser therapy
- p.-d. neodymium:YAG laser
- pulsed-field gel electrophoresis (PFGE)

Pulse-Pak infusion kit
pulse-width analysis

pulsion
- enterocele p.

Pulsolith laser
pulsus
- p. abdominalis
- p. paradoxus

pulverizer
- Thermovac tissue p.

Pulvules
- Cinobac P.
- Compound-65 P.

pump
- Abbott LifeCare p.
- acid p.
- AS-800 p.
- ASID Bonz PP infusion p.
- bile salt export p. (BSEP)
- Biosearch 7000 enteral feeding p.
- Bluemle p.
- calcium ATPase p.
- centrifugal p.
- Companion feeding p.
- Compat 199205 enteral feeding p.
- Cub R-200 enteral feeding p.
- Endolav lavage p.
- Enteroport feeding p.
- Felig insulin p.
- Flexiflo Companion enteral feeding p.
- Flexiflo II enteral feeding p.
- Flocare 500 feeding p.
- Flo-Gard p.
- Frenta Mat feeding p.
- Frenta System II feeding p.
- Harvard p.
- hepatic artery infusion p.
- HK-ATPase proton p.
- Holter Pediatric P. 903, 907
- IMED 430 enteral feeding p.
- Infusaid chemotherapy implantable p.
- Infusaid hepatic p.
- infusion p. (IP)
- Kangaroo 200, 330 enteral feeding p.
- Kangaroo 324 feeding p.
- Keofeed 500 enteral feeding p.
- Keofeed II enteral feeding p.
- KMI 60 enteral feeding p.
- low-compliance perfusion p.
- low-compliance pneumohydraulic p.
- MasterFlex p.
- McGaw volumetric p.
- Nutromat Pad S feeding p.
- peristaltic p.
- pneumatic leg p.
- proton p.
- retroperistaltic p.
- reverse osmosis p.

roller p.
Sarns Siok II blood p.
sodium p.
Space Saver volumetric p.
stomach p.
subcutaneous morphine p. (SQMP)
suction p.
Tonkaflo p.
VTR-300 enteral feeding p.
xenobiotic p.
pumped-dye laser
punch
aortic p.
biopsy p.
p. biopsy
kidney p.
Murphy kidney p.
Turkel p.
punched-out
p.-o. orchidometer
p.-o. ulcer
p.-o. ulceration
punctata
Aeromonas p.
punctate
p. area
p. fluorescence pattern
p. ulcer
puncture
caliceal p.
calix p.
cystic p.
diathermic p.
direct cautery p.
endoscopic fine-needle p.
epididymis percutaneous p.
epigastric p.
Marfan epigastric p.
needle tracheoesophageal p.
pseudocyst p.
suprapubic p.
tracheoesophageal p. (TEP)
pungens
Pseudo-nitzschia p.
pupil
asymmetric p.'s
blown p.
dilated p.
irregular p.
nonreactive p.
pinpoint p.

pure
p. cholestasis
p. cutting current
p. nephrosis
p. pancreatic juice (PPJ)
p. PPoma
p. red cell aplasia (PRCA)
Puregene DNA isolation kit
purgation
purgative
novel tableted p.
purge
oral p.
purging
bingeing and p.
self-induced p.
purified
p. HBeAg
p. protein derivative test (PPD)
p. T cell
Purilon
Comfeel P.
purine
dietary p.
p. synthesis inhibitor
puromycin
p. aminonucleoside
p. aminonucleoside necrosis
p. aminonucleoside nephropathy (PAN)
p. aminonucleoside nephrosis (PAN)
purpose-built silicone rubber multilumen manometric assembly
purpura
p. abdominalis
anaphylactoid p.
Echinacea p.
Henoch-Schönlein p.
idiopathic thrombocytopenic p.
lung p.
Schönlein-Henoch p.
thrombocytopenic p.
thrombotic thrombocytopenic p. (TTP)
purpureum
tinea p.
pursestring
p. ligature
p. suture
pursestringed

NOTES

Pursuer
    P. CBD helical stone basket
    P. minihelical stone basket
purulent
    p. appendicitis
    p. debris
    p. discharge
    p. gastritis
    p. material
    p. pancreatitis
puruloid
pus
    p. collection
    frank p.
push
    complete PEG p.
    p. enteroscope
    p. enteroscopy
    PEG p.
    p. technique
pusher
    p. catheter
    Clarke-Reich knot p.
    Endo-Assist reusable knot p.
    Gazayerli knot p.
    metal-tipped stent p.
    p. tube
push-pull T technique
push-type enteroscopy
pustule
putative
    p. anion transporter (PAT1)
    p. hepatotrophic factors
      insulin/glucagon
    p. host restriction
    p. transmitter
putredinis
    Bacteroides p.
putrefactive diarrhea
putrescine
putty kidney
PUV
    posterior urethral valve type I–IV
PUVT
    paraumbilical vein tumor
PV
    portal vein
P&V
    pyloroplasty and vagotomy
PVA
    partial villous atrophy
PVB
    platinum, Velban, bleomycin
PVC
    polyvinyl chloride
    postvoiding cystogram
      PVC catheter
PVCI
    portal vein congestive index

PVH
    persistent viral hepatitis
PVH-B
    persistent viral hepatitis type B
PVH-NANB
    persistent viral hepatitis non-A, non-B
PVN
    paraventricular nucleus
PVP
    portal venous pressure
PVR
    postvoid residual
PVS
    peritoneovenous shunt
PVT
    portal vein thrombosis
PVV
    portal venous velocity
p21/Waf1 protein
PW-5V
    Olympus spray catheter PW-5V
pyelectasis, pyelectasia
pyelic
pyelitic
pyelitis
    calculous p.
    p. cystica
    defloration p.
    encrusted p.
    p. glandularis
    hematogenous p.
    urogenous p.
pyelocalicotomy
pyelocaliectasis
pyelocalyceal cyst
pyelocystanastomosis
pyelocystitis
pyelocystostomosis
pyelofluoroscopy
pyelogenic renal cyst
pyelogram
    antegrade p.
    dragon p.
    hydrated p.
    intravenous p. (IVP)
    powder p.
    retrograde p. (RPG)
pyelography
    air p.
    antegrade p.
    ascending p.
    p. by elimination
    excretion p.
    infusion p.
    intravenous p. (IVP)
    lateral p.
    percutaneous antegrade p.
    respiration p.
    respiratory p.

retrograde p.
washout p.
pyeloileocutaneous anastomosis
pyelointerstitial
pyelolithotomy
    coagulum p.
    extended p.
    Gil-Vernet extended p.
    laparoscopic p.
    open p.
    standard p.
pyelolymphatic backflow
pyelolysis
pyelometer
pyelometry
pyelonephritis (PN)
    acute nonobstructive p.
    ascending p.
    asymptomatic p.
    chronic p. (CP, CPN)
    chronic bacterial p.
    cryptococcal p.
    emphysematous p.
    fungal p.
    hematogenous p.
    p. of pregnancy
    xanthogranulomatous p. (XGP)
pyelonephrosis
pyelopathy
pyeloplasty
    Anderson-Hynes dismembered p.
    capsular flap p.
    Culp-DeWeerd spiral flap p.
    Culp spiral flap p.
    disjoined p.
    dismembered p.
    Foley Y-plasty p.
    Foley Y-V p.
    laparoscopic dismembered p.
    robotically assisted laparoscopic dismembered p.
    Scardino-Prince vertical flap p.
    Scardino vertical flap p.
    Thompson capsule flap p.
pyeloplication
pyelorenal
    p. backflow
    p. reflux
pyeloscopy
pyelosinus
    p. backflow
    p. extravasation

pyelostomy
    cutaneous p.
pyelotomy
    p. closure
    extended p.
    p. incision
    open p.
    slash p.
pyelotubular
    p. backflow
    p. reflux
pyeloureteral catheter
pyeloureterectasis
pyeloureteritis cystica
pyeloureterogram
pyeloureterography
    antegrade p.
pyeloureterolysis
pyeloureteroplasty
pyeloureterostomy
pyelovenous backflow
pyelovesical stent
pyelovesicostomy
pyemesis
pyemia
    portal p.
Pygeum
    P. africanum
    P. extract
pyknotic nucleus
pyleography
    limited intravenous p.
pylephlebitis
pyloralgia
pylorectomy
    Kocher p.
pylori
    cagA-negative *Helicobacter p.*
    cagA-positive *Helicobacter p.*
    Campylobacter p.
    coccoid form of *Helicobacter p.*
    Helicobacter p. (HP)
    intrafamilial clustering of *Helicobacter p.*
    neutrophil-activating protein of *Helicobacter p.* (HP-NAP)
    taeniae p.
pyloric
    p. atresia
    p. autotransplantation
    p. canal
    p. cap

NOTES

pyloric *(continued)*
- p. channel
- p. channel ulcer
- p. dilation
- p. fullness
- p. gland
- p. insufficiency
- p. intubation
- p. metaplasia (PYME)
- p. mucosa
- p. outlet
- p. outlet obstruction
- p. pressure wave
- p. ring
- p. sphincter
- p. spreader
- p. stenosis
- p. stricture
- p. string sign
- p. tone

pyloricum
- antrum p.
- ostium p.

Pylorid
PyloriScreen test
Pyloriset EIA-G test
PyloriStat assay test
pyloristenosis
PyloriTek
- P. *Helicobacter pylori* test kit
- P. rapid urease test
- P. reagent strip

pylorodiosis
pyloroduodenal
- p. junction
- p. obstruction
- p. perforation
- p. segment

pylorogastrectomy
pyloromyotomy
- Fredet-Ramstedt p.
- Ramstedt p.
- Ramstedt-Fredet p.

pyloroplasty
- double p.
- Finney p.
- Heineke-Mikulicz p.
- Horsley p.
- Jaboulay p.
- Judd p.
- Mikulicz p.
- Ramstedt p.
- reconstructive p.
- truncal vagotomy and p.
- p. and vagotomy (P&V)
- vagotomy and p. (V&P)
- Weinberg modification of p.

pyloroptosis, pyloroptosia
pyloroscopy

pylorospasm
- congenital p.
- persistent p.
- reflex p.

pylorostenosis
pylorostomy
pylorotomy
pylorus
- closed p.
- double p.
- hypertrophic p.
- patulous p.

pylorus-preserving
- p.-p. pancreatoduodenectomy (PPPD)
- p.-p. Whipple modification (PPW)

pylorus-sparing pancreaticoduodenectomy
PYME
- pyloric metaplasia

PyNPase activity
pyocalix
pyocele
pyochezia
pyocystis
pyoderma gangrenosum (PG)
pyogenes
- *Streptococcus* p.

pyogenic
- p. bacterium
- p. cholangitis
- p. granuloma
- p. liver
- p. liver abscess
- p. meningitis
- p. organism

pyohydronephrosis
pyonephritis
pyonephrolithiasis
pyonephrosis
pyonephrotic
pyopneumocholecystitis
pyopneumohepatitis
pyopneumoperitoneum
pyopneumoperitonitis
pyopyelectasis
pyosemia
pyospermia
pyostomatitis vegetans
pyoureter
pyovesiculosis
PYP
- pyrophosphate
- ^{99m}Tc PYP

pyramid
- base of renal p.
- p. of kidney
- Malpighi p.
- medullary p.
- renal p.

pyramidal
    p. muscle
    p. trocar
Pyraminyl
pyramis
pyrantel pamoate
pyrazinamide
pyrazinoisoquinoline
pyrexia
pyrexial
Pyribenzamine
pyridinoline
    serum p.
Pyridium
    P. Plus
    P. test of vaginal drainage
Pyridorin XR
pyridostigmine
pyridoxal
    p. phosphate
    p. 5'-phosphate deficiency
pyridoxamine
pyridoxine

pyrilamine
Pyrilinks-D urinary assay
pyrimethamine
pyrimidine synthesis
pyrogen
    endogenous p.
pyrophosphate (PYP)
    stannous p. (SPP)
pyrosis
pyrrolidinedithiocarbamate
pyruvate
    p. dehydrogenase (PDH)
    p. kinase
PYtest urea breath test
pyuria
    abacterial p.
pyxigraphic device
PYY
    peptide YY
PYY-like immunoreactivity
PZD
    partial zonal dissection

NOTES

Q
Q cell
Q fever
Q200 gastroscope
QAD-1
Doppler QAD-1
QAD-1 sonography unit
QDR 1000 densitometer absorptiometer
QHS
quantitative hepatobiliary scintigraphy
QID
Quantum inflation device
Q-Maxx side-firing laser device
QOL
quality of life
QOLRD
Quality of Life in Reflux and Dyspepsia
QOLRD score
Q-switched
Q-s. alexandrite laser
Q-s. Nd:YAG laser
Q-tip test
Q-TWIST
quality-adjusted time without symptoms or toxicity
Quad-Lumen drain
Quadra-Coil ureteral stent
quadrant
all four q.'s
both lower q.'s (BLQ)
both upper q.'s (BUQ)
left lower q. (LLQ)
left upper q. (LUQ)
right lower q. (RLQ)
right upper q. (RUQ)
quadrant-sampling technique
quadrate
q. lobe
q. lobe of liver
quadriplegia
quadruple therapy
quadruplicate well
qualitative
q. fecal fat test
q. microculture assay
quality
assessment of bowel preparation q.
q. of kidney graft
q. of life (QOL)
q. of life instrument
Q. of Life in Reflux and Dyspepsia (QOLRD)
Q. of Life in Reflux and Dyspepsia score

quality-adjusted time without symptoms or toxicity (Q-TWIST)
quality-of-life parameter
quantified protein excretion
Quantikine quantitative immunoenzymatometric sandwich technique
quantitative
q. angiography
q. fecal fat test
q. hepatobiliary scintigraphy (QHS)
q. liquid hybridization
q. measurement
q. scintigraphic evacuation proctography
q. stool collection
q. ultrasound (QUS)
Quantum
Q. inflation device (QID)
Q. TTC balloon dilator
Q. TTC biliary balloon
quartan malaria
Quartey technique
quartz waveguide
Quarzan
quasispecies
quazepam
queasiness
queasy
quercetin
Quervain abdominal retractor
query
questionnaire
Biliary Symptoms Q. (BSQ)
Bowel Disease Q.
Bowel Disease Q.
Chronic Liver Disease Q. (CLDQ)
q. data
Diabetes Bowel Symptom Q. (DBSQ)
Inflammatory Bowel Disease Q. (IBDQ)
McGill pain q.
Sexual Function Inventory Q. (SFIQ)
Short Inflammatory Bowel Disease Q. (SIBDQ)
Questran
Quetelet BMI index
Queyrat
Quickclip
Quick-Core needle
quick-dissolving crystal
Quick-Tap paracentesis system
Quick test

QuickVue
    Q. *H. pylori* gII test kit
    Q. One-Step *H. pylori* test
Quidel-QuickVue *H. pylori* test
quiescence
    motor q.
quiescent
    q. hepatitis
    q. human fibroblast
Quiess
quiet bowel sounds
quill sheath
quilted suture
Quimby
    Q. method
    Q. pattern
quinacrine
Quinaglute
quinapril
Quincke
    Q. pulse
    Q. triad
quinidine
    q. gluconate
    q. intoxication
    q. sulfate
quinine urea hydrochloride
Quinlan test
quinolone
Quinton
    Q. catheter
    Q. PermCath
    Q. single-port scissor valve
    Q. suction biopsy instrument
    Q. tube
Quinton-Mahurkar dual-lumen peritoneal catheter
Quinton-Scribner shunt
QuinTron
    Q. AlveoSampler
    Q. MicroLyzer
    Q. Microlyzer 12 chromatograph
Quire mechanical finger forceps
Quixil spray
QUS
    quantitative ultrasound
Q-200V
    Olympus EVIS Q-200V

R
> resistance
>> R factor in bacterial antimicrobial resistance

R5
> *Salmonella typhimurium* R5

RA
> renal artery

RAAA
> ruptured abdominal aortic aneurysm

RAAS
> renin-angiotensin-aldosterone system

rabbit stool
rabeprazole sodium
Rabuteau test
RAC
> ranitidine bismuth citrate, amoxicillin, clarithromycin

racephedrine
RackBeta scintillation counter
rac protein
RAD
> reactive airway disease

radial
> r. examination
> r. groove
> r. immunodiffusion
> r. incision
> R. jaw bladder biopsy forceps
> R. jaw hot biopsy forceps
> R. Jaw III Max Capacity 1589 biopsy forceps
> R. Jaw III Max Capacity with needle biopsy forceps
> R. Jaw III single-use biopsy forceps
> r. mode
> r. Ro-resection
> r. suture track

radial-sector scanning echoendoscope
radiata
> corona r.

radiating pain
radiation
> r. cystitis
> r. dosage
> effective dose equivalent r.
> endocavitary r.
> r. enteritis
> r. enterocolitis
> r. enteropathy
> r. esophagitis
> r. exposure
> 5-fluorouracil, mitomycin C r. (FUMIR)
> r. gastritis
> r. hepatopathy
> r. injury
> ionizing r.
> nonionizing r.
> nonparticulate r.
> particulate r.
> r. pneumonitis
> r. proctitis
> r. proctocolitis
> radiotracer half-life r.
> rectosigmoid r.
> r. sensitizer
> r. stenosis
> r. telangiectasia
> r. therapy

radiation-induced
> r.-i. angiosarcoma
> r.-i. angiosclerosis
> r.-i. colitis
> r.-i. disease
> r.-i. obliterative arteritis
> r.-i. sterility
> r.-i. ulceration
> r.-i. ureteral stricture
> r.-i. vesicovaginal fistula

radical
> r. cystectomy
> r. en bloc removal
> free r.
> r. hemorrhoidectomy
> hydroxyl r.
> hydroxyl-free r.
> r. inguinal orchiectomy
> r. nephrectomy
> r. nephroureterectomy
> oxygen r.
> oxygen-derived free r.
> oxygen-free r.
> r. perineal prostatectomy
> r. resection group
> r. retropubic prostatectomy (RRP)
> superoxide r.
> r. surgery
> r. transcoccygeal prostatectomy

radicality
> oncological r.

radices (*pl. of* radix)
radiciform
radicle
> biliary r.
> intrahepatic r.
> right hepatic r.
> tertiary r.

radiculitis

radii (*pl. of* radius)
radioactive
    r. carbon-14 test
    r. cholesterol
    r. detection
    r. iodine-131
    r. seed
    r. seed implantation
radioallergosorbent test (RAST)
radioautography
    thaw-mount r.
radiobiology
radiocephalic fistula
radiochemotherapy
radiochromium-labeled erythrocyte method
radiocolloid
radiocontrast-induced
    r.-i. acute renal failure
    r.-i. renal vasoconstriction
radiocystitis
radiodensity
radioenzymatic assay
radiograph
    plain r.
radiographic
    r. situation
    r. triad
radiography
    abdominal r.
    barium contrast r.
    calculus r.
    double-contrast r.
    kidneys, ureters, bladder r.
    KUB r.
    plain abdominal r.
    postvoid r.
    single-contrast r.
    skeletal r.
radioimmunoassay (RIA)
    Cyclotrac-SP r.
    homogenous r.
    solid-phase r.
    Yang PSA r.
radioimmunodetection
radioimmunoguided surgery (RIGS)
radioimmunoinhibition assay
radioimmunoprecipitation assay
radioiodination
radioisotope
    r. capsule
    r. renal excretion test
    r. renogram test
    r. renography
    r. scan
    r. scanning
    r. scintigraphy
radiolabeled
    r. imaging
    r. leucine
    r. macromolecule
radiologic
    r. biliary stent placement
    r. castration
    r. portacaval shunt
radiological
    r. investigation
    r. study
radiolucent
    r. gallstone
    r. object
Radiometer
    R. GK2803C pH probe
    R. 85 instrument
radionecrosis
radionuclide
    r. cholescintigraphy
    r. cystography
    r. esophageal emptying time
    [^{123}I]iodoamphetamine r.
    r. renal imaging
    r. scan
    r. scintigraphy
    r. ^{99}Tc scintiscanning
    r. therapy
    r. transit study
    r. voiding cystourethrography
radioopaque iodized oil
radiopaque
    r. density
    r. dye
    r. ERCP catheter
    r. marker
    r. pellet
radioresistant gastric plasmacytoma
radioscintigraphy
radioscopically
radiosensitive organ
radiotelemetering capsule
radiotherapy
    infradiaphragmatic r.
    intraluminal r.
    intraoperative r. (IORT)
    intraoperative electron beam r.
radiotracer half-life radiation
radius, pl. radii
    R. enteral feeding tube
    thrombocytopenia-absent r. (TAR)
    r. of varix
radix, pl. radices
    r. penis
RAEB
    refractory anemia with excess blasts
ragged-red fiber
railroading
railroad track scars
RAIR
    rectoanal inhibitory reflex

rake
    r. retractor
    r. ulcer
Ralks adapter
Raman
    R. scattering
    R. spectroscopic system
rami (*pl. of* ramus)
ramification
ramipril
    R. Efficacy in Nephropathy (REIN)
    R. Efficacy in Nephropathy study
Ramirez
    R. shunt
    R. Silastic cannula
Ramond point
ramosum
    Absidia r.
    Clostridium r.
ramotomy
    superior pubic r.
Rampley sponge-holding forceps
Ramstedt
    R. operation
    R. pyloric stenosis dilator
    R. pyloromyotomy
    R. pyloroplasty
Ramstedt-Fredet pyloromyotomy
ramus, pl. **rami**
    pubic r.
ranarum
    Basidiobolus r.
Randall
    R. plaque
    R. stone forceps
Randolph abdominoplasty
random
    r. bladder biopsy
    r. flap
    R. Primed DNA Labeling kit
    r. stool sample
randomized clinical trial data
Rand Short Form-36 survey
Ranfac cholangiographic catheter
range
    arrhythmic frequency r.
    chromatofocusing pH r.
    dilation r.
    hapatotoxic r.
    metabolic r.
    r. of motion
    optimum cooling r.

ranging
    resection syndrome r.
ranitidine
    r. bismuth citrate (RBC)
    r. bismuth citrate, amoxicillin, clarithromycin (RAC)
    r. bismuth citrate, metronidazole, tetracycline (RMT)
    r. hydrochloride
    r. nocte
    r. therapy
rank
    R. operation
    Spearman r.
Rankin clamp
Ransley-Cantwell repair
Ransley procedure
Ranson
    R. acute pancreatitis classification
    R. criteria
    R. criteria for severity of pancreatitis
    R. grading system
RANTES
    regulated upon activation, normal T cells expressed and secreted
RAP
    receptor-associated protein
    recurrent abdominal pain
    robot-assisted laparoscopy
Rapamune
    R. oral solution
    R. tablet
rapamycin
    r. inhibitor
    treatment with r.
raphe
    anococcygeal r.
    r. pallidus
    penile r.
    r. penis
    perineal r.
    r. perinealis
    r. perinei
    r. of perineum
    scrotal r.
    r. scroti
    r. of scrotum
Rapicide
rapid (RPD)
    r. acquisition fast spin-echo sequence

NOTES

rapid *(continued)*
    r. colonic lavage
    r. emptying of dye
    r. enzyme immunoassay
    r. exchange (RX)
    r. exchange technique for therapeutic endoscopy
    r. gastric emptying
    r. pullthrough (RPT)
    r. pullthrough esophageal manometry technique
    r. serum amylase test
    R. Strand implant
    r. urease test (RUT)
    r. urease testing kit
RapidFire multiple-band ligator
Rapid-hyb buffer
rapidly progressive glomerulonephritis (RPGN)
RapiSeal pouch
Rapoport test
Rappaport classification
Rapunzel syndrome
RARS
    refractory anemia with ringed sideroblasts
RAS
    renin-angiotensin system
    RAS blocker
rasburicase
rash
    butterfly r.
    discoid r.
    genital r.
    petechial r.
    scarlatiniform r.
raspatory
    Doyen r.
ras p21 oncogene
ras-**related protein**
RAST
    radioallergosorbent test
rate
    albumin excretion r. (AER)
    alcohol elimination r. (AER)
    allograft survival r.
    amphotericin B-induced reduction glomerular filtration r.
    average flow r.
    basal carbohydrate oxidation r.
    basal metabolic r. (BMR, BRM)
    basal secretory flow r. (BSFR)
    blood flow r. (BFR)
    crude incidence r.
    demonstrated hypertensive r.
    detection r.
    erythrocyte sedimentation r. (ESR)
    exponential r.
    flow r.
    gallbladder ejection r. (GBER)
    glomerular filtration r. (GFR)
    high failure r.
    high false-positive r.
    kidney electrolyte clearance r.
    kidney electrolyte excretion r.
    lipid oxidation r.
    logarithmic r.
    low recurrence r.
    maximum free-flow r.
    maximum urinary flow r.
    mean TIMP-1/GAPDH r.
    metabolic r.
    normalized protein catabolic r. (NPCR)
    operative mortality r.
    optimal shock wave r.
    pancreatic secretory flow r. (PSFR)
    patency r.
    peak flow r. (PFR)
    peak secretory flow r. (PSFR)
    postoperative recurrent bleeding r.
    posttransplantation survival r.
    pressure increment r. (PIR)
    prevalence of low glomerular filtration r.
    protein catabolic r. (PCR)
    r. ratio (RR)
    rebleeding r.
    recurrence r.
    reduced graft survival r.
    reintervention r.
    reoperation r.
    respiratory r.
    retreatment r.
    seroconversion r.
    seroprevalence r.
    single-nephron glomerular filtration r. (SNGFR)
    stone-free r.
    stone recurrent r.
    survival r.
    transcapillary escape r.
    urine flow r.
    voiding flow r.
Rathke
    R. duct
    R. plica
Rating Form of Inflammatory Bowel Disease Patient Concerns (RFIPC)
ratio
    adenoma-hyperplastic polyp r.
    adenoma-nonadenoma r.
    aldosterone-to-renin r.
    amylase/creatinine clearance r.
    androstenedione-to-testosterone r.
    apolipoprotein CII-CIII r.
    AST/ALT r.
    BCAA/AAA plasma r.

bile salt-phospholipid r.
BUN-to-creatinine r.
calcium-creatinine r.
CD4+–CD8+ T-cell r.
chloride-to-phosphate r.
CO_2-CO_2 abundance r.
decreased postprandial-to-fasting power r.
dialysate-to-plasma r.
distribution r. (DR)
D-P urea r.
foveola-gland r.
free-to-total PSA r.
G:D-cell r.
ketone body r. (KBR)
lactulose-mannitol r.
LCA-DCA r.
likelihood r.
lipid-to-protein r.
lithocholic acid-deoxycholic acid r. (LCA-DCA)
mean TIMP-3-GAPDH r.
r. of mucosa to submucosa to muscularis propria
nuclear-to-cytoplasmic size r.
pepsinogen A-C r.
r. of PGF2-alpha PGE2
phospholipid r.
pressure transmission r. (PTR)
presumed circle area r. (PCAR)
rate r. (RR)
renal vein renin r.
serum pepsinogen I/II r.
signal-to-cutoff r.
somatostatin mRNA-D-cell density r.
standardized incidence r. (SIR)
surface-to-volume r.
UA/C r.
urea reduction r. (URR)
urinary protein-urinary creatinine r.
urine-plasma r. (U/P)
Valsalva r.
Xc/R r.

rational allocation strategy
rationing
Ratliff-Blake gallstone forceps
Ratliff-Mayo forceps
rat-tail
    r.-t. appearance on pancreatogram
    r.-t. configuration
    r.-t. sign

rat-tooth Olympus FG 8L grasping forceps
Rauber
    hepatic funiculus of R.
Raudixin
Rautina
Rauval
Rauwolfia
Rauzide
raw
    r. milk-associated diarrhea
    r. surface of liver bed
Rayer disease
Raz
    R. anterior vaginal wall sling
    R. bladder neck suspension
    R. double-prong ligature carrier
    R. four-corner vaginal wall sling
    R. four-quadrant suspension
    R. modification
    R. needle bladder suspension
    R. procedure
    R. sling operation
    R. urethral suspension
razor
    r. blade
    r. blade ingestion
Rb
    rubidium
    Rb influx
    Rb protein
RBC
    ranitidine bismuth citrate
    red blood cells
        technetium-99m pyrophosphate-tagged RBC
RBF
    renal blood flow
***Rb* gene**
RBL
    rubber band ligation
    rubber band ligator
RBP
    retinol-binding protein
RC
    retrograde cystogram
RCC
    renal cell carcinoma
RCCD
    recurrent episodes of *Clostridium difficile* disease

NOTES

RCF
    Ross carbohydrate-free
        RCF formula
RCRC
    recurrent colorectal cancer
RCS
    red color sign
        RCS sign
RCT
    rectal carcinoid tumor
RCU
    recurrent calcium urolithiasis
RDA
    recommended daily allowance
RDG
    retrograde duodenogastroscopy
RDW
    red cell distribution width
RE
    reflux esophagitis
    regional enteritis
Reabilan HN tube feeding formula
reabsorption
    fractional proximal r.
    HCO_3^- r.
    implant r.
    protein tubular r.
    sodium r.
    spontaneous cyst r.
    tubular sodium r.
reactance (Xc)
    r. and resistance (Xc/R)
reaction
    acrosome r.
    allergic r.
    amplification refractory mutation system-polymerase chain r. (ARMS-PCR)
    anaphylactic r.
    Bittorf r.
    cholestatic r.
    desmoplastic r.
    drug r.
    Ehrlich diazo r.
    Feulgen r.
    fixed drug r.
    foreign body r.
    hypersensitivity r.
    immune-mediated r.
    inflammatory r.
    insulin r.
    Jaffe picrate r.
    lichenoid r.
    nonenzymic r.
    one-stage r.
    paradoxical sphincter r.
    periglandular nonspecific inflammatory r.
    Perls r.
    polymerase chain r. (PCR)
    reversed passive hemagglutination r. (RPHA)
    reverse transcriptase r.
    reverse transcriptase-polymerase chain r. (RT-PCR)
    scar tissue r.
    Schmorl r.
    sphincter r.
    T-lymphocyte-mediated cytotoxic r.
    urticarial r.
    van den Bergh r.
    Weiss r.
reactive
    r. airway disease (RAD)
    r. arthritis
    r. hyperemia
    r. inflammatory vascular dermatosis
    r. oxygen metabolite
    r. oxygen species (ROS)
reactivity
    Goodpasture r.
    lectin r.
    p53 r.
reader
    microtitration plate r.
reagent
    ABC r.
    Chemstrip bG r.
    CHOD-PAP cholesterol r.
    Ehrlich r.
    Folin phenol r.
    lipofection r.
    SAB r.
real focus shock wave
real-time
    r.-t. confocal scanning laser microscope
    r.-t. 3-D biplanar transperineal prostate implantation
    r.-t. endoscopic ultrasound-guided fine-needle aspiration
    r.-t. fine-needle aspiration (RTFNA)
    r.-t. gallbladder ultrasound
    r.-t. sonographic unit
    r.-t. spectral analysis
    r.-t. transmission (RTX)
    r.-t. ultrasonography (RUS)
    r.-t. videoprocessor
reanastomosis
    end-to-end branch r.
    laparoscopic ureteral r.
    Roux-en-Y r.
reapproximate
reassignment
    gender r.
Rebetol
    R. capsule
    R. with Intron

Rebetron Combination therapy
rebleeding rate
rebound
    gastric acid r.
    r. pain
    postdialysis urea r.
    r. sign
    r. tenderness
recanalization
    r. of clogged biliary stent
    endoscopic laser r.
    spontaneous r.
    umbilical vein r.
receiver
    Olympus EU-M30S endoscopic ultrasonography r.
receiver-operating characteristic (ROC)
receiving
    external r.
recent
    r. clinical trial
    r. technical modification
    r. work
receptaculum, pl. **receptacula**
    r. chyli
    r. Pecqueti
receptive
    r. anal intercourse
    r. relaxation
receptor
    ability of glucocorticoid r.
    adhesive protein r.
    adrenergic r.
    alpha-adrenergic r.
    alpha-1-adrenergic r.
    alpha-2-adrenergic r.
    androgen r.
    angiotensin II r.
    ANP r.
    antidiuretic arginine vasopressin V2 r. (AVPR2)
    asialoglycoprotein r.
    beta-adrenergic r.
    bladder muscarinic r.
    bombesin r.
    cardiac beta r.
    C3b, C4b r.
    C3, C5 r.
    cell surface r.
    chemokine r.
    cholinergic r.
    ciliary-derived neurotrophic factor r. (CDNF)
    c-*met* r.
    complement r. type 1 (CR1)
    corpus cavernosum muscarinic r.
    r. crosstalk
    endothelin A r.
    epidermal growth factor r. (EGFR)
    estrogen r. (ER)
    EtA r.
    EtB r.
    expression of hemin r.
    fMLP chemoattractant r.
    formyl peptide r.
    gastric mucosal laminin r.
    gastric oxyntic cell r.
    gastrin r.
    gp330 r.
    H2 r.
    high-affinity r.
    histaminergic type 2 r.
    hormone r.
    5-HT3 r.
    5HTM3 r. antagonist
    human motilin r.
    human PDGF r.
    IL-2,-3,-4,-6,-8 r.
    insulin receptor-related r.
    32/67-kD laminin r.
    killer-activating r. (KAR)
    laminin r.
    liver Ah r.
    mesenteric sensory r.
    multiligand r.
    muscarinic r.
    muscle sensory r.
    native pancreatic secretin r.
    natriuretic peptide r. (NPR)
    nerve growth factor r. (NGFR)
    neural growth factor r. (NGFR)
    nicotinic r.
    NK1, NK2 tachykinin r.
    opiate r.
    peptic cell r.
    peroxisome proliferator-activated r. (PPAR)
    phosphorylated growth factor r.
    polyimmunoglobulin r. (pIgR)
    recombinant pancreatic secretin r.
    retinoid X r. (RXR)
    sensory r.
    serotonergic type 3 r.

NOTES

receptor *(continued)*
    r. and signal transduction
    smooth muscle motilin r.
    soluble recombinant complement r. 1
    soluble transferrin r. (sTf-R)
    somatostatin r. (SSR)
    steroid r.
    stretch r.
    T-cell r. (TCR)
    toll-interleukin 1 r. (TIR)
    toll-like r. (TLR)
    transferrin r. (TfR)
    tyrosine kinase growth-factor r.
    umami taste r.
    uroepithelial glycoid r.
    vasopressin type 2 r.
    vitamin D r. (VDR)
receptor-associated
    r.-a. protein (RAP)
    r.-a. protein-glutathione-S-transferase
receptor-blocker
    H2 r.-b.
receptor-mediated endocytosis pathway
recess
    duodenojejunal r.
    splenorenal r.
recession
    clitoral r.
recessive polycystic kidney disease
recessus, pl. **recessus**
recipient
    r. hepatectomy
    kidney transplant r.
    marrow transplant r.
    phase II, III marrow transplant r.
    relationship of r.
    renal allograft r.
    renal transplant r.
    unsensitized transplant r.
recipient-derived anti-HLA antibody
reciprocal ligand
Reclomide
recognition
    ligand r.
recombinant
    r. capsid protein of Norwalk virus (rNV)
    r. HBcAg (rHBcAg)
    r. hepatitis C antigen
    r. HGF
    r. human alfa interferon
    r. human erythropoietin (rh-EPO)
    r. human gelsolin
    r. human relaxin
    r. IL-10
    r. immunoblot assay (RIBA)
    r. immunoblot assay-2
    r. immunoblot assay-2 test
    r. interferon alfa (rIFN-alfa)
    r. interferon alfa-2a, 2b
    r. interleukin-2
    r. methionyl human leptin (r-metHuLeptin)
    r. pancreatic secretin receptor
    r. tissue transglutaminase radioligand assay
    r. tTG radioligand assay
recombination fraction
Recombivax HB
recommendation
    criteria for grading of clinical studies and r.'s
recommended daily allowance (RDA)
reconstruction
    anal sphincter r.
    biliary r.
    Billroth I, II r.
    bladder neck r.
    bladder outlet r.
    corporeal r.
    dural patch r.
    functional r.
    genital r.
    Kropp bladder neck r.
    orthotopic r.
    penile r.
    penis r.
    Roux-en-Y r.
    sphincter r.
    synchronous bladder r.
    Tanagho bladder neck r.
    r. technique
    total anorectal r.
    tubularized bladder neck r.
    urethral surgical r.
    urinary r.
    Young-Dees bladder neck r.
    Young-Dees-Leadbetter bladder neck r.
reconstructive
    r. endourology
    r. phalloplasty
    r. pyloroplasty
    r. surgery
record
    initial in-plan r.
    intragastric pH monitor r.
recorder
    Digitrapper MK III portable digital r.
    multichannel r.
    Narco Bio-Systems rectilinear r.
    portable digital data r.
    Rectigraph-8K r.
    rectilinear r.
    Sandhill-800 TDS chart r.
    Sekomic SS-100F r.

Toshiba ERVF 1A video floppy r.
video r.

recording
bipolar esophageal r.
cutaneous r.
external r.
intraluminal pressure r.
neurophysiologic r.
penile pulse volume r.
pH r.
pulse volume r.

recovery
complete anatomical r.
detrusor r.
improvement in patient r.
postanesthesia r. (PAR)
r. of sexual potency
uneventful r.

recreational drug
recrudescence
recruitment
mononuclear cell r.

recta (*pl. of* rectum)

rectal
r. abscess
r. air suctioning
r. akinesia
r. alimentation
r. ampulla
r. amyloidosis
r. artery
r. augmentation
r. balloon
r. barostat
r. barostat study
r. biopsy
r. bladder urinary diversion
r. bleeding
r. cancer
r. capacity
r. carcinoid tumor (RCT)
r. cell proliferation
r. cisapride
r. coil MRI
r. column
r. compliance
r. compliance measurement
r. cream
r. descensus
r. dilation
r. dilator
r. disease
r. dissection
r. distention
r. emptying
r. endoscopic ultrasonography (REU, REUS)
r. endosonography
r. epithelial cell
r. evacuation
r. evacuatory disorder (RED)
r. examination
r. expander
r. expander-assisted transanal endoscopic microsurgery (RE-TEM)
r. fascia
r. feedback trigger
r. filling
r. fistula
r. fold
r. foreign body
r. fossa
r. gluten challenge
r. gonorrhea
r. hypotonia
r. impaction
r. impedance
r. impedance planimetry
r. incontinence
r. inhibitory reflex
r. injury
r. innervation
r. intussusception
r. laceration
r. leiomyosarcoma
r. linitis plastica (RLP)
r. linitis plastica colorectal carcinoma
r. lumen
r. mass
r. motor complex
r. mucosa
r. mucosectomy
r. muscle cuff
r. myogenic tumor
r. nerve
r. plexus
r. polyp
r. pouch
r. probe
r. probe electroejaculation
r. procidentia
r. prolapse

NOTES

rectal *(continued)*
    r. pulsed irrigation
    r. reservoir
    r. sensation
    r. shelf
    r. sinus
    r. snare
    r. sparing
    r. spasm
    r. speculum
    r. sphincter
    r. stenosis
    r. stricture
    r. stump
    r. suppository
    r. tenderness
    r. tenesmus
    r. thermometer
    r. trauma
    r. tube
    r. ulcer
    r. valve
    r. valvotomy
    r. varix
    r. vault
    r. vein
    r. villous adenoma
    r. visceral sensitivity
rectale
    Eubacterium r.
rectales
    columnae r.
recti
    ampulla r.
    flexura perinealis r.
    flexura sacralis r.
    folliculi lymphatici r.
    procidentia r.
Rectigraph-8K recorder
rectilinear recorder
rectoabdominal
rectoanal
    r. dyssynergia
    r. function
    r. inhibitor
    r. inhibitory reflex (RAIR)
rectocele
    r., cystocele, enterocele
    r. presentation
rectoclysis
rectococcygeus muscle
rectocystotomy
rectogenital septum
rectoischiadic excavation
rectolabial fistula
rectoneovaginal fistula
rectopexy
    abdominal r.
    anterior r.
    Ivalon sponge r.
    laparoscopic suture r.
    Marlex mesh abdominal r.
    posterior r.
    presacral r.
    Ripstein anterior sling r.
    suture r.
    Teflon sling r.
    Wells posterior r.
rectoplasty
    vertical reduction r.
Rector-Gordon-Healey-Mendoza-Spitzer type IV renal tubular acidosis
rectorrhagia
rectosacral
    r. fascia
    r. ligament
rectosigmoid
    r. anastomosis
    r. cancer
    r. colon
    r. function
    r. junction
    r. manometry
    r. radiation
    r. region
    r. varix
rectosigmoidectomy
    Altemeier perineal r.
    perineal r.
rectosigmoidoscopy
rectosphincteric
    r. abnormality
    r. dyssynergia
    r. reflex (RSR)
rectosphincter manometric study
rectotomy
rectourethral
    r. fistula
    r. muscle
rectourethralis muscle
rectourinary fistula
rectouterina
    excavatio r.
rectouterine
    r. pouch
    r. pouch of Douglas
rectovaginal
    r. fistula
    r. pouch
    r. septum
    r. surgery
    r. surgical treatment
rectovesical
    r. center
    r. fascia
    r. fistula
    r. lithotomy

r. pouch
r. septum
rectovesicalis
excavatio r.
rectovestibular fistula
rectovulvar fistula
rectum, pl. **recta**
ampulla of r.
augmented valved r.
benign lymphoma of rectum
bleeding per rectum
blood per rectum (BPR)
bright red blood per rectum (BRBPR)
rectum digital stimulation
gastric mucosal ectopia in rectum (GMER)
Hartmann closure of rectum
horizontal folds of rectum
rectum irrigation
nonrehydrated guaiac examination of rectum
per rectum
prolapsed rectum
transverse folds of rectum
valved rectum
vasa recta
watermelon rectum
rectus
r. abdominis
r. abdominis hematoma
r. abdominis muscle
r. abdominis musculocutaneous flap
r. diastasis
r. fascia
r. fascial wrap
r. fascia sling
r. femoris flap
r. sheath
r. sheath hematoma (RSH)
recurrence
anastomotic r.
local r.
r. rate
short-term prostate-specific antigen r.
source of r.
varicocelectomy r.
Wilms tumor r.
recurrent
r. abdominal pain (RAP)
r. appendicitis
r. bleeding
r. bouts of vomiting
r. calcium-containing stones
r. calcium stone formation
r. calcium urolithiasis (RCU)
r. cholestasis
r. colonic histoplasmosis
r. colorectal cancer (RCRC)
r. cystitis
r. episodes of *Clostridium difficile* disease (RCCD)
r. focal sclerosing glomerulonephritis
r. molar pregnancy
r. pancreatitis
r. pyogenic cholangiohepatitis (RPC)
r. stress incontinence
r. stricture
r. ulcer
r. urinary calculus
r. urinary tract infection
RED
rectal evacuatory disorder
red
r. blood cell cast
r. blood cell count
r. blood cell extravasation
r. blood cell folate
r. blood cell folate level
r. blood cells (RBC)
r. cell distribution width (RDW)
r. color sign (RCS)
r. degeneration of uterine myoma
r. flag sign
pseudocolor fluorescence of Fura r.
r. ring sign
r. rubber Robinson catheter
ruthenium r.
r. wale marking
Reddick cystic duct cholangiogram catheter
Reddick-Saye
R.-S. method
R.-S. screw
Redfield infrared coagulator
Redipen
Redivac suction drain
Rediwash skin cleanser
Redman approach
redness
diffuse r. (DR)

NOTES

Redo intestinal clamp
Redon drain
red-out
redox potential
reduced
    r. graft survival rate
    r. liver transplant (RLT)
    r. motility
    r. rejection episode
reduced-size
    r.-s. graft
    r.-s. liver transplant (RSLT)
reducible hernia
reducing
    r. diet
    r. substance
    r. substances test
reductase
    aldose r. (AR)
    hepatic 3-methylglutaryl coenzyme A r. (HMG-CoA)
    5,10-methylene-tetrahydrofolate r. (MTHFR)
reduction
    air pressure enema r.
    barium enema r.
    dissimilatory sulfate r.
    r. en masse
    gastric acidity r.
    hemorrhoid r.
    hepatic venous pressure gradient r.
    profound acid r.
    proportionate r.
    sigmoid loop r.
    volvulus r.
redundant sac tissue
Redux
Redy hemodialysis system
REE
    resting energy expenditure
reefing
    stomach r.
reentry
reexamined
    retrospectively r.
reexploration
refeeding
    casein r.
    r. syndrome
reference value
referred pain
refill
    capillary r.
    delayed capillary r.
refined carbohydrate complex
refining surgical technique
reflectance
    r. analysis
    endoscopic r.
    r. spectrophotometer
    r. spectrophotometric probe
    r. spectrophotometry
    r. spectroscopy
    r. TS-200 spectrum analyzer
reflecting edge of ligament
reflection
    colon medial r.
    hepatoduodenal r.
    hepatoduodenal-peritoneal r.
    peritoneal r.
    total internal r.
reflex
    absent gag r.
    anal r.
    anocutaneous r.
    axon r.
    Babinski r.
    Barrington third r.
    bladder cooling r.
    blinking r.
    r. bradycardia
    bulbocavernosus r. (BCR)
    cardioesophageal r.
    celiac plexus r.
    consensual r.
    corneal r.
    cremasteric r.
    cutaneous r.
    deep tendon r.
    deglutition r.
    descending inhibitory r.
    detrusodetrusor facilitative r.
    r. detrusor contraction
    detrusosphincteric inhibitory r.
    detrusourethral inhibitory r.
    diminished gag r.
    r. dyspepsia
    emetic r.
    enteric neuronal r.
    enterogastric r.
    epigastric r.
    r. erection
    esophagosalivary r.
    fencing r.
    gag r.
    Galant r.
    gastrocolic r.
    gastroileac r.
    gastroileal r.
    gastropancreatic r.
    glabella r.
    guarding r.
    gustatory-salivary r.
    r. HPV test
    ileogastric r.
    r. incontinence
    infant r.
    inhibitory intestinointestinal r.

intestinogastric r.
intramural secretory r.
intrinsic r.
Landau r.
light r.
masticatory-salivary r.
micturition r.
Moro r.
myenteric r.
r. neurogenic bladder
r. neuropathic bladder
orienting r.
parachute r.
penile r.
penis r.
perineobulbar detrusor facilitative r.
perineobulbar detrusor inhibitory r.
perineodetrusor inhibitory r.
peristaltic r.
polarized standing r.
polysynaptic r.
pontine-sacral r.
primary vesicoureteral r.
pudendal-anal r.
r. pylorospasm
rectal inhibitory r.
rectoanal inhibitory r. (RAIR)
rectosphincteric r. (RSR)
renal r.
renointestinal r.
renorenal r.
Roger r.
rooting r.
scrotal r.
secondary vesicoureteral r.
secretory r.
sexual r.
single lens r. (SLR)
skin-CNS-bladder r.
somatointestinal r.
spinobulbospinal micturition r.
r. splanchnic vasoconstriction
stepping r.
swallowing r.
r. sympathetic dystrophy
sympathetic enteroenteric inhibitory r.
sympathetic sphincter constrictor r.
thermal sphincteric r.
urethrodetrusor facilitative r.
urethrosphincteric guarding r.
urethrosphincteric inhibitory r.
urethrosphincteric recruitment r.
urinary continence r.
vasovagal r.
vesicoanal r.
vesicointestinal r.
virile r.
visceral traction r.
viscerosensory r.
r. voiding
r. voiding dysfunction
von Mering r.
wake r.
wink r.
reflexogenic erection
reflux
acid r.
antiperistaltic r.
bile r.
r. bile gastritis
cecoileal r.
cholangiovenous r.
contralateral r.
delayed vesicoureteral r.
r. disease
duodenal gastroesophageal r. (DGER)
duodenobiliary r.
duodenogastric r. (DGR)
duodenogastroesophageal r. (DGER)
duodenopancreatic r.
r. dyspepsia
ejaculatory duct r.
esophageal r.
r. esophagitis (RE)
r. esophagitis classification I–IV
free r.
gastroesophageal r. (GER)
gastrointestinal r.
hepatojugular r.
Hinman r.
ileal r.
intrarenal r.
r. laryngitis
r. morbidity
nasopharyngeal r.
r. nephropathy
r. neuropathy
nocturnal acid r.
nocturnal gastric r.
nondilating r.
pancreaticobiliary r.
pathologic r.

NOTES

reflux *(continued)*
    peptic r.
    postmyotomy r.
    postoperative r.
    pyelorenal r.
    pyelotubular r.
    Roux gastric r.
    scintigraphic r.
    r. small bowel examination
    r. symptom
    ureterorenal r.
    vesicoileal r.
    vesicoureteral r. (VUR)
    vesicoureteric r.
    vesicourethral r.
refluxant
refluxate
refluxlike dyspepsia
reflux-related stricture
refraction
refractory
    r. anemia with excess blasts (RAEB)
    r. anemia with ringed sideroblasts (RARS)
    r. ascites
    r. duodenal ulcer
    r. esophagitis
    r. hypertension
    r. motor urge incontinence
    r. pouch inflammation
    r. pouchitis
    r. proctosigmoiditis
    r. sideroblastic anemia
    r. sprue
    r. variceal hemorrhage
refrigerant diuretic
Regan isoenzyme
regeneration
    bladder r.
    carbon tetrachloride-induced liver r.
    tubular r.
regenerative cirrhotic nodule
regimen
    antireflux r.
    bismuth triple r.
    bowel-emptying r.
    calcineurin inhibitor-free immunosuppressive r.
    dietetic r.
    immunosuppressive r.
    multidrug r.
    sequential quadruple-drug r.
    Shorr r.
    three-drug r.
region
    abdominal r.
    antropyloroduodenal r.
    capsid-encoding r.
    choledochal r.
    floor of inguinal r.
    gastric pacemaker r.
    genitourinary r.
    hepatic hilar r.
    hydrophobic binding r.
    hypervariable r. 1 (HVR1)
    hypochondriac r.
    hypogastric r.
    ileocecal r.
    inframammary r.
    interpolar r.
    intertriginous r.
    ischiorectal r.
    lateral abdominal r.
    nonpolar r.
    pancreatobiliary r.
    paraaortic r.
    perianal r.
    perineal r.
    periumbilical r.
    polar r.
    rectosigmoid r.
    retroperitoneal r.
    substernal r.
    suprainguinal r.
    suprapubic r.
    umbilical r.
    ureteropelvic r.
    urogenital r.
regional
    r. colitis
    r. enteritis (RE)
    r. enterocolitis
    r. heparinization
    r. ileitis (RI)
    R. Organ Procurement Agency (ROPA)
registration
    transcutaneous r.
registry
    Michigan Kidney R.
Regitine
Reglan
Regressin
regression
    r. analysis
    linear r.
    lymphocele spontaneous r.
    Poisson r.
    spontaneous r.
Regroton
regucalcin
regular diet
regularly
    bowels open r. (BOR)
regulated upon activation, normal T cells expressed and secreted (RANTES)

regulation
    autocrine r.
    follicle-stimulating hormone inhibin r.
    growth r.
regulator
    cystic fibrosis transductance r.
    cystic fibrosis transmembrane conductance r. (CFTR)
regulatory peptide
Regulax SS
regurgitant
regurgitation
    acid r.
    chronic r.
    r. jaundice
    nocturnal r.
    postural r.
    vesicoureteral r.
Regutol
rehabilitation
    pelvic floor r.
    renal r.
    sexual r.
Rehfuss
    R. duodenal tube
    R. method
    R. stomach tube
    R. test
Rehne abdominal retractor
Rehne-Delorme plication
Rehydralyte
rehydrating solution (RS)
rehydration
    oral r.
    r. therapy
Reichel-Pólya
    R.-P. stomach procedure
    R.-P. stomach resection
Reichert
    R. FLPS-series flexible fiberoptic sigmoidoscope
    R. MS-series flexible fiberoptic sigmoidoscope
    R. SC-series flexible fiberoptic sigmoidoscope
Reichmann
    R. disease
    R. rod
    R. syndrome
Reich-Nechtow forceps
Reifenstein syndrome

reimplantation
    aortorenal r.
    Cohen cross-trigonal r.
    end-to-side r.
    extravesical r.
    Leadbetter-Politano r.
    Paquin ureteral r.
    ureteral r.
    ureteric r.
REIN
    Ramipril Efficacy in Nephropathy REIN study
reinforcement
    Gore-Tex sling r.
    responsibility r.
reinforcing suture
Reinke crystal
reinsertion
reintervention rate
reintroduction
reintubation
Reitan Trail-Making test
Reiter
    R. disease
    R. syndrome
Reitman-Frankel test
rejection
    accelerated transplant r.
    acute cellular r.
    acute humoral r. (AHR)
    acute humoral renal allograft r.
    acute vascular r.
    allograft r.
    r. cholangitis
    chronic allograft r.
    chronic transplant r.
    clinical r.
    delayed hyperacute transplant r.
    ductopenic r.
    higher incidence of r.
    hyperacute r.
    incidence of acute r.
    interstitial r.
    no r. (NR)
    renal allograft r.
    renal transplantation r.
    steroid-resistant r.
    subclinical r.
    transmural r.
    transplant r.
    tubulointerstitial r.

NOTES

rejection *(continued)*
    vascular r.
    xenograft r.
relapsing
    r. acute pancreatitis
    r. appendicitis
related
    incontinence r.
    r. living donor (RLD)
relationship
    dyadic r.
    endoscope-body position r.
    intraluminal pH-pressure r.
    r. of recipient
relative
    first-degree r.
    r. sterility
    r. supersaturation (RSs)
relatively minimal complication
relaxant
    cGMP-mediated r.
    musculotropic r.
    smooth muscle r.
relaxation
    adaptive r.
    bladder stress r.
    cardioesophageal r.
    endothelial-dependent r.
    esophageal sphincter r.
    incomplete r.
    LES r.
    lower esophageal sphincter r. (LESR)
    nitric oxide-blocked sphincter r.
    non–swallow-associated r.
    pelvic floor r.
    pelvic girdle r. (PGR)
    receptive r.
    stress r.
    r. suture
    r. technique
    transient LES r.
    transient lower esophageal sphincter r. (TLESR)
    upper esophageal sphincter r. (UESR)
    vagovagally mediated receptive r.
relaxatory response
relaxin
    recombinant human r.
relaxing incision
Relay suture delivery system
release
    extended r. (XL, XR)
    G-cell gastrin r.
    nifedipine extended r.
    paranitroaniline r.
    renin r.
    stimulated r.
    tethered-cord r.
    twin-pulse shock wave r.
Release-NF catheter
relevant gastroduodenal findings
reliability
    interobserver r.
    penile prothesis r.
reliable percutaneous renal access
Relia-Flow device
Reliance urinary control insert
ReliaSeal skin barrier
Relia-Vac drain
relief
    Peptic R.
Reliquet lithotrite
relocation
    polyp r.
REM
    return electrode monitor
REMBL
    retroflexed endoscopic multiple band ligation
Remegel Soft Chewable Antacid
remethylation
Remicade IV infusion
remission of pain
remnant
    cloacal r.
    gastric r.
    mesonephric r.
    müllerian r.
    prostatic mesonephric r.
remodeling reestablished tissue strength
removal
    colonoscopic r.
    cut-and-push method of PEG tube r.
    endoscopic stone r.
    forceps r.
    foreign body r.
    gastric coin r.
    Lithovac stone r.
    percutaneous endoscopic r.
    percutaneous stone r.
    peritoneal dialysis urea r.
    radical en bloc r.
    small polyp r.
    through-the-scope balloon r.
    tube r.
    ureteral stoma r.
remover
    Detachol adhesive r.
    Macaluso stent r.
Renacidin irrigation
Renaflo hollow-fiber dialyzer
Renagel tablet
renal
    r. absorption of calcium
    r. acid excretion

r. adenocarcinoma
r. afferent arteriolar resistance
r. afferent nerve
r. agenesis
r. allograft
r. allograft infection
r. allograft recipient
r. allograft rejection
r. allograft rupture
r. allograft survival
r. aminoaciduria
r. ammonium excretion
r. amyloidosis
r. angiography
r. angiomyolipoma
r. anuria
r. arterial occlusive disease
r. arteriography
r. arteriole
r. arteriovenous fistula
r. artery (RA)
r. artery aneurysm
r. artery cholesterol embolization
r. artery diameter
r. artery embolectomy
r. artery embolism
r. artery graft
r. artery stenosis
r. artery stent
r. artery thrombosis
r. autoregulation
r. autoregulatory ability
r. autoregulatory mechanism
r. autotransplantation
r. baroreceptor
r. biopsy
r. blastema
r. blood flow (RBF)
r. bone disease
r. calcium leak
r. capsular flap
r. capsule
r. capsulotomy
r. carbuncle
r. carcinosarcoma
r. cell carcinoma (RCC)
r. cholesterol embolus
r. clearance
r. coagulation necrosis
r. colic
r. collecting duct cell
r. complication

r. concentrating defect
r. congestion
r. corpuscles
r. cortex
r. corticoadrenal
r. cryoablation
r. cryptococcosis
r. cyst decortication
r. cyst hemorrhage
r. cystic disease
r. cyst infection
r. cyst marsupialization
r. descensus
r. deterioration
r. dialysis
r. duplication
r. ectopia
r. endarterectomy
r. endothelin
r. epistaxis
r. excretion of acid
r. excretion of calcium
r. exploration
r. failure
r. failure index
r. Fanconi-like syndrome
r. fascia
r. fibroma
r. fibromuscular disease
r. function
r. function study (RFS)
r. gallium-67 scintigraphy
r. glomeruli
r. glucosuria
r. hamartoma
r. helical CT (RHCT)
r. helical CT imaging
r. hemangioma
r. hematoma
r. hematuria
r. hemodynamics
r. hemophilia
r. hilar dissection
r. hilum
r. hilus
r. histologic section
r. histopathology
r. homotransplantation
r. hydatid disease
r. hydatidosis
r. hypercalciuria
r. hyperchloremia acidosis

NOTES

renal *(continued)*
- r. hyperfiltration
- r. hypertension
- r. hypertrophy
- r. hypoperfusion
- r. hyposthenuria
- r. hypothermia
- r. impression
- r. impression on liver
- r. injury repair
- r. insufficiency
- r. interstitium
- r. involvement
- r. ischemia
- r. kallikrein-kinin system
- r. labyrinth
- r. lithiasis
- r. lobe
- r. lymphoblastoma
- r. mass
- r. medicine
- r. medulla
- r. messenger ribonucleic acid
- r. messenger ribonucleoprotein acid
- r. morphometric analysis
- r. obstruction
- r. oncocytoma
- r. osteodystrophy
- r. papilla
- r. papillary necrosis (RPN)
- r. parenchyma
- r. parenchymal damage
- r. pathology
- r. pedicle
- r. pelvis
- r. pelvis calculus
- r. percutaneous transluminal angioplasty
- r. perfusion pressure
- r. perfusion pressure-flow study
- r. perfusion scintigraphy
- r. phosphate
- r. phosphate excretion
- r. physiology
- r. plasma flow (RPF)
- r. pouch
- r. preservation
- r. preservation-perfusion system
- r. progression
- r. prostaglandin
- r. proximal tubular cell
- r. proximal tubule preparation
- r. ptosis
- r. pyramid
- r. reflex
- r. rehabilitation
- r. replacement therapy
- r. resistive index
- r. revascularization
- r. rhabdosarcoma
- r. rickets
- r. sarcoidosis
- r. scan
- r. scanning
- r. scarring
- r. segmental renal dysplasia
- r. sinus
- r. sinus cyst
- r. sodium
- r. sodium excretion
- r. sodium retention
- r. sodium wasting
- r. sonography
- r. stab wound
- r. stone
- r. stone formation
- r. structural damage
- r. sympathetic activity
- r. sympathetic nerve
- r. sympathetic nerve activity recording electrode
- R. System HF250 filter
- r. thromboendarterectomy
- r. tissue kallikrein expression
- r. toxicity
- r. transduction pathway
- r. transplant
- r. transplantation
- r. transplantation rejection
- r. transplant patient
- r. transplant recipient
- r. trauma
- r. tuberculosis
- r. tubular acidosis (RTA)
- r. tubular epithelium
- r. tubular fluid
- r. tubular metabolic acidosis
- r. tubular necrosis
- r. tubular sodium handling
- r. tubular type I–IV acidosis (RTA-I–IV)
- r. tubule
- r. tubule epithelial cell
- r. tumorlike pyonephrosis with foreign body
- r. ultrasonogram
- r. vasculitis
- r. vasoconstriction
- r. vasodilation
- r. vasodilator
- r. vasodilator prostaglandin
- r. vein
- r. vein renin
- r. vein renin activity (RVRA)
- r. vein renin assay (RVRA)
- r. vein renin concentration (RVRC)
- r. vein renin ratio
- r. vein thrombosis

r. venogram
r. venography
r. venous outflow compression
vertebral, anal, tracheoesophageal fistula, r. (VATER)
r. volume
r. xanthine oxidase-xanthine dehydrogenase activity

renale
    hilum r.

renales
    columnae r.

renal-hepatic steal syndrome
Renalin dialyzer
renalis
    fascia r.
    hilum r.
    plexus r.

renal-ocular syndrome
renal-retinal syndrome
renal-sparing surgery
Renalyzer
Renatron dialyzer
Renax film-coated caplet
rendezvous
    pancreatic r.
    r. technique
    r. technique for treatment of choledocholithiasis

Rendu-Osler-Weber
    R.-O.-W. disease
    R.-O.-W. syndrome

Renese
renewal
    epithelial restitution and r.
    tissue r.

renicapsule
renicardiac
reniculus, pl. **reniculi**
renin
    active r.
    r. inhibition
    plasma r.
    r. release
    renal vein r.
    r. secretion
    r. stimulation test
    r. synthesis

renin-aldosterone system
renin-angiotensin
    r.-a. system (RAS)
    r.-a. system blocker

renin-angiotensin-aldosterone
    r.-a.-a. axis
    r.-a.-a. system (RAAS)

renin-mediated renovascular hypertension
reninoma
renin-secreting juxtaglomerular cell tumor
renipelvic transitional cell carcinoma
reniportal anastomosis
renipuncture
renis
    capsula adiposa r.
    capsula fibrosa r.
    porta r.
    venulae rectae r.

Rennes variant galactosemia
renocortical
    r. abscess
    r. adenoma
    r. malondialdehyde content
    r. necrosis
    r. scintigraphy
    r. tubule cell

renogastric fistula
Renografin
renogram
    captopril r.
    furosemide washout r.
    isotope r.
    MDT r.

renography
    captopril r.
    captopril-enhanced r.
    diethylenetriamine pentaacetic acid r.
    diuretic nuclear r.
    DTPA r.
    isotope r.
    radioisotope r.

renointestinal reflex
Reno-M contrast medium
renomedullary
    r. carcinoma
    r. interstitial cell (RMIC)

renomegaly
renopathy
renoprival
renoprotective agent
renopulmonary
Renoquid
renorenal reflex

NOTES

renorrhaphy
renotrophic
renotropic
renotropin
renovascular
    r. disease
    r. hypertension
    r. hypertrophy
    r. injury
    r. obstruction
    r. resistance (RVR)
    r. resistance index (RVRI)
    r. surgery
    r. tone
Renovist Injection
Renovue 65
Renu enteral feeding
renzapride
reoperation
    lower abdominal r.
    r. rate
reoperative ureteroneocystostomy
reovirus
reoxygenation
repaglinide
repair (*See also* operation, procedure)
    Alliston GE reflux r.
    Altemeier r.
    anal sphincter r.
    anastomotic r.
    Asopa hypospadias r.
    Barcat-Redman hypospadias r.
    Bassini inguinal hernia r.
    Belsey Mark IV r.
    Belt-Fuqua hypospadias r.
    Boari ureteral flap r.
    Boerema hernia r.
    bulboprostatic r.
    Cantwell-Ransley epispadias r.
    Cecil r.
    cloacal exstrophy one-stage r.
    cloacal exstrophy two-stage r.
    Collis r.
    cross-trigonal r.
    Devine-Horton flip-flap for hypospadias r.
    Devine hypospadias r.
    double-faced island flap for hypospadias r.
    DualMesh hernia r.
    end-to-end anastomotic r.
    epispadias r.
    extracorporeal r.
    first-stage r.
    Halsted-Bassini hernia r.
    hernia r.
    Hill esophageal antireflux r.
    Hill hiatus hernia r.
    Hill median arcuate r.
    Horton-Devine flip-flap hypospadias r.
    hydrocele r.
    intraperitoneal onlay mesh hernia r. (IPOM)
    Judd ventral hernia r.
    Koyanagi technique for hypospadias r.
    laparoscopic renal artery aneurysm r.
    laparoscopic varicocele r.
    LaRoque r.
    Lich-Gregoire r.
    Lichtenstein hernia r.
    Limberg flap r.
    Madden r.
    Marlex hernial r.
    McVay inguinal hernial r.
    Mitchell technique for epispadias r.
    Moschcowitz vaginal prolapse r.
    Mustarde hypospadias r.
    mutation mismatch r. (MMR)
    neonatal exstrophic bladder r.
    Nissen r.
    omphalocele r.
    one-stage hypospadias r.
    Orr rectal prolapse r.
    pants-over-vest hernia r.
    Paquin r.
    paravaginal fascial r.
    postanal r.
    Ransley-Cantwell r.
    renal injury r.
    reverse sigma penoscrotal transposition r.
    Rodney Smith biliary stricture r.
    slipped Nissen r.
    sphincter r.
    Stoppa r.
    TAPP hernia r.
    tension-free cystocele r.
    TEP hernia r.
    Thal esophageal stricture r.
    Thiersch-Duplay r.
    tight Nissen r.
    timing of r.
    totally extraperitoneal hernia r.
    transabdominal preperitoneal hernia r.
    transvaginal mesh cystocele r.
    two-stage r.
    ureteropelvic junction obstruction r.
    vaginal r.
    varicocele r.
    vascular laceration r.
    vest-over-pants hernial r.
    VVF r.
    Young epispadias r.

repeat
- direct r.
- r. exploration
- long terminal r. (LTR)
- r. operation
- r. procedure
- r. sequence
- terminal r. (TR)

repeated complete mole

repens
- *Serenoa r.*

reperfusion injury
reperitonealization
Repetabs
- Trinalin R.

replaced hepatic vessel
replacement
- antegrade stent r.
- bladder r.
- buccal mucosal urethral r.
- r. enzyme protein
- gastric bladder r.
- intestinal ureteral r.
- r. PEG
- tube r.
- tunica r.
- volume r.

Replete liquid nutrition
replication
- r. error phenotype
- gastric epithelial cell r.
- viral r.

replicator
- Steers r.

Repliform dermal allograft
Replogle tube
repopulation
- clonogenic r.

report
- human case r.

Rep-Pred
repreparation
representative electrophoretic mobility shift assay
reprocessor
- American Endoscopy automatic r.
- automatic endoscopic r. (AER)
- Bard automatic r.
- Custom Ultrasonic automatic r.
- ECI automatic r.
- KeyMed automatic r.
- Lutz automatic r.
- Medivator automatic r.
- Olympus automatic r.
- Orr automatic r.
- Steris automatic r.

reproduction
- assisted r.

reproductive
- r. axis
- r. system

reptilase acid
required transfusion
requirement
- analgesic r.
- minimum daily r. (MDR)
- postoperative analgesia r.

re-reflux
rescinnamine
rescue
- fluorouracil, Adriamycin, methotrexate with leucovorin r. (FAMTX)
- leucovorin r.
- r. therapy
- uridine r.

research
- r. application
- biomedical r.

resectable
resection
- abdominoperineal r. (APR)
- abdominosacral r.
- anterior r.
- antral r.
- bladder neck transurethral r.
- bowel r.
- cap-assisted r.
- cold cup r.
- colon cancer r.
- colorectal r.
- colosigmoid r.
- continence-preserving r.
- curative tumor r.
- cutting endoscopic mucosal r. (C-EMR)
- cylindrical mucosal r.
- diathermic r.
- duodenum-preserving pancreatic head r.
- ejaculatory duct transurethral r.
- elective r.
- electrocautery r.
- en bloc endoscopic r.

NOTES

resection *(continued)*
    en bloc vein r.
    endoscopic mucosal r. (EMR)
    endoscopic snare r.
    esophageal r.
    fluidjet technology-assisted mucosal r.
    free r.
    gastric r. (GR)
    hepatic r.
    ileal r. (IR)
    ileocecal r.
    ileocolic r.
    intersphincteric r.
    laparoscopic abdominoperineal r.
    laparoscopically assisted colorectal r.
    laparoscopic ultralow anterior r.
    lift-and-cut endoscopic mucosal r. (LC-EMR)
    liver r.
    Lortat-Jacob hepatic r.
    low anterior r. (LAR)
    Mason abdominotranssphincteric r.
    Miles abdominoperineal r.
    mucosal sleeve r.
    open transurethral r.
    pancreatic tail r.
    Paul-Mikulicz r.
    percutaneous r.
    piecemeal r.
    prostate gland transurethral r.
    Reichel-Pólya stomach r.
    second r.
    segmental colonic r.
    snare r.
    spermatocele r.
    strip r.
    suture rectopexy with sigmoid r.
    r. syndrome ranging
    terminal ileal r.
    r. time
    total transurethral r. of prostate (T-TURP)
    transanal endoscopic microsurgical r.
    transhiatal r.
    transurethral r. (TUR)
    transverse r.
    wedge r.
    Whipple r.
resective colostomy
resectoscopy
resedation
reserpine
    hydrochlorothiazide and r.
reserpine-induced ulcer
reservoir
    Camey r.
    colonic J-pouch r.
    continent cutaneous r.
    continent ileal r.
    detubularized right colon r.
    double-barrel r.
    double J-shaped r.
    double-stapled ileal r.
    fecal r.
    Florida pouch urinary r.
    Hadera continent r.
    Hoffmann-Steinberg gastric r.
    Hunt-Limo-Basto gastric r.
    ileal r.
    ileoanal r.
    ileocecal continent urinary r.
    Indiana continent r.
    intraabdominal ileal r.
    inverted U-pouch ileal r.
    isoperistaltic ileal r.
    J r.
    J-shaped ileal r.
    J-Vac suction r.
    Kock r.
    lateral internal pelvic r.
    Lawrence gastric r.
    Le Bag pouch r.
    Mainz pouch urinary r.
    r. mucosal absorption
    orthotopic colonic r.
    orthotopic continent r.
    orthotopic remodeled ileocolonic r.
    Parks ileal r.
    Parks ileoanal r.
    r. phase
    rectal r.
    S r.
    sigmoid colon r.
    spherical r.
    S-shaped r.
    Studer crossfolded ileal r.
    r. of underdiagnosed and misdiagnosed interstitial cystitis
    W-stapled urinary r.
reset osmostat syndrome
Resident Assessment Protocol for incontinence
residua *(pl. of* residuum)
residual
    r. albuminuria
    r. barium
    r. chordee
    r. fragment
    postvoid r. (PVR)
    r. proteinuria
    r. rectoperineal fistula
    r. stone
    r. stool
    r. urine
    r. urine volume (RUV)

residue
    dibasic amino acid r.
    fecal r.
    food r.
    sialic acid r.
    sialyl r.
residue
    histidine r.
residuum, pl. residua
    gastric r.
resin
    anion exchange r.
    bile salt-binding r.
    cation exchange r.
    Epon 812 r.
    potassium-binding r.
resinifera
    Euphorbia r.
resiniferatoxin therapy
resipump
resistance (R)
    activated protein C r. (APCR)
    amphotericin B r.
    antimicrobial r.
    basal renal vascular r.
    cancer drug r.
    drug r.
    hepatic arterial vascular r.
    insulin r.
    mean electrosurgical r.
    r. monomicrobial biofilm
    peripheral vascular r.
    reactance and r. (Xc/R)
    renal afferent arteriolar r.
    renovascular r. (RVR)
    retrospective analysis of antimicrobial r.
    R factor in bacterial antimicrobial r.
    systemic vascular r. (SVR)
    tissue r.
    transhepatic vascular r.
    urethral r.
    vesical neck r.
    vitamin D r.
resistant
    r. ascites
    r. to electrosurgical perforation
    r. organism
resistin
resistive index (RI)
Resol electrolyte solution

resolution
    spatial r.
    spontaneous r.
resonance
    endoscopic magnetic r. (EMR)
    gadolinium-enhancement magnetic r.
    hydatid r.
    magnetic r.
    nuclear magnetic r. (NMR)
    tympanitic r.
    vesiculotympanitic r.
    wooden r.
resonant abdomen
resorbable thread clip applicator
resorption
    tubular r.
resorptive hypercalciuria
resource
    R. Arginaid powder
    R. Diabetic
    R. Diabetic ready-to-use liquid
    R. enteral feeding
    R. Fruit Beverage
    R. Fruit Beverage ready-to-use liquid
    R. Just for Kids
    R. Just for Kids ready-to-use liquid
    medical r.
    R. oral liquid
    R. Plus
respiration pyelography
respiratory
    r. acidosis
    r. alkalosis
    r. burst
    r. burst activity
    r. depression
    r. distress
    r. distress syndrome
    r. embarrassment
    r. excursion
    r. failure
    r. inversion point (RIP)
    r. pyelography
    r. rate
    r. symptoms (RS)
respiratory-esophageal fistula
response
    alloantigen r.
    ameliorated vasodilating r.
    antibody-directed cytotoxic r.

NOTES

response *(continued)*
    apoptotic r.
    bellow r.
    cell-mediated immunohistological r.
    cellular immune r.
    cytotoxic T-cell r.
    desmoplastic r.
    desmopressin r.
    dysregulated immune r.
    effector r.
    fed r.
    gag r.
    humoral antibody r.
    hypercontractile external sphincter r.
    immune r.
    inflammatory r.
    macrophage-rich inflammatory r.
    maladaptive r.
    paradoxical renal r.
    peak r.
    plateau r.
    r. rate to chemotherapy
    relaxatory r.
    sacral evoked r.
    skin sympathetic r.
    sustained virologic r. (SVR)
    sympathetic skin r.
    Th1 r.
    therapeutic r.
responsibility reinforcement
responsiveness
    vasculature r.
rest
    adrenal r.
    bowel r. (BR)
    ectopic adrenal r.
    gut r.
    Krause arm r.
    nephrogenic r.
    pancreatic r.
    testicular adrenal r.
    total bowel r.
restaging of cancer
restenosis
resting
    r. anal sphincter pressure
    r. energy expenditure (REE)
    r. membrane potential
    r. tremor
    r. urethral pressure profile
restless leg syndrome (RLS)
restoration
    foreskin r.
    voice r.
restorative
    r. proctocolectomy (RP, RPC)
    r. proctocolectomy operation
Restoril

restricted
    HLA class II r.
restriction
    dietary protein r.
    r. endonuclease
    r. enzyme
    fluid r.
    r. fragment length polymorphism (RFLP, RLP)
    intrauterine growth r. (IUGR)
    protein r.
    putative host r.
    sodium r.
result
    contradictory r.
    long-term r.
    medium-term r.
    poor long-term r.
    positive culture r.
    previous in vitro r.
    short-term r.
    Surveillance, Epidemiology, and End R.'s (SEER)
    tactile feedback r.
    r.'s in tissue damage
    tissue destruction r.
    transurethral microwave thermotherapy functional r.
    transurethral resection of prostate functional r.
    TUMT functional r.
    TURP functional r.
resuscitation
    fluid r.
retained
    r. antrum
    r. antrum syndrome
    r. barium
    r. bladder syndrome
    r. feces
    r. foreign body (RFB)
    r. gallstone
    r. testicle
    r. testis
retainer
    Mectra tissue sample r.
retardata
    ejaculatio r.
retardation
    triad of adenoma sebaceum, epilepsy, and mental r.
    Wilms tumor, aniridia, genitourinary abnormalities, and mental r. (WAGR)
retch
retching
rete, pl. **retia**
    r. peg
    r. ridge

r. testis
r. testis adenocarcinoma
RE-TEM
rectal expander-assisted transanal endoscopic microsurgery
retention
acute urinary r. (AUR)
r. band
barium r.
BSP r.
chronic urinary r. (CUR)
crystal r.
r. cyst
r. enema
r. esophagitis
gastric r. (GR)
r. jaundice
r. meal
r. polyp
postoperative urinary r.
renal sodium r.
sodium r.
stool r.
r. suture
r. uremia
urinary r.
r. vomiting
retethering
retia (*pl. of* rete)
retial
reticula (*pl. of* reticulum)
reticularis
formatio r.
zona r.
reticulin antigen
reticulocyte hemoglobin content
reticuloendothelial system
reticulonodular pattern
reticulosis
polymorphic r.
reticulum, pl. **reticula**
endoplasmic r.
sarcoplasmic r.
retinaculum, pl. **retinacula**
Morgagni r.
retinal
r. artery occlusion
r. vein occlusion
retinitis
albuminuric r.
retinoblastoma
retinoic acid

retinoid
acyclic r.
r. chaperone
r. transport
r. X receptor (RXR)
retinoid-binding protein
retinol-binding protein (RBP)
retinol concentration
retinopathy of prematurity
retinyl ester clearance
RET protooncogene
retracted stoma
retractile
r. concealed penis
r. mesenteritis
r. testis
retraction
bladder r.
downward r.
foreskin manual r.
retractor
Airlift balloon r.
Army-Navy r.
Aronson esophageal r.
baby Balfour r.
Balfour abdominal r.
Balfour self-retaining r.
Barr rectal r.
Beardsley esophageal r.
B.E. Glass abdominal r.
Berens esophageal r.
Berkeley-Bonney r.
Bookwalter-Goulet r.
Bookwalter-Hill-Ferguson rectal r.
Bookwalter ring r.
Bookwalter-St. Mark deep pelvic r.
Breisky-Navratil straight r.
Buie-Smith r.
Christie gallbladder r.
Cole duodenal r.
Collin abdominal r.
Collin intestinal r.
Crile angle r.
Crile malleable r.
Cushing vein r.
Deaver r.
DeBakey-Cooley r.
Denis Browne abdominal r.
Doyen abdominal r.
fan elevator r.
fan-type laparoscopic r.
Farabeuf r.

NOTES

retractor *(continued)*
- Ferguson anal r.
- Ferguson-Moon rectal r.
- Finochietto r.
- fixed ring r.
- Foerster abdominal ring r.
- Forder r.
- Foss bifid gallbladder r.
- Foss biliary duct r.
- Franz abdominal r.
- Friedman perineal r.
- Fritsch r.
- gallows-type r.
- Gazayerli endoscopic r.
- Gelpi self-retaining r.
- Gibson-Balfour abdominal r.
- Gil-Vernet r.
- Goelet r.
- Goligher r.
- Gosset appendectomy r.
- Grant gallbladder r.
- Greene r.
- Greishaber self-retaining r.
- handheld r.
- Haney r.
- Harrington Deaver r.
- Harrington splanchnic r.
- Heaney r.
- hilar r.
- Hill-Ferguson rectal r.
- Hill rectal r.
- illuminated St. Mark r.
- Israel r.
- Jansen r.
- Johns Hopkins gallbladder r.
- Kelly abdominal r.
- Kirschner abdominal r.
- Kocher gallbladder r.
- Lone Star r.
- Lowsley r.
- malleable r.
- Mayo abdominal r.
- Mayo-Adams appendectomy r.
- McBurney r.
- Mediflex-Gazayerli r.
- metal bar r.
- Mikulicz r.
- Miller-Senn r.
- Millin bladder r.
- Moon rectal r.
- Murphy gallbladder r.
- Nathanson liver r.
- Nuttall liver r.
- Ochsner r.
- Oettingen abdominal r.
- Omnitract r.
- O'Sullivan-O'Connor abdominal r.
- Parker r.
- Parks r.
- Percy-Wolfson gallbladder r.
- Polytrac Gomez r.
- Pratt bivalve r.
- Quervain abdominal r.
- rake r.
- Rehne abdominal r.
- ribbon r.
- Richards abdominal r.
- Richardson appendectomy r.
- Rigby appendectomy r.
- ring abdominal r.
- Robin-Masse abdominal r.
- Roux r.
- Sawyer rectal r.
- Scott r.
- self-retaining ring r.
- Senn r.
- Senn-Kanavel r.
- Smith-Buie rectal r.
- Smith rectal r.
- Space-OR flexible internal r.
- spoon r.
- spring-wire r.
- Stamey dorsal vein apical r.
- T-bar r.
- Theis self-retaining r.
- Tuffier abdominal r.
- Upper Hands r.
- U.S. Army double-ended r.
- vein r.
- Volkmann rake r.
- Walker gallbladder r.
- Webb-Balfour abdominal r.
- Weinberg vagotomy r.
- Weitlaner r.
- Wesson perineal r.
- Wexler r.
- Wickham r.
- Wilkinson abdominal r.
- Wishbone Omni-Track r.
- Wolfson gallbladder r.
- Wylie splanchnic r.
- Young prostatic r.
- Yu-Holtgrewe prostatic r.

retransplantation

retreatment
- lithotripsy r.
- r. rate

retrieval
- r. balloon
- r. basket
- specimen r.
- spermatozoon r.

retriever
- Positrap r.
- snail-headed catheter r.
- Soehendra stent r.
- stone r.
- three-pronged polyp r.

retrocaval ureter
retrocecal
- r. abscess
- r. appendicitis
- r. appendix

retrocecalis tumor thrombus
retrocolic
- r. anastomosis
- r. end-to-end pancreatojejunostomy
- r. end-to-side choledochojejunostomy
- r. fossa

retroduodenal
- r. artery
- r. artery severance
- r. perforation

retroesophageal abscess
retroflexed
- r. cystoscopy sheath
- r. endoscopic multiple band ligation (REMBL)
- r. scope
- r. uterus
- r. view

retroflexion
- endoscopic r.
- intrarectal r.
- success in r.

retrogastric pseudocyst
retrograde
- r. amnesia
- r. approach
- r. balloon rupture
- r. cannulation
- r. cholangiogram
- r. cholangiography
- r. contrast study
- r. cystogram (RC)
- r. cystography
- r. cystourethrogram
- r. duodenogastroscopy (RDG)
- r. ejaculation
- r. endopyelotomy
- r. fashion
- r. flow on barium enema
- r. genitography
- r. hernia
- r. instrumentation
- r. intrarenal surgery
- r. intussusception
- r. loopography
- r. migration
- r. nephrostomy
- r. occlusion balloon catheter
- r. pancreatocholangiography
- r. pancreatogram
- r. pancreatography
- r. peristalsis
- r. pyelogram (RPG)
- r. pyelography
- r. small bowel examination
- r. sphincterotomy
- r. technique
- r. ureteropyelogram
- r. ureteropyelography
- r. urethrogram (RUG)
- r. urethrography (RUG)
- r. urogram (RU)
- r. urography
- r. vascularization of superior mesenteric artery

retrohepatic vena cava
retroileal
- r. appendicitis
- r. appendix

retroiliac ureter
Retromax endopyelotomy stent
retropancreatic tunnel
retroperistaltic pump
retroperitoneal
- r. abscess
- r. approach
- r. area
- r. calcification
- r. carbon dioxide insufflation study
- r. cavity
- r. cutaneous ureterostomy
- r. fat
- r. fibrosis
- r. fistula
- r. hematoma
- r. hemorrhage
- r. hernia
- r. infection
- r. laparoscopic adrenalectomy for pheochromocytoma
- r. lymphadenectomy
- r. lymph node dissection (RPLD)
- r. lymphoma
- r. neoplasm
- r. perforation
- r. pneumography
- r. pneumoradiography
- r. region
- r. seminoma

NOTES

retroperitoneal *(continued)*
- r. space
- r. surgery
- r. tumor
- r. varicocelectomy

retroperitoneal-iliopsoas abscess
retroperitoneoscopic
- r. adrenalectomy
- r. nephrectomy
- r. vein ligature

retroperitoneoscopy
retroperitoneum sarcoma
retroperitonitis
- idiopathic fibrous r.

retropexy
- abdominal r.

retropneumoperitoneum
retropubic
- r. ascending radical prostatectomy
- r. colposuspension
- r. implant
- r. Lapides-Ball bladder neck suspension
- r. needle suspension procedure
- r. space
- r. urethrolysis
- r. urethroscopy

retrorectal
- r. cyst
- r. lymph node
- r. space

retrospective
- r. analysis
- r. analysis of antimicrobial resistance

retrospectively re-examined
retrosternal
- r. chest pain
- r. hernia

retrourethral catheterization
retroversion
retroverted uterus
retrovesical vesiculectomy
retroviral genome
retrovirus
- r. infection
- porcine endogenous r. (PERV)

retrusive meatus
rettgeri
- *Proteus* r.
- *Providencia* r.

return
- r. electrode monitor (REM)
- total predicted r.

retzii
- cavum r.

Retzius
- space of R.
- R. space
- R. vein

REU, REUS
- rectal endoscopic ultrasonography

reusable
- r. forceps with needle
- r. laparoscopic electrode

reuse syndrome
reuteri
- *Lactobacillus* r.

Reuter suprapubic trocar and cannula system
revascularization
- myocardial r.
- penile r.
- renal r.

revenge
- Montezuma r.

reverberation artifact
Reverdin abdominal spatula
reversal
- r. jejunoileal bypass surgery
- jejunoileal fold pattern r.
- vasectomy r.

reverse
- r. alpha-sigmoid loop
- r. cystotome
- r. dot hybridization
- r. osmosis pump
- r. sigma penoscrotal transposition repair
- r. sphincterotome
- r. transcriptase (RT)
- r. transcriptase-polymerase chain reaction (RT-PCR)
- r. transcriptase reaction
- r. transcription
- r. Trendelenburg position

reversed
- r. anorexia syndrome
- r. Mercedes Benz sign
- r. passive hemagglutination reaction (RPHA)
- r. peristalsis
- r. reimplanted appendicocystostomy

reversible
- r. blockade
- r. vasectomy

review
- comprehensive r.
- r. factor
- metaanalytic r.
- technological r.

Rex-Cantli-Serege line
Reye syndrome
Rezipas
Rezulin
RFB
- retained foreign body

RFIPC
  Rating Form of Inflammatory Bowel Disease Patient Concerns
RFLP
  restriction fragment length polymorphism
RFS
  renal function study
  RFS 2000
rhabdoid Wilms tumor
rhabdomyoblastic differentiation
rhabdomyolysis
  exertional r.
  hypoxia-induced r.
rhabdomyoma
rhabdomyomatous
rhabdomyosarcoma (RMS)
  alveolar r.
  bladder r.
  interlabial r.
  kidney r.
  mixed r.
  paratesticular r.
  pleomorphic r.
  prostate r.
  treatment of r.
rhabdosarcoma
  renal r.
rhabdosphincter
  r. electromyography
  r. muscle
rhagades
rhamnosus
  Lactobacillus r.
rHBcAg
  recombinant HBcAg
RHCT
  renal helical CT
  RHCT imaging
Rheaban
Rhein anthrone
rhenium 186
Rheomacrodex
rh-EPO
  recombinant human erythropoietin
rhesus rotavirus-tetravalent vaccine (RRV-TV)
rheumatica
  scarlatina r.
rheumatic disease
rheumatism
  palindromic r.

rheumatoid
  r. arthritis
  r. vasculitis
Rheumatrex dose pack
rhinosporidiosis
Rhinosporidium seeberi
Rhizopus
rhizotomy
  dorsal r.
  sacral posterior root r.
  selective sacral r.
rhodamine
  alexandrite and r.
  r. 6G dye
  r. 6G dye laser
  r. stain
Rhodesian trypanosomiasis
rhodesiense
  Trypanosoma r.
Rhodes Inventory of Nausea and Vomiting
rhonchus, pl. rhonchi
rho protein
rhubarb test
RHV
  right hepatic vein
rhythm
  biphasic diurnal r.
  circadian r.
  gallop r.
  irregular r.
  midline estimating statistic of r. (MESOR)
  paced r.
  r. strip
  ultradian r.
rhythmicity
  circadian r.
rhythmometry
  cosinor r.
RI
  regional ileitis
  resistive index
RIA
  radioimmunoassay
  RIA kit
RIBA
  recombinant immunoblot assay
  RIBA test
RIBA-2 test
ribavirin
ribavirin 200 mg capsule

NOTES

ribbon
    iridium r.
    r. retractor
    r. stool
rib cutter
riboflavin deficiency
ribonuclease (RNAse, RNase)
    low molecular weight protein r.
ribonucleic acid (RNA)
ribonucleoprotein (RNP)
riboprobe
    complementary single-stranded antisense r.
    ^{35}S antisense fibronectin r.
ribose-1-phosphate
ribose-5-phosphate
ribosome
    free r.
rice-flour breath test
rice-fruit diet
Rice-Lyte
rice-water stool
Richard
    R. abdominal retractor
    R. Wolf model 2271.004 ultrasonic energy rigid device
    R. Wolf Piezolith lithotriptor
    R. Wolf videoresectoscope
Richardson
    R. appendectomy retractor
    R. procedure
Richet fascia umbilicus
Richner-Hanhart syndrome
Richter hernia
Richter-Monroe line
ricin
rickets
    celiac r.
    hypophosphatemic r.
    pseudodeficiency r.
    renal r.
Rickettsia conorii
Rider-Moeller
    R.-M. dilator
    R.-M. glossitis
ridge
    interureteric r.
    nephrogenic r.
    rete r.
    ureteric r.
ridged-convoluted villus
Riedel lobe
Riegel test meal
Rieger syndrome
Riepe-Bard gastric balloon
Rieux hernia
rifabutin
Rifadin
rifampicin
rifampin
rifamycin
rifaximin
rIFN-alfa
    recombinant interferon alfa
Rigaud operation
Rigby appendectomy retractor
Righini procedure
right
    r. anterior oblique position
    r. anterior pararenal space
    r. colon
    r. colonic flexure
    r. colon pouch
    r. gastroomental artery
    r. gutter
    r. hepatic duct
    r. hepatic radicle
    r. hepatic vein (RHV)
    r. inguinal hernia (RIH)
    r. lobe
    r. lower quadrant (RLQ)
    r. ovarian vein syndrome
    r. upper quadrant (RUQ)
    r. ureter
right-angle
    r.-a. clamp
    r.-a. electrode
    r.-a. end-to-side anastomosis
    r.-a. lens
right-sided
    r.-s. clonus
    r.-s. lesion
rigid
    r. abdomen
    r. endoscope
    r. esophagoscopy
    9F r. scope
    r. nephroscope
    r. proctoscopy
    r. proctosigmoidoscopy
    r. scoop
    r. sigmoidoscope
    r. ureteroscope
    r. ureteroscopy
rigidity
    abdominal r.
    boardlike r.
    flexural r.
    involuntary reflex r.
    nuchal r.
Rigiflator handheld inflation/deflation device
Rigiflex
    R. ABD balloon dilatation catheter
    R. achalasia balloon
    R. achalasia dilator
    R. biliary balloon dilatation catheter

R. esophageal TTS balloon catheter
R. OTW balloon dilatation catheter
R. TTS balloon
R. TTS balloon dilatation catheter
R. TTS balloon dilator
RigiScan
R. device
R. measurement
R. penile tumescence and rigidity monitor
R. testing
Rigler
classic triad of R.
R. sign
triad of R.
rigor mortis
RIGS
radioimmunoguided surgery
RIGScan
RIGScan CR49
RIGScan CR49 test for colorectal cancer detection
RIH
right inguinal hernia
Riley-Day
R.-D. syndrome
R.-D. syndrome of familial dysautonomia
rim
r. of fascia
r. nephrogram
r. sign
rima, pl. **rimae**
r. pudenda
r. vulva
Rimactane
rind
ring
A r.
abdominal inguinal r.
r. abdominal retractor
anorectal r.
apex of external r.
B r.
R. biliary drainage catheter
biofragmentable anastomotic r. (BAR)
Cannon r.
Coloplast skin barrier r.
confidence r.
constriction r.
continence r.
deep abdominal r.
distal esophageal r.
elastic O r.
esophageal A, B r.
esophageal contractile r.
esophageal mucosal r.
esophageal muscular r.
estradiol-releasing silicone vaginal r.
Estring estradiol vaginal r.
external abdominal r.
external inguinal r.
finger r.
r. forceps
ilioinguinal r.
iliopsoas r.
inguinal r.
inositol r.
internal abdominal r.
internal inguinal r.
intrahaustral contraction r.
Kayser-Fleischer r.
lower esophageal B r.
lower esophageal contraction r.
lower esophageal mucosal r.
Lyon r.
Maclet magnetic r.
mucosal esophageal r.
muscular esophageal r.
O r.
Ochsner r.
Osbon pressure-point tension r.
pressure-point tension r.
pyloric r.
rust r.
Schatzki r.
r. shadow
Silastic r.
silicone elastomer r.
Smith r.
sphincter contraction r.
superficial abdominal r.
sutureless biofragmentable r.
Ringer lactate
ringlike
r. contraction
r. lesion
r. stricture
ring-type rigidity measuring device
Rink modification of Casale continent catheterizable vesicostomy
rinse
SaliCept oral r.

NOTES

Riopan Plus
RIP
    respiratory inversion point
Ripstein
    R. anterior sling rectopexy
    R. procedure
    R. rectal prolapse operation
risedronate
risk
    r. adjustment
    r. of bacteremia
    r. evaluation
    r. factors of posttransplant diabetes mellitus
    Goldman classification of operative r.
    morbidity r.
    neoplasia r.
    perioperative r.
risk-adjusted mortality
Ritalin
RiteBite biopsy forceps
ritonavir
river blindness
Rives-Stoppa
    R.-S. procedure
    R.-S. technique
RJL Model 10 bioelectrical impedance analyzer
RLD
    related living donor
RLP
    rectal linitis plastica
    restriction fragment length polymorphism
    RLP colorectal carcinoma
RLQ
    right lower quadrant
RLS
    restless leg syndrome
RLT
    reduced liver transplant
r-metHuLeptin
    recombinant methionyl human leptin
RMIC
    renomedullary interstitial cell
RMS
    rhabdomyosarcoma
    Ruvalcaba-Myhre-Smith
    RMS syndrome
    RMS voltage
RMT
    ranitidine bismuth citrate, metronidazole, tetracycline
RNA
    ribonucleic acid
    albumin messenger RNA
    GB virus C/hepatitis G virus RNA (GBV-C/HGV-RNA)
    HCV RNA
    hepatitis C virus RNA
    IGF-1R RNA
    messenger RNA (mRNA)
    RNA probe
RNA-based findings
RNAse, RNase
    ribonuclease
    RNAse digestion
    RNAse inhibitor
RNP
    ribonucleoprotein
rNV
    recombinant capsid protein of Norwalk virus
Roadmapper
    FluoroPlus R.
Roadrunner wire
Robaxisal
Robbers forceps
Roberts
    R. folding esophagoscope
    R. oval esophagoscope
    R. syndrome
Robertson
    R. sign
    R. TM urethroscope
Robin-Masse abdominal retractor
Robinow syndrome
robin's egg-blue gallbladder
Robinson catheter
Robinson-Kepler-Power water test
Robinul Forte
Roboprep G instrument
robot-assisted laparoscopy (RAP)
robotically assisted laparoscopic dismembered pyeloplasty
robotic-automated assist device
Robson
    R. intestinal forceps
    R. point
    R. position
ROC
    receiver-operating characteristic
    ROC XS suture fastener
Rocaltrol
Rocephin IM
Roche
    R. Elecsys free prostate-specific antigen assay
    R. sign
Rochester-Carmalt forceps
Rochester gallstone forceps
Rochester-Mixter forceps
Rochester-Ochsner forceps
Rochester-Péan
    R.-P. forceps
    R.-P. hemostat
Rockey-Davis incision

rod
    colostomy r.
    gram-negative r.
    ileostomy r.
    Meckel r.
    Reichmann r.
    Sur-Fit Natura loop ostomy r.
rod-lens system
rodless end-loop stoma
Rodney Smith biliary stricture repair
Roeder
    R. loop
    R. loop knot
Roenigk
    R. grade
    R. score
roentgen findings
roentgenography
    double-contrast r.
rofecoxib
Roferon-A
Roger
    R. reflex
    R. syndrome
Rokitansky
    R. disease
    R. diverticulum
    R. hernia
    R. kidney
Rokitansky-Aschoff
    R.-A. sinus
    R.-A. sinus hyperplasia
Rokitansky-Cushing ulcer
Rokitansky-Kuster-Hauser syndrome
Rolaids
role
    additional unproven r.
    r. of diet in therapy
    plasmid profile r.
    r. of the resistive index
    r. of ureteroscopy
roll
    iliac r.
    Kraske r.
rollerball electrode
roller pump
rolling hiatal hernia
Romazicon
Rome
    R. criteria I, II
    R. I, II criteria for irritable bowel syndrome

Rommelaere sign
roof
    pseudoaneurysmal r.
    r. strip
rooperi
    Hypoxis r.
Roosevelt clamp
root
    r. abscess
    ginger r.
    r. mean square voltage
    needle r.
    r. neurostimulation
    penile r.
    sacral nerve r.
rooting reflex
rootlet
    ventral sacral r.
ROPA
    Regional Organ Procurement Agency
Ro-resection
    radial R.-r.
ROS
    reactive oxygen species
Rosch-Uchida transjugular liver access set
rose
    r. bengal sodium ^{131}I biliary scan
    r. bengal sodium ^{131}I radioactive agent
    r. bengal test
    r. thorn ulcer
    r. thorn ulcer of mucosa
Rose-Bradford kidney
rosebud stoma
Roseburia
Rosenbach-Gmelin test
Rosenbach sign
Rosen cyst
Rosenthal test
rosette
    r. appearance of anus
    Homer Wright r.
rosetted
    E r.
Rosewater syndrome
Rossbach disease
Rosser crypt hook
Rossetti modification of Nissen fundoplication
rotary shadowing electron microscopy
rotatable Roth retrieval net

NOTES

rotating
   r. Bruel and Kjaer probe
   r. endoprobe
   r. endoscissors
   r. sphincterotome

rotation
   external r.
   internal r.

rotational colonoscope overtube

rotator
   Jarit r.
   R. polypectomy snare

rotavirus
   r. diarrhea
   r. gastroenteritis
   group C r.
   r. infection
   r. tetravalent vaccine

rotavirus-associated diarrhea
Rotazyme test
Roth
   R. Grip-Tip suture guide
   R. polyp retrieval net
   R. spot

Rothmund-Thomson syndrome
roticulator stapling device
Rotolith lithotrite
Rotor syndrome

rotunda
   pityriasis r.

rotund abdomen
roughage
round
   r. ligament
   r. ulcer

roundworm
route
   fecal-oral r.
   paracellular r.
   sodium entry r.

routine
   r. neonatal circumcision
   r. outpatient procedure
   r. ureteral stenting

Roux
   R. gastric reflux
   R. limb
   R. limb emptying
   R. retractor
   R. stasis syndrome

Roux-en-Y
   R.-e.-Y anastomosis
   R.-e.-Y biliary bypass with antrectomy
   R.-e.-Y chimney surgical technique
   R.-e.-Y choledochojejunostomy
   R.-e.-Y cystojejunostomy
   R.-e.-Y distal jejunoileostomy
   R.-e.-Y esophagojejunostomy
   R.-e.-Y gastric bypass
   R.-e.-Y gastroenterostomy
   R.-e.-Y hepaticojejunostomy
   R.-e.-Y jejunal limb
   R.-e.-Y jejunostomy
   R.-e.-Y limb enteroscopy
   R.-e.-Y loop
   R.-e.-Y loop of jejunum
   R.-e.-Y operation
   R.-e.-Y pancreaticojejunostomy
   R.-e.-Y procedure
   R.-e.-Y procedure with vagotomy
   R.-e.-Y reanastomosis
   R.-e.-Y reconstruction

Roux-limb stasis
Roux-type gastroduodenal anastomosis
Roux-Y chimney
Rovighi sign
Rovsing
   R. operation
   R. sign
   R. syndrome

Rowasa enema
Rowland pouch
roxatidine acetate
Roxicodone
roxithromycin
RP
   restorative proctocolectomy

RP3 stain
RPC
   recurrent pyogenic cholangiohepatitis
   restorative proctocolectomy

RPD
   rapid
      Pepcid RPD

RPF
   renal plasma flow

RPG
   retrograde pyelogram

RPGN
   rapidly progressive glomerulonephritis

RPHA
   reversed passive hemagglutination reaction

RPLD
   retroperitoneal lymph node dissection

RPMI-1640 medium
RPN
   renal papillary necrosis

RPT
   rapid pullthrough
      RPT technique

RR
   rate ratio

RRP
   radical retropubic prostatectomy

RRV-TV
   rhesus rotavirus-tetravalent vaccine

RS
 rehydrating solution
 respiratory symptoms
  RS associated with GERD
RSH
 rectus sheath hematoma
RSLT
 reduced-size liver transplant
RSR
 rectosphincteric reflex
RSs
 relative supersaturation
RT
 reverse transcriptase
RTA
 renal tubular acidosis
RTA-I–IV
 renal tubular type I–IV acidosis
RTFNA
 real-time fine-needle aspiration
RT-PCR
 reverse transcriptase-polymerase chain reaction
  PSA RT-PCR
RTX
 real-time transmission automated counter Technicon H.3 RTX
RU
 retrograde urogram
rub
 friction r.
 peritoneal friction r.
 pleural r.
rubber
 r. band ligation (RBL)
 r. band ligation of hemorrhoid
 r. band ligator (RBL)
 r. dam
rubber-sheathed clamp
rubber-shod clamp
rubella
rubeola
rubidium (Rb)
Rubin-Quinton small bowel biopsy tube
Rubinstein-Taybi syndrome
Rubin tube
rubitecan
rubor
 dependent r.
rubra
 miliaria r.

Rubratope-57 radioactive agent
rubrum
 tinea r.
 Trichophyton r.
ructus
Rudd
 R. Clinic hemorrhoidal forceps
 R. Clinic hemorrhoidal ligator
rudiment
 hepatic r.
rudimentary testis syndrome
Rud syndrome
RUG
 retrograde urethrogram
 retrograde urethrography
ruga, pl. **rugae**
 rugae gastricae
 rugae of stomach
 r. of urinary bladder
 rugae zone
rugal
 r. fold
 r. hypertrophy
 r. pattern
rugate
rugitus
rugose, rugous
rule
 Goodsall r.
 Weigert-Meyer r.
ruler catheter
RuLox No. 1, 2
rumble
rumbling bowel sounds
Rumel tourniquet
rumen
rumination
Ruminococcus
 R. lactaris
 R. obeum
 R. productus
runner's diarrhea
running suture
runny stool
runting syndrome
Runyon group III mycobacteria
rupture
 acute hepatic r.
 bladder r.
 catheterization pouch r.
 ERCP-induced splenic r.
 esophageal r.

NOTES

rupture *(continued)*
    extraperitoneal r.
    gastric r.
    hepatic r.
    hydatid cyst intrahepatic r.
    Mallory-Weiss mucosal r.
    mesenteric r.
    penile r.
    renal allograft r.
    retrograde balloon r.
    splenic r.
    spontaneous r.
    traumatic r.
    umbilical hernia r.
    uterine r.
ruptured
    r. abdominal aortic aneurysm (RAAA)
    r. appendiceal cystadenoma
    r. appendix
    r. hepatic tumor
    r. peliotic lesion
    r. pseudoaneurysm
    r. sigmoid diverticulum
RUQ
    right upper quadrant
RUS
    real-time ultrasonography
Rusch stent
Rusconi anus
rush
    peristaltic r.
rushing
Russell
    R. gastrostomy kit
    R. peel-away sheath dilator
    R. percutaneous endoscopic gastrostomy
    R. sign
    R. technique
    R. viper venom test
    R. viper venom time
Russell-Silver syndrome
Russian tissue forceps
rust ring

RUT
    rapid urease test
        RUT kit
ruthenium red
Rutkow sutureless plug and patch
Rutzen ileostomy bag
RUV
    residual urine volume
Ruvalcaba-Myhre-Smith (RMS)
    R.-M.-S. syndrome
Ru-Vert-M
Ruysch
    R. disease
    R. glomeruli
    R. vein
RVR
    renovascular resistance
RVRA
    renal vein renin activity
    renal vein renin assay
RVRC
    renal vein renin concentration
RVRI
    renovascular resistance index
R-wave
    R-w. coordination
    R-w. triggering
RWG
    rye whole-grain
RX
    rapid exchange
    RX Herculink 14
    RX Herculink 14 biliary stent system
    RX Herculink Plus
    RX Herculink Plus biliary stent system
    MagneBind 400 RX
    RX stent delivery system
RXR
    retinoid X receptor
ryanodine binding
rye whole-grain (RWG)
Ryle tube

S
  S cell
  S cord
  S neuron
  S pelvic ileal pouch
  S pouch
  S reservoir
S-100
  S-100 immunohistochemical stain
  S-100 protein
S100 super family
S3 segment
SAA
  serum amyloid A
  splenic artery aneurysm
SAAG
  serum-ascites albumin gradient
Saathoff test
saber stroke
Sabouraud glucose agar
sabre
  coup de s.
  en coup de s.
SAB reagent
saburra
saburral colic
sac
  enterocele s.
  entrapment s.
  fluid-filled s.
  greater peritoneal s.
  hernia s.
  high ligation of hernia s.
  indirect hernia s.
  Lap s.
  lesser peritoneal s.
  peritoneal s.
  Pleatman s.
  wide-mouth s.
  yolk s.
saccharate
saccharin
saccharomyces
  S. boulardii
  S. cerevisiae
  yeast s.
sacciform kidney
Saccomanno
  S. fixative
  S. solution
saccular
  s. aneurysm
  s. colon
sacculated bladder

sacculation
  cecal s.
  colic s.
  s. of colon
  tubular narrowing and s.
saccule
sacculiform
sacculus, pl. sacculi
  sacculi of Beale
Sachse
  S. urethrotome
  S. urethrotomy
Sachs solution
Sacks
  S. QuickStick catheter
  S. Single-Step catheter
Sacks-Vine
  S.-V. feeding gastrostomy tube
  S.-V. gastrostomy kit
  S.-V. PEG system
  S.-V. PEG tube
  S.-V. technique
Sacks-Vine-type PEG
sacral
  s. afferent fiber
  s. agenesis
  s. artery
  s. edema
  s. evoked response
  s. nerve neuromodulation
  s. nerve root
  s. nerve stimulation (SNS)
  s. nerve stimulation therapy
  s. neurostimulation
  s. plexus
  s. posterior root rhizotomy
  s. promontory
  s. reflex arc
  s. root neuromodulation
  s. vein
sacroabdominoperineal pullthrough
sacrococcygeal
  s. pilonidal cyst
  s. pilonidal sinus tract
  s. region germ cell tumor
  s. teratoma
sacrocolpopexy
  abdominal s.
sacrofixation operation
sacroiliitis
sacrospinalis
  s. ligament vaginal fixation
  s. muscle

sacrospinous
    s. ligament
    s. ligament vaginal fixation
sacrotuberous ligament
sacrouterine ligament
sacrum
SAD
    sinoaortic denervation
S-adenosylmethionine (SAMe)
    S-a. deficiency
Saeed
    S. multiband ligator
    S. multiple ligator
    S. six-shooter
    S. six-shooter ligator
    S. technique
    S. ten-shooter
safe
    S. and Dry panty and pad system
    s. gastrocutaneous fistulous tract
Safe-T-Flex enteral feeding container
safe-tract technique
safety
    S. AV fistula needle
    s. pin ingestion
    s. wire
saffron stain
SAGB
    Swedish Adjustable Gastric Band
SAGES
    Society of American Gastrointestinal Endoscoping Surgeons
saginata
    Taenia s.
sagittal
    s. fissure of liver
    s. image
sago-grain stool
sagrada
    cascara s.
Sahli glutoid test
Sahli-Nencki test
saint (St.)
Salem
    S. duodenal sump tube
    S. sump double-lumen polyvinyl tube
SALF
    subacute liver failure
Salflex
SaliCept
    S. freeze-dried dressing
    S. oral rinse
salicylate
    s. abuse
    methyl s.
salicylazosulfapyridine
saline
    buffered s.
    s. cleansing enema
    s. continence test
    s. cystometry
    s. flush
    half-normal s.
    heparinized s.
    hypertonic s.
    iced s.
    indigo carmine-stained normal s.
    s. infusion
    s. injection therapy
    isotonic s.
    s. laxative
    s. load test
    phosphate-buffered s. (PBS)
    s. slush
    s. suppression test
saline-assisted polypectomy (SAP)
saline-epinephrine
    hypertonic s.-e. (HSE)
saline-filled cholangiocatheter
saline-moistened sponge
saliva
    s. bicarbonate
    pooled s.
    s. substitute
salivarius
    Streptococcus s.
Salivart solution
salivary
    s. amylase
    s. calculus
    s. epidermal growth factor (sEGF)
    s. epidermal growth factor-1
    s. gland enlargement
    s. gland scan
    s. hypersecretion
    s. mass
    s. tenderness
    s. testing
salivary-type isoamylase
salivation
Salkowski-Schipper test
Salle procedure
Salmon
    S. backcut incision
    S. law
Salmonella
    S. agona
    S. choleraesuis
    S. colitis
    S. enteritidis
    S. enteritidis orchitis
    S. hartford
    S. heidelberg
    S. hirschfeldii
    S. infantis
    S. newport
    nontyphoidal *S.*

S. *paratyphi* A, B, C
Salmonella food poisoning
S. *stanley*
S. *typhi*
S. *typhimurium*
S. *typhimurium* enterocolitis
S. *typhimurium* R5

salmonellosis
    nontyphoidal s.

salmonicida
    Aeromonas s.

Salomon test
salpingitis
salpinx, pl. **salpinges**
salt
    amphipathic bile s.
    artificial Carlsbad s.
    artificial Kissingen s.
    artificial Vichy s.
    bile s. (BS)
    bismuth s.
    Cheatle s.
    s. consumption
    dihydroxy s.
    fura-2 pentapotassium s.
    gold s.
    low s. (LNaCl)
    magnesium s.
    monohydroxy bile s.
    structural effects of dietary s.
    s. transporting protein
    trihydroxy s.

salt-and-pepper duodenal erosion
salt-losing
    s.-l. nephritis
    s.-l. nephropathy

salt-sensitive hypertension
saluresis
Saluron
Salutensin
salutory
salvage
    s. brachytherapy
    s. cryoablation
    s. cryoablation of prostate
    s. cystectomy
    s. cystoprostatectomy
    s. cytology
    s. cytology technique
    s. prostatectomy
    s. protocol

    s. surgery
    s. therapy

Salvanios pH 10 disinfectant solution
Salvati proctoscope
Salzer test meal
samarium
SAMe
    S-adenosylmethionine
    SAMe nutritional supplement

sample
    arterial blood s.
    aspirated s.
    Bethesda System for cervicovaginal s.
    blood s.
    random stool s.
    serum s.
    stool s.
    urine s.
    venous blood s.

sampling
    adrenal vein aldosterone s.
    arterial stimulation venous s. (ASVS)
    s. gate
    mediastinal lymph node s.
    tissue s.
    transhepatic portal venous s.

Sam Roberts esophagoscope
sand
    hydatid s.
    urinary s.

sandbag
Sanders incision
Sand-Eze EGD pillow
Sandhill-800 TDS chart recorder
Sandhill P32 pH antimony probe
Sandifer syndrome
Sandimmune
Sandostatin LAR depot
Sandoz
    S. Caluso 22F, 28F super PEG
    S. Caluso PEG gastrostomy tube
    S. 22F balloon replacement tube
    S. feeding/suction tube

sandwich
    s. staghorn calculus therapy
    s. technique

sandy skin-prepping paste
sanguineous
    s. drainage
    s. fluid

NOTES

sanguis
    Streptococcus s.
Sani-Pads medicated cleansing pad
Sani-Supp
Sanorex
SANS
    Stoller afferent nerve stimulation
        PerQ SANS
Sansert
Santiani-Stone classification
^{35}**S antisense fibronectin riboprobe**
santonin test
Santorini
    accessory duct of S.
    S. canal
    duct of S.
    S. labyrinth
    papilla of S.
    S. sphincter
    S. venous plexus
santorinicele
SAP
    saline-assisted polypectomy
    serum amyloid P
saphenofemoral junction
saphenous
    s. nerve
    s. vein
saponifiable fecal bile acid
saponification
Sappey
    accessory portal system of S.
Sapporo virus
saprophyticus
    Staphylococcus s.
saprophytism
SAPS
    single-action pumping system
saquinavir
saralasin
sarcocele
sarcocystosis
sarcoidosis
    epididymal s.
    hepatic s.
    pancreatic s.
    renal s.
    urethral s.
sarcoma
    appendiceal Kaposi s.
    bladder s.
    Boeck s.
    botryoid s.
    s. botryoides
    clear cell s.
    Ewing s.
    gastric Kaposi s.
    gastrointestinal Kaposi s.
    granulocytic s.
    hemangioendothelial s.
    intracolonic Kaposi s.
    Ito cell s.
    Kaposi s. (KS)
    kidney clear cell s.
    kidney osteogenic s.
    Kupffer cell s.
    lipoblastic s.
    osteogenic s.
    penis s.
    prostate gland s.
    retroperitoneum s.
    seminal vesicle s.
    testis s.
    vasoablative endothelial s. (VABES)
    s. virus oncogene
sarcomatoid squamous cell carcinoma
sarcomatous
sarcomphalocele
sarcoplasmic reticulum
Sarcoptes scabiei
Sarfeh principle
Sarisol No. 2
Sarns Siok II blood pump
Sarot needle holder
SART
    standard acid reflux test
Sassone score
satellite lesion
Satietrol
satiety
    early s.
    s. test
Satinsky clamp
satisfaction
    patient s.
satisfactory continence
satraplatin
satumomab pendetide
saturated fatty acid (SFA)
saturation
    arterial s.
    s. index (SI)
    oxygen s.
    percent transferrin s.
    s. riboprobe concentration
    transferrin s.
saturnine
    s. colic
    s. nephritis
saturnism
satyri
    Bertiella s.
saucerization
saucerized biopsy
Saundby test
Saunders disease
sausage digit
sausagelike appearance

sausage-string pattern
Savage perineal body
Savary
    S. bougie
    S. bronchoscope
    complete S.
    S. tapered thermoplastic dilator
Savary-Gilliard
    S.-G. esophagitis grade I, II
    S.-G. metal olive
    S.-G. over-the-wire dilator
    S.-G. Silastic flexible bougie
    S.-G. wire-guided bougie
Savary-Miller
    S.-M. criteria
    S.-M. grade I-III erosive esophagitis
    S.-M. grade I-III reflux esophagitis
    S.-M. II grade
saver
    Cell S.
sawtooth
    s. appearance sign
    s. irregularity of bowel contour
sawtoothed appearance
Sawyer
    S. rectal retractor
    S. rectal speculum
saxitoxin
S-B
    Sengstaken-Blakemore S-B tube
S3BA3003
    Glaxo Wellcome protocol S3BA3003
SBE
    small bowel enteroscopy
SBFT
    small bowel followthrough
SBGM
    self blood glucose monitoring
SBO
    small bowel obstruction
SBP
    spontaneous bacterial peritonitis
SBPN
    simultaneous bilateral percutaneous nephrolithotomy
SBT
    skin bleeding time
SC
    secretory component

sieving coefficient
subcutaneous
sulfur colloid
    ^{99m}Tc SC
scabiei
    Sarcoptes s.
scabies
    genital s.
scale
    Charrière s.
    children's coma s.
    ECOG performance status s.
    Flint Colon Injury S. (FCIS)
    French s.
    Gastrointestinal Symptom Rating S. (GSRS)
    Glasgow coma s.
    Goldberg Anorectic Attitude s.
    gray s.
    Hetzel-Dent s.
    Karnofsky performance status s.
    Lanza s.
    Likert s.
    Madsen-Iversen s.
    modified Hetzel-Dent s.
    Perceived Stress S. (PSS)
scaling
    physiologic s.
scalloped
    s. antimesenteric border
    s. bowel lumen
scalpel
    s. blade
    harmonic s.
    LaserSonics Nd:YAG Laserblade s.
    ultrasonic s.
scan
    acetyltriglycine renal s.
    bone s.
    colloid shift on liver-spleen s.
    CT s.
    diethylenetriamine pentaacetic acid renal s.
    dimercaptosuccinic acid renal s.
    dimethyl iminodiacetic acid s.
    DISIDA s.
    DMSA s.
    DTPA renal s.
    dual-energy CT s.
    endoanal ultrasound s.
    esophageal transit s.

NOTES

scan *(continued)*
  fluorescence-activated cell sorter s. (FACScan)
  gallbladder s.
  gallium s.
  gastric emptying s.
  gastroesophageal reflux s.
  GI bleeding s.
  hepatic blood pool s.
  hepatobiliary s.
  HIDA s.
  Hybritech PSA s.
  indium-labeled leukocyte s.
  indium 64-labeled white blood cell s.
  indium leukocyte s.
  intercostal s.
  iodine s.
  iodocholesterol s.
  isotope renal s.
  isotropic s.
  labeled red blood cell s.
  liver s.
  liver-spleen s.
  MAG-3 renal s.
  Meckel s.
  monoclonal antibody scintigraphic s.
  MRI s.
  nuclear bleeding s.
  nuclear isotope s.
  nuclear medicine s.
  peritoneovenous shunt patency s.
  PET s.
  PIPIDA hepatobiliary s.
  positron emission tomography s.
  ProstaScint s.
  radioisotope s.
  radionuclide s.
  renal s.
  rose bengal sodium ^{131}I biliary s.
  salivary gland s.
  SPECT s.
  splenic perfusion measurement by dynamic CT s.
  sulfur colloid liver s.
  tagged red blood cell bleeding s.
  ^{99m}Tc DTPA renal s.
  ^{99m}Tc HMPAO-labeled leukocyte s.
  ^{99m}Tc IDA s.
  ^{99m}Tc MDP nuclear isotope bone s.
  ^{99m}Tc pertechnetate s.
  ^{99m}Tc RBC bleeding s.
  ^{99m}Tc sulfur colloid s.
  technetium-labeled autologous red blood cell s.
  technetium-labeled red blood cell s.
  technetium-99m diethylenetriamine pentaacetic acid s.
  technetium-99m HIDA s.
  technetium radionuclide s.
  s. test
  transabdominal s.
  transrectal s.
  transvesical s.
  UJ13A nuclear isotope bone s.
  ultrasound s.
scan-directed biopsy
scanner
  BladderScan BVI2500 ultrasound s.
  Bruel-Kjaer s.
  conventional static s.
  CT Twin s.
  General Electric Signa s.
  high-resolution real-time s.
  Kretz Combison 330 ultrasound s.
  Kretz 311 ultrasound s.
  linear convex array s.
  Lunar DPX total-body s.
  7.5 MHz sector s.
  MKII automated s.
  Tesla GE Signa whole-body s.
scanning
  captopril-DTPA s.
  s. electron microscope
  s. electron microscopy
  endoscopic magnetic resonance s.
  fluorescent gene s.
  s. force microscopy (SFM)
  iodine hippurate s.
  radioisotope s.
  renal s.
  transrectal ultrasound s. (TRUS)
scaphoid abdomen
scapus penis
scar
  Billroth II anastomotic s.
  chest tube s.
  episiotomy s.
  iridectomy s.
  railroad track s.'s
  sternotomy s.
  thoracotomy s.
  s. tissue formation
  s. tissue reaction
scarce bowel sounds
Scardino
  S. flap
  S. ureteropelvioplasty
  S. vertical flap pyeloplasty
Scardino-Prince
  S.-P. ureteropelvioplasty
  S.-P. vertical flap pyeloplasty
scarf-ring sign
scariasis
scarified duodenum
scarlatinal nephritis
scarlatina rheumatica

scarlatiniform rash
Scarpa
    S. fascia
    S. triangle
scarring
    duodenum deformed by s.
    gastrostomy s.
    kidney s.
    local s.
    postdystrophic s.
    postnecrotic s.
    renal s.
scatoma
scattered fluorescein
scatter factor
scattering
    Raman s.
scavenger
    free radical s.
    hydroxyl radical s.
SCC
    squamous cell carcinoma
S-CCK-Pz
    secretin-cholecystokinin-pancreatozymin
        S-CCK-Pz stimulation
        S-CCK-Pz test
SCE
    specialized columnar epithelium
SCFA
    short-chain fatty acid
Schachowa spiral tube
Schäfer nomogram
Schatzki ring
Schaumann body
Scheffe-F test
schematic diagram
schenckii
    Sporothrix s.
Schiff
    S. biliary cycle
    S. stain
    S. test
Schilder disease
Schiller-Duval body
Schilling test
Schindler
    S. disease
    S. esophagoscope
    S. peritoneal forceps
    S. semiflexible gastroscope
Schistosoma
    S. haematobium
    S. intercalatum
    S. japonica
    S. japonicum
    S. mansoni
    S. mekongi
schistosomal
    s. cervicitis
    s. dysentery
    s. liver disease
    s. pelvic floor myopathy
schistosomiasis
    active s.
    acute s.
    Asiatic s.
    bladder s.
    colon s.
    colonic s.
    ectopic s.
    hepatic s.
    inactive s.
    intestinal s.
    Japanese s.
    s. japonica
    Manson s.
    s. mansoni
    s. mekongi
    Oriental s.
    s. sandy patch
    ureteral s.
    urinary s.
    vesical s.
Schmidt
    S. diet
    S. syndrome
Schmitz bacillus
schmitzii
    Shigella s.
Schmorl reaction
Schneider stent
Schnidt
    S. gall duct forceps
    S. thoracic forceps
Schoemaker
    S. anastomosis
    S. gastroenterostomy
    S. procedure
Schoemaker-Billroth II technique
Schoenberg intestinal forceps
SchonCath chronic dialysis catheter
Schönlein-Henoch
    S.-H. disease
    S.-H. purpura

NOTES

Schramm phenomenon
Schuchardt relaxing incision
Schultz
    S. angina
    S. disease
    S. syndrome
Schwachman syndrome
Schwann
    S. cell
    S. cell lipidosis
schwannian spindle cell
schwannoma
    penile s.
Schwartz
    S. clamp
    S. method
    S. test
Schwartz-Jampel syndrome
Schwartz-Pregenzer
    S.-P. urethropexy procedure
    S.-P. urethroplasty
Schweizer-Foley Y-plasty
SCI
    spinal cord injury
ScI-70 autoantibody
sciatic
    s. hernia
    s. nerve
sciatica
sciatica-like pain
SCID
    severe combined immunodeficiency
science
    biomedical s.
scintigram
    ^{99m}technetium dimercaptosuccinic acid s.
scintigraph
scintigraphic
    s. balloon
    s. balloon topography
    s. diagnosis
    s. emptying study
    s. reflux
scintigraphy
    aberration by s.
    adrenal s.
    antral s.
    dimercaptosuccinic acid s.
    direct vesicoureteral s. (DVS)
    diuretic renal s.
    DMSA s.
    gastric emptying s.
    gastroesophageal s.
    hepatobiliary s.
    OctreoScan s.
    OncoScint CR/OV Bcarcinoma localization s. (OncoScint CR/OV)
    per rectal portal s.
    quantitative hepatobiliary s. (QHS)
    radioisotope s.
    radionuclide s.
    renal gallium-67 s.
    renal perfusion s.
    renocortical s.
    somatostatin receptor s. (SRS)
    tagged erythrocyte s.
    ^{99m}Tc GSA s.
    ^{99m}Tc pertechnetate s.
    technetium-labeled red blood cell s.
    technetium-99m red cell s.
    whole-gut transit s. (WGTS)
scintillation vial
scintiphotosplenoportography
scintirenography
scintiscan
    biliary s.
    false positive s.
    gastroesophageal s.
scintiscanning
    radionuclide ^{99}Tc s.
scintography
    leukocyte s.
scirrhous
    s. adenocarcinoma
    s. carcinoma
    s. lesion
scissors
    Buie rectal s.
    Busch umbilical s.
    Church deep surgery s.
    cold s.
    Crafoord thoracic s.
    curved Mayo s.
    Deaver operating s.
    diathermy s.
    dissection s.
    s. dissection
    Doyen abdominal s.
    Duffield deep surgery s.
    electrosurgical curved s.
    endoscopic s.
    Ferguson abdominal s.
    Graham deep surgery s.
    Harrington-Mayo s.
    Heiss flexible endoscopic s.
    hook s.
    Hooper deep surgery s.
    insulated curved s.
    insulated straight s.
    Kelly fistula s.
    laparoscopic s.
    Lincoln deep surgery s.
    Mayo s.
    Mayo-Noble dissecting s.
    meatotomy s.
    Metzenbaum s.
    Miller rectal s.

Nelson s.
Nu-Tip laparoscopic s.
Panzer gallbladder s.
Penn umbilical s.
Potts s.
Potts-Smith s.
Pratt rectal s.
Snowden-Pencer s.
strabismus s.
Strulle s.
Super-Cut s.
surgical s.
suture s.
Sweet esophageal s.
Thorek-Feldman gallbladder s.
Thorek gallbladder s.
umbilical s.
s. valve
Vezien abdominal s.
Westcott tenotomy s.
Willauer thoracic s.

Scivoletto test
SCIWOA
spinal cord injury without radiographic abnormality
SCJ
squamocolumnar junction
sclera, pl. **sclerae**
anicteric sclerae
icteric sclerae
nonicteric sclerae
scleral icterus
sclerodactyly
scleroderma
s. bowel disease
esophageal s.
s. of esophagus
s. renal crisis
scleroderma sine s.
Scleromate sclerosant
sclerosant
absolute alcohol s.
bucrylate s.
s. dosage
esophageal variceal s.
ethanolamine oleate s.
s. injection
Krazy Glue s.
latex s.
morrhuate s.
polidocanol s.
Scleromate s.

sodium tetradecyl sulfate s.
s. solution
Sotradecol s.
variceal s.
sclerosant-contrast solution
sclerose
sclerosing
s. adenosis
s. agent
s. cholangitis
s. encapsulating peritonitis
s. hepatic carcinoma (SHC)
s. lymphangitis
s. mesenteritis
s. solution
s. therapy
sclerosis
alcohol s.
biliary s.
central hyaline s.
diffuse mesangial s. (DMS)
endoscopic injection s.
esophageal variceal s.
focal s.
gastric s.
global s.
glomerular s.
hepatic s.
hepatoportal s.
injection s.
laser s.
multiple s.
nuclear s.
progressive systemic s. (PSS)
systemic s. (SSc)
systemic duodenal s.
tetracycline s.
tuberous s.
variceal s.
sclerosus
lichen s.
sclerotherapist
sclerotherapy
antegrade scrotal s.
bismuth s.
colonoscopic s.
s. complication
endoscopic s. (ES)
endoscopic injection s. (EIS)
endoscopic retrograde s.
endoscopic variceal s.
esophageal variceal s. (EVS)

NOTES

sclerotherapy *(continued)*
    ethanol s.
    fiberoptic injection s. (FIS)
    hemorrhoidal s.
    injection s.
    intravariceal injection s.
    low-volume s.
    s. needle
    paravariceal s.
    prophylactic s.
    ultralow-volume s.
    variceal s.

sclerotic
    s. atrophy
    s. kidney
    s. stomach
    s. tuft

SCO
    Sertoli-cell-only
    SCO syndrome

scolex, pl. **scoleces**

scoliosis

scombroid fish poisoning

scoop
    Beck abdominal s.
    Desjardins gallbladder s.
    Desjardins gallstone s.
    Ferguson gallstone s.
    Ferris common duct s.
    gallbladder s.
    Klebanoff gallstone s.
    malleable s.
    Mayo common duct s.
    Mayo gallstone s.
    Mayo-Robson gallstone s.
    Moore gallstone s.
    Moynihan gallstone s.
    rigid s.

scope
    baby s.
    7-8F flexible s.
    9F rigid s.
    J turn of s.
    M-scope multibending s.
    Olympus ENF-P2 s.
    Olympus OSF s.
    retroflexed s.
    torquing of s.

Scopinaro pancreaticobiliary bypass

scopolamine

scorbutic dysentery

S cord

score
    activity s.
    APACHE-II s.
    Baylor bleeding s.
    Beppu s.
    Boyarsky BPH symptom s.
    CCKNOW s.
    Child-Pugh s.
    Cleveland Clinic Incontinence S.
    DeMeester acid s.
    Emory s.
    fibrin s.
    fibrosis s.
    Glasgow Dyspepsia Severity S. (GDSS)
    Gleason s.
    hostility s.
    incontinence s.
    International Autoimmune Hepatitis Group s.
    International Prognostic Index s.
    International Prostate Symptom S. (IPSS)
    Johnson and Demeester S.
    Johnson-DeMeester symptom s.
    Karnofsky s.
    Knodell s.
    linear analog pain s.
    Madsen symptom s.
    MELD s.
    PELD s.
    posttest s.
    pretest global rating s.
    QOLRD s.
    Quality of Life in Reflux and Dyspepsia s.
    Roenigk s.
    Sassone s.
    sexual function s.
    SOFA s.
    symptom s.
    total corrected incremental s. (TCIS)

Scott
    S. AMS inflatable penile prosthesis
    S. jejunoileal bypass
    S. operation
    S. retractor

SCP
    squamous cell papilloma

SCr
    serum creatinine

scrapie protein

scraping brush

screen
    Biosafe PSA4 s.
    ChemTrak AccuMeter s.
    ENA s.
    genomewide s.

screening
    cancer s.
    catatonic trypsinogen DNA s.
    colon cancer s.
    colonoscopy s.
    colorectal cancer s.
    s. cystometry

endocrine s.
s. endoscopy
office-based esophageal s.
screw
Reddick-Saye s.
Scribner shunt
scrota (*pl. of* scrotum)
scrotal
s. agenesis
s. angiokeratoma
s. arteriovenous malformation
s. calcification
s. encroachment
s. fat necrosis
s. hemangioma
s. hernia
s. hypospadias
s. lymphangioma
s. mass
s. pain
s. panniculitis
s. pneumatocele
s. pouch operation
s. pouch orchiopexy
s. raphe
s. reflex
s. septum
s. swelling
s. tenderness
s. trauma
s. varicocelectomy
s. violation
scrotal-perineal artery
scrotectomy
total s.
scroti
elephantiasis s.
pruritus s.
raphe s.
scrotitis
scrotocele
scrotoplasty
scrotoscopy
scrotum, pl. **scrota**
acute s.
angiokeratoma of s.
bifid s.
s. calcification
s. cyst
ectopic s.
lymph s.
necrotizing fasciitis of s.

prepenile dislocation of s.
raphe of s.
sebaceous cyst of s.
septum of s.
watering-can s.
scrub
Betadine s.
pHisoHex s.
SCTAT
sex cord tumors with annular tubules
SCTP
solid and cystic tumors of pancreas
Scudder
S. intestinal clamp
S. intestinal forceps
SCUF
slow continuous ultrafiltration
Scultetus position
scybalous stool
scybalum, pl. **scybala**
SDB
sleep-disordered breathing
SDH
sorbitol dehydrogenase
SDH enzyme
SDS
sodium dodecyl sulfate
SDS-PAGE
sodium dodecyl sulfate polyacrylamide gel electrophoresis
SEA
soluble egg antigen
sea anemone ulcer
sea-blue histiocyte syndrome
seabuckthorn seed oil
seal
fibrin s.
Karaya 5 s.
long s. (LS)
sealant
Beriplast fibrin s.
Crosseal fibrin s.
fibrin s.
Hemaseel APR kit fibrin s.
Periplast s.
Tisseel fibrin s.
searcher
stone s.
Sears Wee Alert
sebaceous
s. cyst
s. cyst of scrotum

NOTES

sebaceum
    adenoma s.
seborrheic
    s. dermatitis
    s. keratitis
SEC
    sinusoidal endothelial cell
    superficial esophageal carcinoma
secalin
Secca
    S. procedure
    S. radiofrequency system
Seckel syndrome
secobarbital
secoisolariciresinol
secondary
    s. achalasia
    s. amyloidosis
    s. bacterial peritonitis
    s. bile acid
    s. biliary cirrhosis
    s. biliary fibrosis
    s. case
    s. closure
    s. contraction
    s. cyst
    s. enterocele
    s. hyperaldosteronism
    s. hyperparathyroidism
    s. hypertension
    s. impotence
    s. incontinence
    s. jejunal ulcer
    s. metastatic carcinoma
    s. peristalsis
    s. peristaltic wave
    s. priapism
    s. prophylaxis
    s. pseudoobstruction syndrome
    s. refluxing megaureter
    s. renal calculus
    s. sclerosing cholangitis
    s. spermatocyte
    s. sterility
    s. surgery
    s. suture
    s. syphilis
    s. tumor
    s. ureteropelvic junction obstruction
    s. vesicoureteral reflex
    s. volvulus
second-cuff implantation
second-generation
    s.-g. cephalosporin
    s.-g. enzyme immunoassay (EIA-2)
    s.-g. lithotriptor
    s.-g. recombinant immunoblot assay
second-line drug

second-look
    s.-l. flexible nephroscopy
    s.-l. laparotomy
    s.-l. operation
second resection
second-set phenomenon
secosteroid hormone
SecreFlo
secretagogue
    luminal s.
    mucus s.
    somatostatin s.
secreted
    s. autotransporter toxin
    s. mediator
    regulated upon activation, normal T cells expressed and s. (RANTES)
secretin
    proton-induced release of s.
    s. provocation test
    s. stimulation
    s. stimulation test
    synthetic porcine s.
    s. ultrasonography
secretin-CCK stimulation test
secretin-cholecystokinin-pancreatozymin (S-CCK-Pz)
Secretin-Ferring Powder
secretin-glucagon-vasoactive intestinal peptide family
secretin-pancreozymin stimulation test
secretion
    acid s.
    basal acid s.
    biliary cholesterol s.
    chloride s.
    chylomicron s.
    epididymis s.
    estrogen testicular s.
    follicle-stimulating hormone s.
    gastric acid s.
    gonadotropin-releasing hormone pulsatile s.
    hydrochloric acid s.
    idiopathic gastric acid s.
    intrinsic factor s.
    Leydig cell s.
    macromolecular s.
    meal-stimulated pancreatic s.
    medication-associated suppression of gastric s.
    mucoid s.
    paralytic s.
    pepsin s.
    physiologic role in acid s.
    prostate gland s.
    renin s.
    toxin-mediated intestinal s.

urinalysis sediment microscopy
prostatic s.
vas deferens s.
secretory
s. canaliculus
s. cell
s. coil
s. component (SC)
s. diarrhea
s. IgA (sIgA)
s. immunoglobulin A
s. leukocyte proteinase inhibition (SLPI)
s. product
s. reflex
section
abdominal s.
adrenal gland microscopic s.
distal shave s.
frozen s.
Giemsa-stained s.
perineal s.
permanent s.
prostate gland cross-section
renal histologic s.
ultrathin araldite s.
sectioning
celiac plexus s.
thin shave s.
sector
7.5 MHz s. scanner
Sectral
Securcut aspiration biopsy needle
sedation
benzodiazepine conscious s.
conscious s.
I.V. s.
meperidine conscious s.
midazolam conscious s.
nurse-administered propofol s. (NAPS)
patient-controlled s. (PCS)
terminal s. (TS)
sedation-induced hypoventilation
sedative
anxiolytic s.
gastric s.
intestinal s.
sediment
nephritic s.
spun urine s.
urinary s.

sedimentation
Ficoll-Hypaque gradient s.
sedoanalgesia
seeberi
Rhinosporidium s.
seed
BrachySeed brachytherapy s.
EchoSeed radioactive iodine-125 brachytherapy s.
iodine-125 brachytherapy s.
I-Plant brachytherapy s.
iridium s.
mustard s.
PharmaSeed iodine-125 s.
PharmaSeed palladium-103 s.
L-phenylalanine mustard (L-PAM)
Plantago ovata s.
ProstaSeed I-125 s.
radioactive s.
SeedNet ice s.
Symmetra I-125 brachytherapy s.
seeding
instrument-track s.
malignant s.
needle-track s.
peritoneal s.
tumor s.
SeedNet
S. cryotherapy system
S. gold ultrathin CryoNeedle
S. ice seed
seepage
fecal s.
SEER
Surveillance, Epidemiology, and End Results
sEGF
salivary epidermal growth factor
segment
afferent tubular isoperistaltic s.
Ask-Upmark renal s.
Barrett s.
demucosalized augmentation with gastric s. (DAWG)
digital stream s.
distal nephron s.
ileal s. (IS)
ileocecal s.
midtransverse s.
nephron s.
pyloroduodenal s.

NOTES

segment *(continued)*
    S3 s.
    tumor-bearing s.
segmenta (*pl. of* segmentum)
segmental
    s. appendicitis
    s. bile duct fibrosis
    s. change
    s. colectomy
    s. colonic adenomatous polyposis syndrome
    s. colonic resection
    s. colonic tuberculosis
    s. enteritis
    s. glomerulosclerosis
    s. ileal infarction
    s. intestine
    s. ischemic colitis
    s. liver graft
    s. testicular infarction
    s. ureterectomy
segmentary pancreatitis
segmentation movement
segmentectomy
    hepatic s.
    s. of liver
segmented neutrophil
segment-specific expression pattern
segmentum, pl. **segmenta**
segregator
    Cathelin s.
    Harris s.
    Luy s.
Segura basket
Segura-Dretler laser basket
SeHCAT
    selenium-labeled homocholic acid conjugated with taurine
    SeHCAT test
Seidlitz powder
Seitzinger tripolar cutting forceps
seizure
    autonomic s.
    s. disorder
Sekomic SS-100F recorder
^{75}Se-labeled bile acid test
SelCID
Seldinger
    S. cystic duct catheterization
    S. gastrostomy needle
    S. principle
    S. technique
selectin
selective
    s. bladder activation
    s. catheterization
    s. ductal cannulation
    s. endothelin A
    s. intestinal decontamination (SID)
    s. jejunal hyperalgesia
    s. left gastric arteriography
    s. mesenteric angiography
    s. paracellular conductance
    s. proximal vagotomy (SPV)
    s. sacral rhizotomy
    s. targeting
    s. tubal occlusion procedure (STOP)
selectivity
    charge s.
selenite
    insulin-transferrin-sodium s.
Selenite-F enrichment medium
selenium-75
selenium-labeled homocholic acid conjugated with taurine (SeHCAT)
selenomethionine radioactive agent
self-antigen
self blood glucose monitoring (SBGM)
self-bougienage treatment
self-catheterization
    intermittent s.-c. (ISC)
self-channelization
    urethral s.-c.
self-drainage catheter
self-expandable stainless steel braided endoprosthesis
self-expanding
    s.-e. biliary metal stent
    s.-e. coil stent
    s.-e. metallic (SEM)
    s.-e. metallic stent (SEMS)
self-fulfilling prophecy
self-induced
    s.-i. purging
    s.-i. vomiting
self-injection therapy
self-management
    primary advantage of s.-m.
self-MHC
self-monitoring
    nocturnal tumescence s.-m.
self-obturation
    intermittent s.-o.
self-poisoning
self-retaining
    s.-r. catheter
    s.-r. coil stent
    s.-r. ring retractor
self-retraction clamp
self-retractor
    Lone Star s.-r.
self-test
    Coloscreen S.-t.
self-tightening slip knot
Seltzer
    Bromo S.

SELU
   seromuscular enterocystoplasty lined with urothelium
SEM
   self-expanding metallic
      SEM stent
semantic conditioning
Semb ligature carrier
semen
   s. analysis
   s. analysis test
   s. coagulation
   s. collection
   s. liquefaction
   s. round cell
   s. sperm concentration
   s. viscosity
   s. volume
semenuria
semicircular line of Douglas
semielemental
   s. diet
   s. enteral feeding
semiflexible endoscope
semiformed stool
Semilente insulin
semilunar-shaped fold
seminal
   s. colliculus
   s. fluid
   s. oxidative stress in patient
   s. plasma C3
   s. plasma cholesterol
   s. plasma choline
   s. plasma citrate
   s. plasma citric acid
   s. plasma fructose
   s. plasma Zn-alpha 2-glycoprotein
   s. tract washout
   s. vesicle
   s. vesicle abscess
   s. vesicle adenocarcinoma
   s. vesicle agenesis
   s. vesicle amyloid deposit
   s. vesicle aplasia
   s. vesicle aspiration
   s. vesicle atrophy
   s. vesicle calculus
   s. vesicle carcinoid
   s. vesicle hydatid cyst
   s. vesicle infection
   s. vesicle innervation
   s. vesicle lymphoma
   s. vesicle obstruction
   s. vesicle sarcoma
   s. vesicle weight
   s. vesiculography (SVG)
   s. vesiculotomy
seminalis
   colliculus s.
   ductus excretorius vesiculae s.
   vesicula s.
semination
seminiferous
   s. tubule
   s. tubule blood-testis barrier
   s. tubule epithelium
   s. tubule gonocyte
   s. tubule peritubular structure
   s. tubule Sertoli cell
seminis
   liquor s.
seminogelin
seminologist
seminology
seminoma
   anaplastic s.
   retroperitoneal s.
   testicular s.
seminomatous
seminoprotein
   gamma s.
seminuria
semioblique position
semiopen hemorrhoidectomy
semipedunculated
   s. lesion
   s. tumor
semiquantitative
   s. agglutination SERA-TEK Ames
   s. culture
semirigid
   s. endoscope
   s. fiberoptic ureteroscope
   s. Nottingham introducer
   s. sigmoidoscope
semisolid stool
Semken tissue forceps
SEMS
   self-expanding metallic stent
      membrane-coated SEMS
Senecio
senescence
   accelerated s.

NOTES

senescent cell
Sengstaken-Blakemore (S-B)
    S.-B. esophageal balloon
    S.-B. method
    S.-B. tamponade
    S.-B. tube
    S.-B. tube insertion
senile nephrosclerosis
Senior-Loken syndrome
senktide
senna
    extractum s.
Senn-Kanavel retractor
Senn retractor
Senokot-S
Senokot X-Prep
Sensa
    Hemoccult s.
sensation
    bladder s.
    burning s.
    esophageal globus s.
    foreign body s.
    perineal s.
    rectal s.
    S. Short Throw snare
    threshold of rectal s.
SensiCare synthetic powder-free surgical glove
Sensipar
sensitive and specific ELISA
sensitivity
    anaphylactoid food s.
    culture and s. (C&S, C+S)
    esophageal acid s.
    gluten s.
    interpersonal s.
    penile s.
    rectal visceral s.
    soy protein s.
sensitizer
    radiation s.
sensor
    anal EMG PerryMeter s.
    anterior esophageal s. (AES)
    bladder pressure s.
    Dentsleeve sleeve s.
    fiberoptic s.
    manometric s.
    S. Medics pressure transducer
    sleeve s.
    ultrasonic tactile s.
sensorium change
sensory
    s. biofeedback
    s. findings
    s. loss
    s. nervous terminal
    s. neuron

    s. receptor
    s. urgency
    s. voiding dysfunction
sentinel
    s. clot
    s. fold
    s. hyperplastic polyp
    s. loop
    s. node
    s. pile
    s. tag
sentry system
separate peripheral venipuncture
separation
    peripartum symphysis s.
separator
    Benson pylorus s.
Sephacryl S-300 HR gel
Sepharose 4B-coupled-protein-A column
Seprafilm bioresorbable membrane
Sepramesh
sepsis
    anal s.
    anorectal s.
    biliary s.
    enterococcal s.
    gram-negative s.
    gram-positive s.
    s. intestinalis
    intraabdominal s. (IAS)
    pancreatic s.
    pelvic s.
    perianal s.
    post rubber band s.
    staphylococcal s.
    s. syndrome
Sepsis-Related Organ Failure Assessment (SOFA)
septa (*pl. of* septum)
septal hematoma
Septata intestinalis
septate vagina
septation
    cloaca s.
    internal s.
septectomy
septic
    s. cholangitis
    s. necrosis
    s. shock
    s. wound
septicemia
Septisol
Septopal
    S. bead
    S. implant
septotomy
    endoscopic transpancreatic ampullary s.

Septra DS
septulum, pl. **septula**
    septula testis
septum, pl. **septa**
    s. bulbi urethra
    cloacal s.
    fibrous s.
    s. glandis penis
    s. of glans penis
    interhaustral s.
    pancreaticobiliary s.
    s. pectiniforme
    perforated nasal s.
    rectogenital s.
    rectovaginal s.
    rectovesical s.
    scrotal s.
    s. of scrotum
    s. of testis
    tracheoesophageal s.
    transverse vaginal s.
    urethrovaginal s.
    urorectal s.
sequela, pl. **sequelae**
    clinical s.
sequence
    adenoma-carcinoma s.
    adenomatous polyp-cancer s.
    contrast-enhanced fast s. (CE-FAST)
    dysplasia-to-carcinoma s.
    esophageal manometric s. (EMS)
    flanking s.
    FLASH pulse s.
    genomic s.
    HASTE s.
    leucine zipper s.
    metaplasia-dysplasia-carcinoma s.
    papilloma-carcinoma s.
    phasic wave s.
    rapid acquisition fast spin-echo s.
    repeat s.
    turbo spin-echo s.
    ZIRTL s.
sequenced
    automatically s.
sequence-sequence oligonucleotide hybridization
sequencing
    s. analysis
    molecular cloning and s.

sequential
    s. counterstaining
    s. motility
    s. multiple analyzer (SMA)
    s. quadruple-drug regimen
    s. ultrafiltration hemodialysis
    s. videoconverter
sequestrant
    bile acid s.
sequestration
    fluid s.
sera (*pl. of* serum)
Serenoa
    S. repens
    S. repens extract
Serentil
Sergent white adrenal line
serial
    s. cholangiograms
    s. dilution
series
    acute abdominal s. (AAS)
    gallbladder s. (GBS)
    Gastrografin GI s.
    800 s. KTP/YAG surgical laser system
    liver function s. (LFS)
    motor meal barium GI s.
    upper GI s.
    worldwide clinical s.
serine
    s. protease
    s. protease-activated prorenin
    s. threonine kinase gene 11
Seriola dumerili
seroconversion rate
Serodia commercial kit
seroepidemiological study
seroepidemiology
serologic
    s. diagnosis
    s. marker
    s. test
    s. test for syphilis (STS)
serology
    IgG s.
    specific anti-Hp s.
seromuscular
    s. colocystoplasty
    s. enterocystoplasty lined with urothelium (SELU)
    s. intestinal patch graft

NOTES

seromuscular *(continued)*
    s. layer
    s. Lembert suture
seromyectomy
    duodenal s.
seromyotomy
    laparoscopic s.
seronegative polyarthritis
seropositive
seroprevalence rate
seroprotection
serosa
    cecal s.
    gastric s.
    perispermatitis s.
    tunica s.
serosal
    s. afferent innervation
    s. blood vessel
    s. creeping fat
    s. infiltration
    s. surface
    s. tear
serosanguineous
    s. drainage
    s. fluid
serositis
    uremic s.
serotonergic
    s. drug
    s. type 3 receptor
serotonin (5-HT)
    s. antagonist treatment
    s. cell
    s. receptor antagonist
    s. reuptake transporter (SERT)
    serum s.
    s. stain
serotoninergic neuron
serous
    s. diarrhea
    s. membrane
Serpasil-Esidrix
serpiginous
    s. microcystic duct
    s. ulcer
    s. ulceration
Serpulina
    S. hyodysenteria
    S. innocens
    S. pilosicoli
serrated adenoma
Serratia
    S. liquefaciens
    S. marcescens
serratum
    Lycopodium s.
serratus posterior muscle
serrefine clamp

SERT
    serotonin reuptake transporter
Sertina
Sertoli
    S. cell
    S. cell secretory function
    S. cell tumor
Sertoli-cell-only (SCO)
    S.-c.-o. syndrome
Sertoli-Leydig cell
sertraline serotonin reuptake inhibitor
serum, pl. **sera**
    s. albumin
    s. alpha$_1$-protease inhibitor
    s. ammonia
    s. amylase
    s. amylase test
    s. amyloid A (SAA)
    s. amyloid P (SAP)
    s. amyloid P component
    s. bicarbonate
    s. bile acid measurement
    s. bilirubin
    s. bilirubin test
    s. blocking factor
    s. calcitonin
    s. calcium
    s. calcium concentration
    calibrator s.
    s. carotene
    s. ceruloplasmin
    s. chloride
    s. cholesterol
    s. cholinesterase activity
    s. chromogranin A
    s. core protein
    s. creatinine (SCr)
    s. creatinine test
    s. cytokine analysis
    s. elastase 1
    s. eotaxin level
    familial nephritis s.
    s. ferritin
    s. ferritin concentration
    fetal calf s.
    s. folate
    s. gamma-glutamyltransferase
    s. gastrin
    s. gastrin level
    s. glutamic-oxaloacetic transaminase (SGOT)
    s. glutamic-pyruvic transaminase (SGPT)
    s. haptoglobin
    heat-inactivated fetal calf s.
    s. hepatitis
    s. hyaluronic acid
    immune s. (IS)
    s. interleukin-2

s. interleukin-6
s. interleukin-8
s. iron (SI)
s. iron test
s. kinase
s. leptin level
s. lipase
s. marker
s. metabolic evaluation
s. nephritis
s. noradrenaline
s. osmolarity
s. pepsinogen I/II ratio
s. pepsinogen isoenzyme I, II
s. PG
s. phosphate
s. phospholipid
s. phosphorus
s. protein electrophoresis (SPEP)
s. protein test
s. pyridinoline
s. pyruvate kinase (SPK)
s. RIBA-2 test
s. sample
s. serotonin
s. sickness
s. sicknesslike syndrome
s. testosterone
s. thrombotic accelerator
s. transferrin
s. triglyceride
s. urate level
s. urea nitrogen (SUN)
s. uric acid
s. virus antibody

serum-ascites albumin gradient (SAAG)
serum-free conditional media
Serutan
servomechanism sphincter
sesquioxide
chromium s.
sessile
s. adenoma
s. lesion
s. nodular carcinoma
s. polyp
session
didactic teaching s.
set
Assura deluxe irrigation s.
Assura economy irrigation s.
Boehm rectal diagnostic and treatment s.
Brunner ligature s.
Coloplast ostomy irrigation s.
Conseal ostomy irrigation s.
cytocentrifuge s.
Dansac ostomy irrigation s.
dilating s.
Eliminator nasobiliary catheter s.
Freiburg biopsy s.
French introducer s.
Heyer-Schulte Small-Carrion sizing s.
introducer s.
Jeffrey introducer s.
KeyMed advanced esophageal dilator s.
Lipshultz urology microsurgical s.
mandril s.
no-scalpel vasectomy instrument s.
over-the-wire s.
s. point theory
Rosch-Uchida transjugular liver access s.
Sur-Fit Natura night drainage container s.
Sur-Fit Natura Visi-Flow irrigation starter s.
United Ostomy irrigation s.
urology s.

Setguard antireflux valve
Sethotope radioactive agent
seton
s. management
Penrose s.
silk s.
s. treatment of high anal fistula
setophobia
sevelamer
s. hydrochloride
s. hydrochloride tablet
severance
retroduodenal artery s.
severe
s. aldosterone excess
s. combined immunodeficiency (SCID)
s. erosive esophagitis
s. gastritis
s. hematochezia
s. macrovesicular steatosis
s. morbid illness

NOTES

severe (continued)
    s. pain
    s. recurrent bladder neck contracture
    s. reflux esophagitis
    s. secretory diarrhea
    s. ureteral stricture
    s. variceal bleeding

severity
    Crohn Disease Endoscopic Index of S. (CDEIS)
    leakage s.

sex
    s. accessory tissue
    s. assignment by fetal ultrasonography
    s. cord-mesenchyme tumor
    s. cord tumors with annular tubules (SCTAT)
    s. hormone-binding globulin (SHBG)
    phenotypic s.
    s. reversal syndrome
    s. therapy

sextant
    s. technique
    s. transrectal ultrasound-guided biopsy

sexual
    s. abuse
    s. differentiation
    s. dysfunction androgeny
    s. evaluation
    s. function
    S. Function Index (SFI)
    S. Function Inventory Questionnaire (SFIQ)
    s. function score
    s. infantilism
    s. potency
    s. reflex
    s. rehabilitation
    s. stimulation testing

sexually
    s. related intestinal disease
    s. transmitted colitis
    s. transmitted disease (STD)
    s. transmitted disease contact tracing

Seyd-Neblett perineal template
Sézary syndrome
SF
    sucrose-free
    Isomil SF

SF-9 baculovirus-insect cell system
SFA
    saturated fatty acid
SFI
    Sexual Function Index

SFIQ
    Sexual Function Inventory Questionnaire
SFM
    scanning force microscopy
SFU
    Society for Fetal Urology
Sgambati
    S. reaction test
    S. test for peritonitis
SGOT
    serum glutamic-oxaloacetic transaminase
    SGOT test
SGP-2
    sulfated glycoprotein-2
SGPT
    serum glutamic-pyruvic transaminase
    SGPT test
SH2
    src-homology 2
SH2-binding domain
shadow
    arc s.
    dumbbell-shaped s.
    obliteration of psoas s.
    psoas s.
    ring s.
shadowing
    hyperechoic s.
shaft
    Eder-Puestow dilator s.
shaggy tumor
shagreen patch
sham
    s. feeding
    s. feeding test
    s. injection
    s. surgery
    s. treatment
Shambaugh fistula hook
shape
    double-wing s.
    s. memory alloy (SMA)
    s. memory alloy stent
shaped
    olive s.
sharing
    United Network for Organ S. (UNOS)
shark
    S. disposable biopsy forceps
    s. fin papillotome
shark-tooth forceps
sharp
    s. dissection
    s. spoon
sharp-edged
    s.-e. orifice
    s.-e. tip

Sharpoint
    S. cutting instrument
    S. microsuture
shave biopsy
SHBG
    sex hormone-binding globulin
SHC
    sclerosing hepatic carcinoma
SHE
    subclinical hepatic encephalopathy
shears
    Bethune s.
    harmonic scalpel coagulating s.
    LaparoSonic coagulating s.
    Lebsche s.
    UltraCision harmonic laparoscopic cutting s.
sheath
    Acucise access s.
    Amplatz s.
    anterior rectus s.
    fibrous s.
    Futura resectoscope s.
    miniaturized s.
    nephroscope s.
    overtube s.
    peel-away introducer s.
    perivascular s.
    posterior rectus s.
    quill s.
    rectus s.
    resectoscope s.
    retroflexed cystoscopy s.
    sport s. (SS)
    Teflon s.
    Universal s.
    ureterorenoscope procedure s.
    ureteroscope s.
    Waldeyer s.
    water-filled balloon s.
    working s.
sheathed
    s. cytology brush
    s. flexible sigmoidoscope
shedding
    virus s.
sheet
    Dacron-impregnated Silastic s.
sheetlike adenoma
shelf
    Blumer rectal s.
    mesocolic s.
    rectal s.
shell vial culture
shelving edge of Poupart ligament
shepherd's
    s. hook catheter
    s. hook-shaped angiographic catheter
shield
    Active Living incontinence s.
    CapSure continence s.
    Fuller rectal s.
    syringe s.
shift
    fluid s.
    mediastinal s.
shifting dullness
Shiga
    S. bacillus
    S. dysentery
    S. toxin (Stx)
    S. toxin-producing *Escherichia coli* (STEC)
shigae
    Shigella s.
Shiga-like toxin (SLT)
Shigella
    S. ambigua
    S. boydii
    S. colitis
    S. dysenteriae
    S. dysentery
    S. flexneri
    S. newcastle
    S. paradysenteriae
    S. schmitzii
    S. shigae
    S. sonnei
shigelloides
    Plesiomonas s.
shigellosis
shim
    step-up s.
Shimadzu RF-5301 PC spectrometer
Shiner tube
Shirodkar cervical cerclage
shock
    extracorporeal s.
    hypovolemic s.
    s. liver
    s. number
    s. patient

NOTES

shock *(continued)*
    septic s.
    spinal s.
    s. wave (SW)
    s. wave-gas bubble interaction
    s. wave lithotripsy (SWL)
    s. wave lithotripsy cavitation component
    s. wave lithotripsy failure
    s. wave lithotriptor
    s. wave treatment
Shoemaker intestinal clamp
Shohl-Pedley method
Shohl solution
shooter
Shorr regimen
short
    s. band stenosis
    s. daily dialysis
    s. incubation hepatitis
    S. Inflammatory Bowel Disease Questionnaire (SIBDQ)
    s. urethra
short-bowel syndrome
short-chain fatty acid (SCFA)
short-dwell hypertonic exchange
shortened prep time
short-gut syndrome
short-lasting afterhyperpolarizing potential
short-segment
    s.-s. Barrett epithelium
    s.-s. Barrett esophagus (SSBE)
    s.-s. CLE
    s.-s. lesion
short-term
    s.-t. prostate-specific antigen recurrence
    s.-t. result
    s.-t. survival outcome
sho-saiko-to
shot
    flat low-angle s. (FLASH)
shotty lymph nodes
shoulder
    s. girdle
    s. shrug
Shouldice inguinal herniorrhaphy
shower
    uric acid s.
shrapnel-induced
    s.-i. biliary obstruction
    s.-i. obstructive jaundice
shrug
    shoulder s.
shrunken liver
shunt
    Al-Ghorab modification s.
    Allen-Brown s.
    angiographic portacaval s.
    arterioportal venous s.
    arteriovenous s.
    AV shunt
    biliopancreatic s.
    Brescia-Cimino s.
    Buselmeier s.
    caval-atrial s.
    cavernospongiosum s.
    cerebral fluid s.
    chloride s.
    congenital portacaval s.
    Cordis-Hakim s.
    cystoperitoneal s.
    Denver peritoneovenous s.
    Denver pleuroperitoneal s.
    dialysis s.
    distal splenorenal s. (DSRS)
    Drapanas s.
    end-to-side portacaval s.
    esophageal s.
    extrahepatic s.
    gastric venacaval s.
    gastrorenal s.
    Gott s.
    Hashmat s.
    Hashmat-Waterhouse s.
    hepatofugal arterioportal s.
    hepatofugal portosystemic venous s.
    Hyde s.
    s. index via inferior mesenteric vein (SI-I)
    s. index via superior mesenteric vein (SI-S)
    intrahepatic artery-systemic s.
    jejunoileal s.
    Kasai peritoneal venous s.
    LeVeen ascites s.
    LeVeen peritoneal s.
    LeVeen peritoneovenous s.
    Linton s.
    mesocaval H-graft s.
    mesocaval interposition s.
    s. nephritis
    occluded s.
    pentose phosphate s.
    peritoneal-atrial s.
    peritoneocaval s.
    peritoneojugular s.
    peritoneovenous s. (PVS)
    portacaval s. (PCS)
    portacaval H-graft s.
    portopulmonary s.
    portosystemic s.
    proximal splenorenal s.
    Quinton-Scribner s.
    radiologic portacaval s.
    Ramirez s.
    Scribner s.

    side-to-side s.
    small bowel s.
    splenorenal bypass s.
    spontaneous portosystemic s. (SPSS)
    stenotic s.
    Thomas s.
    transhepatic portacaval s.
    transjugular intrahepatic portosystemic s. (TIPS)
    transjugular intrahepatic portosystemic stent s. (TIPSS)
    s. tubing
    ventriculoperitoneal s.
    vesicoamniotic s.
    VP s.
    Warren splenorenal s.
    Winter s.

shunting
    arterioportal vein s. (APS)
    intrapulmonary s.
    portosystemic s. (PSS)
    surgical portosystemic s.

shuntlike pore
Shwachman-Diamond syndrome
Shwachman syndrome
Shy-Drager syndrome
SI
    saturation index
    serum iron
    SI of bile

SIADH
    syndrome of inappropriate secretion of antidiuretic hormone

sialic
    s. acid
    s. acid residue

sialidase
sialoadenectomy
sialoglycoprotein
sialomucin
    acidic s.

sialorrhea pancreatica
sialosyl-Tn antigen
sialyl
    s. Lewis A
    s. Lewis A antigen
    s. residue

sialylated
    s. derivative
    s. lacto-N-fucopentaose

sialylation
    cell-surface s.

sialyllactose
sialyl-Tn antigen
SIBDQ
    Short Inflammatory Bowel Disease Questionnaire

sibling
    HLA-identical s.

SIBO
    small intestine bacterial overgrowth

sibutramine HCl
sicca
    cholera s.
    s. syndrome

sicchasia
sick
    s. cell syndrome
    s. euthyroid state

sickle
    s. cell anemia
    s. cell disease
    s. cell nephropathy
    s. hemoglobinopathy

sickling
    erythrocyte s.

sickness
    black s.
    Gambian sleeping s.
    s. impact profile
    Indian s.
    Jamaican vomiting s.
    milk s.
    motion s.
    serum s.

SID
    selective intestinal decontamination
    sucrose-isomaltase deficiency

side
    s. branch
    high-lying s.
    host s.
    orad s.

side-effect profile
Side-Fire
    S.-F. laser
    S.-F. reflecting dish

sideroblast
    refractory anemia with ringed s.'s (RARS)

sideropenic dysphagia

NOTES

siderotic
    s. nodule
    s. splenomegaly
side-to-side
    s.-t.-s. anastomosis
    s.-t.-s. isoperistaltic strictureplasty (SSIS)
    s.-t.-s. shunt
side-viewing
    s.-v. endoscope
    s.-v. fiberoptic duodenoscope
    s.-v. fiberscope
    s.-v. videoduodenoscope
sidewall
    pelvic s.
Siegel-Cohen dilating catheter
Siegel stent
Sielaff gastroscope
Siemens
    S. Endo-P endorectal transducer
    S. Lithostar
    S. Lithostar Plus System C lithotriptor
    S. MRI unit
    S. Somatom DRH CT analyzer
    S. Somatom DRH CT analyzer unit
    S. Sonoline ultrasonography
sieving
    s. coefficient (SC)
    dextran s.
    s. effect
    s. function
    Keller hydrodynamic hypothesis of s.
    s. of solid food
sIgA
    secretory IgA
siginata
    Taenia s.
sigma
    S. 34 monoplace hyperbaric chamber
    s. rectum pouch
sigmoid
    s. colon
    s. colon carcinoma
    s. colon reservoir
    s. colon volvulus
    s. conduit
    s. curve
    s. cystoplasty
    s. disease
    s. diverticulitis
    s. diverticulum
    s. enterocystoplasty
    s. flexure
    s. fold
    s. kidney
    s. loop
    s. loop reduction
    s. neobladder
    s. pouch
    s. ulcer
    s. valve
sigmoideae
    arteriae s.
sigmoidectomy
    hand-assisted laparoscopic s.
sigmoid-end colostomy
sigmoideum
    colon s.
sigmoid-loop rod colostomy
sigmoidoanal intussusception
sigmoidocele
sigmoidocystoplasty
sigmoidopexy
    endoscopic s.
sigmoidoproctostomy
sigmoidorectostomy
sigmoidoscope, sigmoscope
    ACMI T-915, TX-915 fiberoptic s.
    adult s.
    American ACMI (S3565, TX-915) flexible fiberoptic s.
    Boehm s.
    Buie s.
    disposable sheathed flexible s.
    ESI fiberoptic s.
    fiberoptic s.
    flexible s.
    Fujinon ES-200ER s.
    Fujinon FS-100ER s.
    Fujinon PRO-PC flexible fiberoptic s.
    Fujinon SIG-E2 fiberoptic s.
    Fujinon SIG-EK-series flexible fiberoptic s.
    Fujinon SIG-E-series flexible fiberoptic s.
    Fujinon SIG-ET-series flexible fiberoptic s.
    Kelly s.
    Lieberman s.
    Lloyd-Davis s.
    Montague s.
    Olympus CF-L-series flexible s.
    Olympus CF-OSF-series flexible s.
    Olympus CF100S s.
    Olympus OSF flexible s.
    Pentax FS-series flexible fiberoptic video s.
    Reichert FLPS-series flexible fiberoptic s.
    Reichert MS-series flexible fiberoptic s.
    Reichert SC-series flexible fiberoptic s.

rigid s.
semirigid s.
sheathed flexible s.
Vernon-David s.
Vision System s.
VSI 2000 s.
Welch Allyn flexible s.

sigmoidoscopy
fiberoptic s.
flexible s.
s. table

sigmoidostomy
sigmoidotomy
sigmoidovesical fistula
sigmoidovesicostomy
transverse retubularized s.

sigmoid-rectum pouch
sigmoscope (*var. of* sigmoidoscope)
sign
Aaron s.
accordion s.
arrowhead s.
auscultatory s.
Babinski s.
Ballance s.
barber pole s.
Battle s.
beading s.
Bergman s.
Blatin s.
blue dot s.
Blumberg s.
Boas s.
bowler hat s.
Boyce s.
Brodie s.
Brudzinski s.
burning drops s.
Carman s.
Carman-Kirklin meniscus s.
Carnett s.
catheter coiling s.
chain-of-lakes s.
Chilaiditi s.
Christmas tree s.
Clark s.
Claybrook s.
closed eyes s.
cobblestoning s.
cobra-head s.
coiled spring s.
Cole s.

colon cutoff s.
colon single-stripe s.
comblike redness s.
comet s.
Cope s.
Courvoisier s.
Cowen s.
Cruveilhier s.
Cruveilhier-Baumgarten s.
Cullen s.
cushion s.
Dance s.
Dew s.
double bubble duodenal s.
double duct s.
double halo s.
drooping lily s.
Duroziez s.
E s.
Earle s.
echo s.
Federici s.
flapping tremor s.
flush-tank s.
Fothergill s.
four lines s.
Fournier s.
Fraley s.
Frostberg reversed-3 s.
Gilbert s.
Gottron s.
Gowers s.
Grey Turner s.
Grocco s.
guarding s.
Guyon s.
Hampton s.
Haudek s.
heliotrope s.
Henning s.
histologic s.
Horn s.
Howship-Romberg s.
iliopsoas s.
inverted-V s.
Kantor string s.
Kehr s.
Kelly s.
Kernig s.
Klemm s.
Lennhoff s.
Leser-Trélat s.

NOTES

sign *(continued)*
lifting s.
ligature s.
liver flap s.
Lloyd s.
lollipop tree s.
malignant meniscus s.
McBurney s.
McCormack gastric mucosal s.
McCort s.
Meltzer s.
meniscus s.
Mercedes Benz s.
Mexican hat s.
moulage s.
multiple concentric rings s.
Murphy s.
Naclerio s.
naked fat s.
niche s.
obturator s.
peritoneal s.
Pfuhl s.
pillow s.
Pitres s.
Poppel s.
Prehn s.
pruning s.
pseudocholangiocarcinoma s.
pseudoparallel channel s.
psoas s.
puddle s.
pyloric string s.
rat-tail s.
RCS s.
rebound s.
red color s. (RCS)
red flag s.
red ring s.
reversed Mercedes Benz s.
Rigler s.
rim s.
s. of rising tide
Robertson s.
Roche s.
Rommelaere s.
Rosenbach s.
Rovighi s.
Rovsing s.
Russell s.
sawtooth appearance s.
scarf-ring s.
Sister Mary Joseph s.
snow-white duodenum s.
Stierlin s.
Stransky s.
Strauss s.
string s.
string-of-beads s.
string-of-pearls s.
Sumner s.
tail s.
tenting s.
Terry fingernail s.
tethered-bowel s.
Thornton s.
thread-and-streaks s.
thumbprinting s.
tissue rim s.
Toma s.
Trimadeau s.
Troisier s.
Turner s.
Uhthoff s.
ureterocele drooping lily s.
vital s.
white ball s.
white nipple s.

Signa
S. Dress Hydrocolloid dressing
S. EXCITE 3.0T MRI system

signal
adenosine s.
adrenergic s.
beta-actin mRNA s.
sodium s.
s. transduction pathway
s. transduction process
transmembrane s.
weaker immunofluorescence s.

signaling cascade
signal-to-cutoff ratio
signet-ring
s.-r. cell
s.-r. cell carcinoma
s.-r. pattern of gastric carcinoma

significance
atypical glandular cells of unknown s. (AGUS)
atypical squamous cells of undetermined s. (ASCUS)
monoclonal gammopathy of undetermined s. (MGUS)
prognostic s.
visible vessel s.

significant
s. benefit
s. clinical history
s. correlation
s. hydronephrosis
s. liver lesion
s. parameter estimate
s. reported complication
statistically s.

SIHC
surgically implanted hemodialysis catheter

SI-I
shunt index via inferior mesenteric vein
Silain-Gel
Silastic
S. catheter
S. collar-reinforced stoma
S. indwelling ureteral stent
S. ring
S. ring vertical gastroplasty
S. silo reduction of gastroschisis
S. sling
Silber
S. technique
S. vasoepididymostomy
sildenafil
s. citrate
s. plus Doppler ultrasonography
silent
s. abdomen
s. aspiration
s. autonephrectomy
s. belch
s. gallstone
s. lupus nephritis
s. prostatism
s. stone
s. thrombosis
s. ulcer
silicate
s. calculus
s. urolithiasis
silicone
s. balloon
s. donut prosthesis
s. elastomer band
s. elastomer ring
s. elastomer ring vertical gastroplasty (SRVG)
s. microimplant particulate s.
s. polymer
s. pressure sensor device
s. rubber Dacron cuffed catheter
s. self-expanding prosthesis
s. sizer
silicone-based oil
silicone-coated metallic self-expanding stent
Silipos
S. arthritic/diabetic gel sock
S. soft-walk gel sock

Silitek Uropass stent
silk
S. Bullet feeding tube
s. jejunal tube
s. ligature
s. Mersilene suture
S. Pill feeding tube
s. pop-off suture
s. seton
S. Tip feeding tube
s. traction suture
Silon tent
silver
s. catheter
s. cell
s. clip
s. nephropathy
s. nitrate
s. probe
s. stain
s. stool
silver-coated stent
Silverman-Boeker needle
Silverman needle
Silybum marianum
Silymarin
SIM
small intestine mesentery
specialized intestinal metaplasia
SIM 2 catheter
Simaal Gel 2
simethicone
aluminum hydroxide, magnesium hydroxide, and s.
calcium carbonate and s.
simian strain
Similac PM 60/40 low-iron formula
similar psychometric properties
Simmons catheter
Simplastic catheter
simple
s. cold storage preservation
s. cystectomy
s. enterocele
s. hydrocele
s. mechanical obstruction
s. nephrectomy
s. neprectomy
s. renal cyst

NOTES

simplex
    exulceratio s.
    herpes s.
simplified nocturnal home hemodialysis (SNHHD)
Simpson endoscope
Sims
    S. anoscope
    S. position
    S. rectal speculum
simulation
    computer graphic s. (CGS)
    s. skill
simulator
    flexible bronchoscopy s.
    heartbeating s.
    inanimate s.
    surgical s.
    validity of surgical s.
    virtual reality s.
Simulect
simultaneous
    s. bilateral extracorporeal shock waves
    s. bilateral percutaneous nephrolithotomy (SBPN)
    s. hemodialysis and hemofiltration
    s. Malone antegrade continent enema and Mitrofanoff procedure
    s. Malone antegrade continent enema and Mitrofanoff procedure using divided appendix
    s. pancreas and kidney transplant
    s. urethral cystometry
simvastatin
sincalide
Sinemet
sinensis
    Clonorchis s.
    Opisthorchis s.
Sinequan
Singer-Blom endoscopic tracheoesophageal puncture technique
single
    s. beta-actin mRNA species
    s. gamma wrap
    s. lens reflex (SLR)
    s. lumen
    s. midline caliceal infundibulum
    s. potential analysis of cavernous electrical activity (SPACE)
    s. potential analysis cavernous electrical activity
    s. stapling
    s. strand conformation polymorphism analysis
single-action pumping system (SAPS)
single-cell keratinization
single-channel
    s.-c. colonoscope
    s.-c. in vivo light dosimeter
    s.-c. wire-guided sphincterotome
single-color direct immunofluorescence study
single-contrast
    s.-c. barium enema
    s.-c. radiography
single-dose
    s.-d. IV Timentin
    s.-d. packet
single-drug therapy
single-fiber
    s.-f. EMG electrode
    s.-f. needle electromyography
single-layer continuous intestinal anastomosis
single-lens reflex camera
single-loop tourniquet
single-lumen Broviac silicone catheter
single-nephron
    s.-n. GFR
    s.-n. glomerular filtration rate (SNGFR)
    s.-n. glomerular transport
single-parameter
    s.-p. DNA
    s.-p. DNA analysis
single-pass hemodialysis
single-photon
    s.-p. emission computed tomography (SPECT)
    s.-p. emission computerized tomography (SPECT)
single-pigtail stent
single-puncture laparoscopy
single-shot voxel projection
single-stage total proctocolectomy
single-stripe colitis (SSC)
single-system ureterocele
single-use maximum-capacity radial jaw with needle
Singley
    S. intestinal forceps
    S. intestinal ring clamp
Singular Oval polypectomy snare
singultation
singultus gastricus nervosus
sinister
    ductus hepaticus s.
    ductus lobi caudati s.
sinistra
    arteria gastrica s.
    arteria gastroomentalis s.
    flexura coli s.
sink-trap malformation

sinoaortic
    s. baroreceptor
    s. denervation (SAD)
sinogram
sinus
    anal s.
    s. anales
    s. bradycardia
    coronary s.
    draining s.
    s. excision
    Forssell s.
    perineal s.
    pilonidal s.
    piriform s.
    pleuroperitoneal s.
    prostatic s.
    rectal s.
    renal s.
    Rokitansky-Aschoff s.
    splenic s.
    subpubic s.
    s. tachycardia
    s. tenderness
    s. tract
    urachal s.
    urogenital s.
sinusoid
    corporeal s.
    erectile s.
    hepatic s.
    liver s.
sinusoidal
    s. capillary pressure
    s. endothelial cell (SEC)
    s. endothelium
    s. endothelium cornucopia
    s. fibrosis
    s. lymphocyte
    s. obstruction syndrome (SOS)
    s. wall
sinusoid lining cell
siphonage
Sipple syndrome
Sippy
    S. diet
    S. esophageal dilator
SIR
    standardized incidence ratio
Siroky
    S. nomogram
    S. nomogram for uroflowmetry

sirolimus
    s. monotherapy
    s. oral solution
    s. tablet
SIRS
    systemic inflammatory response syndrome
SIR-Spheres
SI-S
    shunt index via superior mesenteric vein
Sister
    S. Mary Joseph lymph node
    S. Mary Joseph nodule
    S. Mary Joseph sign
site
    bleeding s.
    crypt-villus s.
    endoscopic biopsy s.
    entry s.
    estrogen binding s. (EBS)
    exit s.
    genomic s.
    injection s.
    internal ribosome entry s. (IRES)
    s. specificity
    stoma s.
    vascular access s.
sitophobia
sitosterolemia
    beta s.
situ
    adenocarcinoma in s.
    bladder carcinoma in s.
    carcinoma in s. (CIS)
    in s.
    squamous cell carcinoma in s.
situation
    radiographic s.
situs
    s. inversus
    s. inversus viscerum
    s. perversus
sitz bath
Sitzmarks
    S. radiopaque marker in gelatin capsule
    S. test
Siurala classification
six-shooter
    Saeed s.-s.
    Wilson-Cook s.-s.
six-wire spiral-tip Segura basket

NOTES

size
- inoculum s.
- kidney s.
- large needle s.
- normal penile s.
- spot s.
- uterine s.

sizer
- silicone s.

Sjögren syndrome (SS)
Sjöqvist method
SJS
- Stevens-Johnson syndrome

skatole
Skelaxin
skeletal
- s. muscle disease
- s. radiography

skeletonize
Skene
- S. duct
- S. gland

skill
- access psychomotor s.
- minimal-access surgical s.
- simulation s.

skin
- anicteric s.
- s. atrophy
- s. bleeding time (SBT)
- s. crease
- s. dimpling
- s. disease
- dry s.
- s. graft
- s. graft imbibition phase
- s. graft inoculation phase
- s. graft neovagina
- icteric s.
- s. inlay urethroplasty
- jaundiced s.
- s. knife
- s. line
- nonicteric s.
- ostomy s.
- s. perfusion
- peristomal s.
- s. staple
- s. stapling
- s. sympathetic response
- s. tag
- s. tube
- s. turgor
- s. xanthoma

skin-CNS-bladder reflex
skinfold
- thickness of s. (TSF)
- s. thickness test

skinny Chiba needle

skinny-needle biopsy
skip
- s. appendicitis
- s. area
- s. lesion

ski position
skipping
- exon s.

Skirrow
- S. agar plate
- S. medium

skirrowii
- *Acrobacter s.*

skullcap
SL
- standard laparoscopy

SL20
- Storz Modulith SL20

SLA
- soluble liver antigen

slash pyelotomy
SLC
- sodium-lithium countertransporter

SLE
- systemic lupus erythematosus

SLED
- slow low-efficiency dialysis
- sustained low-efficiency dialysis

sleep
- s. apnea syndrome
- s. enuresis

sleep-disordered breathing (SDB)
sleeve
- s. advancement
- Assura irrigation s.
- Bard irrigation s.
- Coloplast transparent irrigation s.
- ileal s.
- laparoscopic trocar s.
- Pneumo S.
- s. sensor
- Sur-Fit Natura irrigation s.
- s. technique
- Watzki s.
- Williams overtube s.

sleeve-type circumcision
slice
- coronal s.

slide
- gelatin-subbed s.
- guaiac-impregnated s.
- Hemoccult Sensa s.
- poly-L-lysine-coated glass s.
- s. system

slide-by view
sliding
- s. esophageal hiatal hernia
- s. filament model of contraction
- s. tube

SlimSIGHT gastrointestinal videoscope
sling
    anterior vaginal wall s. (AVWS)
    autologous rectus fascia s.
    BioSling bioabsorbable urethral s.
    Brigham s.
    Burch-Cooper ligament s.
    Cooper ligament s.
    s. failure
    fascia lata suburethral s.
    FortaPerm surgical s.
    intestinal s.
    lyophilized dura mater for pubovaginal s.
    Martius fascial s.
    Mersilene for pubovaginal s.
    s. muscle fiber
    s. operation
    porcine dermis for pubovaginal s.
    s. procedure
    puboprostatic s.
    puborectalis s.
    pubourethral s.
    pubovaginal s.
    Raz anterior vaginal wall s.
    Raz four-corner vaginal wall s.
    rectus fascia s.
    Silastic s.
    Stratasis urethral s.
    suburethral s.
    Suspend s.
    triangular vaginal patch s.
    Vesica s.
sling-and-blanket technique
sling/mesh
    Surgisis s./m.
sling-ring complex
Slip-Coat tip
slippage
    nipple s.
slipped
    s. fundoplication wrap
    s. Nissen fundoplication
    s. Nissen repair
slipper-tipped guidewire
slit
    Cheatle s.
    s. diaphragm
    dorsal s.
    s. lamp
    s. pore length density

SLM-8000 fluorescence spectrophotometer
Slo-bid
slotted
    s. anoscope
    s. instrument
    s. nerve clamp
    s. speculum
sloughed
    s. papilla
    s. urethra syndrome
sloughing of mucosa
slow
    s. bilirubin glucuronidation phenotype
    s. colonic transit
    s. continuous ultrafiltration (SCUF)
    S. Fe
    s. low-efficiency dialysis (SLED)
    s. phasic contraction
    s. wave
    s. wave coupling
Slow-K
slow-transit constipation (STC)
slow-twitch
    s.-t. oxidative
    s.-t. striated muscle fiber
SLPI
    secretory leukocyte proteinase inhibition
SLR
    single lens reflex
SLT
    Shiga-like toxin
    SLT contact MTRL laser
    SLT 7 laser fiber
sludge
    biliary s.
    gallbladder s.
slurry of stool
slush
    ice s.
    saline s.
SMA
    sequential multiple analyzer
    shape memory alloy
    smooth muscle antibody
    superior mesenteric artery
        Doppler sonography of SMA
        SMA formula
        SMA spiral stent
small
    s. bowel

NOTES

small *(continued)*
- s. bowel anastomosis
- s. bowel biopsy
- s. bowel continuity
- s. bowel enema
- s. bowel enteroclysis
- s. bowel enteroscopy (SBE)
- s. bowel erosion
- s. bowel followthrough (SBFT)
- s. bowel infarct
- s. bowel meal
- s. bowel obstruction (SBO)
- s. bowel shunt
- s. bowel thickening
- s. bowel transit time
- s. bowel transplantation
- s. bowel tube
- s. cell tumor
- s. dissecting sponge
- s. granule cell
- s. inflammatory polyp
- s. intestinal Crohn disease
- s. intestinal enterocyte
- s. intestinal infarction
- s. intestinal malignant lymphoma
- s. intestinal membrane
- s. intestinal stenosis
- s. intestinal submucosa
- s. intestinal ulcer
- s. intestinal villus
- s. intestine
- s. intestine bacterial overgrowth (SIBO)
- s. intestine leiomyosarcoma
- s. intestine mesentery (SIM)
- s. intestine trauma
- s. non-cleaved-cell lymphoma
- s. polyp removal
- s. pseudocyst
- s. solitary renal calculus
- s. stomach syndrome

small-caliber
- s.-c. duodenovideoscope
- s.-c. esophagogastroduodenoscopy

Small-Carrion penile prosthesis
small-diameter endosonographic instrument
small-droplet fatty liver
small-duct primary sclerosing cholangitis
smaller gauge needle
SmallHand polypectomy snare
SMA-portogram
SMART
  sperm microaspiration retrieval technique
  SMART anti-CD3
SmartCath esophageal balloon catheter
SMAS
  superior mesenteric artery syndrome
Smead-Jones closure

smear
  buccal s.
  duodenal s.
  KOH s.
  low-grade positive s.
  Papanicolaou s.
  potassium hydroxide s.
smegma praeputii
smegmatis
  Mycobacterium s.
SM-HCV Rapid Test
smiley-face knotting technique
smiling incision
Smith
  S. electrode
  S. method of silver staining
  S. rectal retractor
  S. ring
  S. test
Smith-Boyce operation
Smith-Buie rectal retractor
Smith-Hodge pessary
smithii
  Methanobrevibacter s.
Smith-Lemli-Opitz syndrome
smoker's
  s. palate
  s. tongue
SmokEvac
smooth
  s. diet
  s. muscle
  s. muscle antibody (SMA)
  s. muscle immunological study
  s. muscle isoform actin
  s. muscle motilin receptor
  s. muscle relaxant
  s. tissue forceps
  s. urethral sphincter
SMV
  superior mesenteric vein
  SMV thrombosis
SMX
  sulfamethoxazole
SMX/TMP (*var. of* TMP-SMX)
  sulfamethoxazole and trimethoprim
SMZ
  sulfamethoxazole
snail-headed catheter retriever
snake-skin mucosal pattern
snake-venom converting enzyme-inhibiting action
snap
  s. gauge
  s. gauge band
  s. gauge test
snap-frozen biopsy
Snap-Gauge
Snap-It lubricating jelly

snare
  barbed s.
  Captiflex polypectomy s.
  Captivator polypectomy s.
  s. cautery
  coaxial s.
  colorectal s.
  crescent s.
  diathermal s.
  Douglas rectal s.
  s. electrocoagulation
  electrosurgical s.
  endoscopic s.
  s. excision biopsy
  Frankfeldt rectal s.
  hexagon s.
  incarcerated s.
  lasso s.
  long-nosed retriever s.
  s. loop biopsy
  Nakao s. I, II
  Norwood rectal s.
  Olympus SD-5L semicircular s.
  open electrocautery s.
  oval s.
  s. polypectomy
  polypectomy s.
  Profile pediatric polypectomy s.
  rectal s.
  s. resection
  Rotator polypectomy s.
  Sensation Short Throw s.
  Singular Oval polypectomy s.
  SmallHand polypectomy s.
  standard endoscopy polypectomy s.
  UroSnare cystoscopic tumor s.
  Weston rectal s.
  wire s.
SNGFR
  single-nephron glomerular filtration rate
SNHHD
  simplified nocturnal home hemodialysis
Sn-mesoporphyrin
Snodgrass
  S. incised plate urethroplasty
  S. technique
Snowden-Pencer scissors
Snow procedure
snowstorm effect
snow-white duodenum sign
SNP
  sodium nitroprusside

Sn-protoporphyrin
SNS
  sacral nerve stimulation
  sympathetic nervous system
    SNS therapy
Snyder drain
SO
  sphincter of Oddi
soak
  perianal s.
soap-bubble nephrogram
soapsuds enema (SSE)
soap sudsy appearance
soapy kidney
soar-crash effect
Soave
  S. abdominal pullthrough procedure
  S. endorectal pullthrough
  S. operation
sobria
  Aeromonas s.
society
  S. of American Gastrointestinal
    Endoscoping Surgeons (SAGES)
  S. for Fetal Urology (SFU)
  International Continence S. (ICS)
sock
  polytetrafluoroethylene s.
  Silipos arthritic/diabetic gel s.
  Silipos soft-walk gel s.
SOD
  sphincter of Oddi dysfunction
  superoxide dismutase
sodium
  s. acid urate
  acyclovir s.
  s. anion diarrhea
  s. azide
  s. balance
  s. bicarbonate
  brequinar s.
  butabarbital s.
  Butisol S.
  s. butyrate concentration
  cefazolin s.
  ceftriaxone s.
  s. cellulose phosphate
  cephapirin s.
  s. chloride
  s. citrate
  s. citrate and potassium citrate mixture

NOTES

sodium *(continued)*
   s. cromoglycate
   cromolyn s.
   dalteparin s.
   dantrolene s.
   s. deficiency
   s. deoxycholate
   diclofenac s.
   dietary s.
   docusate s.
   s. dodecyl sulfate (SDS)
   s. dodecyl sulfate polyacrylamide gel electrophoresis (SDS-PAGE)
   Ecabet S. (ES)
   s. electrolyte
   enoxaparin s.
   s. entry route
   epoprostenol s.
   ertapenem s.
   estramustine phosphate s.
   s. exchange
   s. fluorescein (NaF)
   s. flux
   fractional excretion of s. (FENa)
   s. homeostasis
   s. hyaluronate
   s. hyaluronate injection
   s. iodipamide
   s. iodipamide contrast medium
   s. iothalamate
   latamoxef s.
   low s. (LNa)
   luminal s.
   s. meclofenamate
   s. meclofenamate-induced esophageal ulcer
   mesalamine s.
   s. methylglucamine diatrizoate
   s. morrhuate
   s. morrhuate injection
   naproxen s.
   s. nitroprusside (SNP)
   olsalazine s.
   oxychlorosene s.
   pantoprazole s.
   s. pentosan polysulfate
   pentosan polysulfate s.
   peritubular s.
   s. phosphate (NaP)
   s. phosphate-based laxative
   s. phosphate dibasic anhydrous
   s. phosphate monobasic monohydrate
   s. phosphosoda
   s. picosulfate
   piperacillin s.
   s. polystyrene sulfonate
   porfimer s.
   s. pump
   rabeprazole s.
   s. reabsorption
   renal s.
   s. restriction
   s. retention
   s. signal
   sterile ceftriaxone s.
   sulbactam s.
   s. taurocholate
   s. tauroglycocholate
   s. tetradecyl injection
   s. tetradecyl sulfate
   s. tetradecyl sulfate sclerosant
   s. thiosulfate solution spray
   s. transport
   tyropanoate s.
   Urovist S. 300
   s. valproate

sodium-linked process
sodium-lithium countertransporter (SLC)
sodium-loading test
sodium-wasting nephropathy
Soehendra
   S. catheter dilator
   S. catheter system
   S. graduated dilating catheter
   S. stent extractor
   S. stent retrieval device
   S. stent retriever

SOFA
   Sepsis-Related Organ Failure Assessment
   SOFA score

soft
   s. abdomen
   s. balloon method for endoscopic ultrasound
   s. bland diet
   s. diverticuloscope
   s. food dysphagia
   S. Guard XL Skin Barrier
   Modane S.
   s. rubber string
   s. stool
   s. tissue
   s. tissue mass
   s. tissue stranding
   s. x-ray film

softener
   stool s.

softgel
   laxative and stool softener s.

SofTouch vacuum erection device
Softpatch
   Impress S.

soft-tipped wire guide
software
   s. characteristics of treating protocol
   CODAS s.

Cytologic s.
Medtrax urology s.
SPOT mobile 3-D ultrasound system and s.
t-EASE s.
UN-GRAPH computer s.

soilage
peritoneal s.

soiling
colostomy s.
fecal s.

solani
Fusarium s.

solar fever
Solcia classification
solder
laser tissue-welding s.
protein s.

solid
s. bolus challenge
s. and cystic tumors of pancreas (SCTP)
s. egg-white meal
s. emptying
s. evidence
s. food
s. food digestion
s. food dysphagia
s. sphere test
s. teratoma
s. tumor

solid-column esophagogram
solid-phase
s.-p. extraction chromatography
s.-p. radioimmunoassay

solid-state
s.-s. esophageal manometry catheter
s.-s. pressure transducer

solifenacin
solitaire
cholesterol s.

solitarius, pl. **solitarii**
folliculi lymphatici solitarii
nucleus s.
nucleus tractus solitarii

solitary
s. diverticulum
s. hepatic cyst
s. kidney
s. lower pole calculus
s. rectal ulcer syndrome (SRUS)
s. testis

s. ulcer
s. ulcer syndrome

solium
Taenia s.

SoloPass Percuflex biliary stent
SOLO-Surg Colorectal self-retaining retractor system
solubility
solubilization
micellar s.

solubilize
solubilized
s. HLA
s. human leukocyte antigen

Solu-Biloptin contrast medium
soluble
s. CD44 binding
s. egg antigen (SEA)
s. liver antigen (SLA)
s. recombinant complement receptor 1
s. transferrin receptor (sTf-R)

Solu-Medrol
pulsed S.-M.

solute
s. diuresis
s. equilibrium
s. removal index
s. transport

solution
Adcon-P adhesion barrier s.
AIO parenteral s.
Albright s.
amino acid-based dialysate s.
Aminofusin L Forte amino acid s.
BA-EDTA s.
balanced electrolyte s.
balanced salt s. (BSS)
Balance lavage s.
barium sulfate s.
Belzer UW liver preservation s.
betaine anhydrous s.
bile acid-EDTA solution
Block-Ace s.
Bouin fixative s.
Bretschneider histidine tryptophan s.
buffer s.
Burrow s.
Cidex activated dialdehyde s.
Cidex Plus s.
Collins indigo carmine s.
Collins intracellular electrolyte s.

NOTES

solution *(continued)*
    colloid s.
    colonic lavage s.
    commercial dialysis s. (CDS)
    crystalloid s.
    Delflex peritoneal dialysis s.
    Denhardt s.
    diphosphate buffer s.
    Domeboro s.
    Earle s.
    electrolyte flush s.
    electrolyte-polyethylene glycol lavage s.
    Euro-Collins s.
    Extraneal 7.5% peritoneal dialysis s.
    ferumoxides injectable s.
    formaldehyde s.
    FreAmine amino acid s.
    Gastrolyte oral s.
    gelatin Hank buffered salt s. (GHBSS)
    gluten s.
    GoLYTELY s.
    grit-free s.
    Hank balanced salt s. (HBSS)
    Hank buffer s.
    Hartmann s.
    HepatAmine amino acid s.
    HEPES s.
    Hibidil s.
    Hollande s.
    HSE s.
    s. hybridization RNAse protection assay
    hypertonic saline-epinephrine s.
    iced lactated Ringer s.
    icodextrin 7.5% peritoneal dialysis s.
    Intergel adhesion prevention s.
    Intergel irrigating s.
    inulin s.
    Krebs s.
    Krebs-Ringer s.
    Kristalose for oral s.
    lactated Ringer s.
    lactulose s.
    lavage s.
    Liposyn II fat emulsion s.
    LoSo Prep bowel cleansing s.
    Lugol iodine s.
    Lytren electrolyte s.
    Mayer hematoxylin s.
    Mefoxin-saline s.
    Mitrofanoff s.
    mucolytic-antifoam s.
    normal saline s.
    NTZ Long-Acting Nasal S.
    NutraPrep bowel cleansing s.
    oral rehydration s. (ORS)
    Pedialyte RS electrolyte s.
    PEG-3500 s.
    perfusate s.
    phosphate-buffered saline s.
    physiologic pH s.
    physiologic salt s. (PSS)
    podofilox s.
    polyethylene glycol electrolyte lavage s. (PEG-ELS)
    probenecid-containing s.
    Rapamune oral s.
    rehydrating s. (RS)
    Resol electrolyte s.
    Saccomanno s.
    Sachs s.
    Salivart s.
    Salvanios pH 10 disinfectant s.
    sclerosant s.
    sclerosant-contrast s.
    sclerosing s.
    Shohl s.
    sirolimus oral s.
    Soyalac fat emulsion s.
    Sporox disinfectant s.
    Suby G s.
    Synthamin amino acid s.
    taurocholate s.
    Tolerex feeding s.
    Travamulsion fat emulsion s.
    University of Wisconsin s.
    UW s.
    Vamin amino acid s.
    warm saline s.
    whole-gut lavage s.
    Wisconsin s.
    Y-type Dianeal peritoneal dialysis s.
solution-diluted India ink
Solutrast 300 contrast
Soluvite
solvent
    s. drag
    s. infusion
    Nu-Hope cleaning s.
    stone s.
solvent-dehydrated cadaveric fascia lata
SOM
    somatostatin
    sphincter of Oddi manometry
Soma
somatic
    s. allelic deletion
    s. growth
    s. pain
    s. peripheral nerve
    s. teniasis
somatization
somatointestinal reflex

somatomedin C
Somatome DRG CT technique
somatostatin (SOM, SS)
    s. analog
    s. analog octreotide
    s. analog therapy
    antral s.
    s. cell
    s. infusion therapy
    s. mRNA-D-cell density ratio
    s. MRNA level
    s. peptide
    s. prevention
    s. receptor (SSR)
    s. receptor scintigraphy (SRS)
    s. secretagogue
    s. stain
somatostatin-14, -28
somatostatinoma syndrome
somatotropin release-inhibiting factor (SRIF)
somatropin injection
somite
    müllerian duct, unilateral renal agenesis, and anomalies of cervicothoracic s.'s (MURCS)
Somogyi unit
Sonablate
    S. ablation device
    S. 200 system
Sonazoid
Sonde
    S. enteroscope
    S. enteroscopy
Song stent
sonicated albumin
Sonicath endoluminal ultrasound catheter
Sonne-Duval bacillus
Sonne dysentery
sonnei
    Shigella s.
Sonnenberg classification
Sonocath ultrasound probe
sonoelasticity imaging
sonogram
    fatty meal s. (FMS)
    transverse s.
sonographic
    s. gallstone pattern
    s. layer

    s. planning of oncology treatment (SPOT)
sonography
    amplitude-coded color Doppler s.
    catheter s.
    colonic transabdominal s. (CTAS)
    color-coded Doppler s.
    color-coded duplex s.
    3-D s.
    duplex s.
    endoureteral ultrasound s.
    gray-scale s.
    high-frequency ultrasound probe s. (HFUPS)
    high-resolution endoluminal s. (HRES)
    intraaortic endovascular s.
    renal s.
    transabdominal hydrocolonic s.
    transrectal s.
sonography-guided aspiration
sonoguided biopsy
Sonoline SI-200/250 ultrasound imaging system
Sonolith
    S. Praktis
    S. Praktis portable lithotriptor
Sonoprobe
    S. Endoscopic Ultrasonography System
    S. SP-501
Sonotrode
    S. channel
    S. lithotriptor
sonourethrography
Sony Promavica still capture device
SOP
    sphincter of Oddi pressure
sorbent
    s. dialysate regeneration system
    s. hemodialysis
sorbitol
    s. dehydrogenase (SDH)
    s. diarrhea
    s. enema
sorbitol-MacConkey
    s.-M. agar
    s.-M. medium
sordes gastricae
sore
    canker s.

NOTES

sore *(continued)*
    pressure s.
    venereal s.
Soreson pressure transducer
sorter
    fluorescence-activated cell s. (FACS)
SOS
    sinusoidal obstruction syndrome
    Surgitek One-Step
sotalol
soterenol
Sotradecol sclerosant
souffle
    splenic s.
sound
    absent bowel s.'s
    active bowel s.'s
    apical s.
    auscultation of bowel s.'s
    auscultatory s.
    Béniqué s.
    breath s.
    bronchial s.
    Campbell s.
    common duct s.
    crescendoing bowel s.'s
    Davis interlocking s.'s
    diminished bowel s.'s
    distant heart s.'s
    Dittel s.
    esophageal s.
    extra heart s.'s
    Greenwald s.
    gurgling bowel s.'s
    Guyon s.
    high-pitched bowel s.'s
    hyperactive bowel s.'s
    hypoactive bowel s.'s
    Jewett s.
    Klebanoff common duct s.
    LeFort s.
    low-pitched bowel s.'s
    McCrea s.
    metal s.
    musical bowel s.'s
    normoactive bowel s.'s (NABS)
    Otis s.
    positive bowel s.'s
    quiet bowel s.'s
    rumbling bowel s.'s
    scarce bowel s.'s
    succussion s.'s
    tinkling bowel s.'s
    van Buren s.
    Walther s.
sour
    s. brash
    s. stomach

source
    discrete bleeding s.
    endoscopic light s.
    Olympus CLV10 fiberscope light s.
    Olympus CLV-U 20 endoscopic halogen light s.
    s. of recurrence
    xenon light s.
South American trypanosomiasis
Southern
    S. blot
    S. blot analysis
    S. blot hybridization
Souttar tube
soya-induced enteropathy
Soyalac
    S. fat emulsion solution
    S. formula
soy-based formula
soy protein sensitivity
SP
    status post
    substance P
SP-501
    SP-501 gastric lesion staging by endoscopic ultrasonography
    Sonoprobe SP-501
S/P
    status post
SPA
    sperm penetration assay
SPACE
    single potential analysis of cavernous electrical activity
space
    anorectal s.
    Bogros s.
    Bowman s.
    Courtney s.
    dead s.
    deep perineal s.
    deep postanal anorectal s.
    s. of Disse
    epidural s.
    extravascular s.
    intercellular s.
    intercostal s.
    intermediate s.
    intersphincteric anorectal s.
    ischiorectal anorectal s.
    Kiernan s.
    lateral fossa of preputial s.
    Lesgaft s.
    s. of Mall
    perianal anorectal s.
    periglomerular s.
    perisinusoidal s.
    peritoneal s.
    preperitoneal s.

presacral s.
retroperitoneal s.
retropubic s.
retrorectal s.
s. of Retzius
Retzius s.
right anterior pararenal s.
S. Saver volumetric pump
subarachnoid s.
subhepatic s.
subperitoneal s.
subphrenic s.
subumbilical s.
superficial perineal s.
suprahepatic s.
supralevator anorectal s.
supraomental s.
Traube semilunar s.
vesicovaginal s.

Spacemaker balloon dissector
space-occupying
s.-o. disease
s.-o. lesion
Space-OR flexible internal retractor
spacing
third s.
span
hepatic s.
levator s.
liver s.
spansule
SPARC
S. procedure
S. sling system
sparfloxacin
sparing
rectal s.
spark-gap shock wave generator
sparse
s. inflammatory infiltrate
s. polyposis
sparteine
spasm
acid-provoked s.
bladder s.
cervical s.
cricopharyngeal s.
diffuse esophageal s. (DES)
esophageal s.
fecal paradoxical puborectalis s.
glottic s.

muscle s.
rectal s.
spasmodic stricture
Spasmolin
spasmolytic
spastic
s. bowel syndrome
s. colon
s. constipation
s. esophagus
s. gait
s. ileus
s. motor disorder
s. paraparesis
s. pelvic floor syndrome
spastica
cholepathia s.
dysphagia s.
spasticity
spatial
s. change
s. resolution
spatula
Davis s.
electrosurgical s.
Haberer abdominal s.
Pucci-Seed s.
Reverdin abdominal s.
Tuffier abdominal s.
spatulated overlap anastomosis
spatulation
graft s.
ureteral s.
spatula-tip laparoscopic electrode
Spearman
S. rank
S. rank correlation
S. test
specialist
gastrointestinal endoscopic s.
specialized
s. columnar epithelium (SCE)
s. intestinal metaplasia (SIM)
species
Cryptosporidium s.
gastrin mRNA s.
G3PDH mRNA s.
reactive oxygen s. (ROS)
single beta-actin mRNA s.
specific
s. activity
s. algorithm

NOTES

specific *(continued)*
- antigen s.
- s. anti-Hp serology
- s. clinical parameter
- s. gastritis
- s. gravity test
- s. immunotherapy
- s. oligonucleotide
- s. organic acidopathy
- s. red cell adherence test
- s. stone presentation
- s. urethritis

specificity
- LKM s.
- site s.

specimen
- clean-catch urine s.
- clean-voided s. (CVS)
- culture of biopsy s.
- cytologic s.
- esophageal biopsy s.
- intraurethral swab s.
- multiple endoscopic biopsy s.'s
- negative core biopsy s.
- paraffin-embedded s.
- photomicrograph of colonoscopic biopsy s.
- s. retrieval
- s. trap
- yarn-collected s.

speck
- hemorrhagic s.

SPECT
- single-photon emission computed tomography
- single-photon emission computerized tomography
- SPECT scan

spectinomycin
spectometry
- time-of-flight mass s. (TOFMS)

Spectracef
spectral
- s. analysis
- s. broadening

Spectramed transducer
spectrometer
- liquid scintillation s.
- Shimadzu RF-5301 PC s.

spectrometry
- gas isotope ratio mass s.
- laser desorption/ionization mass s.

spectrophotometer
- atomic absorbance s.
- Genetics Systems microplate reader s.
- Hitachi F-2000 fluorescence s.
- model IL 750 AA s.
- Perkin-Elmer model 5000 atomic absorption s.
- reflectance s.
- SLM-8000 fluorescence s.
- Uvidec-77 s.

spectrophotometric analysis
spectrophotometry
- endoscopic reflectance s.
- reflectance s.

spectroscopy
- elastic scattering s.
- fluorescence correlation s. (FCS)
- Fourier transform infrared s. (FTIR)
- gas chromatography/mass s. (GC/MS)
- ^{1}H magnetic resonance s.
- infrared s.
- laser-induced fluorescence s. (LIFS)
- light-induced autofluorescence s.
- magnetic resonance s. (MRS)
- model 3-60 mass s.
- near-infrared Raman s.
- phosphorous-31 magnetic resonance s.
- proton magnetic resonance s.
- reflectance s.
- steady-state autofluorescence s.
- x-ray photoelectron s.

Spectrum silicone Foley catheter
speculum, pl. **specula**
- Barr rectal s.
- Barr-Shuford rectal s.
- beveled s.
- Bodenhammer rectal s.
- Brinkerhoff rectal s.
- Chelsea-Eaton anal s.
- Cook rectal s.
- Czerny rectal s.
- David rectal s.
- Hinkle-James rectal s.
- Hirschmann s.
- Kelly rectal s.
- Killian rectal s.
- Martin-Davis rectal s.
- Mathews rectal s.
- Pennington rectal s.
- Pratt rectal s.
- rectal s.
- Sawyer rectal s.
- Sims rectal s.
- slotted s.
- Vernon-David rectal s.

speech
- garbled s.

speedbander
Speedband Superview ligator
Speed Lok soft stent
Spence procedure

Spencer disease
Spenco padding
SPEP
    serum protein electrophoresis
sperm
    s. aspiration
    s. cryopreservation
    extracted ductal s.
    s. granuloma
    s. immunobead coincubation
    s. microaspiration retrieval technique (SMART)
    microsurgical extraction of ductal s. (MEDS)
    s. motility-inhibiting factor
    muzzled s.
    s. penetration assay (SPA)
    s. survival factor
    s. yield
spermacrasia
spermagglutination
Sperma-Tex preshaped mesh
spermatic
    s. abscess
    s. artery
    s. calculus
    s. cord
    s. cord leiomyosarcoma
    s. cord liposarcoma
    s. cord torsion
    s. fascia
    s. fistula
    s. plexus
    s. vein
    s. vein ligation
    s. vesicle
spermatica
    chorda s.
spermaticide (*var. of* spermicide)
spermaticus
    funiculus s.
    plexus s.
spermatid
spermatin
spermatoblast
spermatocele
    alloplastic s.
    autogenous s.
    s. resection
spermatocelectomy
spermatocidal (*var. of* spermicidal)
spermatocyst
spermatocystectomy
spermatocystitis
spermatocystotomy
spermatocytal
spermatocyte
    primary s.
    secondary s.
spermatocytic
spermatocytogenesis, spermatogeny
spermatogenesis depression
spermatogenic, spermatogenous
    s. arrest
    s. epididymitis
    s. granulomatous orchitis
spermatogeny (*var. of* spermatocytogenesis)
spermatogonium, spermatogone, pl. **spermatogonia**
    s. dark type A
    s. pale type A
    s. type B
spermatogram
spermatoid
spermatology
spermatolysin
spermatolysis
spermatolytic, spermolytic
spermatopoietic
spermatorrhea
spermatoschesis
spermatotoxin, spermatoxin, spermotoxin
spermatozoal
spermatozoon, pl. **spermatozoa**
    acrosome-reacted s.
    s. concentration
    s. cryopreservation
    disordered acrosome reaction of s.
    double-head s.
    double-tail s.
    s. motility
    s. production
    s. retrieval
    s. volume
spermaturia
SpermCheck test
spermectomy
spermia
spermiation
spermicidal, spermatocidal
    s. jelly
spermicide, spermaticide

NOTES

spermidine
   s. uptake
   s. uptake activity
spermiduct
sperm-immunobead binding
spermine
   s. NONOate
   polyamine s.
spermiogenesis
spermoblast
spermolith
spermolytic (*var. of* spermatolytic)
spermophlebectasia
spermosphere
spermotoxic
spermotoxin (*var. of* spermatotoxin)
spherical reservoir
spheroplast
   mycobacterial s.
sphincter
   AMS 700-series double-cuff Silastic artificial urinary s.
   AMS 800-series double-cuff Silastic artificial urinary s.
   anal s. (AS)
   anal ileostomy with preservation of s.
   anorectal s.
   artificial genitourinary s.
   artificial urethral s. (AUS)
   artificial urinary s. (AUS)
   AS-800 artificial s.
   s. atony
   biliary s.
   Boyden s.
   canine s.
   cardiac s.
   cardioesophageal s.
   choledochal s.
   s. contraction ring
   cricopharyngeal s.
   double-cuff urinary s.
   duodenojejunal s.
   s. dysfunction
   s. EMG
   esophageal s.
   external anal s. (EAS)
   external rectal s.
   external striated urinary s.
   external urethral s.
   s. function
   gastroesophageal s.
   Giordano s.
   Glisson s.
   Henle s.
   Hydroflex s.
   hypertensive lower esophageal s.
   Hyrtl s.
   ileocecal s.
   incompetent s.
   inguinal s.
   internal anal s. (IAS)
   internal rectal s.
   intrinsic striated s.
   intrinsic urethral s.
   lesser esophageal s. (LES)
   long anal s.
   lower esophageal s. (LES)
   Lütkens s.
   Nélaton s.
   neoanal s.
   O'Beirne s.
   s. of Oddi (SO)
   s. of Oddi ablation
   s. of Oddi dysfunction (SOD)
   s. of Oddi homogenate
   s. of Oddi manometry (SOM)
   s. of Oddi pressure (SOP)
   pancreatic duct s. (PDS)
   pancreaticobiliary s.
   pharyngoesophageal s.
   preprostatic s.
   prepyloric s.
   presumptive s.
   pyloric s.
   s. reaction
   s. reconstruction
   rectal s.
   s. repair
   Santorini s.
   servomechanism s.
   smooth urethral s.
   stomach s.
   striated detrusor s.
   striated urethral s.
   threshold of internal s.
   s. tone
   upper esophageal s. (UES)
   urethral s.
   urethrovaginal s.
   Wirsung s.
sphincteral achalasia
sphincterectomy
   endoscopic s.
sphincteric
   s. construction
   s. disobedience syndrome
   s. incontinence
   s. mechanism
   s. squeeze
sphincterismus
sphincteritis
sphincteroplasty
   overlapping s.
   pancreatic s.
   transduodenal s.
sphincteroscope
   Kelly s.

sphincteroscopy
sphincterotome
    Autotome rotatable s.
    bipolar s.
    Bitome bipolar s.
    Cotton s.
    DASH s.
    Demling-Classen s.
    Doubilet s.
    double-channel s.
    ERCP s.
    Fluorotome double-lumen s.
    long-nosed s.
    needle-knife s.
    needle-tipped s.
    Olympus s.
    open s.
    precut s.
    reverse s.
    rotating s.
    single-channel wire-guided s.
    Ultratome double-lumen s.
    Ultratome XL triple-lumen s.
    Wilson-Cook double-channel s.
    Wilson-Cook modified wire-guided s.
    wire-guided s.
sphincterotomy
    s. basket
    biliary endoscopic s.
    choledochal s.
    Doubilet s.
    endoscopic s. (ES)
    endoscopic biliary s.
    endoscopic pancreatic s. (EPS)
    endoscopic pancreatic duct s.
    Erlangen pull-type s.
    external s.
    guidewire s.
    internal s.
    lateral s.
    minor papilla s.
    Mulholland s.
    multiple anal s.'s (MAS)
    needle-knife endoscopic pancreatic s.
    pancreatic duct s.
    Parks partial s.
    precut s.
    pull-type s.
    retrograde s.
    stenosed s.
    s. stenosis
    stent-guided s.
    transduodenal s.
    transendoscopic s.
    transpancreatic sphincter precut approach to biliary s.
    transurethral s.
    urethral s.
    zipper s.
sphincter-preserving operation (SPO)
sphincter-saving procedure
sphingolipid derivative
sphingomyelin
SPI
    symptom problem index
spiculated appearance
spiculation on colon
spicule
    bony s.
    s. in profile
spider
    s. angioma
    arterial s.
    colonic arterial s.
    s. nevus
    s. pelvis
    s. telangiectasia
spiderweb appearance
spigelian hernia
spike
    s. burst on electromyogram of colon
    Monoscopy locking trocar with Woodford s.
    s. potential
spike-burst electrical activity
spiking fever
spillage
    fecal s.
    tumor s.
    s. of tumor cells
spina bifida
spinach stool
spinal
    s. anesthesia
    s. cord compression
    s. cord electric stimulation
    s. cord injury (SCI)
    s. cord injury without radiographic abnormality (SCIWOA)
    s. cord necrosis
    s. dysraphism

NOTES

spinal *(continued)*
    s. findings
    s. hemangioblastoma
    s. shock
    s. stenosis
spindle
    s. cell
    s. cell nodule
    s. colonic groove
spine
    s. dysraphism
    iliac s.
spin-echo
    fat-suppressed s.-e. (FSSE)
    half-Fourier acquisition single-shot turbo s.-e. (HASTE)
Spinelli biopsy needle
spinning
    s. top deformity of bladder
    s. top urethra
spinobulbospinal
    s. micturition reflex
    s. micturition reflex inhibition
spinous
    s. aspect
    s. process
    s. tenderness
spiral
    s. bacterium
    s. basket
    s. computed tomography
    s. computed tomography pneumocolon
    s. CT
    s. CT technique
    s. fold
    s. fold of cystic duct
    s. gallstone forceps
    intraprostatic s.
    s. valve
    s. valve of Heister
    s. Z stent
spiralis
    Trichinella s.
    valvula s.
spiral-tip catheter
spiramycin
SpiraStent ureteral stent
spirillar dysentery
spirochetal dysentery
spirochete
    intestinal s.
spirochetosis
SpiroFlo prostate stent
spirometry
    incentive s.
spironazide
spironolactone
    hydrochlorothiazide and s.

Spirozide
Spirulina Pacifica nutritional supplement
Spitzer-Weinstein syndrome
Spivack
    S. operation
    S. valve
SPK
    serum pyruvate kinase
    SPK transplantation
splanchna
splanchnectopia
splanchnemphraxis
splanchnic
    s. afferent fiber
    s. AV fistula
    s. blood flow
    s. capillary pressure
    s. hyperemia
    s. nerve
    s. primary afferent
    s. vasoconstriction
    s. vein
splanchnicectomy
    chemical s.
splanchnicus
    Bacteroides s.
splanchnocele
splanchnodiastasis
splanchnolith
splanchnopathy
splanchnoptosis, splanchnoptosia
splanchnotomy
splanchnotribe
splash
    succussion s.
S-plasty
spleen
    accessory s.
    s. index
    kidneys, liver, s. (KLS)
    s. tip
    trabeculae of s.
splenalgia
splenectomy
    incidental s.
splenic
    s. abscess
    s. agenesis syndrome
    s. angiogram
    s. anlage
    s. arterial embolization
    s. artery
    s. artery aneurysm (SAA)
    s. atrophy
    s. AV fistula
    s. avulsion
    s. capillary hemangiomatosis
    s. capsule
    s. dullness

s. flexure
s. flexure carcinoma
s. flexure colonoscopy
s. flexure syndrome
s. function
s. hilum
s. injury
s. laceration
s. notch
s. penetration
s. perfusion measurement by dynamic CT scan
s. portography
s. pulp
s. rupture
s. sinus
s. souffle
s. tissue
s. trauma
s. vein
s. vein obstruction (SVO)
s. vein thrombosis
s. venography
s. venous blood flow

splenica
arteria s.
pulpa s.

splenicae
penicilli arteriae s.
trabeculae s.

splenici
folliculi lymphatici s.
lymphonoduli s.

splenobronchial fistula
splenocele
splenocleisis
splenocolic ligament
splenodynia
splenogastric omentum
splenogonadal fusion
splenography
splenolaparotomy
splenomegaly, splenomegalia
congenital s.
congestive s.
Egyptian s.
fibrocongestive s.
Gaucher s.
hemolytic s.
infectious s.
infective s.
myelophthisic s.

siderotic s.
spodogenous s.
tropical s.

splenonephroptosis
splenopancreatic ligament
splenopathy
splenopexy
splenoportal
s. hypertension
s. venography

splenoportography
splenorenal
s. angle
s. bypass
s. bypass graft
s. bypass shunt
s. ligament
s. recess
s. venous anastomosis

splenorrhagia
splenorrhaphy
splenosis
splice-cite mutation
splicing
aberrant mRNA s.
alternate mRNA s.

splinting of abdomen
splint/stent
kidney internal s./s. (KISS)

split
s. ileostomy
s. overtube
s. pelvis
s. renal function
s. renal function study (SRFS)
s. renal function test

split-and-roll technique
split-beam coupler for TURP
split-cuff
s.-c. nipple
s.-c. nipple technique

split-liver
s.-l. transplant
s.-l. transplantation

split-nipple
s.-n. technique
s.-n. technique urinary diversion

split-sheath introducer
splitter
Syn-Optics videoimage s.

split-thickness skin graft

NOTES

SPN
  support parenteral nutrition
SPO
  sphincter-preserving operation
spodogenous splenomegaly
spondylitis
  ankylosing s.
sponge
  absorbable gelatin s.
  cherry s.
  s. count
  s. dissector
  Endozime s.
  fibrin s.
  s. forceps
  gauze s.
  gelatin s.
  Ivalon s.
  lap s.
  laparotomy s.
  peanut s.
  polyvinyl alcohol s.
  Prosthex s.
  saline-moistened s.
  small dissecting s.
  s. stick
  s. tent
  Weck-Cel s.
sponge-holding forceps
spongiofibrosis
  periurethral s.
spongioplasty
spongiosa
spongiosal
spongiosi
  tunica albuginea corporis s.
spongiositis
spongiosum
  corpus s.
spongy pattern
spontaneous
  s. ascites filtration
  s. bacterial peritonitis (SBP)
  s. cystometry
  s. cyst reabsorption
  s. dialytic ultrafiltration
  s. dissection
  s. fluctuation
  s. fragment passage
  s. heartburn
  s. partial elimination
  s. penile ischemic necrosis
  s. portosystemic shunt (SPSS)
  s. reactivation of hepatitis
  s. recanalization
  s. regression
  s. resolution
  s. rupture
  s. stone passage

spoon
  Falk appendectomy s.
  s. forceps
  gall duct s.
  Mayo common duct s.
  s. retractor
  sharp s.
  Volkmann pancreatic calculus s.
spoon-tip laparoscopic electrode
Sporacidin disinfectant
sporadic
  s. dysentery
  s. gingival papilloma
  s. hollow visceral myopathy
  s. nonfamilial clear cell carcinoma
spore
  fungal s.
sporocyst
Sporothrix schenckii
Sporox disinfectant solution
sporozoite
sport sheath (SS)
sporulation
  coccidian s.
SPOT
  sonographic planning of oncology treatment
  SPOT mobile 3-D ultrasound system and software
spot
  central s.
  cherry red s. (CRS)
  cold s.
  cotton-wool s. (CWS)
  dark s.
  S. endoscopic marker
  epigastric s.
  Fordyce s.
  gastric red s.
  hematocystic s. (HCS)
  hot s.
  hyperechoic s.
  Koplik s.
  mongolian s.
  Roth s.
  s. size
S pouch
spout
  ileal s.
SPP
  stannous pyrophosphate
  ^{99m}Tc SPP
Spratt curette
spray
  alginate s.
  DDAVP nasal s.
  Maalox s.
  Prevacare total solution skin care s.

Quixil s.
sodium thiosulfate solution s.
thrombin s.
spray-fixed
spraying
    dye s.
    fibrin s.
    magnification endoscopy with acetic acid s.
spreader
    meatal s.
    pyloric s.
spreading fistulation
spring loaded biopsy gun
spring-loaded-type biopsy instrument
spring-wire
    s.-w. coil
    s.-w. retractor
Sprinz-Dubin syndrome
Sprinz-Nelson syndrome
sprue
    celiac s.
    collagenous s.
    nontropical s.
    refractory s.
    subclinical s.
    tropical s.
SPSS
    spontaneous portosystemic shunt
SPT
    station pullthrough
    SPT technique
spun urine sediment
spuria
    hemospermia s.
    melena s.
spurious calculus
spurting blood
sputum, pl. **sputa**
    s. aeroginosum
    green s.
SPV
    selective proximal vagotomy
SQMP
    subcutaneous morphine pump
squamocolumnar
    s. junction (SCJ)
    s. mucosal junction
squamous
    s. cell
    s. cell cancer
    s. cell carcinoma (SCC)
    s. cell carcinoma antigen
    s. cell carcinoma in situ
    s. cell papilloma (SCP)
    s. epithelium
square knot
squeeze
    hot s.
    phasic fluctuation on s.
    s. pressure
    s. pressure profile of anal sphincter test
    sphincteric s.
***src*-homology**
    src-h. 2 (SH2)
    src-h. 2 domain
***src* phosphorylation**
S reservoir
SRFS
    split renal function study
SRH
    stigmata of recent hemorrhage
SRIF
    somatotropin release-inhibiting factor
SRMD
    stress-related mucosal disease
SRS
    somatostatin receptor scintigraphy
SRUS
    solitary rectal ulcer syndrome
SRVG
    silicone elastomer ring vertical gastroplasty
***SRY* gene**
SS
    Sjögren syndrome
    somatostatin
    sport sheath
    Regulax SS
Ssabanejew-Frank
    S.-F. gastrostomy
    S.-F. operation
SSBE
    short-segment Barrett esophagus
SSC
    single-stripe colitis
SSc
    systemic sclerosis
SSE
    soapsuds enema
SSE2-L electrosurgical unit
S-shaped
    S-s. body

NOTES

S-shaped *(continued)*
    S-s. ileal pouch-anal anastomosis
    S-s. pouch
    S-s. reservoir

SSI
    symptom severity index

SSIAM
    Structured and Scaled Interview to Assess Maladjustment

SSIS
    side-to-side isoperistaltic strictureplasty

SSR
    somatostatin receptor

ST
    heat-stable enterotoxin

St.
    saint
        St. John's wort
        St. Mark pudendal electrode
        St. triad

stab
    s. incision
    s. wound

Stabiliplan orthovolt applicator

stability
    detrusor muscle s.
    structural s.

stabilization
    percutaneous bladder neck s. (PBNS)
    Vesica percutaneous bladder neck s.

stabilizer

stable
    s. face
    microsatellite s. (MSS)

stab-wound drain

staccato voiding

Stachrom AT III routine chromogenic method

Stacke meatoplasty

stack-of-coins appearance

Stadol

stage
    s. B, C carcinoma
    Dean s.
    Dukes s.
    Hoehn and Yahr s.
    s. III papillary serous cystadenocarcinoma
    morphologic s.
    post-TNM s. I, II, III, IV
    Tanner s.
    tumor s.

staged orchiopexy

stage-specific embryonic antigen

staghorn
    s. calculus
    s. stone
    s. urolithiasis

staging
    Ann Arbor cancer s.
    Boden-Gibb tumor s.
    s. of cancer
    clinicopathologic s.
    endosonographic s.
    Marshall and Tanner pubertal s.
    neoplasm s.
    neuroblastoma s.
    s. operation
    operative s.
    primary gastric lymphoma s.
    Stanford s.
    TNM system for tumor s.
    transrectal ultrasound s.
    tumor s.

stagnant
    s. bile
    s. loop syndrome

STAI
    State Trait Anxiety Index-I

stain
    19A2 s.
    acid-Schiff s.
    Alcian blue s.
    anti-Schiff s.
    argentaffin s.
    azan s.
    Bryan-Leishman s.
    carbolfuchsin s.
    chromogranin s.
    Congo red s.
    Diff-Quik s.
    elastin s.
    El-Zimaity triple s.
    eosin s.
    esterase s.
    Fite s.
    Fontana-Masson s.
    Fungi-Fluor chitin s.
    gastrin s.
    Genta s.
    Giemsa s.
    Glaxo s.
    glucagon s.
    Gram s.
    Grimelius silver s.
    Grocott methenamine silver s.
    Hale colloidal iron s.
    Hansel s.
    H&E s.
    hematological s.
    hematoxylin and eosin s.
    immunocytochemical s.
    immunohistochemical s.
    immunoperoxidase s.
    indigo carmine s.

insulin s.
Jones silver s.
Ki-67 s.
Kossa s.
lead citrate s.
Lendrum s.
Lugol solution s.
Mallory-Azan s.
Martius scarlet blue s.
Masson-Fontana s.
Masson trichrome s.
Mayer acid alum hematoxylin s.
May-Grünwald-Giemsa s.
methylene blue s.
NADPH diaphorase s.
oil red O s.
Orcein s.
pancreatic polypeptide s.
Papanicolaou s.
PAS s.
periodic acid-Schiff s.
periodic acid-Schiff-Alcian blue combination s.
Perls s.
peroxidase s.
p53 immunohistochemical s.
rhodamine s.
RP3 s.
saffron s.
Schiff s.
serotonin s.
silver s.
S-100 immunohistochemical s.
somatostatin s.
Steiner s.
Sternheimer-Malbin s.
Sudan black B fat s.
Sudan-III s.
sulfated mucin s.
toluidine blue s.
trichrome s.
uranyl acetate s.
vasoactive intestinal polypeptide s.
VIP s.
von Kossa s.
Warthin-Starry silver s.
Wright s.
Wright-Giemsa s.
Ziehl-Neelsen s.

staining
Berlin blue s.
BrDu s.
cytokeratin s.
cytoplasmic s.
endoscopy with iodine s.
ethidium bromide s.
Feulgen s.
Grimelius s.
immunohistochemical s.
immunoperoxidase s.
iodine s.
lectin s.
MIB-1 s.
perinuclear intracellular s.
photomicrograph of specimen s.
p53 nuclear s.
Smith method of silver s.
Steiner modification of Warthin-Starry s.
vimentin s.
vital s.

stainless
s. steel mesh stent
s. steel suture

stairstep air-fluid level

stalk
polyp s.

Stamey
S. classification
S. colosuspension
S. dorsal vein apical retractor
S. needle
S. needle bladder neck suspension
S. open-tip ureteral catheter
S. procedure
S. test
S. tube
S. urethropexy

Stamey-Malecot catheter

Stamey-Martius procedure

Stamm
S. gastroplasty
S. gastrostomy
S. gastrostomy tube

stammering bladder

stand
Mayo s.

standard
s. acid reflux test (SART)
Aub-Dubois s.
s. colonoscope
s. duodenoscope
s. endoscopy polypectomy snare
s. ERCP catheter

NOTES

standard *(continued)*
    s. fatty meal
    s. hemodialysis
    s. laparoscopy (SL)
    s. measurement
    s. orchiopexy
    s. pyelolithotomy
    s. radioenzymatic method
    s. radiological test
    s. silicone manometric assembly
    s. transabdominal ultrasound
standardized
    s. incidence ratio (SIR)
    s. instrument
Stanford
    S. protocol
    S. radical retropubic prostatectomy
    S. staging
stanley
    S. bacillus
    Salmonella s.
stanniocalcin
stannous pyrophosphate (SPP)
stanolone
stanozolol
staphylococcal sepsis
Staphylococcus
    S. albus
    S. aureus
    coagulase-negative *S.*
    S. epidermidis
    S. food poisoning
    growth of coagulase-negative *S.*
    S. saprophyticus
    S. viridans
staple
    absorbable s.
    s. line dehiscence
    metallic s.
    polyglyconate s.
    skin s.
stapled
    s. closure
    s. end-to-end ileoanal anastomosis
    s. hemorrhoidectomy
    s. intestinal anastomosis
    s. pouch-anal anastomosis
    s. strictureplasty
stapler
    anvil portion of EEA s.
    Auto Suture Multifire Endo GIA 30 s.
    Auto Suture Premium CEEA s.
    CEEA s.
    circular s.
    double-headed P190 s.
    s. doughnut
    end-end s.
    Endo-Babcock s.
    Endo GIA 30, 60 s.
    Endo GIA suture s.
    Endo Hernia s.
    Endopath 30, 60 s.
    Endopath EMS hernia s.
    Ethicon CDH29 s.
    Ethicon TLH30 s.
    EZ vascular 35 linear s.
    GIA s.
    hernia s.
    ILA surgical s.
    intraluminal s. (ILS)
    laparoscopic s.
    LDS s.
    ligating and dividing s. (LDS)
    linear s.
    PI-30 s.
    PI-90 double-headed s.
    PI surgical s.
    PLC-50 linear s.
    Poly GIA s.
    Premium CEEA circular s.
    Premium Plus CEEA disposable s.
    ProTack s.
    Proximate flexible linear s.
    Proximate ILS SDH circular s.
    Proximate intraluminal s.
    TA90-BN s.
    TA30, TA55 s.
    TL90 Ethicon s.
    vascular s.
stapling
    gastric s.
    laparoscopic s.
    single s.
    skin s.
    surgical s.
starch
    amylase-resistant s. (ARS)
    s. blocker
    s. granulomatous peritonitis
    wheat s.
Starck dilator
star construction test
Starlix
STAR protein
Starr
    S. plication
    S. technique
stasis, pl. **stases**
    antral s.
    bile s.
    biliary s.
    s. cirrhosis
    s. esophagitis
    fecal s.
    s. gallbladder
    gallbladder s.
    gastric s.

ileal s.
intestinal s.
s. liver
pelvicaliceal s.
postgastrectomy s.
postsurgical gastric s.
Roux-limb s.
s. syndrome
s. ulceration
urinary s.
venous s.
stasis-induced ulceration
STAT!
ImmunoCard STAT!
state
catecholamine excess s.
S. end-to-end anastomosis
gradient recalled acquisition in steady s. (GRASS)
hypercoagulable s.
hypermetabolic s.
hypogonadal s.
neurohumoral excitation s.
proliferating s.
proteinuric s.
sick euthyroid s.
S. Trait Anxiety Index-I (STAI)
utopian s.
statement
evidence-based position s.
Statham
S. external transducer
S. P23 strain gauge
statherin
static
s. closure pressure
s. cystogram
s. cytophotometry
s. image DNA cytometry
station
s. pullthrough (SPT)
s. pullthrough esophageal manometry technique
statistic
nonparametric Wilcoxon s.
preliminary baseline descriptive s.
statistically significant
Stat Simple whole-blood antibody test
status
apical biopsy s.
s. evaluation
fertility s.

s. gastricus
nutritional s.
s. post (SP, S/P)
stone-free s.
ureteroenteric s.
Stat-View computer program
Stauffer syndrome
stavudine
StayErec system
Stay-Put jejunal tube
stay suture
STC
slow-transit constipation
STD
sexually transmitted disease
STDS
stone-tissue detection system
steady pain
steady-state autofluorescence spectroscopy
steakhouse syndrome
steal
arterial s.
steam autoclave
steatohepatitis
nonalcoholic s. (NASH)
steatorrhea, stearrhea
biliary s.
idiopathic s.
intestinal s.
pancreatic s.
steatosis
drug-induced s.
hepatic s.
macrovesicular s.
microvesicular s.
severe macrovesicular s.
toxic s.
Steblay nephritis
STEC
Shiga toxin-producing *Escherichia coli*
Stx 2-producing *Escherichia coli* strain
steely-hair disease
steerable
s. cystoscopy
s. nephroscope
Steers replicator
stegnosis
stegnotic
Steigmann-Goff
S.-G. endoscopic ligator kit
S.-G. endoscopic ligature overtube

NOTES

Steinach operation
Steiner
    S. modification of Warthin-Starry staining
    S. stain
Steinert
    S. disease
    S. myotonic dystrophy
Stein-Leventhal syndrome
Steinmann intestinal forceps
steinstrasse
Stelazine
stellate
    s. cell
    s. venule
stem cell
Stemetic
stemline
    DNA s.
stenosed sphincterotomy
stenosis, pl. **stenoses**
    afferent limb nipple s.
    ampullary s.
    anal s.
    anorectal s.
    antral s.
    aortic valvular s.
    atherosclerotic renal artery s.
    benign papillary s.
    bile duct s.
    canal s.
    choledochoduodenal junctional s.
    congenital esophageal s.
    congenital hypertrophic pyloric s.
    congenital pyloric s.
    cystic duct s.
    delayed ureteral anastomotic s.
    diaphragmlike s.
    distal esophageal s.
    duodenal s.
    esophageal s.
    hypertrophic pyloric s. (HPS)
    idiopathic hypertrophic pyloric s.
    infantile hypertrophic pyloric s. (IHPS)
    infundibular s.
    infundibulopelvic s.
    intestinal s.
    Klatskin s.
    luminal s.
    malignant s.
    meatal s.
    pancreaticojejunostomy s.
    pancreatic papillary s.
    papillary s.
    preputial s.
    pyloric s.
    radiation s.
    rectal s.
    renal artery s.
    short band s.
    small intestinal s.
    sphincterotomy s.
    spinal s.
    stomal s.
    s. of TIPS
    transplant renal artery s. (TRAS)
    tubular s.
    unilateral renal artery s.
    ureteral reimplantation s.
    ureteroileal s.
    urethral s.
    vesical neck s.
    vesicoureteric s.
stenotic
    s. cancer
    s. lesion
    s. shunt
    s. stoma
Stenotrophomonas maltophilia
Stensen duct
stent
    Amsterdam biliary s.
    Angiomed blue s.
    Angiomed Puroflex s.
    antibiotic-coated s.
    antireflux double-J s.
    ASI prostatic s.
    ASI Titan s.
    Bard Memotherm colorectal s.
    Beamer injection s.
    Biliary Spiral Z s.
    biliopancreatic diversion with duodenal s.
    Biofix s.
    bioresorbable s.
    BioSorb resorbable urology s.
    Biostent biliary s.
    Black Beauty ureteral s.
    Braun s.
    Carson internal/external endopyelotomy s.
    C-Flex Amsterdam s.
    C-Flex ureteral s.
    coil s.
    colonic s.
    colonic Z s.
    common bile duct s.
    conventional s.
    Cook s.
    Corinthian s.
    Cotton-Huibregtse double pigtail s.
    Cotton-Leung biliary s.
    covered biliary metal s.
    Cragg Endopro System I s.
    crutched stick-type biliary duct s.
    Cysto Flex s.
    s. deployment

stent · stent

Diamond s.
digestive-respiratory fistula s.
double-J indwelling catheter s.
double-J silicone s.
double-J Surgitek catheter s.
double-J ureteral s.
double-pigtail s.
DoubleStent biliary
  endoprosthesis s.
Dua antireflux s.
Elastalloy esophageal s.
Eliminator biliary s.
Eliminator pancreatic s.
encrustation of s.
encrusted ureteral s.
endobronchial s.
EndoCoil biliary s.
EndoCoil esophageal s.
endopyelotomy s.
endoscopic biliary s.
EsophaCoil self-expanding
  esophageal s.
esophageal I s.
esophageal Strecker s.
esophageal Z stent with Dua
  antireflux s.
s. exchange
expandable esophageal s. (EES)
expandable intrahepatic portacaval
  shunt s.
expandable metallic s.
Fader Tip ureteral s.
Firlit-Kluge s.
Flexima biliary s.
floating s.
forgotten s.
French double-J ureteral s.
s. funnel
future of s.
Gianturco expandable self-expanding
  metallic biliary s.
Gianturco metal urethral s.
Gianturco-Rosch biliary Z s.
Gianturco-Rosch self-expandable
  Z s.
Gianturco-Roubin flexible coil s.
Gianturco Z s.
Gibbon indwelling ureteral s.
Greenen pancreatic s.
helical-ridged ureteral s.
Herculink Plus biliary s.
Heyer-Schulte s.

Horizon prostatic s.
Huibregtse biliary s.
Hydromer-coated polyurethane s.
Hydro Plus s.
ileal artery s.
s. incrustation
indwelling ureteral s.
InStent EsophaCoil s.
internal biliary s.
intracholedochal s.
IntraCoil nitinol s.
intraesophageal s.
intraluminal Silastic esophageal s.
intraprostatic s.
iridium 192 loaded s.
J-Maxx s.
large-bore double-pigtail s.
Lubri-Flex ureteral s.
magnetic internal ureteral s.
main pancreatic duct s.
Mardis soft s.
Megalink biliary s.
membrane-covered s.
Memotherm colorectal s.
Memotherm endoscopic biliary s.
Memotherm Flexx biliary s.
Memotherm nitinol s.
mesh s.
metal s.
metallic biliary s.
metal Z s.
s. migration
modified Z s.
MPD s.
Multi-Flex s.
nephroureteral s.
nephrovesical s.
Nissenkorn s.
nitinol mesh s.
Niti-S s.
Oasis s.
OMNILINK 0.018, 0.035 biliary s.
Palmaz balloon-expandable s.
Palmaz Corinthian s.
Palmaz-Schatz biliary s.
pancreatic duct s.
s. patency
Percuflex Amsterdam s.
Percuflex biliary s.
Percuflex endopyelotomy s.
Percuflex Plus ureteral s.
percutaneous s.

NOTES

stent *(continued)*
    pigtail biliary s.
    polyethylene s.
    Polyflex s.
    polyurethane s.
    polyurethane-covered metallic s.
    Prostacoil s.
    Prostakath urethral s.
    prostatic s.
    pyelovesical s.
    Quadra-Coil ureteral s.
    recanalization of clogged biliary s.
    renal artery s.
    Retromax endopyelotomy s.
    Rusch s.
    Schneider s.
    self-expanding biliary metal s.
    self-expanding coil s.
    self-expanding metallic s. (SEMS)
    self-retaining coil s.
    SEM s.
    shape memory alloy s.
    Siegel s.
    Silastic indwelling ureteral s.
    silicone-coated metallic self-expanding s.
    Silitek Uropass s.
    silver-coated s.
    single-pigtail s.
    SMA spiral s.
    SoloPass Percuflex biliary s.
    Song s.
    Speed Lok soft s.
    spiral Z s.
    SpiraStent ureteral s.
    SpiroFlo prostate s.
    stainless steel mesh s.
    straight s.
    Strecker s.
    Surgitek Tractfinder ureteral s.
    Surgitek Uropass s.
    Tannenbaum s.
    Teflon s.
    thermoexpandable s.
    thermosensitive s.
    s. through wire mesh technique
    Titan s.
    titanium urethral s.
    tracheobronchial Z s.
    transhepatic biliary s.
    transpapillary cystopancreatic s.
    transpapillary insertion of self-expanding biliary metal s.
    T-tube s.
    Ultraflex Diamond s.
    Ultraflex Microvasive s.
    Ultraflex nitinol expandable esophageal s.
    Ultraflex tracheobronchial s.
    uncoated mesh s.
    Universal s.
    ureteral s.
    urethral s.
    UroCoil self-expanding s.
    Uro-Guide s.
    UroLume prostate s.
    UroLume urethral s.
    UroLume Wallstent s.
    Urosoft s.
    Urospiral urethral s.
    U-tube s.
    s. and vent system
    Vistaflex biliary s.
    Wallstent s.
    Wallstent-covered SEM s.
    whistle s.
    Wilson-Cook French s.
    Z s.
    Za-Stent endoscopic biliary s.
    Zilver biliary self-expanding s.
    Zimmon biliary s.

stent after ureteroscopy
stented ureteroscopic lithotripsy
stent-guided sphincterotomy
stent-induced pneumoperitoneum
stenting
    biliary s.
    s. catheter
    endoscopic pancreatic s. (EPS)
    endoscopic papillotomy and s.
    endoscopic retrograde biliary s.
    endovascular s.
    hilar bile duct s.
    indications for s.
    pancreatic transpapillary s.
    routine ureteral s.
    tumor s.
    ureteral s.

stent-related complication
stepladder incision technique
steppage gait
stepping reflex
step-up shim
stepwise regression analysis
steradian
Sterapred
stercolith
stercoraceous
    abdominal s.
    s. abscess
    amebic liver s.
    anal s.
    anorectal s.
    appendiceal s.
    s. appendicitis
    bile duct s.
    biliary s.
    cavernosal s.

cholangitic s.
s. colic
cortical s.
crypt s.
cuff s.
deep interloop s.
diaphragmatic s.
s. diarrhea
distant s.
diverticular s.
Douglas s.
echinococcal liver s.
endoscopic transpapillary drainage of pancreatic s.
entamebic s.
Entamoeba histolytica s.
enteroperitoneal s.
epididymal s.
epiploic s.
fecal s.
filarial s.
s. fistula
s. formation
fungal liver s.
gallbladder wall s.
gas s.
gas-forming liver s.
helminthic s.
hepatic s.
high intermuscular s.
horseshoe s.
interloop s.
intermesenteric s.
intersphincteric perirectal s.
intraabdominal s.
intrahepatic s.
intramesenteric s.
intraperitoneal s.
ischiorectal s.
kidney s.
lacunar s.
liver s.
midabdominal s.
non-gas-forming liver s.
pancreatic pseudocyst s.
paracolic s.
parafrenal s.
paranephric s.
pararectal s.
pelvic s.
pelvirectal s.

percutaneous drainage of epididymal s.
s. perforation
perianal fistula s.
pericecal s.
pericholecystic s.
pericolic s.
perineal s.
perinephric s.
perirectal s.
perirenal s.
peritoneal cavity s.
periureteral s.
periurethral s.
phlegmonous s.
pilonidal perirectal s.
postcecal s.
postoperative s.
preperitoneal s.
prostatic s.
protozoan s.
psoas s.
pyogenic liver s.
rectal s.
renocortical s.
retrocecal s.
retroesophageal s.
retroperitoneal s.
retroperitoneal-iliopsoas s.
root s.
seminal vesicle s.
spermatic s.
splenic s.
stercoraceous s.
stercoraceous s.
sterile s.
subacute s.
subaponeurotic s.
subcapsular hepatic s.
subdiaphragmatic s.
subhepatic s.
subperitoneal s.
subphrenic s.
suprahepatic s.
supralevator perirectal s.
testicular s.
tympanitic s.
s. ulcer
s. ulceration
urachal s.
urethral s.
urinary s.

NOTES

stercoraceous (*continued*)
    urinous s.
    s. vomiting
    s. vomitus
stercoralis
    Strongyloides s.
stercoroma
stercorous
stercus
stereocilium, pl. **stereocilia**
StereoGuide
    Lorad S.
stereomicroscopic view
sterile
    s. abscess
    s. ceftriaxone sodium
    s. cyst
    s. dressing
    s. pancreatic necrosis
    s. peritonitis
sterility
    absolute s.
    aspermatogenic s.
    chemotherapy-induced s.
    dysspermatogenic s.
    male s.
    normospermatogenic s.
    primary s.
    radiation-induced s.
    relative s.
    secondary s.
sterilization
    ETO s.
    gas s.
sterilize
sterilized
    autoclave s.
Steris automatic reprocessor
Steri-Strip
steri-stripped incision
sterna (*pl. of* sternum)
Sternberg paradigm
Sternheimer-Malbin stain
sternocleidomastoid
sternotomy scar
sternum, pl. **sterna**
    bowed s.
sterocoralis
    Strongyloides s.
steroid
    adrenal s.
    anabolic s.
    s. foam enema
    high-dose pulse s.
    s. moiety
    s. receptor
    s. therapy
    s. withdrawal

steroid-dependent
    s.-d. Crohn disease
    s.-d. diet
    s.-d. idiopathic nephrosis
steroid-induced azoospermia
steroidogenic acute regulatory protein
steroid-refractory
    s.-r. Crohn disease
    s.-r. diet
steroid-resistant
    s.-r. idiopathic nephrosis
    s.-r. nephrotic syndrome
    s.-r. rejection
steroid-responsive pancolitis
steroid-sensitive idiopathic nephrosis
sterol
stethoscope
    esophageal s.
Stetten intestinal clamp
Stevens-Johnson syndrome (SJS)
Stewart crypt hook
Stewart-Treves syndrome
sTf-R
    soluble transferrin receptor
STI571
stick
    sponge s.
    s. tie
Stiegmann-Goff
    S.-G. Clearvue endoscopic ligator
    S.-G. technique
    S.-G. variceal ligator
Stierlin sign
Stifcore transbronchial aspiration needle
stiffening
    s. tube
    s. wire
stiff-man syndrome
stigma, pl. **stigmata, stigmas**
    endoscopic s.
    stigmata of recent hemorrhage (SRH)
    syphilitic s.
    Turner s.
stigmatic
stigmatism
stigmatization
still camera
Stille
    S. clamp
    S. elevator
    S. gallstone forceps
Stille-Barraya intestinal forceps
Stilphostrol
stimulant laxative
stimulated
    s. gastric secretion test
    s. gracilis neosphincter
    s. gracilis neosphincter technique

s. gracilplasty
s. release
s. tube
stimulation
    adenyl cyclase s.
    anal electrical s.
    anocutaneous s.
    antigen s.
    central vagal nerve s.
    chronic low-frequency electrical s.
    chronic sacral-spinal nerve s.
    cutaneous electrical field s.
    electrogalvanic s. (EGS)
    extradural electrical s.
    s. fork
    gastric electrical s.
    hilum s.
    interferential electrical s.
    interferon gamma s.
    intraoperative cavernous nerve s.
    intravaginal electrical s.
    magnetic s.
    mitogenic s.
    nociceptive s.
    peak acid output after pentagastrin s. (PAOPg)
    pelvic floor electrical s.
    penile vibratory s.
    s. probe
    rectum digital s.
    sacral nerve s. (SNS)
    S-CCK-Pz s.
    secretin s.
    spinal cord electric s.
    Stoller afferent nerve s. (SANS)
    s. test
    testosterone s.
    transcranial magnetic s. (TCMS)
    transcutaneous electrical nerve s. (TENS)
    transurethral electrical bladder s. (TEBS)
    vagal s.
    vaginal electrical s.
stimulator
    EGS Model 100 electrogalvanic s.
    electrogalvanic s.
    Grass Model S9 s.
    Nicolet SM-300 s.
    URYS 800 nerve s.
stimulus, pl. **stimuli**
    external s.
    mitogenic s.
    osmotic s.
    symbolic s.
STING
    subureteric Teflon injection
Sting procedure
stirrup
    Allen s.'s
    Lloyd-Davies s.'s
    pediatric s.'s
stitch
    baseball s.
    cobbler's s.
    Connell s.
    Gambee s.
    intersymphyseal s.
    lock s.
    marker s.
    tagging s.
    tilt s.
    Z s.
STK11
    STK11 gene
stochastic knotting
Stockholm trial I, II
stoichiometry
    coupling s.
Stokvis
    S. disease
    S. test
Stokvis-Talma syndrome
Stoller
    S. afferent nerve stimulation (SANS)
    S. scoring system
Stoll test
stoma, pl. **stomas, stomata**
    abdominal s.
    anastomotic s.
    appendicoumbilical s.
    bowel s.
    s. cap
    concealed umbilical s.
    continent abdominal wall s.
    diverting s.
    dusky s.
    end s.
    end-loop s.
    flush s.
    gastrointestinal s.
    Gomez horizontal gastroplasty with reinforced s.

NOTES

stoma *(continued)*
    ileostomy s.
    Laws gastroplasty with Silastic collar-reinforced s.
    loop s.
    maturing the s.
    Mitrofanoff catheterizable s.
    Mitrofanoff continent urinary s.
    nippled s.
    permanent s.
    prolapsed s.
    retracted s.
    rodless end-loop s.
    rosebud s.
    Silastic collar-reinforced s.
    s. site
    stenotic s.
    Turnbull loop s.
    ureteral s.
    ureteric s.

stomach
    aberrant umbilical s.
    acid-suppressed s.
    adenomatous polyp of s.
    adenomyoepithelioma of s.
    anacidic s.
    angular notch of s.
    angulus of s.
    antrum of s.
    s. bed
    bilocular s.
    butterflies in s.
    s. calculus
    caliber-persistent artery of s.
    cardia of s.
    cardiac s.
    cascade s.
    cirrhosis of s.
    cup-and-spill s.
    curvature of s.
    dilation of s.
    distal blind s.
    drain-trap s.
    dumping s.
    functional disorder s.
    fundus of s.
    granulocytic sarcoma of s.
    greater curvature of s.
    hourglass s.
    insufflation of s.
    intrathoracic s.
    s. lavage
    leather-bottle s.
    lesser curvature of s.
    middle s.
    mucous lake of s.
    s. neoplasm
    oblique fibers of s.
    s. pump

    s. reefing
    rugae of s.
    sclerotic s.
    sour s.
    s. sphincter
    thoracic s.
    trifid s.
    s. tube
    tympany of s.
    upset s.
    upside-down s.
    vascular coat of s.
    villous folds of s.
    watermelon s. (WS)
    water-trap s.

stomachache
stomachalgia
stomachodynia
Stomahesive
    S. paste
    S. skin barrier wafer

stomal
    s. aperture
    s. bag
    s. duskiness
    s. invagination
    s. prolapse
    s. stenosis
    s. ulcer

stomalike channel
stomas (*pl. of* stoma)
stomata (*pl. of* stoma)
Stomate
    S. decompression tube
    S. extension tube

stomatitis
    aphthous s.
    herpetic s.

stomatoscopy
    diagnostic fiberoptic s.

stomatostatinoma
stone
    ampullary s.
    artificial cystine s.
    s. and basket impaction
    bile duct s.
    biliary tract s.
    bilirubinate s.
    black faceted s.
    black pigment s.
    bladder s.
    branched s.
    brown pigment s.
    s. burden
    calcium bilirubinate s.
    calcium oxalate dihydrate s.
    calcium oxalate monohydrate s.
    carbonate apatite s.
    cholesterol s.

stone · stool

S. clamp applier
s. clearance
s. comminution
common bile duct s. (CBDS)
complex s.
s. composition
S. Cone
S. Cone nitinol stone retrieval device
s. cup
cystic duct s.
cystine s.
s. disease
s. dislodger
endoscopic extraction pancreatic duct s.
s. extraction
extraction bile duct s.
extraction pancreatic s.
s. former
s. fragmentation
gallbladder s.
genuine cystine s.
s. granuloma
s. granuloma formation
hepatic duct s.
hyperoxaluric s.
impacted ampullary s.
impacted ureteral s.
s. impactor
infection s.
S. intestinal clamp
intrahepatic s.
intraluminal s.
kidney s.
large common duct s.
large impacted ureteral s.
lower pole s.
s. management
s. maturation
metabolic s.
mulberry s.
multiple s.'s
noncalcified s.
nonstruvite s.
pancreatic duct s.
pelvic s.
periureteral s.
pigment s.
s. plaque
s. recognition system
recurrent calcium-containing s.'s
s. recurrent rate
renal s.
residual s.
s. retrieval balloon
s. retrieval basket
s. retriever
s. searcher
silent s.
s. solvent
staghorn s.
struvite s.
s. surgery
types of s.'s
ureteral s.
ureteric s.
uric acid s.
urinary s.
s. in urinary diversion
s. variable

stone-forming patient
stone-free
    s.-f. rate
    s.-f. status
stone-grasping forceps
Stone-Holcombe intestinal clamp
stone-holding basket forceps
stonelike debris
stone-prevention program
StoneRisk
    S. citrate test
    S. cystine test
    S. diagnostic monitoring kit
    S. diagnostic profile
    S. diagnostic test
    S. profile test
stone-tissue
    s.-t. detection system (STDS)
    s.-t. recognition system (STR)
stool
    ability to form solid s.
    acholic s.
    s. antigen assay
    bilious s.
    black tarry s.
    blood in s.
    blood admixed with s.
    blood on surface of s.
    blood passed with s.
    blood-streaked s.
    bloody s.
    brown s.
    bulky s.

NOTES

stool *(continued)*
    butter s.
    caddy s.
    s. chromatography
    clay-colored s.
    Clinitest-negative s.
    Clinitest-positive s.
    s. colonization
    s. color
    continent of s.
    s. culture
    currant jelly s.
    s. cytotoxin test
    dark s.
    diarrhea s.
    s. electrolyte
    s. electrolyte test
    s. elimination
    s. evacuation
    fatty s.
    floating s.
    foamy s.
    formed s.
    foul-smelling s.
    frank blood in s.
    frequency of s.
    Gram stain of s.
    green s.
    guaiac-negative s.
    guaiac-positive s.
    hard s.
    heme-negative s.
    heme-positive s.
    impacted s.
    s. incontinence
    lienteric s.
    liquid s.
    loose s.
    mahogany-colored s.
    malodorous s.
    maroon-colored s.
    melenic s.
    mucoid s.
    mucous s.
    mushy s.
    nonbloody s.
    s. for occult blood
    oily s.
    s. osmolality test
    s. osmotic gap
    s. osmotic gap test
    s. for ova and parasites
    pale s.
    palpable s.
    particulate s.
    passage of s.
    pea soup s.
    pelleted s.
    pencillike s.
    pipestem s.
    rabbit s.
    residual s.
    s. retention
    ribbon s.
    rice-water s.
    runny s.
    sago-grain s.
    s. sample
    scybalous s.
    semiformed s.
    semisolid s.
    silver s.
    slurry of s.
    soft s.
    s. softener
    spinach s.
    straining at s.
    tarry black s.
    s. toxin assay
    Trélat s.
    undigested food in s.
    unformed s.
    watery s.
    Wright stain of s.
stooling
stool-softening laxative
STOP
    selective tubal occlusion procedure
stopcock
    three-way s.
Stoppa
    S. operation
    S. repair
storage
    cold s.
    hypothermic s.
store
    hepatic glycogen s.
    iron s.
    liver iron s.
    liver protein s.
Storz
    S. cholangiograsper
    S. cystoscope
    S. esophagoscope
    S. minilaparoscope
    S. Modulith SL20
    S. multifunction valve trocar/cannula system
    S. nephroscope
    S. panendoscope
    S. resectoscope
    S. 27022 SK ureteroscope
    S. syringe
    S. urethrotome
STR
    stone-tissue recognition system
strabismus scissors

Strachan
    S. disease
    S. syndrome
Strachan-Scott syndrome
straddle injury
straight
    s. endoprosthesis
    s. intestine
    s. Maryland forceps
    s. mosquito clamp
    s. stent
    s. venule
straightener
    colonoscopy technique with external s.
    external s.
straightening maneuver
Straight-In
    S.-I. male sling system
    S.-I. surgical system
strain
    Bio-Tract proprietary s.
    Cowan 1 s.
    cystitis-causing s.
    eubacterial s.
    s. gauge transducer
    metronidazole-resistant s.
    precore mutant s.
    simian s.
    Statham P23 s. gauge
    Stx 2-producing *Escherichia coli* s. (STEC)
straining
    s. at stool
    defecatory s.
    excessive s.
    s. for urination
strand
    Billroth s.
    fibrin s.
    internodal s.
    intramembranous particle s.
stranding
    fascial s.
    hyperechoic s.
    mesenteric fat s.
    pericholecystic s.
    perinephric s.
    periureteral s.
    soft tissue s.
strangulated
    s. bowel
    s. bowel obstruction
    s. hemorrhoid
    s. hernia
    s. viscus
strangulation
    s. of bladder
    s. necrosis
strangury, stranguria
S-transferase
    glutathione S-t. (GST)
Stransky sign
strap
    Allen s.
    Montgomery abdominal s.
Strassburg test
strata (*pl. of* stratum)
Stratagene SCS-96 thermocycler
Stratasis urethral sling
strategy
    antisense s.
    rational allocation s.
stratiform
Stratte needle holder
stratum, pl. **strata**
    s. malpighii
    submucous s.
Strauss sign
strawberry
    s. gallbladder
    s. hemangioma
straw-colored
    s.-c. ascites
    s.-c. fluid
streak
    erythematous s.
    s. gonad
    lymphangitic s.
    s. ovary
stream
    curve of s.
Strecker stent
Strelinger colon clamp
strength
    artery weld s.
    detrusor contraction s.
    double s. (DS)
    hemostatic bond s.
    masseter s.
    pelvic muscle s.
    remodeling reestablished tissue s.
    tensile s.

NOTES

streptavidin
    peroxidase-conjugated s.
streptococcal esophagitis
streptococcus, pl. **streptococci**
    S. agalactiae
    alpha-hemolytic s.
    anhemolytic s.
    beta-hemolytic s.
    S. bovis
    S. bovis bacteremia
    S. bovis endocarditis
    S. enteritis
    S. faecalis
    group B s. (GBS)
    hemolytic s.
    S. milleri
    S. mulleri
    nonhemolytic *S.*
    S. pyogenes
    S. salivarius
    S. sanguis
    S. thermophilus
    S. viridans
streptokinase
Streptomyces misakiensis
streptomycin nephropathy
streptozocin, streptozotocin
streptozotocin-induced diabetes mellitus
stress
    s. cystogram
    s. erosion
    s. erythrocytosis
    s. gastritis
    s. hematuria
    s. incontinence type 0, I, II, III
    s. lesion
    oxidative s.
    s. protein
    s. relaxation
    surgical s.
    s. testing
    s. ulcer
    s. ulceration
    s. ulcer hemorrhage
    s. ulcer prophylaxis
    s. urethral pressure profile
    s. urinary incontinence (SUI)
stress-induced gastric ulceration
stress-related
    s.-r. erosive syndrome
    s.-r. mucosal disease (SRMD)
    s.-r. mucosal injury
Stresstein liquid feeding
stretch receptor
stretch-sensitive ion channel
Stretta
    S. catheter
    S. procedure
    S. system
stria, pl. **striae**
    epidermal s.
    Looser-Milkman s.
STRIANT buccal system
striated
    s. detrusor sphincter
    s. muscle innervation
    s. urethral sphincter
Strickler
    S. technique ureterocolonic anastomosis
    S. ureteral anastomosis
stricture
    anal s.
    anastomotic s.
    annular esophageal s.
    antral s.
    avascular s.
    benign bile duct s. (BBDS)
    benign biliary s.
    bile duct s.
    biliary tract s.
    bulbomembranous s.
    bulbourethral s.
    s. cannulation
    caustic s.
    cicatricial s.
    colorectal s.
    complete ureteral s.
    congenital ureteral s.
    congenital urethral s.
    contractile s.
    corrosive esophageal s.
    diaphragmlike s.
    distal esophageal s.
    ductal s.
    esophageal s.
    extrahepatic biliary s.
    filiform s.
    focal s.
    hourglass s.
    Hunner s.
    intestinal s.
    intrahepatic biliary s.
    intrinsic ureteral s.
    irritable s.
    left hepatic duct s.
    longitudinal esophageal s.
    malignant rectal s.
    membraneous urethral s.
    nonsteroidal antiinflammatory drug-induced intestinal s.
    pancreatic duct s.
    pancreaticobiliary s.
    peptic esophageal s.
    postcholangitic s.
    postoperative s.

posttraumatic posterior urethral s.
s. prophylaxis
pyloric s.
radiation-induced ureteral s.
rectal s.
recurrent s.
reflux-related s.
ringlike s.
severe ureteral s.
spasmodic s.
upper tract s.
ureteral s.
ureterocolic s.
ureteroenteric s.
ureteroileal s.
urethral s.
vas deferens s.
vesicoureteral anastomotic s.
vesicourethral anastomotic s.

strictured esophagus
strictureplasty, stricturoplasty (SXPL)
   endoscopic s.
   Finney s.
   Heineke-Mikulicz s.
   isoperistaltic s.
   side-to-side isoperistaltic s. (SSIS)
   stapled s.
   Thal s.
stricturotomy
   endoscopic s.
stridor
strigosus
   Ctenochaetus s.
string
   s. guideline
   s. method for treatment of penile incarceration
   s. operation
   s. sign
   soft rubber s.
   swallowed s.
   s. test
string-of-beads
   s.-o.-b. appearance
   s.-o.-b. appearance of renal medial fibroplasia
   s.-o.-b. sign
string-of-pearls
   s.-o.-p. appearance of gastric body
   s.-o.-p. sign
strip
   Ames Hemastix reagent s.

Bio-Gen urine test s.
s. biopsy
s. biopsy resection technique
DiaScreen 10 Reagent S.
DisIntek reagent s.
ganglion-free muscle s.
Gore-Tex s.
PyloriTek reagent s.
s. resection
rhythm s.
roof s.

stripe
   s. interstitial fibrosis
   properitoneal flank s.
stripping
   mucosal s.
   urethral s.
stroke
   saber s.
stroma, pl. **stromata**
   fibroelastic connective tissue s.
   fibrous s.
   hyalinized s.
   s. ovarii
   prostate gland s.
stromal
   s. invasion
   s. tumor of unknown malignant potential (STUMP)
strong
   s. association
   s. clinical suspicion
   S. Start chewable tablet
Strongyloides
   S. stercoralis
   S. sterocoralis
   S. venezuelensis
strongyloidiasis
   disseminated s.
strongyloid infection
strongyloma
strontium-89 chloride
Strovite Advance caplet
structural
   s. effects of dietary salt
   s. fatigue
   s. property
   s. stability
structure
   biliary s.
   cord s.
   ductular s.

NOTES

structure *(continued)*
    glandular s.
    insular s.
    malignant nuclear s.
    mixed s.
    nociceptive s.
    seminiferous tubule peritubular s.
    trabecular s.
    undifferentiated s.

Structured and Scaled Interview to Assess Maladjustment (SSIAM)

Strulle scissors

struma, pl. **strumae**
    Hashimoto s.
    s. ovarii

strumous bubo

strut
    Mersilene s.

struvite
    s. calculus
    s. crystal formation
    s. stone
    s. urolithiasis

Stryker frame

STS
    serologic test for syphilis
        STS lithotripsy system

stuartii
    Providencia s.

Stucker bile duct dilator

studding
    omental s.
    peritoneal s.

Studer
    S. bladder substitute
    S. crossfolded ileal reservoir
    S. neobladder
    S. pouch
    S. pouch procedure
    S. reservoir urinary diversion

studeri
    Bertiella s.

study
    AEC S.
    A28 immunological s.
    American Endosonography Club S.
    antegrade contrast s.
    anti-DNA immunological s.
    anti-ENA immunological s.
    antihepatitis A-IgM immunological s.
    antinuclear antibody immunological s.
    anti-SSA immunological s.
    anti-SSB immunological s.
    barium s.
    bead-chain s.
    B12 immunological s.
    bladder outlet kinesiologic s.
    bulb-tip retrograde s.
    Candida immunological s.
    Celecoxib Long-Term Arthritis Safety S. (CLASS)
    C3 immunological s.
    cinefluorographic s.
    circulating immunocomplex immunological s.
    Collaborative Transplant S. (CTS)
    colonic transit s.
    colonoscopic s.
    colon transit marker s.
    colorectal physiologic s.
    congruent grade A s.
    dark adaptation s.
    detrusor muscle pressure-flow micturition s.
    diisopropyliminodiacetic acid enterogastroesophageal reflux s.
    DISIDA enterogastroesophageal reflux s.
    diuretic renal quantitative camera s.
    DNCB immunological s.
    double-blind randomized s.
    dynamic urethral profile s.
    ESR immunological study immunological s.
    European retrospective s.
    flow cytometric s.
    gene-blotting s.
    genitocerebral evoked potential s.
    HALT-C s.
    HBeAg immunological s.
    HBsAg immunological s.
    hematologic s.
    HLA typing immunological s.
    HOPE s.
    24-hour ambulatory manometry s.
    24-hour intraesophageal pH s.
    IgA immunological s.
    IgG immunological s.
    IgM immunological s.
    Intergroup Rhabdomyosarcoma S. (IRS)
    intestinal transit s.
    isotope s.
    kinetic gallbladder s.
    light micrographic s.
    luminal contrast s.
    MACH1 s.
    manometric s.
    marker transit s.
    microperfusion s.
    mitochondrial immunological s.
    molecular s.
    multicenter s.
    Multicentre International Liver Tumor S. (MILTS)
    National Cooperative Dialysis S.

nerve conduction s.
nuclear-tagged red blood cell bleeding s.
Nurses' Health s. (NHS)
observational followup s.
one-session crossover s.
ORCHID s.
peak urinary flow s.
perfusion s.
phenotypic s.
Physicians' Health S. I, II (PHS I, II)
pilot s.
polarographic s.
positive secretin stimulation s.
PPD immunological s.
pressure s.
pressure-flow s. (PFS)
pressure-flow electromyography s.
pressure-flow micturition s.
prospective multicenter s.
radiological s.
radionuclide transit s.
Ramipril Efficacy in Nephropathy s.
rectal barostat s.
rectosphincter manometric s.
REIN s.
renal function s. (RFS)
renal perfusion pressure-flow s.
retrograde contrast s.
retroperitoneal carbon dioxide insufflation s.
scintigraphic emptying s.
seroepidemiological s.
single-color direct immunofluorescence s.
smooth muscle immunological s.
split renal function s. (SRFS)
^{99m}Tc-phytate liquid state esophageal transit s.
transurethral prostatic resection s.
Treponema immunofluorescence s.
T-tube s.
upper gastrointestinal barium roentgenographic s.
urodynamic flow s.
videoendoscopic swallowing s. (VESS)
videofluoroscopic swallow s.
videofluorourodynamic s.
voiding s.

Stühmer disease
STUMP
   stromal tumor of unknown malignant potential
stump
   appendiceal s.
   blind s.
   dehiscence of cystic s.
   duodenal s.
   funicular s.
   gastric s.
   s. invagination
   s. ligation
   polypectomy s.
   rectal s.
Sturge-Weber syndrome
stuttering
   s. priapism
   urinary s.
   s. urination
Stx
   Shiga toxin
   Stx 2-producing *Escherichia coli* strain (STEC)
stylet, stylette
   bayonet s.
   S. internal esophageal MRI coil
styloglossus muscle
stylohyoid muscle
stylopharyngeus muscle
S-type amylase
Stypven time test
subacute
   s. abscess
   s. atrophy of liver
   s. cystitis
   s. fatty liver of pregnancy
   s. hepatic necrosis
   s. hepatitis
   s. liver disease
   s. liver failure (SALF)
   s. nephritis
   s. nonspecific peritonitis
subadventitial fibroplasia
subaponeurotic abscess
subarachnoid space
subareolar
subcapsular
   s. hematoma
   s. hemorrhage
   s. hepatic abscess

NOTES

subcarinal
- s. lymph
- s. node

subcecal appendix
subcholangiopancreatoscope
subchronic
- s. atrophy of liver
- s. sacral neuromodulation

subcitrate
- colloidal bismuth s. (CBS)

subclavian
- s. catheter
- s. catheter insertion
- s. position
- s. vein
- s. vein catheterization

subclinical
- s. hepatic encephalopathy (SHE)
- s. hepatitis
- s. rejection
- s. sprue

subconjunctival hemorrhage
subcoronal hypospadias
subcostal
- s. flank incision
- s. margin
- s. nerve
- s. port
- s. transperitoneal incision

subcutaneous (SC)
- s. EGF
- s. emphysema
- s. fat
- s. layer
- s. morphine pump (SQMP)
- s. tissue
- s. urinary diversion

subcuticular suture
subdeterminant
- hepatitis B surface antigen s.

subdiaphragmatic abscess
subendoscope
subendothelial deposit
subepithelial
- s. deposit
- s. hematoma of renal pelvis
- s. hemorrhage

subfertile
subfraction
- uremic serum s.

subfulminant liver failure
subglottic lesion
subgroup F adenovirus
subhepatic
- s. abscess
- s. area
- s. space

subinguinalis
- fossa s.

subinguinal microsurgical varicocelectomy
subjective
- s. improvement
- s. symptom
- s. vertigo

sublingual hyoscyamine
submassive hepatic necrosis
submucosa
- small intestinal s.

submucosal
- s. arterial malformation
- s. artery
- s. calculus
- s. dissection
- s. endothelial angiodysplasia
- s. fat
- s. fibromuscular angiodysplasia
- s. gastric hemorrhage
- s. ileal lipoma
- s. mass
- s. saline injection
- s. saline injection technique
- s. tattoo
- s. Teflon injection
- s. thickening
- s. track
- s. upper gastrointestinal tract lesion
- s. vaginal muscle
- s. vaginal smooth musculofascial layer
- s. vascular dilation
- s. vascular malformation
- s. venous plexus
- s. wound

submucous
- s. cystitis
- s. layer
- s. plexus
- s. stratum
- s. ulcer

submuscular plexus
subparta
- ileus s.

subperitoneal
- s. abscess
- s. appendicitis
- s. fascia
- s. space

subphrenic
- s. abscess
- s. space

subpleural blanketing technique
subpubic sinus
Subrini penile prosthesis
subsalicylate
- bismuth s. (BSS)

subsaturation riboprobe concentration
subscapular

subsegmentectomy
    hepatic s.
subsequent
    s. diagnostic laparoscopy
    s. rejection episode
subserosal
    s. calbindin
    s. disease
    s. layer
subserous
    s. fascia
    s. ganglion
    s. tunnel
subsigmoid fossa
substaging
    pathologic s.
substance
    s. abuse
    s. A, K, S
    caustic s.
    hepatic stimulatory s. (HSS)
    noncholecystokinin s.
    ouabainlike s. (OLS)
    s. P (SP)
    reducing s.
substantial regional difference
substernal region
substitute
    graft s.
    ileal orthotopic bladder s.
    low-pressure bladder s.
    Olestra fat s.
    saliva s.
    Studer bladder s.
substituted benzimidazole
substitution
    bladder s.
    ileal ureteral s.
    orthotopic bladder s.
    s. urethroplasty
substrate
    copolymerized s.
    narrow s.
    s. oxidation
substratum
    cell s.
subsymphyseal epispadias
subtotal
    s. colectomy
    s. gastrectomy
    s. gastric exclusion

    s. pancreatectomy
    s. villous atrophy (SVA)
subtraction angiography
subtrigonal cystectomy
subtunical venule
subtype
    HBsAg s.
subtyping
    HLA-DR2 s.
subumbilical space
subunit
    corticosteroid regulation of amiloride-sensitive sodium channel s.
    glutamylcysteine synthetase heavy s. (GCS-HS)
subureteric Teflon injection (STING)
suburethral
    s. component
    s. epithelial inclusion cyst
    s. rectus fascial sling procedure
    s. sling
suburothelial
    s. infiltrative cancer
    s. nerve plexus
    s. vascular bed
subvesical duct
subxiphoid
Suby G solution
subzonal insemination (SUZI)
succagogue
success
    s. in retroflexion
    s. of surgical treatment
succi (*pl. of* succus)
succimer
succinate
    s. dehydrogenase
    sumatriptan s.
succinylcholine
succorrhea
succulent mesenteric lymph node
succus, pl. **succi**
    s. entericus
    s. gastricus
    s. pancreaticus
succussion
    hippocratic s.
    s. sounds
    s. splash
suck-and-cut
    s.-a.-c. method

NOTES

suck-and-cut (continued)
    s.-a.-c. mucosectomy
    s.-a.-c. technique
sucker
    tonsil s.
sucralfate
    s. retention enema
    s. therapy
sucrose
    iron s.
    s. tolerance test
sucrose-free (SF)
sucrose-isomaltase deficiency (SID)
suction
    s. banding
    s. biopsy
    bulb s.
    S. Buster catheter
    s. channel
    continuous NG s.
    s. cylinder
    s. drain
    s. drainage
    flexible dental s.
    s. foot pedal
    Gomco s.
    Harris tube s.
    lavage and s.
    low intermittent s.
    nasogastric s.
    NG s.
    S. oral brush
    s. pump
    s. tip
    s. tube
    Wangensteen s.
suction-coagulator
    Cameron-Miller s.-c.
suctioning
    intermittent s.
    rectal air s.
Suda classification type I, II, III of papilla
Sudan black B fat stain
Sudan-III stain
sudden
    s. expansion
    s. onset of pain
    s. valve prolapse
Sudeck
    S. atrophy
    S. critical point
sufentanil
sugar
    s. oxime
    s. test
Sugarbaker technique
Sugar-Free
    Citrucel S.-F.

Sugiura
    S. esophageal variceal transection
    S. esophageal varices procedure
    S. paraesophagogastric devascularization
SUI
    stress urinary incontinence
suitable rabbit polyclonal antibody
suite
    endoscopy s.
sulamserod HCl
sulbactam sodium
sulciform
sulcus, pl. **sulci**
    coronal s.
    costovertebral s.
    intersphincteric s.
    s. of umbilical vein
sulfa
sulfacytine
sulfadiazine
sulfamethizole
sulfamethoprim
sulfamethoxazole (SMX, SMZ)
    s. and phenazopyridine
    s. and trimethoprim (SMX/TMP)
Sulfamylon
sulfanilamide
sulfasalazine enema
sulfasalazine-induced oxidative hemolysis
sulfasoxazole
sulfate
    atropine s.
    barium s.
    bleomycin s.
    dehydroepiandrosterone s. (DHAS)
    dermatan s.
    dextran sodium s. (DSS)
    ephedrine s.
    ferrous s.
    gentamicin s.
    hydrazine s.
    hyoscyamine s.
    pentosan s.
    protamine s.
    quinidine s.
    sodium dodecyl s. (SDS)
    sodium tetradecyl s.
    tetradecyl s.
sulfated
    s. glycoprotein-2 (SGP-2)
    s. mucin stain
sulfation
    tyrosine s.
Sulfatrim DS
sulfhydryl donor
sulfinpyrazone
sulfisoxazole and phenazopyridine
sulfolithocholylglycine

sulfolithocholyltaurine
sulfomucin
    acidic s.
sulfonamide nephropathy
sulfonate
    mercaptoethane s.
    polystyrene sodium s.
    sodium polystyrene s.
sulfone syndrome
sulfoxide
    dimethyl s. (DMSO)
sulfur
    s. amino acid metabolism
    s. colloid (SC)
    s. colloid liver scan
sulfuric acid
sulglycotide
sulindac
Sulkowitch test
sulmarin
sulodexide
sulotroban
sulphonylurea
sulpiride
sumatriptan succinate
Sumikoshi classification
summer
    s. cholera
    s. diarrhea
summit of bladder
Sumner
    S. method
    S. sign
sump
    s. drain
    s. nasogastric tube
    s. syndrome
    s. ulcer
Sumycin Oral
SUN
    serum urea nitrogen
superantigen
Super-Bright microsphere
SuperChar
Super-Cut scissors
superfibronectin
superficial
    s. abdominal ring
    s. bladder cancer
    s. bladder tumor
    s. depressed cancer
    s. esophageal carcinoma (SEC)
    s. extension
    s. fascia
    s. fluorescein
    s. gastric carcinoma
    s. gastritis
    s. inguinal pouch
    s. linear ulcer
    s. perineal aponeurosis
    s. perineal space
    s. trigonal muscle
superficialis
    arteria epigastrica s.
    colitis cystica s.
    esophagitis dissecans s.
    fascia penis s.
superficially spreading carcinoma
superimposed alcoholic hepatitis
superinfection
    delta hepatitis s.
    hepatitis D s.
superior
    s. aberrant ductule
    arteria epigastrica s.
    arteria mesenterica s.
    arteria rectalis s.
    ductulus aberrans s.
    s. duodenal fold
    s. extremity
    fascia diaphragmatis pelvis s.
    flexura duodeni s.
    s. hemorrhoidal artery
    s. hypogastric nerve plexus
    s. margin
    s. mesenteric angiography
    s. mesenteric arteriogram
    s. mesenteric artery (SMA)
    s. mesenteric artery syndrome (SMAS)
    s. mesenteric to renal artery saphenous vein bypass graft
    s. mesenteric vein (SMV)
    s. mesenterorenal bypass
    s. mesenterorenal bypass technique
    s. passive fixation
    plica duodenalis s.
    s. pubic ramotomy
    s. rectal vein
    s. rectal venous plexus
    s. vesical artery
supernatant
supernumerary kidney

NOTES

superoxide
- s. dismutase (SOD)
- extracellular s.
- s. production
- s. radical

Super PEG tube
supersaturated bile
supersaturation
- cystine s.
- relative s. (RSs)
- urine s.

superselective
- s. arteriography
- s. transcatheter embolization
- s. vagotomy

supination
supine position
supper
- fat-free s. (FFS)

supplement
- Arginaid dietary s.
- caloric s.
- Cal Power calorie s.
- Casec calcium s.
- Case Power protein s.
- Dent s.
- Enrich protein and calorie s.
- food s.
- Hy-Cal calorie s.
- Impact nutritional s.
- keto acid-amino acid s.
- Maalox Antacid/Calcium s.
- Nepro diet s.
- Polycose glucose s.
- protein s.
- ProXeed dietary s.
- SAMe nutritional s.
- Spirulina Pacifica nutritional s.
- Travasorb MCT s.

supplementation
- calcium s.
- chronic intravenous s.
- citrate s.
- dietary L-arginine s.
- fish oil s.
- prostaglandin s.
- vitamin D s.

support
- artificial hepatic s.
- bladder s.
- imaging bladder s.
- midurethral s.
- nutritional s.
- s. parenteral nutrition (SPN)
- psychological s.
- psychosexual s.
- ventilatory s.

supportive treatment

suppository
- alprostadil urethral s.
- B & O No. 15A, 16A C-II s.
- Canasa s.
- Compro s.
- FIV-ASA s.
- glycerin s.
- intraurethral prostaglandin s. (IPS)
- mesalamine rectal s.
- MUSE urethral s.
- prochlorperazine s.
- rectal s.
- vaginal s.

suppression
- acid s.
- androgen s.
- cell-mediated s.
- hypothalamic s.
- immune s.
- metastasis s.
- s. treatment
- urinary tract infection s.

suppressive
- s. anuria
- s. maneuver

suppressor
- cellular tumor s.
- s. gene
- s. T cell

suppuration
suppurativa
- hidradenitis s.

suppurative
- s. appendicitis
- s. appendix
- s. cholangitis
- s. cortical nephritis
- s. gastritis

supraceliac aorta
supraclavicular
supracolic compartment
supracostal incision
supradiaphragmatic diverticulum
supraduodenal approach
Supra-Foley catheter
supragastric bursoscopy
supraglottic squamous cell carcinoma
suprahepatic
- s. abscess
- s. caval cuff
- s. space
- s. vena cava

suprahilar
- s. disease
- s. lymph node dissection

suprainguinal region
supralevator
- s. anorectal space

s. pelvic exenteration
s. perirectal abscess
Supramid suture
supraomental space
suprapapillary
s. fistula
s. Roux-en-Y duodenojejunostomy
supraphysiological fundoplication
supraprostatectomy
suprapubic
s. aspiration
s. aspiration of bladder
s. cystography
s. cystomy drainage
s. cystostomy
s. cystotomy
s. cystotomy tract urethral atresia
s. lithotomy
s. port
s. prostatectomy
s. puncture
s. region
s. tube
suprarenal
s. area of liver
s. gland
s. Greenfield filter
s. impression
s. medulla
s. plexus
suprarenale
melasma s.
suprarenalectomy
suprarenalis
cortex glandulae s.
medulla glandulae s.
suprarenalism
suprarenalopathy
suprarenogenic syndrome
suprasphincteric fistula
supratrigonal cystectomy
supravesical urinary diversion
sural nerve graft
suramin
!nSure
!nSure fecal immunochemical test
!nSure immunochemical fecal occult blood test
SureBite biopsy forceps
Sure-Cut biopsy needle
Sureseal pressure bandage

Suretys
S. incontinence brief
S. pants
S. panty system
surface
antimesenteric s.
biomaterial s.
bosselated s.
cholesterolosis of mucosal s.
colonic mucosal s.
s. cooling
s. cooling technique
depression s.
s. electrode
s. epithelium
s. membrane actin cytoskeleton complex
s. nodularity
s. nodule
s. pelvic floor electromyography
s. protein
serosal s.
s. thermometer
urethral cooling s.
ventral s.
surface-to-volume ratio
surfactant laxative
Surfak
Sur-Fit
S.-F. auto-lock closed-end pouch with filter
S.-F. Minipouch
S.-F. Natura closed-end pouch, opaque
S.-F. Natura disposable convex insert
S.-F. Natura flange cap
S.-F. Natura flexible wafer and drainable pouch
S.-F. Natura irrigation adapter face plate
S.-F. Natura irrigation sleeve
S.-F. Natura irrigation sleeve tail closure
S.-F. Natura loop ostomy rod
S.-F. Natura night drainage container set
S.-F. Natura night drainage container tubing
S.-F. Natura opaque closed-end pouch with filter
S.-F. Natura urostomy pouch

NOTES

Sur-Fit *(continued)*
    S.-F. Natura Visi-Flow irrigation starter set
    S.-F. Natura Visi-Flow irrigator
    S.-F. Pouch cover
    S.-F. stoma cap
Surgaloy suture
Surgenomic endoscope
surgeon
    colorectal s.
    genitourinary s.
    Society of American Gastrointestinal Endoscoping S.'s (SAGES)
    urogynecologic s.
surgeon-endoscopist
surgeon's knot
surgery
    abdominal s.
    adrenal-sparing s.
    anal s.
    anorectal s.
    antireflux s.
    bariatric s.
    bench s.
    biliopancreatic obesity s.
    colorectal s. (CRS)
    complex reconstructive s.
    concomitant antireflux s.
    cytoreductive s.
    diagnostic s.
    dialysis access s.
    dysphagia after antireflux s.
    extracorporeal s.
    failed antireflux s.
    feminizing s.
    flank s.
    gastric bypass s.
    hand-assisted laparoscopic s. (HALS)
    incontinence s.
    intestinal s.
    invasive s.
    invasiveness of s.
    jejunoileal bypass s.
    laparoscopic adrenal gland s.
    laparoscopic antireflux s. (LARS)
    laparoscopic colorectal cancer s.
    laser s.
    major GI s.
    minimal access s.
    minimally invasive s.
    nephron-sparing s.
    nonbench s.
    open stone s.
    outcome equivalent to open s.
    palliative s.
    parenchymal-sparing s.
    Parietex composite mesh for hernia s.
    pelvic colonic s.
    penile reconstructive s.
    penile venous ligation s.
    PlasmaKinetic s.
    portosystemic shunt s.
    postchemotherapy s.
    primary perineal hypospadias s.
    radical s.
    radioimmunoguided s. (RIGS)
    reconstructive s.
    rectovaginal s.
    renal-sparing s.
    renovascular s.
    retrograde intrarenal s.
    retroperitoneal s.
    reversal jejunoileal bypass s.
    salvage s.
    secondary s.
    sham s.
    stone s.
    systemic s.
    TAAA s.
    telerobotic-assisted laparoscopic s.
    thoracoabdominal aortic aneurysm s.
    transsexual s.
    ureteral reimplantation s.
    urologic s.
    vascular s.
    videoassisted thoracic s. (VATS)
    weight-reduction s.
surgical
    s. abdomen
    s. approach
    s. care
    s. cystgastrostomy
    s. decompression
    s. drain
    s. drape
    s. extirpation
    s. failure
    s. flap
    s. incision
    s. loupe
    s. portosystemic shunting
    s. procedure
    s. scissors
    s. simulation virtual reality laboratory
    s. simulator
    s. stapling
    s. stress
    s. therapy
    s. vagotomy
surgically implanted hemodialysis catheter (SIHC)
Surgicel gauze
Surgilube lubricant

Surgi-PEG replacement gastrostomy feeding system
Surgipro
    S. mesh
    S. suture
Surgisis
    S. Gold hernia repair graft
    Surgisis sling/mesh
Surgitek
    S. button
    S. catheter
    S. Flexi-Flate II penile implant
    S. graduated cystocope GC-16
    S. graduated cystoscope
    S. One-Step (SOS)
    S. One-Step percutaneous endoscopic gastrostomy
    S. Tractfinder ureteral stent
    S. Uropass stent
Surgitite ligating loop
Surgiwip suture ligature
Surpass
surreptitious vomiting
surrogate marker
surveillance
    s. colonoscopy
    s. cystogram
    endoscopic s.
    s. endoscopy
    S., Epidemiology, and End Results (SEER)
    s. program
    s. protocol
survey
    Digestive Health Status Instrument s.
    metabolic bone s.
    National Health and Nutrition Examination S. (NHANES)
    Rand Short Form-36 s.
survival
    allograft s.
    s. analysis
    graft s.
    improved graft s.
    mean allograft s. (MAS)
    overall s. (OS)
    progression-free s.
    s. rate
    renal allograft s.
Susano Elixir
susceptibility
    genetic s.
    higher host s.
    LDL s.
    low-density lipoprotein s.
susceptible population
Suspend sling
suspension
    barium sulfate for s.
    bladder neck s. (BNS)
    Burch iliopectineal ligament urethrovesical s.
    charcoal s.
    colloidal bismuth s.
    Enecat CT concentrated rectal s.
    EntroEase Dry powder for oral s.
    EntroEase oral radiopaque contrast medium s.
    extraperitoneal laparoscopic bladder neck s. (ELBNS)
    Formula EM oral s.
    Gadolite oral s.
    Gittes bladder neck s.
    Gittes-Loughlin bladder neck s.
    laparoscopic bladder neck s.
    leuprolide acetate for injectable s.
    Maalox Anti-Gas Extra-Strength oral s.
    modified Pereyra bladder neck s.
    mycophenolate mofetil oral s.
    needle bladder neck s.
    Nephrox S.
    nystatin s.
    octreotide acetate for injectable s.
    OK432 streptococcal s.
    oral barium s.
    percutaneous bladder neck s. (PBNS)
    percutaneous needle bladder neck s.
    Pereyra bladder neck s.
    Prevacid Packet powder for oral s.
    Raz bladder neck s.
    Raz four-quadrant s.
    Raz needle bladder s.
    Raz urethral s.
    retropubic Lapides-Ball bladder neck s.
    Stamey needle bladder neck s.
    triptorelin pamoate for injectable s.
    urethral s.
    vesicoureteral s.

NOTES

suspension *(continued)*
    vesicourethral s.
    Young-Dees s.
suspensory
    s. bandage
    s. ligament
    s. muscle
suspicion
    strong clinical s.
Sustacal
    S. HC liquid feeding
    S. pudding
Sustagen liquid feeding
sustained
    s. detrusor contraction
    s. low-efficiency dialysis (SLED)
    s. virologic response (SVR)
suture
    absorbable s.
    Albert s.
    Albert-Lembert s.
    anastomotic s.
    anchoring s.
    Appolito s.
    approximation s.
    atraumatic s.
    Bell s.
    black silk s. (BSS)
    bolster s.
    s. bridge
    buried s.
    button s.
    cardinal s.
    chain s.
    chromic catgut s.
    chromic gut s.
    circular s.
    Connell s.
    continuous s.
    corner s.
    cotton s.
    Cushing s.
    s. cutter
    Czerny s.
    Czerny-Lembert s.
    Dacron s.
    dermal s.
    Dermalene s.
    Dermalon s.
    Dexon s.
    Dupuytren s.
    Endoloop s.
    Ethibond s.
    Ethiflex s.
    Ethilon s.
    everting s.
    s. fatigue
    figure-of-eight s.
    furrier s.
    Gambee s.
    Gély s.
    Gould inverted mattress s.
    s. granuloma
    green Mersilene s.
    s. guide
    Gussenbauer s.
    Halsted interrupted mattress s.
    Halsted interrupted quilt s.
    heavy silk s.
    hemostatic s.
    horizontal mattress s.
    Horsley s.
    interrupted manual mucomucosal absorbable s.
    interrupted seromuscular s.
    intracuticular s.
    intradermal s.
    inverting s.
    Ivalon s.
    Jobert de Lamballe s.
    Kessler-Kleinert s.
    Lembert inverting seromuscular s.
    s. ligated
    s. ligature
    s. line
    s. line dehiscence
    s. line ulceration
    locking s.
    lock-stitch s.
    loop s.
    Marshall U-stitch s.
    s. material
    mattress s.
    Maxon s.
    Mersilene s.
    Monocryl s.
    monofilament absorbable s.
    monofilament nylon s.
    nonabsorbable s.
    over-and-over s.
    Parker-Kerr s.
    PDS Vicryl s.
    pericostal s.
    Perma-Hand silk s.
    plain catgut s.
    plain gut s.
    s. plication
    plication s.
    Polydek s.
    polydioxanone s.
    polyglactin s.
    polyglecaprone 25 s.
    polyglycolic acid s.
    polyglyconate s.
    polypropylene s.
    pop-off s.
    primary s.
    Prolene s.

pursestring s.
quilted s.
s. rectopexy
s. rectopexy with sigmoid resection
reinforcing s.
relaxation s.
retention s.
running s.
s. scissors
secondary s.
seromuscular Lembert s.
silk Mersilene s.
silk pop-off s.
silk traction s.
stainless steel s.
stay s.
subcuticular s.
Supramid s.
Surgaloy s.
Surgipro s.
swaged-on s.
Teflon-coated Dacron s.
Tevdek s.
Ti-Cron s.
Tom Jones s.
traction s.
transition s.
s. ulcer
vascular s.
vertical mattress s.
vertical plication s.
Vicryl s.
Z s.

sutured hemorrhoidectomy
sutureless
    s. biofragmentable ring
    s. bowel anastomosis
    s. colostomy closure

suture-release needle
suturing
    s. time
    transoral endoscopic s.
    transvaginal s. (TVS)

suum
    Ascaris s.

SUZI
    subzonal insemination

SVA
    subtotal villous atrophy

SVG
    seminal vesiculography

SVO
    splenic vein obstruction

SVR
    sustained virologic response
    systemic vascular resistance

SVRI
    systemic vascular resistance index

SW
    shock wave
        SW 480 cell

swab
    urethral s.

swaged needle
swaged-on
    s.-o. needle
    s.-o. suture

swallow
    s. apraxia
    barium s.
    dry s.
    Gastrografin s.
    Hypaque s.
    ice-water s.
    modified barium s. (MBS)
    water-soluble contrast esophageal s.
    wet s.

swallowed string
swallowing
    air s.
    s. center
    four phases of s.
    s. mechanism
    s. reflex
    s. threshold

Swan-Ganz
    S.-G. pulmonary artery catheter
    S.-G. thermodilution catheter

swan-neck
    s.-n. deformity
    s.-n. Missouri catheter
    s.-n. pediatric Coil-Cath catheter

sweating
    gustatory s.

sweat test
Swedish
    S. Adjustable Gastric Band (SAGB)
    S. Rectal Cancer Trial

Sween
    S. Cream
    S. Micro Guard powder
    S. Prep

NOTES

Sween-A-Peel skin barrier
sweep
    duodenal s.
Sweet
    S. esophageal scissors
    S. syndrome
swelling
    cell s.
    external s.
    genital s.
    lysosomal s.
    popliteal s.
    scrotal s.
    testicular s.
    uvular s.
Swenson
    S. abdominal pullthrough
    S. operation
    S. papillotome
swimmer's itch
swim-up processing
Swiss
    S. Lithoclast
    S. Lithoclast lithotriptor
    S. Lithoclast Master device
    S. roll embedding technique
switch
    duodenal s.
    optical s.
swivel adapter
SWL
    shock wave lithotripsy
swollen
    s. tongue
    s. turbinate
Swyer syndrome
SXPL
    strictureplasty
Sydney
    S. classification of gastritis
    S. system
    S. system gastritis classification
Syllact
sylvian fistula
symbolic stimulus
Syme external urethrotomy
Symington body
Symlin
Symmetra I-125 brachytherapy seed
symmetric face movement
Symmetry endobipolar generator
sympathetic
    s. chain
    s. cystitis
    s. enteroenteric inhibitory reflex
    s. nervous system (SNS)
    s. nervous system activity
    s. projection
    s. response to vasodilation
    s. skin response
    s. sphincter constrictor reflex
symphyseal bar
symphysis, pl. **symphises**
    s. ossium pubis
    pubic s.
    s. pubica syndrome
    s. pubis
Symphytum
symptom
    alarm s.
    alcohol-induced gastrointestinal s.
    Bristol female lower urinary tract s.
    Candida s.
    S. Checklist-90R
    chronic functional gastrointestinal s.
    s. of chronic heartburn
    chronic prostatitis-like s.
    s. control
    dyspeptic s.
    extraesophageal s.
    s. free
    head s.
    incarceration s.
    intradialytic s.
    irritative s.
    lower urinary tract s. (LUTS)
    Medical Therapy of Prostatic s.'s (MTOPS)
    persistent s.
    postcibal s.
    s. problem index (SPI)
    prodromal s.
    reflux s.
    respiratory s.'s (RS)
    s. score
    s. sensitivity index
    s. severity index (SSI)
    subjective s.
    symptomatic progression of s.'s
    target s.
    tuberculosis s.
    unresponsive s.
    urgency-frequency s.
    urinary s.
    urologic s.
symptomatic
    s. benign prostatic hyperplasia
    s. benign prostatic hypertrophy
    s. fluid gain
    s. gallstone
    s. impotence
    s. progression of symptoms
    s. varicocele
symptomatology
    chronic functional s.
    lower urinary tract s.
symptom-giving PGR

Syms tractor
Synalar Topical
Synalgos-DC Capsules
synapse
    axoaxonic s.
synaptic transmission
synaptogenesis
synchondroseotomy
SynchroMed infusion system intraspinal catheter
SYNCHRON CX-5, CX-7 automated analyzer
synchronous
    s. adenoma
    s. bladder reconstruction
    s. inferior cavography
    s. lesion
    s. neonatal torsion
    s. polyp
    s. superior cavography
    s. urinary tract infection
syncope
    defecation s.
syncytium
syndrome
    Aagenaes s.
    Aarskog s.
    Aarskog-Scott s.
    abdominal compartment s. (ACS)
    abdominal cutaneous nerve entrapment s.
    abdominal muscle deficiency s.
    acquired immunodeficiency s. (AIDS)
    acute flank pain s.
    acute nephritic s.
    acute urethral s.
    Adamantiades-Behçet s.
    Addison s.
    addisonian s.
    adrenogenital s.
    adult respiratory distress s. (ARDS)
    afferent loop s.
    Alagille s.
    Alagille-Watson s.
    Albright s.
    Alcock s.
    Allemann s.
    Allen-Masters s.
    Alport s.
    Alstrom-Edwards s.
    Andersen s.

    androgen insensitivity s.
    androgenital s.
    anorexia-cachexia s.
    anterior abdominal wall s.
    anterior cord s.
    anterior rib impingement s.
    anterior spinal artery s.
    antiandrogen withdrawal s.
    anticardiolipin antibody s.
    antimüllerian derivative s.
    antiphospholipid s.
    Apert s.
    apparent mineral corticoid excess s.
    apple-peel bowel s.
    Arias s.
    Asherson s.
    asplenia s.
    autoimmune deficiency s.
    autoimmune polyglandular s. type 1 (APS-1)
    autosomal-recessive Alport s.
    bacterial overgrowth s.
    Bannayan-Zonana s.
    Banti s.
    Bardet-Biedl s.
    Barrett s.
    Barsony-Polgar s.
    Bartter s.
    basal cell nevus s.
    Bassen-Kornzweig s.
    Baumgarten s.
    Bazex s.
    Bearn-Kunkel-Slater s.
    Beckwith-Wiedemann s.
    Behçet s.
    bent nail s.
    Bernard-Sergent s.
    Bernard-Soulier s.
    Bessauds-Hilmand-Augier s.
    BHD s.
    bilharzial bladder cancer s.
    Birt-Hogg-Dube s. (BHDS)
    Blatin s.
    bleomycin-associated adult respiratory distress s.
    blind loop s. (BLS)
    blue diaper s.
    blue rubber bleb nevus s.
    blue toe s.
    Boerhaave s.
    Bouveret s.
    bowel bypass s.

NOTES

syndrome *(continued)*
    branchio-otorenal s.
    Brennemann s.
    brown bowel s. (BBS)
    Budd s.
    Budd-Chiari s.
    Bürger-Grütz s.
    buried bumper s.
    Burnett s.
    burning feet s.
    burning mouth s. (BMS)
    Byler s.
    Bywaters s.
    Cacchi-Ricci s.
    cafe coronary s.
    Canada-Cronkhite s.
    cancer family s.
    carcinoid s.
    Carignan s.
    Carney s.
    Caroli s.
    Carpenter s.
    Carter-Horsley-Hughes s.
    cast s.
    cat-eye s.
    cauda equina s.
    caudal regression s.
    Cecil urethral stricture s.
    celiac s.
    cerebrohepatorenal s. (CHRS)
    cerebrooculofacial s.
    Charcot s.
    CHARGE s.
    Cheek-Perry s.
    Chilaiditi s.
    Chinese restaurant s. (CRS)
    s. of chloride depletion
    cholestatic s.
    cholesterol emboli s.
    cholinergic s.
    chronic intestinal ischemic s.
    chronic intestinal pseudoobstruction s.
    chronic pelvic pain s. (CPPS)
    chronic prostate pain s. (CPPS)
    chronic prostatitis/pelvic pain s. (CPPS)
    chronic urethral s.
    Churg-Strauss s.
    Cilaidit s.
    Clarke-Hadfield s.
    Cohen s.
    colonic polyposis s.
    colonic pseudoobstruction s.
    colonic solitary ulcer s.
    colorectal cancer s.
    compression s.
    congenital nephrotic s. (CNS)
    Conn s.
    constipation-predominant irritable bowel s.
    Cooke-Apert-Gallais s.
    Cornelia de Lange s.
    Courvoisier-Terrier s.
    couvade s.
    Cowden s.
    CREST s.
    cri du chat s.
    Crigler-Najjar s. type I, II
    Cronkhite-Canada s.
    CRST s.
    crush s.
    Cruveilhier-Baumgarten s.
    Curran s.
    Cushing medicamentosus s.
    cyclic vomiting s. (CVS)
    Danbolt-Closs s.
    Debré-de Toni-Fanconi s.
    Degos s.
    Dejerine-Sottas s.
    del Castillo s.
    dengue shock s.
    Denys-Drash s. (DDS)
    descending perineum s.
    de Toni-Debré-Fanconi s.
    de Toni-Fanconi-Debré s.
    dialysis disequilibrium s.
    dialysis encephalopathy s.
    dialysis equilibrium s.
    diarrhea-predominant irritable bowel s.
    diencephalic s.
    diffuse alveolar hemorrhage s.
    DiGeorge s.
    Diogenes s.
    Down s.
    Drash s.
    Dubin-Johnson s.
    Dubin-Sprinz s.
    Dubowitz s.
    dumping s.
    dyskinetic cilia s.
    dysmetabolic s.
    dysuria-pyuria s.
    Eagle-Barrett s.
    early dumping s.
    Edwards s.
    efferent loop s.
    Ehlers-Danlos s.
    Ellis-van Creveld s.
    empty sella s.
    encephalotrigeminal s.
    eosinophilic gastroenteritis s.
    Epstein s.
    Faber s.
    faciodigital s.
    familial atypical multiple-mole melanoma s.

syndrome · syndrome

familial chylomicronemia s.
familial polyposis s.
FAMM s.
Fanconi s.
Fanconi-de Toni-Debré s.
fatty liver and kidney s. (FLKS)
Fechtner s.
Felty s.
female urethral s.
fertile eunuch s.
Fiessinger-Leroy-Reiter s.
Fitz s.
Fitz-Hugh and Curtis s.
Flood s.
flulike s.
flushing s.
food protein-induced enterocolitis s. (FPIES)
Fraley s.
Fraser s.
frequency-urgency-pain s.
Friderichsen-Waterhouse s.
Fröhlich s.
functional bowel s.
G s.
Galloway-Mowat s. (GMS)
Gardner s. (GS)
Gardner-Diamond s.
gas-bloat s.
Gasser s.
gasserian s.
gastrocardiac s.
gastrointestinal immunodeficiency s.
gastrojejunal loop obstruction s.
GAVE s.
gay bowel s.
Gee-Herter-Heubner s.
Gianotti-Crosti s.
Gilbert s.
Gilbert-Behçet s.
Gilbert-Dreyfus s.
Gitelman s.
glioma-polyposis s.
glucagonoma s.
Goldenhar s.
Goldston s.
Goodpasture s.
Gopalan s.
Gordon s.
Gorlin basal cell nevus s.
Gorlin-Chaudhry-Moss s.
Gowers s.

Guillain-Barré s.
gynecomastia-aspermatogenesis s.
Hadefield-Clarke s.
Hadju-Cheney acroosteolysis s.
Hanot s.
Hanot-Chauffard s.
Hanot-Rössle s.
Hartnup s.
Hawes-Pallister-Landor s.
Heller-Nelson s.
HELLP s.
hematuria-dysuria s.
hemolytic-uremic s. (HUS)
hemorrhagic fever with renal s.
hepatonephoric s.
hepatopulmonary s. (HPS)
hepatorenal s. (HRS)
hereditary flat adenoma s. (HFAS)
hereditary nonpolyposis colorectal cancer s.
Hermansky-Pudlak s.
Heyde s.
Hinman s.
Hinman-Allen s.
Hippel-Lindau s.
Holt-Oram s.
hormone-secreting tumor s.
Horner s.
Howel-Evans s.
HPRC s.
hungry bone s.
hyperammonemic s.
hyperdynamic s.
hypereosinophilia s.
hypertensive lower esophageal sphincter s.
hypoperistalsis s.
iatrogenic immunodeficiency s.
idiopathic hypereosinophilic s. (IHES)
idiopathic nephrotic s.
ileocecal s.
Imerslund s.
immotile cilia s.
impaired regeneration s. (IRS)
s. of inappropriate secretion of antidiuretic hormone (SIADH)
infantile food protein-induced enterocolitis s.
infantile nephrotic s.
inflammatory bowel s. (IBS)
infrequent voider-lazy bladder s.

NOTES

767

syndrome *(continued)*
    inhibitory s.
    inspissated bile s.
    inspissated sump s.
    insulin resistance s.
    intestinal polyposis-cutaneous pigmentation s.
    intestinal stasis s.
    irrigation fluid absorption s.
    irritable bowel s. (IBS)
    irritable colon s.
    irritable gut s.
    irritable pouch s.
    isolated retained antrum s.
    Ivemark s.
    Jadassohn s.
    Jamaican vomiting s.
    jejunal s.
    Jeune s.
    Job s.
    Johanson-Blizzard s.
    Joseph s.
    Joubert s.
    juvenile polyposis s. (JPS)
    Kallmann s.
    Karroo s.
    Kartagener s.
    Katayama s.
    Kaufman s.
    Kawasaki s.
    Kearns-Sayre s. (KSS)
    Kimmelstiel-Wilson s.
    Klinefelter s.
    Klippel-Trenaunay-Weber s.
    Koenig s.
    Koro s.
    Korsakoff s.
    Kunkel s.
    Labbe s.
    Ladd s.
    Lambert-Eaton myasthenic s.
    late dumping s.
    Laubry-Soulle s.
    Launois-Cléret s.
    Laurence-Moon-Bardet-Biedl s.
    Laurence-Moon-Biedl s.
    lazy bladder s.
    LEOPARD s.
    Leriche s.
    Lesch-Nyhan s.
    levator ani s.
    Liddle s.
    Li-Fraumeni s.
    Lightwood s.
    Lignac s.
    Lignac-Fanconi s.
    locker room s.
    Loeffler s.
    loin pain hematuria s. (LPHS)
    Lowe s.
    Lubb s.
    Lucey-Driscoll s.
    Luder-Sheldon s.
    Lyell s.
    lymphadenopathy s. (LAS)
    lymphoproliferative s.
    Lynch s. II
    Mad Hatter s.
    Maffucci s.
    malabsorption s.
    maldigestion-absorption s.
    male Turner s.
    malignant B-cell s.
    malignant carcinoid s.
    Mallory-Weiss s.
    Maranon s.
    Marchiafava-Micheli s.
    Marfan s.
    Marinesco-Sjögren s.
    massive bowel resection s.
    Mayer-Rokitansky s.
    Mayer-Rokitansky-Kuster-Hauser s.
    McArdle s.
    McCune-Albright s.
    Meckel s.
    Meckel-Gruber s.
    meconium plug s.
    megacystic s.
    megacystis-megaureter s.
    megacystis-microcolon-intestinal hypoperistalsis s.
    megasigmoid s.
    Meigs s.
    Melkersson-Rosenthal s.
    MEN I s.
    Menkes s.
    mesenteric steal s.
    metastatic carcinoid s.
    microscopic colitis s.
    milk-alkali s.
    Miller Fisher s.
    mind-bladder s.
    minimal-change nephritic s.
    minimal-change nephrotic s.
    minimal-lesion nephrotic s.
    Mirizzi s.
    mitochondrial neurogastrointestinal encephalomyopathy s.
    Mosse s.
    Muckle-Wells s.
    mucocutaneous pigmentation of Peutz-Jeghers s.
    mucosal prolapse s.
    Muir-Torre s.
    müllerian duct derivation s.
    multiple endocrine neoplasia s. (MENS)
    multiple hamartoma s.

syndrome · syndrome

multiple organ failure s.
Munchausen s.
myoclonus-opsoclonus s.
nail-patella s.
narcotic bowel s.
necrolytic migratory erythema s.
Nelson s.
nephritic s.
nephrotic s.
nerve entrapment s.
Neu-Laxova s.
neurocutaneous s.
Nonnenbruch s.
Noonan s.
obesity hypoventilation s. (OHS)
Ochoa s.
oculocerebrorenal s.
Ogilvie s.
Oldfield s.
oligoteratoasthenozoospermia s.
Opitz-Frias s.
Ormond s.
Osler II s.
Osler-Weber-Rendu s.
osmotic demyelination s.
outlier s.
ovarian hyperstimulation s.
ovarian overstimulation s.
ovarian remnant s.
ovarian vein s.
overlap s.
pain-associated disability s. (PADS)
pain-predominant irritable bowel s.
pancreatic cholera s.
pancreaticohepatic s.
paraneoplastic s.
Paterson-Brown-Kelly s.
Paterson-Kelly s.
Payr s.
Pearson s.
pelvic floor s.
Pento-X s.
pericolic membrane s.
perihepatitis s.
persistent müllerian duct s.
Peutz-Jeghers s. (PJS)
pharyngeal pouch s.
Picchini s.
pickwickian s.
Pierre Robin s.
Plummer-Vinson s.
POEMS s.

Poland s.
Polhemus-Schafer-Ivemark s.
POLIP s.
polyposis s.
polysplenia s.
postcholecystectomy s. (PCS)
postcoagulation s.
postcolonoscopy distention s.
postenteritis s.
postfundoplication s.
postgastrectomy s.
postpolypectomy coagulation s.
postthrombotic s.
posttransurethral microwave thermotherapy prostatitis-like s.
post-TUMT prostatitis-like s.
postvagotomy s.
Potter s.
Prader-Willi s.
primary antiphospholipid s.
s. of primary biliary cirrhosis
primary pseudoobstruction s.
prune-belly s. category I-III
pseudo-Cushing s.
pseudoobstruction s.
pseudopancreatic cholera s.
pseudo-prune-belly s.
puborectalis s.
Rapunzel s.
refeeding s.
Reichmann s.
Reifenstein s.
Reiter s.
renal Fanconi-like s.
renal-hepatic steal s.
renal-ocular s.
renal-retinal s.
Rendu-Osler-Weber s.
reset osmostat s.
respiratory distress s.
restless leg s. (RLS)
retained antrum s.
retained bladder s.
reuse s.
reversed anorexia s.
Reye s.
Richner-Hanhart s.
Rieger s.
right ovarian vein s.
Riley-Day s.
RMS s.
Roberts s.

NOTES

syndrome *(continued)*
- Robinow s.
- Roger s.
- Rokitansky-Kuster-Hauser s.
- Rome I, II criteria for irritable bowel s.
- Rosewater s.
- Rothmund-Thomson s.
- Rotor s.
- Roux stasis s.
- Rovsing s.
- Rubinstein-Taybi s.
- Rud s.
- rudimentary testis s.
- runting s.
- Russell-Silver s.
- Ruvalcaba-Myhre-Smith s.
- Sandifer s.
- Schmidt s.
- Schultz s.
- Schwachman s.
- Schwartz-Jampel s.
- SCO s.
- sea-blue histiocyte s.
- Seckel s.
- secondary pseudoobstruction s.
- segmental colonic adenomatous polyposis s.
- Senior-Loken s.
- sepsis s.
- Sertoli-cell-only s.
- serum sicknesslike s.
- sex reversal s.
- Sézary s.
- short-bowel s.
- short-gut s.
- Shwachman s.
- Shwachman-Diamond s.
- Shy-Drager s.
- sicca s.
- sick cell s.
- sinusoidal obstruction s. (SOS)
- Sipple s.
- Sjögren s. (SS)
- sleep apnea s.
- sloughed urethra s.
- small stomach s.
- Smith-Lemli-Opitz s.
- solitary rectal ulcer s. (SRUS)
- solitary ulcer s.
- somatostatinoma s.
- spastic bowel s.
- spastic pelvic floor s.
- sphincteric disobedience s.
- Spitzer-Weinstein s.
- splenic agenesis s.
- splenic flexure s.
- Sprinz-Dubin s.
- Sprinz-Nelson s.
- stagnant loop s.
- stasis s.
- Stauffer s.
- steakhouse s.
- Stein-Leventhal s.
- steroid-resistant nephrotic s.
- Stevens-Johnson s. (SJS)
- Stewart-Treves s.
- stiff-man s.
- Stokvis-Talma s.
- Strachan s.
- Strachan-Scott s.
- stress-related erosive s.
- Sturge-Weber s.
- sulfone s.
- sump s.
- superior mesenteric artery s. (SMAS)
- suprarenogenic s.
- Sweet s.
- Swyer s.
- symphysis pubica s.
- systemic inflammatory response s. (SIRS)
- Takayasu s.
- TAR s.
- terminal reservoir s.
- testicular feminization s.
- tethered-cord s. (TCS)
- thoracic endometriosis s.
- Thorn salt-depletion s.
- three-week sulfasalazine s.
- thrombocytopenia-absent radius s.
- TINU s.
- tissue matrix s.
- Torres s.
- Townes-Brocks s.
- toxic shock s.
- transurethral resection s.
- tremor-nystagmus-ulcer s.
- triad s.
- tropical diarrhea-malabsorption s. (TDMS)
- Trousseau s.
- tubulointerstitial nephritis and uveitis s.
- tumor lysis s.
- TUR s.
- Turcot s.
- Turner s.
- Ullrich-Turner s.
- uremic s.
- urethral s.
- urethritis s.
- urge s.
- VACTERL s.
- vanished testis s.
- vanishing bile duct s. (VBDS)
- vascular steal s.

VATER s.
venous leak s.
Verner-Morrison s.
vertebral, anal, cardiac, tracheoesophageal fistula, renal, limb s. (VACTERL)
vertebral, anal, tracheoesophageal fistula, renal s. (VATER)
Vinson s.
VIPoma s.
von Hippel-Lindau s.
vulvar vestibulitis s.
VURD s.
WAGR s.
wasting s.
Waterhouse-Friderichsen s.
watery diarrhea, hypokalemia, and achlorhydria s.
Watson-Alagille s.
WDHA s.
Weil s.
Weinstein s.
Welt s.
Wermer s.
Wernicke s.
Wernicke-Korsakoff s.
Whipple s.
Wiedemann-Beckwith s.
Williams s.
Wiskott-Aldrich s.
Wolfram s.
X-linked Alport s. (XLAS)
XX male s.
XYY male s.
Young s.
Youssef s.
Zanca s.
ZE s.
Zellweger s.
Zieve s.
Zollinger-Ellison s. (ZES)

synechia, pl. **synechiae**
    penile s.

synectenterotomy

Synectics
    S. computer program
    S. 6000 digital pH-meter meter
    S. PC Polygraf 16HR
    S. visceral stimulator electronic barostat

Synectics-Dantec
    S.-D. Flo-Lab II uroflowmeter
    S.-D. UD10000 uroflowmeter

synergism
    in vitro s.

synergistic combination

Synergist vacuum erection device

synergy

Syn-Optics videoimage splitter

synorchism, synorchidism

synoscheos

synovial fluid

Synthamin amino acid solution

synthase
    aldosterone s.
    citrate s.
    induced nitric oxide s. (iNOS)

synthesis
    albumin s.
    apolipoprotein s.
    collagen s.
    dihydrotestosterone s.
    DNA s.
    eicosanoid s.
    focal collagen s.
    hepatocyte protein s.
    hormone-stimulated cAMP s.
    impaired lecithin s.
    mucosal prostaglandin s.
    prostaglandin s.
    prostanoid s.
    protein s.
    pyrimidine s.
    renin s.
    urea s.

synthesizer
    deoxyribonucleic acid s.

synthetase
    nitric oxide s.
    paraaminohippuric acid s.

synthetic
    s. ^{13}C-urea
    S.'s dual-channel solid-state Digitrapper
    s. five-channel water-perfused motility catheter
    s. mesh
    s. porcine secretin
    s. porcine secretin for injection
    s. vascular graft

Synthroid

NOTES

syphilis
- anorectal s.
- gastric s.
- primary s.
- secondary s.
- serologic test for s. (STS)
- tertiary s.

syphilitic
- s. gastritis
- s. hepatitis
- s. inguinal adenitis
- s. nephritis
- s. stigma

syphiloma
- Fournier s.

syringe
- Arrow Raulerson s.
- Asepto irrigation s.
- aspiration s.
- Fortuna s.
- LeVeen inflation s.
- Lewy s.
- Luer s.
- Luer-Lok s.
- motor s.
- Neisser s.
- piston-type s.
- s. shield
- Storz s.
- Toomey s.
- tuberculin s.
- Wolff s.

syringocele
- Cowper s.

syringoma
- penis s.

syrosingopine

syrup
- Calcidrine s.
- s. of glycyrrhiza
- ipecac s.

system
- Abbott Lifeshield needleless s.
- Ablatherm HIFU s.
- Advantx digital s.
- AJCC/UICC staging s.
- alimentary s.
- Alliance integrated inflation s.
- American Medical S.'s (AMS)
- Amplatz TractMaster s.
- AMS ProstaJect ethanol injection s.
- Ancure abdominal aortic aneurysm s.
- AneuRx stent graft s.
- anomalous arrangement of pancreaticobiliary ductal s. (AAPBDS)
- antigen-antibody s.
- APACHE-II, -III scoring s.
- AquaSens FMS 1000 fluid monitoring s.
- Arndorfer capillary perfusion s.
- Arndorfer pneumohydraulic capillary infusion s.
- Arrow UserGard injection cap s.
- ASAP Stacker automated multisample biopsy s.
- autofluorescent endsocopic s.
- automatic titration s.
- autonomic nervous s. (ANS)
- Balthazar grading s.
- Bard EndoCinch endoscopic suture s.
- Bard EndoCinch endoscopic suturing s.
- Bard Urolase fiber laser s.
- Baveno portal hypertensive gastropathy grading s.
- Baxter Interline IV s.
- Beamer injection stent s.
- Bergkvist grading s.
- BICAP hemostatic s.
- bicarbonate buffer s.
- BiliBlanket Phototherapy S.
- bioartificial extracorporeal liver support s. (BELS)
- BioLogic-DT s.
- BioLogic-DTPF s.
- Bitome bipolar s.
- B-lymphocyte s.
- Bookwalter retractor s.
- Borrmann gastric cancer typing s. type I–IV
- Boyarsky symptom scoring s.
- Bravo Catheter-Free pH testing s.
- Bridge Assurant biliary stent delivery s.
- Bridge X3 renal stent s.
- Browning and Parks continence grading s. category A, B, C, D
- Bruel-Kjaer 1846 ultrasound s.
- buffer s.
- Caldwell needle/cannula Quick-Tap paracentesis s.
- Can-Opt dual-lumen ERCP s.
- cell analysis s.
- Cell Recovery S. (CRS)
- Cell Soft s.
- central nervous s. (CNS)
- Ceralas PDT 633 diode laser s.
- classification s.
- CLAVE needleless s.
- closed-suction drainage s.
- coculture s.
- collecting s.
- Colormate TLc BiliTest S.
- Colour-Quad-System imaging s.
- Comhaire grading s.

system · system

computer-aided diagnostic s.
computer-controlled sedation infusion s.
computerized image analysis s.
Conseal one-piece continent colostomy s.
contact-tip laser s.
Contrajet ERCP contrast delivery s.
core-cut s.
COSTART s.
cost-conscious healthcare s.
COX enzyme s.
CS-5 cryosurgical s.
CSM Stretta s.
C-Trak surgical guidance s.
cytochrome P450 enzyme s.
Dantec 12-channel Urocolor Video s.
Dantec Menuet s.
DASH s.
daughter endoscopic retrograde cholangiopancreatoscopy s.
da Vinci Surgical S.
Debioclip single-dose delivery s.
Dentsleeve pneumohydraulic perfusion s.
digestive s.
Digitrapper Mark II pH monitoring s.
DIONEX 2000 s.
Director Guidewire s.
DNA Sequencing S.
Doppler Quantum color flow s.
Dornier MPL 9000 electrohydraulic lithotriptor ultrasound focusing s.
double-antibody sandwich s.
Drake-Willock delivery s.
Drake-Willock peritoneal dialysis s.
drug carrier s.
Dual-Port s.
ductal s.
Dukes staging s.
Dumon-Gilliard endoprosthesis s.
Dynalink 0.035 biliary self-expanding stent s.
EdGr s.
Edmondson grading s.
e10 electrosurgery s.
EndoCinch suturing s.
endocrine s.
Endo-Dop transendoscopic Doppler catheter probe s.
endoscopic s.
enteric nervous s. (ENS)
Enterra Therapy implantable neurostimulation s.
ErecAid vacuum s.
EVIS EXERA Video S.
FastPack s.
Fisher Capillary S.
Flexiflo Top-Fill Enteral Nutrition S.
free-beam laser s.
French Pharmacovigilance s.
Fresenius volumetric dialysate balancing s.
Fujinon SP-501 sonoprobe s.
Fujinon videoendoscopy s.
Garden prognostic s.
GaSampler collection s.
GastrograpH ambulatory pH monitoring s.
gastrointestinal s. (GIS)
gastrointestinal therapeutic s. (GITS)
Gatekeeper reflux repair s.
Gatta prognostic s.
GERDcheck ambulatory esophageal pH monitoring s.
Given diagnostic imaging s.
Given videocapsule s.
Gleason grading s.
Grabstald Memorial staging s.
Gynecare TVT support s.
Gyrus endourology s.
HandPort s.
hemi-Kock s.
HepatAssist Liver Support S.
Hewlett-Packard IVUS imaging s.
high-affinity low-capacity s.
high-affinity sodium-dependent phosphate transport s.
Hind-SITE 20/20 s.
H+/K+-ATPase enzyme s.
Hp Chek screening s.
HP7754 pneumohydraulic capillary infusion s.
human cytochrome P-450 enzyme s.
hydraulic capillary infusion s.
Hydra Vision Es urological imaging s.
Hydra Vision IV urology s.

NOTES

system (continued)
  Hydra Vision Plus DR urological imaging s.
  illumination s.
  immune s.
  Impact lithotriptor s.
  implantable neuromodulation s.
  IMx PSA s.
  InCare PRES 9300 s.
  Indigo LaserOptic treatment s.
  Indigo Optima laser s.
  InjecAid s.
  Innova home incontinence therapy s.
  InSIGHT manometry s.
  integrated automatic stone-tissue detection s.
  intensified radiographic imaging s. (IRIS)
  International Biomedical Mode 745-100 microcapillary infusion s.
  intracellular signaling s.
  intrarenal collecting s.
  IsoMed constant-flow infusion s.
  iterative bifid branching s.
  IVAC needleless IV S.
  Jackson staging s.
  Janus S. III
  Jewett staging s.
  Jewett-Strong s.
  Jewett-Whitmore Cancer Staging S.
  Johns Hopkins prostate cancer grading s.
  Joyce-Loebl Magiscan image analysis s.
  Kangaroo Delivery S.
  kidney collecting s.
  Kleinert Safe and Dry panty and pad s.
  Kretz ultrasound s.
  KTP/532 laser s.
  LAGB s.
  Lambda Plus PDL 1, 2 laser s.
  Laparolift s.
  laparoscopic retraction s.
  Laparoshield laparoscopic smoke filtration s.
  Lap-Band adjustable gastric banding s.
  Laser CHRP rigid fiberscope s.
  LifeSite hemodialysis access s.
  Lithostar Plus electromagnetic lithotriptor bidimensional x-ray focusing s.
  liver dialysis s.
  Lorad StereoGuide prone breast biopsy s.
  low-affinity high-capacity s.
  low-compliance perfusion s.
  low-pressure venous s.
  Madsen-Iversen scoring s.
  magnifying endoscopy with narrow-band image s.
  Mayo grading s.
  mechanical assist s.
  MediClenze hygiene and water therapy s.
  Mediflex MD-7 endoscopic video s.
  Medstone IRIS s.
  Medstone STS lithotripsy s.
  MetaFluor s.
  microsomal ethanol oxidizing s. (MEOS)
  Microvasive biliary stent s.
  Microvasive Ultraflex esophageal stent s.
  mitochondrial ethanol oxidase s.
  molecular adsorbents recirculating s. (MARS)
  MOP-Videoplan morphometric s.
  Morganstern aspiration/injection s.
  mother-baby endoscope s.
  mother-baby-scope s.
  mother endoscopic retrograde cholangiopancreatoscopy s.
  Mui Scientific pressurized capillary infusion s.
  Multipulse laser s.
  Mycotrim triphasic culture s.
  myeloperoxidase-H2O2-halide s.
  NA+-linked cotransport s.
  NA+ transport s.
  needleless s.
  Oasis pusher tube s.
  obstructed collecting s.
  OEC-Diasonics 9400 fluoroscopy C-arm s.
  Olympus CLV-series fiberoptic s.
  Olympus endoscopy s. (OES)
  Olympus EVIS color computer chip s.
  Olympus GF-UM3, -UM20 s.
  Olympus MAJ363 FNA needle s.
  Olympus OSP fluorescence measuring s.
  Olympus videoendoscopy s.
  Olympus videourology procedure s.
  Omni-LapoTract support s.
  One Action Stent Introduction S. (OASIS)
  Opmilas 144 Plus laser s.
  optical multichannel analyzer s.
  Ortho Diagnostic S.
  O'Sullivan scoring s.
  oxybutynin transdermal s.
  Oxytrol transdermal s.
  Palco enuretic alarm s.

Palmaz Corinthian biliary stent and delivery s.
pancreaticobiliary ductal s.
P blood group s.
pelvicaliceal s.
Percutaneous Stoller Afferent Nerve Stimulation S.
Performa ultrasound s.
Personal Scanner TM 18 bedside real-time ultrasonography s.
pneumohydraulic capillary infusion s.
Polachrome 35-mm slide s.
portable perfused manometric s.
portal venous s.
Precision office TUNA s.
Precision QID glucose monitoring s.
Precision SpeedTac transvaginal anchor s.
Precision Tack transvaginal anchor s.
Precision Twist transvaginal anchor s.
Prempree modification staging s.
probenecid-inhibited organic anion transport s.
Prolieve microwave therapy s.
Proscan ultrasound imaging s.
Prostalase laser s.
ProstaLund CoreTherm s.
Prostathermer prostatic hyperthermia s.
Prostatron microwave s.
Pugh-Child scoring s.
Quick-Tap paracentesis s.
Raman spectroscopic s.
Ranson grading s.
Redy hemodialysis s.
Relay suture delivery s.
renal kallikrein-kinin s.
renal preservation-perfusion s.
renin-aldosterone s.
renin-angiotensin s. (RAS)
renin-angiotensin-aldosterone s. (RAAS)
reproductive s.
reticuloendothelial s.
Reuter suprapubic trocar and cannula s.
rod-lens s.
RX Herculink 14 biliary stent s.
RX Herculink Plus biliary stent s.
RX stent delivery s.
Sacks-Vine PEG s.
Safe and Dry panty and pad s.
Secca radiofrequency s.
SeedNet cryotherapy s.
sentry s.
800 series KTP/YAG surgical laser s.
SF-9 baculovirus-insect cell s.
Signa EXCITE 3.0T MRI s.
single-action pumping s. (SAPS)
slide s.
Soehendra catheter s.
SOLO-Surg Colorectal self-retaining retractor s.
Sonablate 200 s.
Sonoprobe Endoscopic Ultrasonography S.
sorbent dialysate regeneration s.
SPARC sling s.
StayErec s.
stent and vent s.
Stoller scoring s.
stone recognition s.
stone-tissue detection s. (STDS)
stone-tissue recognition s. (STR)
Storz multifunction valve trocar/cannula s.
Straight-In male sling s.
Straight-In surgical s.
Stretta s.
STRIANT buccal s.
STS lithotripsy s.
Suretys panty s.
Surgi-PEG replacement gastrostomy feeding s.
Sydney s.
sympathetic nervous s. (SNS)
Talent LPS endoluminal stent-graft s.
Targis microwave catheter-based s.
Technos ultrasound s.
telerobotic s.
terminal bifid branching s.
testosterone buccal s.
testosterone transdermal s. (TTS)
Therasonics Lithotripsy S.
ThermoChem-HT s.
ThermoFlex s.
tissue-stone recognition s. (TSRS)
TMx-2000 BPH thermotherapy s.

NOTES

system *(continued)*
    Top Notch automated biopsy s.
    transdermal therapeutic s. (TTS)
    transvaginal suturing s.
    Tricomponent Coaxial S. (TCS)
    triple-lumen perfused catheter s.
    Truelove-Witts grading s.
    TVS s.
    Ultrabag dialysis s.
    UltraPak enteral closed feeding s.
    Ultraseed s.
    Ultra Twin bag s.
    Ultra Y-set s.
    United States Renal Data S. (USRDS)
    Universal sheath s.
    Urocyte diagnostic cytometry s.
    Uro-jet delivery s.
    Urolab Janus S. III
    Uro-Pak s.
    Urotract x-ray s.
    Urovision ultrasound imaging s.
    UroVive self-contained balloon s.
    Vaccine Adverse Event Reporting S.
    vanishing bile duct s.
    varix grading s. F1, F2, F3
    VET-CO vacuum s.
    ViaCath computer-assisted robotic endoluminal s.
    ViaCath endoluminal surgery s.
    Virtual Biopsy S.
    Visick gastric cancer grading s.
    Vision Sciences VSI 2000 flexible sigmoidoscope s.
    VitalStim Therapy electrical stimulation s.
    Vivonex Acutrol Enteral Feeding S.
    Vocare bladder s.
    V-sign single-ear sensory s.
    Welch Allyn videoendoscopy s.
    Whitmore-Jewitt prostate cancer classification s.
    Wolf aspiration/injection s.
    Wolf delivery s.
    wolffian ductal s.
    WuScope s.
    Xillix LIFE-Lung s.
    Y-set s.
    Zeiss fluorescein filter s.
    Zenith AAA endovascular graft s.
    Zenith abdominal aortic aneurysm endovascular graft s.
    Zieve s.
    Z stent esophageal endoprosthesis s.

systematic sextant biopsy
systemic
    s. amyloidosis
    s. arterial pressure
    s. *Candida*
    s. duodenal sclerosis
    s. effect
    s. endotoxemia
    s. hypertension
    s. hypotension
    s. inflammatory response syndrome (SIRS)
    s. lupus erythematosus (SLE)
    s. lupus erythematosus vasculitis
    s. MAP
    s. mast cell disease
    s. mastocytosis
    s. mercury intoxication
    s. radiation therapy
    s. sclerosis (SSc)
    s. surgery
    s. vascular resistance (SVR)
    s. vascular resistance index (SVRI)
    s. venodilation
systolic
    s. click
    s. murmur
Szabo-Berci needle driver
Szabo test

T
- T antigen
- T bandage
- T binder
- T cell-specific protein
- T clamp
- T connector
- T drain
- T effector cell
- T fastener
- T lymphocyte
- T tube
- T tubogram
- T wave

T138 antigen
TA30, TA55 stapler
TA90-BN stapler
TAA
  tumor-associated antigen
TAAA
  thoracoabdominal aortic aneurysm
  TAAA surgery
tabes
  t. dorsalis
  t. mesaraica
  t. mesenterica
tabetic
table
  Aub-Dubois t.
  Dornier Urotract cystoscopy t.
  floating t.
  Gerhardt t.
  lithotripsy t.
  Maquet endoscopy t.
  Multifunctional Opus surgical t.
  Partin t.
  sigmoidoscopy t.
  Urodiagnost x-ray t.
tablet
  alosetron HCl t.
  Asacol delayed-release t.
  Body Fortress Natural Amino t.
  Cal Carb 600 with Vitamin D antacid t.
  Cal Carb 600 with Vitamin D dietary supplement t.
  Chenix T.
  Dairy Ease chewable t.'s
  delayed-release t.
  Hemocyte-F t.
  Hemocyte Plus t.
  hyoscyamine sulfate orally disintegrating t.
  L-carnitine t.
  Lotronex t.
  Maalox Quick Dissolve chewable t.
  Magsal t.
  Monocal t.
  mycophenolate mofetil t.
  NuLev orally disintegrating t.
  Nullo deodorant t.
  Pantoloc t.
  pantoprazole sodium delayed-release t.
  Peptic Relief chewable t.
  Protonix delayed-release t.
  Rapamune t.
  Renagel t.
  sevelamer hydrochloride t.
  sirolimus t.
  Strong Start chewable t.
  tegaserod maleate t.
  Urex t.
  Visicol t.
  Vitelle Nesentials t.
  Vitelle Nestrex t.
  wax-matrix t.
  Zelnorm t.

Tabs
  Hydro-T T.
tabularized incised plate urethroplasty
tabule
  Mediplex Ultra t.
TAC
  total abdominal colectomy
TACE
  transarterial catheter embolization
  transarterial chemoembolization
  transcatheter arterial chemoembolization
tachycardia
  sinus t.
  ventricular t.
tachygastria
tachykinin-bombesin family
tachykinin component
tachyphylaxis
tachypnea
tacked down
tacrolimus
tacrolimus-associated microangiopathy
tactile
  t. feedback result
  t. probe
tactor
Tactyl 1 glove
TACurea
  timed average urea concentration
tadalafil
tadpolelike appearance

TAE
    total abdominal evisceration
    transcatheter arterial embolization
taenia, pl. **taeniae**
    Taeniae coli
    t. libera
    t. mesocolica
    t. omentalis
    taeniae pylori
    T. saginata
    T. siginata
    T. solium
    taeniae of Valsalva
taeniacide
taeniasis
taeniform
taenioides
    Diphyllobothrium t.
tag
    edematous t.
    external skin t.
    hemorrhoidal t.
    H-shaped tilt t.
    perianal skin t.
    perineal skin t.
    sentinel t.
    skin t.
TAG-72 glycoprotein
Tagamet HB
tagatose
tagged
    t. erythrocyte scintigraphy
    t. red blood cell bleeding scan
tagging
    fecal t.
    t. stitch
tail
    t. of pancreas
    t. sign
tailgut cyst (TGC)
tailing defect
Tait law
Takayasu
    T. arteritis
    T. disease
    T. syndrome
takedown
    bilateral ureterostomy t.
    t. of colostomy
    ostomy t.
    t. of pelvic sling procedure
taking down of adhesion
TAL
    thick ascending limb
talc embolus
Talent LPS endoluminal stent-graft system
talin

TALT
    testicular adrenallike tissue
Tamm-Horsfall
    T.-H. mucoprotein (THM)
    T.-H. protein (THP)
tamoxifen
tampon
    Corner t.
    t. tube
tamponade, tamponage
    balloon tube t.
    esophageal balloon t.
    esophagogastric balloon t. (EGBT)
    ferromagnetic t.
    Sengstaken-Blakemore t.
    tract t.
tamponment
tamsulosin HCl
Tanagho
    T. bladder flap urethroplasty
    T. bladder neck reconstruction
tandem
    t. colonoscopy (TC)
    T. thin-shaft transureteroscopic balloon dilatation catheter
    T.'s XL triple-lumen ERCP cannula
Tandem-E-PSA immunoenzymetric assay
Tandem-ERA PSA immuenzymetric assay
Tandem-R
    T.-R assay kit
    T.-R PSA assay
tangential
    t. biopsy
    t. colonic submucosal injection
Tangier disease
tangle of hemorrhoidal veins
Tannenbaum stent
Tanner
    T. operation
    T. stage
tannex
    bisacodyl t.
tannic acid
tantalum-182
tap
    abdominal t.
    peritoneal t.
    t. water enema
TAP2 **peptide transporter gene**
tape
    adhesive t.
    appendectomy t.
    Cath-Secure t.
    circular t.
    Coban t.
    lap t.
    laparotomy t.

t. marker
Mersilene t.
Montgomery t.
polyester-reinforced Dacron t.
tension-free vaginal t. (TVT)
Transpore t.
umbilical t.

tapered
t. common bile duct
t. needle
t. rubber bougie

tapered-tip
t.-t. dilator
t.-t. hydrophilic-coated push catheter

tapeworm
beef t.
Cestoda t.
fish t.
pork t.

TAP **gene**
TAPP
transabdominal preperitoneal
TAPP hernia repair

Taq polymerase
TAR
thrombocytopenia-absent radius
TAR syndrome

Tarceva
tarda
Edwardsiella t.
porphyria cutanea t. (PCT)

tardive
forme t.

target
t. appearance
t. area
t. cell
t. hemocrit value
t. lesion
t. localization
peritoneal dialysis creatinine clearance t.
t. symptom
t. volume (TV)

targeted
t. biopsy
t. cryoablation device
t. microwave thermotherapy

targeting
selective t.

Targis microwave catheter-based system
Tarlov cyst

tarry black stool
tartrate
antimony sodium t.
metoprolol t.
t. nephritis
tolterodine t.
trimeprazine t.

TASI
transperitoneal anterior subcostal incision

TA stapling device
taste perversion
TATA-binding protein
tattoo
colonic t.
colonoscopic t.
endoscopic four-quadrant t.
India ink t.
submucosal t.

tattooing
four-quadrant t.

taurine
t. cotransporter (TCT)
t. cotransporter mRNA
selenium-labeled homocholic acid conjugated with t. (SeHCAT)

taurocholate
sodium t.
t. solution

taurocholic acid
tauroglycocholate
sodium t.

taurolithocholate
Taut cystic duct catheter
taxis
Taxol
Taxoprexin DHA-paclitaxel
Taylor
T. gastric balloon
T. gastroscope

Tazicef
Tazidime
tazobactam
TBA
total bile acid

T bandage
T-bar retractor
TBI
total body irradiation

T binder
TBM
thin basement membrane
tubular basement membrane

NOTES

TBMD
    thin basement membrane disease
TBN
    total body nitrogen
TBW
    total body water
TC
    tandem colonoscopy
    therapeutic concentrate
    transhepatic cholangiography
Tc
    technetium
^{99m}Tc, Tc-99m
    technetium-99m
        ^{99m}Tc albumin colloid
        ^{99m}Tc albumin microsphere
        ^{99m}Tc DISIDA
        ^{99m}Tc DISIDA contrast injection
        ^{99m}Tc DMSA
        ^{99m}Tc DPTA
        ^{99m}Tc DTPA aerosol
        ^{99m}Tc GHP
        ^{99m}Tc GSA scintigraphy
        ^{99m}Tc HIDA
        ^{99m}Tc HMPAO-labeled leukocyte scan
        ^{99m}Tc IDA scan
        ^{99m}Tc lidofenin
        ^{99m}Tc MAA
        ^{99m}Tc MDP
        ^{99m}Tc MDP nuclear isotope bone scan
        ^{99m}Tc medronate
        ^{99m}Tc pertechnetate scan
        ^{99m}Tc pertechnetate scintigraphy
        ^{99m}Tc PIPIDA
        ^{99m}Tc polyphosphate
        ^{99m}Tc PYP
        ^{99m}Tc RBC bleeding scan
        ^{99m}Tc SC
        ^{99m}Tc sodium pertechnetate
        ^{99m}Tc SPP
        ^{99m}Tc sulfur colloid scan
        ^{99m}Tc GSA
        ^{99m}Tc MAG-3 isotope
        ^{99m}Tc SC
        ^{99m}Tc tin colloid
TCA
    tricarboxylic acid
    trichloroacetic acid
    trihydrocoprostanic acid
TCBS
    thiosulfate-citrate-bile salts-sucrose agar
TCCA
    transitional cell cancer-associated
        TCCA virus
TCCB
    transitional cell carcinoma of bladder
TCD/CBDE
    transcystic duct/common bile duct exploration
^{99m}Tc-DTPA renal scan
T84 cell
T-cell
    T-c. activation
    T-c. adhesion
    T-c. antigen receptor/CD3 complex
    T-c. crossmatch
    T-c. cytotoxic therapy
    T-c. depletion by elutriation
    T-c. epitope
    T-c. line
    T-c. lymphoma
    T-c. receptor (TCR)
    T-c. second messenger
    T-c. vaccination
T-cell-dependent mechanism
TCIS
    total corrected incremental score
^{99m}Tc-labeled
    99mTc-l. Amberlite pellet
    99mTc-l. anti-alpha-fetoprotein
    99mTc-l. stannous methylene diphosphonate
T clamp
Tc-99m (*var. of* ^{99m}Tc)
TCMS
    transcranial magnetic stimulation
T-C needle holder
^{99m}Tc-phytate liquid state esophageal transit study
TCR
    T-cell receptor
TCS
    tethered-cord syndrome
    Tricomponent Coaxial System
^{99m}Tc SC
    ^{99m}Tc sulfur colloid
    technetium-99m sulfur colloid
^{99m}Tc-sulfur colloid egg meal
TCT
    taurine cotransporter
        TCT mRNA
TDMS
    tropical diarrhea-malabsorption syndrome
T drain
TDU
    time domain ultrasound
TDX fluorescent polarization immunoassay
TE
    tracheoesophageal
TEA
    tetraethylammonium
tea
    bush t.
Teale gorget

tear
    capsular t.
    diastatic serosal t.
    t. duct
    esophageal t.
    gastric t.
    Mallory-Weiss t.
    mesenteric t.
    mucosal t.
    pharyngeal t.
    pharyngoesophageal t.
    serosal t.

teardrop
    t. bladder
    t. incision
    t. poikilocyte

tearing
    t. pain
    t. through

t-EASE software

TEBS
    transurethral electrical bladder stimulation

TEC
    transpapillary endoscopic cholecystotomy

teceleukin and interferon alfa-2a

TechneScan MAG-3

technetium (Tc)
    t. GSA
    t. imaging
    t. radionuclide scan

^{99m}technetium dimercaptosuccinic acid scintigram

technetium-labeled
    t.-l. autologous red blood cell scan
    t.-l. red blood cell scan
    t.-l. red blood cell scintigraphy

technetium-99m (^{99m}Tc, Tc-99m)
    t.-99m diethylenetriamine pentaacetic acid
    t.-99m diethylenetriamine pentaacetic acid scan
    t.-99m galactosyl-human serum albumin
    t.-99m HIDA scan
    t.-99m iminodiacetic acid
    t.-99m macroaggregated albumin
    t.-99m mercaptoacetythiglycine isotope
    t.-99m 99m Exametazime injection
    t.-99m pertechnetate
    t.-99m pyrophosphate-tagged RBC
    t.-99m red cell scintigraphy
    t.-99m sulfur colloid (^{99m}Tc SC)
    t.-99m tin colloid

technetium-99m diisopropyl iminodiacetic acid

technical
    t. advance
    t. biomaterial

technically elaborate method

technique
    abdominal pressure t.
    abdominal wall lift t.
    anthrone colorimetric t.
    antiperistaltic t.
    antireflux ureteral implantation t.
    aseptic t.
    assisted reproductive t.
    autosuture t.
    avascular cuff t.
    balloon catheter and basket retrieval t.
    band and snare t.
    band-snare t.
    Barcat t.
    Belt t.
    bench surgical t.
    bladder neck-preserving t.
    blind t.
    Brackin ureterointestinal anastomosis t.
    Bricker t.
    Buerhenne stone basket t.
    bulking t.
    buttonhole puncture t.
    Campbell t.
    Cantwell-Ransley t.
    Cape Town t.
    capsule flap t.
    cavernosal alpha blockade t.
    cell separation t.
    cephalotrigonal t.
    clamshell t.
    closed tubule fixation t.
    Coffey t.
    Cohen cross-trigonal t.
    colonic obstruction t.
    combined endoscopic sandwich t.
    continuous pullthrough t.
    Coomassie brilliant blue t.
    cup-patch t.
    Davis t.
    Deisting t.

NOTES

technique *(continued)*
    Denis Browne urethroplasty t.
    de novo needle-knife t.
    diagnostic t.
    diathermy t.
    direct fragmentation t.
    double balloon t.
    double-folded cup-patch t.
    double-staple t.
    double stapling t. (DST)
    dual-endoscope t.
    Dufourmentel t.
    Eisenberger t.
    en bloc t.
    endoscopic esophageal mucosal resection tube t.
    endoscopic magnet-assisted nonsurgical t.
    end-to-side vasoepididymostomy t.
    enuresis alarm t.
    esophageal banding t.
    extraanatomical renal revascularization t.
    extraction balloon t.
    extravesical ureteral reimplantation t.
    Fairley bladder washout localization t.
    fan-shaped biopsy t.
    Ferguson t.
    finger fracture t.
    first-line screening t.
    flap t.
    flip-flap t.
    flow microsphere fluorescent immunoassay t.
    full-bladder t.
    full Monti t.
    Gaur balloon distension t.
    Gil-Vernet t.
    Gittes t.
    Glenn t.
    Glenn-Anderson t.
    Goldschmiedt t.
    gold seed implantation t.
    Goodwin t.
    Goodwin-Hohenfellner t.
    Goodwin-Scott t.
    Graves t.
    gravimetric t.
    Grimelius t.
    guidewire and minisnare t.
    Hale colloidal iron t.
    Hammock t.
    Hartmann reconstruction t.
    Hauri t.
    Heibronn t.
    Hendren t.
    Hippuran clearance t.
    histocytochemical t.
    Hofmeister t.
    hot biopsy t.
    hydrocelectomy plication t.
    hydrogen gas clearance t.
    immunoperoxidase staining t.
    immunostaining t.
    indirect immunolocalization t.
    ^{111}In-leukocyte t.
    interventional t.
    intradermal tattooing t.
    intramural incision t.
    invagination t.
    Jaboulay-Doyen-Winkleman t.
    Jones-Politano t.
    Kaliscinski ureteral folding t.
    Keystone t.
    King t.
    Kock t.
    Kropp t.
    laparoscopic colposuspension t.
    LaRoque t.
    laryngeal jack t.
    laser-assisted tissue-welding t.
    laser welding t.
    lasso t.
    lateral bending t.
    lateral window t.
    Latzko t.
    lawn mower t.
    Lazaro da Silva t.
    Lazarus-Nelson t.
    Leach t.
    Leadbetter and Clarke t.
    Leadbetter modification t.
    Leadbetter tunneling t.
    LeDuc t.
    Lich extravesical t.
    Lich-Gregoire t.
    lift-and-cut t.
    Lotheissen-McVay t.
    Madden t.
    Marlex plug t.
    Masson trichrome staining t.
    Mathieu t.
    Meares-Stamey t.
    membrane catheter t.
    Menghini t.
    Michal II t.
    micropuncture t.
    microtransducer t.
    Mikulicz drain t.
    miniperc t.
    Mitchell t.
    Mitrofanoff continent urinary diversion t.
    modified Cantwell t.
    modified Hassan open t.
    modified Sacks-Vine push-pull t.

modified Thiersch-Duplay t.
modified Vest t.
Mohs microsurgery t.
morcellation t.
Moynihan t.
muscle-splitting t.
Myers bunching t.
nasovesicular catheter t.
needle-knife t.
Nesbit t.
Norfolk t.
onlay t.
onlay-tube-onlay urethroplasty t.
Orandi t.
orbital exenteration gastroscopic access t.
over-the-wire t.
Palomo t.
Paquin t.
patch clamp t.
pelviscopic clip ligation t.
t. of penile disassembly
perfusion hypothermia t.
Pippi-Salle t.
pluck t.
Politano-Leadbetter t.
Pólya t.
Ponsky t.
prograde t.
pullthrough t.
push t.
push-pull T t.
quadrant-sampling t.
Quantikine quantitative immunoenzymatometric sandwich t.
Quartey t.
rapid pullthrough esophageal manometry t.
reconstruction t.
refining surgical t.
relaxation t.
rendezvous t.
retrograde t.
Rives-Stoppa t.
Roux-en-Y chimney surgical t.
RPT t.
Russell t.
Sacks-Vine t.
Saeed t.
safe-tract t.
salvage cytology t.

sandwich t.
Schoemaker-Billroth II t.
Seldinger t.
sextant t.
Silber t.
Singer-Blom endoscopic tracheoesophageal puncture t.
sleeve t.
sling-and-blanket t.
smiley-face knotting t.
Snodgrass t.
Somatome DRG CT t.
sperm microaspiration retrieval t. (SMART)
spiral CT t.
split-and-roll t.
split-cuff nipple t.
split-nipple t.
SPT t.
Starr t.
station pullthrough esophageal manometry t.
stent through wire mesh t.
Stiegmann-Goff t.
stimulated gracilis neosphincter t.
strip biopsy resection t.
submucosal saline injection t.
subpleural blanketing t.
suck-and-cut t.
Sugarbaker t.
superior mesenterorenal bypass t.
surface cooling t.
Swiss roll embedding t.
thermal therapy t.
Thomas t.
Thompson t.
three-loop t.
T-pouch t.
transperineal ultrasonography t.
Traverso-Longmire t.
tube-within-tube t.
tunneled t.
turn-and-suction biopsy t.
Turnbull t.
two-layer latex and Marlex closure t.
two-layer open t.
ultrasound dilution t.
Ussing chamber t.
U-stitch reimplantation t.
ventral bending t.
videofluoroscopic t.

NOTES

technique *(continued)*
- video transurethral resection t.
- Vim-Silverman t.
- VQ t.
- VQQ t.
- Wallace t.
- Warwick and Ashken t.
- Wickham t.
- xenon-washout t.
- Young t.
- Young-Dees t.

technological review

technology
- computed tomography t.
- CryoNeedle t.
- DNA microarray t.
- endoscopic sewing machine t.
- fiberoptic instrument t.
- imaging t.
- interactive video t. (IVT)
- laser t.
- lithotripsy t.
- polymerase chain reaction t.
- vacuum erection t. (VET)
- videographic tool t. (VGTT)
- virtual reality t.

Technomed Sonolith 3000 lithotriptor
Technos ultrasound system
Techstar percutaneous closure device
teeth
- carious t.
- full-surface micromesh t.
- interdigitating t.

TEF
- thermic effect of feeding
- tracheoesophageal fistula

Teflon
- T. ERCP cannula
- T. guiding catheter
- T. injector
- T. nasobiliary drain
- T. nasobiliary tube
- T. paste injection for incontinence
- T. sheath
- T. sling rectopexy
- T. stent

Teflon-coated
- T.-c. Dacron suture
- T.-c. guidewire

Tegaderm dressing
tegaserod
- t. maleate
- t. maleate tablet

Tegretol
teicoplanin
Tektronix digital oscilloscope
tela
- t. subserosa intestini tenuis
- t. subserosa vesicae urinariae

telangiectasia
- calcinosis cutis, Raynaud phenomenon, esophageal motility disorder, sclerodactyly, and t. (CREST)
- calcinosis cutis, Raynaud phenomenon, sclerodactyly, and t. (CRST)
- duodenal t.
- gastrointestinal t.
- hemorrhagic t.
- hepatic t.
- hereditary hemorrhagic t. (HHT)
- Osler-Weber-Rendu t.
- radiation t.
- spider t.
- t. syndrome

telangiectatic
- t. angioma
- t. vessel

telar vesical tenesmus
tele-endoscopy
Telepaque contrast medium
telerobotic-assisted laparoscopic surgery
telerobotic system
telescope
- forward-viewing t.
- t. heater
- Hopkins t.
- Wolff t.

teletherapy
- orthovoltage t.

television
- t. camera
- t. monitor
- t. photography

Telfa dressing
Teline
tellurite resistance loci
telomerase
telomere length
telopeptide
TEM
- transanal endoscopic microsurgery
- transmission electron microscopy
- TEM transanal endoscopy

TEMAC
- tetramethyl ammonium chloride

temafloxacin
Temaril
temazepam
temperature
- actual intraprostatic t.
- core t.
- hand t.
- intraprostatic t.
- laser t.
- urethral t.

template
- Mick prostate t.
- Seyd-Neblett perineal t.

Tempo
temporary
- t. end colostomy
- t. endoprosthetic device
- t. enteroscope
- t. loop ileostomy

temporizing measure
temporomandibular arthritis
TEN
- total enteral nutrition
- toxic epidermal necrolysis
- Vivonex TEN

Tena pouch
Tenckhoff
- T. peritoneal dialysis catheter
- T. two-cuff catheter

tender
- t. liver
- t. thyroid

tenderness
- adnexal t.
- ballottement t.
- bony t.
- cervical motion t.
- costochondral t.
- costovertebral angle t. (CVAT)
- diffuse t.
- exquisite t.
- focal t.
- frontal t.
- generalized abdominal t.
- localizing t.
- palpation t.
- paracervical t.
- percussion t.
- point t.
- popliteal t.
- rebound t.
- rectal t.
- salivary t.
- scrotal t.
- sinus t.
- spinous t.
- thyroid t.
- uterine t.

tendinous
- t. arc
- t. arch of levator ani muscle

tendon
- conjoined t.
- perineal t.
- t. xanthoma

tenesmic
tenesmus
- rectal t.
- telar vesical t.

Tenex
tenia, pl. **teniae**
tenial
teniamyotomy
teniasis
- somatic t.

teniposide (VM-26)
Ten-K
Tenoretic
Tenormin
tenoxicam
TENS
- transcutaneous electrical nerve stimulation
- TENS unit

tense ascites
ten-shooter
- Saeed t.-s.
- Wilson-Cook t.-s.

tensile strength
Tensilon test
tensiometer
tension
- t. myalgia
- t. pneumoperitoneum
- t. pneumothorax
- wall t.

tension-free
- t.-f. anastomosis
- t.-f. closure of abdominal cavity
- t.-f. cystocele repair
- t.-f. vaginal tape (TVT)
- t.-f. vaginal tape procedure

tensor
- t. fascia lata flap
- t. veli palatini muscle

tensostat
tent
- Silon t.
- sponge t.

tenting
- baseline t.
- t. sign

Tenuate

NOTES

tenuis
   Corynebacterium t.
   folliculi lymphatici solitarii intestini t.
   tela subserosa intestini t.

TEP
   totally extraperitoneal
   tracheoesophageal puncture
   TEP hernia repair

TEPA
   thermic effect of physical activity

Tepanil
tepoxalin
teratocarcinoma
teratogenesis
   medication t.

teratogenic medicine
teratoma
   anaplastic malignant t.
   benign cystic t.
   differentiated t.
   gastric t.
   immature t.
   malignant t. (MT)
   mature t.
   ovarian t.
   presacral t.
   sacrococcygeal t.
   solid t.
   testicular t.
   t. testicular cancer
   trophoblastic malignant t.
   undifferentiated malignant t.

teratomatous
teratospermia
terazosin
terbutaline hepatitis
teres
   fissure of ligamentum t.
   ligamentum t.

teretis
   fissura ligamenti t.

terfenadine
terlipressin
terminal
   afferent t.
   t. anuria vesical dialysis
   t. bifid branching system
   t. bile duct
   t. colostomy
   t. deoxynucleotide transferase-mediated deoxyuridine triphosphate
   t. hematuria
   t. ileal disease
   t. ileal pouch
   t. ileal resection
   t. ileitis
   t. ileostomy
   t. ileum
   t. ileum intubation (TII)
   t. ileus
   t. inner medullary collecting duct
   t. repeat (TR)
   t. reservoir syndrome
   t. sedation (TS)
   sensory nervous t.
   t. uridine deoxynucleotide nick-end labeling (TUNEL)

terminus
   amino t.
   duodenal t.
   intrapapillary t.

terms
   Coding Systems for a Thesaurus of Adverse Reaction T. (COSTART)

terodiline
teroxirone
terrestrial organism
Terry fingernail sign
***tert*-buty ether**
tertiary
   t. contraction
   t. hyperparathyroidism
   t. radicle
   t. syphilis

tertium
   Clostridium t.

Terumo
   T. dialyzer
   T. Glidewire
   T. hydrophilic guidewire

Terumo/Meditech guidewire
Terumo-Radiofocus hydrophilic polymer-coated guidewire
Tesberg esophagoscope
TESE
   testicular sperm extraction

Tesla
   T. GE Signa whole-body scanner
   T. Signa MR imager

Teslascan
tesmilifene
test
   Abbott AxSYM antibody to hepatitis C virus lab t.
   abnormal esophageal t.
   Accu-Dx t.
   acid clearance t. (ACT)
   acidemia of stool t.
   acid hemolysis t.
   acidification of stool t.
   acid perfusion t.
   acid reflux t.
   adrenocorticotropic hormone infusion t.
   Advanced Care cholesterol t.
   agglutination t.

air tightness t.
Albarran t.
Albustix t.
alkaline phosphatase t.
alkalinization t.
Allen t.
ALT t.
Althausen t.
Ames t.
aminopyrine breath t.
Amplicor HCV 2.0 RNA t.
angiotensin II infusion t.
anorectal function t.
antiendomysial antibody t.
antigen stool detection t.
anti-Hu t.
antineuronal enteric antibody t.
anti-SLA t.
APC stool t.
APT-Downey alkali denaturation t.
argentaffin reaction t.
artificial erection t.
AST t.
ASTRA profile t.
Aura-Tek FDP t.
AxSYM free PSA t.
Baermann stool t.
balloon expulsion t.
Bard BTA t.
basal secretory flow rate t.
belt t.
bentiromide t.
bentonite flocculation t.
Bernstein acid perfusion t.
beta-2 t.
betazole stimulation t.
bethanechol t.
bile acid breath t.
bile acid tolerance t.
bile solubility t.
BiliCheck t.
bilirubin t.
binder t.
Bio-Enzabead t.
biopsy urease t.
Biotel home screening t.
BioWhittaker assay t.
bladder tumor antigen t.
bolus challenge t.
Bonney t.
Bors ice water t.
Bourne t.

Boyden t.
Boyle and Goldstein saline t.
Bozicevich t.
t. breakfast
breath hydrogen excretion t.
breath pentane t.
Breslow-Day t.
brushing urea breath t.
BSFR t.
BSP t.
BTA stat t.
BTA TRAK t.
BT-PABA t.
buckling t.
CA19-9 t.
calcium infusion t.
Campylobacter t.
Campylobacter-like organism t. (CLOtest)
cancelling A's t.
captopril plasma renin activity t.
carbon-13 urea breath t. (^{13}C-UBT)
carbon-14 urea breath t.
carbon-14 urinary excretion t.
Carnot t.
Casoni skin t.
catheterization t.
^{13}C-bicarbonate breath t.
CBP t.
C^{13} breath t.
C-cholylglycine breath excretion t.
CEA t.
cephalin-cholesterol flocculation t.
^{14}C-glycocholate breath t.
C-glycocholic acid breath t.
7C Gold urine t.
chew-and-spit t.
Chiron RIBA HCV t.
Choice2 t.
cholecystokinin t.
C of Hosmer-Lemeshow ratio t.
citrate t.
^{13}C-labeled cholesteryl octanoate breath t.
C-lactose t.
Clinitest stool t.
clomiphene t.
clonidine suppression t.
Coat-A-Count Free PSA IRMA t.
CO_2 breath t.
Cochran-Mantel-Haenszel t.

NOTES

test (*continued*)
   ^{13}C-octanoic acid gastric emptying breath t.
   Cohen t.
   Colaris genetic susceptibility t.
   Colaris molecular diagnostic t.
   cold stress t.
   ColoCARE fecal occult blood t.
   colonic transit t.
   combined intracavernous injection and stimulation t.
   complement fixation t.
   complete blood count t.
   Coombs t.
   copper-binding protein t.
   cornflake esophageal motility t.
   Cortrosyn stimulation t.
   cosyntropin stimulation t.
   cotton swab t.
   cough stress t.
   Cox-Mantel t.
   CP t.
   cracker t.
   creatinine t.
   C&S t.
   CSF glutamine t.
   ^{14}C-triolein breath t.
   culture and sensitivity t.
   ^{14}C urea breath t.
   deferoxamine mesylate infusion t.
   dexamethasone suppression t.
   diabetes home screening t.
   Diagnex Blue t.
   differential renal function t.
   differential ureteral catheterization t.
   dilute Russell viper venom t. (DRVVT)
   Dimension Free prostate-specific antigen Flex reagent cartridge t.
   t. dinner
   direct immunobead t.
   direct immunofluorescence t. (DIF-test)
   Doppler flow t. (DFT)
   duodenal secretin t. (DST)
   D-xylose absorption t.
   dye-exclusion t.
   E t.
   edrophonium t.
   egg yolk-cobalamin absorption t. (EYCAT)
   Einhorn string t.
   Eitest MONO P-II t.
   Ektachem slide t.
   ELISA-I, -II, -III t.
   endomysial antibody t.
   Enzygnost anti-HIV 1+2 t.
   Enzymun t.
   ergonovine t.
   erythrocyte sedimentation rate t.
   esophageal acid infusion t.
   esophageal function t.
   Fairley bladder washout t.
   FDL t.
   fecal alpha-1-antitrypsin t.
   fecal fat t.
   fecal leukocyte count t.
   fecal occult blood t. (FOBT)
   fingerprick latex agglutination t.
   Fisher exact probability t.
   Fisher two-tailed exact t.
   Fishman-Doubilet t.
   FlexSure HP t.
   FlexSure whole-blood t.
   fluorescein dilaurate t.
   fluorescein string t.
   fluorescent treponemal antibody absorption t.
   FoodSCAN food allergy t.
   Fouchet t.
   four-glass t.
   Fowler-Stephens t.
   Francis t.
   FTA-ABS t.
   gallbladder function t.
   GAP t.
   gastric accommodation t.
   gastric emptying breath t. (GEBT)
   gastric function t.
   gastric secretory t.
   gastrin stimulation t.
   Gastroccult t.
   gastrointestinal blood loss t.
   Gerhardt t.
   GGT t.
   GGTP liver function t.
   Ghedini-Weinberg serologic t.
   Glahn t.
   Glazyme APF-EIA-TEST t.
   glucose t.
   Glucose Analyzer II t.
   glutamine t.
   glycopyrrolate t.
   glycyltryptophan t.
   Gmelin t.
   gonadotropin-releasing hormone t.
   graded esophageal balloon distention t.
   Graham t.
   Gram stain of stool t.
   Griess t.
   Gross t.
   guaiac t.
   Guenzberg t.
   Ham t.
   Hanger t.
   Harrison spot t.
   hatching t.

Hay t.
H2 breath t.
HCV DupliType t.
HCV ELISA t.
HCV QuantaSure Plus t.
heel tap t.
Helicobacter pylori breath excretion t.
Helicoblot 2.1 t.
Helisal rapid blood t.
Hematest t.
HemaWipe t.
heme t.
Hemoccult II t.
Hemoccult Sensa t.
HemoQuant fecal blood t.
HemoSelect t.
Hepaplastin t.
hepatitis C virus DupliType t.
HEPTIMAX hepatitis C viral load t.
Herzberg t.
Histalog stimulation t.
histamine t.
HM-CAP serological t.
Hoesch t.
Hollander t.
home screening t.
HomeSelect t.
24-hour ambulatory pH t.
72-hour fecal fat t.
24-hour gastric acidity t.
12-hour home pad t.
Howard t.
Hpfast rapid urease t.
HpSA t.
H. pylori SA t.
5-HT t.
human lymphocyte chromosomal aberration t.
Hunt t.
Hybritech Tandem PSA ratio t.
hydrochloric acid t.
hydrogen breath t.
ICA t.
ice water t.
ICG t.
iliopsoas t.
immunoblot t.
ImmunoCard serum antibody t.
ImmunoCard STAT! Rotavirus t.
ImmunoCyt t.

immunodiffusion t.
immunofluorescent antibody t.
Immuno I complex PSA t.
immunological fecal occult blood t. (IFOBT)
immunological rapid urease t.
^{111}indium-labeled autologous leukocyte t.
intracavernous injection and stimulation t.
intraductal secretin t. (IDST)
intraesophageal acid t.
intraesophageal pH t.
intravenous secretin t.
Inutest t.
invasive diagnostic t.
Jacoby t.
Jaffe t.
Jaksch t.
Jatrox *Helicobacter pylori* t.
Jaworski t.
jejunal gas infusion t.
Jolles t.
Kapsinow t.
Kashiwado t.
Kato t.
Kelling t.
ketone body t.
KidneyScreen at Home t.
Kolmogorov-Smirnov t.
Krokiewicz t.
Kruskal-Wallis t.
Kveim t.
lactose tolerance t.
lactulose breath t. (LBT)
lactulose-mannitol permeability t.
Lange t.
LAP t.
Lapides t.
last-generation serologic ELISA t.
latex fixation t.
LDH t.
LDL Direct t.
Leo t.
leucine aminopeptidase t.
leukocyte adherence inhibition t.
leukocyte alkaline phosphatase t.
leukocyte esterase t.
levulose t.
Ligat t.
lipase t.
litmus milk t.

NOTES

test (continued)
  locally made rapid urease t. (LRUT)
  log-rank t.
  Lundh t.
  Macdonald t.
  Machado-Guerreiro t.
  MacLean t.
  magnetic susceptibility t.
  Mann-Whitney rank sum t.
  Mantel-Haenszel t.
  Mardi t.
  Marechal-Rosen t.
  Marshall t.
  Marshall-Bonney t.
  Marshall-Marchetti t.
  Masset t.
  McNemar ascites t.
  t. meal
  measurement t.
  Meltzer-Lyon t.
  methyl red t.
  metyrapone stimulation t.
  Micral urine dipstick t.
  Mitscherlich t.
  Mohr t.
  monoethylglycinexylidide liver function t.'s
  morphine-neostigmine t.
  motility t.
  Moynihan t.
  Myers-Fine t.
  Mylius t.
  Nakayama t.
  Nardi t.
  N-benzoyl-L-tyrosyl-P-aminobenzoic acid excretion t.
  NBT-PABA t.
  Neubauer and Fischer t.
  Neukomm t.
  nitrite t.
  nitrogen partition t.
  nitrogen retention t.
  NMP22 BladderChek t.
  noninvasive diagnostic t.
  noninvasive urodynamic t.
  nonradioactive ^{13}C t.
  Normotest t.
  number connection t. (NCT)
  Nymox urinary t.
  obturator t.
  octanoic acid breath t.
  omeprazole t.
  one-hour office pad t.
  one-minute endoscopy room t.
  O&P t.
  Oresus Potentest t.
  PABA t.
  pad urinary incontinence t.
  palmin t., palmitin t.
  pancreatic secretory t.
  Papanicolaou t.
  paracetamol absorption t.
  PAS t.
  peak secretory flow rate t.
  pentagastrin gastric secretory t.
  pentagastrin infusion t.
  pentagastrin provocative t.
  pentagastrin stimulated analysis t.
  Peptavlon stimulation t.
  percutaneous pressure ureteral perfusion t.
  perineal nerve terminal motor latency t.
  periodic acid-Schiff t.
  peripheral nerve evaluation t.
  peritoneal equilibration t. (PET)
  Pettenkofer t.
  pH t.
  Phadebas angiotensin-I t.
  phenoltetrachlorophthalein t.
  phentolamine t.
  physiologic reflux t. (PRT)
  pineapple t.
  plasma renin activity captopril t.
  PNE t.
  POA t.
  Posner attention t.
  postage stamp penile tumescence t.
  postcoital t.
  post hoc t.
  postural stimulation t. (PST)
  posture t.
  potassium sensitivity t. (PST)
  PPD t.
  Premier Platinum HpSA t.
  Prentice-Wilcoxon t.
  proteinuria t.
  Protocult t.
  provocative t.
  PSA4 prostate cancer t.
  PSFR t.
  psychometric t.
  purified protein derivative t. (PPD)
  PyloriScreen t.
  Pyloriset EIA-G t.
  PyloriStat assay t.
  PyloriTek rapid urease t.
  PYtest urea breath t.
  Q-tip t.
  qualitative fecal fat t.
  quantitative fecal fat t.
  Quick t.
  QuickVue One-Step *H. pylori* t.
  Quidel-QuickVue *H. pylori* t.
  Quinlan t.
  Rabuteau t.

radioactive carbon-14 t.
radioallergosorbent t. (RAST)
radioisotope renal excretion t.
radioisotope renogram t.
rapid serum amylase t.
rapid urease t. (RUT)
Rapoport t.
recombinant immunoblot assay-2 t.
reducing substances t.
reflex HPV t.
Rehfuss t.
Reitan Trail-Making t.
Reitman-Frankel t.
renin stimulation t.
rhubarb t.
RIBA t.
RIBA-2 t.
rice-flour breath t.
Robinson-Kepler-Power water t.
rose bengal t.
Rosenbach-Gmelin t.
Rosenthal t.
Rotazyme t.
Russell viper venom t.
Saathoff t.
Sahli glutoid t.
Sahli-Nencki t.
saline continence t.
saline load t.
saline suppression t.
Salkowski-Schipper t.
Salomon t.
santonin t.
satiety t.
Saundby t.
scan t.
S-CCK-Pz t.
Scheffe-F t.
Schiff t.
Schilling t.
Schwartz t.
Scivoletto t.
secretin-CCK stimulation t.
secretin-pancreozymin stimulation t.
secretin provocation t.
secretin stimulation t.
SeHCAT t.
^{75}Se-labeled bile acid t.
semen analysis t.
serologic t.
serum amylase t.
serum bilirubin t.

serum creatinine t.
serum iron t.
serum protein t.
serum RIBA-2 t.
Sgambati reaction t.
SGOT t.
SGPT t.
sham feeding t.
Sitzmarks t.
skinfold thickness t.
SM-HCV Rapid T.
Smith t.
snap gauge t.
sodium-loading t.
solid sphere t.
Spearman t.
specific gravity t.
specific red cell adherence t.
SpermCheck t.
split renal function t.
squeeze pressure profile of anal sphincter t.
Stamey t.
standard acid reflux t. (SART)
standard radiological t.
star construction t.
Stat Simple whole-blood antibody t.
stimulated gastric secretion t.
stimulation t.
Stokvis t.
Stoll t.
StoneRisk citrate t.
StoneRisk cystine t.
StoneRisk diagnostic t.
StoneRisk profile t.
stool cytotoxin t.
stool electrolyte t.
stool osmolality t.
stool osmotic gap t.
Strassburg t.
string t.
Stypven time t.
sucrose tolerance t.
sugar t.
Sulkowitch t.
!nSure fecal immunochemical t.
!nSure immunochemical fecal occult blood t.
sweat t.
Szabo t.
Tensilon t.

NOTES

test (*continued*)
    Tes-Tape urine glucose t.
    TIBC t.
    tilt t.
    Töpfer t.
    Torquay t.
    total fecal weight t.
    total iron-binding capacity t.
    Trail t.
    Trail-Making T.
    transferrin t.
    transmucosal electrical potential t.
    transvesical potassium sensitivity t.
    triceps skinfold thickness t.
    triolein C-14 breath t.
    Trousseau t.
    tuberculin t.
    tubular reabsorption of phosphate t.
    Tukey t.
    Tuttle t.
    two-stage triolein t.
    two-tailed Fisher t.
    two-tailed McNemar t.
    t. type
    Tyson t.
    UBT breath t.
    Udranszky t.
    Uffelmann t.
    ultrasound t.
    Ultzmann t.
    Uni-Gold *Helicobacter pylori* t.
    uPM3 urine t.
    urea breath t. (UBT)
    urea nitrogen t.
    urease t.
    Urecholine supersensitivity t.
    uric acid t.
    urinary nitrite t.
    urine chloride t.
    urine concentration t.
    Uriscreen t.
    van den Bergh t.
    ViraPap HPV dot blot hybridization t.
    vitamin A, B_{12} absorption t.
    Voges-Proskauer t.
    von Jaksch t.
    Wagner t.
    washout t.
    water-gurgle t.
    water-nutrient t.
    water-recovery t.
    water-restriction t.
    water-sipping t.
    water-soluble contrast esophageal swallow t.
    Watson-Schwartz t.
    whiff t.
    Whipple triad t.
    Whitaker pressure-perfusion t.
    Winckler t.
    Witz t.
    Woldman t.
    Wolff-Junghans t.
    Woolf t.
    xylose absorption t.
    xylose tolerance t.
    Yang Pros-Check PSA t.
    Z t.
    Zappacosta t.
    zona hamster egg t.

testalgia
Tes-Tape urine glucose test
testectomy
testes (*pl. of* testis)
testicle
    maldescended t.
    retained t.
testicular
    t. abscess
    t. adenocarcinoma
    t. adenofibromyoma
    t. adenomatoid tumor vacuole
    t. adrenallike tissue (TALT)
    t. adrenal rest
    t. androgen-binding protein
    t. angioma
    t. artery
    t. biopsy
    t. carcinoma
    t. cyst
    t. descent
    t. feminization syndrome
    t. fibroma
    t. Hodgkin disease
    t. hypothermia device
    t. implant
    t. interstitial fluid (TIF)
    t. leiomyoma
    t. leukemia
    t. lymphoma
    t. mass
    t. microlithiasis
    t. pain
    t. plexus
    t. prosthesis
    t. seminoma
    t. sperm extraction (TESE)
    t. swelling
    t. teratoma
    t. torsion
    t. tuberculosis
    t. tubular adenoma
    t. tubule
testicularis
    plexus t.
testiculoma
testiculus, pl. **testiculi**

Testim 1%
testing
    anorectal physiology t.
    breath alkane t.
    fecal occult blood t.
    histocompatibility t.
    lactose hydrogen breath t. (LHBT)
    multiple data t.
    nucleic acid t. (NAT)
    pad t.
    penile injection t.
    pH-metric t.
    physiology t.
    provocative t.
    psychophysiologic t.
    RigiScan t.
    salivary t.
    sexual stimulation t.
    stress t.
    urea breath t.
    urodynamic t.
    viability t.
    vibrotactile stimulation t.
    videourodynamic t.
    visual sexual stimulation t.
testis, pl. **testes**
    abdominal t.
    aberratio t.
    adenocarcinoma of infantile t.
    albuginea t.
    appendix t.
    t. cancer
    t. carcinoid
    Cooper irritable t.
    descensus aberrans t.
    descensus paradoxus t.
    dorsum of t.
    dystopia transversa externa t.
    dystopia transversa interna t.
    ectopic t.
    femoral t.
    fibroma of t.
    free-floating t.
    fungus t.
    high t.
    interstitial cell tumor of t.
    inverted t.
    irritable t.
    lobuli t.
    mediastinum t.
    mottled t.
    movable t.
    t. muliebris
    obstructed t.
    peeping t.
    prosthetic t.
    pulpy t.
    retained t.
    rete t.
    retractile t.
    t. sarcoma
    septula t.
    septum of t.
    solitary t.
    torsion of t.
    tunica albuginea t.
    tunica vaginalis t.
    undescended t.
    unilateral palpable right t.
    vanishing t.
testis-determining factor
testitis
testitoxicosis
Testoderm
    T. patch
    T. TTS
testoid
testolactone
testopathy
testosterone
    basal t.
    t. buccal system
    t. cypionate
    t. deficiency
    t. enanthate
    free t.
    t. gel 1%
    t. patch
    t. plasma concentration
    t. propionate
    serum t.
    t. stimulation
    t. transdermal system (TTS)
    t. transdermal therapy
    undecenoate of t.
testosterone-binding globulin
testosterone-estrogen-binding globulin
testosterone-repressed prostate message-2 (TRPM-2)
testotoxicosis
Testred C-III
Test-Size orchidometer
test-yolk buffer cryopreservation agent

NOTES

tetani
    Clostridium t.
tetanus globulin
tetany
    gastric t.
tether circulating leukocyte
tethered-bowel sign
tethered-cord
    t.-c. release
    t.-c. syndrome (TCS)
tethered spinal cord
tethering of mucosa
tetracaine lozenge
Tetracap
tetrachloride
    carbon t.
tetracycline
    bismuth, metronidazole, t. (BMT)
    t. hydrochloride
    t. nephropathy
    ranitidine bismuth citrate, metronidazole, t. (RMT)
    t. sclerosis
tetracycline-induced spongiotic esophagitis
tetradecapeptide
tetradecyl sulfate
tetraethylammonium (TEA)
Tetragastrin-NS
tetrahydrocannabinol (THC)
tetrahydrochloride
    3′,3-diaminobenzidine t.
tetrahydrozoline
tetralogy
    Fallot t.
Tetram
tetramethyl ammonium chloride (TEMAC)
tetrapalmitate
    maltose t.
tetraplegia
tetraploid cell
tetrapyrrol compound
tetrathiomolybdate
tetrazolium
    nitroblue t. (NBT)
tetrodotoxin (TTX)
tetroxide
    osmium t.
Teucrium chamaedrys
Tevdek suture
Texas-style two-piece catheter
Texas trauma
texture
    heterogeneous t.
    homogenous t.
tezacitabine
T fastener
TFE-coated wire guide

TFF
    trefoil factor family
TFF1
TFF2
TFF3
    intestinal peptide TFF3
TfR
    transferrin receptor
TF/UF
    tubular fluid:ultrafiltrate
TGC
    tailgut cyst
TGE
    transgastrostomic enteroscopy
TG ELISA
TGF
    transforming growth factor
    tubuloglomerular feedback
    human recombinant TGF
TGF-alpha
    transforming growth factor alpha
TGF-beta
    transforming growth factor beta
TGF-beta-1
    transforming growth factor beta-1
    TGF-beta-1 gene
TGF-beta-2
    transforming growth factor beta-2
TGF-beta-3
    transforming growth factor beta-3
TGHA
    thyroglobulin antibody
Th1 response
Thal
    T. esophageal stricture repair
    T. esophagogastroscopy
    T. esophagogastrostomy
    T. fundic patch operation
    T. fundoplasty
    T. strictureplasty
thalidomide
Thalitone
thallium
    t. imaging
    t. poisoning
thallium-201
thamuria
thaw-mount radioautography
Thaysen disease
THC
    tetrahydrocannabinol
    transhepatic cholangiography
tHcy
    total homocysteine
THE
    transhepatic embolization
Theis self-retaining retractor
thelium, pl. **thelia**
T-helper precursor

thenar eminence
theophylline
- t. clearance
- t. ethylenediamine
- t. level
- t. olamine enema
- t. toxicity

theory
- Dieulafoy t.
- Freter t.
- hyperfiltration t.
- overflow t.
- peripheral arterial vasodilation t.
- set point t.

TheraCLEC
TheraCys
Theradex
Theradigm-HBV
Theragyn
Theralax
therapeutic
- t. angiography
- t. colonoscopy
- t. concentrate (TC)
- t. endoscope
- t. endourology
- t. laparoscopy
- t. modality
- t. option
- t. pancreaticobiliary endoscopy
- t. plasmapheresis
- t. response
- t. side-viewing duodenoscope
- t. upper endoscopy
- t. value

therapy
- ablative laser t.
- acid suppression t. (AST)
- adjuvant drug t.
- adrenalin injection t.
- alarm t.
- alfa-interferon t.
- alimentary t.
- alkaline citrate t.
- alpha-blocker t.
- alpha-receptor blockade t.
- amoxicillin-tinidazole-ranitidine t.
- amphotericin B t.
- ampullary ablative t.
- androgen ablation t. (AAT)
- androgen deprivation t.
- androgen withdrawal endocrine t.
- antibiotic t.
- anticholinergic medicine t.
- anticoagulation t.
- antilymphocyte t.
- antimicrobial t.
- antioncogene t.
- antireflux t.
- antisecretory t.
- argon laser t.
- autolymphocyte t.
- Aza-Pred t.
- azole t.
- balloon photodynamic t.
- beta-blocker t.
- bile acid t.
- biofeedback t.
- biologic response modifier t.
- bismuth-free triple t.
- bismuth triple t.
- bridging t.
- bright light t. (BLT)
- broad-spectrum t.
- bubble t.
- buprenorphine narcotic analgesic t.
- chemoradiation t. (CRT)
- cholestyramine t.
- CIFN t.
- clarithromycin triple t.
- coagulative laser t.
- combined chemoradiation t.
- conditioning t.
- conformal radiation t.
- continuous renal replacement t. (CRRT)
- corticosteroid t.
- cost effectiveness of t.
- cytokine t.
- cytolytic t.
- debulking t.
- dendritic cell t.
- diclofenac analgesic t.
- diet t.
- dilation t.
- diltiazem t.
- dose optimized t. (DOT)
- doxycycline-metronidazole-bismuth subcitrate triple t.
- drug t.
- Emitasol nasal t.
- endocrine t.
- endoscopic Doppler ultrasound-guided injection t.

NOTES

therapy *(continued)*
- endoscopic hemoclip t.
- endoscopic hemostatic t.
- endoscopic injection t.
- endoscopic laser t. (ELT)
- endoscopic pancreatic t.
- enterostomal t. (ET)
- Enterra T.
- enzyme replacement t.
- eradication t.
- erythropoietin t.
- esophageal photodynamic t.
- estrogen replacement t. (ERT)
- ethanol injection t.
- external-beam radiation t. (EBRT)
- external vacuum t.
- ex vivo liver-directed gene t.
- fluid replacement t.
- fluoroquinolone t.
- flutamide t.
- foscarnet t.
- gamma globulin t.
- gene t.
- gene-transfer t.
- H2-antagonist t.
- heat t.
- heater probe t.
- Helidac t.
- hematoporphyrin derivative t.
- hemofiltration t. (HFT)
- hemostatic t.
- highly active antiretroviral t. (HAART)
- homeostatic t.
- hormonal t.
- H2-receptor antagonist t.
- hydrocelectomy scleral t.
- hydrostatic pressure t.
- hyperbaric oxygen t. (HBOT)
- hyperfractionated radiation t.
- IFN alfa t.
- IFN alfa-2b t.
- image-guided t.
- immunomodulatory gene t.
- immunosuppressive t.
- initial broad-spectrum t.
- injection t.
- instillation t.
- intensity-modulated proton t. (IMPT)
- intensity-modulated radiation t. (IMRT)
- interferon alpha t.
- interferon alpha-2b t.
- intermittent calcitriol t.
- intermittent hormone t.
- International Association for Enterostomal T.
- interstitial photodynamic t.
- intracavernosal injection t. (ICIT)
- intracavernous injection t.
- intracavitary radiation boost t.
- intracavitary topical t.
- intracorporeal injection t.
- intraoperative radiation t. (IORT)
- I.V. fluid t.
- ketoprofen analgesic t.
- laser t.
- lifestyle t.
- medical t.
- metabolic t.
- methyl-*tert*-butyl ether t.
- metronidazole, amoxicillin, clarithromycin, *H. pylori*, one-week t. (MACH1)
- microwave t.
- minimally invasive t.
- monoclonal antibody t.
- morphine narcotic analgesic t.
- MTBE t.
- Nd:YAG laser t.
- neoadjuvant androgen derivation t.
- neoadjuvant hormonal ablation t.
- neodymium:YAG laser t.
- Nexium triple t.
- nutritional t.
- omeprazole t.
- omeprazole-clarithromycin-amoxicillin t.
- oral rehydration t. (ORT)
- OssaTron shock wave t.
- palliative t.
- pancreatic enzyme replacement t.
- pancreatic intraluminal radiation t.
- PARIET t.
- PEI t.
- penile injection t.
- penile vein occlusion t.
- percutaneous embolization t.
- percutaneous ethanol injection t.
- periurethral injection t.
- phosphate binder t.
- photodynamic t. (PDT)
- photoradiation t.
- physiologic testosterone-replacement t.
- placebo t.
- polidocanol injection t.
- polyestradiol phosphate t.
- postoperative anticoagulation t.
- posttransplant immunosuppression t.
- PPI triple t.
- preventive intravesical t.
- Prevpac triple t.
- probiotic t.
- prokinetic t.
- proton pump inhibition t.
- psychosexual t.

pulsed-dye laser t.
quadruple t.
radiation t.
radionuclide t.
ranitidine t.
Rebetron Combination t.
rehydration t.
renal replacement t.
rescue t.
resiniferatoxin t.
role of diet in t.
sacral nerve stimulation t.
saline injection t.
salvage t.
sandwich staghorn calculus t.
sclerosing t.
self-injection t.
sex t.
single-drug t.
SNS t.
somatostatin analog t.
somatostatin infusion t.
steroid t.
sucralfate t.
surgical t.
systemic radiation t.
T-cell cytotoxic t.
testosterone transdermal t.
TheraSphere t.
thermal t.
three-dimensional conformal radiation t. (3-DCRT)
thrombolytic t.
Trager t.
transcatheter arterial embolization t.
transpapillary t.
transurethral collagen injection t.
transvaginal t.
triple t. (TT)
triple eradication t.
tumor suppressor gene t.
ultrasound-guided shock wave t.
universally accepted t.
unresponsiveness to standard t.
valproic acid t.
YAG laser t.

TheraSeed
Therasonics
    T. Lithotripsy System
    T. lithotriptor
TheraSphere therapy
Theratope vaccine

Therevac Plus
Therevac-SB
Therma
    T. Jaw disposable hot biopsy forceps
    T. Jaw hot urologic forceps
thermal
    t. ablation
    t. blocking
    t. burn
    t. imaging
    t. sphincteric reflex
    t. therapy
    t. therapy technique
thermally active method
TherMatric hyperthermia device
TherMatrx
    T. DOT
    T. TMx-2000 device
Thermex-II transurethral prostate heating device
thermic
    t. effect of feeding (TEF)
    t. effect of physical activity (TEPA)
thermoablation
    transurethral hot-water balloon t.
ThermoChem-HT system
thermocoagulation
    endoscopic heater probe t.
    heater probe t.
    heat probe t.
    HP t.
    KeyMed heater probe t.
    laser t.
thermocoagulator
    Olympus CD-Z-series heat probe t.
thermocycler
    Stratagene SCS-96 t.
thermodisinfector
    endoscopic t.
thermodynamic solubility product
thermoexpandable stent
ThermoFlex
    T. system
    T. thermotherapy unit
thermogenesis
    adaptive t. (AT)
thermography
    Primus transrectal t.
thermomechanical

NOTES

thermometer
- air t.
- alcohol t.
- Celsius t.
- centigrade t.
- Fahrenheit t.
- gas t.
- oral t.
- rectal t.
- surface t.

thermometry
- magnetic resonance imaging t.

thermophilus
- *Streptococcus* t.

thermoreceptor
thermosensitive stent
thermosensor
thermotherapy
- biological predictors for treatment outcome of transurethral microwave t.
- cooled catheter transurethral microwave t.
- different t.
- high-energy transurethral microwave t. (HE-TUMT)
- low-energy transurethral microwave t. (LE-TUMT)
- microwave t.
- 30-minute transurethral microwave t.
- periurethral transurethral microwave t. (P-TUMT)
- targeted microwave t.
- transurethral microwave t. (TUMT)
- Urowave t.
- water-induced t. (WIT)

Thermovac tissue pulverizer
Thermus
- *T. aquaticus*
- *T. aquaticus* DNA ligase

thetaiotaomicron
- *Bacteroides* t.

thiabendazole
thiacetazone
thiamine deficiency
thiazide diuretic
thiazide-induced hyponatremia
thick
- t. adhesion
- t. ascending limb (TAL)
- t. bile

thickened
- t. gallbladder wall
- t. nail

thickening
- apical t.
- hypoechoic t.
- mediastinal t.
- plaquelike t.
- small bowel t.
- submucosal t.
- wall t.

thick-loop transurethral resection of prostate
thickness
- esophageal wall t. (EWT)
- mucous gel t.
- t. of skinfold (TSF)
- triceps skinfold t.

thick-walled gallbladder
Thiersch
- T. anal incontinence operation
- T. graft
- T. procedure
- T. tube

Thiersch-Duplay
- T.-D. proximal tube procedure
- T.-D. repair
- T.-D. tube graft
- T.-D. tubularization
- T.-D. urethroplasty

thiethylperazine
thigh graft arteriovenous fistula
thimble
- bladder t.
- t. bladder

thin
- t. adhesion
- t. basement membrane (TBM)
- t. basement membrane disease (TBMD)
- Cutinova Hydro T.
- t. descending limb
- t. glomerular basement membrane disease
- t. shave sectioning

thin-layer chromatography (TLC)
thin-needle percutaneous cholangiogram
ThinPrep Processor
thin-walled
- t.-w. diverticulum
- t.-w. gallbladder
- t.-w. vascular channel

thiocyanate
- guanidine t.

thiol
- exogenous t.
- t. intermediate

Thiola
thiopental
Thioplex
thiopropazate
thioridazine hydrochloride
thiosulfate-citrate-bile salts-sucrose agar (TCBS)
Thiosulfil
thiotepa

thiothixene
thiourea-resorcinol method
thiphenamil
thiram
third-generation
    t.-g. cephalosporin
    t.-g. lithotriptor
third spacing
thirst
    t. fever
    osmotic threshold for t.
Thiry fistula
Thiry-Vella fistula (TVF)
thistle
    milk t.
THM
    Tamm-Horsfall mucoprotein
Thomas
    T. shunt
    T. technique
Thompson
    T. capsule flap pyeloplasty
    T. lithotrite
    T. procedure
    T. technique
Thomsen-Friedenreich antigen
thoracic
    t. aortic pathology
    t. aortorenal bypass
    t. duct
    t. endometriosis syndrome
    t. esophagus
    t. fistula
    t. inlet
    t. kidney
    t. stomach
thoracoabdominal
    t. aortic aneurysm (TAAA)
    t. aortic aneurysm surgery
    t. collateral vein
    t. esophagogastrectomy
    t. extrapleural approach
    t. incision
    t. intrapleural approach
    t. retroperitoneal lymphadenectomy
thoracolaparotomy
thoracoscopic transdiaphragmatic adrenalectomy
thoracotomy
    esophagectomy with t.
    t. scar
Thorazine

Thorek
    T. gallbladder aspirator
    T. gallbladder forceps
    T. gallbladder scissors
Thorek-Feldman gallbladder scissors
Thorek-Mixter gallbladder forceps
thorium
    colloidal t.
    t. dioxide
Thorn salt-depletion syndrome
Thornton sign
Thorotrast contrast medium
THP
    Tamm-Horsfall protein
thread-and-streaks sign
thread-locking device
threadworm
    nondisseminated intestinal t.
thready pulse
three-armed basket forceps
three-dimensional (3-D)
    t.-d. conformal radiation therapy (3-DCRT)
    t.-d. CT pancreatography (3-DCTP)
    t.-d. linear endosonography
    t.-d. pelvicaliceal endocast
three-drug regimen
three-field
    t.-f. dissection
    t.-f. lymphadenectomy
three-finger grip
three-limb S pouch
three-loop
    t.-l. ileal pouch
    t.-l. technique
three-pronged
    t.-p. grasper
    t.-p. grasping forceps
    t.-p. polyp retriever
three-quarter circle electrode
three-space dissection
three-trocar technique for laparoscopic cholecystectomy
three-way
    t.-w. irrigating catheter
    t.-w. stopcock
three-week sulfasalazine syndrome
threonine
threshold
    gastric mechanosensory t.
    t. of internal sphincter
    median detection t. (MDT)

NOTES

threshold *(continued)*
    pH t.
    t. potential
    t. of rectal sensation
    swallowing t.
    urethral sensory t.
thrifty colon
thrive
    failure to t.
thrombectomy
thrombi *(pl. of* thrombus*)*
thrombic lesion
thrombin
    bovine t.
    t. spray
    topical bovine t.
thrombin-antithrombin
    t.-a. III
    t.-a. III complex
Thrombinar
Thrombin-JMI
thrombocytopenia
    heparin-induced t. (HIT)
thrombocytopenia-absent
    t.-a. radius (TAR)
    t.-a. radius syndrome
thrombocytopenic purpura
thrombocytosis
thromboelastography
thromboembolic
    t. disease
    t. event
thromboembolism
    venous t. (VTE)
thromboendarterectomy
    renal t.
Thrombogen
thrombolytic
    t. agent
    t. therapy
thrombomodulin
thrombophlebitis
    puerperal septic pelvic vein t.
thrombopoietin (TPO)
thrombosed
    t. internal and external hemorrhoids
    t. pile
thrombosis, pl. **thromboses**
    arterial t.
    bilateral renal vein t.
    bland t.
    deep venous t.
    glomerular microvascular t.
    hepatic artery t. (HAT)
    hepatic vein t.
    inferior vena cava t.
    intracapillary t.
    intrarenal vascular t.
    intravascular t.
    mesenteric arterial t.
    mesenteric vein t. (MVT)
    nonocclusive mesenteric t.
    peripheral venous t.
    portal vein t. (PVT)
    renal artery t.
    renal vein t.
    silent t.
    SMV t.
    splenic vein t.
    venous t.
thrombospondin
thrombotic
    t. microangiopathy
    t. risk factor
    t. thrombocytopenic purpura (TTP)
thromboxane A_2
thrombus, pl. **thrombi**
    bile t.
    mural t.
    portal vein t.
    retrocecalis tumor t.
    t. tumor
    white t.
through
    tearing t.
through-and-through appearance
through-the-scope (TTS)
    t.-t.-s. balloon
    t.-t.-s. balloon dilation
    t.-t.-s. balloon removal
    t.-t.-s. bougie
    t.-t.-s. catheter probe
    t.-t.-s. dilator
    t.-t.-s. injection needle
thrush
    t. esophagitis
    oral t.
thumbnail image
thumbprinting
    t. of mucosa
    t. sign
thymalfasin
thymic
    t. EC
    t. hypoplasia
thymidine
thymidine-labeling index
Thymitaq
thymocyte NA+/H+ exchanger
Thymoglobulin
thymol crystal
thymosin
thymoxamine
thymus
thymus-derived
    t.-d. cell
    t.-d. lymphocyte
thyreoideus impar plexus

thyroarytenoid muscle
thyroglobulin antibody (TGHA)
thyrohyoid muscle
thyroid
    t. autoimmunity
    t. disease
    t. hormone
    t. hormone response element (TRE)
    t. hormone serum concentration
    medullary carcinoma of t. (MCT)
    t. microsomal antibody
    t. nodule
    tender t.
    t. tenderness
thyroiditis
    autoimmune t.
    Hashimoto t.
thyroidization
thyroid-stimulating hormone level
thyromegaly
thyroplasty
thyrotoxicosis
    gestational t.
thyrotropin-releasing hormone
thyroxine
    free t. (FT4)
thyroxine-binding globulin
TI
    tubulointerstitial
TIBC
    total iron-binding capacity
    TIBC test
ticarcillin
tic douloureux of bladder
Tice
ticklish
ticlopidine
Ti-Cron, Tycron
    T.-C. suture
    T.-C. tie
ticrynafen-induced jaundice
tidal drainage
tide
    sign of rising t.
tie
    free t.
    stick t.
    Ti-Cron t.
Tielle Plus hydropolymer dressing
tie-over dressing
TIF
    testicular interstitial fluid

Tigan
tight
    t. abdomen
    t. junction membrane protein
    t. junction permeability
    t. Nissen repair
    t. perirectal adhesion
tigroid appearance
TII
    terminal ileum intubation
TIL
    tumor-infiltrating lymphocyte
tilt
    t. stitch
    t. test
Timberlake obturator
time
    abdominopelvic orocecal transit t.
    activated partial thromboplastin t. (aPTT)
    activated thromboplastin t.
    ascites euglobulin lysis t. (AELT)
    bleeding t.
    caliceal filling t.
    cancer doubling t.
    clotting t.
    coagulation t.
    cold ischemia t. (CIT)
    colonic transit t.
    dextrinizing t.
    t. domain ultrasound (TDU)
    doubling t.
    duration t.
    esophageal transit t.
    explosive doubling t.
    gastric bleeding t. (GBT)
    gastric emptying t. (GET)
    gastric transit t.
    mean dissolution t. (MDT)
    mean input t. (MIT)
    mean resistance t. (MRT)
    mean transit t. (MTT)
    median operative t.
    nucleation t. (NT)
    operative t.
    orocecal transit t. (OCTT)
    partial thromboplastin t. (PTT)
    pH holding t.
    post-UUO t.
    preservation t.
    pro t.
    prothrombin t. (PT)

NOTES

time *(continued)*
    prothrombin time/partial thromboplastin t. (PT/PTT)
    PSA doubling t.
    radionuclide esophageal emptying t.
    resection t.
    Russell viper venom t.
    shortened prep t.
    skin bleeding t. (SBT)
    small bowel transit t.
    suturing t.
    T-1/2 t. of gastric emptying
    transit t. (TT)
    warm ischemia t.

time-activity curve

Timecaps
    Levsinex T.

time-concentration curve

timed
    t. average urea concentration (TACurea)
    t. voiding

time-dependent variable

Timentin
    double-dose IV T.
    single-dose IV T.

time-of-flight mass spectometry (TOFMS)

timer
    video t.

timing of repair

Tim knot

timolol

timori
    Brugia t.

TIMP
    tissue metalloproteinase

TIMP-2
    tissue inhibitor of metalloproteinase-2

TIN
    tubulointerstitial nephritis

tincture
    t. of belladonna
    t. of benzoin

Tindal

tinea
    t. cruris
    t. purpureum
    t. rubrum

tinidazole

tinkling bowel sounds

TINU
    tubulointerstitial nephritis and uveitis
    TINU syndrome

tiopronin

tip
    Andrews suction t.
    atraumatic t.
    Buie rectal suction t.
    filiform t.
    Frazier suction t.
    oblique mucosectomy device t.
    open-end flow-through radiopaque t.
    papillary t.
    sharp-edged t.
    Slip-Coat t.
    spleen t.
    suction t.
    tulip t.
    vessel t.
    villus t.
    weighted t.

TIPPB
    transperineal interstitial permanent prostate brachytherapy

TIPS
    transjugular intrahepatic portosystemic shunt
    occlusion of TIPS
    TIPS procedure
    stenosis of TIPS

TIPSS
    transjugular intrahepatic portosystemic stent shunt

TIR
    toll-interleukin 1 receptor

TIRAP
    toll-interleukin 1 receptor domain-containing adapter protein

Tis disease

Tisseel
    T. fibrin sealant
    T. fibrin sealant injection

tissue
    acinar t.
    adipose t.
    ampullary granulation t.
    t. approximation
    bronchus-associated lymphoepithelial t. (BALT)
    chromaffin t.
    cicatricial t.
    t. coagulation
    connective t.
    cryostat t.
    t. culture
    t. culture assay
    t. cushion
    t. destruction result
    t. expansion vaginoplasty
    extraperitoneal t.
    exuberant granulation t.
    fatty t.
    fibroadipose t.
    fibrocollagenous t.
    fibroelastic t.
    fibrous t.
    t. fixation

t. forceps
formalin-fixed t.
t. fusion
gastrointestinal-associated lymphoid t. (GALT)
t. glue
gut-associated lymphoepithelial t. (GALT)
gut-associated lymphoid t. (GALT)
hilar structure scar t.
t. inhibitor of metalloproteinase
t. inhibitor of metalloproteinase-2 (TIMP-2)
t. kallikrein
lipomalike t.
lipomatous t.
t. manifestation
t. matrix syndrome
mesorectal t.
t. metalloproteinase (TIMP)
t. monomer
t. morcellator
mucosa-associated lymphoid t. (MALT)
t. necrosis
necrotic t.
neoplastic t.
noninflamed peripheral t.
nontarget t.
nonviable t.
paracancerous t.
paraffin-embedded t.
parenchymal t.
periadvential t.
perinephric t.
periprostatic t.
t. plasminogen activator (TPA, tPA)
t. polypeptide antigen
proliferation of prostastic t.
redundant sac t.
t. renewal
t. resistance
t. rim sign
t. sampling
sex accessory t.
soft t.
t. spectrum analyzer TS-200
splenic t.
subcutaneous t.
T. Tek-II cryostat
testicular adrenallike t. (TALT)

t. transglutaminase (tTG)
t. transglutaminase ELISA treated t.
TissueMend soft tissue repair matrix
tissue-specific gene expression
tissue-stone recognition system (TSRS)
tissue-type plasminogen activator
Titan
   T. endoprosthesis
   T. stent
titanium
   t. clip
   t. urethral stent
titanous chloride
titer
   anti-HSV IgM Ab t.
   antineutrophil cytoplasmic antibody t.
   antistreptolysin-O t.
   ELISA t.
   end-point dilution t.
   IgM-HEV antibody t.
   viral serologic t.
title peritoneal dialysis (TPD)
Titralac Plus
titratable acidity
TJF-100, -130 large-channel duodenoscope
TJF-10, -20 videoduodenoscope
TL90 Ethicon stapler
TLA
   transperitoneal laparoscopic adrenalectomy
TLC
   thin-layer chromatography
TLESR
   transient lower esophageal sphincter relaxation
TLI
   total lymphoid irradiation
TLN
   transperitoneal laparoscopic nephrectomy
TLR
   toll-like receptor
T-lymphocyte activation
T-lymphocyte-mediated cytotoxic reaction
Tm
   tubular maximal
TMD
   transmural drainage
TME
   total mesorectal excision

NOTES

TMPD
: transmucosal potential difference

TMP-SMX, SMX/TMP
: trimethoprim-sulfamethoxazole
  lomefloxacin TMP-SMX

TMx-2000 BPH thermotherapy system

TNF
: tumor necrosis factor

TNF-alpha
: tumor necrosis factor alpha
  TNF-alpha assay
  TNF-alpha gene

TNM
: tumor, nodes, metastases
  TNM carcinoma classification
  TNM classification of carcinoma
  TNM system for tumor staging

TNTC
: too numerous to count

toast
: bananas, rice, cereal, applesauce, and t. (BRAT)
  bananas, rice, cereal, applesauce, tea, and t. (BRATT)

tobacco dose exposure
tobramycin
tocainide hydrochloride
tocodynamometer
: guard-ring t.
  Nihon t.

TODAY
: Treatment Options for Type 2 Diabetes in Adolescents and Youths

Todd cirrhosis
toddler's diarrhea
toe
: clubbing of fingers and t.'s

TOFMS
: time-of-flight mass spectometry

Tofranil
Tofranil-PM
toilet
: peritoneal t.

tolazamide
tolazoline hydrochloride
tolbutamide-induced cholestasis
tolcapone
Toldt
: line of T.
  T. membrane
  white line of T.

tolerability data
tolerance
: glucose t.
  oral t.
  transplantation t.

tolerated
: diet as t. (DAT)

toleration
: maximal t. (MT)

Tolerex feeding solution
tolerogenic dendritic cell
tolevamer
toll-interleukin
: t.-i. 1 receptor (TIR)
  t.-i. 1 receptor domain-containing adapter protein (TIRAP)

toll-like receptor (TLR)
tolmetin
tolnaftate
tolterodine
: t. tartrate
  t. tartrate capsule

toluidine
: t. blue
  t. blue stain

Tom
: T. Jones closure
  T. Jones suture

Toma sign
Tomenius gastroscope
Tomocat
tomodensitometric examination
tomodensitometry
: computed t.

tomography
: computed t. (CT)
  computerized t. (CT)
  contrast-enhanced computed t.
  dual-phase helical computed t.
  electron-beam computerized t. (EBCT)
  endoscopic optical coherence t.
  F-18 fluorodeoxyglucose positron emission t.
  helical computed t.
  noncontrast computerized t.
  noncontrast helical computed t. (NCCT)
  optical coherence t. (OCT)
  positron emission t. (PET)
  single-photon emission computed t. (SPECT)
  single-photon emission computerized t. (SPECT)
  spiral computed t.
  ultrafast computerized t.
  ultrasonic t.
  unenhanced helical computed t.

Tonalin
tone
: anal sphincter t.
  bowel t.
  cardiac sympathovagal t.
  gastric t.
  lower esophageal sphincter t.
  pyloric t.

renovascular t.
sphincter t.
tongs
tongue
bifid t.
black hairy t.
t. deviation
fissured t.
geographic t.
hairy t.
t. movement
mucosal t.
smoker's t.
swollen t.
t. of tumor
tongue-shaped villus
tonic
t. contraction
t. neck
tonicity
low t.
plasma t.
Tonkaflo pump
tonometry
tonsil
t. clamp
t. forceps
orange-colored t.
t. sucker
tonsillar enlargement
tonsillectomy
tool
prognostic t.
Toomey
T. evacuator
T. syringe
too numerous to count (TNTC)
toothed tissue forceps
TOPA
topical oropharyngeal anesthesia
Töpfer test
Top-Fill enteral feeding bag
topical
t. anesthetic
t. antibiotic
t. betamethasone
t. bovine thrombin
t. neuropathy
t. nifedipine
t. oropharyngeal anesthesia (TOPA)
Synalar T.

t. treatment
t. Xylocaine
topic effect
Topicort Cream
Topiglan
topiramate
Top Notch automated biopsy system
topogram
balloon t.
topography
scintigraphic balloon t.
topoisomerase I inhibitor
toposcopic catheter
topotecan
Toprol
Toradol
Torbot
T. cement
T. faceplate
Torecan
Torek
T. operation
T. orchiopexy
toremifene
tori (*pl. of* torus)
Toronto-Western catheter
torovirus
Torquay test
torque
t. catheter
translation of t.
t. vise
t. wire
torquing of scope
torrential hemorrhage
Torres syndrome
torsemide
torsion
adnexal t.
t. of appendage
appendix testis t.
biliary tract t.
cryptorchidism t.
extravaginal t.
t. of gallbladder
gallbladder t.
intravaginal t.
penile t.
perinatal t.
spermatic cord t.
synchronous neonatal t.
testicular t.

NOTES

torsion *(continued)*
    t. of testis
    ureteral t.
torso crease
torticollis
tortuous
    t. esophagus
    t. ureter
    t. venous ectasia
torulopsis
    T. glabrata
    t. infection
torus, pl. **tori**
    t. palatinus
    t. ureter
Toshiba
    T. ERVF 1A video floppy recorder
    T. Sal 38B real-time ultrasonography
    T. Sonolayer SSA250A transrectal ultrasonography
    T. TCE-M-series colonoscope
    T. videoendoscope
Tosoh assay
Tostrex
Totacillin
total
    t. abdominal colectomy (TAC)
    t. abdominal evisceration (TAE)
    t. anorectal reconstruction
    t. bilateral vagotomy
    t. bile acid (TBA)
    t. bilirubin
    t. body irradiation (TBI)
    t. body nitrogen (TBN)
    t. body water (TBW)
    t. bowel rest
    t. colonoscopy
    t. corrected incremental score (TCIS)
    t. cystectomy
    t. cystourethrectomy
    t. descent
    t. dose infusion
    t. enteral nutrition (TEN)
    t. fasting
    t. fecal weight test
    t. gastrectomy
    t. gastric wrap
    t. glutathione content
    t. hematuria
    t. hemolytic complement
    t. homocysteine (tHcy)
    t. homocysteine plasma concentration
    t. infarction
    t. internal reflection
    t. iron-binding capacity (TIBC)
    t. iron-binding capacity test
    t. lymphocyte (TTL)
    t. lymphoid irradiation (TLI)
    t. measured renal cortex
    t. mesorectal excision (TME)
    t. pancreatectomy
    t. parenteral alimentation
    t. parenteral nutrition (TPN)
    t. parenteral nutrition line
    t. pelvic exenteration
    t. perineal prostatectomy
    t. peripheral parenteral nutrition (TPPN)
    t. peroral intraoperative enteroscopy
    t. predicted return
    t. prostatoseminal vesiculectomy
    t. protein
    t. protein concentration
    t. PSA (tPSA)
    t. scrotectomy
    t. serum prostatic acid phosphatase (TSPAP)
    t. slit pore length
    t. transurethral resection of prostate (T-TURP)
totalis
    varicosis coli t.
totally
    t. extraperitoneal (TEP)
    t. extraperitoneal hernia repair
    t. stapled restorative proctocolectomy (TSRPC)
touch
    t. cytology
    T. preparation
Toupet
    T. hemifundoplication
    T. partial posterior fundoplication
    T. procedure
tour de maitre
tourniquet
    double-loop t.
    Dupuytren t.
    Gill renal t.
    t. occlusion
    Rumel t.
    single-loop t.
towel clip
Townes-Brocks syndrome
toxemia
    hepatic t.
    t. of pregnancy
toxic
    t. appearance
    t. cirrhosis
    t. colitis
    t. diarrhea
    t. dilatation of bowel
    t. dilation of colon

t. epidermal necrolysis (TEN)
t. gastritis
t. glomerulopathy
t. hepatitis
t. megacolon
t. metabolite
t. nephropathy
t. shock syndrome
t. steatosis

toxicity
acetaminophen t.
acute hepatic t.
aluminum t.
ammonia t.
bleomycin t.
calcineurin inhibitor t.
chloroform t.
chlorzoxazone t.
cyclosporine t.
direct tubular t.
hyperbaric oxygen t.
octreotide-induced hepatic t.
potential t.
progressive t.
protein-mediated tubular t.
quality-adjusted time without symptoms or t. (Q-TWIST)
renal t.
theophylline t.
vitamin A t.

Toxicodendron **dermatitis**
toxicosis
toxicum
erythema t.
toxigenic
t. bacterium
t. diarrhea
toxin
t. A, B
t. assay
botulinum t. (BTX)
cholera t.
Coley t.
cytoskeleton-altering t.
t. exposure
heat-labile t. (LT)
industrial t.
occupational t.
pertussin t.
secreted autotransporter t.
Shiga t. (Stx)
Shiga-like t. (SLT)
VacA t.

toxin-mediated intestinal secretion
Toxocara canis
toxocariasis
Toxoplasma gondii
toxoplasmosis
TP-400t pressure transducer
TP40 **gene**
TP53 **gene**
Tp53-**mutated carcinoma**
TPA, tPA
12-O-tetradecanoylphorbol-13-acetate
tissue plasminogen activator
phorbol ester TPA
TPD
title peritoneal dialysis
TPH
transrectal prostatic hyperthermia
TPN
total parenteral nutrition
TPN line
TPO
thrombopoietin
T-pouch technique
TPPN
total peripheral parenteral nutrition
tPSA
total PSA
TPSV
tumor peak systolic velocity
TR
terminal repeat
trabecula, pl. trabeculae
trabeculae of corpora cavernosa of penis
trabeculae corporis spongiosi penis
trabeculae corporum cavernosorum penis
trabeculae of corpus spongiosum of penis
trabeculae lienis
trabeculae of spleen
trabeculae splenicae
trabecular
t. bone fracture
t. sinusoidal pattern
t. structure
trabecularism
trabeculate
trabeculated bladder

NOTES

trabeculation
    t. of bladder dome
    detrusor muscle t.
Trabucco double balloon catheter
trace-gas analysis
tracer
    focal accumulation of t.
    t. Hybrid wire guide
    T. ST wire
tracheal
    t. bifurcation
    t. deviation
    t. ulceration
trachelocystitis
tracheobronchial
    t. aspiration
    t. malacia
    t. Z stent
tracheoesophageal (TE)
    t. fistula (TEF)
    t. junction
    t. puncture (TEP)
    t. septum
tracheostomy
Trach-Eze closed suction catheter
trachomatis
    Chlamydia t.
tracing
    Narco Bio-Systems MMS 200 physiograph t.
    sexually transmitted disease contact t.
track
    horseshoe t.
    radial suture t.
    submucosal t.
Tracker catheter
tract
    alimentary t.
    allantoic t.
    benign mesothelioma of genital t.
    biliary t.
    digestive t.
    t. dilation
    double-contrast barium examination of upper gastrointestinal t. (DCGI)
    drilling t.
    fistula t.
    fistulous t.
    gastrocutaneous fistulous t.
    gastrointestinal t. (GIT)
    genital t.
    genitourinary t.
    GI t.
    hepatic outflow t.
    ileal inflow t.
    ileal outflow t.
    infected t.
    intestinal t.
    intramural fistulous t.
    Lewis classification for vascular anomalies of the gastrointestinal t.
    Moore classification for vascular anomalies of gastrointestinal t.
    needle t.
    nephrostomy t.
    nucleus of solitary t.
    ororespiratory t.
    outflow t.
    pancreaticobiliary t.
    perineal sinus t.
    portal t.
    sacrococcygeal pilonidal sinus t.
    safe gastrocutaneous fistulous t.
    sinus t.
    t. tamponade
    transsphincteric fistulous t.
    T-tube t.
    upper gastrointestinal t.
    urinary t.
    Z t.
traction
    caudal t.
    cephalad t.
    t. diverticulum
    enterocele t.
    postinflammatory t.
    t. suture
tractor
    Lowsley t.
    Syms t.
    Young prostatic t.
trafficking
    leukocyte t.
    membrane t.
Trager therapy
Trail-Making Test
Trail test
trainer
    Personal EMG t.
training
    bladder t.
    endourological t.
    pelvic muscle t.
    pubococcygeal muscle t.
trait
    X-linked recessive t.
tramadol
tramazoline
tram-line calcification
Trandate
tranexamic
    t. acid
    t. acid enema
Tranilast
tranquilizer

transabdominal
    t. Burch urethropexy
    t. cholangiography
    t. hydrocolonic sonography
    t. preperitoneal (TAPP)
    t. preperitoneal hernia repair
    t. scan
transactivator
    classical t.
transaminase
    glutamate pyruvate t. (GLPT)
    glutamic-oxaloacetic t. (GOT)
    glutamic-pyruvic t. (GPT)
    serum glutamic-oxaloacetic t. (SGOT)
    serum glutamic-pyruvic t. (SGPT)
transampullary
transanal
    t. anastomosis
    t. catheter
    t. endoscopic microsurgery (TEM)
    t. endoscopic microsurgical resection
    t. excision
    t. ultrasonography
transaortic endarterectomy
transarterial
    t. catheter embolization (TACE)
    t. chemoembolization (TACE)
    t. perfusion cooling
transballoon cystometry
transblotting cell
transcapillary
    t. diffusion
    t. escape rate
    t. hydrostatic pressure gradient
transcarbamylase
    heterozygous ornithine t. (HOTC)
transcatheter
    t. arterial chemoembolization (TACE)
    t. arterial embolization (TAE)
    t. arterial embolization therapy
    t. arterial infusion
    t. embolotherapy
    t. hepatic arterial embolization
    t. perfusion
    t. splenic arterial embolization (TSAE)
    t. treatment
    t. variceal embolization

transcellular
    t. absorption
    t. pathway
transcoccygeal vesiculectomy
transcolonic endoscopy
transcranial magnetic stimulation (TCMS)
transcriptase
    avian myeloblastosis virus reverse t.
    t. polymerase chain reaction assay
    reverse t. (RT)
transcription
    t. factor
    t. factor AP1
    reverse t.
transcutaneous
    t. biopsy
    t. electrical nerve stimulation (TENS)
    t. nerve
    t. registration
    t. sacral neurostimulation
    t. sonogram endoscope
    t. ultrasonography
    t. ultrasound
    t. ultrasound imaging
transcystic duct/common bile duct exploration (TCD/CBDE)
transdermal
    t. oxybutynin for urinary incontinence
    t. therapeutic system (TTS)
transdermal therapeutic system (TTS)
Transderm-Nitro
transducer
    antral pressure t.
    bifocal multiplane rectal t.
    Bruel-Kjaer axial t.
    t. catheter
    Dantec Etude uroflow t.
    electromagnetic flow t.
    Elema-Siemens AB pressure t.
    external pressure t.
    GF-UM2 radial-sector scan t.
    GF-UM3 radial-sector scan t.
    GF-UM20 radial-sector scan t.
    Gould pressure t.
    intracavitary t.
    linear-array t.
    LSC 7000 curved-array t.
    3.5–10 MHz curved-array t.

NOTES

transducer *(continued)*
    35-MHz linear-array t.
    Nellcor Durasensor adult oxygen t.
    Olympus intracavity t.
    P23b Statham pressure t.
    piezoelectric t.
    pressure t.
    Sensor Medics pressure t.
    Siemens Endo-P endodrectal t.
    solid-state pressure t.
    Soreson pressure t.
    Spectramed t.
    Statham external t.
    strain gauge t.
    TP-400t pressure t.
    transrectal multiplane three-dimensional t.
    ultrasound t.
    Unisensor strain-gauge t.
    volume displacement t.

transduction
    downstream signal t.
    t. pathway
    receptor and signal t.

transduodenal
    t. approach
    t. drainage
    t. endoscopic decompression
    t. injection
    t. sphincteroplasty
    t. sphincterotomy

transection
    bladder t.
    t. and devascularization operation
    esophageal t.
    high t.
    Sugiura esophageal variceal t.

transendoscopic
    t. electrocoagulation
    t. laser photocoagulation
    t. sphincterotomy
    t. ultrasound

transepithelial tubular transport

transesophageal
    t. endoscopy
    t. ligation
    t. ligation of varix

transfected
    cell t.

transfemoral liver biopsy

transfer
    t. dysfunction
    t. dysphagia
    t. factor
    gamete intrafallopian t. (GIFT)
    unidirectional t.

transferase
    aspartate t.
    glucuronyl t.
    glutathione t.
    phenylethylamine N-methyl t. (PNMT)

transferrin
    t. receptor (TfR)
    t. saturation
    t. saturation level
    serum t.
    t. test

transformary mass

transformation
    blastoid t.
    Eadie-Hofstee t.
    giant cell t. (GCT)
    neoplastic t.
    nodular t.
    t. zone

transforming
    t. growth factor (TGF)
    t. growth factor alpha (TGF-alpha)
    t. growth factor beta (TGF-beta)
    t. growth factor beta-1 (TGF-beta-1)
    t. growth factor beta-2 (TGF-beta-2)
    t. growth factor beta-3 (TGF-beta-3)

transfuse

transfusion
    autologous t.
    blood t.
    donor-specific t. (DST)
    t. hepatitis
    intraoperative autologous t.
    t. nephritis
    peritoneal t.
    platelet t.
    postoperative autologous t.
    required t.
    type-specific blood t.

transfusional iron overload
transfusion-associated hepatitis
transfusion-related chronic liver disease
transfusion-transmitted virus (TTV)

transgastric
    t. cholangiogram
    t. drainage
    t. esophageal bougienage
    t. fine-needle aspiration biopsy
    t. ligation
    t. plication

transgastrostomic enteroscopy (TGE)
transgastrostomy

transgenesis
    mammalian t.

transglomerular hydrostatic filtration pressure

transglutaminase
    tissue t. (tTG)

trans-Golgi network
transhepatic
- t. antegrade biliary drainage procedure
- t. biliary drainage
- t. biliary stent
- t. catheterization
- t. cholangiogram
- t. cholangiography (TC, THC)
- t. embolization (THE)
- t. portacaval shunt
- t. portal venous sampling
- t. portography
- t. vascular resistance

transhiatal
- t. blunt esophagectomy
- t. radical esophagectomy
- t. resection
- t. simple esophagectomy

transient
- t. cholangitis
- t. discontinuation
- t. gastroparesis
- t. LES relaxation
- t. lower esophageal sphincter relaxation (TLESR)
- t. proteinuria
- t. relaxation of LES

transileostomy manometry
transilluminate
transillumination
- kidney t.

transilluminator
- UV t.

transistor
- ion-sensitive field-effect t.

transit
- delayed colonic t.
- gastrointestinal t.
- ileocolonic t.
- mean colonic t. (MCT)
- slow colonic t.
- t. time (TT)
- whole-gut t.

transition
- t. mutation
- t. suture
- t. zone index
- t. zone volume

transitional
- t. cell
- t. cell cancer-associated (TCCA)
- t. cell carcinoma
- t. cell carcinoma of bladder (TCCB)
- t. epithelium
- t. feeding
- t. zone
- t. zone biopsy

transitory block
transjugular
- t. intrahepatic portacaval shunt procedure
- t. intrahepatic portosystemic shunt (TIPS)
- t. intrahepatic portosystemic stent shunt (TIPSS)
- t. liver biopsy
- t. portal venography

translation of torque
translumbar inferior vena cava catheter
transluminal
- t. pseudocyst drainage
- t. ultrasonography

transmembrane
- t. beta-subunit
- t. electrical potential difference
- t. hydraulic pressure
- t. protein
- t. signal

transmesenteric plication
transmission
- bloodborne t.
- t. electron microscopy (TEM)
- fecal t.
- fecal-oral t.
- horizontal t.
- oral t.
- real-time t. (RTX)
- synaptic t.
- vertical t.

transmittable disease
transmitter
- NANC inhibitory t.
- nonadrenergic noncholinergic inhibitory t.
- putative t.

transmucosal
- t. electrical potential test
- t. potential difference (TMPD)

transmural
- t. approach
- t. burn
- t. colitis

NOTES

transmural *(continued)*
- t. drainage (TMD)
- t. endoscopy
- t. fibrosis
- t. hydrostatic pressure gradient
- t. ileocolitis
- t. inflammation
- t. rejection

transnasal
- t. bile duct catheterization
- t. endoluminal ultrasonography
- t. pancreaticobiliary drain
- t. videogastroscope

Transonics
- T. laser-Doppler flowmeter
- T. Systems flow probe

transoral endoscopic suturing

transpancreatic sphincter precut approach to biliary sphincterotomy

transpapillary
- t. approach
- t. biopsy
- t. cannulation
- t. catheterization
- t. cystopancreatic stent
- t. drain
- t. drainage
- t. endoscopic cholecystotomy (TEC)
- t. endoscopic endoprosthesis
- t. insertion of self-expanding biliary metal stent
- t. therapy

transparent elastic band ligating device

transpeptidase
- gamma-glutamyl t. (GGTP)
- glutamyl t. (GTP)

transperineal
- t. interstitial permanent prostate brachytherapy (TIPPB)
- t. palladium-103
- t. seed implant
- t. ultrasonography
- t. ultrasonography technique
- t. ultrasound-guided template biopsy
- t. vesiculectomy

transperitoneal
- t. anterior subcostal incision (TASI)
- t. laparoscopic adrenalectomy (TLA)
- t. laparoscopic nephrectomy (TLN)
- t. laparoscopic nephroureterectomy

transplant
- acute rejection of liver t.
- allogenic kidney t.
- auxiliary t.
- cadaveric intestinal t.
- cadaveric renal t.
- combined kidney and pancreas t. (CKPT)
- t. consideration
- Domino t.
- failed t.
- Gallie t.
- heart t.
- heart-kidney t.
- hypercholesterolemic cadaveric renal t.
- kidney t.
- liver t.
- living donor t.
- t. nephrectomy
- orthotopic liver t. (OLT)
- pancreas-kidney t.
- reduced liver t. (RLT)
- reduced-size liver t. (RSLT)
- t. rejection
- renal t.
- t. renal artery stenosis (TRAS)
- simultaneous pancreas and kidney t.
- split-liver t.

transplantation
- ABO-incompatible living donor kidney t.
- anhepatic stage of liver t.
- t. antigen
- auxiliary heterotopic liver t. (AHLT)
- auxiliary partial orthotopic liver t. (APOLT)
- auxiliary partial orthotopic living donor t.
- bone marrow t. (BMT)
- cadaveric renal t.
- chronic rejection after renal t.
- en bloc kidney t.
- future role of target of rapamycin inhibitors in renal t.
- heart t.
- hematopoietic cell t.
- hepatocyte t.
- infection after renal t.
- kidney t.
- liver t.
- living donor liver t. (LDLT)
- nonmyeloablative allogeneic peripheral blood stem cell t.
- organ t.
- pancreas t.
- pancreatic islet cell t.
- pancreaticoduodenal t.
- piggyback liver t.
- renal t.
- small bowel t.
- SPK t.
- split-liver t.

t. tolerance
warrant t.
xenograft t.
transplantectomy
transplanted cancer
Transpore tape
transport
    active t.
    t. aminoaciduria
    bolus t.
    cation t.
    chyme t.
    conditions of impaired sodium t.
    convective t.
    diffusive t.
    fluid t.
    glucose t.
    lymphatic t.
    nephron t.
    peritoneal membrane t.
    peritoneal solute t.
    retinoid t.
    single-nephron glomerular t.
    sodium t.
    solute t.
    transepithelial tubular t.
    urine t.
transporter
    glucose t.
    low-affinity t.
    multispecific organic anion t.
    polarized glucose t.
    putative anion t. (PAT1)
    serotonin reuptake t. (SERT)
transporterlike
    zinc-iron regulated t. (ZIRTL)
transposition
    buttonhole preputial t.
    gastric t.
    gluteus maximus t.
    ileocecal segment t.
    penoscrotal t.
    portacaval t. (PCT)
transpubic incision
transpyloric
    t. feeding
    t. tube
transrectal
    t. multiplane three-dimensional transducer
    t. probe
    t. prostatic hyperthermia (TPH)
    t. prostatic ultrasonography
    t. scan
    t. sonography
    t. ultrasonography (TRUS)
    t. ultrasonography-guided biopsy
    t. ultrasound (TRUS)
    t. ultrasound-guided sextant biopsy
    t. ultrasound scanning (TRUS)
    t. ultrasound staging
    t. vasography
transscrotal
transsection
    nerve t.
transseptal orchiopexy
transsexual surgery
transsphincteric
    t. anal fistula
    t. fistulous tract
transthoracic
    t. esophagectomy
    t. resection of esophageal carcinoma
transthyretin
transtubular potassium gradient (TTKG)
transudative ascites
transureteral endoscopic manipulation
transureteropyelostomy
transureteroureteral anastomosis
transureteroureterostomy (TUU)
transurethral
    t. ablative prostatectomy
    t. balloon dilation
    t. balloon laserthermia prostatectomy
    t. catheter
    t. collagen injection therapy
    t. electrical bladder stimulation (TEBS)
    t. electrovaporization
    t. electrovaporization of prostate (TUVP, TVP)
    t. evaporation of prostate (TUEP)
    t. grooving of prostate
    t. hot-water balloon thermoablation
    t. incision (TUI)
    t. incision of bladder neck (TUIBN)
    t. incision of prostate (TUIP)
    t. laser incision of prostate
    t. microwave thermotherapy (TUMT)

NOTES

transurethral *(continued)*
    t. microwave thermotherapy functional result
    t. needle ablation (TUNA)
    t. needle ablation of prostate
    t. prostatic resection study
    t. rectal ultrasound
    t. resection (TUR)
    t. resection of bladder tumor (TURBT)
    t. resection of prostate (TURP)
    t. resection of prostate functional result
    t. resection syndrome
    t. resectoscope
    t. sphincterotomy
    t. ultrasound-guided laser-induced prostatectomy (TULIP)
    t. unroofing
    t. ureterorenoscopy (URS)
    t. vaporization of prostate (TUVP)
    t. vaporization-resection of prostate (TUVRP)

transvaginal
    t. bone anchor
    t. Burch procedure
    t. mesh cystocele repair
    t. sacrospinous colpopexy
    t. suturing (TVS)
    t. suturing system
    t. therapy
    t. trocar
    t. ultrasound (TVUS)
    t. urethrolysis

transvenous
    t. liver biopsy
    t. perfusion

transversa
    plica vesicalis t.

transversalis fascia

transverse
    t. abdominis muscle
    t. colectomy
    t. colon
    t. colostomy
    t. colostomy effluent
    t. duodenotomy
    t. fissure
    t. folds of rectum
    t. image
    t. loop
    t. process
    t. resection
    t. retubularized ileovesicostomy
    t. retubularized sigmoidovesicostomy
    t. retubularized sigmoidovesicostomy continent urinary diversion to umbilicus
    t. semilunar skin incision
    t. sonogram
    t. testicular ectopia
    t. ulceration
    t. umbilical line
    t. vaginal septum
    t. view

transverse-loop rod colostomy
transversion mutation
transversostomy
transversourethralis
transversum
    colon t.

transversus
    t. abdominis muscle
    t. perinei muscle

transvesical
    t. laparoscopic approach
    t. laparoscopic detachment
    t. potassium sensitivity test
    t. scan
    t. vesiculectomy

transwell
    cell culture t.

Tranxene
tranylcypromine
trap
    Endodynamics suction polyp t.
    specimen t.

trapezoid method
trapped
    t. basket
    t. penis
    t. penis after circumcision
    t. prostate gland

trapping
    penoscrotal t.

TRAS
    transplant renal artery stenosis

Tratner catheter
Traube semilunar space
trauma
    autoerotic rectal t.
    bile duct t.
    birth t.
    bladder t.
    blunt abdominal t.
    blunt liver t.
    blunt pancreatic t.
    colonic t.
    colorectal t.
    diaphragmatic hernia t.
    duodenal t.
    esophageal t.
    external t.
    foreign body t.
    functional t.
    gallbladder t.
    t. of gallbladder
    gastric t.

trauma · treatment

hepatic t.
homosexual rectal t.
iatrogenic pancreatic t.
liver t.
management of adult urinary tract t.
pancreatic t.
penetrating abdominal t.
penetrating pancreatic t.
perineal impact t.
rectal t.
renal t.
scrotal t.
small intestine t.
splenic t.
Texas t.

TraumaCal enteral feeding
Traum-Aid HBC enteral feeding
traumatic
t. appendicitis
t. corporeal venoocclusive dysfunction
t. diaphragmatic hernia
t. grasping forceps
t. inflammation
t. lesion
t. locking grasper
t. masturbation
t. orchitis
t. proctitis
t. renal mass
t. rupture

Travamulsion fat emulsion solution
Travasol amino acid
Travasorb
T. Hepatic Diet
T. HN powdered feeding
T. MCT liquid feeding
T. MCT supplement
T. Renal Diet
T. STD liquid feeding

traveler
t. chemoprophylaxis
t. diarrhea

Traverso-Longmire technique
tray
Urine Meter Foley t.

trazodone
TRE
thyroid hormone response element
treated tissue
treating physician

treatment
acorn t.
add-back t.
adjuvant t.
alpha-blocker t.
alpha interferon t.
alternate-day t.
amoxicillin-omeprazole t.
anabolic steroid t.
anoplasty t.
anti-*Helicobacter pylori* t.
antihypertensive t.
t. balloon
behavioral t.
t. of bladder cancer
BrachySeed prostate cancer t.
Candida t.
t. channel
cholecystectomy t.
chronic anoplasty t.
conventional t.
corticosteroid t.
CyPat t.
dialytic t.
downregulation after furosemide t.
endoscopic t.
endovascular t.
esophageal dilation t.
t. failure
famotidine maintenance t.
first-line t.
fixed and dynamic urethral compression t.
foscarnet t.
Gelfoam particle transarterial embolization t.
glucocorticoid t.
hemangioma laser t.
Hypertension Optimal T. (HOT)
initial t.
interferon t.
intracavernosal injection t.
intralesional t.
intraprostatic temperature-guided t.
KTP/Nd:YAG laser t.
lipiodol transarterial embolization t.
lower energy t.
maintenance t.
mercury bougienage t.
microwave nonsurgical t.
Milligan-Morgan technique for hemorrhoid t.

NOTES

treatment *(continued)*
    minimally invasive t.
    mitomycin transarterial
      embolization t.
    t. morbidity
    Murphy t.
    neoadjuvant antiandrogenic t.
    t. of neurogenic refractory urge
    t. of nonspecific inflammatory
      injury
    Ochsner t.
    T. Options for Type 2 Diabetes in
      Adolescents and Youths
      (TODAY)
    oxandrolone t.
    pharmacological t.
    photocoagulation t.
    Plummer t.
    preoperative tumor t.
    prophylactic antibiotic t. (PAT)
    ProstaLund feedback t.
    prostatic thermal t.
    ProstRcision t.
    t. protocol
    rectovaginal surgical t.
    t. of renal calculus
    t. of rhabdomyosarcoma
    self-bougienage t.
    serotonin antagonist t.
    sham t.
    shock wave t.
    sonographic planning of
      oncology t. (SPOT)
    success of surgical t.
    supportive t.
    suppression t.
    topical t.
    transcatheter t.
    t. with rapamycin
tree
    biliary t.
    cannulation of biliary t.
    Croton lechleri t.
    hepatobiliary t.
    pancreatic t.
    pancreaticobiliary t.
    phylogenetic t.
trefoil
    t. deformity
    t. domain
    t. factor
    t. factor family (TFF)
    t. peptide
trehalose
Treitz
    T. arch
    T. fossa
    T. hernia
    ligament of T.

Trélat stool
Trelex mesh
Trelstar
    T. Depot
    T. LA
tremor
    resting t.
tremor-nystagmus-ulcer syndrome
trench nephritis
Trendelenburg
    T. gait
    T. position
Trental
trephine biopsy
Treponema
    T. immunofluorescence study
    T. pallidum
tretinoin
Treves
    T. fold
    plane of T.
Trexall
TRI
    intracytoplasmic tuboreticular inclusion
    tubuloreticular inclusion
triad
    t. of adenoma sebaceum, epilepsy,
      and mental retardation
    Andersen t.
    Borchardt t.
    Charcot t.
    Currarino t.
    Dieulafoy t.
    hepatic t.
    portal t.
    Quincke t.
    radiographic t.
    t. of Rigler
    St. t.
    t. syndrome
    Whipple t.
triaditis
    portal t.
trial
    T. AG
    aggressive therapeutic t.
    AIPRI t.
    Angiotensin-Converting Enzyme
      Inhibition in Progressive Renal
      Insufficiency t.
    T. Antacid
    Antihypertensive and Lipid-
      Lowering Treatment to Prevent
      Heart Attack T. (ALLHAT)
    Antioxidant Polyp Prevention T.
    calcitriol t.
    cisapride-functional dyspepsia t.
    clinical t.
    direct-current electrotherapy t.

domperidone-functional dyspepsia t.
HOT t.
Hypertension Optimal Treatment t.
IRS-IV t.
Medical Therapy of Prostatic Symptoms t.
Modification of Diet in Renal Disease t.
MTOPS t.
multicenter prospective t.
placebo-controlled t.
prospective clinical t.
prospective multicenter randomized t.
prospective randomized controlled t.
Prostate Cancer Intervention Versus Observation T. (PCIVOT, PIVOT)
published comparative t.
recent clinical t.
Stockholm t. I, II
Swedish Rectal Cancer T.
T. Using Medicinal Microbiotic Yogurt (TUMMY)
VIGOR t.
Vioxx Gastrointestinal Outcomes Research t.
t. without catheter (TWOC)

triamcinolone cream
Triamonide 40
triamterene
    t. calculus
    hydrochlorothiazide and t.
    t. urolithiasis

triangle
    anal t.
    Calot t.
    cardiohepatic t.
    Charcot t.
    cystohepatic t.
    digastric t.
    t. of doom
    femoral t.
    gastrinoma t.
    T. gelatin-sealed sling material
    Grynfeltt t.
    Henke t.
    Hesselbach t.
    inguinal t.
    Killian t.
    Labbe t.
    Lesgaft t.
    Livingston t.
    lumbocostoabdominal t.
    mesenteric t.
    t. of pain
    Petit t.
    Scarpa t.
    urogenital t.

triangle-tipped knife
triangular
    t. ligament
    t. vaginal patch sling

triangulation stapling method
triazolam
tricarboxylic
    t. acid (TCA)
    t. acid cycle

triceps
    t. skinfold thickness
    t. skinfold thickness test

trichilemmoma
Trichinella
    T. paupae
    T. pseudospiralis
    T. spiralis

trichinosis, trichinelliasis, trichinellosis, trichiniasis
trichiura
    Trichuris t.

trichlormethiazide
trichloroacetic acid (TCA)
trichloroethylene
trichobezoar
trichocyst
trichomonal balanitis
Trichomonas
    T. hominis
    T. vaginalis

trichomoniasis
    vaginal t.

trichomycosis
trichophagia
trichophytobezoar
Trichophyton
    T. mentagrophytes
    T. rubrum

Trichosporon
    T. beigelli
    T. capitatum

Trichostrongylus
trichrome
    Masson t.
    t. stain

trichuriasis

NOTES

Trichuris
    T. muris
    T. trichiura
tricitrate
trickle perfusion
TriClip endoscopic clipping device
triclosan 0.1%
Tricomponent Coaxial System (TCS)
tricyclamol
tricyclic antidepressant
tridecapeptide
tridihexethyl chloride
Tridrate bowel preparation
triene
    macrocyclic t.
triethylenethiophosphoramide
trifid stomach
trifluoperazine
triflupromazine
trifurcation variant
trigeminy
Trigesic
trigger
    t. point injection
    rectal feedback t.
    urethral feedback t.
    t. voiding
triggering
    R-wave t.
triglyceride
    t. enzyme deficiency
    long-chain t. (LCT)
    medium-chain t. (MCT)
    serum t.
    VLDL t.
triglyceride-rich lipoprotein (TRL)
triglyceride-rich protein
trigona (*pl. of* trigonum)
trigonal plate
trigone
    bladder t.
    deep t.
    fascia of urogenital t.
trigonitis
trigonotome
trigonum, pl. **trigona**
    t. urogenitale
    t. vesicae
    t. vesicae lieutaudi
trihexyphenidyL
trihydrate
    amoxicillin t.
trihydrocoprostanic acid (TCA)
trihydroxy salt
triiodobenzene
Trilafon
trilobar
    t. hyperplasia
    t. hypertrophy

Trilogy low-profile balloon dilatation catheter
Tri-Lyte
Trimadeau sign
Trimazide
Trimedyne
    T. Flex MAX fiber
    T. holmium laser
    T. Optilase 1000 device
trimeprazine tartrate
trimer
trimetaphan
trimethidinium
trimethobenzamide
trimethoprim
    sulfamethoxazole and t. (SMX/TMP)
trimethoprim-sulfamethoxazole (TMP-SMX, SMX/TMP)
    t.-s. DS
trimethylsilyl ether
trimetrexate glucuronate
Trimox
Trimpex
Trinalin Repetabs
trinitrate
    glyceryl t. (GTN)
Trinovin
Trinsicon
triolein C-14 breath test
triopathy
trioxide
    antimony t.
tripelennamine
tripeptide
    disaccharide t.
triphasic cystometric curve
triphosphatase
    adenosine t. (ATPase)
    hydrogen adenosine t.
triphosphate
    adenosine t. (ATP)
    guanosine t. (GTP)
    inositol t.
    terminal deoxynucleotide transferase-mediated deoxyuridine t.
1,4,5-triphosphate
    inositol 1,4,5-t. (IP3)
triple
    t. eradication therapy
    t. intussusception
    t. rubber band ligation
    t. therapy (TT)
triple-balloon probe
triple-lobe hepatectomy
triple-loop pouch
triple-lumen
    t.-l. manometry catheter

t.-l. perfused catheter system
t.-l. Sengstaken-Blakemore tube
triple-phosphate crystal
triplet
neurofilament protein t.
triple-voiding cystography
triplication
triploid cell
tripod
t. grasper
t. grasping forceps
triprolidine
triptorelin pamoate for injectable suspension
trip wire
triradiate cecal fold
trisegmentectomy
Tris HCl
tris(hydroxymethyl)aminomethane
trisilicate
aluminum hydroxide and magnesium t.
magnesium t.
trismus presentation
trisodium
mangafodipir t.
trisomy 13, 18, 21
Tritec
Triton tumor
TRL
triglyceride-rich lipoprotein
trocar
accessory t.
Beardsley cecostomy t.
Campbell t.
conical t.
Cook urological t.
t. cystostomy
disposable t.
ensheathing t.
Ethicon t.
gallbladder t.
Hasson t.
Landau t.
Ochsner gallbladder t.
Origin t.
pyramidal t.
transvaginal t.
trochanter
troglitazone
Troisier
T. ganglion

T. node
T. sign
troleandomycin
Trombovar
tromethamine
carboprost t.
fosfomycin t.
ketorolac t.
Tronolane
Tropheryma whipplei
trophic
t. change
t. lesion
trophoblastic
t. malignant teratoma
malignant teratoma, t. (MTT)
trophozoite form
tropical
t. calcific pancreatitis
t. diarrhea
t. diarrhea-malabsorption syndrome (TDMS)
t. hyphema
t. mesangiocapillary glomerulonephritis
t. nephropathy
t. spastic paraparesis
t. splenomegaly
t. sprue
tropicalis
Candida t.
tropomyosin
troponin
baseline t. T
trospium hydrochloride
trota
Aeromonas t.
Trousseau
T. esophageal bougie
T. syndrome
T. test
Troutman rectus forceps
trovafloxacin
Trovan/Zithromax Compliance Pak
TRPM-2
testosterone-repressed prostate message-2
Tru-Cut
T.-C. biopsy needle
T.-C. needle biopsy
Truelove-Witts
T.-W. grading system
T.-W. index

NOTES

trumpet
    nasal t.
truncal
    t. vagotomy
    t. vagotomy and gastroenterostomy
    t. vagotomy and pyloroplasty
truncus, pl. trunci
    t. celiacus
    trunci intestinales
trunk
    bicarotid t.
    celiac t.
    lumbosacral t.
    portal t.
TRUS
    transrectal ultrasonography
    transrectal ultrasound
    transrectal ultrasound scanning
truss
Tru Taper Ethalloy needle
Trypan blue-stained cell
Trypanosoma
    T. congolense
    T. cruzi
    T. rhodesiense
trypanosomiasis
    American t.
    Rhodesian t.
    South American t.
trypsin
    bovine t.
    t. inhibitor
trypsinization
trypsinogen
    t. activation peptide
    immunoreactive t. (IRT)
tryptic soy broth
tryptophan metabolism
TS
    terminal sedation
TS1
    tuberous sclerosis gene TS1
TS2
    tuberous sclerosis gene TS2
TS-200
    tissue spectrum analyzer TS-200
TSAE
    transcatheter splenic arterial embolization
TSC
    tuberous sclerosis complex
TSF
    thickness of skinfold
TSPAP
    total serum prostatic acid phosphatase
TSRPC
    totally stapled restorative proctocolectomy
TSRS
    tissue-stone recognition system

TT
    transit time
    triple therapy
        TT virus (TTV)
TT-3 needle
TTC
    T-tube cholangiogram
tTG
    tissue transglutaminase
        IgA tTG
TTKG
    transtubular potassium gradient
TTL
    total lymphocyte
TTP
    thrombotic thrombocytopenic purpura
TTS
    testosterone transdermal system
    through-the-scope
    transdermal therapeutic system
        TTS balloon dilation
        TTS dilator
        Testoderm TTS
T-tube
    T-t. cholangiogram (TTC)
    T-t. cholangiography
    T-t. drain
    T-t. drainage
    T-t. stent
    T-t. study
    T-t. tract
    T-t. tract choledochofiberoscopy
    T-t. tract choledochoscopy
T-TURP
    total transurethral resection of prostate
TTV
    transfusion-transmitted virus
    TT virus
TTX
    tetrodotoxin
tuaminoheptane
tubal
    t. ectopic pregnancy
    t. infertility
    t. ligation
tube
    Abbott t.
    Abbott-Miller t.
    Abbott-Rawson double-lumen gastrointestinal t.
    Adson suction t.
    All-Silicone Side-Eye EPT feeding t.
    Anderson gastric t.
    Argyle chest t.
    Argyle-Salem sump t.
    ascites drainage t.
    aspiration and dissection t.
    Aspisafe nasogastric t.

Atkinson silicone rubber t.
Axiom double sump t.
Baker intestinal decompression t.
Baker jejunostomy t.
Bard gastrostomy feeding t.
Bard PEG t.
Bilbao-Dotter t.
Blakemore t.
Blakemore-Sengstaken t.
Bower PEG t.
Boyce modification of Sengstaken-Blakemore t.
Broncho-Cath double-lumen endotracheal t.
Buie rectal suction t.
button-type G t.
Caluso PEG gastrostomy t.
Cantor t.
castlike t.
Cattell T t.
t. cecostomy
Celestin esophageal t.
Celestin latex rubber t.
chest t.
COBED t.
collecting t.
conical centrifuge t.
Cope loop nephrostomy t.
Corflo enteral feeding t.
Corflo PEG t.
Corpak feeding t.
Corpak weighted-tip self-lubricating t.
Council-tip t.
cuffed endotracheal t.
cystostomy t.
Davol colon t.
Davol feeding t.
decompression t.
t. decompression
Dennis colorectal t.
Dennis intestinal t.
Diamond t.
digestive t.
direct percutaneous jejunostomy t.
Dobbhoff gastrectomy feeding t.
Dobbhoff gastric decompression t.
Dobbhoff PEG t.
double-lumen t.
DPJ t.
drainage t.
Dreiling t.
dual percutaneous gastrostomy t.
Dumon-Gilliard prosthesis pushing t.
duodenal t.
Duo-Tube feeding t.
Edlich gastric lavage t.
endoscopic gastrostomy t.
endothelial t.
endotracheal t. (ET)
ENDO-Tube nasojejunal feeding t.
t. enlargement
EnteraFlo feeding t.
enteroclysis t.
t. enteroscope
t. enterostomy
EntriStar feeding t.
EntriStar polyurethane PEG t.
Eppendorf t.
esophageal t.
t. esophagogram
Ethox feeding t.
Ewald t.
fallopian t.
t. feeding
feeding gastrostomy t.
Ferrein t.
Flexiflo Inverta-PEG t.
Flexiflo stoma-creator t.
Flexiflo Stomate low-profile gastrostomy t.
Flexiflo tungsten weighted feeding t.
Flexiflo Versa-PEG t.
Flow-Thru feeding t.
four-lumen t.
20F PEG t.
Frazier suction t.
Frederick-Miller t.
French T t.
gastric aspiration t.
gastric augment and single-pedicle t. (GASP)
gastric lavage t.
gastrostomy t.
Gilman-Abrams gastric t.
Glasser gastrostomy t.
Gomco suction t.
Gott t.
t. graft
guttered T t.
Haldane-Priestly t.
Harris t.

NOTES

tube *(continued)*
    Hodge intestinal decompression t.
    insertion t.
    jejunal feeding t.
    jejunostomy t.
    K t.
    Kangaroo gastrostomy t.
    Kaslow intestinal t.
    Kehr T t.
    Keofeed II feeding t.
    Killian suction t.
    large-bore gastric lavage t.
    t. leakage
    Levin t.
    Linton-Nachlas t.
    long intestinal t.
    Malecot gastrostomy t.
    Malecot nephrostomy t.
    marked t.
    Medena t.
    mediastinal t.
    Medina t.
    Medoc-Celestin pulsion t.
    mercury-weighted t.
    metal-weighted Silastic feeding t.
    MIC gastroenteric t.
    MIC gastrostomy t.
    MIC-Key G gastrostomy t.
    MIC-Key J gastrostomy t.
    MIC-TJ transgastric jejunal t.
    t. migration
    Mikulicz gastrostomy t.
    Miller-Abbott intestinal t.
    Minnesota t.
    Mitrofanoff t.
    modified Minnesota t.
    Montgomery salivary bypass t.
    Moss G t.
    Moss gastrostomy t.
    Moss Mark IV t.
    Mousseau-Barbin prosthetic t.
    myringotomy t.
    Nachlas gastrointestinal t.
    nasobiliary t.
    nasocystic drainage t.
    nasoduodenal feeding t.
    nasoenteric feeding t.
    nasogastric t. (NGT)
    nasogastric feeding t.
    nasoileal t.
    nasojejunal feeding t.
    negative-pressure t.
    negative pressure-controlled t.
    nephrostomy t.
    nephrotomy t.
    NJ feeding t.
    Nuport PEG t.
    Nyhus-Nelson gastric decompression and jejunal feeding t.
    Olympus one-step button gastrostomy t.
    orogastric Ewald t.
    oropharyngeal t.
    t. overgrowth
    Panda gastrostomy feeding t.
    Paul-Mixter t.
    pediatric feeding t.
    pediatric nasogastric t.
    Pedi PEG t.
    Pee Wee low-profile gastrostomy t.
    PEG t.
    PEG-400 t.
    PEJ t.
    percutaneous endoscopic gastrostomy and jejunal extension t. (PEG-JET)
    percutaneous endoscopic placement of jejunal t.
    photomultiplier t.
    pigtail nephrostomy t.
    t. placement
    pleural t.
    polyethylene t.
    Poole suction t.
    postpyloric feeding t.
    Proctor-Livingston t.
    pusher t.
    Quinton t.
    Radius enteral feeding t.
    rectal t.
    Rehfuss duodenal t.
    Rehfuss stomach t.
    t. removal
    t. replacement
    Replogle t.
    Rubin t.
    Rubin-Quinton small bowel biopsy t.
    Ryle t.
    Sacks-Vine feeding gastrostomy t.
    Sacks-Vine PEG t.
    Salem duodenal sump t.
    Salem sump double-lumen polyvinyl t.
    Sandoz Caluso PEG gastrostomy t.
    Sandoz 22F balloon replacement t.
    Sandoz feeding/suction t.
    Schachowa spiral t.
    Sengstaken-Blakemore t.
    Shiner t.
    Silk Bullet feeding t.
    silk jejunal t.
    Silk Pill feeding t.
    Silk Tip feeding t.
    skin t.
    sliding t.
    small bowel t.
    Souttar t.

Stamey t.
Stamm gastrostomy t.
Stay-Put jejunal t.
stiffening t.
stimulated t.
stomach t.
Stomate decompression t.
Stomate extension t.
suction t.
sump nasogastric t.
Super PEG t.
suprapubic t.
T t.
tampon t.
Teflon nasobiliary t.
Thiersch t.
transpyloric t.
triple-lumen Sengstaken-Blakemore t.
Vacutainer t.
venting percutaneous gastrostomy t.
Vivonex Moss t.
Wangensteen suction t.
Willscher t.
Wilson-Cook nasobiliary t.
Wilson-Cook NJFT-series feeding t.
wire-guided J t.
Wookey skin t.
woven Dacron t.
Wurbs-type nasobiliary t.
Yankauer suction t.
Young-Dees t.

tubed
t. free skin graft
t. groin flap
t. urethroplasty

tube-fed patient
tubeless lithotriptor
tubercle
pubic t.

tubercular
t. diarrhea
t. involvement

tuberculin
t. syringe
t. test

tuberculocele
tuberculoid
tuberculoma
cavitating t.

tuberculosis
adrenal t.
bladder t.
colonic t.
duodenal t.
esophageal t.
gastric t.
genital t.
genitourinary t.
ileocecal t.
intestinal t.
t. of kidney and bladder
miliary t.
Mycobacterium t.
penile t.
peritoneal t.
t. polyp
primary t.
prostatic t.
renal t.
segmental colonic t.
t. symptom
testicular t.
ureteral t.
urethral t.

tuberculous
t. colitis
t. enteritis
t. gastritis
t. ileocolitis
t. infectious esophagitis
t. nephritis
t. peritonitis
t. prostatitis

tuberosity
ischial t.
omental t.

tuberous
t. sclerosis
t. sclerosis angiomyolipoma
t. sclerosis complex (TSC)
t. sclerosis gene TS1
t. sclerosis gene TS2

tube-within-tube technique
tubi (*pl. of* tubus)
tubing
t. clamp
large-bore Tygon t.
Nu-Hope t.
polyvinyl t.
shunt t.
Sur-Fit Natura night drainage container t.

NOTES

tubing *(continued)*
    Tygon venovenous bypass t.
    Y-connecting t.

tubogram
    T t.

tubular
    t. adenoma of Pick
    t. atrophy
    t. basement membrane (TBM)
    t. carcinoma
    t. cell desquamation
    t. cell dysfunction
    t. colonic duplication
    t. damage
    t. diuresis
    t. epithelial cell
    t. epithelial cell injury
    t. excretory mass
    t. fluid flow
    t. fluid:ultrafiltrate (TF/UF)
    t. iron accumulation
    t. ischemia
    t. maximal (Tm)
    t. morphologic injury
    t. narrowing and sacculation
    t. necrosis
    t. nephropathy
    t. obstruction
    t. polyp
    t. proteinuria
    t. reabsorption of phosphate test
    t. reabsorption of phosphorus
    t. regeneration
    t. resorption
    t. sodium handling
    t. sodium reabsorption
    t. stenosis
    t. vertical gastroplasty

tubularization
    bladder neck t.
    Thiersch-Duplay t.

tubularized
    t. bladder neck reconstruction
    t. cecal flap
    t. incised plate urethroplasty

tubule
    Albarran t.
    Bellini t.
    collecting t.
    connecting t.
    cortical collecting t.
    distal t. (DT)
    distal convoluted t. (DCT)
    epididymal t.
    epithelium-lined t.
    Ferrein t.
    Henle t.
    human proximal t. (HPT)
    immunostaining of transversely sectioned t.
    isolated cortical t. (ICT)
    lumen of seminiferous t.
    mesonephric t.
    metanephric t.
    nonischemic t.
    proximal convoluted t. (PCT)
    proximal straight t. (PST)
    renal t.
    seminiferous t.
    sex cord tumors with annular t.'s (SCTAT)
    testicular t.
    urine-collecting t.
    uriniferous t.
    uriniparous t.

tubuli *(pl. of* tubulus*)*

tubulin

tubulitis
    mild t.

tubulocystic

tubulogenesis
    vitronectin-inhibiting HGF-induced t.

tubulogenic

tubuloglomerular
    t. feedback (TGF)
    t. feedback mechanism

tubulointerstitial (TI)
    t. disease
    t. fibrosis
    t. inflammation
    t. injury
    t. nephritis (TIN)
    t. nephritis and uveitis (TINU)
    t. nephritis and uveitis syndrome
    t. nephropathy
    t. rejection

tubulointerstitium

tubulopathy
    cyclosporine t.

tubuloreticular inclusion (TRI)

tubulorrhexis

tubulosaccular

tubulotoxic effect

tubulous

tubulovesicle

tubulovillar lesion

tubulovillous
    t. adenoma
    t. polyp

tubulus, pl. **tubuli**

tubus, pl. **tubi**
    t. digestorius

tuck
    dorsal tunical t.
    T.'s ointment

Tucker
    T. esophagoscope
    T. spindle-shaped dilator
TUEP
    transurethral evaporation of prostate
Tuffier
    T. abdominal retractor
    T. abdominal spatula
    T. operation
tuft
    t. adhesion
    glomerular t.
    sclerotic t.
    vascular t.
tufting disease
TUI
    transurethral incision
TUIBN
    transurethral incision of bladder neck
TUIP
    transurethral incision of prostate
Tukey test
TULIP
    transurethral ultrasound-guided laser-induced prostatectomy
tulip tip
tumefaction
    mesenteric t.
tumescence
    t. monitoring
    nocturnal penile t. (NPT)
tumeur pileuse
TUMMY
    Trial Using Medicinal Microbiotic Yogurt
tumor
    abdominal desmoid t.
    t. ablation
    Abrikosov t.
    adenomatoid t.
    adnexal t.
    adrenal cortex estrogen-secreting t.
    adrenal cortex testosterone-secreting t.
    adrenal gland metastatic t.
    adrenal rest t.
    alcohol injection of t.
    ampullary t.
    anaplastic Wilms t.
    t. angiogenesis
    angiomatoid t.
    benign t.
    bifurcation t.
    bilateral renal t.
    bilateral Wilms t.
    biliary tract t.
    bismuth t.
    bladder t. (BT)
    bladder nonepithelial t.
    bladder yolk sac t.
    bleeding t.
    Bolande t.
    brain t.
    branch duct-type t.
    Brenner t.
    burned-out t.
    Buschke-Löwenstein t.
    t. cachexia
    carcinoid t.
    Castleman t.
    celiac t.
    t. cell
    t. cell lysis
    chemotherapy of primary t.
    chromophobe cell t.
    colorectal t.
    core of t.
    cystic Wilms t.
    t. debulking
    depressed t.
    dermatological t.
    desmoid t.
    diagnosis of testicular t.
    diploid t.
    t. displacement
    ductectatic t.
    duodenal t.
    embryonal t.
    encapsulated carcinoid t.
    t. encapsulation
    enterochromaffin-like gastric carcinoid t. (ECLoma)
    epithelial t.
    esophageal t.
    extracapsular t.
    fecal t.
    focal t.
    t. focus
    focus of t.
    gastric carcinoid t.
    gastrin-secreting non beta islet cell t.
    gastroenteropancreatic t.
    gastrointestinal autonomic nerve t.

NOTES

tumor *(continued)*
- gastrointestinal stromal t. (GIST)
- germ cell t.
- gestational trophoblastic t. (GTT)
- glomus t.
- glycoprotein-producing t.
- t. grade
- t. grading
- granular cell t. (GCT)
- granulosa cell t.
- granulosa-theca cell t.
- Grawitz t.
- gritty t.
- hepatic t.
- high-grade t.
- histopathologic nature of t.
- hypersecreting t.
- t. infiltration
- ingrowth of t.
- internist t.
- interstitial cell t. of testis
- intraabdominal desmoid t.
- intractable t.
- intraductal mucin-producing t.
- intraductal papillary t. (IPT)
- intraductal papillary and mucinous t.'s
- intraductal papillary-mucinous t. (IPMT)
- intramesenteric desmoid t.
- intraparenchymal t.
- islet cell t.
- juxtaglomerular apparatus t.
- kidney ossifying t.
- Klatskin t.
- Krukenberg t.
- Leydig cell t.
- t. location
- luteinized granulosa-theca cell t.
- lymphoid t.
- t. lysis syndrome
- malignant mesenchymal t.
- t. marker
- MCF-7 t.
- mediastinal t.
- mediastinum germ cell t.
- metachronous t.
- mixed germ cell t.
- mixed germ cell-sex cord stromal t.
- mucin-hypersecreting t.
- mucinous cystic t.
- mucinous pancreatic t.
- mucin-producing t.
- multifocal bladder t.
- myogenic t.
- t. necrosis
- t. necrosis factor (TNF)
- t. necrosis factor alpha (TNF-alpha)
- t. necrosis factor-alpha assay
- neuroendocrine t. (NET)
- neurogenic t.
- 4-nitroquinolin-1-oxide-induced t. (4NOQ)
- t., nodes, metastases (TNM)
- nonaneuploid t.
- non-B islet cell t.
- nonfunctional pituitary t.
- noninvasive t.
- nonsecreting pituitary t.
- nonseminomatous germ cell t. (NSGCT)
- notification of t.
- null cell t.
- t. overgrowth
- pancreatic islet cell t.
- pancreatic polypeptide-secreting t. (PPoma)
- paratesticular t.
- paraumbilical vein t. (PUVT)
- parenchymal t.
- t. peak systolic velocity (TPSV)
- periampullary duodenal t.
- persistent postmolar gestational trophoblastic t.
- pituitary t.
- polypoid t.
- prepubertal testicular t. (PPTT)
- presacral t.
- primary staging of testicular t.
- primitive neuroectodermal t. (PNET)
- t. probe
- t. proliferative index
- rectal carcinoid t. (RCT)
- rectal myogenic t.
- renin-secreting juxtaglomerular cell t.
- retroperitoneal t.
- rhabdoid Wilms t.
- ruptured hepatic t.
- sacrococcygeal region germ cell t.
- secondary t.
- t. seeding
- semipedunculated t.
- Sertoli cell t.
- sex cord-mesenchyme t.
- shaggy t.
- small-cell t.
- solid t.
- t. spillage
- t. stage
- t. staging
- t. stenting
- superficial bladder t.
- t. suppressor gene
- t. suppressor gene therapy
- thrombus t.

tongue of t.
transurethral resection of bladder t. (TURBT)
Triton t.
upper GI submucosal t.
upper tract urothelial t.
ureteral t.
urethral t.
urothelial t.
t. vaccine
various types of malignant t.'s
vasoactive intestinal peptide-secreting t. (VIPoma, vipoma)
vasoactive intestinal polypeptide t. (VIPoma, vipoma)
villous t.
virilizing t.
von Recklinghausen t.
Wilms t.
yolk sac t.
Zollinger-Ellison t.

tumoral calcinosis
tumor-associated antigen (TAA)
tumor-bearing segment
tumor-derived angiogenic inhibitor
tumorigenesis
t. activity
colorectal t.
tumorigenic
tumor-infiltrating lymphocyte (TIL)
tumorlet
Wilms t.
tumorous
t. epithelium
t. pseudopodia
tumor-rejection antigen
Tums
TUMT
transurethral microwave thermotherapy
cooled catheter TUMT
TUMT functional result
high-energy TUMT
low-energy TUMT
30-minute TUMT
TUNA
transurethral needle ablation
tunable
t. dye laser lithotripsy
t. pulsed-dye laser
TUNEL
terminal uridine deoxynucleotide nick-end labeling

tunic
t. cyst
epididymal t.
fibrous t.
mucous t.
muscular t.
pharyngeal t.
pharyngobasilar t.
proper t.
t. of spermatic cord

tunica
t. adventitia
t. albuginea
t. albuginea corporis spongiosi
t. albuginea corporum cavernosorum
t. albuginea cyst
t. albuginea ovarii
t. albuginea plication
t. albuginea testis
t. fibrosa
t. mucosa
t. muscularis
t. propria
t. replacement
t. serosa
t. spongiosa urethrae feminae
t. vaginalis blanket wrap
t. vaginalis testis
t. vasculosa

tunnel
t. creation
t. disease
extravesical seromuscular t.
t. infection
retropancreatic t.
subserous t.
ureteral t.
t. vision
Witzel feeding jejunostomy t.

tunneled
t. technique
t. technique urinary diversion

tunneler
Davol t.

Tuohy-Borst
T.-B. adapter
T.-B. connector

TUR
transurethral resection
TUR syndrome
videomonitored TUR

Turapy device

turbid
  t. bile
  t. peritoneal fluid
turbidity
  urinalysis t.
  urine t.
turbinate
  swollen t.
turbo spin-echo sequence
TURBT
  transurethral resection of bladder tumor
turbulent flow
Türck zone
Turcot syndrome
TUR-Cue photometer
turgescence
  penile t.
turgor
  skin t.
turista
Turkel punch
turn-and-suction
  t.-a.-s. biopsy technique
  t.-a.-s. method
Turnbull
  T. colostomy
  T. end-loop ileostomy
  T. loop stoma
  T. multiple ostomy operation
  T. technique
Turner
  T. sign
  T. stigma
  T. syndrome
Turner-Warwick
  T.-W. incision
  T.-W. inlay
  T.-W. needle
  T.-W. operation
  T.-W. stone forceps
  T.-W. urethroplasty
TURP
  transurethral resection of prostate
  bipolar TURP
  direct-beam coupler for TURP
  TURP functional result
  split-beam coupler for TURP
turpentine enema
Turrell-Wittner rectal forceps
Tuttle test
TUU
  transureteroureterostomy
TUVP
  transurethral electrovaporization of prostate
  transurethral vaporization of prostate
TUVRP
  transurethral vaporization-resection of prostate

TV
  target volume
TVF
  Thiry-Vella fistula
TVP
  transurethral electrovaporization of prostate
TVS
  transvaginal suturing
    TVS system
TVT
  tension-free vaginal tape
    TVT procedure
TVUS
  transvaginal ultrasound
Tween 20
Twinheads shock wave lithotripter
twin-pulse shock wave release
Twinrix IM injection
twisted beta-pleated sheet fibril
TWOC
  trial without catheter
two-channel endoscope
two-devices-in-one-channel method
two-dimensional flow cytometric analysis
two-field lymphadenectomy
two-finger grip
two-layer
  t.-l. enteroenterostomy
  t.-l. interrupted intestinal anastomosis
  t.-l. latex and Marlex closure technique
  t.-l. open technique
two-loop J-shaped ileal pouch
two-piece ostomy pouch
two-stage
  t.-s. repair
  t.-s. triolein test
two-step
  Aztec t.-s.
  t.-s. orchiopexy
two-tailed
  t.-t. Fisher test
  t.-t. McNemar test
two-wing Malecot drain
TxA2 receptor antagonist
Tycron (*var. of* Ti-Cron)
Tygon venovenous bypass tubing
Tylenol
tylosis
  t. palmaris
  t. palmaris et plantaris
Tylox
tymazoline
tympanites
  false t.
  uterine t.

tympanitic
    t. abdomen
    t. abscess
    t. dullness
    t. resonance
tympany
    abdominal t. (AT)
    t. of stomach
type
    t. A, B antral gastritis
    t. A, B gastritis
    t. 1, 2 autoimmune hepatitis
    biomaterial t.
    blood t.
    t. C cirrhosis
    t. C, D ulcer
    cell t.
    chronic-continuous t.
    t. 2 diabetes mellitus
    diffuse vasculitis of polyarteritis nodosa t.
    DR2 1501 HLA-DRB tissue t.
    DR2 1502 HLA-DRB tissue t.
    DR2 1601 HLA-DRB tissue t.
    DR2 1602 HLA-DRB tissue t.
    DR1 HLA-DRB tissue t.
    DR3 HLA-DRB tissue t.
    DR4 HLA-DRB tissue t.
    DR7 HLA-DRB tissue t.
    DR9 HLA-DRB tissue t.
    DRw8 HLA-DRB tissue t.
    DRw10 HLA-DRB tissue t.
    DRw11 HLA-DRB tissue t.
    DRw12 HLA-DRB tissue t.
    DRw13 HLA-DRB tissue t.
    DRw14 HLA-DRB tissue t.
    t. II cryoglobulinemia
    t. III cholangiocarcinoma
    t. III glycogenosis
    t. I, II pseudohypoaldosteronism
    t. I interferon
    t. I mesangiocapillary glomerulonephritis
    t. IV amyloidosis
    phage t.
    t. 3 serotonin receptor antagonist
    t.'s of stones
    test t.
typed blood
type-specific blood transfusion
typhi
    Salmonella t.
typhimurium
    Salmonella t.
typhlectasis
typhlectomy
typhlitis, typhlenteritis
    neutropenic t.
typhlodicliditis
typhloempyema
typhlolithiasis
typhlomegaly
typhlopexy, typhlopexia
typhlorrhaphy
typhlostenosis
typhlostomy
typhlotomy
typhloureterostomy
typhoid
    abdominal t.
    t. fever
typing
    HLA t.
    HLA-DQ t.
    HLA-DR DNA t.
    molecular t.
tyramine
tyremesis
tyropanoate
    t. contrast medium
    t. sodium
tyrosine
    t. kinase activity
    t. kinase growth-factor receptor peptide t.
    t. phosphorylation
    t. protein kinase
    t. sulfation
tyrosinemia
    hereditary t.
tyrosinuria
tyrosis
Tyshak catheter
Tyson test

NOTES

UA
    urinalysis
UA/C
    urinary albumin to creatinine
        UA/C ratio
ubiquitination
UBM
    urothelial basement membrane
UBT
    urea breath test
        UBT breath test
        ^{14}C UBT
UC
    ulcerative colitis
    urethral catheterization
UCB
    unconjugated bilirubin
UCHL-1 monoclonal antibody
UCLA catheterization pouch
UCP
    ultrasound catheter probe
UD
    urethral discharge
UDC
    ursodeoxycholate
UDCA
    ursodeoxycholic acid
UDI
    Urogenital Distress Inventory
UDP
    uridine 5'-diphosphate
UDPglucuronyltransferase
UDPGT
    uridine diphosphate
      glucuronosyltransferase
        UDPGT deficiency
Udranszky test
UES
    upper esophageal sphincter
UESR
    upper esophageal sphincter relaxation
UF
    ultrafiltration
Uffelmann test
UFT/leucovorin calcium
UG
    urogenital
UGI
    upper gastrointestinal
        UGI endoscope
        UGI endoscopy
UGIB
    upper gastrointestinal bleeding
UGIE
    upper gastrointestinal endoscopy

UGIH
    upper GI hemorrhage
Uhthoff sign
UIBC
    unbound iron-binding capacity
UICC tumor classification
UJ13A nuclear isotope bone scan
UKM
    urea kinetic modeling
UKTSSA
    United Kingdom Transplant Support Service Authority
ulcer
    acid peptic u.
    active duodenal u.
    agranulocytic u.
    Allingham u.
    amebic u.
    anastomotic u.
    anastomotic-stomal u.
    anterior duodenal u.
    anterior wall antral u.
    antral u.
    antroduodenal u.
    aphthoid u.
    aphthous u.
    apical duodenal u.
    Barrett u.
    u. base
    bear claw u.
    u. bed
    benign gastric u.
    bladder u.
    bleeding u.
    Bouveret u.
    Bouveret-Duguet u.
    bulbar peptic u.
    Cameron u.
    cecal u.
    cervical u.
    chronic u.
    CMV-related u.
    coalescent u.
    u. collar
    collar-buttonlike u.
    colonic u.
    colorectal u.
    complication of benign gastric u.
    corneal u.
    u. crater
    Crohn duodenal u.
    Cruveilhier u.
    Curling u.
    Cushing u.
    Cushing-Rokitansky u.

ulcer *(continued)*
  cysteamine-induced duodenal u.
  decubitus u.
  Dieulafoy u.
  distention u.
  drug-induced u.
  duodenal u. (DU)
  duodenal ulceroinflammatory u.
  u. duodenum
  u. dyspepsia
  elusive u.
  esophageal u.
  Fenwick-Hunner u.
  flat u.
  focal colonic mucosal u.
  Forrest classification of gastroduodenal u.
  gastric u.
  gastroduodenal double u.
  general peptic u.
  genital u.
  giant gastric u. (GGU)
  giant peptic u.
  greater curvature u.
  healed u.
  herpetic u.
  Hunner u.
  idiopathic esophageal u. (IEU)
  indolent radiation-induced rectal u.
  intractable u.
  jejunal u.
  juxtapyloric u.
  kissing u.'s
  Kocher dilatation u.
  lesser curvature u.
  linear gastric u.
  longitudinal u.
  malignant u.
  Mann-Williamson u.
  marginal u.
  Martorell hypertensive u.
  mucosal gastric u.
  nonhealing u.
  open u.
  oral u.
  Palmer acid test for peptic u.
  penetrating u.
  peptic u.
  perforated acid peptic u.
  perforating u.
  perineal u.
  phantom u.
  postbulbar duodenal u.
  posterior duodenal u.
  postligation u.
  postsurgical recurrent u.
  prepyloric gastric u.
  punched-out u.
  punctate u.
  pyloric channel u.
  rake u.
  rectal u.
  recurrent u.
  refractory duodenal u.
  reserpine-induced u.
  Rokitansky-Cushing u.
  rose thorn u.
  round u.
  sea anemone u.
  secondary jejunal u.
  serpiginous u.
  sigmoid u.
  silent u.
  small intestinal u.
  sodium meclofenamate-induced esophageal u.
  solitary u.
  stercoraceous u.
  stomal u.
  stress u.
  submucous u.
  sump u.
  superficial linear u.
  suture u.
  type C, D u.
  vaginal u.
  u. vessel
  virgin u.
  V-shaped u.
  u. with heaped-up edge
ulcera *(pl. of* ulcus)
ulcerating
  u. adenocarcinoma
  u. carcinoma
ulceration
  anal u.
  anastomotic u.
  ASA-induced gastric u.
  CMV-associated u.
  CMV-induced esophageal u.
  collar-button u.
  duodenal u.
  esophageal u.
  fissurelike u.
  flat polycyclic u.
  gastric u.
  labial u.
  linear u.
  necrotic u.
  patchy colonic u.
  pouch u.
  punched-out u.
  radiation-induced u.
  serpiginous u.
  stasis u.
  stasis-induced u.
  stercoraceous u.
  stress u.

stress-induced gastric u.
suture line u.
tracheal u.
transverse u.

ulcerative
    u. colitis (UC)
    u. enteritis
    u. gastritis
    u. jejunitis
    u. jejunitis jejunocecostomy
    u. lymphoma
    u. proctitis
    u. reflux esophagitis

ulcerlike dyspepsia
ulcerogenic fistula
ulcer-prone personality
ulcus, pl. **ulcera**
    u. penetrans
    u. simplex vesicae
    u. ventriculi

Uldall subclavian hemodialysis catheter
Ulex europeus I antigen
Ullrich-Turner syndrome
ulnar deviation
ultimate fistula formation
Ultra
    U. Twin bag system
    U. Y-set system

Ultrabag dialysis system
UltraCision harmonic laparoscopic cutting shears
ultradian rhythm
ultrafast
    u. computerized tomography
    u. MRI

Ultrafem pants
ultrafiltrate
    glomerular u.
    plasma u.

ultrafiltration (UF)
    u. coefficient
    continuous arteriovenous u. (CAVU)
    dialytic u. (DU)
    extracorporeal u. (ECU)
    glomerular u.
    u. hemodialyzer
    hydrostatic u.
    slow continuous u. (SCUF)
    spontaneous dialytic u.

Ultraflex
    U. Diamond stent

    U. esophageal prosthesis
    U. Microvasive stent
    U. nitinol expandable esophageal stent
    U. tracheobronchial stent

ultrahigh-magnification endoscopy
UltraKlenz skin cleanser
Ultralente insulin
UltraLine
    U. fiber
    U. laser
    Lasersonic ACMI U.

ultralow anastomosis
ultralow-volume sclerotherapy
UltraPak enteral closed feeding system
Ultraseed system
Ultrase MT20, MT24
ultrasmall superparamagnetic iron oxide (USPIO)
ultrasonic
    u. aspirator and dissector
    u. cytoreduction
    u. diagnosis
    u. dissection
    u. endoscope
    u. fragmentation
    u. lithotresis
    u. lithotripsy
    u. lithotriptor
    u. lithotriptor probe
    u. oscillating bur
    u. scalpel
    u. tactile sensor
    u. tomography

ultrasonogram
    renal u.

ultrasonographic findings
ultrasonography
    prenatal u.

ultrasonography
    abdominal u.
    bladder u.
    B-mode u.
    catheter probe-assisted endoluminal u. (CP-EUS)
    color Doppler u.
    contrast-enhanced endoscopic u. (CE-EUS)
    Doppler u.
    ejaculatory duct u.
    endoluminal rectal u. (ELUS)
    endoscopic u. (EUS)

NOTES

ultrasonography (continued)
    endoscopic color Doppler u.
    u. estimate
    EUS-AD gastric lesion staging by endoscopic u.
    EUS-M gastric lesion staging by endoscopic u.
    EUS-SM gastric lesion staging by endoscopic u.
    gray-scale u.
    high-intensity focused u.
    high-resolution u.
    intraductal u. (IDUS)
    intraoperative u. (IOUS)
    intraportal endovascular u. (IPEUS)
    intrarectal u.
    laparoscopic contact u. (LCU)
    pelvic u.
    penile duplex u.
    pharmacoduplex u.
    real-time u. (RUS)
    rectal endoscopic u. (REU, REUS)
    secretin u.
    sex assignment by fetal u.
    Siemens Sonoline u.
    sildenafil plus Doppler u.
    SP-501 gastric lesion staging by endoscopic u.
    Toshiba Sal 38B real-time u.
    Toshiba Sonolayer SSA250A transrectal u.
    transanal u.
    transcutaneous u.
    transluminal u.
    transnasal endoluminal u.
    transperineal u.
    transrectal u. (TRUS)
    transrectal prostatic u.

ultrasound
    abdominal u.
    u. ablation
    u. basket extraction
    BladderScan u.
    U. Bone Analyzer
    u. catheter probe (UCP)
    catheter probe u.
    colonoscopic endoluminal u.
    colorectal endoluminal u.
    compression u. (CUS)
    condom catheter endoscopic u.
    u. dilution technique
    Doppler u. (DUS)
    dual-plane catheter-based u.
    endoanal u. (EAUS)
    endoluminal ureteral u.
    endorectal u. (ERUS)
    u. endoscope
    endoscopic u. (EUS)
    u. gastrointestinal fiberscope
    gray-scale u.
    high-frequency intraluminal u.
    high-intensity focused u. (HFU, HIFU)
    hydrogen peroxide u. (HPUS)
    intraductal u. (IDUS)
    intraluminal u. (ILUS)
    intravascular u. (IVUS)
    laparoscopic u. (LUS)
    laparoscopic intracorporeal u. (LICU)
    piezoelectrically generated u.
    power Doppler u.
    pulsed Doppler u.
    quantitative u. (QUS)
    real-time gallbladder u.
    u. scan
    soft balloon method for endoscopic u.
    standard transabdominal u.
    u. test
    time domain u. (TDU)
    transcutaneous u.
    u. transducer
    transendoscopic u.
    transrectal u. (TRUS)
    transurethral rectal u.
    transvaginal u. (TVUS)
    u. wand

ultrasound-assisted
    u.-a. PEG placement
    u.-a. percutaneous endoscopic gastrostomy

ultrasound-guided
    u.-g. anterior subcostal liver biopsy
    u.-g. laser
    u.-g. shock wave therapy
    u.-g. systematic sextant biopsy

ultrastiff wire
ultrastructural basket-weave change
UltraTag RBC kit
ultrathin
    u. araldite section
    u. endoscope
    u. endoscopy
    u. needle brachytherapy-style delivery renal application
    u. pancreatoscope

ultratome
    U. double-lumen sphincterotome Microvasive
    U. XL triple-lumen sphincterotome

ultraviolet (UV)
    u. irradiation

Ultravist 300
Ultrex
    U. cylinder
    U. Plus penile prosthesis

Ultroid

Ultzmann test
umami taste receptor
umbilical
    u. artery
    u. cord
    u. fissure
    u. fistula
    u. granuloma
    u. hernia
    u. hernia rupture
    u. ligament
    u. port
    u. port grasper
    u. portography
    u. region
    u. scissors
    u. tape
    u. vein
    u. vein catheterization
    u. vein recanalization
umbilicalis
    plica u.
umbilicated angioma
umbilication
umbilici (*pl. of* umbilicus)
umbilicoplasty
umbilicovesical fascia
umbilicus, pl. **umbilici**
    everted u.
    Richet fascia u.
    transverse retubularized sigmoidovesicostomy continent urinary diversion to u.
umbrella
    Mobin-Uddin u.
UMCL
    upper midclavicular line
UN
    urea nitrogen
Unasyn
UNaV
    urinary sodium excretion
unbanded gastroplasty
unbound iron-binding capacity (UIBC)
UNC
    urine net charge
uncentrifuged urine
unciform pancreas
uncinate
    u. process
    u. process of pancreas
uncoated mesh stent

uncomplicated
    u. appendectomy
    u. cystitis
    u. urinary tract infection
unconjugated
    u. bilirubin (UCB)
    u. hyperbilirubinemia
unconscious incontinence
uncorrected
    u. maternal morbidity
    u. reflux morbidity
uncoupling
    actual gastric myoelectric u.
undecapeptide
    amino-terminal u.
undecenoate of testosterone
underactivity
    detrusor muscle u.
underdosing
    Nephron u.
underfilling
    arterial u.
underlying
    u. chronic renal insufficiency
    u. muscularis propria
undersurface of liver
underwater spark gap
underwear
    Prevail protective u.
undescended testis
undifferentiated
    u. adenoma
    u. cell
    u. embryonal sarcoma of liver
    u. malignant teratoma
    u. structure
undigested food in stool
undiversion
    urinary u.
unenhanced
    u. helical computed tomography
    u. helical CT
unequal calf diameter
uneventful recovery
unexplained findings
unextractable gallstone
unfavorable infundibular width
unformed stool
UN-GRAPH computer software
ungual fibroma
unguliformis
unicameral cyst

NOTES

unicornuate uterus
unidirectional transfer
Uni-Flate 1000 penile prosthesis
uniformis
    Bacteroides u.
uniform loading
Uni-Gold *Helicobacter pylori* test
unilateral
    u. fused kidney
    u. megaureter
    u. nephrectomy
    u. palpable right testis
    u. periorbital emphysema
    u. renal artery stenosis
    u. renal hypoplasia
    u. renin production
    u. subcostal incision
    u. ureteral calculus
    u. ureteral obstruction (UUO)
unilobular cirrhosis
unilocular
    u. hydatid disease
    u. ovarian cyst
uninhibited
    u. neurogenic bladder
    u. overactive bladder
union
    anomalous pancreaticobiliary u. (APBU)
    anomalous pancreaticobiliary ductal u. (APBDU)
    U. Internationale Contre le Cancer
unipapillary kidney
uniplanar imaging
unipolar
    u. glass electrode
    u. neuron
unique esophageal feature
Unisensor strain-gauge transducer
unit
    amylase u.
    arbitrary u. (AU)
    biceps femoris musculocutaneous u.
    Bodansky u.
    Bovie electrocoagulation u.
    Cameron electrosurgical u.
    Cameron-Miller electrocoagulation u.
    Century bicarbonate dialysis control u.
    colony-forming u. (CFU)
    crypt-villus u.
    densitometric u.
    Diasonics DRF ultrasound u.
    duodenal cluster u.
    electrosurgical u. (ESU)
    ERBE electrocautery u.
    Erbotom F2 electrocoagulation u.
    good performance u.
    GPL u.
    gracilis musculocutaneous u.
    Grass Model SIU5A stimulation isolation u.
    HemoTherapies liver dialysis u.
    Hounsfield u. (HU)
    image-processing u.
    international androgen u.
    Karmen u.
    KeyMed u.
    King-Armstrong u.
    liver dialysis u.
    Olympus heater probe u.
    OSMO reverse osmosis u.
    u. of packed red blood cells (UPRBC)
    Proscan ultrasound u.
    QAD-1 sonography u.
    real-time sonographic u.
    Siemens MRI u.
    Siemens Somatom DRH CT analyzer u.
    Somogyi u.
    SSE2-L electrosurgical u.
    TENS u.
    ThermoFlex thermotherapy u.
    UroCystom u.
    Valleylab E3B cautery u.
    Valleylab SSE-2 cautery u.
Unitary inflatable penile prosthesis
United
    U. Bongort Lifestyle pouch
    U. Kingdom Transplant Support Service Authority (UKTSSA)
    U. Max-E drainable pouch
    U. Network for Organ Sharing (UNOS)
    U. Ostomy Association (UOA)
    U. Ostomy irrigation set
    U. Skin Prep
    U. States Renal Data System (USRDS)
    U. Surgical Bongort Lifestyle pouch
    U. Surgical Convex insert
    U. Surgical Featherlite ileostomy pouch
    U. Surgical Hypalon faceplate
    U. Surgical Seal-Tite gasket
    U. Surgical Shear Plus drainable pouch
    U. Surgical Soft & Secure pouch
    U. XL 14 skin barrier
univariate analysis
Universal
    U. esophagoscope
    U. gastroscope
    U. sheath
    U. sheath system
    U. stent

universale
  angiokeratoma corporis diffusum u.
universally accepted therapy
University
  U. of Wisconsin preservation fluid
  U. of Wisconsin solution
unobstructed patient
UNOS
  United Network for Organ Sharing
unreconstructable obstructive azoospermia
unrelenting
  u. diarrhea
  u. pain
unrelieved pain
unremitting pain
unresectable hepatocellular carcinoma
unresolved urinary tract infection
unresponsiveness to standard therapy
unresponsive symptom
unrest
  peristaltic u.
unroofing
  u. of diverticulum
  transurethral u.
unsaturated fatty acid
unsensitized transplant recipient
unsporulated coccidian
unstable
  u. bladder
  u. colon
  u. urethra
unsteady gait
untethering procedure
unweighted
UOA
  United Ostomy Association
Uosm
  urine osmolarity
U/P
  urine-plasma ratio
UPEP
  urine protein electrophoresis
UPJ
  ureteropelvic junction
uPM3 urine test
U pouch
U-pouch construction
UPP
  urethral pressure profile
upper
  u. alimentary endoscopy
  u. arm flap
  u. endoscopy and colonoscopy
  u. esophageal sphincter (UES)
  u. esophageal sphincter relaxation (UESR)
  u. gastrointestinal (UGI)
  u. gastrointestinal angioma
  u. gastrointestinal barium roentgenographic study
  u. gastrointestinal bleeding (UGIB)
  u. gastrointestinal endoscopy (UGIE)
  u. gastrointestinal panendoscopy
  u. gastrointestinal procedure
  u. gastrointestinal tract
  u. GI endoscope
  u. GI hemorrhage (UGIH)
  u. GI series
  u. GI submucosal tumor
  u. GI tract foreign body
  U. Hands retractor
  u. midclavicular line (UMCL)
  u. motor neuron
  u. tract dilation
  u. tract disease
  u. tract stricture
  u. tract urothelial tumor
  u. ureter
  u. urinary tract calculus
UPRBC
  unit of packed red blood cells
upregulation
  u.-r. of monocyte chemoattractant protein-1 genecytoplasm of cell
Uprima
upsaliensis
  Campylobacter u.
upset stomach
upside-down stomach
upstream pancreatic duct
upstroke
  delayed u.
uptake
  glucose u.
  hepatic u.
  [^{3}H]thymidine u.
  spermidine u.
URA
  urethral resistance factor
Urabeth Tabs
urachal
  u. abscess

NOTES

urachal *(continued)*
    u. adenocarcinoma
    u. cyst
    u. disorder
    u. diverticulum
    u. fistula
    u. sinus
urachus
    patent u.
uracil/tegafur
uragogue
uranyl
    u. acetate
    u. acetate stain
urate
    u. calculus
    u. crystal
    monosodium u.
    u. nephropathy
    u. renal excretion
    sodium acid u.
uraturia
urea
    u. adequacy
    u. breath test (UBT)
    u. breath testing
    u. channel
    u. clearance
    u. cycle
    u. distribution volume
    hepatic u.
    u. hydrolysis
    u. kinetic modeling (UKM)
    u. kinetics
    Kt/V u.
    u. nitrogen (UN)
    u. nitrogen test
    percent reduction in u. (PRU)
    u. permeability
    plasma u.
    u. reduction ratio (URR)
    u. splitting organism
    u. synthesis
urea-derived cyanate
urea-impermeable membrane
urealyticum
    Ureaplasma u.
Ureaplasma
    U. urealyticum
    U. urethritis
urease
    cytoplasmic u.
    mucosal u.
    u. test
urease-producing bacterium
urea splitting
urecchysis
Urecholine supersensitivity test
uredema, uroedema

Urelief
uremia, urinemia
    extrarenal u.
    retention u.
uremic
    u. acidosis
    u. breath
    u. cardiomyopathy
    u. colitis
    u. encephalopathy
    u. gastritis
    u. gastrointestinal lesion
    u. medullary cystic disease
    u. PMN
    u. pruritus
    u. serositis
    u. serum subfraction
    u. syndrome
ureolyticus
    Bacteroides u.
ureter
    abdominal u.
    aberrant u.
    bifid u.
    circumcaval u.
    u. contractility
    u. creep
    dilemma of distal u.
    distal u.
    u. duplication anomaly
    ectopic u.
    en bloc u.
    extraperitoneal excision of lower one-third of u.
    ileal u.
    impassable u.
    u. implantation
    intramural u.
    juxtavesical u.
    left u.
    lower u.
    middle u.
    pelvic u.
    postcaval u.
    proper transurethral resection of intramural u.
    retrocaval u.
    retroiliac u.
    right u.
    tortuous u.
    torus u.
    upper u.
ureteral
    u. anastomosis
    u. atony
    u. bladder augmentation
    u. bud
    u. calculi in pregnancy
    u. *Candida*

u. carcinoma
u. catheterization
u. colic
u. dissection
u. ectopia
u. electromyography
u. encasement
u. hernia
u. injury
u. jet
u. jet into bladder
u. meatoscopy
u. meatotomy
u. muscle cell
u. neocystostomy
u. obstruction
u. occlusion balloon catheter
u. orifice
u. patch procedure
u. peristalsis second messenger
u. pressure
u. reimplantation
u. reimplantation stenosis
u. reimplantation surgery
u. schistosomiasis
u. scoping basketing
u. spatulation
u. split-cuff nipple
u. stent
u. stenting
u. stent placement
u. stoma
u. stoma removal
u. stone
u. stricture
u. torsion
u. tuberculosis
u. tumor
u. tunnel
ureteralgia
uretercystoscope
ureterectasia
ureterectomy
distal u.
segmental u.
ureteric
u. bud
u. calcification
u. calculus
u. diverticulum
u. obstruction
u. plexus
u. reimplantation
u. retrieval net
u. ridge
u. stoma
u. stone
uretericus
plexus u.
ureteritis
u. cystica
u. glandularis
ureterocalicostomy
ureterocele
u. cobra-head deformity
u. drooping lily sign
ectopic u.
intravesical u.
orthotopic u.
u. prolapse
single-system u.
ureterocelectomy
ureterocelorraphy
ureterocervical
ureterocolic
u. fistula
u. stricture
ureterocolonic anastomosis
ureterocolostomy
ureterocutaneostomy
ureterocutaneous fistula
ureterocystanastomosis
ureterocystoneostomy
ureterocystoplasty
ureterocystoscope
ureterocystostomy
ureteroduodenal
ureteroendoscopic disconnection
ureteroendoscopy
ureteroenteric
u. status
u. stricture
ureteroenteroanastomosis
ureteroenterostomy
ureterogram
bulb-tip retrograde u.
ureterography
ureteroheminephrectomy
ureterohydronephrosis
ureteroileal
u. anastomosis
u. neocystostomy
u. stenosis
u. stricture

NOTES

ureteroileocecoproctostomy
ureteroileoneocystostomy
ureteroileostomy
    Bricker u.
ureteroinfundibuloplasty
ureterointestinal
    u. anastomosis
    u. implantation
ureterolith
ureterolithiasis
ureterolithotomy
    laparoscopic u.
ureterolysis
    combined u.
    extravesical u.
    intravesical u.
    laparoscopic u.
    Lich-Gregoire u.
    Pacquin u.
    Politano-Leadbetter u.
ureteromeatotomy
ureteroneocystostomy
    Cohen u.
    Glenn-Anderson u.
    u. herniation
    Leadbetter-Politano u.
    modified Lich-Gregoir u.
    Politano-Leadbetter u.
    reoperative u.
ureteroneopyelostomy
ureteronephrectomy
ureteronephrosis
ureteropathy
ureteropelvic
    u. fungus ball
    u. junction (UPJ)
    u. junction obstruction
    u. junction obstruction repair
    u. ligament
    u. region
ureteropelvioneostomy (*var. of* ureteropyeloneostomy)
ureteropelvioplasty
    Culp u.
    Culp-DeWeerd u.
    Foley Y-type u.
    Foley Y-V u.
    Scardino u.
    Scardino-Prince u.
ureterophlegma
ureteroplasty
    ileal patch u.
ureteroproctostomy
ureteropyelitis
ureteropyelogram
    retrograde u.
ureteropyelography
    retrograde u.
ureteropyeloneostomy, ureteropelvioneostomy
ureteropyelonephritis
ureteropyelonephrostomy
ureteropyeloplasty
ureteropyeloscope
    Karl Storz flexible u.
ureteropyeloscopy
    flexible u.
ureteropyelostomy
ureteropyosis
ureterorectostomy
ureterorenal reflux
ureterorenoscope procedure sheath
ureterorenoscopy
    flexible u.
    transurethral u. (URS)
ureterorrhagia
ureterorrhaphy
ureteroscope
    Circon-ACMI MR-6, MR-9 u.
    flexible u.
    Gautier u.
    Micro-6 u.
    offset-lens u.
    Olympus URF type P2 flexible u.
    Panoview rod-lens u.
    rigid u.
    semirigid fiberoptic u.
    u. sheath
    Storz 27022 SK u.
    Wolf u.
    working-port u.
ureteroscopic
    u. approach
    u. endopyelotomy
    u. intracorporeal electrohydraulic lithotripsy
ureteroscopy
    rigid u.
    role of u.
    stent after u.
ureterosigmoid anastomosis
ureterosigmoidostomy
    ileocecal u.
    Mainz-type u.
    Maydl u.
ureterostenosis, ureterostegnosis, ureterostenoma
ureterostoma
ureterostomosis
ureterostomy
    cutaneous loop u.
    Davis intubated u.
    high-loop cutaneous u.
    low-loop cutaneous u.
    retroperitoneal cutaneous u.
ureterotome
    optical u.

ureterotomy
    Davis intubated u.
    intubated u.
ureterotrigonoenterostomy
ureterotrigonosigmoidostomy
ureterotubal anastomosis
ureteroureteral anastomosis
ureteroureterostomy
ureterouterine fistula
ureterovaginal fistula
ureterovesical
    u. junction (UVJ)
    u. obstruction
ureterovesicoplasty
    Leadbetter-Politano u.
ureterovesicostomy
urethra, pl. **urethrae**
    accessory phallic u.
    anterior u.
    AS-800 male bulbous u.
    u. blowout injury
    bulbar u.
    bulbomembranous u.
    bulbus urethrae
    compressor u.
    devastated u.
    u. duplication
    u. feminina
    fixed drain pipe u.
    fossa of male u.
    fossa navicularis urethrae
    hemispherium bulbi u.
    intrinsic striated muscle of u.
    isthmus u.
    labium u.
    lacuna of u.
    membranous u.
    u. muliebris
    native u.
    patent u.
    pendulous u.
    penile u.
    posterior u.
    preprostatic u.
    prostatic u.
    septum bulbi u.
    short u.
    spinning top u.
    unstable u.
    u. virilis
urethral
    u. abscess
    u. apoplexy
    u. artery
    u. arthritis
    u. atresia
    u. calculus
    u. cancer
    u. carcinoma
    u. caruncle
    u. catheterization (UC)
    u. catheter movement
    u. closure mechanism
    u. closure pressure
    u. closure pressure profile
    u. cooling
    u. cooling surface
    u. crest
    u. cyst
    u. dilation
    u. discharge (UD)
    u. diverticulectomy
    u. diverticulum
    u. electrical conductance
    u. feedback trigger
    u. fistula
    u. gland
    u. hemangioma
    u. hematuria
    u. hemi-Kock
    u. hypermobility
    u. lacuna
    u. meatus
    u. obstruction
    u. occlusion
    u. plate
    u. plate division
    u. plug
    u. pressure measurement
    u. pressure profile (UPP)
    u. pressure profilometry
    u. prolapse
    u. pseudodiverticulum
    u. pseudotumor
    u. reconstruction complication
    u. resistance
    u. resistance factor (URA)
    u. sarcoidosis
    u. self-channelization
    u. sensory threshold
    u. sphincter
    u. sphincterotomy
    u. stenosis
    u. stent

NOTES

urethral *(continued)*
    u. stent prosthesis
    u. stricture
    u. stripping
    u. surgical reconstruction
    u. suspension
    u. swab
    u. syndrome
    u. temperature
    u. tuberculosis
    u. tumor
    u. valve
    u. vein
urethralgia
urethralis
    annulus u.
    crista u.
urethrameter
urethratresia
urethrectomy
urethremorrhagia, urethrorrhagia
urethremphraxis
urethreurynter
Urethrin
urethrism, urethrismus
urethritis
    acute u.
    atrophic u.
    chlamydia u.
    u. cystica
    u. glandularis
    gonococcal u. (GU)
    gonorrheal u.
    gouty u.
    u. granulosa
    hypoestrogenic u.
    mycoplasma u.
    nongonococcal u.
    nonspecific u. (NSU)
    u. orificii externi
    u. petrificans
    polypoid u.
    prophylactic u.
    specific u.
    u. syndrome
    Ureaplasma u.
    u. venerea
urethrobalanoplasty
urethroblennorrhea
urethrocavernous fistula
urethrocele
urethrocutaneous fistula
urethrocystitis
urethrocystocele
urethrocystography
urethrocystometrography
urethrocystometry
urethrocystopexy
urethrocystoscopy
urethrodetrusor facilitative reflex
urethrodynia
urethrogram
    ascending u.
    retrograde u. (RUG)
urethrograph
urethrography
    positive-pressure u. (PPUG)
    retrograde u. (RUG)
urethrohymenal fusion
urethrolysis
    retropubic u.
    transvaginal u.
urethromeatal erythema
urethrometer
urethrometry
urethropelvic ligament
urethropenile
urethroperineal
urethroperineoscrotal
urethropexy
    Gittes u.
    laparoscopic Burch u.
    Lapides-Ball u.
    Marshall-Marchetti-Krantz u.
    Stamey u.
    transabdominal Burch u.
urethrophraxis
urethrophyma
urethroplasty
    anastomotic u.
    augmented anastomotic u.
    buccal mucosal substitution u.
    Cantwell-Ransley u.
    Cecil u.
    long-term outcome of u.
    modified Young u.
    one-stage u.
    onlay island flap u.
    patch graft u.
    pedicled penile skin u.
    pedicle flap u.
    Schwartz-Pregenzer u.
    skin inlay u.
    Snodgrass incised plate u.
    substitution u.
    tabularized incised plate u.
    Tanagho bladder flap u.
    Thiersch-Duplay u.
    tubed u.
    tubularized incised plate u.
    Turner-Warwick u.
    ventral patch u.
urethroprostatic
urethrorectal fistula
urethrorrhagia *(var. of* urethremorrhagia*)*
urethrorrhaphy
urethrorrhea

urethroscope
   Robertson TM u.
urethroscopic
urethroscopy
   retropubic u.
urethroscrotal
urethrospasm
urethrosphincteric
   u. guarding reflex
   u. inhibitory reflex
   u. recruitment reflex
urethrostaxis
urethrostenosis
urethrostomy
   perineal u.
urethrotome
   u. knife
   Otis u.
   Sachse u.
   Storz u.
urethrotomy
   core-through optical u.
   direct-vision internal u. (DVIU)
   endoscopic optical u.
   external u.
   internal u.
   Otis u.
   perineal u.
   Sachse u.
   Syme external u.
urethrotrigonitis
urethrovaginal
   u. fistula
   u. septum
   u. sphincter
urethrovesical
   u. anastomosis
   u. junction
urethrovesicopexy
uretic
Urex tablet
URF-P2 choledochoscope
urge
   u. to defecate
   u. incontinence
   u. syndrome
   treatment of neurogenic refractory u.
urgency
   defecatory u.
   u. incontinence
   motor u.
   sensory u.
   urinary u.
urgency-frequency symptom
urgent colonoscopy
uric
   u. acid
   u. acid calculus
   u. acid crystal
   u. acid infarct
   u. acid level
   u. acid nephropathy
   u. acid shower
   u. acid stone
   u. acid test
   u. acid urolithiasis
uricaciduria
uricometer
uricosuria
uricosuric
Uricult dipslide
uridine
   u. 5'-diphosphate (UDP)
   u. diphosphate glucuronosyltransferase (UDPGT)
   u. diphosphate glucuronosyltransferase deficiency
   u. phosphorylase
   u. rescue
Uridium
uridyltransferase
   galactose-1-phosphate u.
Urifon-Forte
Urigen
Uri-Kit culture kit
Urimar-T
Urimax
urinable
urinacidometer
urinae
   accelerator u.
   ardor u.
   detrusor u.
   incontinentia u.
urinal
   condom u.
   Millie female u.
   Uro-Tex McGuire male u.
   URSEC u.
urinalysis (UA)
   chemical u.
   u. color
   u. dipstick

NOTES

urinalysis *(continued)*
    midstream u.
    u. pH
    u. sediment microscopy
    u. sediment microscopy bacterium
    u. sediment microscopy cast
    u. sediment microscopy cell
    u. sediment microscopy crystal
    u. sediment microscopy parasite
    u. sediment microscopy prostatic secretion
    u. sediment microscopy yeast
    u. specific gravity
    u. turbidity
urinaria, pl. **urinariae**
    fundus vesicae urinariae
    tela subserosa vesicae urinariae
    vertex vesicae urinariae
    vesica u.
urinarius
    meatus u.
urinary
    u. abscess
    u. acidity
    u. albumin to creatinine (UA/C)
    u. alkalinization
    u. amylase
    u. anion gap
    u. ascites
    u. bicarbonate
    u. bilirubin
    u. bladder
    u. cachexia
    u. calcium
    u. calculus
    u. catecholamine
    u. catheterization
    u. cGMP level
    u. chloride
    u. chloride excretion
    u. citrate
    u. composition
    u. concentration
    u. conduit
    u. continence
    u. continence reflex
    u. continuity
    u. control urethral insert
    u. cortisol
    u. crystal
    u. cyclic AMP
    u. cyst
    u. dribbling
    u. exertional incontinence
    u. extravasation
    u. extraversion
    u. fibronectin
    u. flow
    u. frequency
    u. glucose
    u. glycosaminoglycan excretion
    u. hesitancy
    u. incontinence episode
    u. indican
    u. intestinal diversion
    u. kallikrein
    u. kallikrein excretion
    u. ketone
    u. leukocyte esterase
    u. lithiasis
    u. lithogenesis
    u. marker protein
    u. 3-methylhistidine
    u. nitrite test
    u. obstruction
    u. output
    u. oxalate
    u. oxalate excretion
    permanent u.
    u. pH
    u. protein excretion
    u. protein-urinary creatinine ratio
    u. reconstruction
    u. retention
    u. sand
    u. schistosomiasis
    u. sediment
    u. sediment cast
    u. sediment yeast
    u. sodium excretion (UNaV)
    u. specific gravity
    u. stasis
    u. stone
    u. stress incontinence
    u. stuttering
    u. symptom
    u. tract
    u. tract anomaly
    u. tract disease
    u. tract four-glass evaluation
    u. tract infection (UTI)
    u. tract infection suppression
    u. tract reconstruction augmentation cystoplasty
    u. trypsin inhibitor
    u. trypsinogen activation peptide
    u. umbilical fistula
    u. undiversion
    u. urea nitrogen excretion (UUN)
    u. urgency
    u. urobilinogen
urination
    precipitant u.
    straining for u.
    stuttering u.
urine
    u. acidification
    anemic u.

u. ascites
barium sediment in u.
Bence Jones u.
u. bilirubin
black u.
u. chloride test
chylous u.
u. color
u. composition
concentrated u.
u. concentration
u. concentration test
crude u.
u. culture
u. cytokine analysis
u. cytology
dark concentrated u.
diabetic u.
u. dipstick
dyspeptic u.
u. extravasation
febrile u.
u. flow rate
u. glitter cell
gouty u.
hyperosmotic u.
hypoosmotic u.
U. Meter Foley tray
midstream specimen of u. (MSU)
milky u.
nebulous u.
nervous u.
u. net charge (UNC)
u. osmolality
u. osmolarity (Uosm)
postvoid dribbling of u.
postvoid residual u.
u. protein electrophoresis (UPEP)
residual u.
u. sample
u. specific gravity
u. supersaturation
u. transport
u. turbidity
uncentrifuged u.
u. urea nitrogen (UUN)
u. urobilinogen
voided u.
urine-based enzyme-linked immunosorbent assay
urine-collecting tubule
urinemia (*var. of* uremia)
urine-plasma ratio (U/P)
uriniferous
    u. pseudocyst
    u. tubule
uriniparous tubule
urinocryoscopy
urinogenous
urinoglucosometer
urinologist (*var. of* urologist)
urinology (*var. of* urology)
urinoma
urinometer, urometer
urinometry
urinosexual
urinous abscess
Uriscreen test
Urised
Urisedamine
UriSite urine collection kit
Urispas
Uri-Three culture kit
Urizole
uroanthelone
Urobak
urobilin complex
urobilinogen
    fecal u.
    urinary u.
    urine u.
urobilinogenuria
urobilinuria
Uro-Bond skin adhesive
Urocam videocamera
Urocath external catheter
urocele, uroscheocele
urocheras
urochezia
urochrome
urochromogen
Urocit
Urocit-K
uroclepsia
UroCoil self-expanding stent
urocortin
urocrisis
urocriterion
urocyanogen
urocyst
Urocystin
urocystitis
UroCystom unit

NOTES

Urocyte diagnostic cytometry system
urocytogram
UROD
    uroporphyrinogen decarboxylase
urodeum
Urodiagnost x-ray table
urodialysis
urodochium
urodynamic
    ambulatory u.'s
    u. assessment
    u. catheter
    u. dysfunction
    u. evaluation
    u. flow study
    u. investigation
    u. obstruction
    u. parameter
    u. testing
urodynamically
urodynia
urodysfunction
uroedema (*var. of* uredema)
uroenterone
uroepithelial glycoid receptor
uroerythrin
uroflavin
uroflow
    u. index
    peak u.
uroflowmeter
    Dantec Urodyn 1000 u.
    Drake u.
    Synectics-Dantec Flo-Lab II u.
    Synectics-Dantec UD10000 u.
uroflowmetry
    Bristol nomogram for u.
    home u.
    Siroky nomogram for u.
urofuscin
urofuscohematin
urogastrone
urogenital (UG)
    u. abnormality
    u. diaphragm
    U. Distress Inventory (UDI)
    u. fistula
    u. prolapse
    u. region
    u. sinus
    u. sinus anomaly
    u. sinus mobilization
    u. sphincter muscle
    u. triangle
urogenitale
    trigonum u.
urogenous pyelitis
Urogesic
uroglaucin

Urografin 290 contrast medium
urogram
    constant infusion excretory u. (CIXU)
    excretory u. (XU)
    intravenous u. (IVU)
    retrograde u. (RU)
urograph
    Disa 5500 u.
urography
    antegrade u.
    cystoscopic u.
    descending u.
    excretory u. (EU, EXU)
    high-dose intravenous u.
    intravenous u. (IVU)
    magnetic resonance u. (MRU)
    one-shot intravenous u.
    percutaneous antegrade u.
    retrograde u.
Uro-Guide stent
urogynecologic surgeon
urogynecologist
urogynecology
urohematin
urohematonephrosis
urohematoporphyrin
urohypertensin
Uro-jet delivery system
urokinase plasminogen activator
urokinetic
Uro-KP-Neutral
urokymography
Urolab Janus System III
Urolase
    Bard U.
    CR Bard U.
    U. laser
    U. neodymium:YAG laser fiber
Urolene Blue
urolith
urolithiasis
    ammonium acid urate u.
    asymptomatic u.
    calcium oxalate u.
    calcium phosphate u.
    u. in childhood
    cystine u.
    dihydroxyadenine u.
    iatrogenic u.
    magnesium ammonium phosphate u.
    matrix u.
    miscellaneous u.
    pediatric u.
    recurrent calcium u. (RCU)
    silicate u.
    staghorn u.
    struvite u.
    triamterene u.

uric acid u.
xanthine u.
urolithic
urolithology
urolithotomy
urologic (*var. of* urological)
urological, urologic
    u. aspect
    u. condition
    u. disease
    u. drug compendium
    u.'s intervention
    u. surgery
    u. symptom
    u. system cancer
urological
urologist, urinologist
    general-practice u.
urology, urinology, uronology
    Brief Male Sexual Function Inventory for U.
    u. clinic
    geriatric u.
    laparoscopic surgery in pediatric u.
    laparoscopy in pediatric u.
    pediatric u.
    perinatal u.
    u. set
    Society for Fetal U. (SFU)
Uroloop
UroLume
    U. endoprosthesis
    U. Endourethral Wallstent prosthesis
    U. prostate stent
    U. urethral prosthesis
    U. urethral stent
    U. Wallstent
    U. Wallstent stent
urolutein
Uro-Mag
uromancy
uromantia
Uromat dilation
UroMax II high-pressure balloon catheter
uromelanin
urometer (*var. of* urinometer)
uromodulin gene
uromucoid
uronate
    glycosaminoglycans u. (GAGUA)
    macromolecular u. (MMUA)

uroncus
uronephrosis
uronic acid-rich protein
uronology (*var. of* urology)
urononcometry
uronophile
uronoscopy (*var. of* uroscopy)
Uro-Pak system
uropathogen
uropathogenic bacterium
uropathologist
uropathy
    chronic obstructive u.
    congenital u.
    obstructive u.
    positional obstructive u.
uropenia
uropepsinogen
urophanic
urophein
urophosphometer
uroplania
Uroplus DS, SS
uropoiesis
uropoietic
uropontin
uroporphyria
uroporphyrinogen decarboxylase (UROD)
uropsammus
uropterin
uropyonephrosis
uropyoureter
Uroquid-Acid
uroradiology
    diagnostic u.
    interventional u.
urorectal septum
urorhythmography
urorubin
urorubrohematin
Uro-San Plus external catheter
uroscheocele (*var. of* urocele)
uroschesis
uroscopy, uronoscopy
urosemiology
urosepsin
urosepsis
uroseptic
UROS infuser
urosis
UroSnare cystoscopic tumor snare
Urosoft stent

NOTES

urospectrin
Urospiral urethral stent
urostalagmometry
urostealith calculus
urostomy
Uro-Tex McGuire male urinal
urothelial
    u. augmentation
    u. basement membrane (UBM)
    u. cancer
    u. carcinoma
    u. dysplasia
    u. mucosa
    u. neoplasm
    u. tumor
urothelium
    seromuscular enterocystoplasty lined with u. (SELU)
urotherapy
urotoxia
Urotract x-ray system
uroureter
Urovac bladder evacuator
Urovision ultrasound imaging system
Urovist
    U. Cysto
    U. Meglumine
    U. Sodium 300
UroVive self-contained balloon system
UroVysion assay
Urowave thermotherapy
uroxanthin
Uroxatral
URR
    urea reduction ratio
URS
    transurethral ureterorenoscopy
URSEC urinal
ursi
    Diphyllobothrium u.
Ursinus Inlay-Tabs
Urso 250
ursodeoxycholate (UDC)
ursodeoxycholic acid (UDCA)
ursodiol
urticarial
    u. fever
    u. reaction
urticaria pigmentosa
URYS 800 nerve stimulator
U.S. Army double-ended retractor
use
    long-term catheter u.
U-shaped skin flap
USPIO
    ultrasmall superparamagnetic iron oxide
USRDS
    United States Renal Data System
Ussing
    U. chamber
    U. chamber technique
U-stitch reimplantation technique
uteri (*pl. of* uterus)
uterine
    u. artery
    u. colic
    u. coring
    u. enlargement
    u. fibroid
    u. lateral fusion defect
    u. rupture
    u. size
    u. tenderness
    u. tympanites
utero
    hydronephrosis in u.
uterocele
uterolysis
    laparoscopic u.
uterosacral ligament
uteroscope
uterus, pl. uteri
    anteflexed u.
    anteverted u.
    bicornuate u.
    descensus uteri
    u. didelphys
    double u.
    duplicate u.
    enlarged u.
    gravid u.
    u. masculinus
    pregnant u.
    preservation of u.
    retroflexed u.
    retroverted u.
    unicornuate u.
UTI
    urinary tract infection
utopian state
utricle
    prostatic u.
utriculitis
utriculocele
utriculus
    u. masculinus
    u. prostaticus
    u. vestibuli
U-tube stent
U-turn maneuver
UUN
    urinary urea nitrogen excretion
    urine urea nitrogen
UUO
    unilateral ureteral obstruction
UV
    ultraviolet

UV linked
UV transilluminator
uveitis
    tubulointerstitial nephritis and u. (TINU)
UV-Flash ultraviolet germicidal exchange device
Uvidec-77 spectrophotometer
UVJ
    ureterovesical junction
UV linked

uvomorulin
uvula, pl. **uvulae**
    u. of bladder
    Lieutaud u.
    u. vesicae
uvular
    u. deviation
    u. swelling
uvularis
UW solution

NOTES

299v
 Lactobacillus plantarum 299v
VAB
 Velban, actinomycin D, bleomycin
VAB-6 chemotherapy protocol
VABES
 vasoablative endothelial sarcoma
VAB-II
 Velban, actinomycin D, bleomycin, platinum
VAB-VI
 cyclophosphamide, Velban, actinomycin D, bleomycin, platinum
VAC
 vincristine, Adriamycin, cyclophosphamide
VacA
 vacuolating toxin gene A
  VacA cytotoxin
  VacA toxin
vaccination
 T-cell v.
vaccine
 V. Adverse Event Reporting System
 BCG v.
 edible v.
 GVAX pancreatic cancer v.
 Helivax v.
 hepatitis A inactivated & hepatitis B recombinant v.
 hepatitis B virus v. (HBVV)
 irradiated tumor v.
 JT1001 prostate cancer v.
 mucosal v.
 OraVax v.
 rhesus rotavirus-tetravalent v. (RRV-TV)
 rotavirus tetravalent v.
 Theratope v.
 tumor v.
 yeast-recombinant hepatitis B v.
VACTERL
 vertebral, anal, cardiac, tracheoesophageal fistula, renal, limb
 VACTERL syndrome
vacuolar
 v. H+-ATPase
 v. nephrosis
vacuolar-type proton pump immunocytochemistry
vacuolating
 v. toxin gene A (VacA)
 v. toxin gene A cytotoxin

vacuole
 pinocytosis v.
 testicular adenomatoid tumor v.
vacuolization
 isometric tubular v.
Vacutainer
 V. bag
 V. bottle
 V. tube
vacuum
 v. constriction device (VCD)
 v. constriction erection
 v. entrapment device
 v. erection device (VED)
 v. erection technology (VET)
 v. extraction device
 v. tumescence device
VAD
 vincristine, doxorubicin, dexamethasone
VAG
 vascular access graft
vagal
 v. efferent outflow
 v. input neuron
 v. preganglionic neuron
 v. stimulation
vagina, pl. vaginae
 atrophic v.
 high-ending v.
 passage of flatus per v.
 septate v.
vaginal
 v. atresia
 v. bleeding
 v. *Candida*
 v. celiotomy
 v. cone
 v. cone biopsy
 v. cone for pelvic floor exercise
 v. construction
 v. cuff
 v. cuff cellulitis
 v. cutback
 v. descent
 v. discharge
 v. electrical stimulation
 v. estrogen deficiency
 v. eversion
 v. fistula
 v. fistula cup
 v. flap
 v. flap reconstruction and pubovaginal sling procedure
 v. foreign body
 v. hiatus

vaginal *(continued)*
    v. inflammation
    v. lithotomy
    v. mass
    v. morcellation
    v. mucosa
    v. needle suspension procedure
    v. prolapse
    v. repair
    v. suppository
    v. trichomoniasis
    v. ulcer
    v. vesicostomy
    v. wall approach
    v. wall sling procedure
vaginalis
    Gardnerella v.
    patent processus v.
    processus v.
    Trichomonas v.
    vestigium processus v.
vaginalitis
vaginate
vaginectomy
vaginoplasty
    cutback-type v.
    posterior flap v.
    tissue expansion v.
vaginoscopy
vaginosis
    bacterial v.
vaginourethroplasty
vagosympathetic balance
vagotomy
    bilateral v.
    hemigastrectomy and v. (H&V)
    highly selective v.
    laparoscopic v.
    laser laparoscopic v.
    medical v.
    parietal cell v. (PCV)
    proximal gastric v. (PGV)
    pyloroplasty and v. (P&V)
    v. and pyloroplasty (V&P)
    Roux-en-Y procedure with v.
    selective proximal v. (SPV)
    superselective v.
    surgical v.
    total bilateral v.
    truncal v.
vagovagally mediated receptive relaxation
vagus nerve
valacyclovir
Valcyte
valerian
valethamate bromide
valganciclovir
validity of surgical simulator

valine
Valium
vallate papilla
vallecula, pl. **valleculae**
vallecular
    v. dysphagia
    v. pooling
Valleylab
    V. E3B cautery unit
    V. II generator
    V. SSE-2 cautery unit
    V. SSE2L generator
V-alpha gene
Valpin 50
valproate
    sodium v.
valproic
    v. acid
    v. acid hepatotoxicity
    v. acid therapy
Valsalva
    V. leak-point pressure (VLPP)
    V. leak-point pressure concept
    V. maneuver
    V. ratio
    taeniae of V.
valsalviana
    dysphagia v.
Valtrac BAR
valuable additional parameter
value
    F v.
    negative predictive v. (NPV)
    positive predictive v. (PPV)
    predictive v.
    reference v.
    target hemocrit v.
    therapeutic v.
valva, pl. **valvae**
    v. ilealis
    v. ileocaecalis
valve
    v. ablation
    Amussat v.
    anal v.
    anterior urethral v.
    antireflux v.
    Ball v.
    Bauhin v.
    v. of Bauhin
    Benchekroun hydraulic ileal v.
    v. bladder
    blunting of v.
    Braune v.
    v. of colon
    competent ileocecal v.
    continent v.
    esophageal v. (ESV)

esophageal Z Stent with Dua antireflux v.
failed nipple v.
flap v.
frenulum of ileocolic v.
Gerlach v.
gonadal vein v.
v. of Guerin
Heister v.
Holter v.
Houston v.
v. of Houston
ileal intestinal antireflux v.
ileal nipple v.
ileocecal intestinal antireflux v.
incompetent ileocecal v.
intestinal antireflux v.
intussuscepted nipple v.
v. of Kerckring
Kock nipple v.
Kohlrausch v.
LeVeen v.
lipomatous ileocecal v.
Lopez enteral v.
v. of Macalister
Mitrofanoff v.
modified ileocecal v.
Morgagni v.
nipple v.
nonintussuscepted v.
posterior urethral v. type I–IV (PUV)
v. prolapse
Quinton single-port scissor v.
rectal v.
scissors v.
Setguard antireflux v.
sigmoid v.
spiral v.
Spivack v.
urethral v.
v. of Varolius

valved
v. rectum
v. voice prosthesis

valvotomy
rectal v.

valvula, valvule, pl. **valvulae**
Amussat v.
valvulae anales
valvulae conniventes
v. fossae navicularis
v. processus vermiformis
v. spiralis

valvular heart disease
valvulectomy
Vamin amino acid solution
van
V. Bogaert disease
v. Buren disease
v. Buren sound
V. de Kamer fecal fat procedure
v. den Bergh disease
v. den Bergh reaction
v. den Bergh test
v. Hees Activity Index (VHAI)
v. Hees index
v. Hook operation
V. Slyke formula
v. Sonnenberg gallbladder catheter
v. Sonnenberg sump drain

Vanceril inhaler
Vancocin HCl
Vancoled
vancomycin hydrochloride
vancomycin/nalidixic acid agar
vancomycin-resistant enterococcus (VRE)
vanillacetic acid (VLA)
vanilloid agent
vanillylmandelic acid (VMA)
vanished testis syndrome
vanishing
v. bile duct syndrome (VBDS)
v. bile duct system
v. gonad
v. testis

Vanquish Analgesic Caplets
Vansil
Vantin
Vapor Cut loop
vaporization
benign prostatic hyperplasia transurethral v.
contact laser v.
laser v.

VaporTome
VaporTrode electrode
Vaqta
Varco gallbladder forceps
vardenafil HCl
variability
variable
v. nuclear crowding
v. stiffness endoscope

NOTES

variable (continued)
    v. stiffness enteroscope
    stone v.
    time-dependent v.

Varian
    V. BrachyTherapy
    V. model 3600 gas chromatography

variance
    geographic v.
    hypovolemic v.
    isovolemic v.
    Kruskal-Wallis analysis of v.

variant
    kidney v.
    trifurcation v.
    Wilms tumor clear cell sarcoma v.
    Wilms tumor multilocular cyst v.
    Wilms tumor rhabdomyosarcoma v.

variation
    coefficient of v.
    diurnal v.
    intraprostatic characteristic v.
    phasic-free tone v.

Varibar oral contrast media

variceal
    v. banding
    v. band ligation
    v. bleeding
    v. column
    v. decompression
    v. hemorrhage
    v. ligator
    v. pressure
    v. pressure measuring device
    v. sclerosant
    v. sclerosis
    v. sclerotherapy
    v. sclerotherapy in esophagus
    v. size inclusion criteria
    v. wall

varicella-zoster
    v.-z. infection
    v.-z. virus (VZV)

varices (*pl. of* varix)

varicocele, varicole
    v. embolization
    v. repair
    symptomatic v.

varicocelectomy
    inguinal v.
    laparoscopic v.
    microsurgical inguinal v.
    v. recurrence
    retroperitoneal v.
    scrotal v.
    subinguinal microsurgical v.

Varicoscreen

varicosis coli totalis

varicosity

variegate
    v. coproporphyria
    v. porphyria (VP)

Variject needle

varioliform
    v. gastritis
    v. gastropathy

varioliformis
    gastritis v.

variolosa
    orchitis v.

various types of malignant tumors

VariSeed 7.0 software computer program

varix, pl. **varices**
    actively bleeding v.
    alcoholic v.
    anorectal v.
    bar-type esophageal v.
    bleeding gastric v. (BGV)
    blue v.
    v. of colon
    colonic v.
    common bile duct v.
    downhill esophageal v.
    duodenal v.
    ectopic v.
    EEA stapling of v.
    endoscopic band ligation of v.
    esophageal v.
    esophagogastric v.
    familial colonic v.
    fundal v.
    fundic v.
    gallbladder v.
    gastric v.
    gastroesophageal v. type 1, 2
    v. grading system F1, F2, F3
    idiopathic v.
    ileal v.
    isolated gastric varices type 1, 2 (IGV)
    jejunal v.
    v. ligation
    mesenteric v.
    obliterated v.
    Okuda transhepatic obliteration of v.
    paraesophageal v.
    percutaneous transhepatic obliteration of esophageal v.
    peristomal v.
    radius of v.
    rectal v.
    rectosigmoid v.
    transesophageal ligation of v.

Varolius
    valve of V.

varying degrees of certainty
vas, pl. **vasa**
    v. aberrans
    v. afferens glomeruli
    vasa afferentia
    v. deferens
    v. deferens obstruction
    v. deferens secretion
    v. deferens stricture
    v. efferens glomeruli
    v. epididymidis
    vasa recta
    vasa recta bundle
    vasa vasorum
vasalgia
vasal pedicle orchiopexy
Vas-Cath
Vasclip alternative to vasectomy
vascopressin
    hydroosmotic action of v.
vascular
    v. abnormality
    v. access
    v. access complication
    v. access failure
    v. access graft (VAG)
    v. access site
    v. anastomosis
    v. bruit
    v. cachexia
    v. cecal fold
    v. cell adhesion molecule-1 (VCAM-1)
    v. cirrhosis
    v. clamp
    v. coat of stomach
    v. collateral network
    v. compromise
    v. disease
    v. ectasia
    v. endothelial growth factor (VEGF)
    v. hemangioma
    v. injury
    v. insufficiency
    v. invasion
    v. laceration
    v. laceration repair
    v. lamina
    v. lesion
    v. malformation
    v. malformation of bladder
    v. neoplasm
    v. nephritis
    v. nephropathy
    v. parameter
    v. pattern
    v. pedicle
    peripheral v.
    v. permeability factor (VPF)
    v. permeation of tumor cell
    v. plasminogen activator (v-PA)
    v. plexus
    v. rejection
    v. renal mass
    v. smooth muscle
    v. smooth muscle cell (VSMC)
    v. stapler
    v. steal syndrome
    v. surgery
    v. suture
    v. tuft
vascularity
vascularization
    intraprostatic v.
vasculature
    appearance of normal colon v.
    intraprostatic v.
    kidney v.
    preglomerular v.
    v. responsiveness
vasculitic
    v. lesion
    v. neuropathy
vasculitis
    allergic v.
    ANCA-associated systemic v.
    antineutrophilic cytoplasmic autoantibody-small vessel v. (ANCA-SVV)
    extrarenal v.
    leukocytoclastic v.
    lymphocytic v.
    mesenteric v.
    necrotizing bowel v.
    renal v.
    rheumatoid v.
    systemic lupus erythematosus v.
    visceral v.
vasculogenic impotence
vasculopathy
    acute renal transplant v.
    noncerebral v.

NOTES

vasculopathy (continued)
    portal hypertensive intestinal v. (PHIV)
vasculosa
    tunica v.
vasculum aberrans
vasectomized
vasectomy
    Casale v.
    crossover v.
    no-scalpel v.
    open-ended v.
    percutaneous v.
    v. reversal
    reversible v.
    Vasclip alternative to v.
Vaseline gauze
vasiform
vasitis nodosa
vasoablative endothelial sarcoma (VABES)
vasoactive
    v. drug
    v. intestinal peptide (VIP)
    v. intestinal peptide distribution
    v. intestinal peptide-secreting tumor (VIPoma, vipoma)
    v. intestinal polypeptide (VIP)
    v. intestinal polypeptide binding
    v. intestinal polypeptide immunoreactivity (VIP-IR)
    v. intestinal polypeptide stain
    v. intestinal polypeptide tumor (VIPoma, vipoma)
    v. peptide-cytokine interaction
vasoconstriction
    afferent arteriolar v.
    baroreceptor-mediated mesenteric arterial v.
    radiocontrast-induced renal v.
    reflex splanchnic v.
    renal v.
    splanchnic v.
vasoconstrictor peptide
vasocutaneous fistula
vasodilatation
    peripheral v.
vasodilation
    endothelium-dependent v.
    v. of portasystemic collateral
    renal v.
    sympathetic response to v.
vasodilator
    renal v.
vasoepididymography
vasoepididymostomy
    ASSI METE-5168 end-to-end v.
    Goldstein Microspike approximator clamp for v.
    Silber v.
vasoformative
vasography
    fine-needle v.
    percutaneous v.
    transrectal v.
vasoligation
Vasomax
vasomotor disorder
vasoorchidostomy
vasopressin
    arginine v. (AVP)
    1-deamino-8-d-arginine v.
    fetal arginine v.
    v. infusion
    neonatal arginine v.
    v. type 2 receptor
    v. with nitroglycerin
vasopressinase
vasopressin-induced cAMP
vasopuncture
vasorelaxation
vasoresection
vasorrhaphy
vasorum
    vasa v.
vasosection
vasospasm
vasospasmolytic
vasospastic
vasostomy
Vasotec
vasotomy
vasovagal reflex
vasovasostomy
    Goldstein Microspike approximator clamp for v.
vasovasotomy
    cross v.
    multiple v.'s
vasovesiculectomy
vasovesiculitis
vasovesiculography
Vasoxyl
vastus lateralis muscle flap
VATER
    vertebral, anal, tracheoesophageal fistula, renal
        VATER syndrome
Vater
    ampulla of V.
    invaginating ampulla of V.
    papilla of V.
VATS
    videoassisted thoracic surgery
vault
    rectal v.

Vaxcel dialysis catheter
VBDS
    vanishing bile duct syndrome
V-beta gene
VBG
    vertical banded gastroplasty
VCA
    antiviral capsid antigen
VCAM-1
    vascular cell adhesion molecule-1
VCD
    vacuum constriction device
        Dacomed Catalyst VCD
        Mentor-Piston VCD
        Mentor Response VCD
        Mentor-Touch VCD
        Osbon ErecAid VCD
        Pos-T-Vac VCD
VCD, VED
    Mission VCD, VED
VCG
    voiding cystogram
VCR
    vincristine
VCUG
    vesicoureterogram
    voiding cystourethrogram
Vd
    volume of distribution
VDR
    vitamin D receptor
VDRL
    Venereal Disease Research Laboratory
V-echinocandin
Vectastain ABC kit
vector
    amplitude-acrophase v.
    bacterial v.
    V. volume measurement
vectorial delivery
Vectra hemodialysis access graft
vecuronium
VED
    vacuum erection device
Veetids
vegetable
    allium v.
    cruciferous v.
vegetans
    pyostomatitis v.
vegetarian diet
vegetative lesion

VEGF
    vascular endothelial growth factor
veil
    Jackson v.
vein
    aberrant obturator v.
    accessory saphenous v.
    adrenal v.
    arcuate v.
    arterialization of portal v.
    azygos v.
    bladder v.
    Burow v.
    cardinal v.
    cavernosal v.
    cavernous transformation of portal v. (CTPV)
    circumflex v.
    common iliac v.
    crural v.
    deep dorsal v.
    dilated v.
    dorsal v.
    esophageal collateral v. (ECV)
    external spermatic v.
    extrahepatic portal v.
    gastric v.
    gonadal v.
    gubernacular v.
    hepatic v. (HV)
    iliac v.
    inferior adrenal v.
    inferior mesenteric v. (IMV)
    inferior rectal v.
    interlobar v.
    internal iliac v.
    internal pudendal v.
    Krukenberg v.
    left hepatic v. (LHV)
    lumbar v.
    mesenteric v.
    middle hepatic v. (MHV)
    middle rectal v.
    muscularization of v.
    obturator v.
    omental v.
    palisade-type v.
    pancreaticoduodenal v.
    paraesophageal collateral v.
    paraumbilical v.
    v. patch
    periesophageal collateral v.

NOTES

vein (continued)
    peripheral acinar v.
    peritoneal v.
    periurethral v.
    portal v. (PV)
    pudendal v.
    rectal v.
    renal v.
    v. retractor
    Retzius v.
    right hepatic v. (RHV)
    Ruysch v.
    sacral v.
    saphenous v.
    shunt index via inferior mesenteric v. (SI-I)
    shunt index via superior mesenteric v. (SI-S)
    spermatic v.
    splanchnic v.
    splenic v.
    subclavian v.
    sulcus of umbilical v.
    superior mesenteric v. (SMV)
    superior rectal v.
    tangle of hemorrhoidal v.'s
    thoracoabdominal collateral v.
    umbilical v.
    urethral v.
    vesical v.

Velban
    V., actinomycin D, bleomycin (VAB)
    V., actinomycin D, bleomycin, platinum (VAB-II)
    cisplatin, methotrexate, V. (CMV)

Vella fistula

velocimetry
    laser Doppler v.

velocity
    angular v.
    dorsal nerve conduction v.
    v. measurement
    portal blood v.
    portal vein blood flow v. (PFV)
    portal venous v. (PVV)
    prostate-specific antigen v. (PSAV)
    tumor peak systolic v. (TPSV)

velopharyngeal insufficiency (VPI)

Velosef

Velpeau hernia

vena, pl. **venae**
    v. cava
    v. cava hiatus
    venae cavernosae penis
    v. cavography
    v. marginalis epididymis of Haberer

venacavogram

venacavography

venae (*pl. of* vena)

venerea
    urethritis v.

venereal
    v. bubo
    v. disease
    V. Disease Research Laboratory (VDRL)
    v. proctocolitis
    v. sore
    v. wart

venereum
    lymphogranuloma v. (LGV)
    papilloma v.

veneris
    mons v.

venezuelensis
    Strongyloides v.

venipuncture
    separate peripheral v.

venlafaxine

venodilation
    nitrate-induced v.
    systemic v.

Venofer

venogenic impotence

venogram
    hepatic v.
    renal v.
    weeping willow appearance on v.

venography
    adrenal v.
    hepatic v.
    pedal control v.
    renal v.
    splenic v.
    splenoportal v.
    transjugular portal v.

venoocclusive
    v. disease of liver
    v. dysfunction
    v. liver disease

venoperitoneostomy

venosi
    fissura ligamenti v.

venosum
    fissure of ligamentum v.
    ligamentum v.

venosus
    plexus v.

venous
    v. blood sample
    v. circulation
    v. ectasia
    v. engorgement
    v. hum
    v. invasion
    v. leakage

v. leak impotence
v. leak syndrome
v. outflow obstructive disease
v. pattern
v. pooling
v. stasis
v. thromboembolism (VTE)
v. thrombosis
v. web
v. web disease
venovenous
    v. access
    v. bypass
    v. continuous hemodialysis
    v. hemofiltration
venter propendens
ventilation
    mechanical v.
ventilatory support
venting
    v. percutaneous gastrostomy (VPG)
    v. percutaneous gastrostomy tube
Ventolin
ventral
    v. apron prepuce
    v. bending technique
    v. bud
    v. celiotomy
    v. chronic calcific pancreatitis
    v. hernia
    v. herniorrhaphy
    v. meatotomy
    v. mesogastrium
    v. patch urethroplasty
    v. posterior inferior (VPI)
    v. sacral rootlet
    v. surface
    v. transperitoneal laparoscopic approach
ventralis
ventricle
ventricular
    v. canal
    v. cerebrospinal
    v. tachycardia
ventriculare
    corpus v.
ventricularis
    fundus v.
ventriculoperitoneal (VP)
    v. shunt
ventriculus, pl. ventriculi

    anadenia ventriculi
    caecus minor ventriculi
    corpus ventriculi
    descensus ventriculi
    fibrae obliquae ventriculi
    fibromatosis ventriculi
    fundus ventriculi
    polyposis ventriculi
    ulcus ventriculi
ventrocystorrhaphy
ventroscopy
ventrotomy
ventrum
    v. of penis
    v. penis flap
venula, pl. venulae
    venulae rectae renis
venular
venule
    collecting v.
    hepatic v.
    portal v.
    stellate v.
    straight v.
    subtunical v.
VePesid, ifosfamide (with mesna rescue), Platinol (VIP)
vera
    hemospermia v.
    melena v.
    polycythemia v.
verapamil
Veratrum alkaloid
Veress
    V. cannula
    V. needle
verge
    anal v.
Vergon
veritas
    in vivo v.
vermicular
    v. appendage
    v. colic
    v. movement
vermicularis
    Enterobius v.
vermiform
    v. appendix
    v. body

NOTES

vermiformis
    ostium appendicis v.
    valvula processus v.

verminous
    v. appendicitis
    v. colic
    v. ileus

Vermox

Verner-Morrison syndrome

Vernon-David
    V.-D. proctoscope
    V.-D. rectal speculum
    V.-D. sigmoidoscope

verruca vulgaris

verruciform xanthoma

verrucous
    v. carcinoma
    v. gastritis

Versabran
    Modane V.

VERSANT HCV RNA qualitative assay

Versa-PEG gastrostomy kit

VersaPulse
    V. PowerSuite dual-wavelength laser
    V. PowerSuite holmium laser
    V. Select laser

Versed

vertebra, pl. **vertebrae**
    picture-frame v.

vertebral
    v., anal, cardiac, tracheoesophageal fistula, renal, limb (VACTERL)
    v., anal, tracheoesophageal fistula, renal (VATER)

vertex, pl. **vertices**
    v. of urinary bladder
    v. vesicae urinariae

vertical
    v. banded gastroplasty (VBG)
    v. fold
    v. mattress suture
    v. midline incision
    v. plication suture
    v. reduction rectoplasty
    v. ring gastroplasty (VRG)
    v. Silastic ring gastroplasty
    v. strip-pattern breast examination
    v. transmission
    v. vesicomyotomy (VVM)

vertigo
    gastric v.
    objective v.
    subjective v.

verum
    diverticulum ilei v.

verumontanitis

verumontanum

very
    v. late activation (VLA)
    v. low birth weight infant
    v. low calorie diet (VLCD)
    v. low density lipoprotein (VLDL)
    v. low density lipoprotein cholesterol

vesica, pl. **vesicae**
    v. biliaris
    bullous edema V.
    ectopia vesicae
    endometriosis vesicae
    v. fellea
    v. ileale pouch
    malacoplakia vesicae
    V. percutaneous bladder neck stabilization
    V. percutaneous bladder neck suspension kit
    v. prostatica
    V. sling
    V. sling procedure
    trigonum vesicae
    ulcus simplex vesicae
    v. urinaria
    uvula vesicae

vesical
    v. artery
    v. calculus
    v. compliance
    v. diverticulectomy
    v. diverticulum
    v. exstrophy
    v. external sphincter dyssynergia (VSD)
    v. fibrosis
    v. fistula
    v. hematuria
    v. ligament
    v. lithotomy
    v. neck
    v. neck resistance
    v. neck stenosis
    v. plexus
    v. prostatism
    v. schistosomiasis
    v. vein

vesicale
    plexus v.

vesicalis
    anus v.
    plexus v.

vesical-sacral-sphincter loop

Vesicare

vesicle
    brush-border membrane v. (BBMV)
    endocytotic v.
    Golgi v.
    v. hernia

vesicle · vesiculography

    leiomyoma of seminal v.
    metanephric v.
    prechylomicron transport v.
    seminal v.
    spermatic v.
vesicoamniotic shunt
vesicoanal reflex
vesicocavernous
vesicocele
vesicocervical
vesicoclysis
vesicocolic fistula
vesicocolonic fistula
vesicocutaneous fistula
vesicoenteric fistula
vesicofixation
vesicoileal reflux
vesicointestinal
    v. fistula
    v. reflex
vesicolithiasis
vesicomyectomy
vesicomyotomy
    circular v. (CVM)
    vertical v. (VVM)
vesicopelvic fascia
vesicoperineal
vesicoprostatic
    v. calculus
    v. plexus
vesicopubic
vesicopustule
vesicorectal fistula
vesicorectostomy
vesicorenal
vesicosalpingovaginal fistula
vesicosigmoid
vesicosigmoidostomy
vesicosphincteric dyssynergia
vesicospinal
vesicostomy
    Blocksom v.
    Casale v.
    continent v.
    cutaneous v.
    Lapides v.
    preputial continent v.
    Rink modification of Casale continent catheterizable v.
    vaginal v.
vesicotomy
vesicoumbilical fistula

vesicourachal diverticulum
vesicoureteral
    v. anastomotic stricture
    v. reflux (VUR)
    v. regurgitation
    v. suspension
vesicoureteric
    v. reflux
    v. stenosis
vesicoureterogram (VCUG)
vesicourethral
    v. anastomosis
    v. anastomotic stricture
    v. canal
    v. reflux
    v. reflux and renal dysplasia (VURD)
    v. suspension
vesicouterina
    excavatio v.
vesicouterine
    v. fistula
    v. pouch
vesicouterinum
    cavum v.
vesicouterovaginal
vesicovaginal
    v. fistula (VVF)
    v. Holter
    v. lithotomy
    v. space
vesicovaginorectal fistula
vesicovaginostomy
vesicula
    v. bilis
    v. fellea
    v. seminalis
vesiculase
vesiculectomy
    prostatoseminal v.
    retrovesical v.
    total prostatoseminal v.
    transcoccygeal v.
    transperineal v.
    transvesical v.
vesiculitis
vesiculobullous disorder
vesiculocavernous
vesiculodeferential artery
vesiculogram
vesiculography
    seminal v. (SVG)

NOTES

vesiculoprostatitis
vesiculotomy
    seminal v.
vesiculotubular
vesiculotympanitic resonance
Vespore disinfectant
Vesprin
VESS
    videoendoscopic swallowing study
Vess chair
vessel
    accessory v.
    blood v.
    caliber-persistent v.
    capsular blood v.
    chyliferous v.
    cremasteric v.
    v. dilator
    dysmorphic v.
    ectatic v.
    feeding v.
    gastroepiploic blood v.
    gonadal v.
    hypogastric v.
    hypoplastic blind-ending spermatic v.
    ileal blood v.
    ileocolic v.
    internal spermatic v.
    lacteal v.
    lymphatic v.
    mesocolonic v.
    nonbleeding visible v. (NBVV)
    pudendal v.
    replaced hepatic v.
    serosal blood v.
    telangiectatic v.
    v. tip
    ulcer v.
    visible v.
    visible ulcer v.
vestibular gland
vestibularis
    anus v.
vestibule
    laryngeal v.
vestibuli
    utriculus v.
vestibulourethral
vestige
vestigial
vestigium processus vaginalis
vest-over-pants
    v.-o.-p. hernial repair
    v.-o.-p. herniorrhaphy
VET
    vacuum erection technology
VET-CO vacuum system
Vezien abdominal scissors

VFC
    Actis venous flow controller
VFEND
V-flap meatoplasty
VGTT
    videographic tool technology
VHAI
    van Hees Activity Index
VHL gene
VIABIL biliary endoprosthesis
viability
    intestinal v.
    v. testing
ViaCath
    V. computer-assisted robotic endoluminal system
    V. endoluminal surgery system
Viadur
Viagra
    esprolol plus V.
vial
    Port-A-Germ anaerobic transport v.
    scintillation v.
Vibramycin
Vibrio
    V. *alginolyticus*
    V. *cholerae*
    V. *cholerae* biotype *albensis*
    V. *cholerae* biotype *eltor*
    V. *cholerae* biotype *proteus*
    V. *cholera O1*
    V. *cholera O139*
    V. *eltor*
    V. *fetus* infection
    V. *fluvialis*
    V. *furnissii*
    V. *hollisae*
    V. *metschnikovii*
    V. *parahaemolyticus*
    V. *vulnificus*
vibriocidal
vibrotactile stimulation testing
Vickers M85a microdensitometer
Vicodin
Vicryl
    V. mesh
    V. suture
VID
    vitellointestinal duct
Vidal operation
vidarabine
video
    V. Image Processor model 450
    v. monitor
    v. pressure flow electromyography
    v. push enteroscope
    v. recorder
    v. small bowel enteroscopy

v. timer
v. transurethral resection technique
videoassisted thoracic surgery (VATS)
videocamera
    Urocam v.
videocapsule
    v. endoscopy
    Given M2A endoscopic v.
videocholangioscope
videocholangioscopy
videocolonoscope
    EVE Fujinon v.
    forward-viewing v.
    Fujinon EC7-CM2 v.
    Fujinon EVC-M v.
    Olympus CF-1T100L v.
    Olympus CF-100TL v.
    Olympus CF-TL-series forward-viewing v.
    Olympus EVIS v.
    Olympus PCF-130L v.
    Welch Allyn videocolonoscope 8451
videoconverter
    sequential v.
videocystourethrography
videodensitometry
videoduodenoscope
    Fujinon ED7-XU2 v.
    Fujinon EVD-XL v.
    Fujinon 310XU v.
    Olympus JF-series v.
    Olympus JF-V-series v.
    Olympus JT-series v.
    side-viewing v.
    TJF-10, -20 v.
videoelectroscope
    Fujinon CEG-FP-series v.
videoendoscope
    double-channel v.
    Fujinon UGI-FP-series v.
    infrared v.
    JF-200 side-viewing v.
    Olympus EVIS 140 Q v.
    Olympus GF-series v.
    Olympus GIF-series double-channel therapeutic v.
    Olympus GIF-SQ-series v.
    Olympus GIF-T-series v.
    Olympus GIF-200Z v.
    Olympus JF-series v.
    Olympus Q200 v.
    Pentax EC-series v.
    Pentax FD-series v.
    Toshiba videoendoscope
    Welch Allyn videoendoscope
videoendoscopic swallowing study (VESS)
videoendoscopy
    dynamic fluorescence v.
    Lugol-combined upper gastrointestinal v.
    zoom v.
videoenteroscope
    Olympus SIG-100L v.
    Olympus SSIF-series v.
    Olympus XSIF-series v.
videoesophagoscopy
videoesophagram
videofluoroscopic
    v. swallow study
    v. technique
videofluoroscopy
videofluorourodynamic study
videogastroscope
videogastroscope
    Fujinon 400-series super image v.
    Olympus GIF-XQ200 v.
    Olympus GIF-XQ230 v.
    Olympus GIF-XQ240 v.
    Pentax EG-2900 v.
    transnasal v.
videographic tool technology (VGTT)
videoinstrument
    XQ v.
videolaseroscopy cholecystectomy
videomonitored TUR
videoprocessor
    real-time v.
videoproctography
videoresectoscope
    continuous-flow v.
    Foroblique v.
    Iglesias fiberoptic v.
    v. loop
    OES 4000 v.
    Olympus continuous flow v.
    Richard Wolf v.
    v. sheath
    Storz v.
    transurethral v.
    Wolf v.

NOTES

videoscope
    CV-1 v.
    SlimSIGHT gastrointestinal v.
videosigmoidoscope
videourodynamic
    v. evaluation
    v. testing
view
    en face v.
    longitudinal v.
    postevacuation v.
    retroflexed v.
    slide-by v.
    stereomicroscopic v.
    transverse v.
vigabatrin
vigorous achalasia
VIGOR trial
villi (*pl. of* villus)
villiferous
villoglandular
    v. adenoma
    v. polyp
villous, villose
    v. arteritis
    v. arthritis
    v. atrophy
    v. coat of small intestine
    v. colorectal adenoma
    v. effacement
    v. epithelium
    v. folds of stomach
    v. papilloma
    v. polyp
    v. tumor
villous-tip cell
villus, pl. **villi**
    v. cell
    colonic v.
    duodenal v.
    fingerlike v.
    intestinal v.
    jejunal v.
    leaflike v.
    ridged-convoluted v.
    small intestinal v.
    v. tip
    tongue-shaped v.
vimentin staining
Vim-Silverman
    V.-S. biopsy needle
    V.-S. technique
    V.-S. technique for liver biopsy
vinblastine
    v., actinomycin D, bleomycin (mini-VAB)
    cisplatin, methotrexate, v. (CMV)
    doxorubicin, bleomycin sulfate, v. (ABV)
    methotrexate, cisplatin, v. (MCV)
Vincent curtsy
vincristine (VCR)
    v., Adriamycin, cyclophosphamide (VAC)
    v., doxorubicin, dexamethasone (VAD)
Vindelov method flow cytometry analysis
vinorelbine
Vinson syndrome
Viokase
violaceous
violation
    scrotal v.
violet
    gentian v.
violin-string adhesion
Vioxx Gastrointestinal Outcomes Research trial
VIP
    vasoactive intestinal peptide
    vasoactive intestinal polypeptide
    VePesid, ifosfamide (with mesna rescue), Platinol
    voluntary interruption of pregnancy
    VIP antiserum
    VIP stain
VIP-IR
    vasoactive intestinal polypeptide immunoreactivity
VIPoma, vipoma
    vasoactive intestinal peptide-secreting tumor
    vasoactive intestinal polypeptide tumor
    VIPoma syndrome
VIP-secreting neuronoma
Virag
    V. injector
    V. operation
viral
    v. cholangitis
    v. colitis
    v. culture
    v. cystitis
    v. diarrhea
    v. dysentery
    v. enteritis
    v. gastritis
    v. gastroenteritis
    v. glycoprotein
    v. hemorrhagic fever
    v. hepatitis
    v. hepatitis marker
    v. hepatitis type A, B
    v. inclusion body
    v. infection

viral · virus

v. membrane fusion
v. oncoprotein
v. replication
v. serologic titer
ViraPap HPV dot blot hybridization test
Virazole
Virchow sentinel node
Virchow-Troisier node
viremia
    hepatitis C v.
virgin
    v. lymphocyte
    v. ulcer
viridans
    alpha *Streptococcus* v.
    Staphylococcus v.
    Streptococcus v.
virile
    membrum v.
    v. reflex
virilis
    crista urethralis v.
    orificium urethrae externum v.
    urethra v.
virilism
    adrenal v.
virilization
virilizing tumor
Virilon
virion
    HBV v.
virological
virology
virtual
    V. Biopsy system
    v. colonoscopy Side Fire APC probe
    v. cystoscopy
    v. endoscopy
    v. enteroscopy
    v. focus shock wave
    v. nephroureteroscopy
    v. reality simulator
    v. reality technology
    V. Vision
    V. Vision audiovisual system for EGD and colonoscopy
virucidal agent
virulence
    encoding v.

enhanced v.
v. factor
virulent diarrhea
virus
    v. A, B hepatitis
    adenoassociated v. (AAV)
    Aichi v.
    antibody to hepatitis A v. (anti-HAV)
    antibody to hepatitis C v. (anti-HCV)
    antibody to hepatitis D v. (anti-HDV)
    delta v.
    dengue v.
    Epstein-Barr v. (EBV)
    esophageal condyloma v.
    GB virus C/hepatitis G v. (GBV-C/HGV)
    Hawaii v.
    hepatitis A v. (HAV)
    hepatitis B v. (HBV)
    hepatitis B-like DNA v.
    hepatitis C v. (HCV)
    hepatitis D v. (HDV)
    hepatitis delta v. (HDV)
    hepatitis E v. (HEV)
    hepatitis G v. (HGV)
    herpes simplex v. (HSV)
    herpes zoster v.
    human immunodeficiency v. (HIV)
    human T-cell leukemia v. type I (HTLV-I)
    human T-cell lymphotrophic v. type I, II
    influenza v.
    live attenuated v.
    v. load
    Manchester v.
    Marburg v.
    molluscum contagiosum v. (MCV)
    mother-to-infant transmission of hepatitis C v.
    neutropic v.
    Norwalk v.
    Norwalk-like v. (NLV)
    recombinant capsid protein of Norwalk v. (rNV)
    Sapporo v.
    v. shedding
    TCCA v.
    transfusion-transmitted v. (TTV)

NOTES

virus *(continued)*
  TT v. (TTV)
  varicella-zoster v. (VZV)
viruslike
  v. action (VLA)
  v. particle (VLP)
Viruzilin
viscera *(pl. of* viscus*)*
visceral
  v. angiography
  v. arteriography
  v. dysfunction
  v. hyperalgesia
  v. hypersensitivity
  v. ischemia
  v. larva migrans
  v. leishmaniasis
  v. muscle
  v. neuropathy
  v. pain
  v. peritoneum
  v. traction reflex
  v. vasculitis
visceralgia
visceralis
  fascia pelvis v.
visceromegaly
visceromotor, viscerimotor
visceroparietal
visceroptosis, visceroptosia
viscerosensory reflex
viscerotomy
viscerotrophic
viscerotropic
viscerum
  situs inversus v.
viscid bile
viscidosis
viscoelastic
  v. collagen fiber
  v. gel
viscoelasticity
  bladder v.
viscometer
viscosity
  plasma v.
  semen v.
viscous
  v. bile
  v. lidocaine
  v. lidocaine premedication
  v. Xylocaine gargle
viscus, pl. **viscera**
  abdominal v.
  hollow v.
  intraabdominal v.
  intraperitoneal v.
  perforated v.
  strangulated v.

vise
  torque v.
visible
  v. abdominal distention
  v. peristalsis
  v. ulcer vessel
  v. vessel
  v. vessel significance
visible-light lithotripsy
Visicath endoscope
Visick
  V. dysphagia classification
  V. gastric cancer grading system
Visicol tablet
Visilex mesh
vision
  direct v.
  V. Sciences VSI 2000 flexible sigmoidoscope system
  V. System EndoSheath
  V. System sigmoidoscope
  tunnel v.
  Virtual V.
Visiport device
Visken
Vistaflex biliary stent
Vistaril
Vistide
visual
  v. endoscopically controlled laser
  v. evoked potential
  v. laser ablation
  v. laser ablation of prostate (VLAP)
  v. laser-assisted prostatectomy (VLAP)
  v. sexual stimulation testing
visualization
  enhanced v.
  improved v.
vital
  V. HN feeding
  v. sign
  v. staining
VitalStim Therapy electrical stimulation system
vitamin
  v. A, B_{12} absorption test
  v. A, D deficiency
  v. A toxicity
  v. B_{12}
  v. B_6
  v. B_{12} malabsorption
  v. C
  v. D-binding protein (DBP)
  v. D-dependent calbindin-D9k
  v. D receptor (VDR)
  v. D resistance
  v. D supplementation

v. E
fat-soluble v.
hydroxylated v. D
v. K2
Maxisal with v. C
water-soluble v.
Vitaneed
V. feeding
V. tube feeding formula
Vitaxin
Vitelle
V. Irospan
V. Nesentials tablet
V. Nestrex tablet
vitelline
v. duct
v. duct anomaly
vitellointestinal
v. cyst
v. duct (VID)
vitiligo
vitro
in v.
vitronectin-inhibiting HGF-induced tubulogenesis
Vitros
V. Immunodiagnostic Products HBsAg Confirmatory Kit
V. Immunodiagnostic Products HBsAg Reagent Pack and Calibrator
Vittaforma corneae
Vivactil
viverrini
Opisthorchis v.
vividialysis
vividiffusion
vivo
ex v.
in v.
Vivonex
V. Acutrol Enteral Feeding System
V. HN powdered feeding
V. Moss tube
V. TEN
V. TEN feeding
VLA
vanillacetic acid
very late activation
viruslike action

VLAP
visual laser ablation of prostate
visual laser-assisted prostatectomy
VLCD
very low calorie diet
VLDL
very low density lipoprotein
VLDL cholesterol
VLDL triglyceride
VLP
viruslike particle
VLPP
Valsalva leak-point pressure
VM-26
teniposide
VMA
vanillylmandelic acid
VMC
von Meyenburg complex
vocal cord
Vocare bladder system
Vogel operation
Voges-Proskauer test
voice restoration
voided
v. urine
v. volume
voiding
alarm clock v.
v. biofeedback
classic high-pressure low-flow v.
v. cystogram (VCG)
v. cystometrography
v. cystometry
v. cystourethrogram (VCUG)
v. cystourethrography
v. diary
dysfunctional v.
v. dysfunction classification
v. dysfunctionrole of prostate stem cell antigen
v. flow rate
fractionated v.
good v.
incomplete v.
v. initiation
orthotopic v.
v. parameter
v. pressure
reflex v.
staccato v.
v. study

NOTES

voiding *(continued)*
    timed v.
    trigger v.
    v. urethral pressure measurement (VUPM)
    v. urine cytology (VUC)
Voillemier point
vol
    volume
volar
Volhard-Fahr method
Volhard nephritis
Volkmann
    V. operation
    V. pancreatic calculus spoon
    V. rake retractor
    V. spoon for pancreatic calculus
voltage
    RMS v.
    root mean square v.
voltage-dependent anion channel
voltage-gated channel
Voltaren
volume (vol)
    bladder v.
    v. displacement transducer
    v. of distribution (Vd)
    drain v.
    effective arterial blood v. (EABV)
    emptying delta v.
    v. expansion
    extracellular fluid v. (ECV)
    fiber bundle v. (FBV)
    flow v.
    functional hepatic v.
    gallbladder v.
    gastric v.
    interstitial v.
    intragastric v.
    intraperitoneal v.
    intravascular v.
    liver v.
    maximum tolerable v. (MTV)
    mean corpuscular v. (MCV)
    mean prostatic v.
    mean renal v.
    v. overload
    pelvic ileal reservoir v.
    PET dialysate v.
    plasma v.
    prostate v.
    prostatic v.
    renal v.
    v. replacement
    residual urine v. (RUV)
    semen v.
    spermatozoon v.
    target v. (TV)
    transition zone v.
    urea distribution v.
    voided v.
    weight-based peritoneal exchange v.
volumetric data
voluminous hiatus hernia
voluntarily stopping eating and drinking (VSED)
voluntary
    v. guarding
    v. interruption of pregnancy (VIP)
    v. sphincter contraction
volunteer
    normal asymptomatic v.
volvulated Meckel diverticulum
volvulus
    cecal v.
    v. of colon
    colonic v.
    gastric v.
    idiopathic v.
    intestinal v.
    mesenteroaxial gastric v.
    midgut v.
    v. neonatorum
    nongangrenous sigmoid v.
    Onchocerca v.
    organoaxial gastric v.
    v. reduction
    secondary v.
    sigmoid colon v.
vomica
    nux v.
vomicus
vomit
    Barcoo v.
    bilious v.
    black v.
    coffee-grounds v.
vomiting
    bilious v.
    v. center
    chemotherapy-induced v.
    concealed v.
    cyclic v.
    cyclical v.
    diarrhea and v. (D&V)
    dry v.
    epidemic v.
    episodic v.
    erotic v.
    explosive v.
    fecal v.
    hysterical v.
    intractable v.
    ipecac-induced v.
    nausea and v. (N&V)
    nervous v.
    periodic v.
    perioperative v.

pernicious v.
persistent v.
postoperative v.
postprandial v.
posttussive v.
profuse v.
projectile v.
psychogenic v.
recurrent bouts of v.
retention v.
Rhodes Inventory of Nausea and V.
self-induced v.
stercoraceous v.
surreptitious v.
winter v.

vomition
vomitive
vomito negro
vomitory
vomiturition
vomitus
Barcoo v.
bile-stained v.
black v.
bloody v.
bright red v.
coffee-grounds v.
v. cruentes
feculent v.
v. marinus
v. matutinus
v. niger
nonbilious v.
stercoraceous v.

von
V. Andel dilating catheter
v. Ebner gland
v. Gierke disease
V. Haberer-Finney anastomosis
v. Hansemann cell
v. Hippel-Lindau cerebellar hemangioblastomatosis
v. Hippel-Lindau disease
v. Hippel-Lindau gene
v. Hippel-Lindau syndrome
v. Jaksch test
v. Kossa stain
v. Kupffer cell
v. Mering reflex
v. Meyenburg complex (VMC)
v. Petz clamp
v. Petz suture clip
v. Petz suturing apparatus
v. Recklinghausen disease
v. Recklinghausen gastric neurofibroma
v. Recklinghausen neurofibromatosis
v. Recklinghausen tumor
v. Rokitansky disease
v. Willebrand disease
v. Willebrand factor

vontrol programme
voracious appetite
voriconazole
Voronoff operation
VP
variegate porphyria
ventriculoperitoneal
VP shunt

VP-16
V&P
vagotomy and pyloroplasty
VP4 protein conservation
v-PA
vascular plasminogen activator
VPF
vascular permeability factor
VPG
venting percutaneous gastrostomy
VPI
velopharyngeal insufficiency
ventral posterior inferior
Coloscreen VPI
VPI nonadhesive open-end pouch
V/Q mismatch
VQQ technique
VQ technique
VRE
vancomycin-resistant enterococcus
VRG
vertical ring gastroplasty
VSD
vesical external sphincter dyssynergia
VSED
voluntarily stopping eating and drinking
V-shaped ulcer
V sign of Naclerio
V-sign single-ear sensory system
VSI 2000 sigmoidoscope
VSMC
vascular smooth muscle cell
VTC biliary catheter

NOTES

VTE
    venous thromboembolism
VTR-300 enteral feeding pump
VTU-1 vacuum erection device
VUC
    voiding urine cytology
vulgaris
    acne v.
    pemphigus v.
    Proteus v.
    verruca v.
vulgatus
    Bacteroides v.
vulnificus
    Vibrio v.
vulva, pl. vulvae
    rima v.
vulvar
    v. carcinoma
    v. vestibulitis syndrome
vulvitis
vulvoplasty
vulvorectal fistula
vulvovaginal
    v. anus
    v. candidiasis

vulvovaginoplasty
    Williams v.
VUPM
    voiding urethral pressure measurement
VUR
    vesicoureteral reflux
VURD
    vesicourethral reflux and renal dysplasia
        VURD syndrome
VVF
    vesicovaginal fistula
        VVF repair
VVM
    vertical vesicomyotomy
V-Y
    V-Y plasty
    V-Y sliding skin graft
Vygon Nutricath S catheter
Vysis UroVysion DNA probe assay
VZV
    varicella-zoster virus

W
  W. pelvic ileal pouch
  W. pouch
Wacker Sil-Gel 604 silicone cement
wafer
  Stomahesive skin barrier w.
Wagner test
WAGR
  Wilms tumor, aniridia, genitourinary abnormalities, and mental retardation
  WAGR syndrome
wait-and-see approach
wake reflex
Waldenström macroglobulinemia
Waldeyer
  W. fascia
  pelvic colon of W.
  W. sheath
Wales rectal bougie
Walker gallbladder retractor
walking stick phenomenon
wall
  abdominal w.
  anterior abdominal w.
  bowel w.
  capillary w.
  colonic w.
  esophageal w.
  gallbladder w.
  gas-forming organism in bowel w.
  glomerular capillary w. (GCW)
  hydrocele w.
  midabdominal w.
  pharyngeal w.
  posterior abdominal w.
  sinusoidal w.
  w. tension
  thickened gallbladder w.
  w. thickening
  variceal w.
Wallace
  W. anastomosis
  W. technique
  W. technique urinary diversion
Wallstent
  W. delivery device
  W. endoprosthesis
  W. esophageal prosthesis
  W. stent
  Urolume W.
Wallstent-covered SEM stent
Wallstent-I
Walsh
  W. procedure

  W. radical retropubic prostatectomy
  W. surgical modification
Walther
  W. dilator
  W. sound
Waltz endoscopic lithotriptor
wand
  ultrasound w.
wandering
  w. gallbladder
  w. liver
Wangensteen
  W. anastomosis clamp
  W. colostomy
  W. drain
  W. drainage
  W. incision
  W. operation
  W. suction
  W. suction apparatus
  W. suction tube
Wappler
  W. cystoscope with microlens optics
  W. microlens cystourethroscope
warfarin
warfarin-associated subcapsular hematoma
warm
  w. ischemia
  w. ischemia time
  w. saline solution
war nephritis
warrant transplantation
Warren splenorenal shunt
wart
  anal w.
  cervical w.
  exophytic w.
  genital w.
  intraanal w.
  perianal w.
  venereal w.
Warthin-Starry
  W.-S. method
  W.-S. silver stain
Warwick and Ashken technique
wash
  povidone-iodine w.
washer
  Olympus Europe ETD automated endoscope w.
washing
  bladder w.
  w. catheter

washout
    w. cannula
    w. factor
    high rectal w.
    mucosal w.
    w. pyelography
    seminal tract w.
    w. test
Wassilieff disease
wastage
    pregnancy w.
waste
    w. nitrogen excretion
    nitrogenous w.
wastebasket
    w. diagnosis
    w. pouchitis
wasting
    muscle w.
    renal sodium w.
    w. syndrome
water
    w. balance
    body w.
    w. brash
    w. channel
    contamination of w.
    w. cushion lithotriptor
    w. cystometry
    degassed w.
    w. displacing balloon
    w. diuresis
    w. excretion
    fecal contamination of w.
    w. immersion
    insensible loss of w.
    w. loading
    w. permeability
    w. pot perineum
    w. probe
    total body w. (TBW)
water-filled balloon sheath
water-gurgle test
Waterhouse-Friderichsen syndrome
water-induced thermotherapy (WIT)
water-infusion esophageal manometry catheter
watering-can
    w.-c. perineum
    w.-c. scrotum
water-losing nephritis
watermelon
    w. cecum
    w. colon
    w. rectum
    w. stomach (WS)
water-nutrient test
water-perfused catheter

Waterpik
    endoscopic W.
    W. lavage
water-recovery test
water-restriction test
watershed area
water-sipping test
water-soluble
    w.-s. bilirubin
    w.-s. contrast
    w.-s. contrast enema
    w.-s. contrast esophageal swallow
    w.-s. contrast esophageal swallow test
    w.-s. contrast medium
    w.-s. vitamin
Waterston method
water-trap stomach
watery
    w. diarrhea
    w. diarrhea, hypokalemia, and achlorhydria (WDHA)
    w. diarrhea, hypokalemia, and achlorhydria syndrome
    w. diarrhea, hypokalemia, and hypovolemia (WDHH)
    w. diarrhea with hypokalemic alkalosis (WDHA)
    w. stool
Watson
    W. capsule
    W. capsule biopsy
Watson-Alagille syndrome
Watson-Schwartz test
wattage
Watzki sleeve
Waugh-Clagett
    W.-C. operation
    W.-C. pancreaticoduodenostomy
wave
    abdominal fluid w.
    w. analyzer
    clustered w.'s (CW)
    clustered jejunal w.'s
    double-peaked w.
    duodenal pressure w.
    extracorporeal shock w.
    flipped T w.
    fluid w.
    focused shock w.
    w. form
    mechanical stress w.
    w. number
    peristaltic w.
    piezoelectric shock w.
    primary peristaltic w.
    propulsive w.
    pyloric pressure w.
    real focus shock w.

secondary peristaltic w.
shock w. (SW)
simultaneous bilateral extracorporeal shock w.'s
slow w.
T w.
virtual focus shock w.

waveform
blend w.
coagulase w.
cut w.
electrical w.
low-pulsatility arterial w.

waveguide
quartz w.

wavelength
wavenumber
waveshape
Wavicide disinfectant
wax-matrix
w.-m. slow-release form
w.-m. tablet

wax-tipped bougie
WBC
white blood cell count
white blood cells
WBC band
WBC basophil
WBC differential
elevated WBC
WBC immature forms
WBC leukocyte
WBC lymphocyte
WBC monocyte
WBC neutrophil

WCE
wireless capsule endoscopy

WD
Whipple disease
Wilson disease

WDHA
watery diarrhea, hypokalemia, and achlorhydria
watery diarrhea with hypokalemic alkalosis
WDHA syndrome

WDHH
watery diarrhea, hypokalemia, and hypovolemia

WDPM
well-differentiated papillary mesothelioma

weaker immunofluorescence signal
weakness
extremity w.
proximal muscle w.

weaning brash
web
antral w.
duodenal w.
endoscopic resection of antral w.
esophageal w.
hepatic w.
intestinal w.
mucosal w.
postcricoid w.
venous w.

Webb-Balfour abdominal retractor
webbed penis
webbing
penoscrotal w.

Weber-Christian disease
Weck
W. clip
W. High-Flow laparoflator

Weck-Cel sponge
weddellite calculus
wedge
W. electrosurgical resection device
W. loop
w. pressure
w. resection

wedged hepatic venous pressure (WHVP)
weekly
W. Stress Inventory (WSI)
W. Stress Inventory-Event (WSI-E)
W. Stress Inventory-Impact (WSI-I)

weeping willow appearance on venogram
Weerda endoscope
Wegener granulomatosis
Weibel-Palade granule
Weigert-Meyer
W.-M. law
W.-M. rule

weighing
gravimetric w.

weight (wt)
actual w. (AW)
actual body w. (ABW)
body w. (BW)
desirable body w. (DBW)
dry w.

NOTES

weight *(continued)*
    Femina vaginal w.
    w. gain
    ideal body w. (IBW)
    kidney w. (KW)
    w. loss
    w. loss with hyperphagia
    low molecular w. (LMW)
    molecular w. (mol wt)
    seminal vesicle w.
    W. Watchers diet
weight-based peritoneal exchange volume
weighted
    T1-w. image
    T2-w. image
weighted tip
weight-reduction surgery
Weil
    W. disease
    W. syndrome
Weinberg
    W. modification of pyloroplasty
    W. vagotomy retractor
Weinstein syndrome
Weiss reaction
Weitlaner retractor
Welch
    W. Allyn flexible sigmoidoscope
    W. Allyn videocolonoscope 8451
    W. Allyn videoendoscope
    W. Allyn videoendoscopy system
welchii
    Clostridium w.
Welchol
weld
    laser tissue w.
welding
    chromophore-enhanced laser w.
    laser tissue w.
well
    W. operation for rectal prolapse
    quadruplicate w.
well-defined anatomical entry criteria
well-differentiated
    w.-d. adenoma
    w.-d. papillary mesothelioma (WDPM)
Wellferon
well-known virulence factor
well-matched organ
Wells posterior rectopexy
Welt syndrome
Werdnig-Hoffman disease
Wermer syndrome
Wernicke
    W. encephalopathy
    W. syndrome
Wernicke-Korsakoff syndrome

Wesson perineal retractor
Westcott tenotomy scissors
Western
    W. blot
    W. blot analysis
    W. blotting
    W. diet
Weston rectal snare
Westphal
    W. gall duct forceps
    W. hemostat
Westphal-Strümpell disease
wet
    w. colostomy
    w. swallow
Wexler retractor
WGTS
    whole-gut transit scintigraphy
Wharton duct
wheal
wheat
    w. amylase inhibitor
    w. gliadin
    w. gluten
    w. starch
Wheeless method
Wheelhouse operation
w hernia
whewellite calculus
whiff test
Whipple
    W. bacillus
    W. disease (WD)
    W. operation
    W. pancreatectomy
    W. pancreaticoduodenectomy
    W. pancreaticoduodenostomy
    W. procedure
    W. resection
    W. syndrome
    W. triad
    W. triad test
whipplei
    Tropheryma w.
whipworm infection
whispered pectoriloquy
whistle stent
whistle-tip ureteral catheter
Whitaker
    W. hook
    W. perfusion pressure
    W. pressure-perfusion test
white
    w. anococcygeal line
    w. atrophy
    w. ball sign
    w. bile
    w. blood cell blast
    w. blood cell cast

w. blood cell count (WBC)
w. blood cells (WBC)
w. blood count differential
w. diarrhea
w. line of Toldt
w. nipple sign
W. operation
w. patch
w. thrombus

Whitehead
W. classification
W. deformity
W. operation

whitish exudate

Whitmore
W. bag
W. classification of prostate cancer

Whitmore-Jewitt prostate cancer classification system

WHO
World Health Organization
WHO gastric carcinoma classification

whole
w. blood
w. body cooling
w. crypt mitotic count

whole-blood
w.-b. clearance
w.-b. trough level

whole-cell oxygen consumption

whole-grain
rye w.-g. (RWG)

whole-gut
w.-g. irrigation
w.-g. lavage solution
w.-g. transit
w.-g. transit scintigraphy (WGTS)

whole-kidney fractional excretion

WHVP
wedged hepatic venous pressure

Wickham
W. retractor
W. technique

wide
w. albumin gradient ascites
w. elliptical anastomosis
w. pubic diastasis

wide-angled loupe
wide-lumen stapled anastomosis
wide-mouth sac

widening
mediastinal w.
width
infundibular w.
red cell distribution w. (RDW)
unfavorable infundibular w.
Wiedemann-Beckwith syndrome
Wilkie disease
Wilkins-Chalgren agar
Wilkinson abdominal retractor
Willauer thoracic scissors
Williams
W. intestinal forceps
W. needle
W. overtube sleeve
W. syndrome
W. varix injection overtube
W. vulvovaginoplasty
Willis
antrum of W.
W. pancreas
W. pouch
Willscher
W. catheter
W. tube
Wilms
W. tumor
W. tumor angiography
W. tumor, aniridia, genitourinary abnormalities, and mental retardation (WAGR)
W. tumor capsule invasion
W. tumor clear cell sarcoma variant
W. tumorlet
W. tumor multilocular cyst variant
W. tumor recurrence
W. tumor rhabdomyosarcoma variant
W. tumor tubuloglomerular pattern
Wilpowr
Wilson
W. disease (WD)
W. muscle
Wilson-Cook
W.-C. dilating balloon
W.-C. double-channel sphincterotome
W.-C. endoprosthesis
W.-C. esophageal balloon
W.-C. feeding tube kit

NOTES

Wilson-Cook *(continued)*
- W.-C. fine-needle aspiration catheter
- W.-C. French stent
- W.-C. gastric balloon
- W.-C. ligator 4, 6, 10 band
- W.-C. mechanical lithotriptor
- W.-C. modified wire-guided sphincterotome
- W.-C. nasobiliary tube
- W.-C. NJFT-series feeding tube
- W.-C. papillotome
- W.-C. plastic prosthesis
- W.-C. prosthesis introducer
- W.-C. Protector guidewire
- W.-C. Quantum TTC esophageal balloon dilatation catheter
- W.-C. six-shooter
- W.-C. ten-shooter
- W.-C. THSF-series guidewire
- W.-C. Tracer guidewire

Wiltek papillotome
Winckler test
wind colic
window
- w. of Deaver
- gastric w.
- mesenteric w.
- peritoneal w.
- zinc selenide w.

windowed esophageal balloon
wind-sock appearance
winged
- w. catheter
- w. steel needle

wink
- anal w.
- w. reflex

Winslow
- foramen of W.
- W. pancreas

winter
- w. acidosis
- w. gastroenteritis
- W. procedure
- W. shunt
- W. shunt for priapism
- w. vomiting

wire *(See also* guidewire)
- bypass w.
- cesium-137 w.
- Cope w.
- cutting w.
- diathermy w.
- w. electrode
- Extra Stiff Amplatz w.
- hydrophilic w.
- ^{192}Ir w.
- J w.
- lead w.
- w. loop connector
- memory w.
- monofilament snare w.
- needle-knife w.
- nitinol w.
- Pathfinder w.
- protector plus w.
- Roadrunner w.
- safety w.
- w. snare
- stiffening w.
- torque w.
- Tracer ST w.
- trip w.
- ultrastiff w.

wire-guided
- w.-g. balloon-assisted endoscopic biliary stent exchange
- w.-g. cytology
- w.-g. hydrostatic balloon
- w.-g. J tube
- w.-g. metal spiral retrieval device
- w.-g. placement
- w.-g. polyvinyl bougie
- w.-g. sphincterotome

wireless
- w. capsule endoscope
- w. capsule endoscopy (WCE)

wire-loop lesion
Wire-Wrap
wiring
- jaw w.

Wirsung
- canal of W.
- W. dilation
- duct of W.
- W. sphincter

Wirthlin splenorenal clamp
Wisconsin solution
Wishbone Omni-Track retractor
Wiskott-Aldrich syndrome
Wistar-Kyoto heart
WIT
- water-induced thermotherapy

withdrawal
- w. of cyclosporine
- steroid w.

Witzel
- W. closure
- W. duodenostomy
- W. enterostomy
- W. enterostomy catheter
- W. feeding jejunostomy tunnel
- W. gastrostomy
- W. jejunostomy
- W. pneumatic dilator

Witz test
WNT/wingless signaling pathway

Woldman test
Wolf
    W. aspiration/injection system
    W. delivery system
    W. lithotrite
    W. percutaneous universal nephroscope
    W. Piezolith 2300 lithotripsy device
    W. Piezolith 2300 lithotriptor
    W. resectoscope
    W. rigid panendoscope
    W. Sonolith lithotriptor
    W. ureteroscope
Wolfe miniscope
Wolff
    duct of W.
    W. syringe
    W. telescope
wolffi
    corpus w.
    ductus W.
wolffian
    w. duct
    w. ductal system
Wolff-Junghans test
Wolf-Henning gastroscope
Wolf-Knittlingen gastroscope
Wolfram syndrome
Wolf-Schindler semiflexible gastroscope
Wolfson
    W. gallbladder retractor
    W. intestinal clamp
Wolinella
Wolman
    W. disease
    W. xanthomatosis
Womack procedure
Women's Gentle Laxative
Wood
    W. lamp
    W. operation
wooden
    w. belly
    w. resonance
Woodward
    W. esophagogastroscopy
    W. esophagogastrostomy
Wookey skin tube
wool ball

Woolf
    W. method
    W. test
work
    neuromodulation w.
    recent w.
working-port ureteroscope
working sheath
workload
    emergency-to-elective w.
workstation
    Dornier MFL 5000 urological w.
World Health Organization (WHO)
worldwide clinical series
worm
    bilharzial w.
    bladder w.
    w. colic
    herring w.
    kidney w.
wort
    St. John's w.
wound
    anal w.
    w. approximation
    aseptic w.
    w. closure
    w. dehiscence
    w. drainage
    w. healing
    w. healing disorder
    w. hematoma
    w. infection
    open w.
    penetrating w.
    renal stab w.
    septic w.
    stab w.
    submucosal w.
woven Dacron tube
W-pouch configuration
wrap
    antireflux w.
    double gracilis w.
    floppy Nissen fundic w.
    gamma split-sling w.
    gastric fundus w.
    Kerlix w.
    Nissen fundoplication w.
    rectus fascial w.
    single gamma w.
    slipped fundoplication w.

NOTES

wrap *(continued)*
    total gastric w.
    tunica vaginalis blanket w.
wrapping
    fat w.
    omental w.
Wright
    W. stain
    W. stain of stool
Wright-Giemsa stain
writer
    laser w.
WS
    watermelon stomach
W-shaped
    W-s. forceps
    W-s. ileal pouch-anal anastomosis
    W-s. pouch
WSI
    Weekly Stress Inventory
WSI-E
    Weekly Stress Inventory-Event
WSI-I
    Weekly Stress Inventory-Impact
W-stapled
    W-s. ileal neobladder
    W-s. urinary reservoir
wt
    weight
    mol wt
WTI gene
Wuchereria bancrofti
Wurbs-type nasobiliary tube
WuScope system
Wyamine
Wyamycin E, S
Wyanoids Relief Factor
Wylie
    W. hypogastric clamp
    W. splanchnic retractor
Wymox

Xanax
xanthelasma
xanthic calculus
xanthine
 x. calculus
 x. dehydrogenase (XDH)
 x. oxidase
 x. oxidation
 x. oxidoreductase activity
 x. urolithiasis
xanthinuria
xanthogranuloma
 juvenile x.
xanthogranulomatous
 x. cholecystitis
 x. cystitis
 x. pyelonephritis (XGP)
xanthoma
 bladder x.
 x. cell
 gastric x.
 planar x.
 skin x.
 tendon x.
 verruciform x.
xanthomatosis
 biliary hypercholesterolemia x.
 cerebrotendinous x.
 familial hypercholesteremic x.
 gastric x.
 Wolman x.
Xanthomonas maltophilia
Xatral OD
XC
 excretory cystogram
Xc
 reactance
X-CGD
 X-linked chronic granulomatous disease
Xc/R
 reactance and resistance
  Xc/R ratio
XDH
 xanthine dehydrogenase
Xenical
xenoantigen
xenobiotic
 x. absorption
 x. glutathione conjugate
 x. pump
xenograft
 x. rejection
 x. transplantation

xenon
 x. lamp
 x. light source
xenon-washout technique
xenopi
 Mycobacterium x.
xenoreactive antibody
xenotransplantation
Xeroform gauze
xerophthalmia
xerostomia
xerotica
 balanitis x.
XGIF-MR30
 nonferromagnetic MR endoscope XGIF-MR30
XGP
 xanthogranulomatous pyelonephritis
Xillix LIFE-Lung system
xiphisternum
xiphoid appendix
xiphoid-to-pubis midline abdominal incision
xiphoid-to-umbilicus incision
XL
 extended release
  Ditropan XL
  Procardia XL
XL1-Blue cell
XLAS
 X-linked Alport syndrome
XLH
 X-linked hypophosphatemia
X-linked
 X-l. Alport syndrome (XLAS)
 X-l. chronic granulomatous disease (X-CGD)
 X-l. hypophosphatemia (XLH)
 X-l. infantile agammaglobulinemia
 X-l. recessive NDI
 X-l. recessive nephrolithiasis (XRN)
 X-l. recessive trait
Xpeedior catheter
X-Prep
 X-P. bowel preparation
 Senokot X-P.
XQ230 Olympus gastroscope
XQ videoinstrument
XR
 extended release
  Cipro XR
  Pyridorin XR
x-ray
 x-r. analysis
 x-r. beam

x-ray *(continued)*
    x-r. crystallography
    x-r. diffractometry
    x-r. photoelectron spectroscopy
XRN
    X-linked recessive nephrolithiasis
XTRAX DNA commercial extraction kit
XU
    excretory urogram
XX
    XX male mosaicism
    XX male syndrome

X, Y chromosome
xylene
Xylocaine
    X. jelly
    topical X.
    X. topical anesthetic
xylometazoline
xylose
    x. absorption test
    x. tolerance test
Xyotax
XYY male syndrome

Y
  Y adapter
YAG
  yttrium-aluminum-garnet
   YAG 1064
   YAG laser
   Laserscope YAG 1064
   YAG laser therapy
Yang
  Y. needle
  Y. polyclonal assay
  Y. Pros-Check PSA assay
  Y. Pros-Check PSA test
  Y. PSA radioimmunoassay
Yang-Monti
  Y.-M. conduit
  Y.-M. ileovesicostomy
  Y.-M. principle
Yangtze Valley fever
Yankauer
  Y. esophagoscope
  Y. suction tube
yarn-collected specimen
Yates correction
Y-connecting tubing
yeast
  y. balanitis
  y. overgrowth
  y. saccharomyces
  y. strain mannan
  urinalysis sediment microscopy y.
  urinary sediment y.
yeast-recombinant hepatitis B vaccine
Yellolax
yellow
  y. atrophy of liver
  y. nodule
  y. phosphorus hepatotoxicity
Yeoman rectal biopsy forceps
Yeoman-Wittner rectal forceps
Yersinia
  Y. enteritis
  Y. *enterocolitica*
  Y. *enterocolitica* colitis
  Y. *frederiksenii*
  Y. *intermedia*
  Y. *kristensenii*
  Y. *pestis*
  Y. *pseudotuberculosis*
yersiniosis
yield
  diagnostic y.
  sperm y.
Yocon

yogurt
  Trial Using Medicinal Microbiotic Y. (TUMMY)
yohimbine hydrochloride
Yohimex
yokogawai
  Metagonimus y.
yolk
  y. sac
  y. sac carcinoma
  y. sac tumor
York-Mason procedure
Yoshi-864 antineoplastic alkylating agent
Young
  Y. cystoscope
  Y. enucleator
  Y. epispadias repair
  Y. intestinal forceps
  Y. needle holder
  Y. operation
  Y. prostatic retractor
  Y. prostatic tractor
  Y. syndrome
  Y. technique
Young-Dees
  Y.-D. bladder neck reconstruction
  Y.-D. operation
  Y.-D. procedure
  Y.-D. suspension
  Y.-D. technique
  Y.-D. tube
Young-Dees-Leadbetter
  Y.-D.-L. bladder neck reconstruction
  Y.-D.-L. operation
Youssef syndrome
youth
  maturity-onset diabetes of y. (MODY)
  Treatment Options for Type 2 Diabetes in Adolescents and Y.'s (TODAY)
yo-yo weight-fluctuation phenomenon
Y-plasty
  Foley Y-p.
  Schweizer-Foley Y-p.
Y-port connector
Y-set system
Y-shaped incision
yttrium-90
yttrium-aluminum-garnet (YAG)
  y.-a.-g. laser
Y-type Dianeal peritoneal dialysis solution
Yu-Holtgrewe prostatic retractor

Y-V

- Y-V anoplasty
- Y-V meatotomy
- Y-V plasty
- Y-V sliding skin graft

YY

- beta-endorphin peptide YY
- peptide YY (PYY)

Z
- Z line
- Z stent
- Z stent esophageal endoprosthesis system
- Z stitch
- Z suture
- Z test
- Z tract

Zachary Cope-DeMartel clamp
zacopride
Zacutex
Zadaxin
zafirlukast
Zagam
Zahn
- anomaly of Z.
- Z. infarct

zalcitabine
Zamboni fixative
Zanca syndrome
Zanosar
zanoterone
Zantac
- Z. EFFERdose
- Z. GELdose

Zappacosta test
Zaroxolyn
Za-Stent endoscopic biliary stent
ZCE 025 antibody
ZE
- Zollinger-Ellison
- ZE cap
- ZE syndrome

zebra
- z. body
- Z. exchange guidewire

Zebrax
Zefazone
Zeiss
- Z. Axiophot microscope
- Z. fluorescein filter system
- Z. IDO3 phase-contrast microscope
- Z. morphomate M30
- Z. S9 electron microscope

Zellweger syndrome
Zelmac
Zelnorm tablet
Zenapax
Zenith
- Z. AAA endovascular graft system
- Z. abdominal aortic aneurysm endovascular graft system

Zenker
- Z. diverticulum
- Z. leiomyoma
- Z. pouch

Zeppelin clamp
ZES
- Zollinger-Ellison syndrome

Zestril
Zeta probe nylon filter
Zichen-Oppenheim (ZO)
zidovudine
Ziehl-Neelsen stain
Zieve
- Z. syndrome
- Z. system

zileuton
Zilver biliary self-expanding stent
zilverstent
Zimmon
- Z. biliary stent
- Z. papillotome/sphincterotome

zinc
- bacitracin z.
- z. colic
- z. deficiency
- z. finger
- z. selenide window

zinc-iron regulated transporterlike (ZIRTL)
zinc-requiring enzyme
zipper
- leucine z.
- z. sphincterotomy

Zipser penile clamp
ZIRTL
- zinc-iron regulated transporterlike
- ZIRTL sequence

Zixoryn
Z-Med catheter
Zn-alpha-2-glycoprotein
- seminal plasma Zn-a.-2-g.

ZO
- Zichen-Oppenheim
- Zuelzer-Ogden

Zocor
Zoladex implant
zoledronic
- z. acid
- z. acid for injection

Zolicef
Zollinger-Ellison (ZE)
- Z.-E. syndrome (ZES)
- Z.-E. tumor

zomepirac
Zometa for injection
zona, pl. **zonae**
- z. fasciculata

zona *(continued)*
    z. glomerulosa
    z. hamster egg test
    z. pellucida (ZP)
    z. reticularis
zonal gastritis
zone
    abdominal z.
    adrenal cortex z.
    anal transitional z. (ATZ)
    border z.
    calcified z.
    claudin-2-positive z.
    cooled antenna z.
    electric z.
    epigastric z.
    hemorrhoidal z.
    high-pressure z. (HPZ)
    hyperemic border z.
    hypogastric papillary z.
    nephrogenic z.
    peripheral z.
    portal z.
    prostate gland peripheral z.
    prostate gland periurethral z.
    prostate gland transition z.
    prostate-specific antigen density of transition z. (PSA-TZ)
    rugae z.
    transformation z.
    transitional z.
    Türck z.
zonula, pl. **zonulae**
    z. occludens

zoom videoendoscopy
Zoon
    balanitis of Z.
    Z. erythroplasia
zoonotic food-borne pathogen
zoospermia
Zorbtive powder for subcu injection
zoster
    herpes z.
Zovirax
ZP
    zona pellucida
Z-plasty anastomosis
Z-type deformity
Zuckerkandl
    organ of Z.
Zuelzer-Ogden (ZO)
Zyderm
Zygomycetes
zygomycosis
zygote
Zyloprim
Zymase
zymogen
    z. granule
    lab z.
zymogenic cell
zymosan
    opsonized z.
zymosis gastrica
Zypan
ZZ phenotype

Appendix 1
Anatomical Illustrations

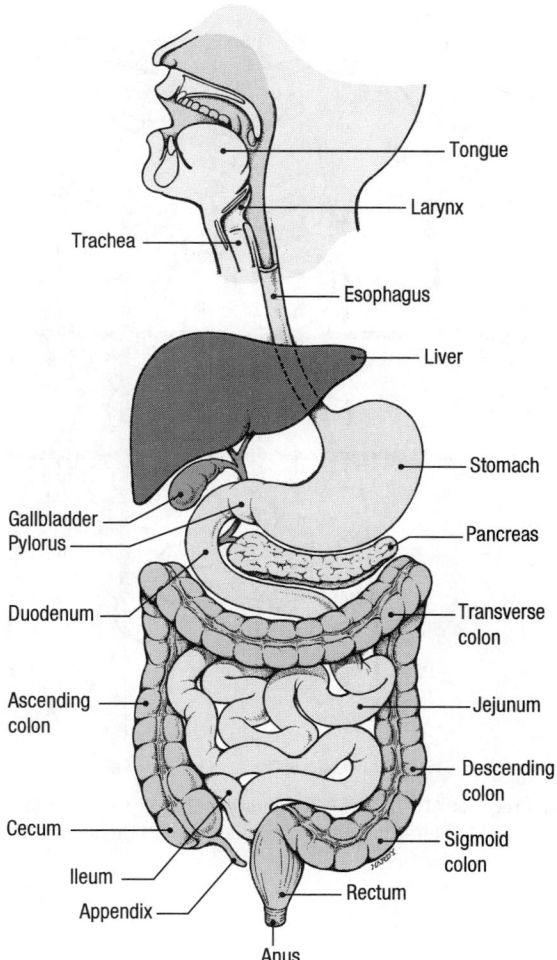

Figure 1. Digestive organs and associated structures.

Appendix 1

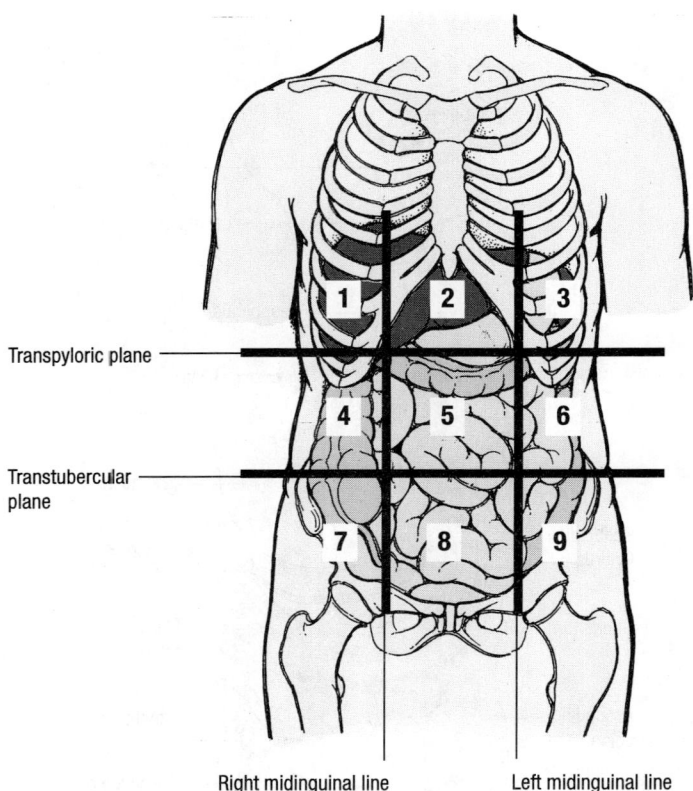

Figure 2. Abdominal regions. (1) Right hypochondriac. (2) Epigastric. (3) Left hypochondriac. (4) Right lateral (lumbar). (5) Umbilical. (6) Left lateral (lumbar). (7) Right iliac. (8) Hypogastric (suprapubic). (9) Left iliac.

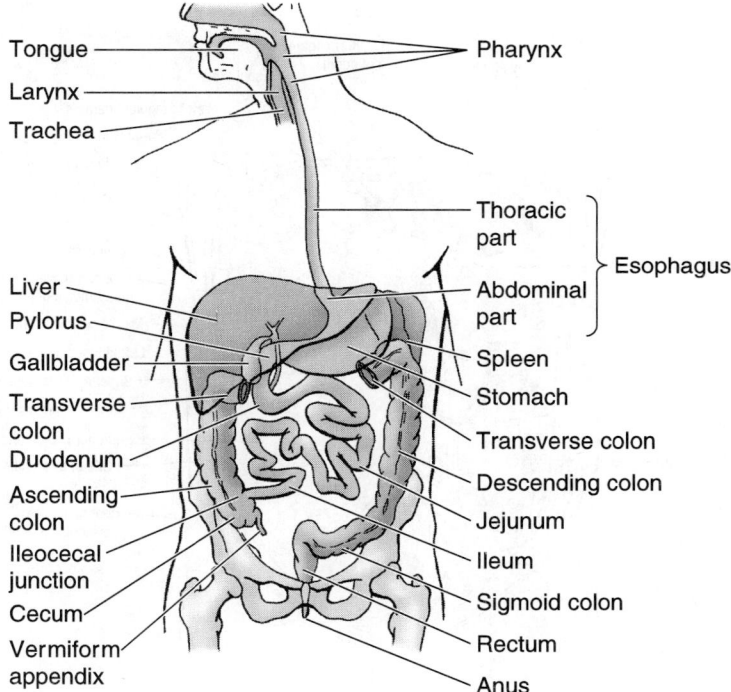

Figure 3. Small and large intestine in situ. Diagrammatic orientation drawing of the digestive system, extending from the lips to the anus.

Appendix 1

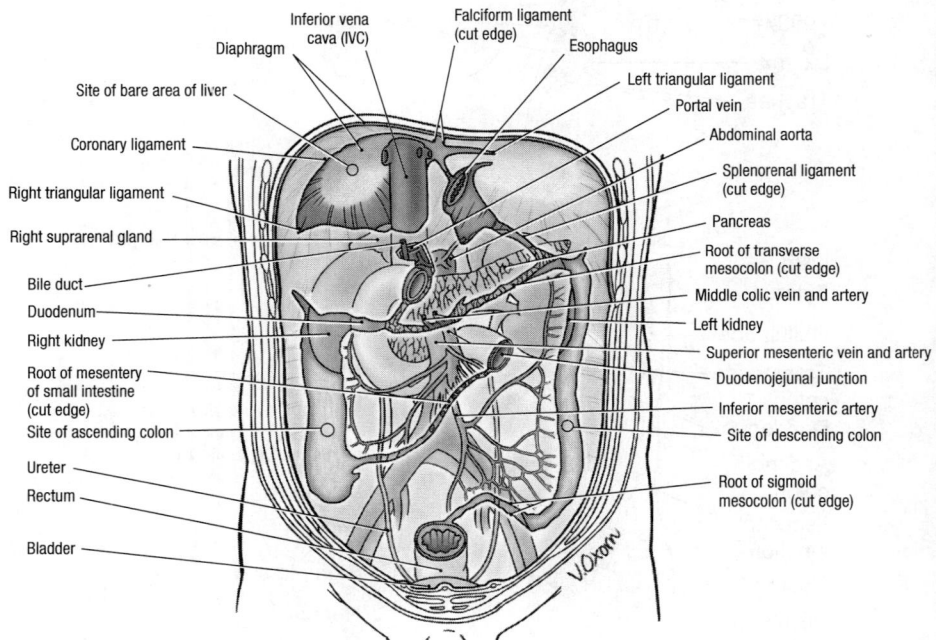

Figure 4. Small and large intestine, arteries, and mesenteries.

Anatomical Illustrations

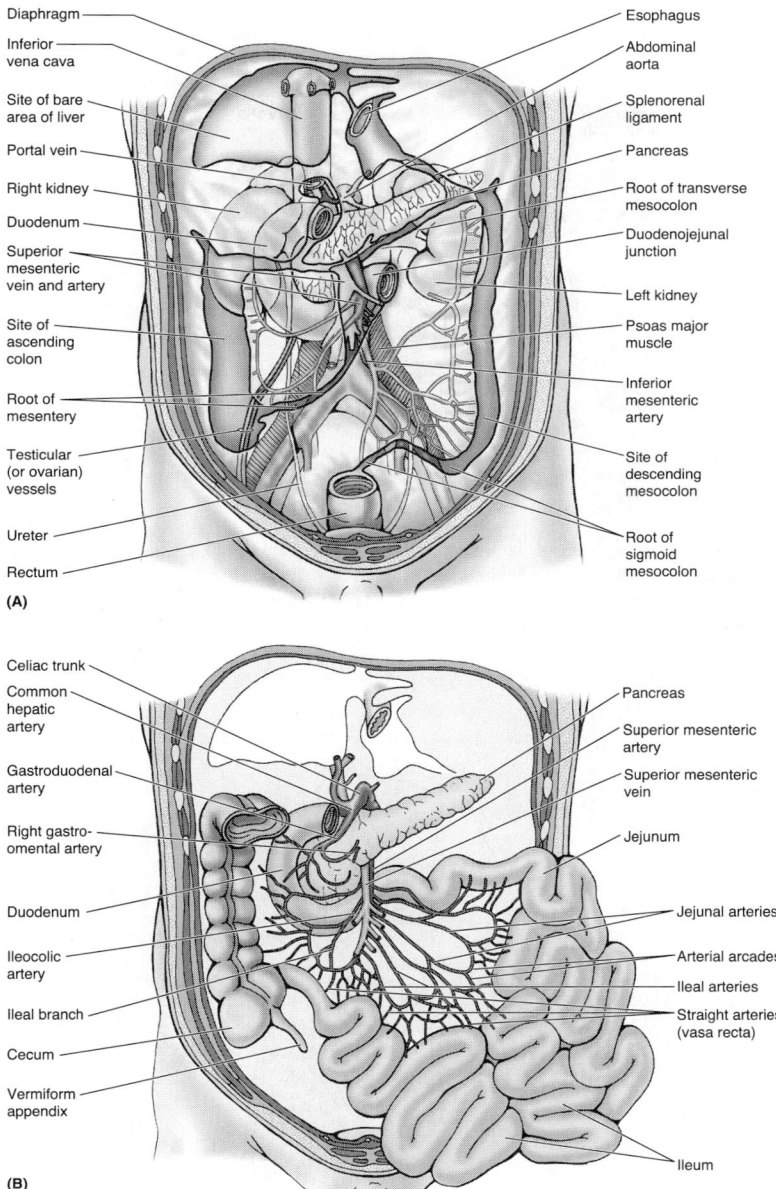

Figure 5. Arterial supply and mesentery of the intestine. (A) Arterial supply to the large intestine. The roots (cut) of mesocolon of transverse and sigmoid and mesentery of the jejunum and ileum are also illustrated. (B) Arterial supply and venous drainage of the small intestine. The superior mesenteric artery (SMA) supplies the jejunoileum, and the superior mesenteric vein (SMV) draws blood from the intestine into the portal vein.

Appendix 1

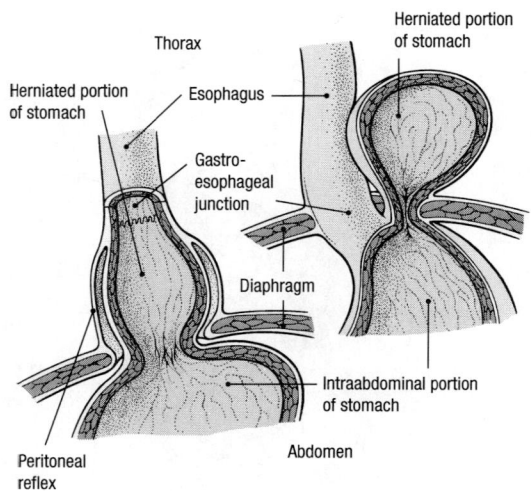

Figure 6. Sliding esophageal and paraesophageal hernias. In sliding esophageal hernias (left), the upper stomach and cardioesophageal junction slide in and out of the thorax; in paraesophageal hernias (right), all or part of the stomach pushes through diaphragm next to gastroesophageal junction.

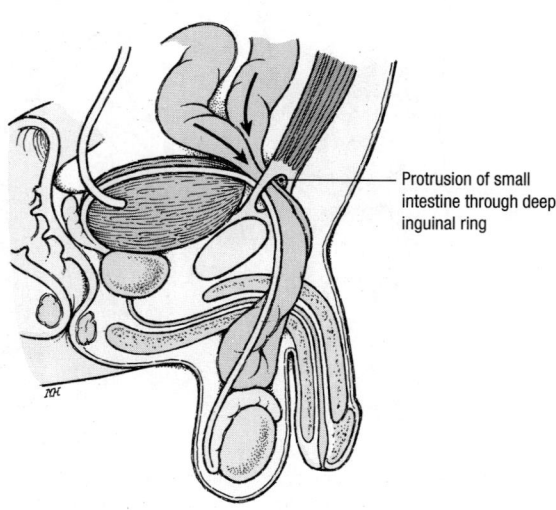

Figure 7. Indirect inguinal hernia.

Anatomical Illustrations

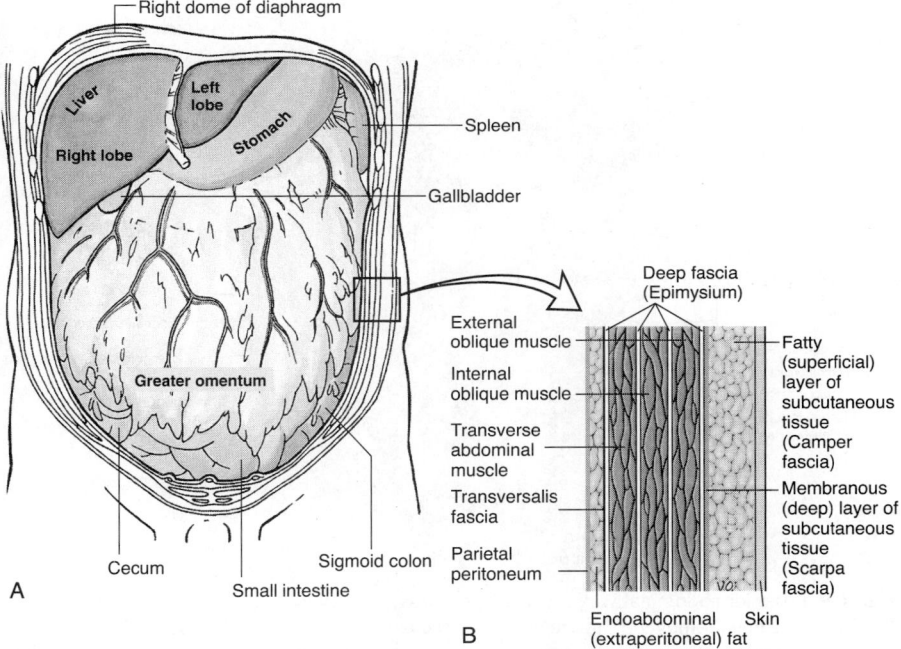

Figure 8. Layers of the anterolateral abdominal wall. (A) Orientation drawing, anterior view. The anterior abdominal wall is cut away. Most of the intestine is covered by the greater omentum. (B) Longitudinal section showing the layers of the inferior part of the wall.

A7

Appendix 1

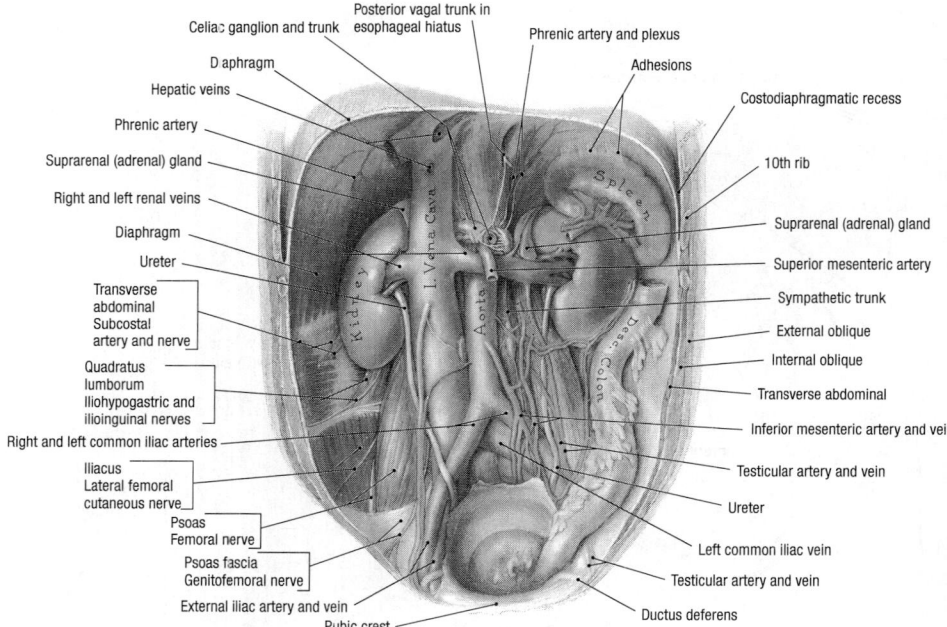

Figure 9. Posterior abdominal wall showing great vessels, kidneys, and suprarenal glands. Most of the fascia has been removed. The ureter crosses the external iliac artery just beyond the common iliac bifurcation and the testicular vessels cross anterior to the ureter and join the ductus deferens (vas deferens) to enter the inguinal canal. Note that the renal arteries are not seen because they lie posterior to the renal veins. Note also that the left renal vein is compressed between the aorta posteriorly and the superior mesenteric artery (SMA), which bears the weight of the intestine.

Anatomical Illustrations

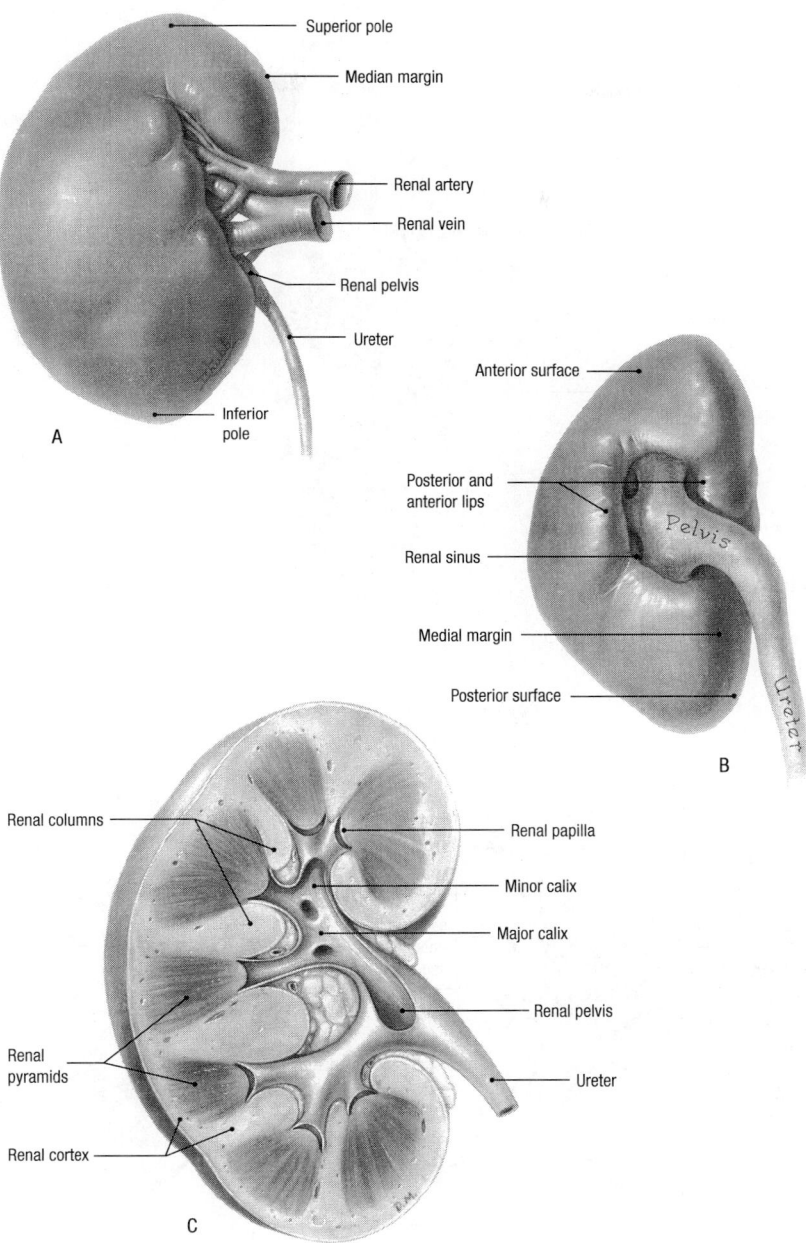

Figure 10. Kidney. (A) Right kidney, anterior view. (B) Sinus of kidney, anteromedial view. (C) Kidney, coronal view.

Appendix 1

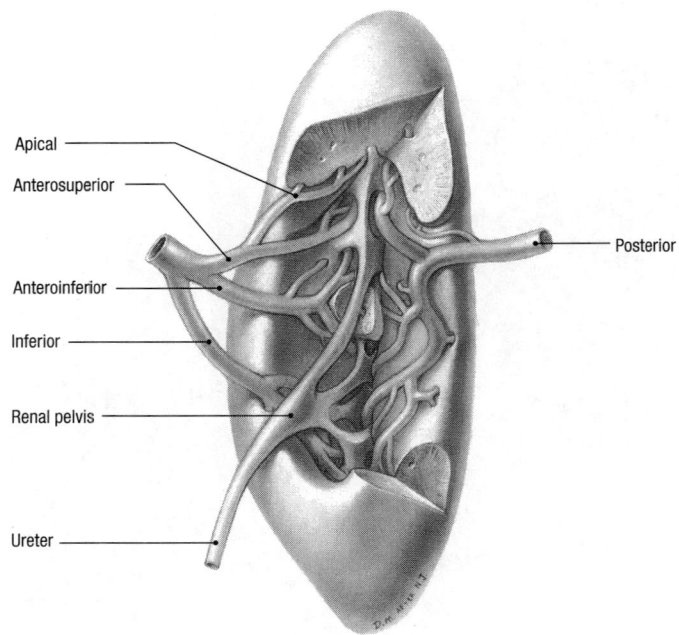

Figure 11. Branches of renal artery within renal sinus, medial view.

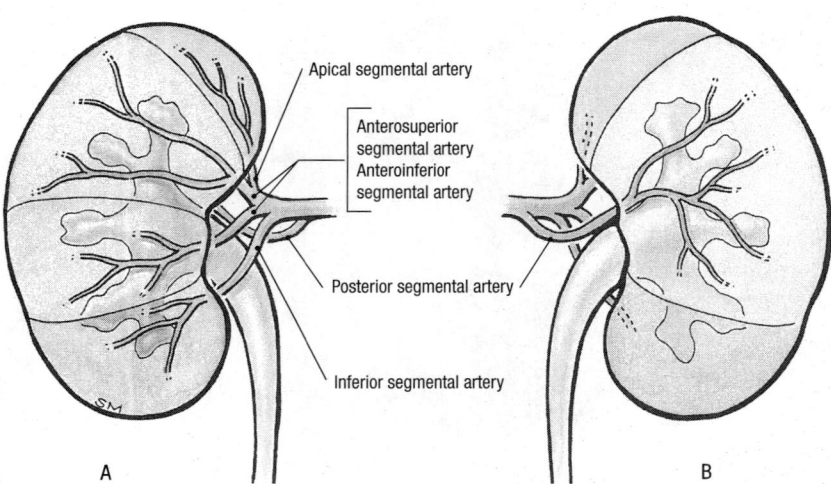

Figure 12. Segmental arteries. (A) Anterior view. (B) Posterior view.

Anatomical Illustrations

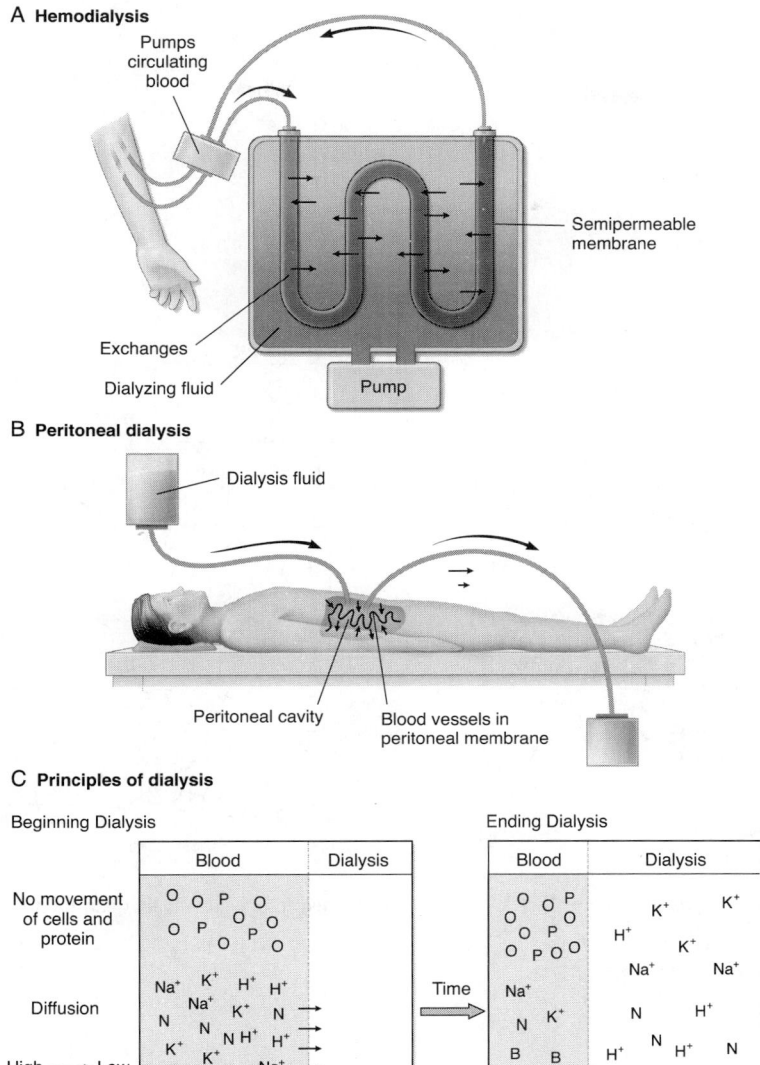

Figure 13. Dialysis or artificial kidney. (A) Hemodialysis; (B) Peritoneal dialysis; (C) Principles of dialysis.

Appendix 1

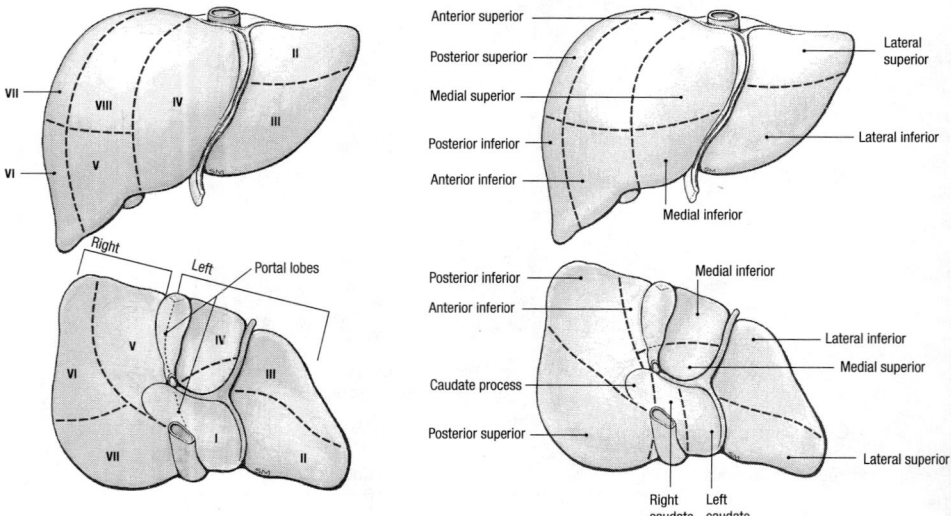

Figure 14. Segments of liver. Each of the lobes is divided into segments that can be numerically identified, as shown (left).

Anatomical Illustrations

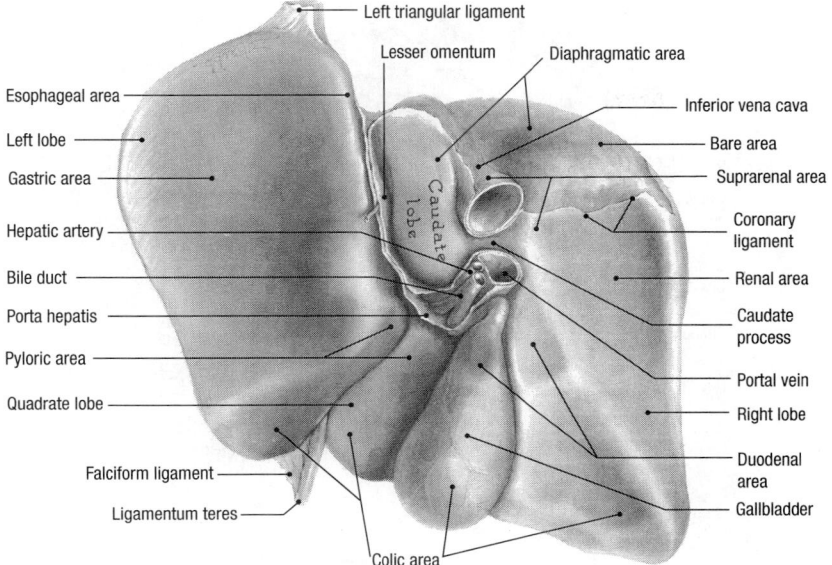

Figure 15. Inferior and posterior surfaces of liver.

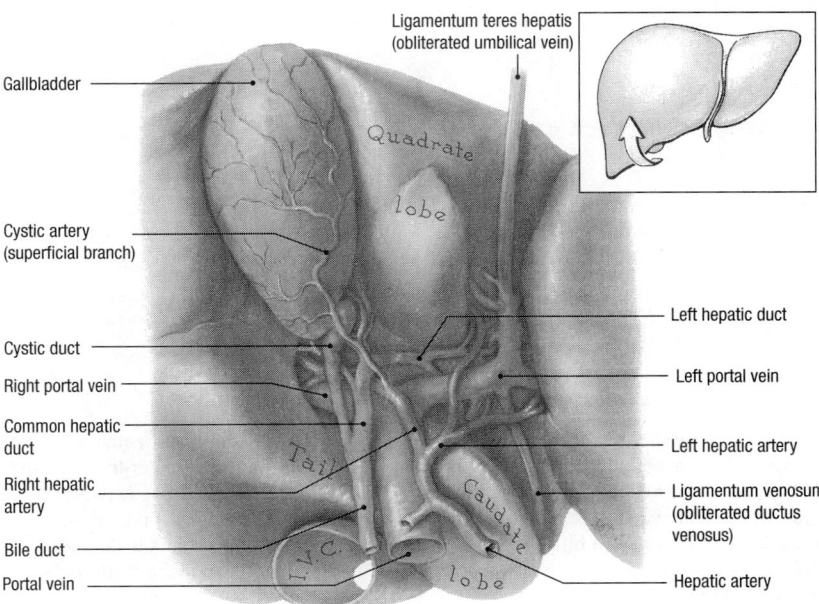

Figure 16. Porta hepatis and cystic artery, posterior view.

A13

Appendix 1

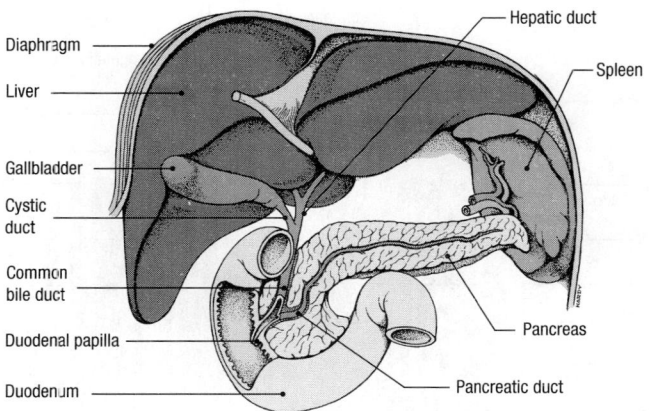

Figure 17. Gallbladder, liver, and biliary system.

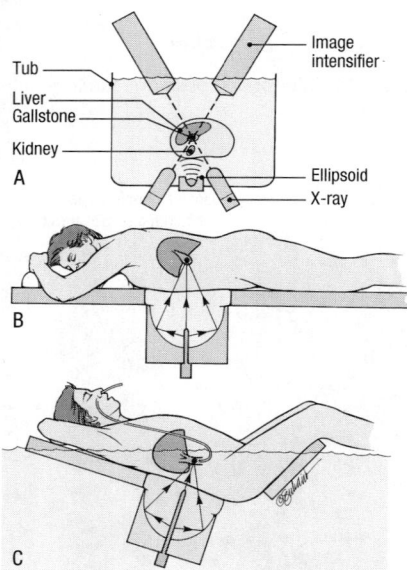

Figure 18. Extracorporeal shock wave lithotripsy. (A) Gallbladder stone is localized by imaging; shock waves are generated in ellipsoid reflector and transmitted through water to stone. (B) Positioning of patient for treatment of stones located in gallbladder; fluid-filled bag is recessed in table and transmits shock wave from generator to patient's skin. (C) Positioning of patient for treatment of stones located in common bile duct; the patient is partially submerged in a water bath; nasobiliary tube is used to introduce contrast material to permit visualization and localization of stone and to decompress biliary tree.

Anatomical Illustrations

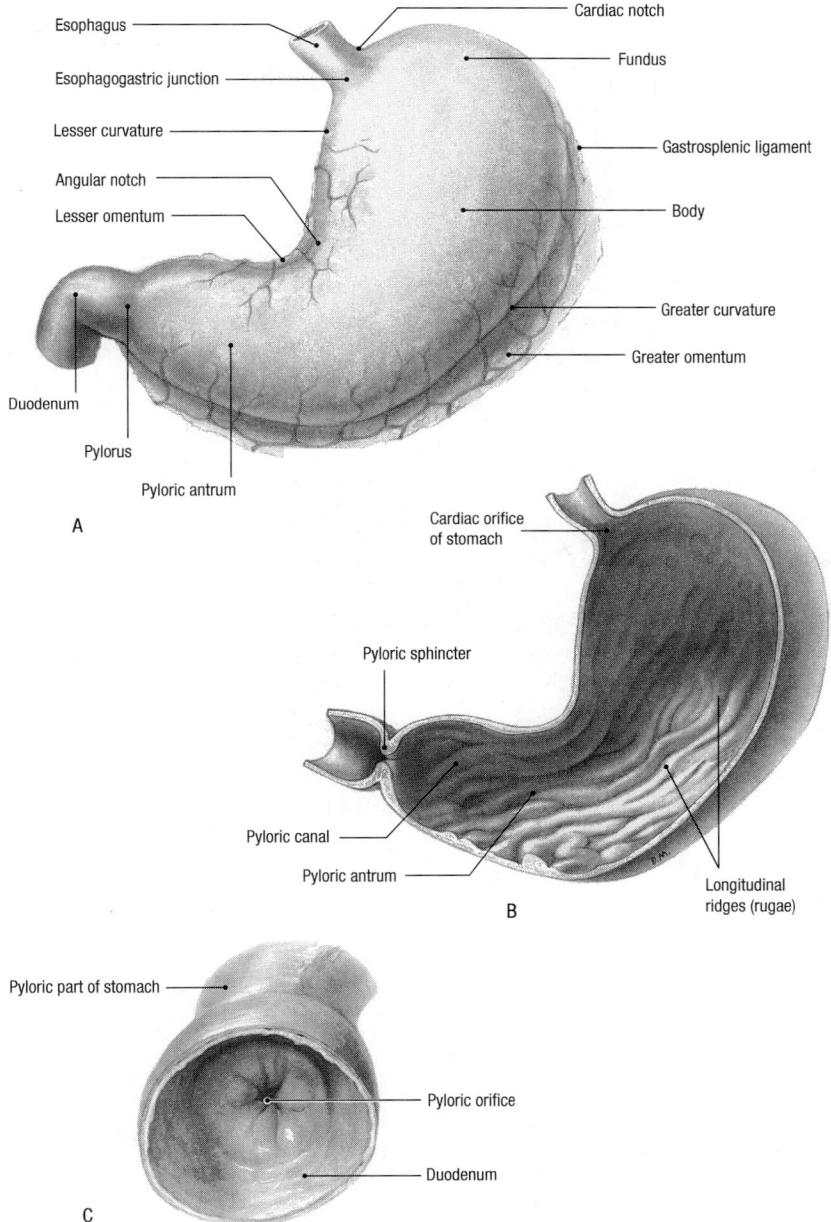

Figure 19. Stomach. (A) External surface, anterior view. (B) Internal surface (mucous membrane), anterior wall removed. (C) Pylorus, viewed from the duodenum.

Appendix 1

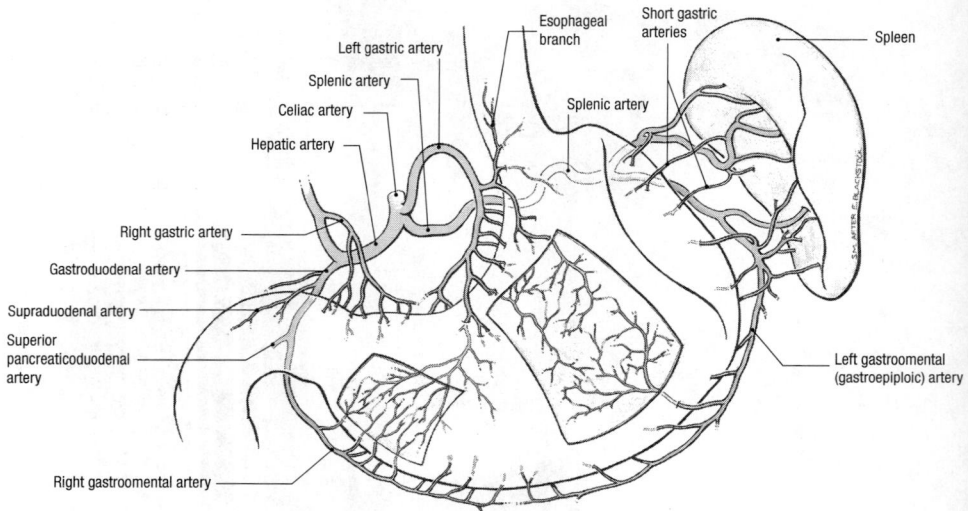

Figure 20. Arteries of stomach and spleen, anterior view.

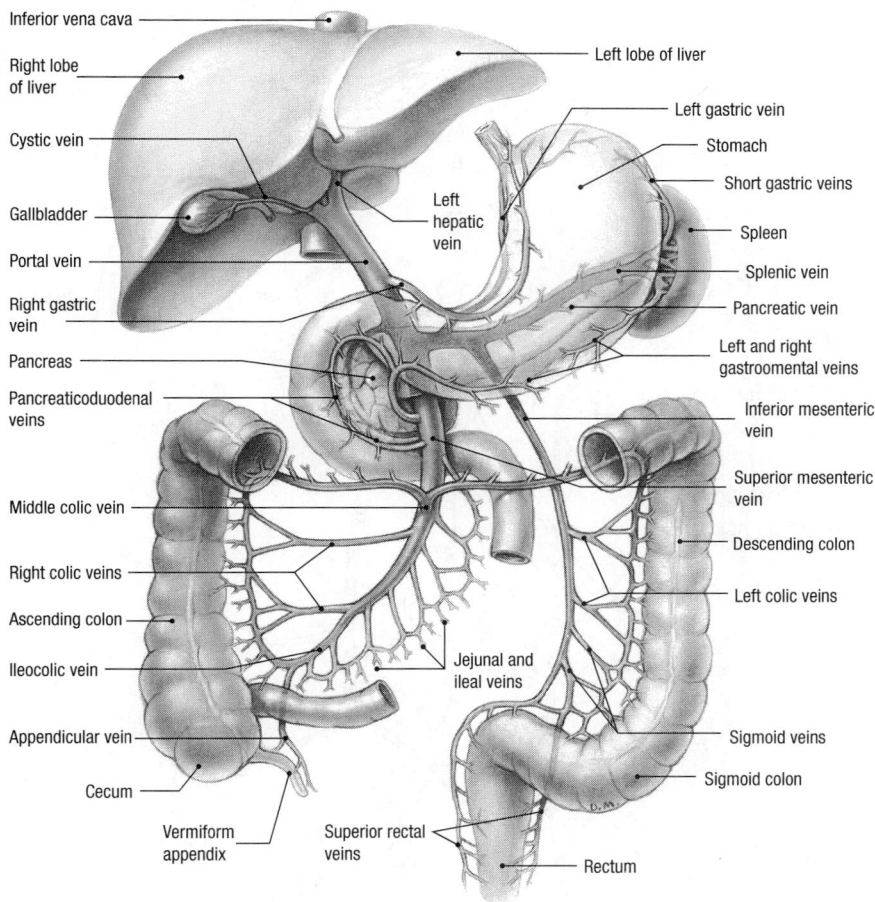

Figure 21. Portal venous system, anterior view.

Appendix 1

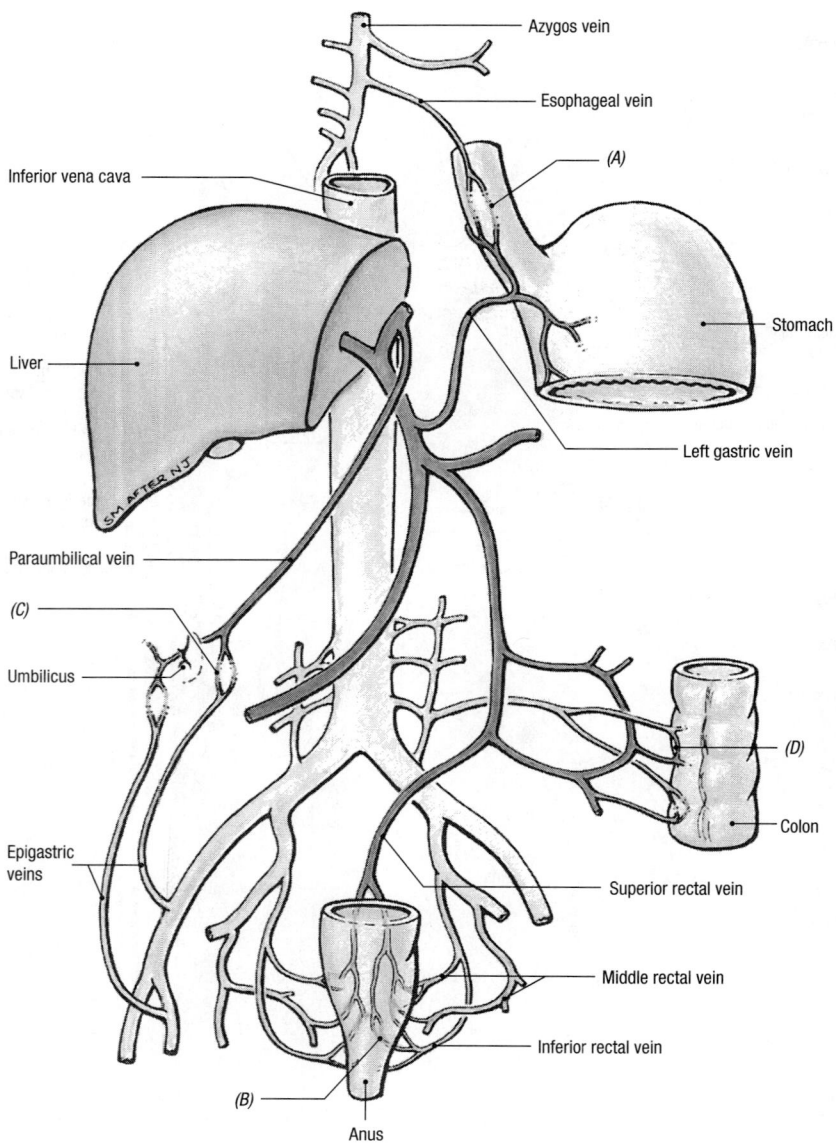

Figure 22. Portacaval system, anterior view. Portal tributaries are shown in dark gray; systemic tributaries and communicating veins are shown in light gray. Sites of anastomosis: *A, B, C,* and *D.*

Anatomical Illustrations

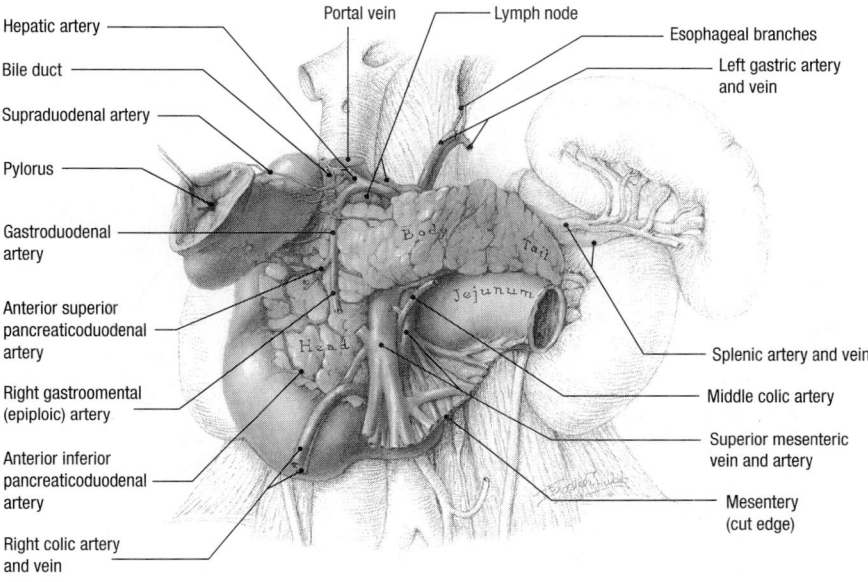

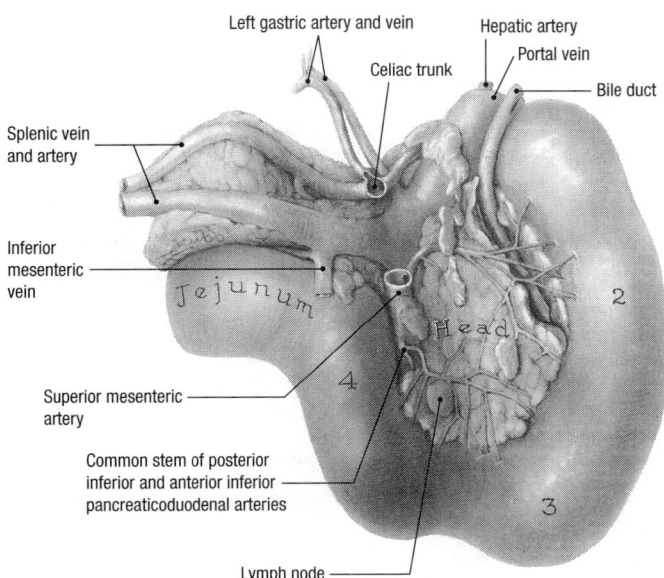

Figure 23. Duodenum and pancreas. Anterior view (top). Posterior view (bottom).

A19

Appendix 1

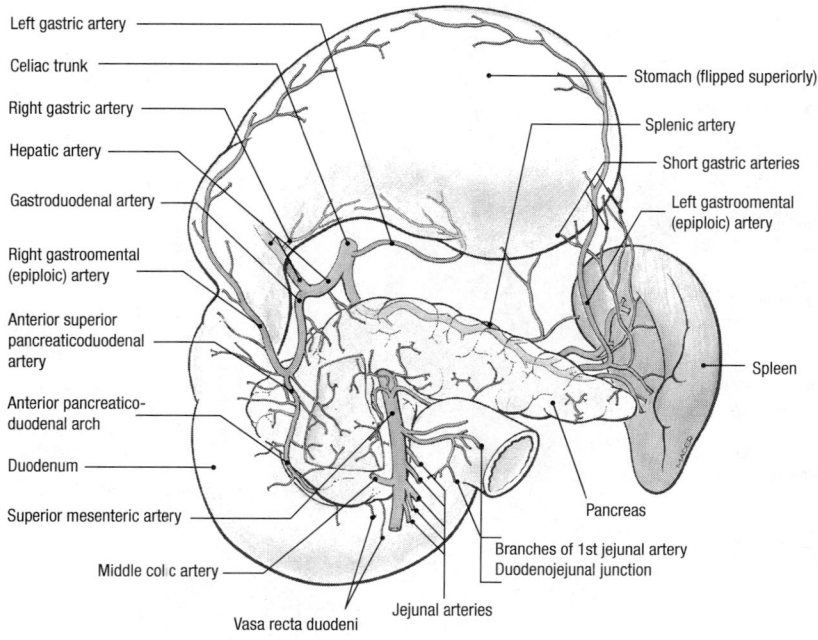

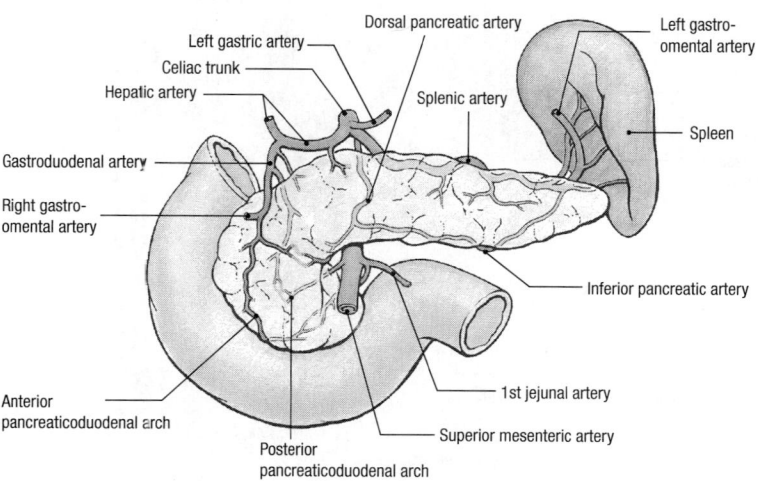

Figure 24. Blood supply to the pancreas, duodenum, and spleen, anterior views. Celiac trunk and superior mesenteric artery (top). Pancreatic and pancreaticoduodenal arteries (bottom).

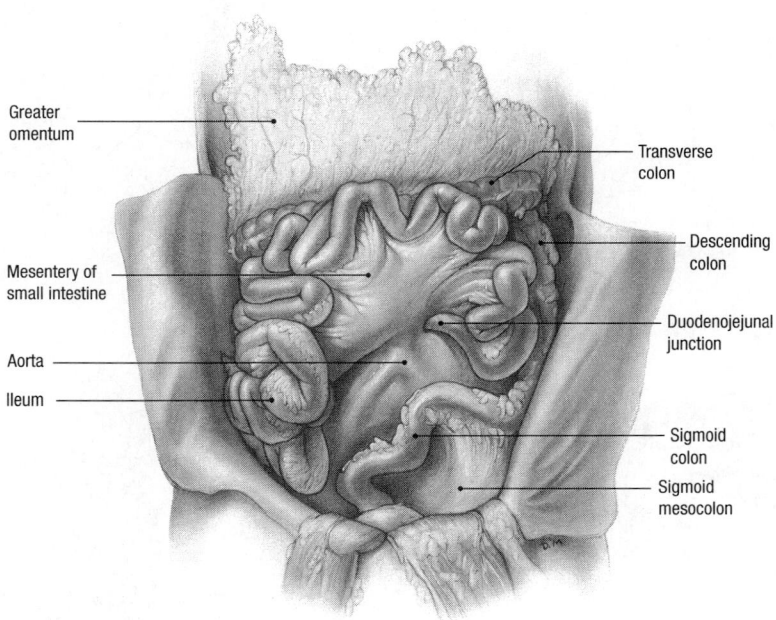

Figure 25. Descending and sigmoid colon and mesentery of small intestine.

Appendix 1

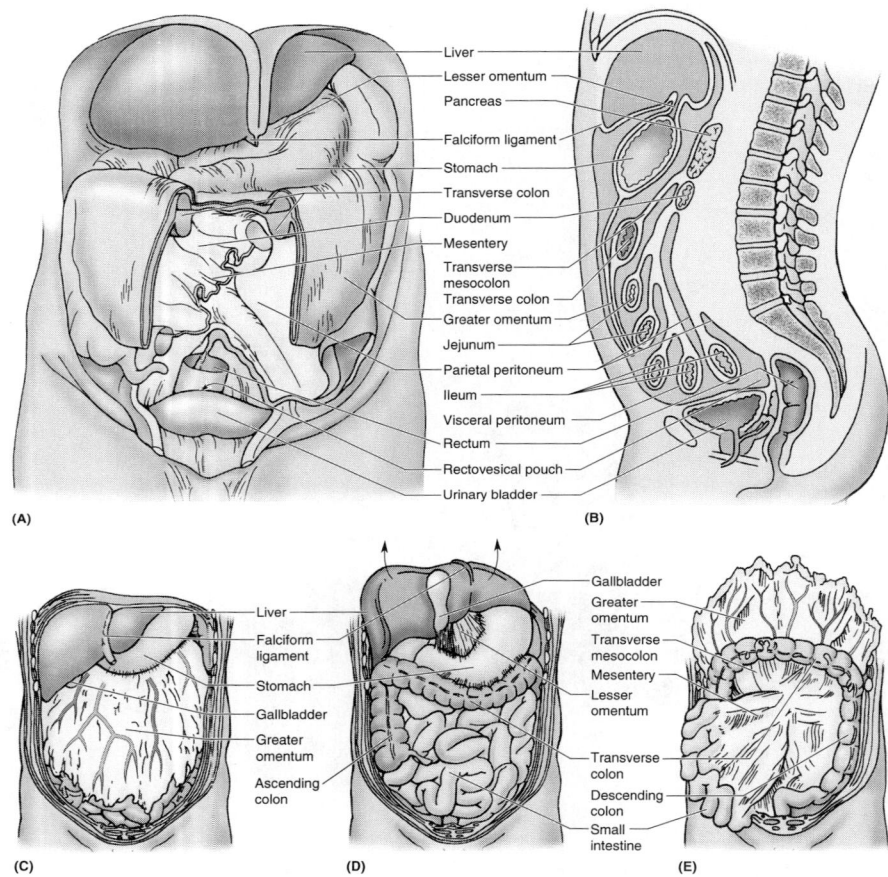

Figure 26. Principal parts of the peritoneum. (A) Anterior view of the opened peritoneal cavity. Parts of the greater omentum, transverse colon, and small intestine have been cut away to reveal deep structures and the layers of the mesenteric structures. The mesentery of the jejunum and ileum (small intestine) and sigmoid mesocolon have been cut close to their parietal attachments. (B) Sagittal section of the abdominopelvic cavity of a male, showing the relationships of the peritoneal attachments. (C) The greater omentum is shown in its "normal" position covering most of the abdominal viscera. (D) The lesser omentum, attaching the liver to the lesser curvature of the stomach, is shown by reflecting the liver and gallbladder superiorly. The greater omentum has been removed from the greater curvature of the stomach to reveal the intestines. (E) The greater omentum has been reflected superiorly and the small intestine has been retracted to the right side to reveal the mesentery of the small intestine.

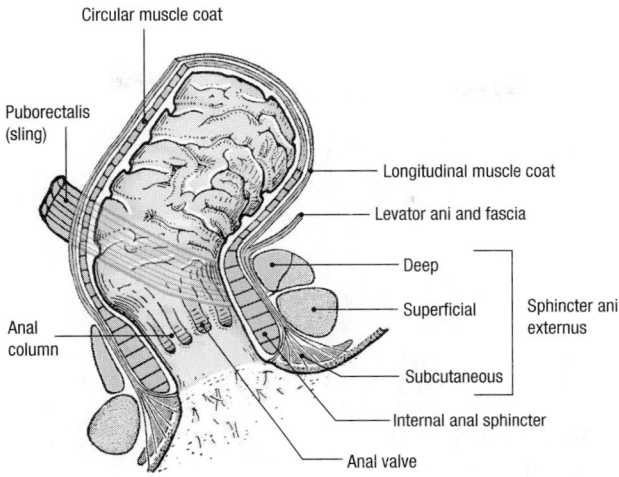

Figure 27. Rectum, anal canal, and anal sphincter.

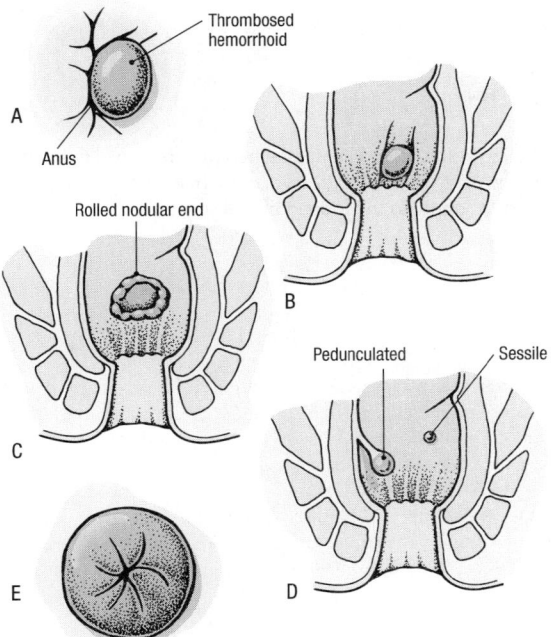

Figure 28. Anal and rectal masses. (A) External hemorrhoid. (B) Internal hemorrhoid. (C) Rectal tumor. (D) Rectal polyps. (E) Rectal prolapse.

Appendix 1

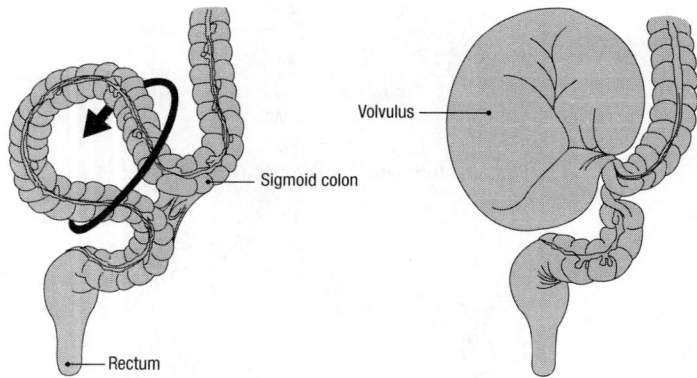

Figure 29. Volvulus of sigmoid colon. The unattached loop of bowel twists (left image), causing the bowel lumen to become obstructed (right image), which leads to the inability of stool to pass and compression of the blood supply to the looped bowel segment.

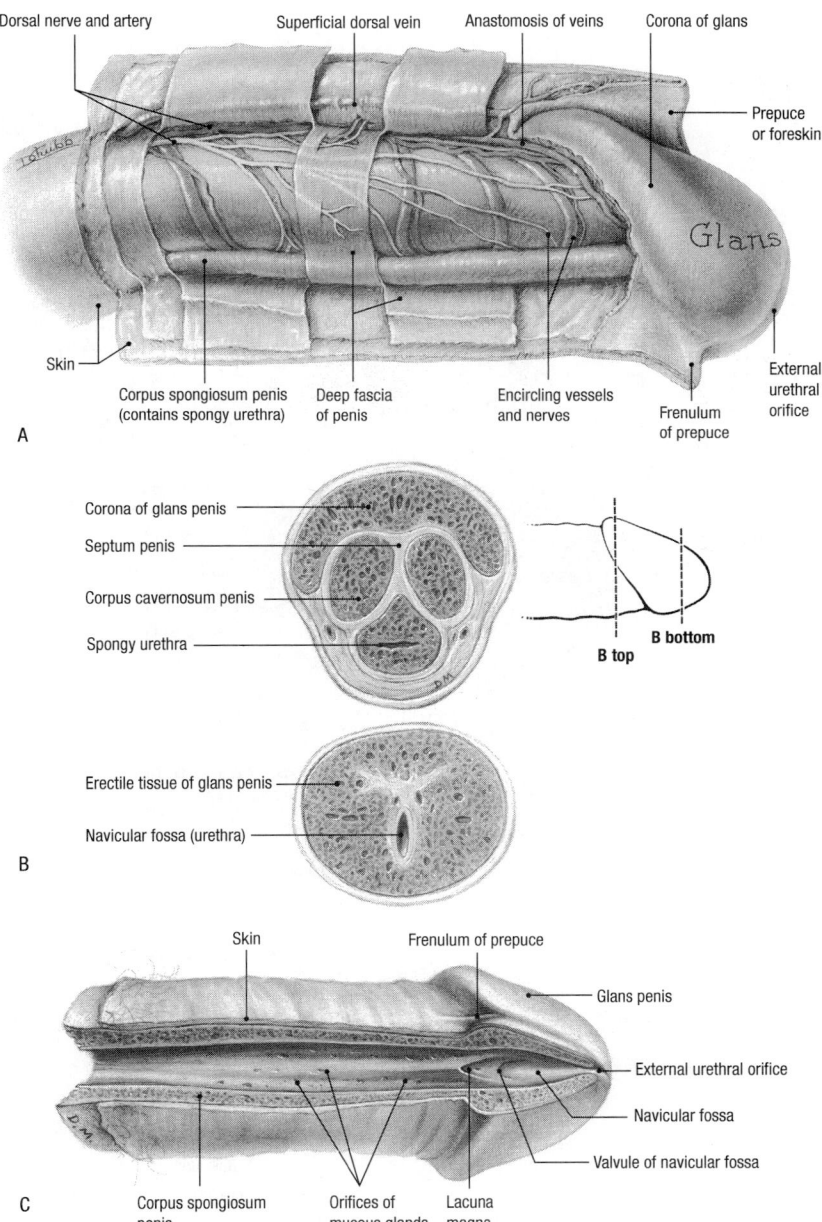

Figure 30. Penis. (A) Lateral view. (B) Transverse sections. (C) Spongy urethra, interior.

Appendix 1

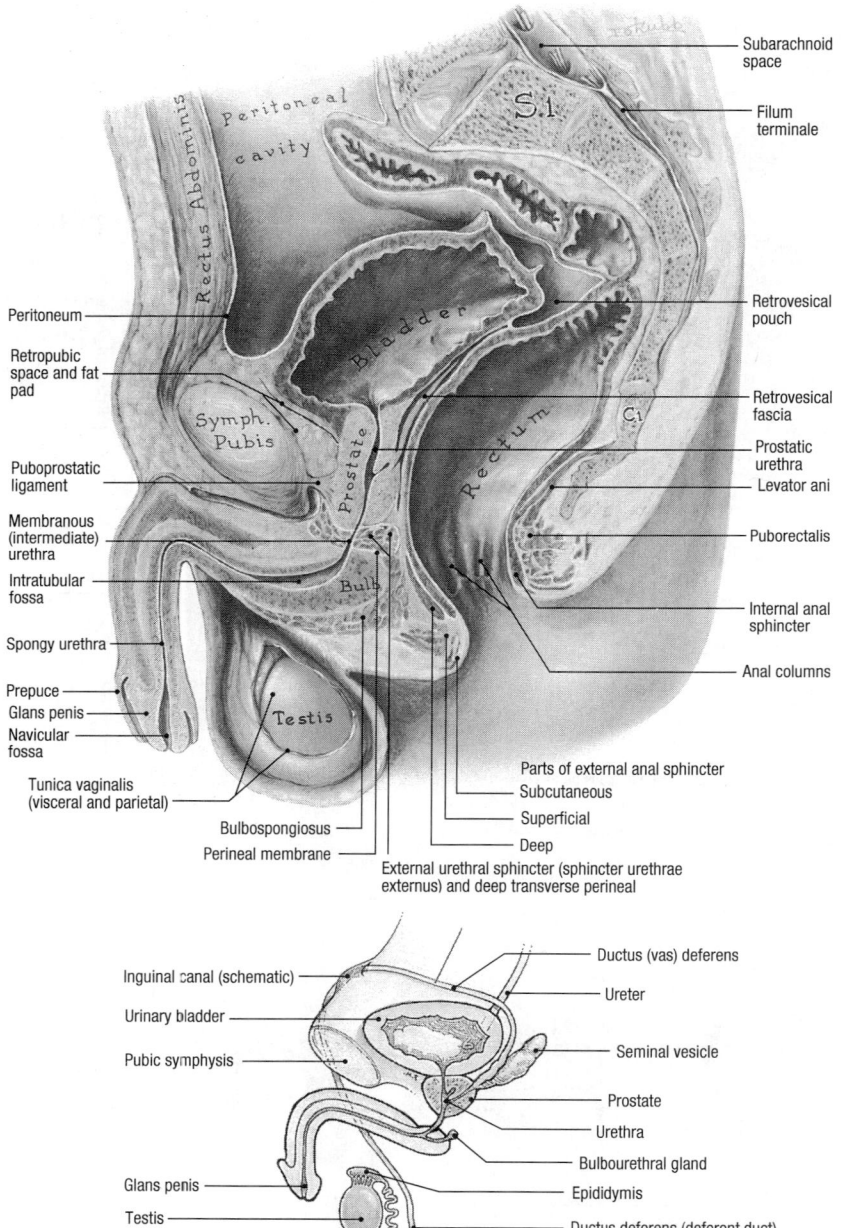

Figure 31. Male pelvis. Median section (top). Overview of urogenital system, median section (bottom).

Anatomical Illustrations

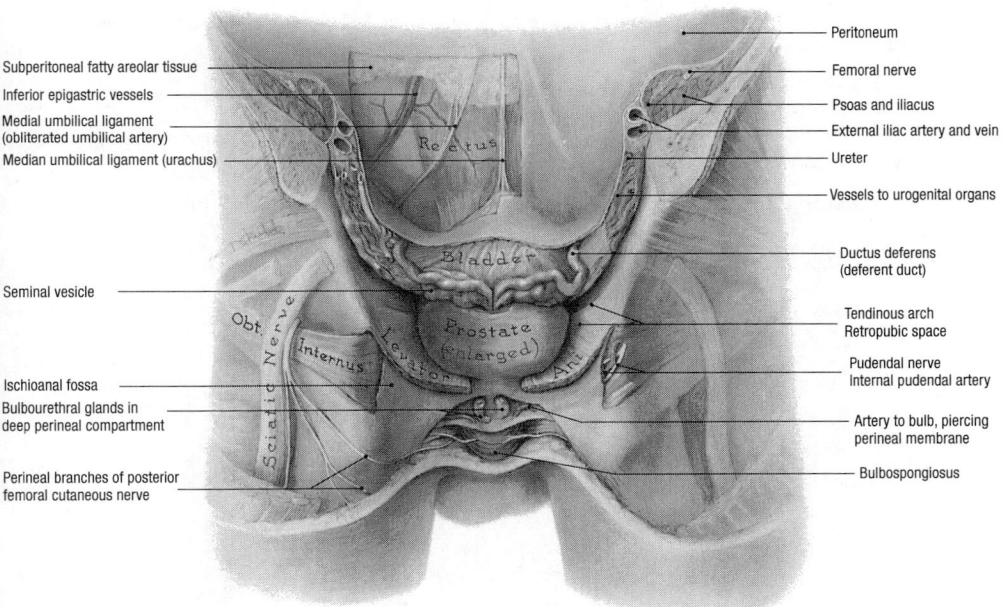

Figure 32. Male pelvis, view of anterior portion from behind.

Appendix 1

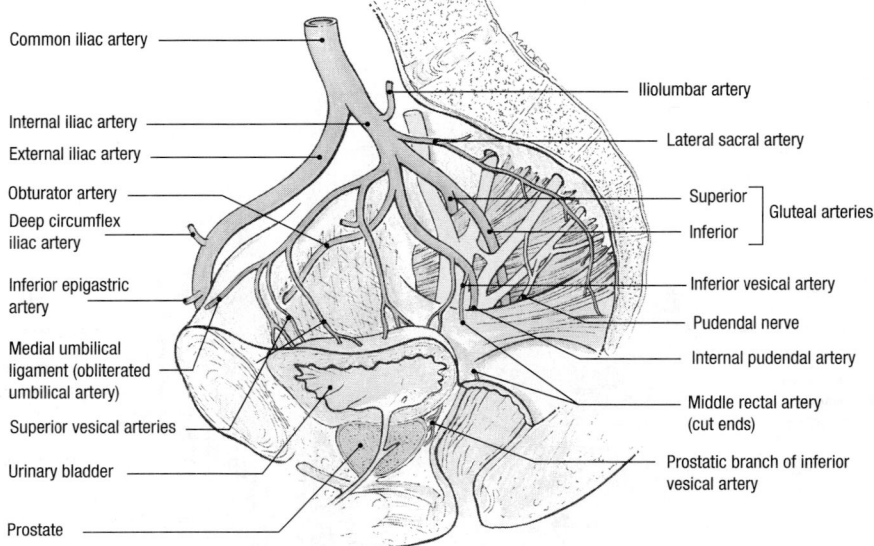

Figure 33. Arteries of the pelvis. Male pelvis, median section.

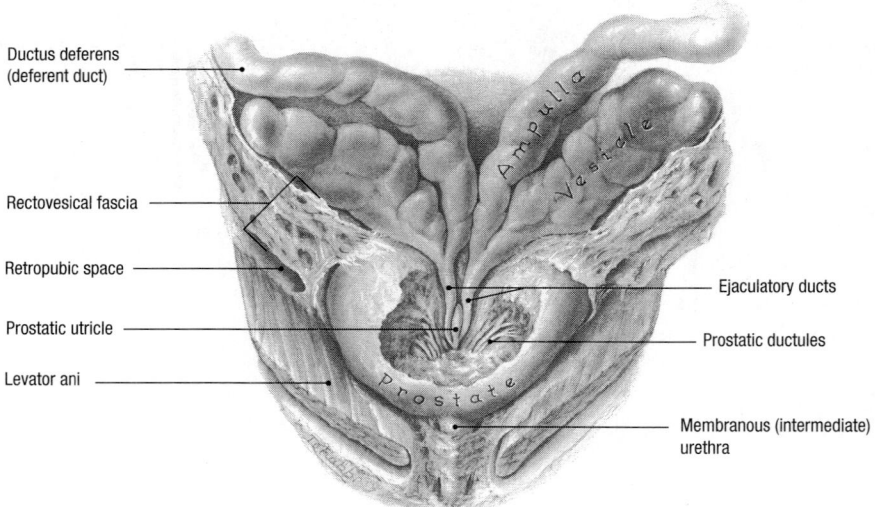

Figure 34. Prostate, posterior view.

Anatomical Illustrations

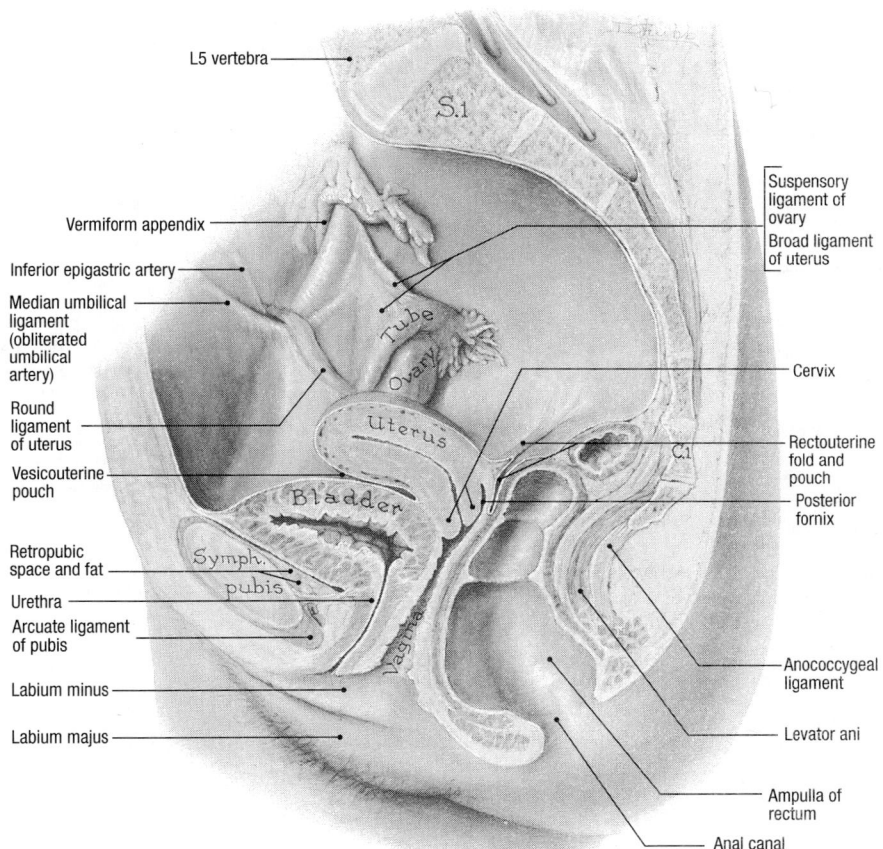

Figure 35. Female pelvis, median section.

Appendix 1

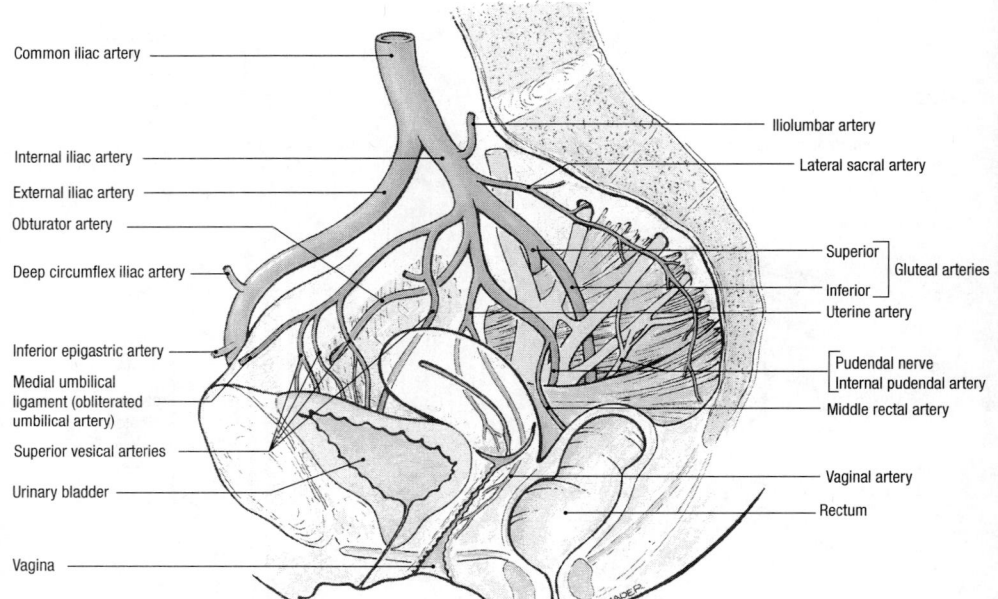

Figure 36. Arteries of the pelvis. Female pelvis, median section.

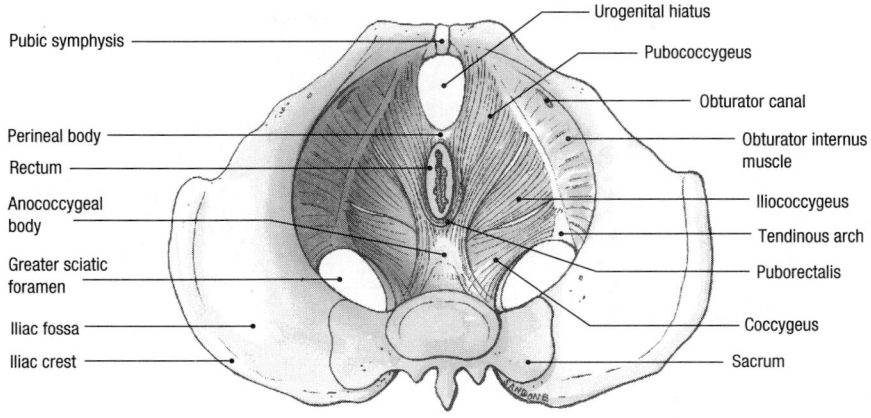

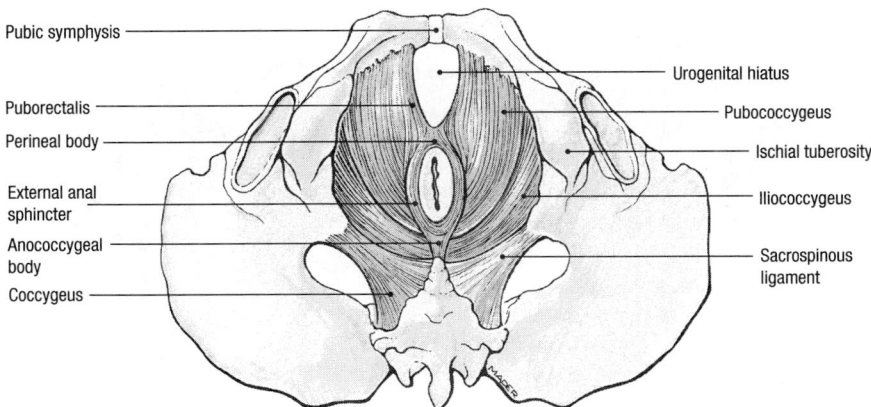

Figure 37. Muscles of pelvic walls and floors. Superior view (top) and inferior view (bottom).

Appendix 1

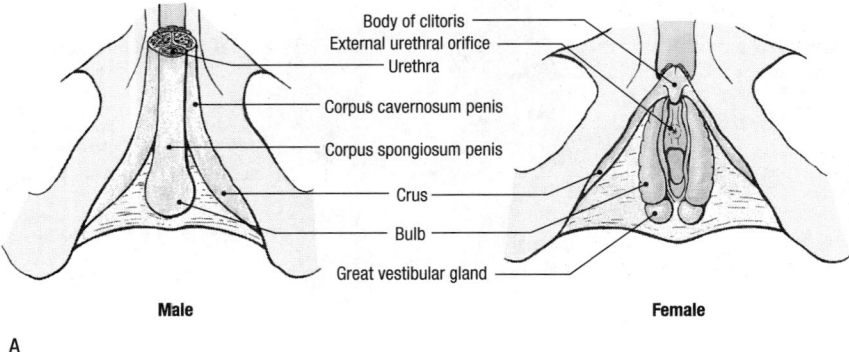

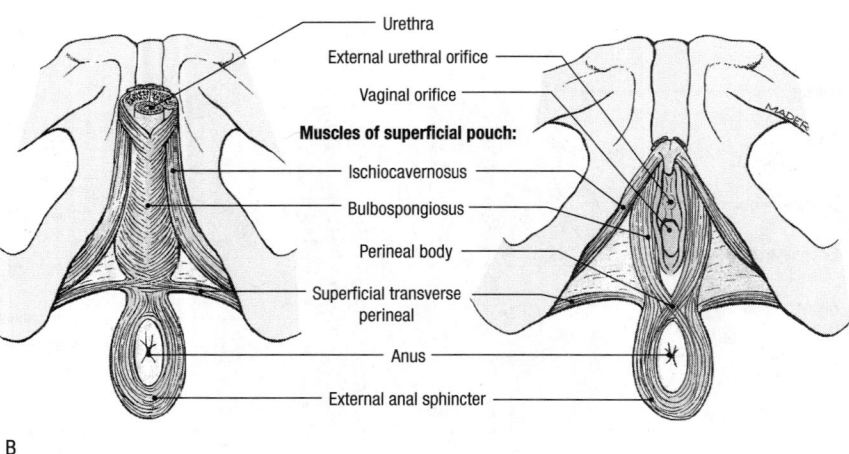

Figure 38. Male and female perineum, inferior views. (A) Crura and bulb of penis and clitoris. (B) Muscles of superficial perineal compartment.

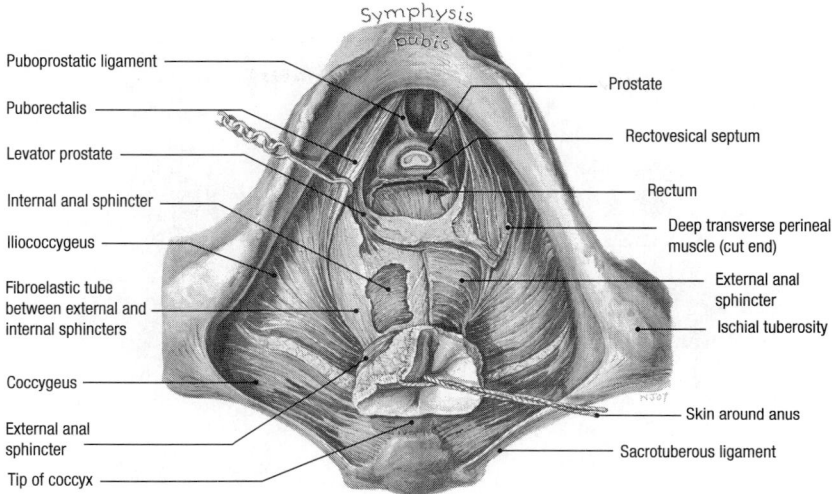

Figure 39. Dissection of male perineum. Levator ani and coccygeus muscles, and exposure of prostate, inferior view.

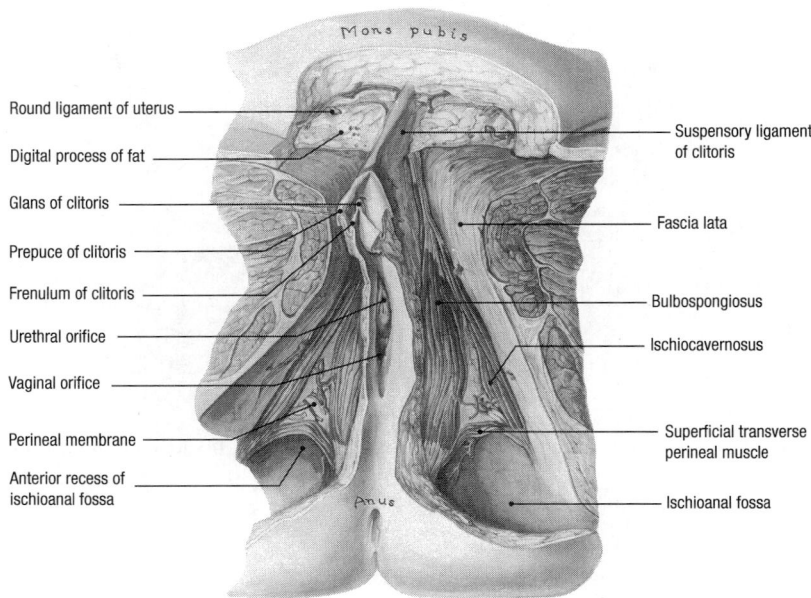

Figure 40. Female perineum, inferior view.

Appendix 1

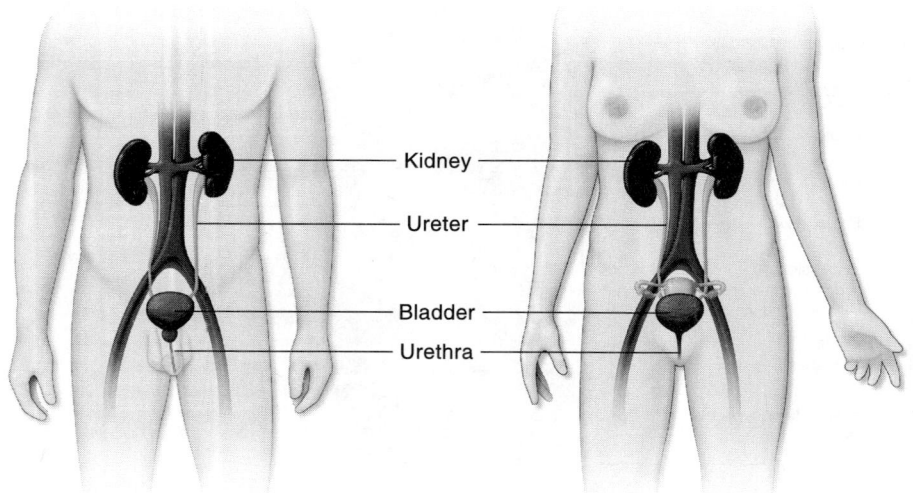

A **Anterior view**

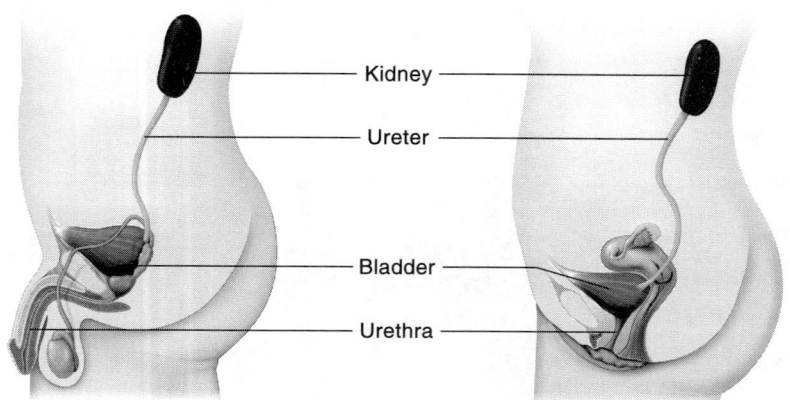

B **Lateral view**

Figure 41. Components of the urinary system in men and women. (A) Anterior view; (B) Lateral view.

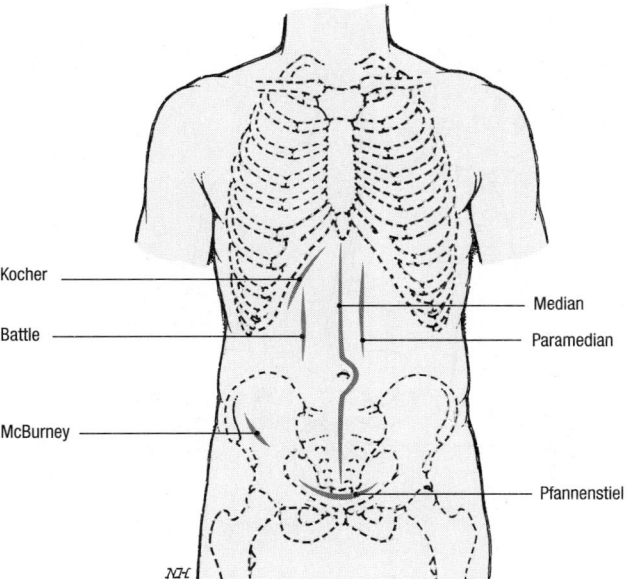

Figure 42. Surgical incisions.

Appendix 1

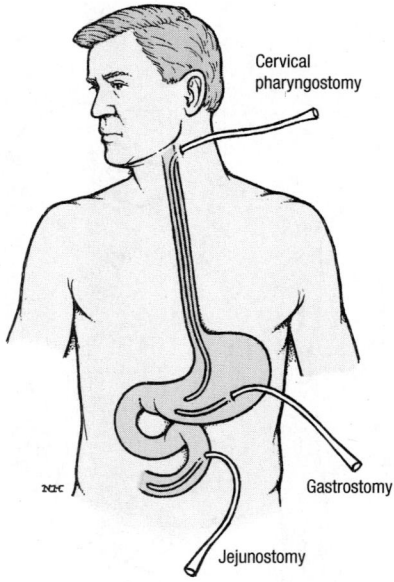

Figure 43. Enterostomy tubes. Flexible tubes passing through surgical openings into selected portions of the gastrointestinal tract, providing access for liquid food.

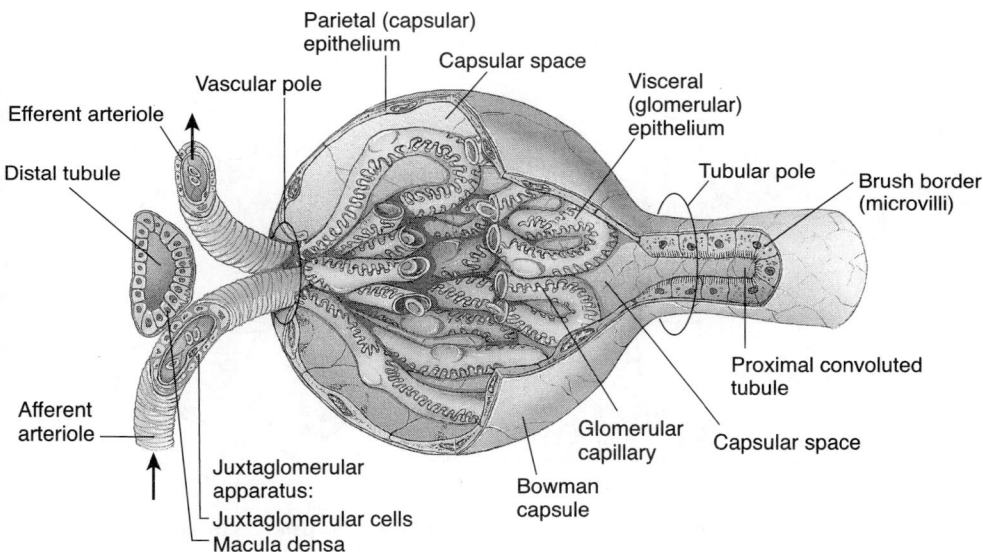

Figure 44. Juxtaglomerular apparatus.

Appendix 1

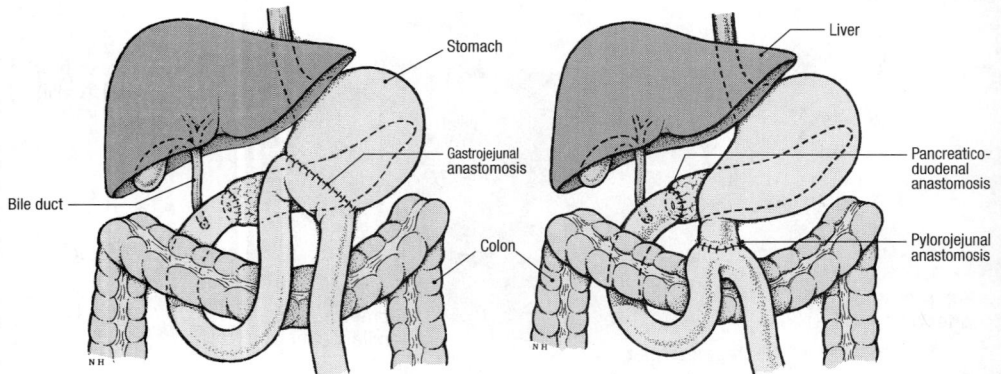

Figure 45. Pancreatoduodenectomy. Excision of all or part of the pancreas together with the duodenum and usually the distal stomach. Whipple operation (left). Pylorus-saving Whipple procedure (right).

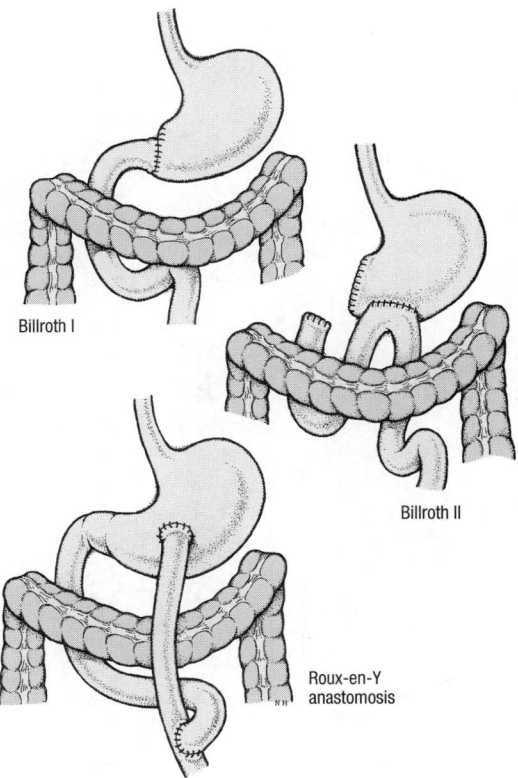

Figure 46. Gastroenterostomy.

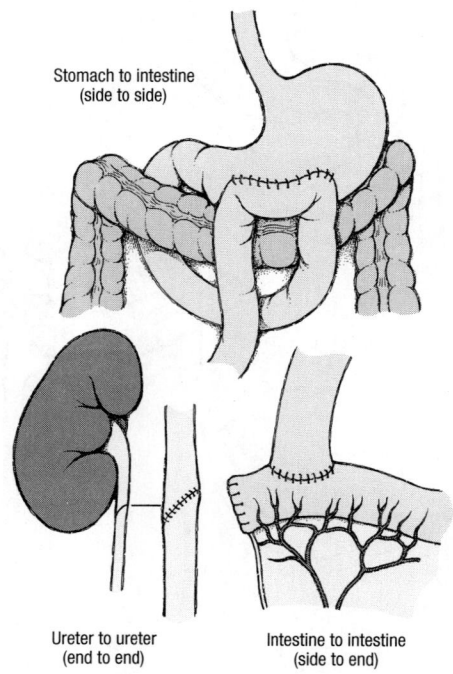

Figure 47. Surgical anastomoses.

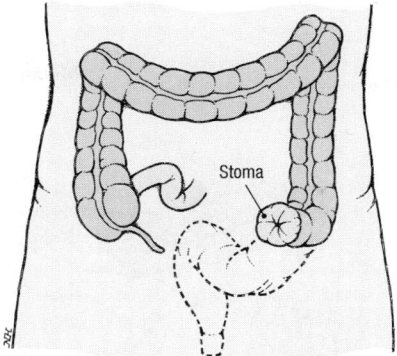

Figure 48. Colostomy. Stoma opens on anterior abdominal wall.

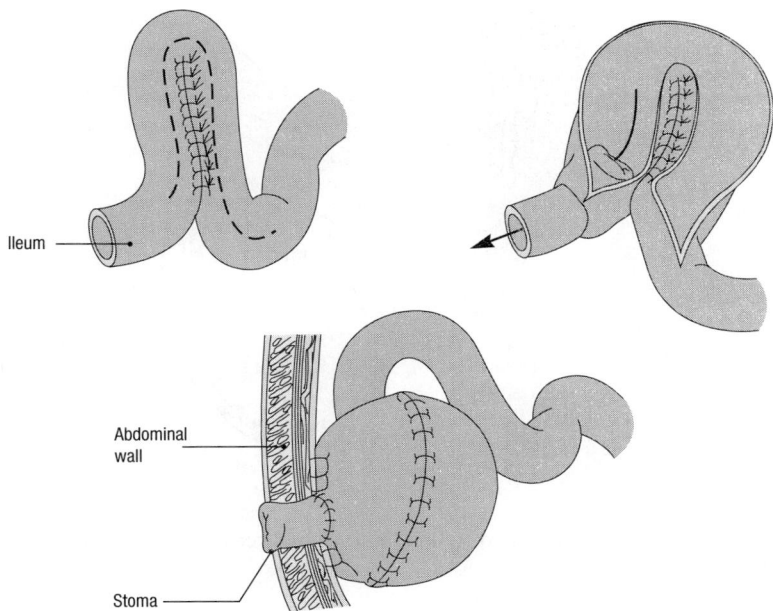

Figure 49. Three-part illustration showing section of intestine undergoing procedure for creating a continent ileostomy. Bowel segment anastomosed (top). Pouch is formed (center). Pouch shown in place with stoma (bottom).

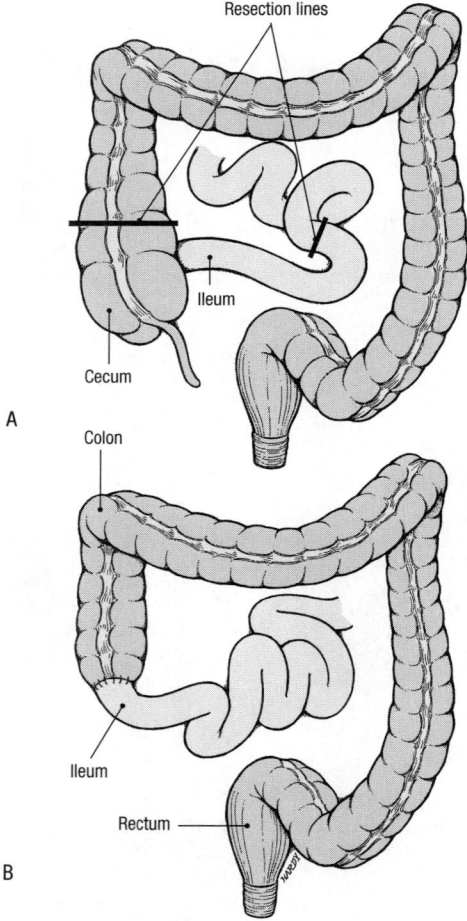

Figure 50. Ileocolostomy. (A) Diseased portions of ileum and cecum resected. (B) Resected ends anastomosed.

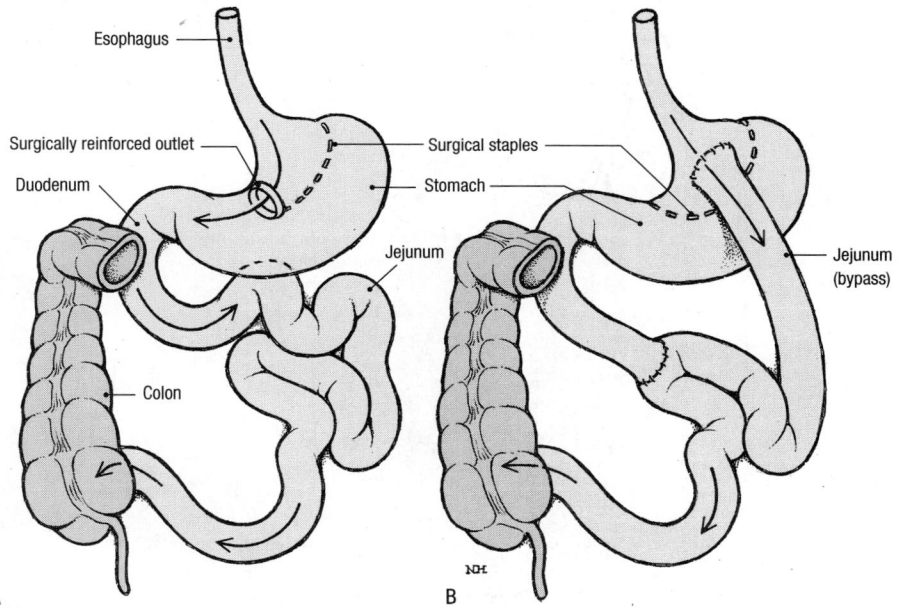

Figure 51. Surgical procedures to control morbid obesity. (A) Vertical banded gastroplasty. (B) Gastric bypass (gastrojejunostomy). In both procedures, the reduction in gastric capacity leads to early satiety and, thus, favors consumption of smaller meals.

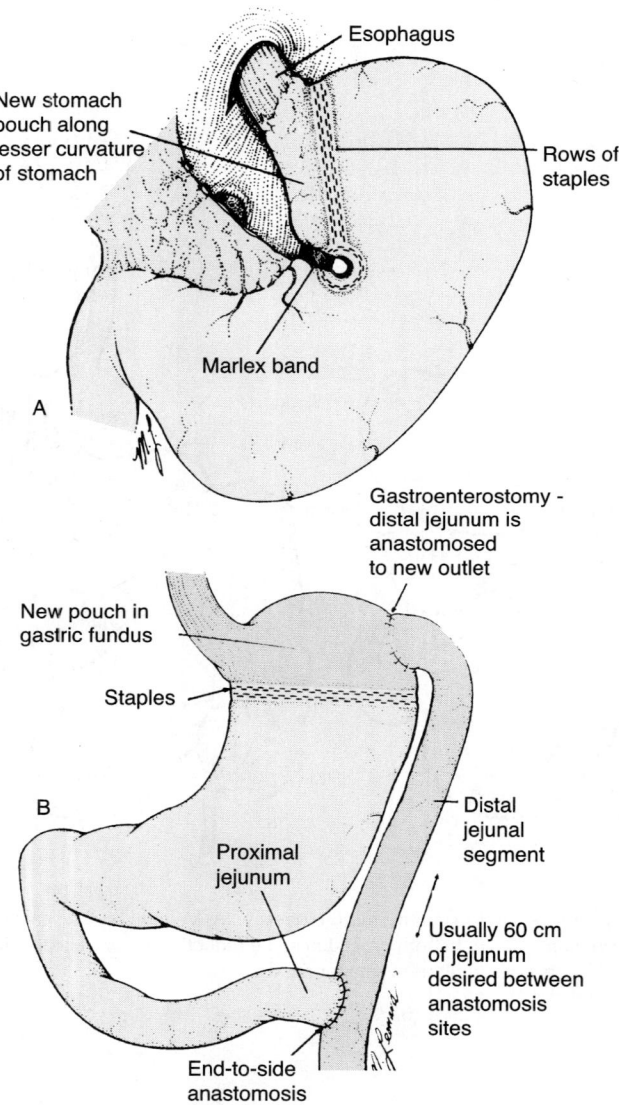

Figure 52. (A) Gastroplasty with vertical banding; (B) Gastric bypass with Roux-en-Y anastomosis.

Appendix 2
Normal Lab Values

Tests	Conventional Units	SI Units
*bilirubin, serum		
adult		
conjugated	0.0–0.3 mg/dL	0–5 μmol/L
unconjugated	0.1–1.1 mg/dL	1.7–19 μmol/L
delta	0–0.2 mg/dL	0–3 μmol/L
total	0.2–1.3 mg/L	3–22 μmol/L
neonates		
conjugated	0–0.6 mg/dL	0–10 μmol/L
unconjugated	0.6–10.5 mg/dL	10–180 μmol/L
total	1.5–12 mg/dL	1.7–180 μmol/L
urine, qualitative	negative	negative
calcium, urine		
low-calcium diet	50–150 mg/24 h	1.25–3.75 mmol/24 h
usual diet; trough	100–300 mg/24 h	2.50–7.50 mmol/24 h
catecholamines, urine		
dopamine	65–400 μg/24 h	425–2610 nmol/24 h
epinephrine	0–20 μg/24 h	0–109 nmol/24 h
norepinephrine	15–80 μg/24 h	89–473 nmol/24 h
*creatinine clearance, serum or plasma and urine		
male	94–140 mL/min/1.73 m^2	0.91–1.35 mL/s/m^2
female	72–110 mL/min/1.73 m^2	0.69–1.06 mL/s/m^2
cyclic AMP		
plasma (EDTA)		
male	4.6–8.6 ng/mL	14–26 nmol/L
female	4.3–7.6 ng/mL	13–23 nmol/L
urine, 24 h	0.3–3.6 mg/d or 0.29–2.1 mg/g creatinine	100–723 μmol/d or 100–723 μmol/mol creatinine
cystine or cysteine, urine, qualitative	negative	negative
phosphorus, urine	0.4–1.3 g/24 h	12.9–42 mmol/24 h
porphobilinogen, urine		
qualitative	negative	negative
quantitative	<2.0 mg/24 h	<9 μmol/24 h
porphyrin, urine		
coproporphyrin	34–230 μg/24 h	52–351 nmol/ 24 h
uroporphyrin	27–52 μg/24 h	32–63 nmol/ 24 h
potassium		
urine, 24 h	25–125 mmol/d; varies with diet	25–125 mmol/d; varies with diet

Appendix 2

*prostate-specific antigen (PSA), serum		
male	<4.0 ng/mL	<4.0 µg/L
*protein, serum		
total	6.4–8.3 g/dL	64–83 g/L
albumin	3.9–5.1 g/dL	39–51 g/L
globulin		
$alpha_1$	0.2–0.4 g/dL	2–4 g/L
$alpha_2$	0.4–0.8 g/dL	4–8 g/L
beta	0.5–1.0 g/dL	5–10 g/L
gamma	0.6–1.3 g/dL	6–13 g/L
urine		
qualitative	negative	negative
quantitative	50–80 mg/24 h (at rest)	50–80 mg/24 h (at rest)
sodium		
urine, 24 h	40–220 mEq/d (diet dependent)	40–220 mmol/d (diet dependent)
urea nitrogen, serum	6–20 mg/dL	2.1–7.1 mmol urea/L
urea nitrogen/creatinine ratio, serum	12:1 to 20:1	48–80 urea/creatinine mole ratio
*uric acid		
serum, enzymatic		
male	4.5–8.0 mg/dL	0.27–0.47 mmol/L
female	2.5–6.2 mg/dL	0.15–0.37 mmol/L
child	2.0–5.5 mg/dL	0.12–0.32 mmol/L
urine	250–750 mg/24 h (with normal diet)	1.48–4.43 mmol/24 h (with normal diet)
urobilinogen, urine	0.1–0.8 EU/2 h 0.5–4.0 EU/d	0.1–0.8 EU/2 h 0.5–4.0 EU/d

* Test values are method dependent.

Appendix 3
Herbs Used to Treat GI/GU Conditions

Herb	Condition
African plum	Benign prostatic hyperplasia
alder buckthorn	See *buckthorn bark*
aloe	Short-term treatment of occasional constipation
angelica root	Loss of appetite, peptic discomfort such as mild spasm of the gastrointestinal tract, feeling of fullness, and flatulence
artichoke leaf	Liver dysfunction, bloating, nausea, and impairment of digestion; lipid-lowering agent
asparagus root	Irrigation therapy for inflammatory diseases of the urinary tract and for prevention of kidney stones; also used as a diuretic and laxative
basil	Reduction of gas, resolution of stomach cramps, and constipation
bilberry fruit	Nonspecific, acute diarrhea and local therapy for mild inflammation of the mucous membranes of the mouth and throat
blessed thistle	Loss of appetite, dyspepsia, and for the increase of gastric juice secretion
boldo leaf	Mild dyspepsia and spastic gastrointestinal complaints, gallstones, liver ailments, and cystitis
bottlebrush	See *horsetail*
box holly	See *butcher's broom*
brewer's yeast/Hansen CBS 5926	Symptomatic treatment of acute diarrhea; prophylactic and symptomatic treatment of traveler's diarrhea; diarrhea occurring while tube feeding
bromelain	In combination with pancreatic extracts of titrated trypsin; suggested as treatment for dyspepsia symptoms and exocrine hepatic insufficiency
buckthorn bark	Stool softener
butcher's broom	Itching and burning of hemorrhoids
cascara	Constipation; stool softener
cascara sagrada bark	See *cascara*
cassia (cassia cinnamon)	See *Chinese cinnamon bark*
catnip	Relief of diarrhea; used as a tea
cayenne	Healing effect on ulcers; used to treat stomach aches, cramps, gas, indigestion, loss of appetite, and diarrhea
cranberry	Treatment of urinary tract infection
ceylon cinnamon	See *cinnamon bark*
chamomile flower	Used internally as symptomatic treatment of digestive ailments such as dyspepsia, epigastric bloating, impaired digestion, and

Appendix 3

	flatulence; used externally for irritation of the mouth and gums, and for hemorrhoids
Chinese cinnamon bark	Loss of appetite, gastrointestinal tract spasm, nausea, diarrhea, bloating, flatulence, colic or dyspepsia
chittem bark	See *cascara*
cinnamon bark	Loss of appetite, dyspeptic complaints such as mild spastic conditions of the gastrointestinal tract, bloating, and flatulence
coriander seed/fruit	Dyspeptic complaints and loss of appetite
couch grass	Cystitis, urethritis, prostatitis, enlarged prostate gland, kidney stones and gravel, healing action on the mucosa of the bladder and associated organs, enuresis, nervous incontinence
dandelion	Loss of appetite, dyspepsia, constipation, cholecystitis, and prevention of renal gravel
dandelion root	Disturbances in bile flow, stimulation of diuresis, loss of appetite, and dyspepsia
devil's claw root	Loss of appetite and dyspepsia
dill weed	Antispasmodic, carminative, diuretic; used for stomach ache and colic
echinacea herb/root	Administered orally in supportive therapy for infections of the urinary tract
fennel oil/seed	Dyspepsia, fullness, and flatulence
fenugreek seed	Anorexia, dyspepsia, gastritis
flaxseed/flax	Chronic constipation, colon damage from laxative abuse, irritable colon, diverticulitis; mucilage for gastritis and enteritis
frangula	See *buckthorn bark*
garlic	As an adjuvant to dietetic management in treatment of hyperlipidemia
gentian root	Loss of appetite, fullness, and flatulence
ginger	Prophylaxis of nausea and vomiting associated with motion sickness, postoperative nausea, and seasickness
goldenrod/European goldenrod	Irrigation therapy for inflammatory diseases of the lower urinary tract, urinary calculi, and kidney gravel; prophylaxis for urinary calculi and kidney gravel
goldenseal	A potent remedy for disorders of the stomach and intestines such as irritable bowel syndrome, colitis, ulcers, and gastritis and internal parasites
holy thistle	See *blessed thistle*
horehound/white horehound	Loss of appetite, bloating, and flatulence
horsetail	Inflammation of the lower urinary tract and renal gravel, urinary and prostatic disease
huckleberry	See *bilberry fruit*

Herbs Used to Treat GI/GU Conditions

hydrangea	Inflamed or enlarged prostate, urinary calculus with gravel and cystitis, and acute nephritis
juniper berry/common juniper	Bladder and kidney conditions
lemon balm/common balm	Gastrointestinal complaints
licorice root	Gastric or duodenal ulcers
linseed	See *flaxseed/flax*
marshmallow root	Used internally for gastroenteritis, peptic and duodenal ulceration, common and ulcerative colitis, and enteritis; used topically as a mouthwash or gargle for inflammation of the mouth and pharynx
melissa	See *lemon balm*
milk thistle fruit/ St. Mary's thistle	Chronic inflammatory liver disease and hepatic cirrhosis
mint oil	Flatulence, as well as functional, gastrointestinal, and gallbladder disorders
oak bark	Nonspecific, acute diarrhea and local treatment of mild inflammation of the genital and anal areas
orange peel/bitter orange peel	Loss of appetite and dyspeptic ailments
onion	Loss of appetite
parsley herb and root	Flushing out the urinary tract and preventing and treating kidney gravel, dysuria, and flatulent dyspepsia
peppermint leaf	Spastic complaints of the gastrointestinal tract, gallbladder, and bile duct
peppermint oil	Spastic discomfort of the upper gastrointestinal and bile duct; irritable bowel syndrome
psyllium seed	Bulk-forming laxative used for treatment of chronic and temporary constipation, irritable bowel syndrome, and constipation related to duodenal ulcer or diverticulitis; also used as a stool softener after anorectal surgery and for patients with hemorrhoids
pumpkin seed	Irritable bladder and micturition problems of benign prostatic hyperplasia stages 1 and 2, functional disorders of the bladder, difficult urination, childhood enuresis nocturna, and irritable bladder; also used successfully to eradicate tapeworms
rhubarb root	Short-term treatment of occasional constipation
rye pollen	Treatment of outflow tract obstruction due to benign prostatic hyperplasia
sacred bark	See *cascara*
sage leaf	Dyspeptic symptoms, stomatitis
saw palmetto berry	Urinary problems in benign prostatic hyperplasia stages 1 and 2, testicular atrophy, sex hormone disorders, and prostatic enlargement

Appendix 3

senna leaf/fruit	Short-term treatment of occasional constipation
shave grass	See *horsetail*
slippery elm	Crohn disease and ulcerative colitis
South African star grass	Benign prostatic hyperplasia
soy lecithin/phospholipid	Hypercholesterolemia
sparrowgrass	See *asparagus root*
stinging nettle herb/leaf	Irrigation therapy for inflammatory diseases of the lower urinary tract; prevention and treatment of kidney gravel
stone root	Treatment and prevention of stones in the urinary tract and gallbladder, enteric and bowel disease, kidney stones, hemorrhoids
sweet balm	See *lemon balm*
turmeric root	Treatment of acid, flatulent, or atonic dyspepsia
uva ursi leaf	Inflammatory disorders of the efferent urinary tract
wild gentian	See *gentian root*
witch hazel	Local inflammation of hemorrhoids
whortleberry	See *bilberry fruit*
yarrow	Mild spastic discomfort of the gastrointestinal tract
yellow gentian	See *gentian root*
yohimbine	Erectile dysfunction

Appendix 4
Sample Reports and Dictation

CHOLECYSTENTERIC FISTULA REPAIR, OPERATIVE REPORT

INDICATIONS FOR PROCEDURE: A fistulous tract was observed during a routine laparoscopic cholecystectomy, located between the gallbladder and the transverse colon.

DESCRIPTION OF PROCEDURE: The patient was prepped and draped in routine fashion for laparoscopic cholecystectomy. The abdomen was entered without incident.

The gallbladder was contracted, with dense adhesions noted to be extending to the omentum. Combining blunt and sharp dissection, the adhesions were freed. The gallbladder fundus was identified and isolated from adjacent fibrous tissue. A small window was created, and the gallbladder was grasped and elevated with gentle traction. An Endo GIA 35-mm stapling device was then inserted across the fistulous connection. The fistula was successfully removed. Then, the gallbladder was removed in standard laparoscopic fashion without complication.

All instruments were removed and air was expelled from the abdomen. Band-Aids were placed over the wounds, and the patient was taken to the recovery room in satisfactory condition.

Sponge, needle, and instrument counts were correct ×3.

If the patient does well, she will be discharged to home tomorrow morning.

GASTRIC ULCER, HISTORY AND PHYSICAL

CHIEF COMPLAINT: Midepigastric pain, severe.

HISTORY OF PRESENT ILLNESS: This 14-year-old boy was brought to the emergency room with the onset of severe midepigastric pain approximately 6 hours before presentation. This was followed by several episodes of vomiting, with the inability to drink or eat. There is no history of hematemesis or bloody diarrhea. According to his mother, he has taken ibuprofen several times per week for approximately 6 months for aching muscles that are the result of sports activities. He took an 800-mg dose yesterday after football practice. He denies a history of steroid or illicit drug use.

Appendix 4

PAST MEDICAL HISTORY: The patient had an adenotonsillectomy when he was 5 years old and a fracture of the left tibia last year. He recovered from both without complication.

FAMILY HISTORY: Father died of cancer last year. Mother reports that the patient appears to be adjusting fairly well. He is the oldest child with 2 younger sisters, both in good health.

PHYSICAL EXAMINATION: VITAL SIGNS: Temperature 101 F, pulse 120, blood pressure 130/80. GENERAL: The patient is sitting upright, with his knees flexed. He avoids sudden movement, and guards his abdominal area. HEENT: Negative. CHEST: Heart is normal sinus rhythm. Lungs reveal clear breath sounds. ABDOMEN: Bowel sounds are diminished. There is exquisite tenderness in the midepigastric area, and there is slight tenderness in the right lower quadrant. Rovsing and obturator signs are negative. Heel drop is positive. GENITALIA: Normal for age. RECTAL: Stool is heme negative.

X-RAY AND LABORATORY DATA: Abdominal x-rays in the emergency room reveal air-fluid levels, and there is free air under the right hemidiaphragm. White count is reported to be 24,000; hematocrit 39.2. Blood type is O negative.

IMPRESSION: We are most likely dealing with a perforated gastric ulcer in this young man.

PLAN: The patient is admitted for workup, with possible surgery for repair of the ulcer.

GUNSHOT WOUND TO ABDOMEN, HISTORY AND PHYSICAL

HISTORY OF PRESENT ILLNESS: The patient is a 25-year-old male who was shot twice in the abdomen at close range with a .38-caliber handgun. The incident occurred outside a nightclub after an argument between the patient and another male. The patient was transported by ambulance, hemodynamically stable, awake and alert, and complaining of abdominal pain.

PAST MEDICAL HISTORY: He denies a past history of medical problems or history of surgery. He is on no prescribed medications, and he denies the use of illicit drugs. No medication allergies are known.

SOCIAL HISTORY: He is single and is a college student. He works as a retail clerk in a department store. He does not smoke and consumes alcohol on occasion. He states that he and some friends had had a few drinks at the nightclub this evening.

PHYSICAL EXAMINATION: GENERAL: The patient is awake and alert and in mild distress secondary to pain. VITAL SIGNS: Blood pressure 110/74; pulse 118; respirations 20, temperature 37.2 C. HEENT: No abnormalities. NECK: No tenderness, wounds, or deformities. CHEST: Nontender. Bilateral breath sounds are present; no crepitation. ABDOMEN: Bowel sounds are very quiet. There is tenderness in the right upper quadrant. Two entrance wounds are present in the right upper quadrant and flank. BACK: No tenderness or deformity. PELVIS: Stable, without tenderness. GENITOURINARY: Normal adult male. RECTAL: Sphincter tone is normal. No occult blood is noted. NEUROLOGIC: Awake and alert x3. Glasgow Coma Score is 15. Sensory and motor examinations are normal. EXTREMITIES: Pulses are 2+ and symmetrical bilaterally.

DIAGNOSIS: Gunshot wounds to the abdomen.

TREATMENT PLAN: The patient has been admitted from the emergency department for probable emergency surgery.

HERNIATION OF FORAMEN OF WINSLOW, DISCHARGE SUMMARY

HISTORY OF PRESENT ILLNESS: The patient, a 42-year-old black male, came to our office complaining of chronic pain in the right upper quadrant. The pain would wax and wane and would, at times, awaken him from sleep. It did not seem to be made worse by certain foods, nor would physical activity exacerbate it. The patient had not had removal of the appendix or gallbladder. There was no history of constipation.

PHYSICAL EXAMINATION: There was no organomegaly on physical examination, and rectal exam was negative for unusual findings.

STUDIES: Ultrasound and HIDA scan revealed no abnormalities. CT scan revealed cholelithiasis with central intrahepatic biliary duct ectasia. The extrahepatic biliary tree was normal, as was the liver itself. An abdominal CT revealed what appeared to be a lesion in the proximal transverse colon, and there were multiple stones. A barium enema suggested a 4-cm constricting lesion involving the distal ascending colon. A subsequent colonoscopy was done. The colonoscope could not be advanced past the hepatic flexure; however, no lesion was observed.

HOSPITAL COURSE: The patient was admitted for exploratory laparotomy. Findings included an ascending colon that was herniated through the foramen of Winslow into the lesser sac. This caused a partial large bowel obstruction. By dividing adhesions that held the cecum and distal ileum in the epiploic foramen of Winslow, the hernia

that held the cecum and distal ileum in the epiploic foramen of Winslow, the hernia was reduced. The greater omentum was placed in the foramen of Winslow, thus removing the potential hernia sac.

Cholecystectomy was performed without complication, as was an incidental appendectomy. Appendectomy was felt necessary to prevent the possibility of future diagnostic confusion due to a displaced appendix.

The patient's hospital course was uneventful, and he is discharged on the 4th postoperative day in good condition. He is moving about without difficulty and is eating a normal diet without a problem. He was given a prescription for Darvocet-N 100 to take as needed for discomfort, and he will be seen in the office in 1 week for postoperative check, sooner if needed.

LIVER BIOPSY, OPERATIVE REPORT

PREOPERATIVE DIAGNOSIS: Melanoma, with liver metastasis.

POSTOPERATIVE DIAGNOSIS: Melanoma, with liver and omental metastases.

PROCEDURES PERFORMED: Liver biopsy. Resection of omental implants.

ANESTHESIA: General.

INDICATIONS FOR PROCEDURE: The patient is a 33-year-old female who underwent resection of melanoma of the maxillary sinus approximately 1 year ago. She received radiation therapy and interferon after the surgery. She was recently discovered to have liver metastasis. No other lesions were detected on preoperative staging workup.

DESCRIPTION OF PROCEDURE: The patient was brought to the surgical suite, placed in the supine position, and prepped and draped in the usual sterile manner. A Kocher incision was made and extended in the midline.

A single lesion was identified in the right lateral lobe of the liver. There were no other identifiable lesions of the liver. A wedge biopsy was taken for tissue confirmation.

Several small, 1- to 2-mm nodules were noted in the greater omentum. There was also a small nodule identified on the transverse colon. Two of the nodules were resected and sent to pathology for frozen section.

Because resection of the liver lesion would not be beneficial, we closed the midline fascia with 2-0 running nylon after assuring hemostasis. The posterior rectus sheath was then closed with 1 Vicryl running suture, and the anterior rectus sheath was closed with 2 running nylon. The skin was approximated with 4-0 Vicryl subcuticular suture. Steri-Strips and a dry, sterile gauze dressing were placed on the wound.

The patient tolerated the procedure well. She was taken to the recovery suite for postoperative recovery and care.

PERCUTANEOUS ENDOSCOPIC GASTROSTOMY (PEG) TUBE COMPLICATION, DISCHARGE SUMMARY

HISTORY OF PRESENT ILLNESS: The patient is a 65-year-old widowed white male. He is cared for at a local nursing home because of a history of cerebrovascular accident approximately 2 years ago. He has also been treated in the past for carcinoma of the prostate, with radical prostatectomy performed three years ago. Because of progressive weakness and increasing inability to take food orally, he has received enteral feedings via percutaneous endoscopic gastrostomy (PEG) tube. On the day of admission to the emergency department, the patient had developed hematemesis.

PHYSICAL EXAMINATION: Initial examination revealed him to be hemodynamically stable, with a pulse rate of 70 per minute. Blood pressure was 150/85. Temperature was normal at 98.6 F.

HOSPITAL COURSE: We attempted to lavage the stomach via the PEG tube, but this was unsuccessful. Placement of a nasogastric tube resulted in a return of 600 mL of bloody fluid. Two liters of normal saline were used to lavage the stomach until it was clear. Endoscopy of the upper GI tract revealed a portion of gangrenous bowel protruding through the pylorus.

An emergent laparotomy was performed, revealing an enlarged duodenum and stomach. Approximately 30 cm of jejunum was in retrograde intussusception around the balloon of the PEG tube and was extending through the duodenum and into the stomach. After we reduced the duodenum, it was viable; however, the intussuscepted jejunum was necrotic. Therefore, approximately 40 cm of jejunum were resected, beginning 4 cm distal to the ligament of Treitz. Primary anastomosis and gastrojejunostomy tube placement completed the procedure.

The patient did remarkably well. Bowel function returned on postoperative day 6. He is being discharged to the nursing home today, postoperative day 12. His primary care physician will provide instruction for follow-up care.

Appendix 4

Phytobezoar, Emergency Department Note

History of Present Illness: The patient is a 12-year-old female, who is brought to the emergency department by her parents. They report that the patient was well until this morning when she began to experience nausea and vomiting after ingestion of the peel of an orange. The patient states that she prefers eating the peel rather than the orange and that she has been ingesting them daily for some time. She also complains of abdominal discomfort. There is no history of hematemesis.

Physical Examination: Exam reveals a pale, thin female. She is mildly mentally retarded but is able to answer questions and converse. Vital signs are within normal limits. Heart and lungs are normal. There is tenderness of the epigastric area.

Emergency Room Treatment: An abdominal ultrasound reveals a phytobezoar in the stomach. Gastric lavage and suction were successful in fragmenting and removing it. It was sent to pathology for analysis.

Plan: The parents were advised to keep the child from eating orange peels. They are to follow up with her pediatrician next week.

Pneumococcal Sepsis, Death Summary

History of Present Illness: The patient was a 30-year-old male who had a history of intravenous drug use and history of splenectomy due to gunshot wound to the abdomen in 1992. He was admitted with a 2-day history of fever, chills, nausea, vomiting, anorexia, and muscle aches. He reported having a mild frontal headache but denied photophobia, shortness of breath, or neck stiffness. Before the sudden onset of symptoms, the patient reported that he had been feeling relatively well.

Past Medical History: His past medical history was significant for the gunshot wound and splenectomy. He had a history of gonorrhea and syphilis that had been treated, and he had been diagnosed with hepatitis C in 1999.

Social History: The patient admitted to daily use of heroine. His last use was 1 day before admission. He denied smoking or alcohol intake.

Family History: One sister died of AIDS. Father and mother were both deceased.

Physical Examination: The patient was cachectic and ill appearing. Temperature was 39 degrees C, pulse 120, blood pressure 130/90, respirations 25; oxygen saturation was 93% on room air. Heart revealed tachycardia. S1 and S2 were normal sinus rhythm. Abdomen was soft and nontender. Extremities were normal, with 2+ peripheral pulses.

HOSPITAL COURSE: Blood cultures were positive at 5 hours of incubation with Quellung positive, gram-positive diplococci. The patient was placed on cefotaxime and vancomycin, but his condition rapidly deteriorated. Unfortunately, he suffered cardiopulmonary arrest and despite heroic measures, he died.

CAUSE OF DEATH: Pneumococcal sepsis.

SPASTIC NEUROGENIC BLADDER, SOAP NOTE

SUBJECTIVE: "I am having more trouble with urinary incontinence. I need to wear a pad all the time now."

OBJECTIVE: The patient is a 30-year-old female who has had the diagnosis of multiple sclerosis for approximately 4 years. During the past year, she has experienced an increasing number of urinary tract infections, and it has become more difficult for her to control voluntary emptying of her bladder.

ASSESSMENT: Outpatient studies, including ultrasound and cystography, reveal increased bladder spasticity.

PLAN: We discussed options, including a trial of antispasmodic medication and condom catheterization. The patient wishes to try medication, and I believe this is appropriate. I gave her a prescription for imipramine 50 mg, and she is to report her progress in 10 days or so.

STERILE SEROSITIS, DISCHARGE SUMMARY

HISTORY OF PRESENT ILLNESS: The patient is a 30-year-old Asian female who was admitted with vomiting, diarrhea, and generalized abdominal pain. She was diagnosed with systemic lupus erythematosus (SLE) approximately 2 years ago. At the time of her diagnosis, ANA and anti-dsDNA were positive, with decreased C3, C4, and CH50.

PHYSICAL EXAMINATION: At the time of admission, she was cushingoid in appearance. On abdominal examination, there was exquisite pain with rebound tenderness, and bowel sounds were absent. Admission and immediate exploratory laparotomy were advised because of the acute abdomen.

Appendix 4

HOSPITAL COURSE: Because of findings of acute abdomen, the patient underwent emergent laparotomy. At surgery she was found to have turbid ascitic fluid; the small bowel appeared to be normal. There was no growth from the culture of the ascitic fluid.

She did well postoperatively and is discharged to home on postoperative day 4. Her daily dose of prednisolone was increased to 40 mg. She will be seen in the office in 2 weeks, sooner if necessary.

DIAGNOSIS: Sterile serositis.

Appendix 5
Common Terms by Procedures

Cholecystenteric Fistula Repair, Operative Report
blunt and sharp dissection
dense adhesion
Endo GIA 35-mm stapling device
fibrous tissue
fistulous tract
gallbladder fundus
gentle traction
laparoscopic cholecystectomy
omentum
prepped and draped in routine fashion
sponge, needle, and instrument counts were correct ×3
stapling device
transverse colon

Gastric Ulcer, History and Physical
air-fluid level
bloody diarrhea
exquisite tenderness
hematemesis
heme negative
hemidiaphragm
midepigastric pain
obturator sign
perforated gastric ulcer
Rovsing sign

Gunshot Wound to Abdomen, History and Physical
abdominal pain
awake and alert
bowel sounds
flank
gunshot wound
hemodynamically stable
mild distress
right upper quadrant
sphincter tone

Herniation of Foramen of Winslow, Discharge Summary
appendectomy
appendix
ascending colon
barium enema
biliary duct
bowel obstruction
cecum
cholecystectomy
cholelithiasis
colonoscope
colonoscopy
constipation
constricting lesion
CT scan
Darvocet-N 100
distal ascending colon
distal ileum
epiploic foramen of Winslow
exacerbate
exploratory laparotomy
extrahepatic biliary tree
foramen of Winslow
gallbladder
greater omentum
hepatic flexure
hernia sac
HIDA scan
intrahepatic biliary duct ectasia
large bowel obstruction
organomegaly
partial large bowel obstruction
proximal transverse colon
rectal exam
right upper quadrant

transverse colon
ultrasound
wax and wane

Liver Biopsy, Operative Report
anterior rectus sheath
dry, sterile gauze dressing
frozen section
interferon
Kocher incision
liver biopsy
liver metastasis
melanoma
midline fascia
nodule
omental implant
omental metastasis
posterior rectus sheath
radiation therapy
recovery suite
rectus sheath
resection
right lateral lobe of the liver
2-0 running nylon
staging workup
Steri-Strips
supine position
tissue confirmation
transverse colon
1 Vicryl running suture
4-0 Vicryl subcuticular suture
wedge biopsy

Percutaneous Endoscopic Gastrostomy (Peg) Tube Complication, Discharge Summary
bloody fluid
bowel function
carcinoma of the prostate
cerebrovascular accident
duodenum
emergent laparotomy
endoscopy
enlarged duodenum
enteral feeding
postoperative day
gangrenous bowel
gastrointestinal (GI)
gastrojejunostomy tube placement
GI tract
hematemesis
hemodynamically stable
jejunum
laparotomy
lavage
ligament of Treitz
nasogastric tube
necrotic
normal saline
PEG tube
percutaneous endoscopic gastrostomy (PEG)
postoperative day
primary anastomosis
progressive weakness
pylorus
radical prostatectomy
upper GI tract

Phytobezoar, Emergency Department Note
abdominal discomfort
abdominal ultrasound
epigastric area
gastric lavage
hematemesis
ingestion
nausea and vomiting
phytobezoar

Pneumococcal Sepsis, Death Summary
cachectic
cardiopulmonary arrest

cefotaxime
fever, chills, nausea, vomiting, anorexia, and muscle aches
frontal headache
gram-positive diplococcus
gunshot wound
heroic measures
ill appearing
intravenous drug use
neck stiffness
normal sinus rhythm
peripheral pulse
photophobia
pneumococcal sepsis
Quellung positive
shortness of breath
splenectomy
sudden onset of symptoms
tachycardia
vancomycin

Spastic Neurogenic Bladder, Soap Note
antispasmodic medication
bladder spasticity
condom catheterization
cystography
imipramine
multiple sclerosis
outpatient study
ultrasound
urinary incontinence
urinary tract infection
voluntary emptying of bladder

Sterile Serositis, Discharge Summary
abdominal examination
acute abdomen
anti-dsDNA
antinuclear antibody (ANA)
ascitic fluid
bowel sounds
CH50
complement 3 (C3)
complement 4 (C4)
cushingoid appearance
emergent laparotomy
exploratory laparotomy
exquisite pain
hemolytic complement (CH50)
postoperative day
prednisolone
rebound tenderness
small bowel
sterile serositis
systemic lupus erythematosus (SLE)
turbid ascitic fluid
vomiting, diarrhea, and generalized abdominal pain

Appendix 6
Drugs by Indication

ABDOMINAL DISTENTION (POSTOPERATIVE)
Hormone, Posterior Pituitary
  Pitressin® [US]
  Pressyn® AR [Can]
  Pressyn® [Can]
  vasopressin

ABETALIPOPROTEINEMIA
Vitamin, Fat Soluble
  Amino-Opti-E® [US-OTC]
  Aquasol A® [US]
  Aquasol E® [US-OTC]
  E-Complex-600® [US-OTC]
  E-Vitamin® [US-OTC]
  Palmitate-A® [US-OTC]
  vitamin A
  vitamin E
  Vita-Plus® E Softgels® [US-OTC]
  Vitec® [US-OTC]
  Vite E® Creme [US-OTC]

ACHALASIA
Adrenergic Agonist Agent
  Brethine® [US]
  Bricanyl® [Can]
  terbutaline
Calcium Channel Blocker
  Adalat® CC [US]
  Adalat® XL® [Can]
  Apo®-Nifed [Can]
  Apo®-Nifed PA [Can]
  Nifedical™ XL [US]
  nifedipine
  Novo-Nifedin [Can]
  Nu-Nifed [Can]
  Procardia® [US/Can]
  Procardia XL® [US]
Vasodilator
  Apo®-ISDN [Can]
  Cedocard®-SR [Can]
  Dilatrate®-SR [US]
  Gen-Nitro [Can]
  Isordil® [US]
  isosorbide dinitrate
  Minitran™ [US/Can]
  Nitrek® [US]
  Nitro-Bid® Ointment [US]
  Nitro-Dur® [US/Can]
  Nitrogard® [US]
  nitroglycerin
  Nitrolingual® [US]
  Nitrong® SR [Can]
  NitroQuick® [US]
  Nitrostat® [US/Can]
  Nitro-Tab® [US]
  NitroTime® [US]
  Novo-Sorbide [Can]
  PMS-Isosorbide [Can]
  Rho-Nitro® Pumpspray [Can]
  Transderm-Nitro® [Can]

ACHLORHYDRIA
Gastrointestinal Agent, Miscellaneous
  Feracid® [US]
  glutamic acid

ALPHA-1 ANTITRYPSIN DEFICIENCY (CONGENITAL)
Antitrypsin Deficiency Agent
  alpha-1 proteinase inhibitor
  Aralast™ [US]
  Prolastin® [US/Can]
  Zemaira™ [US]

AMEBIASIS
Amebicide
  Apo®-Metronidazole [Can]
  Diodoquin® [Can]

Diquinol® [US]
Flagyl ER® [US]
Flagyl® [US/Can]
Florazole ER® [Can]
Humatin® [US/Can]
iodoquinol
MetroCream® [US/Can]
metronidazole
Noritate® [US/Can]
Novo-Nidazol [Can]
paromomycin
Trikacide® [Can]
Yodoxin® [US]
Aminoquinoline (Antimalarial)
Aralen® Phosphate [US/Can]
chloroquine phosphate

AMMONIACAL URINE
Urinary Acidifying Agent
　K-Phos® Original [US]
　potassium acid phosphate

AMMONIA INTOXICATION
Ammonium Detoxicant
　Acilac [Can]
　Apo®-Lactulose [Can]
　Cholac® [US]
　Constilac® [US]
　Constulose® [US]
　Enulose® [US]
　Generlac® [US]
　Kristalose™ [US]
　lactulose
　Laxilose [Can]
　PMS-Lactulose [Can]
　ratio-Lactulose [Can]

AMYLOIDOSIS
Mucolytic Agent
　acetylcysteine
　Acys-5® [US]
　Mucomyst® [US/Can]
　Parvolex® [Can]

ANEMIA
Anabolic Steroid
　Anadrol® [US]
　oxymetholone
Androgen
　Deca-Durabolin® [Can]
　Durabolin® [Can]
　nandrolone
Antineoplastic Agent
　cyclophosphamide
　Cytoxan® [US/Can]
　Neosar® [US]
　Procytox® [Can]
Colony-Stimulating Factor
　Aranesp™ [US/Can]
　darbepoetin alfa
　epoetin alfa
　Epogen® [US]
　Eprex® [Can]
　Procrit® [US]
Electrolyte Supplement, Oral
　Apo®-Ferrous Gluconate [Can]
　Apo®-Ferrous Sulfate [Can]
　Dexferrum® [US]
　Dexiron™ [Can]
　Fe-40® [US-OTC]
　Femiron® [US-OTC]
　Feosol® Tablet [US-OTC]
　Feostat® [US-OTC]
　Feratab® [US-OTC]
　Fer-Gen-Sol [US-OTC]
　Fergon® [US-OTC]
　Fer-In-Sol® Drops [US/Can]
　Fer-Iron® [US-OTC]
　Ferodan™ [Can]
　Feronate® [US-OTC]
　Ferro-Sequels® [US-OTC]
　ferrous fumarate
　ferrous gluconate
　ferrous sulfate
　Fe-Tinic™ 150 [US-OTC]
　Hemocyte® [US-OTC]

Hytinic® [US-OTC]
INFeD® [US]
Infufer® [Can]
Ircon® [US-OTC]
iron dextran complex
Nephro-Fer™ [US-OTC]
Niferex® 150 [US-OTC]
Niferex® [US-OTC]
Novo-Ferrogluc [Can]
Nu-Iron® 150 [US-OTC]
Palafer® [Can]
polysaccharide-iron complex
Slow FE® [US-OTC]
Growth Factor
　Aranesp™ [US/Can]
　darbepoetin alfa
Immune Globulin
　BayGam® [US/Can]
　immune globulin (intramuscular)
Immunosuppressant Agent
　Apo®-Cyclosporine [Can]
　Atgam® [US/Can]
　cyclosporine
　Gengraf™ [US]
　lymphocyte immune globulin
　Neoral® [US/Can]
　Restasis™ [US]
　Rhoxal-cyclosporine [Can]
　Sandimmune® [US/Can]
Iron Salt
　iron sucrose
　Venofer® [US/Can]
Recombinant Human Erythropoietin
　Aranesp™ [US/Can]
　darbepoetin alfa
Vitamin
　Fero-Grad 500® [US-OTC]
　ferrous sulfate and ascorbic acid
　ferrous sulfate, ascorbic acid, and vitamin B-complex
　ferrous sulfate, ascorbic acid, vitamin B-complex, and folic acid
　Iberet-Folic-500® [US]
　Iberet®-Liquid 500 [US-OTC]
　Iberet®-Liquid [US-OTC]
　Vitelle™ Irospan® [US-OTC]
Vitamin, Water Soluble
　Apo®-Folic [Can]
　Cobal® [US]
　Cobolin-M® [US]
　cyanocobalamin
　folic acid
　Nascobal® [US]
　Neuroforte-R® [US]
　Scheinpharm B12 [Can]
　Twelve Resin-K® [US]
　Vita® #12 [US]
　Vitabee® 12 [US]

ANESTHESIA (GENERAL)
Barbiturate
　Brevital® Sodium [US/Can]
　methohexital
General Anesthetic
　Amidate® [US/Can]
　desflurane
　Diprivan® [US/Can]
　enflurane
　Ethrane® [US]
　etomidate
　Forane® [US]
　halothane
　isoflurane
　Ketalar® [US/Can]
　ketamine
　propofol
　sevoflurane
　Sevorane AF™ [Can]
　Suprane® [US/Can]
　Ultane® [US]

ANESTHESIA (LOCAL)
Local Anesthetic
　AK-T-Caine™ [US]
　Alcaine® [US/Can]
　Americaine® Anesthetic Lubricant [US]

Americaine® [US-OTC]
Ametop™ [Can]
Anestacon® [US]
Band-Aid® Hurt-Free™ Antiseptic Wash [US-OTC]
benzocaine
benzocaine, butyl aminobenzoate, tetracaine, and benzalkonium chloride
benzocaine, gelatin, pectin, and sodium carboxymethylcellulose
Benzodent® [US-OTC]
Betacaine® [Can]
bupivacaine
Burnamycin [US-OTC]
Carbocaine® [Can]
Cetacaine® [US]
cetylpyridinium
cetylpyridinium and benzocaine
chloroprocaine
Citanest® Forte [Can]
Citanest® Plain [US/Can]
cocaine
Cylex® [US-OTC]
Detane® [US-OTC]
dibucaine
Diocaine® [Can]
dyclonine
ethyl chloride
ethyl chloride and dichlorotetrafluoroethane
Fleet® Pain Relief [US-OTC]
Fluoracaine® [US]
Fluro-Ethyl® Aerosol [US]
Foille® Medicated First Aid [US-OTC]
Foille® Plus [US-OTC]
Foille® [US-OTC]
hexylresorcinol
Hurricaine® [US]
Isocaine® HCl [US]
LidaMantle® [US]
lidocaine
lidocaine and epinephrine
Lidoderm® [US/Can]
L-M-X™ 4 [US-OTC]
L-M-X™ 5 [US-OTC]
Marcaine® Spinal [US]
Marcaine® [US/Can]
mepivacaine
Mycinettes® [US-OTC]
Naropin™ [US/Can]
Nesacaine®-CE [Can]
Nesacaine®-MPF [US]
Nesacaine® [US]
Novocain® [US/Can]
Nupercainal® [US-OTC]
Ophthetic® [US]
Opticaine® [US]
Orabase®-B [US-OTC]
Orabase® With Benzocaine [US-OTC]
Orajel® Maximum Strength [US-OTC]
Orajel® [US-OTC]
Orasol® [US-OTC]
Parcaine® [US]
Phicon® [US-OTC]
Polocaine® MPF [US]
Polocaine® [US/Can]
Pontocaine® [US/Can]
Pontocaine® With Dextrose [US]
PrameGel® [US-OTC]
pramoxine
Prax® [US-OTC]
Premjact® [US-OTC]
prilocaine
procaine
ProctoFoam® NS [US-OTC]
proparacaine
proparacaine and fluorescein
ropivacaine
tetracaine
tetracaine and dextrose
Topicaine® [US-OTC]
Trocaine® [US-OTC]
Tronolane® [US-OTC]

Tronothane® [US-OTC]
Xylocaine® MPF [US]
Xylocaine® [US/Can]
Xylocaine® Viscous [US]
Xylocaine® With Epinephrine
 [US/Can]
Xylocard® [Can]
Zilactin®-B [US/Can]
Zilactin® [Can]
Zilactin-L® [US-OTC]
Local Anesthetic, Amide Derivative
 Chirocaine® [US/Can]
 levobupivacaine

ANTITHROMBIN III DEFICIENCY (HEREDITARY)
Blood Product Derivative
 antithrombin III
 Thrombate III™ [US/Can]

ASCARIASIS
Anthelmintic
 albendazole
 Albenza® [US]

ASCITES
Diuretic, Loop
 Apo®-Furosemide [Can]
 bumetanide
 Bumex® [US/Can]
 Burinex® [Can]
 Demadex® [US]
 Edecrin® [Can]
 ethacrynic acid
 Furocot® [US]
 furosemide
 Lasix® Special [Can]
 Lasix® [US/Can]
 torsemide
Diuretic, Miscellaneous
 Apo®-Chlorthalidone [Can]
 Apo®-Indapamide [Can]
 chlorthalidone

Gen-Indapamide [Can]
indapamide
Lozide® [Can]
Lozol® [US/Can]
metolazone
Mykrox® [US/Can]
Novo-Indapamide [Can]
Nu-Indapamide [Can]
PMS-Indapamide [Can]
Thalitone® [US]
Zaroxolyn® [US/Can]
Diuretic, Potassium Sparing
 Aldactone® [US/Can]
 Novo-Spiroton [Can]
 spironolactone
Diuretic, Thiazide
 Apo®-Hydro [Can]
 Aquacot® [US]
 Aquatensen® [US/Can]
 Aquazide® H [US]
 bendroflumethiazide
 chlorothiazide
 Diuril® [US/Can]
 Enduron® [US/Can]
 hydrochlorothiazide
 HydroDIURIL® [Can]
 Metatensin® [Can]
 methyclothiazide
 Microzide™ [US]
 Naqua® [US/Can]
 Naturetin® [US]
 Oretic® [US]
 polythiazide
 Renese® [US]
 Trichlorex® [Can]
 trichlormethiazide
 Zide® [US]

BEHÇET SYNDROME
Immunosuppressant Agent
 Alti-Azathioprine [Can]
 Apo®-Azathioprine [Can]
 Apo®-Cyclosporine [Can]

azathioprine
cyclosporine
Gen-Azathioprine [Can]
Gengraf™ [US]
Imuran® [US/Can]
Neoral® [US/Can]
ratio-Azathioprine [Can]
Restasis™ [US]
Rhoxal-cyclosporine [Can]
Sandimmune® [US/Can]

BENIGN PROSTATIC HYPERPLASIA (BPH)
Alpha-Adrenergic Blocking Agent
alfuzocin
Alti-Doxazosin [Can]
Apo®-Doxazosin [Can]
Apo®-Prazo [Can]
Apo®-Terazosin [Can]
Cardura® [US/Can]
doxazosin
Flomax® [US/Can]
Gen-Doxazosin [Can]
Hytrin® [US/Can]
Minipress® [US/Can]
Novo-Doxazosin [Can]
Novo-Prazin [Can]
Novo-Terazosin [Can]
Nu-Prazo [Can]
Nu-Terazosin [Can]
prazosin
ratio-Terazosin [Can]
tamsulosin
terazosin
Uroxatral™ [US]
Xatral® [Can]
Antiandrogen
finasteride
Proscar® [US/Can]
Antineoplastic Agent, Anthracenedione
Avodart™ [US]
dutasteride

BLADDER IRRIGATION
Antibacterial, Topical
acetic acid

BOWEL CLEANSING
Laxative
castor oil
Citro-Mag® [Can]
Colyte® [US/Can]
Emulsoil® [US-OTC]
Fleet® Enema [US/Can]
Fleet® Phospho-Soda® Accu-Prep™ [US-OTC]
Fleet® Phospho®-Soda [US/Can]
GoLYTELY® [US]
Klean-Prep® [Can]
Lyteprep™ [Can]
magnesium citrate
MiraLax™ [US]
Neoloid® [US-OTC]
NuLytely® [US]
PegLyte® [Can]
polyethylene glycol-electrolyte solution
Purge® [US-OTC]
sodium phosphates
Visicol™ [US]

BOWEL STERILIZATION
Aminoglycoside (Antibiotic)
neomycin
Neo-Rx [US]

BRUCELLOSIS
Antibiotic, Aminoglycoside
streptomycin
Antitubercular Agent
streptomycin
Tetracycline Derivative
Adoxa™ [US]
Alti-Minocycline [Can]
Apo®-Doxy [Can]
Apo®-Doxy Tabs [Can]
Apo®-Minocycline [Can]

Appendix 6

Apo®-Tetra [Can]
Brodspec® [US]
Declomycin® [US/Can]
demeclocycline
Doryx® [US]
Doxy-100® [US]
Doxycin [Can]
doxycycline
Dynacin® [US]
EmTet® [US]
Gen-Minocycline [Can]
Minocin® [US/Can]
minocycline
Monodox® [US]
Novo-Doxylin [Can]
Novo-Minocycline [Can]
Novo-Tetra [Can]
Nu-Doxycycline [Can]
Nu-Tetra [Can]
oxytetracycline
ratio-Doxycycline [Can]
ratio-Minocycline [Can]
Rhoxal-minocycline [Can]
Sumycin® [US]
Terramycin® I.M. [US/Can]
tetracycline
Vibramycin® [US]
Vibra-Tabs® [US/Can]
Wesmycin® [US]

CACHEXIA
Progestin
Apo®-Megestrol [Can]
Lin-Megestrol [Can]
Megace® OS
Megace® [US/Can]
megestrol acetate
Nu-Megestrol [Can]

CELIAC DISEASE
Electrolyte Supplement, Oral
Alcalak [US-OTC]
Alka-Mints® [US-OTC]
Amitone® [US-OTC]
Apo®-Cal [Can]
Apo®-Ferrous Gluconate [Can]
Apo®-Ferrous Sulfate [Can]
Calbon® [US]
Calcarb 600 [US-OTC]
Cal Carb-HD® [US-OTC]
Calci-Chew™ [US-OTC]
Calci-Mix™ [US-OTC]
Calcionate® [US-OTC]
Calciquid® [US-OTC]
Cal-Citrate® 250 [US-OTC]
calcium carbonate
calcium citrate
calcium glubionate
calcium lactate
Cal-Gest [US-OTC]
Cal-Lac® [US]
Cal-Mint [US-OTC]
Caltrate® 600 [US/Can]
Chooz® [US-OTC]
Citracal® [US-OTC]
Fe-40® [US-OTC]
Femiron® [US-OTC]
Feosol® Tablet [US-OTC]
Feostat® [US-OTC]
Feratab® [US-OTC]
Fer-Gen-Sol [US-OTC]
Fergon® [US-OTC]
Fer-In-Sol® Drops [US/Can]
Fer-Iron® [US-OTC]
Ferodan™ [Can]
Feronate® [US-OTC]
Ferro-Sequels® [US-OTC]
ferrous fumarate
ferrous gluconate
ferrous sulfate
Florical® [US-OTC]
Hemocyte® [US-OTC]
Ircon® [US-OTC]
Mallamint® [US-OTC]
Mylanta® Children's [US-OTC]
Nephro-Calci® [US-OTC]
Nephro-Fer™ [US-OTC]

Novo-Ferrogluc [Can]
Os-Cal® 500 [US/Can]
Oysco 500 [US-OTC]
Oyst-Cal 500 [US-OTC]
Oystercal® 500 [US]
Palafer® [Can]
Ridactate® [US]
Rolaids® Extra Strength [US-OTC]
Slow FE® [US-OTC]
Titralac™ Extra Strength [US-OTC]
Titralac™ [US-OTC]
Tums® 500 [US-OTC]
Tums® E-X Extra Strength Tablet [US-OTC]
Tums® E-X [US-OTC]
Tums® Smooth Dissolve [US-OTC]
Tums® Ultra [US-OTC]
Tums® [US-OTC]
Vitamin
Fero-Grad 500® [US-OTC]
ferrous sulfate and ascorbic acid
ferrous sulfate, ascorbic acid, and vitamin B-complex
ferrous sulfate, ascorbic acid, vitamin B-complex, and folic acid
Iberet-Folic-500® [US]
Iberet®-Liquid 500 [US-OTC]
Iberet®-Liquid [US-OTC]
Vitelle™ Irospan® [US-OTC]
Vitamin, Fat Soluble
AquaMEPHYTON® [US/Can]
Mephyton® [US/Can]
phytonadione

CHOLELITHIASIS
Gallstone Dissolution Agent
Actigall® [US]
Moctanin® [US/Can]
monoctanoin
ursodiol
Urso® [US/Can]

CHOLESTASIS
Vitamin, Fat Soluble

AquaMEPHYTON® [US/Can]
Mephyton® [US/Can]
phytonadione

CIRRHOSIS
Bile Acid Sequestrant
cholestyramine resin
Novo-Cholamine [Can]
Novo-Cholamine Light [Can]
PMS-Cholestyramine [Can]
Prevalite® [US]
Questran® Light [US/Can]
Questran® Powder [US/Can]
Chelating Agent
Cuprimine® [US/Can]
Depen® [US/Can]
penicillamine
Electrolyte Supplement, Oral
Alcalak [US-OTC]
Alka-Mints® [US-OTC]
Amitone® [US-OTC]
Apo®-Cal [Can]
Calbon® [US]
Calcarb 600 [US-OTC]
Cal Carb-HD® [US-OTC]
Calci-Chew™ [US-OTC]
Calci-Mix™ [US-OTC]
Calcionate® [US-OTC]
Calciquid® [US-OTC]
Cal-Citrate® 250 [US-OTC]
calcium carbonate
calcium citrate
calcium glubionate
calcium lactate
Cal-Gest [US-OTC]
Cal-Lac® [US]
Cal-Mint [US-OTC]
Caltrate® 600 [US/Can]
Chooz® [US-OTC]
Citracal® [US-OTC]
Florical® [US-OTC]
Mallamint® [US-OTC]
Mylanta® Children's [US-OTC]

Nephro-Calci® [US-OTC]
Os-Cal® 500 [US/Can]
Oysco 500 [US-OTC]
Oyst-Cal 500 [US-OTC]
Oystercal® 500 [US]
Ridactate® [US]
Rolaids® Extra Strength [US-OTC]
Titralac™ Extra Strength [US-OTC]
Titralac™ [US-OTC]
Tums® 500 [US-OTC]
Tums® E-X Extra Strength Tablet [US-OTC]
Tums® E-X [US-OTC]
Tums® Smooth Dissolve [US-OTC]
Tums® Ultra [US-OTC]
Tums® [US-OTC]
Immunosuppressant Agent
  Alti-Azathioprine [Can]
  Apo®-Azathioprine [Can]
  azathioprine
  Gen-Azathioprine [Can]
  Imuran® [US/Can]
  ratio-Azathioprine [Can]
Vitamin D Analog
  Calciferol™ [US]
  Drisdol® [US/Can]
  ergocalciferol
  Ostoforte® [Can]
Vitamin, Fat Soluble
  AquaMEPHYTON® [US/Can]
  Aquasol A® [US]
  Mephyton® [US/Can]
  Palmitate-A® [US-OTC]
  phytonadione
  vitamin A

COLITIS
5-Aminosalicylic Acid Derivative
  Alti-Sulfasalazine [Can]
  Asacol® [US/Can]
  Azulfidine® EN-tabs® [US]
  Azulfidine® Tablet [US]
  Canasa™ [US]
  mesalamine
  Mesasal® [Can]
  Novo-ASA [Can]
  Pentasa® [US/Can]
  Quintasa® [Can]
  ratio-Sulfasalazine® [Can]
  Rowasa® [US/Can]
  Salazopyrin® [Can]
  Salazopyrin EN-Tabs® [Can]
  Salofalk® [Can]
  S.A.S.™ [Can]
  sulfasalazine

COLITIS (ULCERATIVE)
Adrenal Corticosteroid
  Emo-Cort® [Can]
  hydrocortisone (rectal)
5-Aminosalicylic Acid Derivative
  Alti-Sulfasalazine [Can]
  Asacol® [US/Can]
  Azulfidine® EN-tabs® [US]
  Azulfidine® Tablet [US]
  balsalazide
  Canasa™ [US]
  Colazal™ [US]
  Dipentum® [US/Can]
  mesalamine
  Mesasal® [Can]
  Novo-ASA [Can]
  olsalazine
  Pentasa® [US/Can]
  Quintasa® [Can]
  ratio-Sulfasalazine® [Can]
  Rowasa® [US/Can]
  Salazopyrin® [Can]
  Salazopyrin EN-Tabs® [Can]
  Salofalk® [Can]
  S.A.S.™ [Can]
  sulfasalazine
Antiinflammatory Agent
  balsalazide
  Colazal™ [US]

COLONIC EVACUATION
Laxative
    Alophen® [US-OTC]
    Apo®-Bisacodyl [Can]
    Bisac-Evac™ [US-OTC]
    bisacodyl
    Correctol® [US-OTC]
    Doxidan® (reformulation) [US-OTC]
    Dulcolax® [US/Can]
    Femilax™ [US-OTC]
    Fleet® Bisacodyl Enema [US-OTC]
    Fleet® Stimulant Laxative [US-OTC]
    Modane Tablets® [US-OTC]
    ratio-Bisacodyl [Can]

CONDYLOMA ACUMINATUM
Antiviral Agent
    interferon alfa-2b and ribavirin combination pack
    Rebetron™ [US/Can]
Biological Response Modulator
    Alferon® N [US/Can]
    interferon alfa-2a
    interferon alfa-2b
    interferon alfa-2b and ribavirin combination pack
    interferon alfa-n3
    Intron® A [US/Can]
    Rebetron™ [US/Can]
    Roferon-A® [US/Can]
Immune Response Modifier
    Aldara™ [US/Can]
    imiquimod
Keratolytic Agent
    Condyline™ [Can]
    Condylox® [US]
    Podocon-25™ [US]
    Podofilm® [Can]
    podofilox
    podophyllum resin
    Wartec® [Can]

CONSTIPATION
Laxative
    Acilac [Can]
    Agoral® Maximum Strength Laxative [US-OTC]
    Alophen® [US-OTC]
    Apo®-Bisacodyl [Can]
    Apo®-Lactulose [Can]
    Arlex® [US]
    Bisac-Evac™ [US-OTC]
    bisacodyl
    calcium polycarbophil
    castor oil
    Cholac® [US]
    Citrucel® [US-OTC]
    Constilac® [US]
    Constulose® [US]
    Correctol® [US-OTC]
    Doxidan® (reformulation) [US-OTC]
    Dulcolax® [US/Can]
    Emulsoil® [US-OTC]
    Enulose® [US]
    Equalactin® [US-OTC]
    Evac-U-Gen [US-OTC]
    Ex-Lax® Maximum Strength [US-OTC]
    Ex-Lax® [US-OTC]
    Femilax™ [US-OTC]
    Fiberall® [US-OTC]
    FiberCon® [US-OTC]
    FiberEase™ [US-OTC]
    Fiber-Lax® [US-OTC]
    FiberNorm™ [US-OTC]
    Fleet® Babylax® [US-OTC]
    Fleet® Bisacodyl Enema [US-OTC]
    Fleet® Enema [US/Can]
    Fleet® Glycerin Suppositories Maximum Strength [US-OTC]
    Fleet® Glycerin Suppositories [US-OTC]

Appendix 6

Fleet® Liquid Glycerin Suppositories [US-OTC]
Fleet® Phospho-Soda® Accu-Prep™ [US-OTC]
Fleet® Phospho®-Soda [US/Can]
Fleet® Stimulant Laxative [US-OTC]
Fletcher's® Castoria® [US-OTC]
Generlac® [US]
Genfiber® [US-OTC]
glycerin
Hydrocil® [US-OTC]
Konsyl-D® [US-OTC]
Konsyl® Easy Mix [US-OTC]
Konsyl® Orange [US-OTC]
Konsyl® Tablets [US-OTC]
Konsyl® [US-OTC]
Kristalose™ [US]
lactulose
Laxilose [Can]
Mag-Gel® 600 [US]
magnesium hydroxide
magnesium hydroxide and mineral oil emulsion
magnesium oxide
magnesium sulfate
Mag-Ox® 400 [US-OTC]
malt soup extract
Maltsupex® [US-OTC]
Metamucil® Smooth Texture [US-OTC]
Metamucil® [US-OTC]
methylcellulose
Modane® Bulk [US-OTC]
Modane Tablets® [US-OTC]
Neoloid® [US-OTC]
Osmoglyn® [US]
Perdiem® Fiber Therapy [US-OTC]
Phillips'® Fibercaps [US-OTC]
Phillips'® Milk of Magnesia [US-OTC]
Phillips' M-O® [US-OTC]
PMS-Lactulose [Can]
psyllium
Purge® [US-OTC]
ratio-Bisacodyl [Can]
ratio-Lactulose [Can]
Reguloid® [US-OTC]
Sani-Supp® [US-OTC]
Senexon® [US-OTC]
senna
Senna-Gen® [US-OTC]
Sennatural™ [US-OTC]
Senokot® Children's [US-OTC]
Senokot® [US-OTC]
SenokotXTRA® [US-OTC]
Serutan® [US-OTC]
sodium phosphates
sorbitol
Uro-Mag® [US-OTC]
Visicol™ [US]
X-Prep® [US-OTC] Agoral® Maximum Strength Laxative [US-OTC]
Laxative, Stimulant
  docusate and senna
  Peri-Colace® (reformulation) [US-OTC]
  Senokot-S® [US-OTC]
Stool Softener
  Colace® [US/Can]
  Colax-C® [Can]
  Diocto® [US-OTC]
  docusate
  docusate and senna
  Docusoft-S™ [US-OTC]
  DOS® Softgel® [US-OTC]
  D-S-S® [US-OTC]
  ex-lax® Stool Softener [US-OTC]
  Fleet® Sof-Lax® [US-OTC]
  Genasoft® [US-OTC]
  Novo-Docusate [Can]
  Peri-Colace® (reformulation) [US-OTC]
  Phillips'® Stool Softener Laxative [US-OTC]
  PMS-Docusate Calcium [Can]

PMS-Docusate Sodium [Can]
ratio-Docusate Calcium [Can]
ratio-Docusate Sodium [Can]
Regulex® [Can]
Selax® [Can]
Senokot-S® [US-OTC]
Soflax™ [Can]
Surfak® [US-OTC]

COPROPORPHYRIA
Beta-Adrenergic Blocker
  Apo®-Propranolol [Can]
  Inderal® LA [US/Can]
  Inderal® [US/Can]
  InnoPran XL™ [US]
  Nu-Propranolol [Can]
  propranolol
  Propranolol Intensol™ [US]

CROHN DISEASE
5-Aminosalicylic Acid Derivative
  Alti-Sulfasalazine [Can]
  Asacol® [US/Can]
  Azulfidine® EN-tabs® [US]
  Azulfidine® Tablet [US]
  Canasa™ [US]
  Dipentum® [US/Can]
  mesalamine
  Mesasal® [Can]
  Novo-ASA [Can]
  olsalazine
  Pentasa® [US/Can]
  Quintasa® [Can]
  ratio-Sulfasalazine® [Can]
  Rowasa® [US/Can]
  Salazopyrin® [Can]
  Salazopyrin En-Tabs® [Can]
  Salofalk® [Can]
  S.A.S.™ [Can]
  sulfasalazine
Monoclonal Antibody
  infliximab
  Remicade® [US]

CRYPTORCHIDISM
Gonadotropin
  chorionic gonadotropin (human)
  Novarel™ [US]
  Pregnyl® [US/Can]
  Profasi® HP [Can]
  Profasi® [US]

CYSTINURIA
Chelating Agent
  Cuprimine® [US/Can]
  Depen® [US/Can]
  penicillamine

CYSTITIS (HEMORRHAGIC)
Antidote
  mesna
  Mesnex™ [US/Can]
  Uromitexan™ [Can]

DIABETIC GASTRIC STASIS
Gastrointestinal Agent, Prokinetic
  Apo®-Metoclop [Can]
  metoclopramide
  Nu-Metoclopramide [Can]
  Reglan® [US]

DIARRHEA
Analgesic, Narcotic
  opium tincture
  paregoric
Anticholinergic Agent
  Donnapectolin-PG® [US]
  hyoscyamine, atropine, scopolamine, kaolin, and pectin
  hyoscyamine, atropine, scopolamine, kaolin, pectin, and opium
  Kapectolin PG® [US]
Antidiarrheal
  Apo®-Loperamide [Can]
  attapulgite
  bismuth

Children's Kaopectate®
(reformulation) [US-OTC]
Colo-Fresh™ [US-OTC]
Devrom® [US]
Diamode® [US-OTC]
Diarr-Eze [Can]
difenoxin and atropine
Diotame® [US-OTC]
diphenoxylate and atropine
Imodium® A-D [US-OTC]
Imodium® [US/Can]
Imogen® [US]
Imotil® [US]
Imperim® [US-OTC]
Kaodene® A-D [US-OTC]
Kaodene® NN [US-OTC]
kaolin and pectin
Kaolinpec® [US-OTC]
Kao-Paverin® [US-OTC]
Kaopectate® Extra Strength [US-OTC]
Kaopectate® [US-OTC]
Kao-Spen® [US-OTC]
Kapectolin® [US-OTC]
K-Pec® II [US-OTC]
Lomocot® [US]
Lomotil® [US/Can]
Lonox® [US]
loperamide
Lopercap [Can]
Motofen® [US]
Novo-Loperamide [Can]
Pepto-Bismol® Maximum Strength [US-OTC]
Pepto-Bismol® [US-OTC]
PMS-Loperamine [Can]
Rhoxal-loperamine [Can]
Riva-Loperamine [Can]
Gastrointestinal Agent, Miscellaneous
Bacid® [US/Can]
calcium polycarbophil
Equalactin® [US-OTC]
Fermalac [Can]

FiberCon® [US-OTC]
Fiber-Lax® [US-OTC]
FiberNorm™ [US-OTC]
Kala® [US-OTC]
Konsyl® Tablets [US-OTC]
Lactinex® [US-OTC]
Lactobacillus
Megadophilus® [US-OTC]
MoreDophilus® [US-OTC]
Phillips'® Fibercaps [US-OTC]
Probiotica® [US-OTC]
Superdophilus® [US-OTC]
Somatostatin Analog
octreotide
Sandostatin LAR® [US/Can]
Sandostatin® [US/Can]

DIARRHEA (BACTERIAL)
Aminoglycoside (Antibiotic)
neomycin
Neo-Rx [US]

DIARRHEA (BILE ACIDS)
Bile Acid Sequestrant
cholestyramine resin
Novo-Cholamine [Can]
Novo-Cholamine Light [Can]
PMS-Cholestyramine [Can]
Prevalite® [US]
Questran® Light [US/Can]
Questran® Powder [US/Can]

DIARRHEA (TRAVELERS)
Antidiarrheal
bismuth
Children's Kaopectate®
(reformulation) [US-OTC]
Colo-Fresh™ [US-OTC]
Devrom® [US]
Diotame® [US-OTC]
Kaopectate® Extra Strength [US-OTC]
Kaopectate® [US-OTC]

Pepto-Bismol® Maximum Strength [US-OTC]
Pepto-Bismol® [US-OTC]

DIVERTICULITIS
Aminoglycoside (Antibiotic)
　AKTob® [US]
　Alcomicin® [Can]
　Apo®-Tobramycin [Can]
　Diogent® [Can]
　Garamycin® [US/Can]
　Gentak® [US]
　gentamicin
　Nebcin® [US/Can]
　PMS-Tobramycin [Can]
　ratio-Gentamicin [Can]
　tobramycin
　Tobrex® [US/Can]
Antibiotic, Miscellaneous
　Alti-Clindamycin [Can]
　Apo®-Clindamycin [Can]
　Apo®-Metronidazole [Can]
　Azactam® [US/Can]
　aztreonam
　Cleocin HCl® [US]
　Cleocin Pediatric® [US]
　Cleocin Phosphate® [US]
　Cleocin T® [US]
　Cleocin® [US]
　Clindagel™ [US]
　Clindamax [US]
　clindamycin
　Clindets® [US]
　Clindoxyl® Gel [Can]
　Dalacin® C [Can]
　Dalacin® T [Can]
　Flagyl ER® [US]
　Flagyl® [US/Can]
　Florazole ER® [Can]
　MetroCream® [US/Can]
　MetroGel® Topical [US/Can]
　MetroGel-Vaginal® [US]
　MetroLotion® [US]
　metronidazole
　Nidagel™ [Can]
　Noritate® [US/Can]
　Novo-Clindamycin [Can]
　Novo-Nidazol [Can]
　ratio-Clindamycin [Can]
　Trikacide® [Can]
Carbapenem (Antibiotic)
　imipenem and cilastatin
　Primaxin® [US/Can]
Cephalosporin (Second Generation)
　Cefotan® [US/Can]
　cefotetan
　cefoxitin
　Mefoxin® [US/Can]Penicillin
　ampicillin
　ampicillin and sulbactam
　Apo®-Ampi [Can]
　Marcillin® [US]
　Novo-Ampicillin [Can]
　Nu-Ampi [Can]
　piperacillin and tazobactam sodium
　Principen® [US]
　Tazocin® [Can]
　ticarcillin and clavulanate potassium
　Timentin® [US/Can]
　Unasyn® [US/Can]
　Zosyn® [US]

DUODENAL ULCER
Antacid
　calcium carbonate and simethicone
　Iosopan® Plus [US]
　Lowsium® Plus [US]
　magaldrate and simethicone
　Mag-Gel® 600 [US]
　magnesium hydroxide
　magnesium oxide
　Mag-Ox® 400 [US-OTC]
　Phillips'® Milk of Magnesia [US-OTC]
　Titralac® Plus Liquid [US-OTC]
　Uro-Mag® [US-OTC]

Antibiotic, Macrolide Combination
  Hp-PAC® [Can]
  lansoprazole, amoxicillin, and
    clarithromycin
  Prevpac™ [US/Can]
Antibiotic, Penicillin
  Hp-PAC® [Can]
  lansoprazole, amoxicillin, and
    clarithromycin
  Prevpac™ [US/Can]
Gastric Acid Secretion Inhibitor
  Aciphex™ [US/Can]
  lansoprazole
  Losec® [Can]
  omeprazole
  Pariet® [Can]
  Prevacid® [US/Can]
  Prilosec OTC™ [US-OTC]
  Prilosec® [US]
  rabeprazole
Gastrointestinal Agent, Gastric or
    Duodenal Ulcer Treatment
  Apo®-Sucralate [Can]
  Carafate® [US]
  Novo-Sucralate [Can]
  Nu-Sucralate [Can]
  PMS-Sucralate [Can]
  sucralfate
  Sulcrate® [Can]
  Sulcrate® Suspension Plus [Can]
Gastrointestinal Agent, Miscellaneous
  Hp-PAC® [Can]
  lansoprazole, amoxicillin, and
    clarithromycin
  Prevpac™ [US/Can]
Histamine H2 Antagonist
  Alti-Ranitidine [Can]
  Apo®-Cimetidine [Can]
  Apo®-Famotidine [Can]
  Apo®-Nizatidine [Can]
  Apo®-Ranitidine [Can]
  Axid® AR [US-OTC]
  Axid® [US/Can]
  cimetidine
  famotidine
  Gen-Cimetidine [Can]
  Gen-Famotidine [Can]
  Gen-Nizatidine [Can]
  Gen-Ranitidine [Can]
  nizatidine
  Novo-Cimetidine [Can]
  Novo-Famotidine [Can]
  Novo-Nizatidine [Can]
  Novo-Ranidine [Can]
  Nu-Cimet® [Can]
  Nu-Famotidine [Can]
  Nu-Nizatidine [Can]
  Nu-Ranit [Can]
  Pepcid® AC [US/Can]
  Pepcid® [US/Can]
  PMS-Cimetidine [Can]
  PMS-Nizatidine [Can]
  ranitidine hydrochloride
  ratio-Famotidine [Can]
  ratio-Ranitidine [Can]
  Rhoxal-famotidine [Can]
  Tagamet® HB 200 [US/Can]
  Tagamet® [US]
  Zantac® 75 [US-OTC]
  Zanta [Can]
  Zantac® [US/Can]

DYSURIA
Analgesic, Urinary
  Azo-Gesic® [US-OTC]
  Azo-Standard® [US]
  Phenazo™ [Can]
  phenazopyridine
  Prodium® [US-OTC]
  Pyridium® [US/Can]
  ReAzo [US-OTC]
  Uristat® [US-OTC]
  UTI Relief® [US-OTC]
Antispasmodic Agent, Urinary
  Apo®-Flavoxate
  flavoxate

Urispas® [US/Can]
Sulfonamide
　sulfisoxazole and phenazopyridine

ENURESIS
Anticholinergic Agent
　belladonna
Antidepressant, Tricyclic (Tertiary Amine)
　Apo®-Imipramine [Can]
　imipramine
　Tofranil-PM® [US]
　Tofranil® [US/Can]
Antispasmodic Agent, Urinary
　Ditropan® [US/Can]
　Ditropan® XL [US]
　Gen-Oxybutynin [Can]
　Novo-Oxybutynin [Can]
　Nu-Oxybutyn [Can]
　oxybutynin
　Oxytrol™ [US]
　PMS-Oxybutynin [Can]
Vasopressin Analog, Synthetic
　Apo®-Desmopressin [Can]
　DDAVP® [US/Can]
　desmopressin acetate
　Minirin® [Can]
　Octostim® [Can]
　Stimate™ [US]

ERECTILE DYSFUNCTION (ED)
Androgen
　Android® [US]
　Methitest® [US]
　methyltestosterone
　Testred® [US]
　Virilon® [US]
Phosphodiesterase (Type 5) Enzyme Inhibitor
　Levitra® [US]
　sildenafil
　vardenafil

Viagra® [US/Can]

EROSIVE ESOPHAGITIS
Proton Pump Inhibitor
　esomeprazole
　Nexium™ [US]

ERYTHROPOIETIC PROTOPORPHYRIA (EPP)
Vitamin, Fat Soluble
　A-Caro-25® [US]
　B-Caro-T™ [US]
　beta-carotene
　Lumitene™ [US]

ESOPHAGEAL VARICES
Hormone, Posterior Pituitary
　Pitressin® [US]
　Pressyn® AR [Can]
　Pressyn® [Can]
　vasopressin
Sclerosing Agent
　Ethamolin® [US]
　ethanolamine oleate
　sodium tetradecyl
　Trombovar® [Can]
　Tromoject® [Can]
Variceal Bleeding (Acute) Agent
　somatostatin (Canada only)
　Stilamin® [Can]

ESOPHAGITIS
Gastric Acid Secretion Inhibitor
　lansoprazole
　Losec® [Can]
　omeprazole
　Prevacid® [US/Can]
　Prilosec OTC™ [US-OTC]
　Prilosec® [US]

FAMILIAL ADENOMATOUS POLYPOSIS
Nonsteroidal Antiinflammatory Drug (NSAID), COX-2 Selective

Celebrex® [US/Can]
celecoxib

GAG REFLEX SUPPRESSION
Analgesic, Topical
  lidocaine
  Xylocaine® Viscous [US]
Local Anesthetic
  Americaine® [US-OTC]
  benzocaine
  benzocaine, butyl aminobenzoate, tetracaine, and benzalkonium chloride
  Benzodent® [US-OTC]
  Cepacol® Maximum Strength [US-OTC]
  dyclonine
  Hurricaine® [US]
  Orabase®-B [US-OTC]
  Orajel® Maximum Strength [US-OTC]
  tetracaine
  Zilactin®-B [US/Can]

GAS PAINS
Antiflatulent
  Alka-Seltzer® Gas Relief [US-OTC]
  aluminum hydroxide, magnesium hydroxide, and simethicone
  Baby Gasz [US-OTC]
  calcium carbonate and simethicone
  Diovol Plus® [Can]
  Flatulex® [US-OTC]
  Gas-X® Extra Strength [US-OTC]
  Gas-X® [US-OTC]
  Genasyme® [US-OTC]
  Iosopan® Plus [US]
  Lowsium® Plus [US]
  Maalox® Anti-Gas (New Formulation) [US-OTC]
  Maalox® Fast Release Liquid [US-OTC]
  Maalox® Max [US-OTC]
  magaldrate and simethicone
  Mylanta® [Can]
  Mylanta™ Double Strength
  Mylanta™ Extra Strength [Can]
  Mylanta® Extra Strength Liquid [US-OTC]
  Mylanta® Gas Maximum Strength [US-OTC]
  Mylanta® Gas [US-OTC]
  Mylanta® Liquid [US-OTC]
  Mylanta™ Regular Strength [Can]
  Mylicon® Infants [US-OTC]
  Mylicon® [US-OTC]
  Ovol® [Can]
  Phazyme® [Can]
  Phazyme® Quick Dissolve [US-OTC]
  Phazyme® Ultra Strength [US-OTC]
  simethicone
  Titralac® Plus Liquid [US-OTC]

GASTRIC ULCER
Antacid
  calcium carbonate and simethicone
  Iosopan® Plus [US]
  Lowsium® Plus [US]
  magaldrate and simethicone
  Mag-Gel® 600 [US]
  magnesium hydroxide
  magnesium oxide
  Mag-Ox® 400 [US-OTC]
  Phillips'® Milk of Magnesia [US-OTC]
  Titralac® Plus Liquid [US-OTC]
  Uro-Mag® [US-OTC]
Histamine H2 Antagonist
  Alti-Ranitidine [Can]
  Apo®-Cimetidine [Can]
  Apo®-Famotidine [Can]
  Apo®-Nizatidine [Can]
  Apo®-Ranitidine [Can]

Axid® AR [US-OTC]
Axid® [US/Can]
cimetidine
famotidine
Gen-Cimetidine [Can]
Gen-Famotidine [Can]
Gen-Nizatidine [Can]
Gen-Ranitidine [Can]
nizatidine
Novo-Cimetidine [Can]
Novo-Famotidine [Can]
Novo-Nizatidine [Can]
Novo-Ranidine [Can]
Nu-Cimet® [Can]
Nu-Famotidine [Can]
Nu-Nizatidine [Can]
Nu-Ranit [Can]
Pepcid® AC [US/Can]
Pepcid® [US/Can]
PMS-Cimetidine [Can]
PMS-Nizatidine [Can]
ranitidine hydrochloride
ratio-Famotidine [Can]
ratio-Ranitidine [Can]
Rhoxal-famotidine [Can]
Tagamet® HB 200 [US/Can]
Tagamet® [US]
Zantac® 75 [US-OTC]
Zanta [Can]
Zantac® [US/Can]
Prostaglandin
Apo®-Misoprostil [Can]
Cytotec® [US/Can]
misoprostol
Novo-Misoprostol [Can]

GASTRITIS
Antacid
aluminum hydroxide and magnesium hydroxide
Diovol® [Can]
Diovol® Ex [Can]
Gelusil® [Can]
Gelusil® Extra Strength [Can]
Maalox® TC (Therapeutic Concentrate) [US-OTC]
Maalox® [US-OTC]
Univol® [Can]
Histamine H2 Antagonist
Alti-Ranitidine [Can]
Apo®-Cimetidine [Can]
Apo®-Ranitidine [Can]
cimetidine
Gen-Cimetidine [Can]
Gen-Ranitidine [Can]
Novo-Cimetidine [Can]
Novo-Ranidine [Can]
Nu-Cimet® [Can]
Nu-Ranit [Can]
PMS-Cimetidine [Can]
ranitidine hydrochloride
ratio-Ranitidine [Can]
Tagamet® HB 200 [US/Can]
Tagamet® [US]
Zantac® 75 [US-OTC]
Zanta [Can]
Zantac® [US/Can]

GASTROESOPHAGEAL REFLUX DISEASE (GERD)
Cholinergic Agent
bethanechol
Duvoid® [Can]
Myotonachol™ [Can]
PMS-Bethanechol [Can]
Urecholine® [US]
Gastric Acid Secretion Inhibitor
Aciphex™ [US/Can]
lansoprazole
Losec® [Can]
omeprazole
Pariet® [Can]
Prevacid® [US/Can]
Prilosec OTC™ [US-OTC]
Prilosec® [US]
rabeprazole

Gastrointestinal Agent, Prokinetic
  Apo®-Metoclop [Can]
  cisapride
  metoclopramide
  Nu-Metoclopramide [Can]
  Propulsid® [US]
  Reglan® [US]
Histamine H2 Antagonist
  Alti-Ranitidine [Can]
  Apo®-Cimetidine [Can]
  Apo®-Famotidine [Can]
  Apo®-Nizatidine [Can]
  Apo®-Ranitidine [Can]
  Axid® AR [US-OTC]
  Axid® [US/Can]
  cimetidine
  famotidine
  Gen-Cimetidine [Can]
  Gen-Famotidine [Can]
  Gen-Nizatidine [Can]
  Gen-Ranitidine [Can]
  nizatidine
  Novo-Cimetidine [Can]
  Novo-Famotidine [Can]
  Novo-Nizatidine [Can]
  Novo-Ranidine [Can]
  Nu-Cimet® [Can]
  Nu-Famotidine [Can]
  Nu-Nizatidine [Can]
  Nu-Ranit [Can]
  Pepcid® AC [US/Can]
  Pepcid® [US/Can]
  MS-Cimetidine [Can]
  PMS-Nizatidine [Can]
  ranitidine hydrochloride
  ratio-Famotidine [Can]
  ratio-Ranitidine [Can]
  Rhoxal-famotidine [Can]
  Tagamet® HB 200 [US/Can]
  Tagamet® [US]
  Zantac® 75 [US-OTC]
  Zanta [Can]
  Zantac® [US/Can]

Proton Pump Inhibitor
  Panto™ IV [Can]
  Pantoloc™ [Can]
  pantoprazole
  Protonix® [US/Can]

GENITAL HERPES
Antiviral Agent
  famciclovir
  Famvir™ [US/Can]
  valacyclovir
  Valtrex® [US/Can]

GENITAL WART
Immune Response Modifier
  Aldara™ [US/Can]
  imiquimod

GIARDIASIS
Amebicide
  Apo®-Metronidazole [Can]
  Flagyl ER® [US]
  Flagyl® [US/Can]
  Florazole ER® [Can]
  Humatin® [US/Can]
  metronidazole
  Noritate® [US/Can]
  Novo-Nidazol [Can]
  paromomycin
  Trikacide® [Can]
Anthelmintic
  albendazole
  Albenza® [US]

GONORRHEA
Antibiotic, Macrolide
  Rovamycine® [Can]
  spiramycin (Canada only)
Antibiotic, Miscellaneous
  spectinomycin
  Trobicin® [US]
Antibiotic, Quinolone
  gatifloxacin
  Tequin® [US/Can]

Zymar™ [US]
Cephalosporin (Second Generation)
  Apo®-Cefuroxime [Can]
  cefoxitin
  Ceftin® [US/Can]
  cefuroxime
  Mefoxin® [US/Can]
  ratio-Cefuroxime [Can]
  Zinacef® [US/Can]
Cephalosporin (Third Generation)
  cefixime
  ceftriaxone
  Rocephin® [US/Can]
  Suprax® [Can]
Quinolone
  Apo®-Oflox [Can]
  ciprofloxacin
  Cipro® [US/Can]
  Cipro® XR [US/Can]
  Floxin® [US/Can]
  ofloxacin
Tetracycline Derivative
  Adoxa™ [US]
  Apo®-Doxy [Can]
  Apo®-Doxy Tabs [Can]
  Apo®-Tetra [Can]
  Brodspec® [US]
  Doryx® [US]
  Doxy-100® [US]
  Doxycin [Can]
  doxycycline
  EmTet® [US]
  Monodox® [US]
  Novo-Doxylin [Can]
  Novo-Tetra [Can]
  Nu-Doxycycline [Can]
  Nu-Tetra [Can]
  ratio-Doxycycline [Can]
  Sumycin® [US]
  tetracycline
  Vibramycin® [US]
  Vibra-Tabs® [US/Can]
  Wesmycin® [US]

GRAM-NEGATIVE INFECTION

Aminoglycoside (Antibiotic)
  AKTob® [US]
  Alcomicin® [Can]
  amikacin
  Amikin® [Can]
  Apo®-Tobramycin [Can]
  Diogent® [Can]
  Garamycin® [US/Can]
  Genoptic® [US]
  Gentacidin® [US]
  Gentak® [US]
  gentamicin
  kanamycin
  Kantrex® [US/Can]
  Nebcin® [US/Can]
  PMS-Tobramycin [Can]
  ratio-Gentamicin [Can]
  TOBI® [US/Can]
  tobramycin
  Tobrex® [US/Can]
Antibiotic, Carbapenem
  ertapenem
  Invanz™ [US/Can]
Antibiotic, Miscellaneous
  Apo®-Nitrofurantoin [Can]
  Azactam® [US/Can]
  aztreonam
  colistimethate
  Coly-Mycin® M [US/Can]
  Furadantin® [US]
  Macrobid® [US/Can]
  Macrodantin® [US/Can]
  nitrofurantoin
  Novo-Furantoin [Can]
Antibiotic, Penicillin
  pivampicillin (Canada only)
  Pondocillin® [Can]
Antibiotic, Quinolone
  gatifloxacin
  Levaquin® [US/Can]

levofloxacin
Quixin™ Ophthalmic [US]
Tequin® [US/Can]
Zymar™ [US]
Carbapenem (Antibiotic)
  imipenem and cilastatin
  meropenem
  Merrem® I.V. [US/Can]
  Primaxin® [US/Can]
Cephalosporin (First Generation)
  Ancef® [US]
  Apo®-Cefadroxil [Can]
  Apo®-Cephalex [Can]
  Biocef® [US]
  cefadroxil
  cefazolin
  cephalexin
  cephalothin
  cephradine
  Ceporacin® [Can]
  Duricef® [US/Can]
  Keflex® [US]
  Keftab® [US/Can]
  Novo-Cefadroxil [Can]
  Novo-Lexin® [Can]
  Nu-Cephalex® [Can]
  Velosef® [US]
Cephalosporin (Second Generation)
  Apo®-Cefaclor [Can]
  Apo®-Cefuroxime [Can]
  Ceclor® CD [US]
  Ceclor® [US/Can]
  cefaclor
  Cefotan® [US/Can]
  cefotetan
  cefoxitin
  cefpodoxime
  cefprozil
  Ceftin® [US/Can]
  cefuroxime
  Cefzil® [US/Can]
  Mefoxin® [US/Can]
  Novo-Cefaclor [Can]
  Nu-Cefaclor [Can]
  PMS-Cefaclor [Can]
  ratio-Cefuroxime [Can]
  Vantin® [US/Can]
  Zinacef® [US/Can]
Cephalosporin (Third Generation)
  Cedax® [US]
  cefixime
  Cefizox® [US/Can]
  cefotaxime
  ceftazidime
  ceftibuten
  ceftizoxime
  ceftriaxone
  Claforan® [US/Can]
  Fortaz® [US/Can]
  Rocephin® [US/Can]
  Suprax® [Can]
  Tazicef® [US]
  Tazidime® [US/Can]
Cephalosporin (Fourth Generation)
  cefepime
  Maxipime® [US/Can]
Genitourinary Irrigant
  neomycin and polymyxin B
  Neosporin® Cream [Can]
  Neosporin® G.U. Irrigant [US/Can]
Macrolide (Antibiotic)
  Apo®-Erythro Base [Can]
  Apo®-Erythro E-C [Can]
  Apo®-Erythro-ES [Can]
  Apo®-Erythro-S [Can]
  azithromycin
  Biaxin® [US/Can]
  Biaxin® XL [US/Can]
  clarithromycin
  Diomycin® [Can]
  dirithromycin
  Dynabac® [US]
  E.E.S.® [US/Can]
  Erybid™ [Can]
  Eryc® [US/Can]
  EryPed® [US]

Ery-Tab® [US]
Erythrocin® [US]
erythromycin and sulfisoxazole
erythromycin (systemic)
Eryzole® [US]
Nu-Erythromycin-S [Can]
PCE® [US/Can]
Pediazole® [US/Can]
PMS-Erythromycin [Can]
Tao® [US]
troleandomycin
Zithromax® [US/Can]
Z-PAK® [US/Can]
Penicillin
  Alti-Amoxi-Clav® [Can]
  amoxicillin
  amoxicillin and clavulanate potassium
  Amoxicot® [US]
  Amoxil® [US]
  ampicillin
  ampicillin and sulbactam
  Apo®-Amoxi [Can]
  Apo®-Amoxi-Clav® [Can]
  Apo®-Ampi [Can]
  Apo®-Pen VK [Can]
  Augmentin ES-600™ [US]
  Augmentin® [US/Can]
  Augmentin XR™ [US]
  Bicillin® C-R 900/300 [US]
  Bicillin® C-R [US]
  Bicillin® L-A [US]
  carbenicillin
  Clavulin® [Can]
  Gen-Amoxicillin [Can]
  Geocillin® [US]
  Lin-Amox [Can]
  Marcillin® [US]
  Moxilin® [US]
  Nadopen-V® [Can]
  Novamoxin® [Can]
  Novo-Ampicillin [Can]
  Novo-Pen-VK® [Can]
  Nu-Amoxi [Can]
  Nu-Ampi [Can]
  Nu-Pen-VK® [Can]
  penicillin G benzathine
  penicillin G benzathine and procaine combined
  penicillin G procaine
  penicillin V potassium
  Permapen® Isoject® [US]
  piperacillin
  piperacillin and tazobactam sodium
  Pipracil® [Can]
  PMS-Amoxicillin [Can]
  Principen® [US]
  PVF® K [Can]
  ratio-AmoxiClav
  Suspen® [US]
  Tazocin® [Can]
  ticarcillin
  ticarcillin and clavulanate potassium
  Ticar® [US]
  Timentin® [US/Can]
  Trimox® [US]
  Truxcillin® [US]
  Unasyn® [US/Can]
  Veetids® [US]
  Wycillin® [US/Can]
  Zosyn® [US]
Quinolone
  Apo®-Norflox [Can]
  Apo®-Oflox [Can]
  Ciloxan® [US/Can]
  Cinobac® [US/Can]
  cinoxacin
  ciprofloxacin
  Cipro® [US/Can]
  Cipro® XR [US/Can]
  Floxin® [US/Can]
  lomefloxacin
  Maxaquin® [US]
  nalidixic acid
  NegGram® [US/Can]
  norfloxacin

Noroxin® [US/Can]
Novo-Norfloxacin [Can]
Ocuflox® [US/Can]
ofloxacin
PMS-Norfloxacin [Can]
Riva-Norfloxacin [Can]
sparfloxacin
Zagam® [US]
Sulfonamide
  Apo®-Sulfatrim [Can]
  Bactrim™ DS [US]
  Bactrim™ [US]
  erythromycin and sulfisoxazole
  Eryzole® [US]
  Gantrisin® Pediatric Suspension [US]
  Novo-Trimel [Can]
  Novo-Trimel D.S. [Can]
  Nu-Cotrimox® [Can]
  Pediazole® [US/Can]
  Septra® DS [US/Can]
  Septra® [US/Can]
  sulfadiazine
  sulfamethoxazole and trimethoprim
  Sulfatrim® DS [US]
  Sulfatrim® [US]
  sulfisoxazole
  sulfisoxazole and phenazopyridine
  Sulfizole® [Can]
  Truxazole® [US]
Tetracycline Derivative
  Adoxa™ [US]
  Alti-Minocycline [Can]
  Apo®-Doxy [Can]
  Apo®-Doxy Tabs [Can]
  Apo®-Minocycline [Can]
  Apo®-Tetra [Can]
  Brodspec® [US]
  Doryx® [US]
  Doxy-100® [US]
  Doxycin [Can]
  doxycycline
  Dynacin® [US]
  EmTet® [US]
  Gen-Minocycline [Can]
  Minocin® [US/Can]
  minocycline
  Monodox® [US]
  Novo-Doxylin [Can]
  Novo-Minocycline [Can]
  Novo-Tetra [Can]
  Nu-Doxycycline [Can]
  Nu-Tetra [Can]
  oxytetracycline
  Periostat® [US]
  ratio-Doxycycline [Can]
  ratio-Minocycline [Can]
  Rhoxal-minocycline [Can]
  Sumycin® [US]
  Terramycin® I.M. [US/Can]
  tetracycline
  Vibramycin® [US]
  Vibra-Tabs® [US/Can]
  Wesmycin® [US]

HEARTBURN

Antacid
  Alcalak [US-OTC]
  Alka-Mints® [US-OTC]
  Amitone® [US-OTC]
  Apo®-Cal [Can]
  Calcarb 600 [US-OTC]
  Cal Carb-HD® [US-OTC]
  Calci-Chew™ [US-OTC]
  Calci-Mix™ [US-OTC]
  calcium carbonate
  calcium carbonate and simethicone
  Cal-Gest [US-OTC]
  Cal-Mint [US-OTC]
  Caltrate® 600 [US/Can]
  Chooz® [US-OTC]
  famotidine, calcium carbonate, and magnesium hydroxide
  Florical® [US-OTC]
  Mallamint® [US-OTC]
  Mylanta® Children's [US-OTC]
  Nephro-Calci® [US-OTC]

Os-Cal® 500 [US/Can]
Oysco 500 [US-OTC]
Oyst-Cal 500 [US-OTC]
Oystercal® 500 [US]
Pepcid® Complete [US-OTC]
Rolaids® Extra Strength [US-OTC]
Titralac™ Extra Strength [US-OTC]
Titralac® Plus Liquid [US-OTC]
Titralac™ [US-OTC]
Tums® 500 [US-OTC]
Tums® E-X Extra Strength Tablet [US-OTC]
Tums® E-X [US-OTC]
Tums® Smooth Dissolve [US-OTC]
Tums® Ultra [US-OTC]
Tums® [US-OTC]
Histamine H2 Antagonist
  Apo®-Cimetidine [Can]
  cimetidine
  famotidine, calcium carbonate, and magnesium hydroxide
  Gen-Cimetidine [Can]
  Novo-Cimetidine [Can]
  Nu-Cimet® [Can]
  Pepcid® Complete [US-OTC]
  PMS-Cimetidine [Can]
  Tagamet® HB 200 [US/Can]
  Tagamet® [US]
Proton Pump Inhibitor
  Panto™ IV [Can]
  Pantoloc™ [Can]
  pantoprazole
  Protonix® [US/Can]

HELICOBACTER PYLORI INFECTION

Antibiotic, Miscellaneous
  Apo®-Metronidazole [Can]
  Flagyl ER® [US]
  Flagyl® [US/Can]
  Florazole ER® [Can]
  metronidazole
  Noritate® [US/Can]
  Novo-Nidazol [Can]
  Trikacide® [Can]
Antidiarrheal
  bismuth
  bismuth subsalicylate, metronidazole, and tetracycline
  Children's Kaopectate® (reformulation) [US-OTC]
  Colo-Fresh™ [US-OTC]
  Devrom® [US]
  Diotame® [US-OTC]
  Helidac™ [US]
  Kaopectate® Extra Strength [US-OTC]
  Kaopectate® [US-OTC]
  Pepto-Bismol® Maximum Strength [US-OTC]
  Pepto-Bismol® [US-OTC]
Macrolide (Antibiotic)
  Biaxin® [US/Can]
  Biaxin® XL [US/Can]
  clarithromycin
Penicillin
  amoxicillin
  Amoxicot® [US]
  Amoxil® [US]
  Apo®-Amoxi [Can]
  Gen-Amoxicillin [Can]
  Lin-Amox [Can]
  Moxilin® [US]
  Novamoxin® [Can]
  Nu-Amoxi [Can]
  PMS-Amoxicillin [Can]
  Trimox® [US]
Tetracycline Derivative
  Apo®-Tetra [Can]
  Brodspec® [US]
  EmTet® [US]
  Novo-Tetra [Can]
  Nu-Tetra [Can]
  Sumycin® [US]
  tetracycline
  Wesmycin® [US]

HEMORRHOID
Adrenal Corticosteroid
  Anusol-HC® Suppository [US]
  Colocort™ [US]
  Cortifoam® [US/Can]
  Emo-Cort® [Can]
  Hycort® [US]
  hydrocortisone (rectal)
  Proctocort™ Rectal [US]
  ProctoCream ® HC Cream [US]
Anesthetic/Corticosteroid
  Analpram-HC® [US]
  Corticaine® [US]
  dibucaine and hydrocortisone
  Enzone® [US]
  Epifoam® [US]
  Pramosone® [US]
  Pramox® HC [Can]
  pramoxine and hydrocortisone
  ProctoFoam®-HC [US/Can]
  Zone-A Forte® [US]
  Zone-A® [US]
Astringent
  Preparation H® Cleansing Pads [Can]
  Tucks® [US-OTC]
  witch hazel
Local Anesthetic
  Americaine® Anesthetic Lubricant [US]
  Americaine® [US-OTC]
  Ametop™ [Can]
  Anusol® [US-OTC]
  benzocaine
  dibucaine
  Fleet® Pain Relief [US-OTC]
  Foille® Medicated First Aid [US-OTC]
  Foille® Plus [US-OTC]
  Foille® [US-OTC]
  Nupercainal® [US-OTC]
  Pontocaine® [US/Can]
  PrameGel® [US-OTC]
  pramoxine
  Prax® [US-OTC]
  ProctoFoam® NS [US-OTC]
  tetracaine
  Tronolane® [US-OTC]
  Tronothane® [US-OTC]

HEPATIC CIRRHOSIS
Diuretic, Potassium Sparing
  amiloride
  Midamor® [US/Can]

HEPATITIS A
Immune Globulin
  BayGam® [US/Can]
  immune globulin (intramuscular)
Vaccine, Inactivated Virus
  Avaxim® [Can]
  Epaxal Berna® [Can]
  Havrix® [US/Can]
  hepatitis A vaccine
  VAQTA® [US/Can]

HEPATITIS B
Antiretroviral Agent, Non-nucleoside Reverse Transcriptase Inhibitor (NNRTI)
  adefovir
  Hepsera™ [US]
Antiviral Agent
  Epivir-HBV® [US]
  Epivir® [US]
  Heptovir® [Can]
  interferon alfa-2b and ribavirin combination pack
  lamivudine
  Rebetron™ [US/Can]
  3TC® [Can]
Biological Response Modulator
  interferon alfa-2b
  interferon alfa-2b and ribavirin combination pack
  Intron® A [US/Can]
  Rebetron™ [US/Can]

Immune Globulin
  BayHep B™ [US/Can]
  hepatitis B immune globulin
  Nabi-HB® [US]
Vaccine, Inactivated Virus
  Comvax® [US]
  Engerix-B® [US/Can]
  Haemophilus B conjugate and hepatitis B vaccine
  hepatitis B vaccine
  Recombivax HB® [US/Can]

HEPATITIS C
Antiviral Agent
  interferon alfa-2b and ribavirin combination pack
  Rebetron™ [US/Can]
Biological Response Modulator
  interferon alfa-2b
  interferon alfa-2b and ribavirin combination pack
  Intron® A [US/Can]
  Rebetron™ [US/Can]
Interferon
  Infergen® [US/Can]
  interferon alfacon-1
  Pegasys® [US]
  peginterferon alfa-2a
  peginterferon alfa-2b
  PEG-Intron™ [US]

HEREDITARY TYROSINEMIA
4-Hydroxyphenylpyruvate Dioxygenase Inhibitor
  nitisinone
  Orfadin® [US]

HERPES SIMPLEX
Antiviral Agent
  acyclovir
  Apo®-Acyclovir [Can]
  Cytovene® [US/Can]
  famciclovir
  Famvir™ [US/Can]
  foscarnet
  Foscavir® [US/Can]
  ganciclovir
  Gen-Acyclovir [Can]
  Nu-Acyclovir [Can]
  trifluridine
  Viroptic® [US/Can]
  Vitrasert® [US/Can]
  Zovirax® [US/Can]
Antiviral Agent, Topical
  Abreva™ [US-OTC]
  docosanol

HERPES ZOSTER
Analgesic, Topical
  Antiphlogistine Rub A-535 Capsaicin [Can]
  ArthriCare® for Women Extra Moisturizing [US-OTC]
  ArthriCare® for Women Silky Dry [US-OTC]
  Capsagel® [US-OTC]
  capsaicin
  Capzasin-HP® [US-OTC]
  TheraPatch® Warm [US-OTC]
  Zostrix®-HP [US/Can]
  Zostrix® [US/Can]
Antiviral Agent
  acyclovir
  Apo®-Acyclovir [Can]
  famciclovir
  Famvir™ [US/Can]
  Gen-Acyclovir [Can]
  Nu-Acyclovir [Can]
  valacyclovir
  Valtrex® [US/Can]
  Zovirax® [US/Can]

HIATAL HERNIA
Antacid
  calcium carbonate and simethicone
  Iosopan® Plus [US]
  Lowsium® Plus [US]

Appendix 6

magaldrate and simethicone
Titralac® Plus Liquid [US-OTC]

HICCUPS
Phenothiazine Derivative
chlorpromazine
Largactil® [Can]
Thorazine® [US]

HOOKWORMS
Anthelmintic
albendazole
Albenza® [US]
Combantrin™ [Can]
mebendazole
Pin-X® [US-OTC]
pyrantel pamoate
Reese's® Pinworm Medicine [US-OTC]
Vermox® [US/Can]

HYPERACIDITY
Antacid
Alcalak [US-OTC]
Alka-Mints® [US-OTC]
ALternaGel® [US-OTC]
Alu-Cap® [US-OTC]
aluminum hydroxide
aluminum hydroxide and magnesium carbonate
aluminum hydroxide and magnesium hydroxide
aluminum hydroxide, magnesium hydroxide, and simethicone
Amitone® [US-OTC]
Amphojel® [Can]
Apo®-Cal [Can]
Basaljel® [Can]
Brioschi® [US-OTC]
Calcarb 600 [US-OTC]
Cal Carb-HD® [US-OTC]
Calci-Chew™ [US-OTC]
Calci-Mix™ [US-OTC]
calcium carbonate

calcium carbonate and magnesium hydroxide
calcium carbonate and simethicone
Cal-Gest [US-OTC]
Cal-Mint [US-OTC]
Caltrate® 600 [US/Can]
Chooz® [US-OTC]
Diovol® [Can]
Diovol® Ex [Can]
Diovol Plus® [Can]
Florical® [US-OTC]
Gaviscon® Extra Strength [US-OTC]
Gaviscon® Liquid [US-OTC]
Gelusil® [Can]
Gelusil® Extra Strength [Can]
Iosopan® Plus [US]
Lowsium® Plus [US]
Maalox® Fast Release Liquid [US-OTC]
Maalox® Max [US-OTC]
Maalox® TC (Therapeutic Concentrate) [US-OTC]
Maalox® [US-OTC]
magaldrate and simethicone
Mag-Gel® 600 [US]
magnesium hydroxide
magnesium oxide
Mag-Ox® 400 [US-OTC]
Mallamint® [US-OTC]
Mylanta® [Can]
Mylanta® Children's [US-OTC]
Mylanta™ Double Strength
Mylanta™ Extra Strength [Can]
Mylanta® Extra Strength Liquid [US-OTC]
Mylanta® Gelcaps® [US-OTC]
Mylanta® Liquid [US-OTC]
Mylanta™ Regular Strength [Can]
Mylanta® Supreme [US-OTC]
Mylanta® Tablets [US-OTC]
Mylanta® Ultra Tablet [US-OTC]
Nephro-Calci® [US-OTC]
Neut® [US]

Os-Cal® 500 [US/Can]
Oysco 500 [US-OTC]
Oyst-Cal 500 [US-OTC]
Oystercal® 500 [US]
Phillips'® Milk of Magnesia [US-OTC]
Rolaids®, Extra Strength [US-OTC]
Rolaids® [US-OTC]
sodium bicarbonate
Titralac™ Extra Strength [US-OTC]
Titralac® Plus Liquid [US-OTC]
Titralac™ [US-OTC]
Tums® 500 [US-OTC]
Tums® E-X Extra Strength Tablet [US-OTC]
Tums® Smooth Dissolve [US-OTC]
Tums® Ultra [US-OTC]
Tums® [US-OTC]
Univol® [Can]
Uro-Mag® [US-OTC]
Electrolyte Supplement, Oral
Calbon® [US]
calcium lactate
Cal-Lac® [US]
Ridactate® [US]

HYPERAMMONEMIA
Ammonium Detoxicant
Acilac [Can]
Apo®-Lactulose [Can]
Cholac® [US]
Constilac® [US]
Constulose® [US]
Enulose® [US]
Generlac® [US]
Kristalose™ [US]
lactulose
Laxilose [Can]
PMS-Lactulose [Can]
ratio-Lactulose [Can]
sodium phenylacetate and sodium benzoate
Ucephan® [US]

HYPERURICEMIA
Enzyme
Elitek™ [US]
rasburicase
Uricosuric Agent
Apo®-Sulfinpyraz [Can]
Benuryl™ [Can]
Nu-Sulfinpyrazone [Can]
probenecid
sulfinpyrazone
Xanthine Oxidase Inhibitor
allopurinol
Aloprim™ [US]
Apo®-Allopurinol [Can]
Zyloprim® [US/Can]

HYPOGONADISM
Androgen
Andriol® [Can]
Androderm® [US]
AndroGel® [US/Can]
Android® [US]
Delatestryl® [US/Can]
Depo®-Testosterone [US]
Methitest® [US]
methyltestosterone
Striant™ [US]
Testim™ [US]
Testoderm® [US]
Testoderm® with Adhesive [US]
Testopel® [US]
testosterone
Testred® [US]
Virilon® [US]
Diagnostic Agent
Factrel® [US]
gonadorelin
Lutrepulse™ [Can]
Estrogen Derivative
Alora® [US]
Cenestin™ [US/Can]
Climara® [US/Can]
Congest [Can]

Appendix 6

Delestrogen® [US/Can]
Depo®-Estradiol [US/Can]
diethylstilbestrol
Esclim® [US]
Estinyl® [US]
Estrace® [US/Can]
Estraderm® [US/Can]
estradiol
Estring® [US/Can]
Estrogel® [Can]
estrogens (conjugated A/synthetic)
estrogens (conjugated/equine)
estrogens (esterified)
estrone
estropipate
ethinyl estradiol
Femring™ [US]
Gynodiol® [US]
Honvol® [Can]
Kestrone® [US/Can]
Menest® [US]
Oesclim® [Can]
Oestrilin [Can]
Ogen® [US/Can]
Ortho-Est® [US]
Premarin® [US/Can]
Vagifem® [US/Can]
Vivelle-Dot® [US]
Vivelle® [US/Can]

HYPOKALEMIA
Diuretic, Potassium Sparing
  Aldactone® [US/Can]
  amiloride
  Dyrenium® [US]
  Midamor® [US/Can]
  Novo-Spiroton [Can]
  spironolactone
  triamterene
Electrolyte Supplement, Oral
  Apo®-K [Can]
  Effer-K™ [US]
  Glu-K® [US-OTC]

K+ 10® [US]
Kaon-Cl-10® [US]
Kaon-Cl® [US]
Kaon® [US]
Kay Ciel® [US]
K+ Care® ET [US]
K+ Care® [US]
K-Dur® 10 [US/Can]
K-Dur® 20 [US/Can]
Klor-Con® 8 [US]
Klor-Con® 10 [US]
Klor-Con®/25 [US]
Klor-Con®/EF [US]
Klor-Con® [US]
K-Lor™ [US/Can]
Klotrix® [US]
K-Lyte/Cl® [US/Can]
K-Lyte® DS [US]
K-Lyte® [US/Can]
K-Phos® MF [US]
K-Phos® Neutral [US]
K-Phos® No. 2 [US]
K-Tab® [US]
Micro-K® 10 Extencaps® [US]
Micro-K® Extencaps [US/Can]
Neutra-Phos®-K [US]
Neutra-Phos® Powder [US]
potassium acetate
potassium acetate, potassium bicarbonate, and potassium citrate
potassium bicarbonate
potassium bicarbonate and potassium chloride, effervescent
potassium bicarbonate and potassium citrate, effervescent
potassium chloride
potassium gluconate
potassium phosphate
potassium phosphate and sodium phosphate
Roychlor® [Can]
Rum-K® [US]
Slow-K® [Can]

Tri-K® [US]
Uro-KP-Neutral® [US]

IMPOTENCY
Androgen
    Android® [US]
    Methitest® [US]
    methyltestosterone
    Testred® [US]
    Virilon® [US]
Phosphodiesterase (Type 5) Enzyme Inhibitor
    Levitra® [US]
    sildenafil
    vardenafil
    Viagra® [US/Can]
Vasodilator
    ethaverine
    Ethavex-100® [US]

INFERTILITY
Antigonadotropic Agent
    ganirelix
    Orgalutran® [Can]
Ovulation Stimulator
    Follistim® [US]
    follitropin alfa
    follitropin beta
    Gonal-F® [US]

INFERTILITY (FEMALE)
Ergot Alkaloid and Derivative
    Apo® Bromocriptine [Can]
    bromocriptine
    Parlodel® [US/Can]
    PMS-Bromocriptine [Can]
Gonadotropin
    chorionic gonadotropin (human)
    menotropins
    Novarel™ [US]
    Pergonal® [US/Can]
    Pregnyl® [US/Can]
    Profasi® HP [Can]
    Profasi® [US]
    Repronex® [US/Can]
Ovulation Stimulator
    Clomid® [US/Can]
    clomiphene
    Serophene® [US/Can]
Progestin
    Crinone® [US/Can]
    Prochieve™ [US]
    Progestasert® [US]
    progesterone
    Prometrium® [US/Can]

INFERTILITY (MALE)
Gonadotropin
    chorionic gonadotropin (human)
    menotropins
    Novarel™ [US]
    Pergonal® [US/Can]
    Pregnyl® [US/Can]
    Profasi® HP [Can]
    Profasi® [US]
    Repronex® [US/Can]

INFLAMMATORY BOWEL DISEASE
5-Aminosalicylic Acid Derivative
    Alti-Sulfasalazine [Can]
    Asacol® [US/Can]
    Azulfidine® EN-tabs® [US]
    Azulfidine® Tablet [US]
    Canasa™ [US]
    Dipentum® [US/Can]
    mesalamine
    Mesasal® [Can]
    Novo-ASA [Can]
    olsalazine
    Pentasa® [US/Can]
    Quintasa® [Can]
    ratio-Sulfasalazine® [Can]
    Rowasa® [US/Can]
    Salazopyrin® [Can]
    Salazopyrin EN-Tabs® [Can]
    Salofalk® [Can]

S.A.S.™ [Can]
sulfasalazine

INTERSTITIAL CYSTITIS
Analgesic, Urinary
  Elmiron® [US/Can]
  pentosan polysulfate sodium
Urinary Tract Product
  dimethyl sulfoxide
  Kemsol® [Can]
  Rimso®-50 [US/Can]

INTESTINAL ABSORPTION (DIAGNOSTIC)
Diagnostic Agent
  d-xylose
  Xylo-Pfan® [US-OTC]

IRRITABLE BOWEL SYNDROME (IBS)
Anticholinergic Agent
  Antispas® Tablet [US]
  Apo®-Chlorax [Can]
  atropine
  belladonna
  Bentylol® [Can]
  Bentyl® [US]
  clidinium and chlordiazepoxide
  Dicyclocot® [US]
  dicyclomine
  Donnatal Extentabs® [US]
  Donnatal® [US/Can]
  Formulex® [Can]
  Haponal® [US]
  Hyonatol® [US]
  hyoscyamine, atropine, scopolamine, and phenobarbital
  Hypersed® [US]
  Librax® [US/Can]
  Lomine [Can]
  Propanthel™ [Can]
  propantheline

Antispasmodic Agent, Gastrointestinal
  Apo®-Trimebutine [Can]
  Modulon® [Can]
  trimebutine (Canada only)
Calcium Antagonist
  Dicetel® [Can]
  pinaverium (Canada only)
Gastrointestinal Agent, Miscellaneous
  Dicetel® [Can]
  pinaverium (Canada only)
5-HT-3 Receptor Antagonist
  alosetron
  Lotronex® [US]
Laxative
  Fiberall® [US-OTC]
  Genfiber® [US-OTC]
  Hydrocil® [US-OTC]
  Konsyl-D® [US-OTC]
  Konsyl® Easy Mix [US-OTC]
  Konsyl® Orange [US-OTC]
  Konsyl® [US-OTC]
  Metamucil® Smooth Texture [US-OTC]
  Metamucil® [US-OTC]
  Modane® Bulk [US-OTC]
  Perdiem® Fiber Therapy [US-OTC]
  psyllium
  Reguloid® [US-OTC]
  Serutan® [US-OTC]
Serotonin 5-HT-4 Receptor Agonist
  tegaserod
  Zelnorm™ [US/Can]

KIDNEY STONE
Alkalinizing Agent
  citric acid, sodium citrate, and potassium citrate
  Cytra-3 [US]
  K-Citra® [Can]
  Polycitra®-LC [US]
  Polycitra® [US]
  potassium citrate
  Urocit®-K [US]

Chelating Agent
  Cuprimine® [US/Can]
  Depen® [US/Can]
  penicillamine
Electrolyte Supplement, Oral
  K-Phos® MF [US]
  K-Phos® Neutral [US]
  K-Phos® No. 2 [US]
  Neutra-Phos®-K [US]
  Neutra-Phos® Powder [US]
  potassium phosphate
  potassium phosphate and sodium phosphate
  Uro-KP-Neutral® [US]
Irrigating Solution
  citric acid bladder mixture
  Renacidin® [US]
Urinary Tract Product
  Calcibind® [US/Can]
  cellulose sodium phosphate
  Thiola™ [US/Can]
  tiopronin
Xanthine Oxidase Inhibitor
  allopurinol
  Aloprim™ [US]
  Apo®-Allopurinol [Can]
  Zyloprim® [US/Can]

LACTOSE INTOLERANCE
Nutritional Supplement
  Dairyaid® [Can]
  Lactaid® Extra Strength [US-OTC]
  Lactaid® Ultra [US-OTC]
  Lactaid® [US-OTC]
  lactase
  Lactrase® [US-OTC]

MALABSORPTION
Trace Element
  Iodopen® [US]
  Molypen® [US]
  M.T.E.-4® [US]
  M.T.E.-5® [US]
  M.T.E.-6® [US]
  M.T.E.-7® [US]
  Multitrace™-4 Neonatal [US]
  Multitrace™-4 Pediatric [US]
  Multitrace™-4 [US]
  Multitrace™-5 [US]
  Neotrace-4® [US]
  Pedtrace-4® [US]
  P.T.E.-4® [US]
  P.T.E.-5® [US]
  Selepen® [US]
  trace metals
Vitamin, Fat Soluble
  Aquasol A® [US]
  Palmitate-A® [US-OTC]
  vitamin A

MALNUTRITION
Electrolyte Supplement, Oral
  Orazinc® [US-OTC]
  Rivasol [Can]
  Zincate® [US]
  zinc sulfate
Nutritional Supplement
  cysteine
  glucose polymers
  Moducal® [US-OTC]
  Polycose® [US-OTC]
Trace Element
  Iodopen® [US]
  Molypen® [US]
  M.T.E.-4® [US]
  M.T.E.-5® [US]
  M.T.E.-6® [US]
  M.T.E.-7® [US]
  Multitrace™-4 Neonatal [US]
  Multitrace™-4 Pediatric [US]
  Multitrace™-4 [US]
  Multitrace™-5 [US]
  Neotrace-4® [US]
  Pedtrace-4® [US]
  P.T.E.-4® [US]
  P.T.E.-5® [US]
  Selepen® [US]
  trace metals

zinc chloride
Vitamin
- ADEKs [US-OTC]
- Advanced NatalCare® [US]
- Anemagen™ OB [US]
- Centrum® Kids Rugrats™ Complete [US-OTC]
- Centrum® Kids Rugrats™ Extra Calcium [US-OTC]
- Centrum® Kids Rugrats™ Extra C [US-OTC]
- Centrum® Performance™ [US-OTC]
- Centrum® Silver® [US-OTC]
- Centrum® [US-OTC]
- Chromagen® OB [US]
- Citracal® Prenatal Rx [US]
- Duet® [US]
- Flintstones® Complete [US-OTC]
- Flintstones® Original [US-OTC]
- Flintstones® Plus Calcium [US-OTC]
- Flintstones® Plus Extra C [US-OTC]
- Flintstones® Plus Iron [US-OTC]
- Folgard® [US-OTC]
- folic acid, cyanocobalamin, and pyridoxine
- Foltx® [US]
- Geritol® Tonic [US-OTC]
- Iberet®-500 [US-OTC]
- Iberet-Folic-500® [US]
- Iberet® [US-OTC]
- Infuvite® Adult [US]
- Infuvite® Pediatric [US]
- M.V.I.®-12 [US]
- M.V.I® Pediatric [US]
- My First Flintstones® [US-OTC]
- NataChew™ [US]
- NataFort® [US]
- NatalCare® GlossTabs™ [US]
- NatalCare® PIC Forte [US]
- NatalCare® PIC [US]
- NatalCare® Plus [US]
- NatalCare® Rx [US]
- NatalCare™ Three [US]
- NataTab™ CFe [US]
- NataTab™ FA [US]
- NataTab™ Rx [US]
- Nestabs® CBF [US]
- Nestabs® FA [US]
- Nestabs® RX [US]
- Niferex®-PN Forte [US]
- Niferex®-PN [US]
- Obegyn™ [US]
- One-A-Day® 50 Plus Formula [US-OTC]
- One-A-Day® Active Formula [US-OTC]
- One-A -Day® Essential Formula [US-OTC]
- One-A-Day® Kids Bugs Bunny and Friends Complete [US-OTC]
- One-A-Day® Kids Bugs Bunny and Friends Plus Extra C [US-OTC]
- One-A-Day® Kids Extreme Sports [US-OTC]
- One-A-Day® Kids Scooby-Doo! Complete [US-OTC]
- One-A-Day® Kids Scooby Doo! Plus Calcium [US-OTC]
- One-A-Day® Maximum Formula [US-OTC]
- One-A-Day® Men's Formula [US-OTC]
- One-A-Day® Today [US-OTC]
- One-A-Day® Women's Formula [US-OTC]
- Poly-Vi-Flor® [US]
- Poly-Vi-Flor® With Iron [US]
- Poly-Vi-Sol® [US-OTC]
- Poly-Vi-Sol® with Iron [US-OTC]
- Pramilet® FA [US]
- Prenatal MR 90 Fe™ [US]
- Prenatal MTR with Selenium [US]
- Prenatal Plus [US]
- Prenatal Rx 1 [US]
- Prenatal Z [US]

Prenate GT™ [US]
Soluvite-F [US]
StrongStart™ [US]
Stuartnatal® Plus 3™ [US-OTC]
Stuart Prenatal® [US-OTC]
Theragran® Heart Right™ [US-OTC]
Theragran-M® Advanced Formula [US-OTC]
Tri-Vi-Flor® [US]
Tri-Vi-Flor® with Iron [US]
Tri-Vi-Sol® [US-OTC]
Tri-Vi-Sol® with Iron [US-OTC]
Ultra NatalCare® [US]
Vicon Forte® [US]
Vicon Plus® [US-OTC]
Vi-Daylin® ADC + Iron [US-OTC]
Vi-Daylin® ADC [US-OTC]
Vi-Daylin® Drops [US-OTC]
Vi-Daylin®/F ADC + Iron [US]
Vi-Daylin®/F ADC [US]
Vi-Daylin®/F + Iron [US]
Vi-Daylin®/F [US]
Vi-Daylin® + Iron Drops [US-OTC]
Vitaball® [US-OTC]
Vitacon Forte [US]
vitamin (multiple/injectable)
vitamin (multiple/oral)
vitamin (multiple/pediatric)
vitamin (multiple/prenatal)
Vitamin, Fat Soluble
  Amino-Opti-E® [US-OTC]
  Aquasol A® [US]
  Aquasol E® [US-OTC]
  E-Complex-600® [US-OTC]
  E-Vitamin® [US-OTC]
  Palmitate-A® [US-OTC]
  vitamin A
  vitamin E
  Vita-Plus® E Softgels® [US-OTC]
  Vitec® [US-OTC]
  Vite E® Creme [US-OTC]
Vitamin, Water Soluble
  Aminoxin® [US-OTC]
  Apatate® [US-OTC]
  Betaxin® [Can]
  Gevrabon® [US-OTC]
  Mega B® [US-OTC]
  Orexin® [US-OTC]
  Penta/3B® [Can]
  pyridoxine
  Thiamilate® [US]
  thiamine
  Vita 3B [Can]
  vitamin B complex

MAPLE SYRUP URINE DISEASE
Vitamin, Water Soluble
  Betaxin® [Can]
  Thiamilate® [US]
  thiamine

MASTOCYTOSIS
Histamine H2 Antagonist
  Alti-Ranitidine [Can]
  Apo®-Cimetidine [Can]
  Apo®-Famotidine [Can]
  Apo®-Ranitidine [Can]
  cimetidine
  famotidine
  Gen-Cimetidine [Can]
  Gen-Famotidine [Can]
  Gen-Ranitidine [Can]
  Novo-Cimetidine [Can]
  Novo-Famotidine [Can]
  Novo-Ranidine [Can]
  Nu-Cimet® [Can]
  Nu-Famotidine [Can]
  Nu-Ranit [Can]
  Pepcid® AC [US/Can]
  Pepcid® [US/Can]
  PMS-Cimetidine [Can]
  ranitidine hydrochloride
  ratio-Famotidine [Can]
  ratio-Ranitidine [Can]

Rhoxal-famotidine [Can]
Tagamet® HB 200 [US/Can]
Tagamet® [US]
Zantac® 75 [US-OTC]
Zanta [Can]
Zantac® [US/Can]
Mast Cell Stabilizer
   Apo®-Cromolyn [Can]
   Crolom® [US]
   cromolyn sodium
   Gastrocrom® [US]
   Intal® [US/Can]
   Nalcrom® [Can]
   Nasalcrom® [US-OTC]
   Nu-Cromolyn [Can]
   Opticrom® [US/Can]

MECONIUM ILEUS
Mucolytic Agent
   acetylcysteine
   Acys-5® [US]
   Mucomyst® [US/Can]
   Parvolex® [Can]

NAUSEA
Anticholinergic Agent
   Scopace™ [US]
   scopolamine
Antiemetic
   Aloxi™ [US]
   aprepitant
   Benzacot® [US]
   dronabinol
   droperidol
   Emend® [US]
   Emetrol® [US-OTC]
   Especol® [US-OTC]
   Formula EM [US-OTC]
   fructose, dextrose, and phosphoric acid
   Inapsine® [US]
   Kalmz [US-OTC]
   Marinol® [US/Can]
   Nausea Relief [US-OTC]
   Nausetrol® [US-OTC]
   palonosetron
   Tigan® [US/Can]
   trimethobenzamide
Antihistamine
   Apo®-Dimenhydrinate [Can]
   dimenhydrinate
   Dramamine® Oral [US-OTC]
   Gravol® [Can]
   Novo-Dimenate [Can]
   TripTone® Caplets® [US-OTC]
Gastrointestinal Agent, Prokinetic
   Apo®-Metoclop [Can]
   metoclopramide
   Nu-Metoclopramide [Can]
   Reglan® [US]
Phenothiazine Derivative
   Anergan® [US]
   Apo®-Perphenazine [Can]
   chlorpromazine
   Compazine® [US/Can]
   Compro™ [US]
   Largactil® [Can]
   Nu-Prochlor [Can]
   perphenazine
   Phenergan® [US/Can]
   prochlorperazine
   promethazine
   Stemetil® [Can]
   Thorazine® [US]
Selective 5-HT-3 Receptor Antagonist
   Aloxi™ [US]
   granisetron
   Kytril™ [US/Can]
   ondansetron
   palonosetron
   Zofran® ODT [US/Can]
   Zofran® [US/Can]

NEPHROLITHIASIS
Alkalinizing Agent
   K-Citra® [Can]
   potassium citrate

Urocit®-K [US]

NEPHROPATHIC CYSTINOSIS
Urinary Tract Product
   Cystagon® [US]
   cysteamine

NEPHROTIC SYNDROME
Adrenal Corticosteroid
   Acthar® [US]
   A-HydroCort® [US]
   A-methapred® [US]
   Apo®-Prednisone [Can]
   Aristocort® Forte Injection [US]
   Aristocort® Intralesional Injection [US]
   Aristocort® Tablet [US/Can]
   Aristospan® Intraarticular Injection [US/Can]
   Aristospan® Intralesional Injection [US/Can]
   Betaject™ [Can]
   betamethasone (systemic)
   Betnesol® [Can]
   Celestone® Phosphate [US]
   Celestone® Soluspan® [US/Can]
   Celestone® [US]
   Cel-U-Jec® [US]
   Cortef® Tablet [US/Can]
   corticotropin
   cortisone acetate
   Cortone® [Can]
   Decadron®-LA [US]
   Decadron® [US/Can]
   Decaject-LA® [US]
   Decaject® [US]
   Deltasone® [US]
   Depo-Medrol® [US/Can]
   Depopred® [US]
   dexamethasone (systemic)
   Dexasone® L.A. [US]
   Dexasone® [US/Can]
   Dexone® LA [US]
   Dexone® [US]
   Hexadrol® [US/Can]
   H.P. Acthar® Gel [US]
   hydrocortisone (systemic)
   Kenalog® Injection [US/Can]
   Medrol® Dosepak™ [US/Can]
   Medrol® Tablet [US/Can]
   methylprednisolone
   Orapred™ [US]
   Pediapred® [US/Can]
   PMS-Dexamethasone [Can]
   Prednicot® [US]
   prednisolone (systemic)
   Prednisol® TBA [US]
   prednisone
   Prednisone Intensol™ [US]
   Prelone® [US]
   ratio-Dexamethasone [Can]
   Solu-Cortef® [US/Can]
   Solu-Medrol® [US/Can]
   Solurex L.A.® [US]
   Sterapred® DS [US]
   Sterapred® [US]
   Tac™-3 Injection [US]
   Triam-A® Injection [US]
   triamcinolone (systemic)
   Triam Forte® Injection [US]
   Winpred™ [Can]
Antihypertensive Agent, Combination
   Aldactazide® [US/Can]
   Apo®-Triazide [Can]
   Dyazide® [US]
   hydrochlorothiazide and spironolactone
   hydrochlorothiazide and triamterene
   Maxzide®-25 [US]
   Maxzide® [US]
   Novo-Spirozine [Can]
   Novo-Triamzide [Can]
   Nu-Triazide [Can]
Antineoplastic Agent
   chlorambucil
   cyclophosphamide
   Cytoxan® [US/Can]

Appendix 6

    Leukeran® [US/Can]
    Neosar® [US]
    Procytox® [Can]
  Diuretic, Loop
    Apo®-Furosemide [Can]
    bumetanide
    Bumex® [US/Can]
    Burinex® [Can]
    Demadex® [US]
    Furocot® [US]
    furosemide
    Lasix® Special [Can]
    Lasix® [US/Can]
    torsemide
  Diuretic, Miscellaneous
    Apo®-Chlorthalidone [Can]
    Apo®-Indapamide [Can]
    chlorthalidone
    Gen-Indapamide [Can]
    indapamide
    Lozide® [Can]
    Lozol® [US/Can]
    metolazone
    Mykrox® [US/Can]
    Novo-Indapamide [Can]
    Nu-Indapamide [Can]
    PMS-Indapamide [Can]
    Thalitone® [US]
    Zaroxolyn® [US/Can]
  Diuretic, Thiazide
    Apo®-Hydro [Can]
    Aquacot® [US]
    Aquatensen® [US/Can]
    Aquazide® H [US]
    bendroflumethiazide
    chlorothiazide
    Diuril® [US/Can]
    Enduron® [US/Can]
    hydrochlorothiazide
    HydroDIURIL® [Can]
    Metatensin® [Can]
    methyclothiazide
    Microzide™ [US]
    Naqua® [US/Can]
    Naturetin® [US]
    Oretic® [US]
    Trichlorex® [Can]
    trichlormethiazide
    Zide® [US]
  Immunosuppressant Agent
    Alti-Azathioprine [Can]
    Apo®-Azathioprine [Can]
    Apo®-Cyclosporine [Can]
    azathioprine
    cyclosporine
    Gen-Azathioprine [Can]
    Gengraf™ [US]
    Imuran® [US/Can]
    Neoral® [US/Can]
    ratio-Azathioprine [Can]
    Restasis™ [US]
    Rhoxal-cyclosporine [Can]
    Sandimmune® [US/Can]

NEPHROTOXICITY (CISPLATIN-INDUCED)
Antidote
  amifostine
  Ethyol® [US/Can]

NEUROGENIC BLADDER
Antispasmodic Agent, Urinary
  Ditropan® [US/Can]
  Ditropan® XL [US]
  Gen-Oxybutynin [Can]
  Novo-Oxybutynin [Can]
  Nu-Oxybutyn [Can]
  oxybutynin
  Oxytrol™ [US]
  PMS-Oxybutynin [Can]

NOCTURIA
Antispasmodic Agent, Urinary
  Apo®-Flavoxate
  flavoxate
  Urispas® [US/Can]

ORAL LESION
Local Anesthetic
    benzocaine, gelatin, pectin, and sodium carboxymethylcellulose
    Orabase® With Benzocaine [US-OTC]

ORGAN REJECTION
Immunosuppressant Agent
    daclizumab
    Zenapax® [US/Can]

ORGAN TRANSPLANT
Immunosuppressant Agent
    Apo®-Cyclosporine [Can]
    basiliximab
    CellCept® [US/Can]
    cyclosporine
    Gengraf™ [US]
    muromonab-CD3
    mycophenolate
    Neoral® [US/Can]
    Orthoclone OKT® 3 [US/Can]
    Prograf® [US/Can]
    Protopic® [US]
    Rapamune® [US/Can]
    Restasis™ [US]
    Rhoxal-cyclosporine [Can]
    Sandimmune® [US/Can]
    Simulect® [US/Can]
    sirolimus
    tacrolimus

OSTOMY CARE
Protectant, Topical
    A and D® Ointment [US-OTC]
    Baza® Clear [US-OTC]
    Clocream® [US-OTC]
    vitamin A and vitamin D

OVERACTIVE BLADDER
Anticholinergic Agent
    Detrol® LA [US]
    Detrol® [US/Can]
    tolterodine
    Unidet® [Can]

PAIN (ANOGENITAL)
Anesthetic/Corticosteroid
    Analpram-HC® [US]
    Enzone® [US]
    Epifoam® [US]
    Pramosone® [US]
    Pramox® HC [Can]
    pramoxine and hydrocortisone
    ProctoFoam®-HC [US/Can]
    Zone-A Forte® [US]
    Zone-A® [US]
Local Anesthetic
    benzocaine
    dibucaine
    dyclonine
    Fleet® Pain Relief [US-OTC]
    Foille® [US-OTC]
    Hurricaine® [US]
    Mycinettes® [US-OTC]
    Nupercainal® [US-OTC]
    Pontocaine® [US/Can]
    pramoxine
    Prax® [US-OTC]
    ProctoFoam® NS [US-OTC]
    tetracaine
    Trocaine® [US-OTC]
    Tronolane® [US-OTC]
    Tronothane® [US-OTC]

PANCREATIC EXOCRINE INSUFFICIENCY
Enzyme
    Cotazym® [Can]
    Creon® 5 [US/Can]
    Creon® 10 [US/Can]
    Creon® 20 [US/Can]
    Creon® 25 [Can]
    Ku-Zyme® HP [US]
    Lipram 4500 [US]
    Lipram-CR [US]

Lipram-PN [US]
Lipram-UL [US]
Pancrease® MT 4 [US/Can]
Pancrease® MT 10 [US/Can]
Pancrease® MT 16 [US/Can]
Pancrease® MT 20 [US/Can]
Pancrease® [US]
Pancrecarb MS-4® [US]
Pancrecarb MS-8® [US]
pancrelipase
Pangestyme™ CN
Pangestyme™ EC
Pangestyme™ MT
Pangestyme™ UL
Ultrase® MT12 [US/Can]
Ultrase® MT18 [US/Can]
Ultrase® MT20 [US/Can]
Ultrase® [US/Can]
Viokase® [US/Can]

PANCREATIC EXOCRINE INSUFFICIENCY (DIAGNOSTIC)
Diagnostic Agent
  SecreFlo™ [US]
  secretin

PANCREATITIS
Anticholinergic Agent
  Propanthel™ [Can]
  propantheline

PARALYTIC ILEUS (PROPHYLAXIS)
Gastrointestinal Agent, Stimulant
  dexpanthenol
  Panthoderm® [US-OTC]

PEPTIC ULCER
Antibiotic, Miscellaneous
  Apo®-Metronidazole [Can]
  Flagyl ER® [US]
  Flagyl® [US/Can]
  Florazole ER® [Can]
  metronidazole
  Noritate® [US/Can]
  Novo-Nidazol [Can]
  Trikacide® [Can]
Anticholinergic Agent
  Anaspaz® [US]
  Antispas® Tablet [US]
  Apo®-Chlorax [Can]
  atropine
  belladonna
  Cantil® [US/Can]
  clidinium and chlordiazepoxide
  Cystospaz-M® [US]
  Cystospaz® [US/Can]
  Donnatal Extentabs® [US]
  Donnatal® [US/Can]
  glycopyrrolate
  Haponal® [US]
  Hyonatol® [US]
  hyoscyamine
  hyoscyamine, atropine, scopolamine, and phenobarbital
  Hyosine [US]
  Hypersed® [US]
  Levbid® [US]
  Levsinex® [US]
  Levsin/SL® [US]
  Levsin® [US/Can]
  Librax® [US/Can]
  mepenzolate
  methscopolamine
  NuLev™ [US]
  Pamine® Forte [US]
  Pamine® [US/Can]
  Propanthel™ [Can]
  propantheline
  Robinul® Forte [US]
  Robinul® [US]
  Spacol T/S [US]
  Spacol [US]
  Symax SL [US]

Symax SR [US]
Antidiarrheal
  bismuth
  bismuth subsalicylate, metronidazole, and tetracycline
  Children's Kaopectate® (reformulation) [US-OTC]
  Colo-Fresh™ [US-OTC]
  Devrom® [US]
  Diotame® [US-OTC]
  Helidac™ [US]
  Kaopectate® Extra Strength [US-OTC]
  Kaopectate® [US-OTC]
  Pepto-Bismol® Maximum Strength [US-OTC]
  Pepto-Bismol® [US-OTC]
Gastric Acid Secretion Inhibitor
  lansoprazole
  Losec® [Can]
  omeprazole
  Prevacid® [US/Can]
  Prilosec OTC™ [US-OTC]
  Prilosec® [US]
Gastrointestinal Agent, Gastric or Duodenal Ulcer Treatment
  Apo®-Sucralate [Can]
  Carafate® [US]
  Novo-Sucralate [Can]
  Nu-Sucralate [Can]
  PMS-Sucralate [Can]
  sucralfate
  Sulcrate® [Can]
  Sulcrate® Suspension Plus [Can]
Histamine H2 Antagonist
  Alti-Ranitidine [Can]
  Apo®-Cimetidine [Can]
  Apo®-Famotidine [Can]
  Apo®-Nizatidine [Can]
  Apo®-Ranitidine [Can]
  Axid® AR [US-OTC]
  Axid® [US/Can]
  cimetidine
  famotidine
  Gen-Cimetidine [Can]
  Gen-Famotidine [Can]
  Gen-Nizatidine [Can]
  Gen-Ranitidine [Can]
  nizatidine
  Novo-Cimetidine [Can]
  Novo-Famotidine [Can]
  Novo-Nizatidine [Can]
  Novo-Ranidine [Can]
  Nu-Cimet® [Can]
  Nu-Famotidine [Can]
  Nu-Nizatidine [Can]
  Nu-Ranit [Can]
  Pepcid® AC [US/Can]
  Pepcid® [US/Can]
  PMS-Cimetidine [Can]
  PMS-Nizatidine [Can]
  ranitidine hydrochloride
  ratio-Famotidine [Can]
  ratio-Ranitidine [Can]
  Rhoxal-famotidine [Can]
  Tagamet® HB 200 [US/Can]
  Tagamet® [US]
  Zantac® 75 [US-OTC]
  Zanta [Can]
  Zantac® [US/Can]
Macrolide (Antibiotic)
  Biaxin® [US/Can]
  Biaxin® XL [US/Can]
  clarithromycin
Penicillin
  amoxicillin
  Amoxicot® [US]
  Amoxil® [US]
  Apo®-Amoxi [Can]
  Gen-Amoxicillin [Can]
  Lin-Amox [Can]
  Moxilin® [US]
  Novamoxin® [Can]
  Nu-Amoxi [Can]
  PMS-Amoxicillin [Can]
  Trimox® [US]

PERIANAL WART
Immune Response Modifier
 Aldara™ [US/Can]
 imiquimod

PINWORM
Anthelmintic
 Combantrin™ [Can]
 mebendazole
 Pin-X® [US-OTC]
 pyrantel pamoate
 Reese's® Pinworm Medicine [US-OTC]
 Vermox® [US/Can]

PROCTITIS
5-Aminosalicylic Acid Derivative
 Asacol® [US/Can]
 Canasa™ [US]
 mesalamine
 Mesasal® [Can]
 Novo-ASA [Can]
 Pentasa® [US/Can]
 Quintasa® [Can]
 Rowasa® [US/Can]
 Salofalk® [Can]

PROCTOSIGMOIDITIS
5-Aminosalicylic Acid Derivative
 Asacol® [US/Can]
 Canasa™ [US]
 mesalamine
 Mesasal® [Can]
 Novo-ASA [Can]
 Pentasa® [US/Can]
 Quintasa® [Can]
 Rowasa® [US/Can]
 Salofalk® [Can]

PROSTATITIS
Quinolone
 Apo®-Oflox [Can]
 Floxin® [US/Can]
 ofloxacin
Sulfonamide
 Apo®-Sulfatrim [Can]
 Bactrim™ DS [US]
 Bactrim™ [US]
 Novo-Trimel [Can]
 Novo-Trimel D.S. [Can]
 Nu-Cotrimox® [Can]
 Septra® DS [US/Can]
 Septra® [US/Can]
 sulfamethoxazole and trimethoprim
 Sulfatrim® DS [US]
 Sulfatrim® [US]

PROTEIN UTILIZATION
Dietary Supplement
 l-lysine
 Lysinyl® [US-OTC]

PROTOZOAL INFECTION
Antiprotozoal
 Apo®-Metronidazole [Can]
 Flagyl ER® [US]
 Flagyl® [US/Can]
 Florazole ER® [Can]
 metronidazole
 NebuPent® [US]
 Noritate® [US/Can]
 Novo-Nidazol [Can]
 Pentacarinat® [Can]
 Pentam-300® [US]
 pentamidine
 Trikacide® [Can]

PYELONEPHRITIS
Antibiotic, Carbapenem
 ertapenem
 Invanz™ [US/Can]
Antibiotic, Quinolone
 gatifloxacin
 Tequin® [US/Can]
 Zymar™ [US]

RENAL ALLOGRAFT REJECTION
Immunosuppressant Agent
  antithymocyte globulin (rabbit)
  Thymoglobulin® [US]

RENAL COLIC
Analgesic, Nonnarcotic
  Apo®-Ketorolac [Can]
  ketorolac
  Novo-Ketorolac [Can]
  ratio-Ketorolac [Can]
  Toradol® [US/Can]
Anticholinergic Agent
  Antispas® Tablet [US]
  Donnatal Extentabs® [US]
  Donnatal® [US/Can]
  Haponal® [US]
  Hyonatol® [US]
  hyoscyamine, atropine, scopolamine, and phenobarbital
  Hypersed® [US]

ROUNDWORM
Anthelmintic
  Combantrin™ [Can]
  mebendazole
  Pin-X® [US-OTC]
  pyrantel pamoate
  Reese's® Pinworm Medicine [US-OTC]
  Vermox® [US/Can]

SALIVATION (EXCESSIVE)
Anticholinergic Agent
  Anaspaz® [US]
  atropine
  Cantil® [US/Can]
  Cystospaz-M® [US]
  Cystospaz® [US/Can]
  glycopyrrolate
  hyoscyamine
  Hyosine [US]
  Levbid® [US]
  Levsinex® [US]
  Levsin/SL® [US]
  Levsin® [US/Can]
  mepenzolate
  NuLev™ [US]
  Robinul® Forte [US]
  Robinul® [US]
  Sal-Tropine™ [US]
  scopolamine
  Spacol T/S [US]
  Spacol [US]
  Symax SL [US]
  Symax SR [US]

STOMATITIS
Local Anesthetic
  Cepacol® Maximum Strength [US-OTC]
  dyclonine
  Sucrets® [US-OTC]

SYPHILIS
Antibiotic, Miscellaneous
  chloramphenicol
  Chloromycetin® Parenteral [US/Can]
  Diochloram® [Can]
  Pentamycetin® [Can]
Penicillin
  Bicillin® L-A [US]
  penicillin G benzathine
  penicillin G (parenteral/aqueous)
  penicillin G procaine
  Permapen® Isoject® [US]
  Pfizerpen® [US/Can]
  Wycillin® [US/Can]
Tetracycline Derivative
  Adoxa™ [US]
  Apo®-Doxy [Can]
  Apo®-Doxy Tabs [Can]
  Apo®-Tetra [Can]
  Brodspec® [US]
  Doryx® [US]
  Doxy-100® [US]

Appendix 6

Doxycin [Can]
doxycycline
EmTet® [US]
Monodox® [US]
Novo-Doxylin [Can]
Novo-Tetra [Can]
Nu-Doxycycline [Can]
Nu-Tetra [Can]
Periostat® [US]
ratio-Doxycycline [Can]
Sumycin® [US]
tetracycline
Vibramycin® [US]
Vibra-Tabs® [US/Can]
Wesmycin® [US]

TAPEWORM INFESTATION
Amebicide
   Humatin® [US/Can]
   paromomycin

TENESMUS
Analgesic, Narcotic
   belladonna and opium
   B&O Supprettes® [US]

THREADWORM (NONDISSEMINATED INTESTINAL)
Antibiotic, Miscellaneous
   ivermectin
   Stromectol® [US]

ULCER (DUODENAL)
Proton Pump Inhibitor
   Panto™ IV [Can]
   Pantoloc™ [Can]
   pantoprazole
   Protonix® [US/Can]

ULCER (GASTRIC)
Proton Pump Inhibitor
   Panto™ IV [Can]
   Pantoloc™ [Can]
   pantoprazole
   Protonix® [US/Can]

UPPER GASTROINTESTINAL MOTILITY DISORDER
Dopamine Antagonist
   Apo®-Domperidone [Can]
   domperidone (Canada only)
   Motilium® [Can]
   Novo-Domperidone [Can]
   Nu-Domperidone [Can]
   PMS-Domperidone [Can]
   ratio-Domperidone [Can]

URINARY BLADDER SPASM
Anticholinergic Agent
   Propanthel™ [Can]
   propantheline

URINARY RETENTION
Antispasmodic Agent, Urinary
   Ditropan® [US/Can]
   Ditropan® XL [US]
   Gen-Oxybutynin [Can]
   Novo-Oxybutynin [Can]
   Nu-Oxybutyn [Can]
   oxybutynin
   Oxytrol™ [US]
   PMS-Oxybutynin [Can]
Cholinergic Agent
   bethanechol
   Duvoid® [Can]
   Myotonachol™ [Can]
   neostigmine
   PMS-Bethanechol [Can]
   Prostigmin® [US/Can]
   Urecholine® [US]

URINARY TRACT INFECTION
Antibiotic, Carbacephem
   Lorabid™ [US/Can]

loracarbef
Antibiotic, Miscellaneous
   Apo®-Nitrofurantoin [Can]
   Apo®-Trimethoprim [Can]
   Azactam® [US/Can]
   aztreonam
   Dehydral® [Can]
   fosfomycin
   Furadantin® [US]
   Hiprex® [US/Can]
   Macrobid® [US/Can]
   Macrodantin® [US/Can]
   Mandelamine® [US/Can]
   methenamine
   Monurol™ [US/Can]
   nitrofurantoin
   Novo-Furantoin [Can]
   Primsol® [US]
   Proloprim® [US/Can]
   trimethoprim
   Urasal® [Can]
   Urex® [US/Can]
   Vancocin® [US/Can]
   Vancoled® [US]
   vancomycin
Antibiotic, Penicillin
   pivampicillin (Canada only)
   Pondocillin® [Can]
Antibiotic, Quinolone
   gatifloxacin
   Levaquin® [US/Can]
   levofloxacin
   Quixin™ Ophthalmic [US]
   Tequin® [US/Can]
   Zymar™ [US]
Antibiotic, Urinary Antiinfective
   Atrosept® [US]
   Dolsed® [US]
   methenamine, phenyl salicylate, atropine, hyoscyamine, benzoic acid, and methylene blue
   UAA® [US]
   Uridon Modified® [US]
   Urised® [US]
   Uritin® [US]
Cephalosporin (First Generation)
   Ancef® [US]
   Apo®-Cefadroxil [Can]
   Apo®-Cephalex [Can]
   Biocef® [US]
   cefadroxil
   cefazolin
   cephalexin
   cephalothin
   cephradine
   Ceporacin® [Can]
   Duricef® [US/Can]
   Keflex® [US]
   Keftab® [US/Can]
   Novo-Cefadroxil [Can]
   Novo-Lexin® [Can]
   Nu-Cephalex® [Can]
   Velosef® [US]
Cephalosporin (Second Generation)
   Apo®-Cefaclor [Can]
   Apo®-Cefuroxime [Can]
   Ceclor® CD [US]
   Ceclor® [US/Can]
   cefaclor
   Cefotan® [US/Can]
   cefotetan
   cefoxitin
   cefpodoxime
   cefprozil
   Ceftin® [US/Can]
   cefuroxime
   Cefzil® [US/Can]
   Mefoxin® [US/Can]
   Novo-Cefaclor [Can]
   Nu-Cefaclor [Can]
   PMS-Cefaclor [Can]
   ratio-Cefuroxime [Can]
   Vantin® [US/Can]
   Zinacef® [US/Can]
Cephalosporin (Third Generation)

Appendix 6

    Cedax® [US]
    cefixime
    Cefizox® [US/Can]
    cefotaxime
    ceftazidime
    ceftibuten
    ceftizoxime
    ceftriaxone
    Claforan® [US/Can]
    Fortaz® [US/Can]
    Rocephin® [US/Can]
    Suprax® [Can]
    Tazicef® [US]
    Tazidime® [US/Can]
Cephalosporin (Fourth Generation)
    cefepime
    Maxipime® [US/Can]
Genitourinary Irrigant
    neomycin and polymyxin B
    Neosporin® Cream [Can]
    Neosporin® G.U. Irrigant [US/Can]
Irrigating Solution
    citric acid bladder mixture
    Renacidin® [US]
Penicillin
    Alti-Amoxi-Clav® [Can]
    amoxicillin
    amoxicillin and clavulanate potassium
    Amoxicot® [US]
    Amoxil® [US]
    ampicillin
    ampicillin and sulbactam
    Apo®-Amoxi [Can]
    Apo®-Amoxi-Clav® [Can]
    Apo®-Ampi [Can]
    Apo®-Cloxi [Can]
    Apo®-Pen VK [Can]
    Augmentin ES-600™ [US]
    Augmentin® [US/Can]
    Augmentin XR™ [US]
    Bicillin® C-R 900/300 [US]
    Bicillin® C-R [US]
    Bicillin® L-A [US]
    carbenicillin
    Clavulin® [Can]
    cloxacillin
    dicloxacillin
    Gen-Amoxicillin [Can]
    Geocillin® [US]
    Lin-Amox [Can]
    Marcillin® [US]
    Moxilin® [US]
    Nadopen-V® [Can]
    nafcillin
    Novamoxin® [Can]
    Novo-Ampicillin [Can]
    Novo-Cloxin [Can]
    Novo-Pen-VK® [Can]
    Nu-Amoxi [Can]
    Nu-Ampi [Can]
    Nu-Cloxi® [Can]
    Nu-Pen-VK® [Can]
    oxacillin
    penicillin G benzathine
    penicillin G benzathine and procaine combined
    penicillin G (parenteral/aqueous)
    penicillin G procaine
    penicillin V potassium
    Permapen® Isoject® [US]
    Pfizerpen® [US/Can]
    piperacillin
    piperacillin and tazobactam sodium
    Pipracil® [Can]
    PMS-Amoxicillin [Can]
    Principen® [US]
    PVF® K [Can]
    ratio-AmoxiClav
    Suspen® [US]
    Tazocin® [Can]
    ticarcillin and clavulanate potassium
    Timentin® [US/Can]
    Trimox® [US]
    Truxcillin® [US]
    Unasyn® [US/Can]

Veetids® [US]
Wycillin® [US/Can]
Zosyn® [US]
Quinolone
   Apo®-Norflox [Can]
   Apo®-Oflox [Can]
   Cinobac® [US/Can]
   cinoxacin
   Floxin® [US/Can]
   lomefloxacin
   Maxaquin® [US]
   nalidixic acid
   NegGram® [US/Can]
   norfloxacin
   Noroxin® [US/Can]
   Novo-Norfloxacin [Can]
   Ocuflox® [US/Can]
   ofloxacin
   PMS-Norfloxacin [Can]
   Riva-Norfloxacin [Can]
   sparfloxacin
   Zagam® [US]
Sulfonamide
   Apo®-Sulfatrim [Can]
   Bactrim™ DS [US]
   Bactrim™ [US]
   Gantrisin® Pediatric Suspension [US]
   Novo-Trimel [Can]
   Novo-Trimel D.S. [Can]
   Nu-Cotrimox® [Can]
   Septra® DS [US/Can]
   Septra® [US/Can]
   sulfadiazine
   sulfamethoxazole and trimethoprim
   Sulfatrim® DS [US]
   Sulfatrim® [US]
   sulfisoxazole
   sulfisoxazole and phenazopyridine
   Sulfizole® [Can]
   Truxazole® [US]
Urinary Tract Product
   acetohydroxamic acid
   Atrosept® [US]
   Dolsed® [US]
   Lithostat® [US]
   methenamine, phenyl salicylate, atropine, hyoscyamine, benzoic acid, and methylene blue
   UAA® [US]
   Uridon Modified® [US]
   Urised® [US]
   Uritin® [US]

VENEREAL WART
Biological Response Modulator
   Alferon® N [US/Can]
   interferon alfa-n3

VOMITING
Anticholinergic Agent
   Scopace™ [US]
   scopolamine
   Transderm Scop® [US]
   Transderm-V® [Can]
Antiemetic
   Aloxi™ [US]
   Anergan® [US]
   ANX® [US]
   Apo®-Hydroxyzine [Can]
   aprepitant
   Atarax® [US/Can]
   Benzacot® [US]
   dronabinol
   droperidol
   Emend® [US]
   hydroxyzine
   Inapsine® [US]
   Marinol® [US/Can]
   Novo-Hydroxyzin [Can]
   palonosetron
   Phenergan® [US/Can]
   PMS-Hydroxyzine [Can]
   promethazine
   Tigan® [US/Can]
   trimethobenzamide

Vistacot® [US]
Vistaril® [US/Can]
Antihistamine
  Apo®-Dimenhydrinate [Can]
  dimenhydrinate
  Dramamine® Oral [US-OTC]
  Gravol® [Can]
  Novo-Dimenate [Can]
  TripTone® Caplets® [US-OTC]
Phenothiazine Derivative
  Apo®-Perphenazine [Can]
  chlorpromazine
  Compazine® [US/Can]
  Compro™ [US]
  Largactil® [Can]
  Nu-Prochlor [Can]
  perphenazine
  prochlorperazine
  Stemetil® [Can]
  Thorazine® [US]
Selective 5-HT-3 Receptor Antagonist
  Aloxi™ [US]
  palonosetron

WHIPWORM
Anthelmintic
  mebendazole
  Vermox® [US/Can]

ZOLLINGER-ELLISON SYNDROME
Antacid
  calcium carbonate and simethicone
  Iosopan® Plus [US]
  Lowsium® Plus [US]
  magaldrate and simethicone
  Mag-Gel® 600 [US]
  magnesium hydroxide
  magnesium oxide
  Mag-Ox® 400 [US-OTC]
  Phillips'® Milk of Magnesia [US-OTC]
  Titralac® Plus Liquid [US-OTC]
  Uro-Mag® [US-OTC]
Antineoplastic Agent
  streptozocin
  Zanosar® [US/Can]
Gastric Acid Secretion Inhibitor
  Aciphex™ [US/Can]
  lansoprazole
  Losec® [Can]
  omeprazole
  Pariet® [Can]
  Prevacid® [US/Can]
  Prilosec OTC™ [US-OTC]
  Prilosec® [US]
  rabeprazole
Histamine H2 Antagonist
  Alti-Ranitidine [Can]
  Apo®-Cimetidine [Can]
  Apo®-Famotidine [Can]
  Apo®-Ranitidine [Can]
  cimetidine
  famotidine
  Gen-Cimetidine [Can]
  Gen-Famotidine [Can]
  Gen-Ranitidine [Can]
  Novo-Cimetidine [Can]
  Novo-Famotidine [Can]
  Novo-Ranidine [Can]
  Nu-Cimet® [Can]
  Nu-Famotidine [Can]
  Nu-Ranit [Can]
  Pepcid® AC [US/Can]
  Pepcid® [US/Can]
  PMS-Cimetidine [Can]
  ranitidine hydrochloride
  ratio-Famotidine [Can]
  ratio-Ranitidine [Can]
  Rhoxal-famotidine [Can]
  Tagamet® HB 200 [US/Can]
  Tagamet® [US]
  Zantac® 75 [US-OTC]
  Zanta [Can]

Zantac® [US/Can]
Prostaglandin
  Apo®-Misoprostil [Can]
  Cytotec® [US/Can]
  misoprostol
  Novo-Misoprostol [Can]

ZOLLINGER-ELLISON SYNDROME (DIAGNOSTIC)
Diagnostic Agent
  SecreFlo™ [US]
  secretin